Essentials of Nursing Informatics

Notice

Essentials of Nursing Informatics

SIXTH EDITION

Virginia K. Saba, EdD, RN, FAAN, FACMI

CEO and President
SabaCare, Inc.
Arlington, Virginia
Distinguished Scholar, Emeritus
Georgetown University
Washington, District of Columbia
Professor, Adjunct
Uniformed Services University
Bethesda, Maryland

Kathleen A. McCormick, PhD, RN, FAAN, FACMI, FHIMSS

Principal/Owner
SciMind, LLC
North Potomac, Maryland

McGraw Hill
Education

New York • Chicago • San Francisco • Athens • London • Madrid • Mexico City
Milan • New Delhi • Singapore • Sydney • Toronto

Essentials of Nursing Informatics, Sixth Edition

A chapter in this book was written by Lynn McQueen in her private capacity. No official support or endorsement by the US Department of Health and Human Services, Substance Abuse and Mental Health Services Administration (SAMHSA) is intended or should be inferred.

2 3 4 5 6 7 8 9 0   DOC/DOC   19 18 17 16

ISBN 978-0-07-182955-7
MHID 0-07-182955-5

This book was set in Warnock Pro 9/11 pt by MPS Limited.
The editors were Andrew Moyer and Christina M. Thomas.
The production supervisor was Rick Ruzycka.
Project management was provided by Asheesh Ratra, MPS Limited.
The cover designer was Thomas De Pierro.
RR Donnelley was the printer and binder.

This book is printed on acid-free paper.

Library of Congress Cataloging-in-Publication Data
Essentials of nursing informatics / [edited by] Virginia K. Saba, Kathleen
A. McCormick. — Sixth edition.
      p. ; cm.
  Includes bibliographical references and index.
  ISBN-13: 978-0-07-182955-7 (pbk. : alk. paper)
  ISBN-10: 0-07-182955-5 (pbk. : alk. paper)
  I. Saba, Virginia K., editor. II. McCormick, Kathleen A., editor.
  [DNLM: 1. Nursing Informatics. WY 26.5]
  RT50.5
  610.730285—dc23
                      2014034815

CONTENTS

CONTRIBUTORS

Kathleen A. McCormick, PhD, RN, FAAN, FACMI, FHIMSS
Principal/Owner
SciMind, LLC
North Potomac, Maryland

Virginia K. Saba, EdD, RN, FAAN, FACMI
CEO and President
SabaCare, Inc.
Arlington, Virginia
Distinguished Scholar, Emeritus
Georgetown University
Washington, DC
Professor, Adjunct
Uniformed Services University
Bethesda, Maryland

SECTION EDITORS/AUTHORS

Gail E. Latimer, MSN, RN, FACHE, FAAN
Vice President and Chief Nursing Officer
Siemens Medical Solutions, Inc.
USA Health Services
Malvern, Pennsylvania

Jacqueline Ann Moss, PhD, RN, FAAN
Chair and Assistant Dean for Clinical
Simulation and Technology
School of Nursing
University of Alabama at Birmingham
Birmingham, Alabama

Susan K. Newbold, PhD, RN-BC, FAAN, FHIMSS, CHTS-CP
Owner
Newbold Consulting
Franklin, Tennessee

Diane J. Skiba, PhD, FACMI, FAAN
Professor and Informatics Specialty
Coordinator
University of Colorado College of Nursing
Aurora, Colorado

Kathleen Smith, BSN, MScEd, RN-BC, FHIMSS
Managing Partner
Informatics Consulting and Continuing
Education, LLC
Weeki Wachee, Florida

FOREWORD CONTRIBUTORS

Kelly Aldrich, DNP, RN-BC
Informatics Nurse Specialist
Chief Nursing Informatics Officer and Assistant
Vice President
Hospital Corporation of America (HCA)
Nashville, Tennessee

Jane D. Englebright, PhD, RN, CENP, FAAN
Chief Nursing Officer, Patient Safety Officer,
and Vice President, Clinical Services Group
HCA
Nashville, Tennessee

John P. Glaser, PhD, FACMI, FCHIME, FHIMSS
CEO, Siemens Health Services
Siemens Healthcare
Malvern, Pennsylvania

Gail E. Latimer, MSN, RN, FACHE, FAAN
Vice President and CNO, Siemens Health Services
Siemens Healthcare
Malvern, Pennsylvania

Jonathan B. Perlin, MD, PhD, MSHA, FACP, FACMI
President, Clinical Services Group
Chief Medical Officer
Hospital Corporation of America (HCA)
Nashville, Tennessee

AUTHORS AND CO-AUTHORS

Dana Alexander, MSN, RN, MBA, FAAN, FHIMSS
Vice President, Integrated Care Delivery & CNO
Caradigm
Castle Rock, Colorado

Gregory L. Alexander, PhD, MHA, MIS, RN
Associate Professor
University of Missouri
Sinclair School of Nursing
Columbia, Missouri

Patricia E. Allen, Ed D, RN, CNE, ANEF, FAAN
Professor
Texas Tech University Health Sciences Center
Lubbock, Texas

Ida M. Androwich, PhD, RN-BC-NI
Professor and Director of Health Systems Management
Loyola University Chicago
La Grange Park, Illinois

Myrna L. Armstrong , EdD MS, BSN, ANEF, FAAN
Nursing Consultant, Professor Emerita
Texas Tech University Health Sciences Center
School of Nursing
Lubbock, Texas

Martha K. Badger, MSN, RN-BC, CPHIMS
Research Scientist
Knowledge-Based Nursing Department
Aurora Health Care
Milwaukee, Wisconsin

Dixie B. Baker, PhD, MS, MS, BS
Senior Partner
Martin, Blanck and Associates
Redondo Beach, California

Khadija Bakrim, Ed D
Instructional Designer
Texas Tech University Health Sciences Center
School of Nursing
Lubbock, Texas

Emily B. Barey, MSN, RN
Director of Nursing Informatics
Epic
Verona, Wisconsin

Mary Lee Barron, PhD, APRN, FNP-BC, FAANP
Associate Professor
Southern Illinois University-Edwardsville
Edwardsville, Illinois

Amy J. Barton, PhD, RN, FAAN
Professor and Associate Dean for Clinical and Community Affairs
College of Nursing
University of Colorado
Aurora, Colorado

Claudia C. Bartz, PhD, RN, FAAN
Coordinator, ICN eHealth Programme
University of Wisconsin-Milwaukee
Milwaukee, Wisconsin

Capt. Margaret S. Beaubien, NC, USN, MSN, RN, MS, CPHIMS
Acting Deputy Director, HIT
Deputy CIO
Defense Health Agency
Falls Church, Virginia

Murielle S. Beene, DNP, RN-BC, MBA, MPH, MS, PMP
Chief Nursing Informatics Officer
Department of Veterans Affairs
Veterans Health Administration
Office of Informatics and Analytics Health Informatics
Office of the Chief Nursing Informatics Officer
Washington, DC

Carol J. Bickford, PhD, RN-BC, CPHIMS
Senior Policy Fellow
Department of Nursing Programs
American Nurses Association
Silver Spring, Maryland

Derryl E. Block, PhD, RN, MPH
Dean, College of Health and Human Sciences
Northern Illinois University
DeKalb, Illinois

Christine Boltz, MA, MS, RN-BC, CPHIMS
Capt., NC, USN (Ret.)/Online Instructor
Excelsior College, School of Nursing
Alexandria, Virginia

Heidi Bossley, MSN, MBA
Independent Healthcare Consultant
Alexandria, Virginia

Enola Boyd (Deceased), EdD, MS
Texas Tech University Health Sciences Center
Lubbock, Texas

Kathleen A. Calzone, PhD, RN, APNG, FAAN
Senior Nurse Specialist, Research
National Institutes of Health, National Cancer Institute, Center for Cancer Research, Genetics Branch
Bethesda, Maryland

Heather Carter-Templeton, PhD, RN-BC
Assistant Professor
The University of Alabama
Tuscaloosa, Alabama

Marian Celli, MS, RN C, FHIMSS
Senior Consultant
Beacon Healthcare Consulting
Potomac, Maryland

Kathleen G. Charters, PhD, RN, CPHIMS
Nurse Consultant
Defense Health Agency
Falls Church, Virginia

Thomas R. Clancy, PhD, MBA, RN, FAAN
Clinical Professor and Assistant Dean, Partnerships, Practices, Professional Development
School of Nursing
University of Minnesota
Minneapolis, Minnesota

Amy Coenen, PhD, RN, FAAN
Professor
University of Wisconsin-Milwaukee
College of Nursing
Milwaukee, Wisconsin
Director of International Classification for Nursing Practice Programme, International Council of Nurses
Geneva, Switzerland

Helen R. Connors, PhD, RN, FAAN
Professor
University of Kansas School of Nursing and Center for Health Informatics
Kansas City, Kansas

Marina Douglas, MS, BSN
Principal, Beacon Healthcare Consulting
Nokesville, Virginia

Patricia C. Dykes, PhD, RN, MA
Senior Nurse Scientist, Director
Center for Patient Safety Research and Practice
Brigham & Women's Hospital
Boston, Massachusetts

Veronica D. Feeg, PhD, RN, FAAN
Gitenstein Professor, Associate Dean
Division of Nursing
Molloy College
Rockville Centre, New York

Beth B. Franklin, MS, RN-BC, CPEHR, CPHIT
Senior Consultant
Beacon Healthcare Consulting
Nokesville, Virginia

Barbara B. Frink, PhD, RN, FAAN
Vice President, Chief Nursing Information Officer
MedStar Health
Columbia, Maryland
Associate Faculty
Johns Hopkins University School of Nursing
Baltimore, Maryland

Judy D. Gibson, MSN, RN
Manager
JD Gibson Consulting, LLC
Atlanta, Georgia

Matthew C. Grissinger, RPh, FISMP, FASCP
Director, Error Reporting Programs
Institute for Safe Medication Practices
Horsham, Pennsylvania

**Elizabeth Casey Halley, BSN, MBA
(RN FHIMSS)**
Principal Advisor
The MITRE Corporation
McLean, Virginia

Kathryn J. Hannah, PhD, RN, FACMI
Health Informatics Advisor, Canadian Nurses
Association
Professor (Adjunct)
School of Nursing
University of Victoria
Calgary, Alberta, Canada

Nicholas R. Hardiker, BSc (Hons), MSc, PhD
Professor of Nursing and Health Informatics
Associate Head, Research & Innovation School of
Nursing, Midwifery, Social Work &
Social Sciences
The University of Salford
Salford, United Kingdom

Director, eHealth Programme, International
Council of Nurses
Geneva, Switzerland
Professor (Adjunct)
College of Nursing, University of Colorado
Denver, Colorado

Lee Ann Harford, MS, RN
Healthcare Informaticist, Project Manager
SBG Technology Solutions
Washington, DC

Eileen Healy, DNP, APRN, ANP-BC
Instructor,
Saint Louis University
School of Nursing
Independent Consultant
New York, New York

Michelle L. L. Honey, RN, PhD, FCNA (NZ)
Senior Lecturer
University of Auckland
Auckland, New Zealand

**Evelyn J. S. Hovenga, PhD, RN, B App Sc,
MHA, FACS**
Professor, CEO, Director, Trainer
eHealth Education Pty Ltd,
Rockhampton, Qld, Australia

Kathleen M. Hunter, PhD, RN-BC, CNE
Dean, MSN Indirect Care Tracks
Chamberlain College of Nursing
Downers Grove, Illinois

**Elizabeth (Liz) O. Johnson, MSN, BSN, RN,
FCHIME, FHIMSS, CPHIMS, RN-BC**
Chief Clinical Informaticist
Vice President, Applied Clinical Informatics
Tenet Health Care
Dallas, Texas

R. Renee Johnson-Smith, BSN, RN, BS, MBA
Risk Manager
VA Medical Center
Indianapolis, Indiana

Irene Joos, PhD, RN, MSIS
Professor, Information and Technology Department
Adjunct, Department of Nursing (Former Director of
Online Learning)
La Roche College
Pittsburgh, Pennsylvania

Virpi Jylhä, MSc, PT
Researcher
Nursing Research Foundation
Helsinki, Finland

**Margaret Ann Kennedy, PhD, MN, BScN,
RN, CPHIMS-CA, PMP**
Atlantic Branch Manager
Senior Consultant in Business Analysis
Clinical SME
Global Village Consulting, Inc.
Halifax, Nova Scotia, Canada

Rosemary Kennedy, PhD, RN, MBA, FAAN
CEO
eCare Informatics, LLC
Frazer, Pennsylvania

Karlene M. Kerfoot, PhD, MS, BSN, NEA-BC, FAAN
Chief Clinical Integration Officer
API Healthcare, a GE Company
Hartford, Wisconsin

Tae Youn Kim, PhD, RN
Associate Professor
University of California Davis
Betty Irene Moore School of Nursing
Sacramento, California

Kathleen C. Kimmel, BSN, MBA, MHA
Senior Instructor
University of Colorado School of Nursing
Denver, Colorado

Ulla-Mari Kinnunen, RN, PhD
University Teacher
University of Eastern Finland
Department of Health and Social Management
Kuopio, Finland

Eija Kivekäs, PhD (c), RN, MSc
Project Coordinator
University of Eastern Finland
Department of Health and Social Management,
RECEPS
Kuopio, Finland

Sarah Knapfel, BSN, RN, CCRN
iTEAM Project Coordinator
University of Colorado
College of Nursing
Aurora, Colorado

Margaret Ross Kraft, PhD, RN
Assistant Professor
Niehoff School of Nursing
Loyola University
Chicago, Illinois

Darlene Lacy, PhD, RN-C, CNE
Assistant Professor, Director of RN-BSN Program
Texas Tech University Health Sciences Center,
School of Nursing
Kingsland, Texas (Telecommuter—Primary campus
Lubbock, Texas)

Laura Heermann Langford, PhD, RN
Director, Nursing Informatics
Intermountain Healthcare
Director/Assistant Professor
Nursing Informatics Program
University of Utah

Mary Ann Lavin, DSc, APRN, ANP-BC, FNI, FAAN
Emerita, Saint Louis University School of Nursing
Consultant, Founder of Network for Language in
Nursing Knowledge Systems (nlinks.org)
St. Louis, Missouri

Chanmi Lee, BSN, RN
Research Assistant
University of Colorado
College of Nursing
Aurora, Colorado

June Levy, MLS
Vice President
Cinahl Information Systems
Glendale, California

LTC Mike Ludwig, MS, RN-BC, CPHIMS
Officer in Charge
Medical Evaluation and Treatment Unit
Falls Church, Virginia
Walter Reed National Military Medical Center
Bethesda, Maryland

Susan H. Lundquist, BSN
Director of Patient Care Solutions
Siemens Healthcare
Malvern, Pennsylvania

Michelle M. Mandrack, RN, MSN
Director of Consulting Services
Institute for Safe Medication Practices
Horsham, Pennsylvania

Heimar de Fatima Marin, PhD, RN, MS, FACMI
Full Professor, Vice Dean, Director of the Graduate
Program in Health Informatics
Nursing School, Universidade Federal de São Paulo
São Paulo (SP), Brazil

Daniel F. Marsh, MSN, RN-BC
Nursing Informatics Specialist
VHA, Office of Informatics & Analytics - Health
Informatics (10P2A) - Applied Informatics
Deployment
Silver Spring, Maryland

Andrea Mazzoccoli, PhD, RN, MSN, MBA, FAAN
Chief Nursing Officer and Senior Vice President
Bon Secours Health System
Center for Clinical Excellence and Innovation
Baltimore, Maryland

Mary L. McHugh, BSN, MSN, PhD
Provost and Dean of Nursing
Angeles College
Los Angeles, California

Lynn McQueen, DrPH, MS, MPH, RN
Performance Officer
US Department of Health and Human Services
Substance Abuse and Mental Health Services
Administration
Rockville, Maryland

**Bernadette Mazurek Melnyk, PhD, RN,
CPNP/PMHNP, FAANP, FNAP, FAAN**
Associate Vice President for Health Promotion
University Chief Wellness Officer
Dean and Professor, College of Nursing
Professor of Pediatrics & Psychiatry
College of Medicine
The Ohio State University
Columbus, Ohio

Susan Meyer, B Soc Sc (Nurs), Dip Paed Nurs
RN, RM, Community Health Nurse,
IT Manager
Addington Hospital
Durban, South Africa

Irene van Middelkoop, Hons BA (Cur)
RN, RM, Nurse Administrator
Community Health Nurse
Durban, South Africa

Judy Murphy, RN, BSN, FACMI, FHIMSS, FAAN
Chief Nursing Officer
Office of the National Coordinator for Health IT
Washington, DC

Lynn M. Nagle, PhD, RN, MScN, BN
Assistant Professor
University of Toronto
Toronto, Ontario, Canada

Eun-Shim Nahm, PhD, RN, FAAN
Professor
University of Maryland
School of Nursing
Baltimore, Maryland

Ramona Nelson, PhD, MN, MSIS, RN-BC, ANEF, FAAN
Professor Emerita, Consulting
Slippery Rock University
President, Ramona Nelson Consulting
Allison Park, Pennsylvania

Hyeoun-Ae Park, PhD, RN, FAAN
Dean and Professor
College of Nursing, Seoul National University
Seoul, Korea

Joel L. Parker, PhD, MS, MA, BSN, PMP
Capt., NC, USN, Chief Nurse Informatics Officer
Enterprise Information Integration
Bureau of Medicine/ Information Delivery Division
Defense Health Agency
Bureau of Medicine and Surgery/Office of the Navy
Medicine CIO (M6)
Falls Church, Virginia

COL Katherine Taylor Pearson, MA, MS, RN-BC, CPHIMS
Assistant Chief of Staff and
Chief Information Officer
Southern Regional Medical Command
San Antonio, Texas

Diane S. Pravikoff, RN, PhD, FAAN
Director of Research
Cinahl Information Systems
Glendale, California

Capt. Stephanie J. Raps, BSN, RN-BC
Workflow Deputy Division Chief (Air Force Medical
Support Agency/SG6W)
Defense Health Headquarters
Falls Church, Virginia

Janise Richards, PhD, MPH, MS
Senior Informatics Advisor
Centers for Disease Control and
Prevention (CDC)
Atlanta, Georgia

Theresa A. Rienzo, MS, RN, BSN, MLIS
Associate Librarian, Health Sciences
Molloy College
Rockville Centre, New York

Juliet Rubini, RN-BC, MSN, MSIS
Lead Program Analyst
Mathematica Policy Research
Oakland, California

Sandra Festa Ryan, MSN, RN, CPNP, FCPP, FAANP, FAAN
Chief Clinical Officer and Robert Wood Johnson
Foundation Executive Nurse Fellow
CareCam Health Systems
West Conshohocken, Pennsylvania

Kaija Saranto, PhD, RNT, RN, FACMI, FAAN
Professor, Academic Coordinator
University of Eastern Finland
Department of Health and Social Management
Kuopio, Finland

Joanne M. Seasholtz, MSN, BSN, WMV, PhD, FACHE
Practice Director, Strategic Consulting Siemens,
Siemens Healthcare Solutions, Strategic Consulting
Malvern, Pennsylvania

Patricia P. Sengstack, DNP, RN-BC, CPHIMS
Chief Nursing Informatics Officer
Bon Secours Health System
Marriottsville, Maryland

Joyce Sensmeier, MS, RN-BC, CPHIMS, FHIMSS, FAAN
Vice President, Informatics
HIMSS
Chicago, Illinois

Theresa J. Settergren, MHA, MA, RN-BC
Director, Nursing Informatics
Cedars-Sinai Health System
Los Angeles, California

Roy L. Simpson, DNP, RN, DPNAP, FAAN
Vice President, Nursing
Cerner Corporation
Kansas City, Missouri
Professor, Emory University Nell Hodgson
Woodruff School of Nursing
Atlanta, Georgia

Capt. Lynn A. Slepski, PhD, RN, PHCNS-BC, FAAN
Senior Public Health Advisor
United States Public Health Service
Washington, DC

Frances (Fran) M. Spivak, MS, RN, CPHIMS
Director, Health Informatics
Walgreens, Health Care Clinics
Deerfield, Illinois

Arunkumar Srinivasan, PhD
Computer Scientist
Centers for Disease Control and Prevention
Atlanta, Georgia

Mark D. Sugrue, BSN, RN-BC, FHIMSS, CPHIMS
Chief Nursing Informatics Officer
Lahey Hospital and Medical Center
Burlington, Massachusetts

Michelle R. Troseth, MSN, RN, DPNAP, FAAN
Chief Professional Practice Officer
Elsevier Clinical Solutions
Amsterdam, The Netherlands

Denise D. Tyler, MSN/MBA, RN-BC
Senior Systems Consultant, Xerox
Adjunct Faculty, Excelsior
House Supervisor, Kaweah Delta Health Care
District (Per Diem)
Visalia, California

Judith J. Warren, PhD, RN, FAAN, FACMI
Professor Emeritus
University of Kansas School of Nursing
Kansas City, Kansas

Charlotte A. Weaver, PhD, RN, MSPH, FAAN
Senior Vice President, Chief Clinical Officer
Gentiva® Health Services, Inc.
Atlanta, Georgia

Elizabeth (Betsy) Weiner, PhD
Senior Associate Dean for Informatics
Centennial Independence Foundation
Professor of Nursing and Biomedical Informatics
Vanderbilt University
Nashville, Tennessee

**Lucy A. Westbrooke, RN, DipNg, PGDipBus
(Health Informatics)**
Telehealth Programme Manager
Auckland District Health Board
Auckland, New Zealand

Bonnie L. Westra, PhD, RN, FAAN, FACMI
Associate Professor and Director
Center for Nursing Informatics
University of Minnesota
School of Nursing & Institute for
Health Informatics
Minneapolis, Minnesota

David J. Whitten, MCS
Medical Informaticist
Central Regional Hospital
Department of Health and Human Services
Butner, North Carolina

Luann Whittenburg, PhD, RN, FNP
Chief Nursing Informatics Officer
Medicomp Systems
Alexandria, Virginia

Marisa L. Wilson, DNSc, MHSc, CPHIMS, RN-BC
Assistant Professor
The Johns Hopkins University
School of Nursing
Baltimore, Maryland

Patricia B. Wise, RN, MS, MA, FHIMSS
COL (USA retired)
Vice President, Health Information Systems
HIMSS
Chicago, Illinois

FOREWORD 1

A Turning Point in U.S. Healthcare

The last edition of this book heralded the recent enactment of the Patient Protection and Affordable Care Act (commonly called the Affordable Care Act or ACA), sweeping legislation intended to reduce the numbers of uninsured and make healthcare accessible to all Americans. As of 2014, over 7 million enrolled for coverage via the healthcare insurance exchange marketplace mandated in the ACA—surpassing all expectations.

Experts predict that these newly insured will increase the use of medical services, particularly prescription drugs and physician and clinical services. By 2022, the numbers of uninsured will drop by 30 million, signaling to healthcare providers that a transformation in healthcare delivery models must begin now if we are to care for the newly insured while making significant progress in improving care quality and reducing costs.

Adding to the challenges created by broader insurance coverage are simple and complex demographics: by 2040, the 65 and over population will double. This population is also the segment with the highest incidence of chronic diseases. Chronic diseases account for 80% of healthcare costs, not just in the United States but in Europe and developing countries—chronic diseases are no longer the particular scourges of the wealthier western nations. It is a global wave that threatens to overwhelm healthcare systems unless we find new ways to manage patients and deliver care over the long term.

In the United States, we have specific issues that may or may not be a product of the current healthcare system but that clearly further galvanize the case for change. In the United States, it is worth noting that 45% of healthcare costs are driven by 3% to 5% of the population—the sickest individuals. But, the next tier of patients, those considered to be at the 20% to 30% risk level consumes 35% of healthcare costs. And consider that one in three Medicare patients is re-admitted within 30 days of an initial hospitalization, largely due to not receiving or complying with recommended follow-up care—and that penalties for such re-admissions are now in effect. Most sobering is that 33% of care expenses do not contribute to improving the health of an individual.

Healthcare organizations have begun the transformation of care delivery already, taking on risk-sharing models and forming Accountable Care Organizations, which now number over 600; patient-centered homes; and population health management functions. This necessitates a shift, not only in the physical care setting approach but also in how providers approach care delivery overall:

- As fee-for-service becomes less the norm, providers will move from a care volume to an outcomes orientation.
- Demographics and the costs of treating chronic diseases over time will necessitate a move from the acute-centric environment to multiple venues, including outpatient clinics and home-based care.
- Evidence-based medicine—and the ability to manage volumes of clinical evidence through sophisticated HIT systems—will mean that providers can tailor treatment for the individual and intervene earlier to keep patients well.
- New care delivery models require a transition from individual care providers to collaborative teams.
- We will move from a "sick care" system to one that focuses on keeping the individual and identified populations of patients (such as those with diabetes) healthy.
- Instead of avoiding care for the chronically ill until it becomes acute, provider organizations will seek out these populations. Population Health Management is intended to deliver specific care protocols aimed at managing these conditions and improving the health status of each individual through monitoring and early intervention. This will not only improve health status but also will reduce costs and reduce re-admissions.
- Patient—and family—engagement will become a critical component in the care process, particularly in population health management.

Such shifts require an equally dramatic shift in healthcare information systems, evolving Electronic Health Record, clinical, and administrative systems from those that support the care "transaction" to those that provide intelligence-based support to:

- Guide clinical diagnostic and therapeutic decisions
- Ensure that the sequence of care activities conform to the evidence-based practices and performance contract requirements
- Monitor the execution of core clinical processes
- Capture, report, and integrate into EHRs quality and performance measures
- Support the interactions of the care team
- Identify, assess, stratify, and select target populations
- Provide care management interventions for individuals and populations
- Provide tools that support and promote patient and family engagement
- Guide the delivery of high-quality care across multiple care settings
- Monitor, predict, report, and improve on quality performance measures

From treating the individual to caring for communities or populations of patients to implementing pay-for-performance and quality measures, HIT systems will move from support of clinical operations to sophisticated tools integral to the delivery of care and management of the health of individuals and populations. Population health management and care coordination systems will help bend the cost and outcomes curves, enabling more effective, efficient care management of an entire population and helping ensure that those individuals dealing with a chronic condition do not join the 3%–5% comprising the sickest patients.

Nursing professionals are at the center of the new care delivery models and care coordination and population health management strategies. Always the foundation of care delivery, the nursing community is the integrator of care and in this role will increasingly require advanced knowledge and expert use of healthcare information technology. To the authors, editors, and publishers of the Sixth Edition of *Essentials of Nursing Informatics*—and to all of the Nursing Informatics professionals, our appreciation for leading the way.

John P. Glaser, PhD, FACMI, FCHIME, FHIMSS
CEO, Siemens Health Services
Siemens Healthcare

Gail E. Latimer, MSN, RN, FACHE, FAAN
Vice President and CNO, Siemens Health Services
Siemens Healthcare

FOREWORD 2

In the previous edition of *Essentials of Nursing Informatics*, we predicted that 2010 would be a watershed year for accelerating the implementation of electronic health records in the United States. The prediction that the "HITECH Act" would forever change health informatics in the United Sates has now been confirmed by multiple sources, including data from the Office of the National Coordinator for Health Information Technology showing that over 84% of eligible hospitals and 69% of eligible providers met Stage 1 of "meaningful use" as of October 2013.

A significant outcome of this widespread adoption and use of health information technology is an increasing focus on nursing informatics. There is a steadily growing recognition of the need for nurse informaticists in the transformation of healthcare delivery. Nurse informaticists are healthcare leaders for the twenty-first century, exemplars in the right place at the right time, masterfully employing education, nursing practice, experience, and leadership skills to help create effective partnerships. Their role is a key one in advancing value and science-driven healthcare—moving healthcare information technology from arduous implementation to ubiquitous practice, and healthcare informatics from data management to decision support.

The accelerating demands of gathering and using data for patient care has increased awareness of informatics as a core skill and intensified the need for all nurses and clinicians to better understand how they can utilize technology. This updated edition incorporates teaching aids to help educators show and teach others, developing more sophisticated users of technology who can collaborate to improve processes and workflow that result in safer, more effective, and efficient patient care.

For decades, primary communication among team members has been accomplished through notes written in the patient chart. Yet, this represented one of the major roadblocks to the most effective and efficient care, as the best patient care is dependent on up-to-date data and timely information sharing among the healthcare team members, including the patient. Access to the most accurate and complete information remains vital, and as we move from paper charts to mobile devices, nursing informaticists are at the center of much of the work being done to improve the speed, accuracy, and utility of patient information. With nearly instant access to patient data and evidence-based decision support, nurses, physicians, and other clinicians will be able make better decisions about a patient's care. Health systems are already progressing toward this goal by embracing new technology that provides real-time notifications and provides clinical staff with intervention-level patient data to drive improvement in both patient experience and the interaction of caregivers.

The challenge for the informatics community is to ensure the new technologies are seamlessly integrated and that use by caregivers improves the patient experience. It is critical that the electronic health record is transformed into a system that provides output, rather than one primarily receiving input. The appropriate use of information structure, information processes, and information technology can support consumers, patients, nurses, and other providers in their decision-making in all roles and settings. While we have not yet built a nationwide network that supports exchange of both clinical and administrative health information, that vision is now coming into sharper focus and is increasingly achievable. When that network is complete, our ability to put it to good use will have been enhanced by decades of preparation by nurse informaticists.

Nurse informaticists have been and will continue to be leaders in the partnerships between information technology providers, clinicians, and health administrators. The crucial role of nurse informaticists in the development, implementation, and optimization of clinical applications, including nursing clinical documentation, computerized provider order entry (CPOE), and electronic medical/health records (EMR/EHR), seems to be confirmed by the results of the HIMSS 2014 Nursing Informatics Workforce Survey. The survey indicates the specialty is increasingly recognized as adding value, and it continues to thrive. Salaries are rising, more nurse informaticists are seeking accredited certification, and increasing demand is drawing some nurses from the bedside.

As the specialty that integrates nursing science, computer science, and information science to manage and communicate data, information, knowledge—and ultimately, wisdom—into nursing practice, nursing informatics is uniquely positioned to help lead the building of inter-professional healthcare teams that will effectively support healthcare transformation. The vision for the future of technology in healthcare will rely heavily on these teams to use data to coordinate care and improve outcomes, from real-time data mining to recognizing population health patterns to using social media to drive awareness.

A decade has passed since the call for ubiquitous electronic health records was first made in the 2004 Presidential State of the Union message. These 10 years represent a very long time in the lifespan of health information technology, and one who has witnessed a rapid evolution of healthcare systems. During this time, nursing informatics has provided tremendous energy, insight and leadership, not only helping to establish the necessary infrastructure but also in driving gains in healthcare technology competency, information literacy, and better healthcare outcomes. On the basis of this history, we

believe even more strongly that our future and the future of nursing informatics hold even more promise.

Jonathan B. Perlin, MD, PhD, MSHA, FACP, FACMI
President, Clinical Services Group and
Chief Medical Officer
Hospital Corporation of America (HCA)

Jane D. Englebright, PhD, RN, CENP, FAAN
Chief Nursing Officer, Patient Safety Officer
and Vice President, Clinical Services Group
Hospital Corporation of America (HCA)

Kelly Aldrich, DNP, RN-BC
Informatics Nurse Specialist
Chief Nursing Informatics Officer and
Assistant Vice President
Hospital Corporation of America (HCA)

PREFACE

This sixth edition of *Essentials of Nursing Informatics* was initiated in response to requests by educators for a digital version of the publication, a guide for faculty to use in the development of their course work, and by nurse users of the fifth edition. Because of these requests we have expanded the content primarily in the areas: Nursing Informatics Technologies—(a) *Computer Hardware,* (b) *Advanced Hardware and mHealth,* (c) *Computer Software,* (d) *Data and Data Processing,* (e) *System Life Cycle,* (f) *System Life Cycle Tools,* (g) *System and Functional Testing.*

Seven section editors edited the sixth edition content: *Nursing Informatics Technologies*—Jacqueline Ann Moss; *System Life Cycle, Informatics Theory, Standards, Foundations of Nursing Informatics, and Research Applications*—Virginia K. Saba; *Nursing Informatics Leadership*—Kathleen Smith; *Advanced Nursing Informatics Practice*—Gail E. Latimer; *Nursing Informatics—Complex Applications, Big Data Initiatives*—Kathleen A. McCormick; *Educational Applications*—Diane Skiba; and *International Perspectives*—Susan K. Newbold.

In addition, this book includes new content that focuses on innovative expansions in Professional Practice using Nursing Informatics such as (a) *The Role of the Nurse Executive in Information Technology Decision-Making,* (b) *Care Delivery Across the Continuum: Hospital-Community-Home,* (c) *Foundations of a Nursing Plan of Care Standard,* (d) *Health Information Technology,* (e) *Striving to Improve Patient Safety,* (f) *Federal Health Care Sector Nursing Informatics,* (g) *Nurse Scheduling and Credentialing Systems,* (h) *Establishing Nursing Informatics in Public Policy,* (i) *Nursing Informatics in Retail Clinics, Safety, Global Initiatives,* and (j) *Big Data.* We welcomed new authors who have expanded the scope of this book and added unique expertise in Nursing Informatics.

Updates of many other chapters include new references and new policies, new concepts, and skills required by nurses in informatics. All Six continents describing International Perspectives updated their unique chapters.

Because a gap still exists with students, faculty, and nurse users' understanding the meaning and scope of the content, a companion book (*Essentials of Nursing Informatics Study Guide*/ISBN: 978-0071845892, edited by Juliana and Jack Brixey, Virginia Saba, and Kathleen McCormick) is available that outlines the chapters and includes sample test questions for every chapter. A companion, online faculty resource has also been created to support both books (accessible at www.EssentialsofNursingInformatics.com), providing online PowerPoint slides for chapters, which include objectives, key words, outlines, and tables/figures.

With each new edition, we have responded to those who teach Nursing Informatics, and who have focused the content where they identified areas that they thought would be most helpful in the profession. Our goal in expanding this edition is to increase the number of professional nurses who are prepared in Nursing Informatics to work to improve Quality and Outcomes in Healthcare. There are 6,000 nurses who consider themselves Nurses in Informatics, and 3,000 credentialed in Nursing Informatics. We cannot achieve the goals in healthcare and HITECH without more nurses prepared in Informatics. It is also our goal to keep all nurses in Informatics up-to-date in the field, and to entice those nurses who are looking for first or second careers in nursing to consider the breadth of areas in Nursing Informatics.

Dr. Virginia K. Saba
Dr. Kathleen A. McCormick

ACKNOWLEDGMENTS

This sixth edition book is dedicated to all of the section editors, chapter authors and their co-authors. Each of these prestigious contributors was extremely busy implementing policies, systems, and educational programs to support Nursing Informatics in the United States and abroad. The nurses who are credentialed by the American Nurses Association, Certification in Nursing Informatics, all 3,000 of them deserve recognition, as well as the 6,000 nurses in informatics in the United States. We acknowledge our international colleagues in nursing informatics. We also acknowledge the McGraw-Hill Education staff who contributed to editing the book, completing the production of this book, and supporting the expansion of the book with new resources. The authors also acknowledge their families because without them encouraging this effort, the book would not be a reality. We thank the Lord in giving us the opportunity to embark on a sixth edition and for the help in completing it.

Dr. Virginia K. Saba
Dr. Kathleen A. McCormick

The authors would like to sincerely thank the following for content in the fifth edition that has been updated in the sixth edition.

Nursing Informatics Technologies

Jacqueline Ann Moss

Historical Perspectives of Nursing Informatics

Virginia K. Saba / Bonnie L. Westra

• OBJECTIVES

1. Describe the historical perspective of nursing informatics.
2. Explore lessons learned from the pioneers in nursing informatics.
3. Describe the types of nursing standards initiatives.
4. Review the historical perspectives of electronic health records.
5. List the major landmark events and milestones of nursing informatics.

• KEY WORDS

Computers
Computer literacy
Computer systems
Data standards
Electronic Health Records (EHR)
Healthcare Information Technology (HIT)
Information systems
Internet
Nursing informatics

OVERVIEW

Nursing Informatics (NI) is a title that evolved from the French word "informatics" which referred to the field of applied computer science concerned with the processing of information such as nursing information (Nelson, 2013). The computer was seen as a tool that could be used in many environments. In the early 1960s, the computer was introduced into healthcare facilities for the processing of basic administrative tasks. Thus the computer revolution in healthcare began and led to today's healthcare information technology (HIT) and/or electronic health record (EHR) systems.

The importance of the computer as an essential tool in HIT systems and in the delivery of contemporary healthcare is indisputable. HIT is an all-encompassing term referring to technology that captures, processes, and generates healthcare information. Computerization and/or electronic processing affect all aspects of healthcare delivery including (a) provision and documentation of patient care, (b) education of healthcare providers, (c) scientific research for advancing healthcare delivery, (d) administration of healthcare delivery services, (e) reimbursement for patient care, (f) legal and ethical implications, as well as (d) safety and quality issues.

Since its inception there has been a shift from the use of mainframe, mini- or microcomputers (PCs) toward integrating multiple technologies and telecommunication devices such as wireless, handheld, mobile computers, and cell phones designed to support the continuity of care across healthcare settings and HIT systems. There has also been a dramatic shift from visible to invisible storage devices such as cloud storage, and from developing instructions for old software programs to today's icon, user-friendly, menu-driven, touch-screen manipulation methods for activating software programs.

Today, computers in nursing are used to manage patient care information, monitor quality, and evaluate outcomes. Computers and networks are also being used for communicating (sending and receiving) data and messages via the Internet, accessing resources, and interacting with patients on the Web. Nurses are increasingly becoming involved with systems used for planning, budgeting, and policy-making for patient care services, as well as enhancing nursing education and distance learning with new media modalities. Computers are also used to document and process real-time plans of care, support nursing research, test new systems, design new knowledge databases, develop data warehouses, and advance the role of nursing in the healthcare industry and nursing science.

This chapter is an updated and revised version of the Chapter 2 "Historical Perspectives of Nursing Informatics" (Saba & Westra, 2011) published in the fifth edition of *Essentials of Nursing Informatics* (Saba & McCormick, 2011). In this chapter, the significant events influencing the growth of NI as a nursing specialty are analyzed according to (1) **Seven Time Periods**, (2) a synthesis of lessons learned from 33 videotaped interviews with **Nursing Informatics Pioneers**, (3) **Nursing Standards Initiatives** including nursing practice and education, nursing content standards, and confidentiality and security standards, (4) **Electronic Health Records from a Historical Perspective**, and (5) **Landmark Events in Nursing and Computers** with Table 1.2 listing those events that influenced the introduction of computers into the nursing profession including key "computer/informatics" nurse(s) that directed the activity.

MAJOR HISTORICAL PERSPECTIVES OF NURSING AND COMPUTERS

Seven Time Periods

Prior to 1960s. Computers were first developed in the late 1930s to early 1940s, but their use in the healthcare industry occurred in the 1950s and 1960s. During this time, there were only a few experts nationally and internationally who formed a cadre of pioneers that attempted to adapt computers to healthcare and nursing. At that time the nursing profession was also undergoing major changes. The image of nursing was evolving, the number of educational programs and nurses increasing, and nursing practices and services were expanding in scope, autonomy, and

complexity from physicians' handmaidens to professional status. These events provided the impetus for the profession to embrace computers—a new technological tool.

Computers were initially used in healthcare facilities for basic office administrative and financial accounting functions. These early computers used punch cards to store data and card readers to read computer programs, sort, and prepare data for processing. They were linked together and operated by paper tape using teletypewriters to print their output. As computer technology advanced, the healthcare technologies also advanced. The major advances are listed chronologically in Table 1.2.

1960s. During the 1960s, the uses of computer technology in healthcare settings began to be explored. Questions such as "Why use computers?" and "What should be computerized?" were discussed. Nursing practice standards were reviewed, and nursing resources were analyzed. Studies were conducted to determine how computer technology could be utilized effectively in the healthcare industry and what areas of nursing should be automated. The nurses' station in the hospital was viewed as the hub of information exchange, the most appropriate center for the development of computer applications.

By the mid-1960s, clinical practice presented nurses with new opportunities for computer use. Increasingly complex patient care requirements and the proliferation of intensive care units required that nurses become super users of computer technology as nurses monitored patients' status via cardiac monitors and instituted treatment regimens through ventilators and other computerized devices. A significant increase in time spent by nurses documenting patient care, in some cases estimated at 40% (Sherman, 1965; Wolkodoff, 1963), as well as a noted rise in medication administration errors prompted the need to investigate emerging hospital computer-based information systems.

1970s. During the late 1960s through the 1970s, hospitals began developing computer-based information systems which initially focused on physician order entry and results reporting, pharmacy, laboratory, and radiology reports, information for financial and managerial purposes, and physiologic monitoring systems in the intensive care units, and a few systems started to include care planning, decision support, and interdisciplinary problem lists. While the content contained in early hospital information systems frequently was not specific to nursing practice, a few systems did provide a few pioneer nurses with a foundation on which to base future nursing information systems (Blackmon et al., 1982; Collen, 1995; Ozbolt & Bakken, 2003; Romano, McCormick, & McNeely, 1982; Van Bemmel & Munsen, 1997). Regardless of the focus, which remained primarily on medical practice, nurses often were involved in implementing HIT systems.

Interest in computers and nursing began to emerge in public and home health services and education during the 1960s to 1970s. Automation in public health agencies began as a result of pressure to standardize data collection procedures and provide state-wide reports on the activities and health of the public (Parker, Ausman, & Overdovitz, 1965). In the 1970s, conferences sponsored by the Division of Nursing (DN), Public Health Service (PHS), and the National League for Nursing (NLN) helped public and home health nurses understand the importance of nursing data and their relationship to new Medicare and Medicaid legislation, passed in 1966, requirements. The conferences provided information on the usefulness of computers for capturing and aggregating home health and public health information. Additional government-sponsored conferences focused on educational uses of computers for nurses (Public Health Service, 1976). At the same time as hospitals and public health agencies embarked on investigating computers and nursing, the opportunity to improve education using computer technology also began. Bitzer (1966) reported on one of the first uses of a computerized teaching system called PLATO, which was implemented to teach classes in off-campus sites as an alternative to traditional classroom education.

The early nursing networks, which were conceived at health informatics organizational meetings, helped expand nursing awareness of computers and the impact HIT could have on practice. The state of technology initially limited opportunities for nurses to contribute to the HIT design, but as technology evolved toward the later part of the 1970s and as nurses provided workshops nationally, nurses gained confidence that they could use computers to improve practice. The national nursing organization's federal agencies (Public Health Service, Army Nurse Corps) and several university schools of nursing provided educational conferences and workshops on the state-of-the-art regarding computer technology and its influence on nursing. During this time, the Clinical Center at the National Institutes of Health implemented the TDS computer system; one of the earliest clinical information systems (called Eclipsys and now Allscripts) was the first system to include nursing practice protocols (Romano et al., 1982).

1980s. In the 1980s, the field of nursing informatics exploded and became visible in the healthcare industry and nursing. Technology challenged creative professionals in the use of computers in nursing, which became revolutionary. As computer systems were implemented, the needs of nursing took on a cause-and-effect modality; that is, as new computer technologies emerged and as computer architecture advanced, the need for nursing software evolved.

It became apparent that the nursing profession needed to update its practice standards and determine its data standards, vocabularies, and classification schemes that could be used for the computer-based patient record systems.

Starting in 1981, national and international conferences and workshops were conducted by a few nursing pioneers to help nurses understand and get involved in this new emerging nursing specialty. Also during the 1980s, invitational conferences were conducted to develop nursing data sets and vocabularies as well as numerous workshops were conducted at universities to introduce this new specialty into nursing education.

During this period, many mainframe healthcare information systems (HISs) emerged with nursing subsystems. These systems documented several aspects of the patient record, namely, provider order entry and results reporting, the Kardex reporting, vital signs, and other systems-documented narrative nursing notes using word-processing software packages. Discharge planning systems were developed and used as referrals to community, public, and home healthcare facilities for the continuum of care.

In the 1980s, the microcomputer or personal computer (PC) emerged. This revolutionary technology made computers more accessible, affordable, and usable by nurses and other healthcare providers. The PC brought computing power to the workplace and, more importantly, to the point of care. Also the PCs served as dumb terminals linked to the mainframe computers and as stand-alone systems (workstations). The PCs were user-friendly and allowed nurses to design and program their own applications.

Nurses began presenting at multidisciplinary conferences and formed their own working groups within HIT organizations, such as the first Nursing Special Interest Group on Computers which met for the first time during SCAMC (Symposium on Computer Applications in Medical Care) in 1981. As medical informatics evolved, nursing began focusing on what was unique about nursing within the context of informatics. Resolutions were passed by the American Nurses Association (ANA) regarding computer use in nursing and in 1985, the ANA approved the formation of the Council on Computer Applications in Nursing (CCAN). One of the first activities the CCAN executive board initiated was to solicit several early pioneers to develop monographs on the status of computers in nursing practice, education, research, and management. The CCAN board developed a yearly *Computer Nurse Directory* on the known nurses involved in the field, conducted computer applications demonstrations at the ANA Annual conferences, and shared information with their growing members in the first CCAN newsletter *Input-Output*. During this time, Nursing Informatics newsletters, journals were being introduced including several books, such as the first edition of this book published in 1986. These were being used for educational courses introduced in the academic nursing programs, and workshops being conducted on computers and nursing. The CCAN became a very powerful force in integrating computer applications into the nursing profession.

1990s. By the 1990s, large integrated healthcare delivery systems evolved, further creating the need for information across healthcare facilities within these large systems to standardize processes, control costs, and assure quality of care (Shortliffe, Perreault, Wiederhold, & Pagan, 2003). Advances in relational databases, client-server architectures, and new programming methods created the opportunity for better application development at lower costs. Legislative activity in the mid-1990s paved the way for EHRs through the Health Insurance Portability and Accountability Act (HIPAA) of 1996 (public-law 104-191), emphasizing standardized transactions, and privacy and security of patient-identifiable information (Gallagher, 2010). The complexity of technology, workflow analysis, and regulations shaped new roles for nursing.

In 1992, the ANA recognized Nursing Informatics as a new nursing specialty with a separate *Scope of Nursing Informatics Practice Standards*, and also established a specific credentialing examination for it (ANA, 2010). Numerous local, national, and international organizations provided a forum for networking and continuing education for nurses involved with informatics (Sackett & Erdley, 2002). The demand for NI expertise increased in the healthcare industry and other settings where nurses functioned, and the technology revolution continued to impact the nursing profession.

The need for computer-based nursing practice standards, data standards, nursing minimum data sets, and national databases emerged concurrent with the need for a unified nursing language, including nomenclatures, vocabularies, taxonomies, and classification schemes (Westra, Delaney, Konicek, & Keenan, 2008). Nurse administrators started to demand that the HITs include nursing care protocols and nurse educators continued to require use of innovative technologies for all levels and types of nursing and patient education. Also, nurse researchers required knowledge representation, decision support, and expert systems based on standards that allowed for aggregated data (Bakken, 2006).

In 1997, the ANA developed the *Nursing Information and Data Set Evaluation Standards* (NIDSEC) to evaluate and recognize nursing information systems (ANA, 1997). The purpose was to guide the development and selection of nursing systems that included standardized nursing terminologies integrated throughout the system whenever it was appropriate. There were four high-level standards: (a) inclusion of ANA-recognized terminologies;

(b) linkages among concepts represented by the terminologies were retained in a logical and reusable manner; (c) data were included in a clinical data repository; and (d) general system characteristics. The Certification Commission for Health Information Technology (CCHIT) had similar criteria for the EHR certification, which was later adopted by the Office of the National Coordinator (ONC); however, nursing data was no longer included. ANA was ahead of its time in their thinking and development. The criteria are now under revision by the ANA to support nurses to advocate their requirements for the emerging HIT systems.

Technology rapidly changed in the 1990s, increasing its use within and across nursing units, as well as across healthcare facilities. Computer hardware—PCs—continued to get smaller and computer notebooks were becoming affordable, increasing the types of computer technology available for nurses to use. Linking computers through networks both within hospitals and health systems as well as across systems facilitated the flow of patient information to provide better care. By 1995, the Internet began providing access to information and knowledge databases to be integrated into bedside systems. The Internet moved into the mainstream social milieu with electronic mail (e-mail), file transfer protocol (FTP), Gopher, Telnet, and World Wide Web (WWW) protocols greatly enhanced its usability and user-friendliness (Saba, 1996; Sparks, 1996). The Internet was used for High-Performance Computing and Communication (HPCC) or the "Information Superhighway" and facilitated data exchange between computerized patient record systems across facilities and settings over time. The Internet led to improvements in networks and a browser, World Wide Web (WWW), allowed organizations to communicate more effectively and increased access to information that supported nursing practice. The World Wide Web (WWW) also became integral part of the HIT systems and the means for nurses to browse the Internet and search worldwide resources (Nicoll, 1998; Saba, 1995).

2000s. A change occurred in the new millennium as more and more healthcare information became digitalized and newer technologies emerged. In 2004, an Executive Order 13335 established the Office of the National Coordinator for Healthcare Information Technology (ONC) and issued a recommendation calling for all healthcare providers to adopt interoperable EHRs by 2014–2015. This challenged nurses to get involved in the design of systems to support their workflow as well as in the integration of information from multiple sources to support nurses' knowledge of technology. In late 2000s, as hospitals became "paperless," they began employing new nurses who had never charted on paper.

Technological developments that influenced healthcare and nursing included data capture and data sharing technological tools. Wireless, point-of-care, regional database projects, and increased IT solutions proliferated in healthcare environments, but predominately in hospitals and large healthcare systems. The use of bar coding and radio-frequency identification (RFID) emerged as a useful technology to match "right patient with the right medication" to improve patient safety. The RFID also emerged to help nurses find equipment or scan patients to assure all surgical equipment is removed from inside patients before surgical sites are closed (Westra, 2009). Smaller mobile devices with wireless or Internet access such as notebooks, tablet PCs, personal digital assistants (PDAs), and smart cellular telephones increased access to information for nurses within hospitals and in the community. The development and subsequent refinement of voice over Internet protocol (VoIP) provided voice cost-effective communication for healthcare organizations.

The Internet provided a means for development of clinical applications. Databases for EHRs could be hosted remotely on the Internet, decreasing costs of implementing EHRs. Remote monitoring of multiple critical care units from a single site increased access for safe and effective cardiac care (Rajecki, 2008). Home healthcare increasingly partnered with information technology for the provision of patient care. Telehealth applications, a recognized specialty for nursing since the late 1990s, provided a means for nurses to monitor patients at home and support specialty consultation in rural and underserved areas. The NI research agenda promoted the integration of nursing care data in HIT systems that would also generate data for analysis, reuse, and aggregation.

2010s. A historical analysis of the impact of the Nursing Minimum Data Set (NMDS) demonstrated that continued consensus and effort was needed to bring to fruition the vision and implementation of minimum nursing data into clinical practice (Hobbs, 2011). The NMDS continues to be the underlining focus in the newer HIT systems.

A new NI research agenda for 2008–2018 (Bakken, Stone, & Larson, 2012) emerged as critical for this specialty. The new agenda is built on the one originally developed and published by the National Institute for Nursing Research (NINR) in 1993 (NINR, 1993). The authors focused on the new NI research agenda on "3 aspects of context—genomic health care, shifting research paradigms, and social (Web2.0) technologies" (p. 280).

A combination of the economic recession along with the escalating cost of healthcare resulted in the American Recovery and Reinvestment Act of 2009 (ARRA) and the Healthcare Information Technology for Economic and Clinical Health (HITECH) Act of 2009 with funding to implement HIT and/or EHR systems, support healthcare information exchange, enhance community and university-based informatics education, and support leading edge research to improve the use of HIT (Gallagher, 2010). During 2010, the ONC convened two national committees, (a) National

Committee on Health Policy and (b) National Committee on Health Standards, which outlined and designed the focus for the "Meaningful Use" (MU) legislation. Meaningful Use was designed to be implemented in at least three stages, each consisting of regulations which built onto each other with the ultimate goal of implementing a complete and interoperable EHR and/or HIT system in all US hospitals. For each stage, regulations were proposed by the national committees, and developed and reviewed by the public before they were finalized by the Centers for Medicaid and Medicare (CMS) and submitted to the healthcare facilities for implementation.

In 2011–2012 MU Stage 1 was initiated focusing primarily on the Computerized Physician Order Entry (CPOE) initiative for physicians. Hospitals that implemented this MU regulation successfully received federal funds for their HIT systems. In 2012–2013 MU Stage 2 was introduced focusing primarily on the implementation of Quality Indicators that required electronic data to be collected, measured, and used to demonstrate that a specific quality indicator was an integral component in the HIT systems. The Quality Indicators are used to guide hospitals in patient safety and if not implemented used as indicators subject to financial penalties. It is anticipated that MU Stage 3 will begin to be implemented in 2015–2016 and will primarily focus on care Outcome Measures and tentatively proposed Care Plans that encompass clinical specialty Plans of Care such as Nursing and Treatment Plans (see Chapter 16 "Nursing Informatics and Healthcare Policy" for MU details).

The billions of dollars invested are intended to move the health industry forward toward complete digitalization of healthcare information. Meanwhile the Center for Medicare & Medicaid Services (CMS) plans to increase reimbursement for the implementation of "MU" regulations in their HIT and/or EHR systems through 2015, and may even penalize eligible providers and facilities who do not meet the proposed MU criteria.

Nurses are involved with all phases of MU, from implementation of systems to assuring usage and adaptation to the evolving health policy affecting the HIT and/or EHR systems. Thus, the field of Nursing Informatics continues to grow due to the MU regulations which continue to impact on every inpatient hospital in the country. As a result, to date the majority of hospitals in the country has established HIT departments and has employed at least one nurse to serve as a NI Expert to assist with the implementation of MU requirements. As the MU requirements increase they will impact on the role of the NI experts in hospitals and ultimately on the roles of all nurses in the inpatient facilities, making NI an integral component of all professional nursing services.

Consumer-Centric Healthcare System. Another impact of the escalating cost of healthcare is a shift toward a Consumer-Centric Healthcare System. Consumers are encouraged to be active partners in managing their own health. A variety of technologies have evolved to enable consumers to have access to their health information and choose whether to share this across healthcare providers and settings. Personal health records multiplied as either stand-alone systems or those tethered to EHRs. Consumers are increasing in healthcare information literacy as they demand to become more involved in managing their own health.

NURSING INFORMATICS PIONEERS

History Project

In 1995, Saba initiated a history of NI at the National Library of Medicine that consisted of the collection of archival documents from the NI pioneers. The History Project was initiated based on a recommendation by Dr. Morris Collen who published the *History of Medical Informatics* in 1995 (Colleen, 1995). However, it was not until 2001 that the Nursing Informatics Working Group (NIWG) of the American Medical Informatics Association (AMIA) became involved and the NI History Committee was established to take on this project. The committee solicited archival material from the known NI pioneers for a History of Nursing Informatics to be housed in the NLM as part of its History Collection (Newbold, Berg, McCormick, Saba, & Skiba, 2012).

Beginning in 2004, the rich stories of pioneers in NI were captured through a project sponsored by the American Medical Informatics Association Nursing Informatics Working Group (AMIA-NIWG). The AMIA-NIWG History Committee developed an evolving list of pioneers and contributors to the history of NI. Pioneers were defined as those who "opened up" a new area in NI and provided a sustained contribution to the specialty (Newbold & Westra, 2009; Westra & Newbold, 2006). Through multiple contacts and review of the literature, the list grew to 145 pioneers and contributors who shaped NI since the 1950s. Initially, each identified pioneer was contacted to submit their nonpublished documents and/or historical materials to the National Library of Medicine (NLM) to be indexed and archived for the Nursing Informatics History Collection. Approximately, 25 pioneers submitted historical materials that were cataloged with a brief description.

Currently, the cataloged document descriptions can be searched online: www.nlm.nih.gov/hmd/manuscripts/accessions.html. The documents can also be viewed by visiting the NLM. Eventually each archived document will be indexed and available online in the NI History Collection. Also from the original list, a convenience sample of pioneers was interviewed over a 4-year period at various NI meetings. Videotaped stories from 33 pioneers were recorded and are now available on the AMIA Web site: www.amia.org/niwg-history-page.

Videotaped Interviews. The AMIA Nursing Informatics History page contains a wealth of information. The 33 videotaped interviews are divided into two libraries. The full interviews are available in Library 1: Nursing Informatics Pioneers. For each pioneer, a picture, short biographical sketch, transcript of the interview, and MP3 audio file are included in addition to the videotaped interview. In Library 2: Themes from Interviews, selected segments from the interviews are shared for easy comparison across the pioneers. The themes include the following:

- Nursing Informatics—what it is, present, future, what nursing brings to the table
- Significant events that have shaped the field of nursing informatics
- Pioneers' paths—careers that lead up to involvement in (nursing) informatics
- When they first considered themselves informatics nurses
- Pioneers' first involvement—earliest events they recall
- Informatics—its value, pioneers' realizations of the value of informatics, how they came to understand the value of informatics
- Demography of pioneers including names, educational backgrounds, and current positions
- Personal aspirations and accomplishments, overall vision that guided the pioneers' work, people the pioneer collaborated with to accomplish their visions, and goals
- Pioneers' lessons learned that they would like to pass on

The Web site also provides "use cases" for ideas about how to use the information for teaching and learning more about the pioneers. These resources are particularly useful for courses in informatics, leadership, and research. They also are useful for nurses in the workforce who want to learn more about NI history.

Backgrounds. The early pioneers came from a variety of backgrounds as nursing education in NI did not exist in the 1960s. Almost all of the pioneers were educated as nurses, though a few were not. A limited number of pioneers had additional education in computer science, engineering, epidemiology, and biostatistics. Others were involved with anthropology, philosophy, physiology, and public health. Their career paths varied considerably (Branchini, 2012). Some nursing faculty saw technology as a way to improve education. Others worked in clinical settings and were involved in "roll-outs" of information systems. Often these systems were not designed to improve nursing work, but the pioneers had a vision that technology could make nursing practice better. Other pioneers gained experience through research projects or working for software vendors. The commonality for all the pioneers is they saw various problems and inefficiencies in nursing and they had a burning desire to use technology to "make things better."

Lessons Learned. What are some of the lessons learned from the pioneers? Pioneers by definition are nurses who forged into the unknown and had a vision of what was possible, even if they did not know how to get there. One of the pioneers advised, "Don't be afraid to take on something that you've never done before. You can learn how to do it. The trick is in finding out who knows it and picking their brain and if necessary, cornering them and making them teach you!" Another said, "Just do it, rise above it [barriers], and go for it…you are a professional, and…you have to be an advocate for yourself and the patient." Many of the pioneers described the importance of mentors, someone who would teach them about informatics or computer technology, but it was still up to them to apply their new knowledge to improve nursing. Mentors were invaluable by listening, exchanging ideas, connecting to others, and supporting new directions. Networking was another strong theme for pioneers. Belonging to professional organizations, especially interprofessional organizations, was key for success. At meetings, the pioneers networked and exchanged ideas, learning from others what worked and, more importantly, what did not work. They emphasized the importance of attending social functions at organizational meetings to develop solid relationships so they could call on colleagues later to further network and exchange ideas.

Nursing informatics did not occur in a vacuum; a major effort was made to promote the inclusion of nurses in organizations affecting health policy decisions such as the ONC's Technology Policy and Standards Committees. The nursing pioneers influenced the evolution of informatics as a specialty from granular-level data through health policy and funding to shape this evolving and highly visible specialty in nursing.

NURSING STANDARDS INITIATIVES

The third significant historic perspective concerns standards initiatives focusing on nursing practice, education, nursing content, and confidentiality and security, as well as federal legislation that impacts the use of computers for nursing. These standards have influenced the nursing profession and its need for computer systems with appropriate nursing content or terminologies. Legislative acts during the early stages significantly influenced the use of computers to collect federally required data, carry out reimbursement,

measure quality, and evaluate outcomes. This section only highlights briefly the critical initiatives "to set the stage" for more information in other chapters of this book.

Nursing Practice Standards

Nursing Practice Standards have been developed and recommended by the ANA, the official professional nursing organization. The ANA published *Nursing: Scope and Standards of Practice* (ANA, 2008) that focused not only on the organizing principles of clinical nursing practice but also on the standards of professional performance. The six standards/phases of the nursing process serve as the conceptual framework for the documentation of nursing practice. The updated *Nursing Informatics: Scope and Standards of Practice* (ANA, 2010) builds on clinical practice standards, outlining further the importance of implementing standardized content to support nursing practice by specialists in NI.

Nursing Education Standards

The NLN has been the primary professional organization that accredits undergraduate nursing programs. Since the NLN's Nursing Forum on Computers in Healthcare and Nursing (NFCHN) was formed in 1985, it has supported the integration of computer technology in the nursing curriculum. The American Association of Colleges of Nursing (AACN), which also accredits nursing education programs, revised *The Essentials for Doctoral Education for Advanced Nursing Practice* (AACN, 2006) and *The Essentials of Baccalaureate Education for Professional Nursing Practice* (AACN, 2011) to require the use of computers and informatics for both baccalaureate and graduate education. These new requirements for informatics competencies prepare nurses to use HITs successfully and to contribute to the ongoing design of technologies that support the cognitive work of nurses (AACN, 2011).

Nursing Content Standards

The nursing process data elements in EHRs are essential for the exchange of nursing information across information systems and settings. The original data elements and the historic details of nursing data standards are described in Chapter 7 of this book. Standardization of healthcare data began in 1893 with the *List of International Causes of Death* (World Health Organization, 1992) for the reporting of morbidity cases worldwide, whereas the standardization of nursing began with Florence Nightingale's six Cannons in her "Notes on Nursing" (1959). However, it was not until 1955 that Virginia Henderson published her 14 Daily Patterns of Living as the list of activities and conditions that became the beginning of nursing practice standards in this country. But it was not until 1970 when the American

Nurses Association (ANA) accepted the Nursing Process as the professional standards for nursing practice, which was followed by the standardization of nursing content—data elements—in 1973 (Westra et al., 2008). Prior to that time nursing theorists proposed concepts, activities, tasks, goals, and so forth, as well as frameworks as a theoretical foundation for the practice of nursing, which could not be processed by computer. Since 1973 several nursing organizations, educational institutions, and vendors developed nursing data sets, classifications, or terminologies for the documentation of nursing practice. These nursing terminologies were developed at different times by different organizations or universities. They vary in content (representing one or more nursing process data elements), most appropriate setting for use, and level of access in the public domain.

Currently, the ANA has "recognized" 12 nursing terminologies (see Chapter 8 "Standardized Nursing Terminologies" for their descriptions). The ANA is also responsible for determining whether a terminology meets the criteria they established. They ANA selected six of the ANA-"recognized" nursing languages for inclusion in the National Library of Medicine's (NLM) Metathesaurus of the Unified Medical Language System (UMLS) (Humphreys & Lindberg, 1992; Saba, 1998) and also for inclusion in the Systematized Nomenclature of Medicine—Clinical Terms (SNOMED-CT). In 2002, SNOMED-CT became the International Health Terminology Standards Development Organization (IHTSDO) (Wang, Sable, & Spackman, 2002) with its headquarters in Europe. However, SNOMED-CT is still distributed, at no cost, by the NLM which is now the US member of IHTSDO and which continues to maintain the Metathesaurus of the UMLS (http://www.nlm.nih.gov/research/umls/SNOMED.snomed_main.html).

There are a large number of standards organizations that impact healthcare data content as well as healthcare technology systems, including their architecture, functional requirements, and certification. They also impact on heath policy which in turn impacts on standardized nursing practice (Hammond, 1994). They are being discussed in Chapter 7 "Health Data Standards: Development, Harmonization, and Interoperability."

Confidentiality and Security Standards

Increasing access through the electronic capture and exchange of information raised concerns about the privacy and security of personal healthcare information (PHI). Provisions for strengthening the original HIPAA legislation were included in the 2009 HITECH Act (Gallagher, 2010). Greater emphasis was placed on patient consent, more organizations handling PHI were included in the legislation, and penalties were increased for security breaches.

ELECTRONIC HEALTH RECORDS FROM A HISTORICAL PERSPECTIVE

In 1989, the Institute of Medicine (IOM) of the National Academy of Sciences convened a committee and asked the question, "Why is healthcare still predominantly using paper-based records when so many new computer-based information technologies are emerging?" (Dick & Steen, 1991). The IOM invited representatives of major stakeholders in healthcare and asked them to define the problem, identify issues, and outline a path forward. Two major conclusions resulted from the committee's deliberations. First, computerized patient record (CPR) is an essential technology for healthcare and is an integral tool for all professionals. Second, the committee after hearing from numerous stakeholders recognized that there was no national coordination or champion for CPRs. As a result, the IOM committee recommended the creation of an independent institute to provide national leadership. The Computer-Based Patient Record Institute (CPRI) was created in 1992 and given the mission to initiate and coordinate the urgently needed activities to develop, deploy, and routinely use CPRs to achieve improved outcomes in healthcare quality, cost, and access.

A CPRI Work Group developed the CPR Project Evaluation Criteria in 1993 modeled after the Baldridge Award. These criteria formed the basis of a self-assessment that could be used by organizations and outside reviewers to measure and evaluate the accomplishments of CPR projects. The four major areas of the initial criteria—(a) management, (b) functionality, (c) technology, and (d) impact—provided a framework through which to view an implementation of computerized records. The criteria, which provided the foundation for the Nicholas E. Davies Award of Excellence Program, reflect the nation's journey from paper-based to electronic capture of health data. The Davies Award of Excellence Program evolved through multiple revisions and its terminology updated from the computerized patient record, to the electronic medical record (EMR), and more recently to the electronic health record (EHR).

Today, under HIMSS management, the Davies Award of Excellence Program is offered in four categories: Enterprise (formerly Organizational or Acute Care), first offered in 1995; Ambulatory Care, started in 2003; Public Health, initiated in 2004; and Community Health Organizations (CHO), first presented in 2008 (http://apps.himss.org/davies/index.asp).

LANDMARK EVENTS IN NURSING AND COMPUTERS

Major Milestones

Computers were introduced into the nursing profession over 40 years ago. Major milestones of nursing are interwoven with the advancement of computer and information technologies, the increased need for nursing data, development of nursing applications, and changes making the nursing profession an autonomous discipline.

The landmark events were also categorized and described in the chapter "Historical Perspectives of Nursing Informatics" (Saba & Westra, 2011) published in the fifth edition of *Essentials of Nursing Informatics* (Saba & McCormick, 2011). In this edition, the major landmark milestones have been updated in Table 1.2. The milestone events are listed in chronological order including for the first time the key NI Pioneer or Expert involved in the event as well as the first time a key event occurred, which may be ongoing. Many other events may have occurred but this table represents the most complete history of the NI specialty movement.

There are currently several key events in which the NI community participates, and many of them are held annually. The conferences, symposia, institutes, and workshops provide an opportunity for NI novices and experts to network and share their experiences. They also provide the latest information, newest exhibits, and demonstrations on this changing field and are shown in Table 1.1.

SUMMARY

Computers, and subsequently information technology, emerged during the past five decades in the healthcare industry. Hospitals began to use computers as tools to update paper-based patient records. Computer systems in healthcare settings provided the information management capabilities needed to assess, document, process, and communicate patient care. As a result, the "human–machine" interaction of nursing and computers has become a new and lasting symbiotic relationship (Blum, 1990; Collen, 1994; Kemeny, 1972).

The history of informatics from the perspective of the pioneers was briefly described in this chapter. The complete video, audio, and transcripts can be found on the AMIA Web site (www.amia.org/niwg-history-page). Over the last 40 years, nurses have used and contributed to the evolving HIT or EHR systems for the improved practice of nursing.

Innumerable organizations sprang up in an attempt to set standards for nursing practice and education, standardize the terminologies, create standard structures for EHRs, and attempt to create uniformity for the electronic exchange of information. This chapter highlighted a few key organizations.

The last section focuses on Landmark Events in Nursing Informatics, including major milestones in national and international conferences, symposia, workshops, and organizational initiatives contributing to the computer literacy of nurses in Table 1.2. The success of

TABLE 1.1	Major Events for Nursing Informatics Community

A. Conferences and Workshops

- **American Medical Informatics Association (AMIA) Annual Symposium**
  - Nursing Informatics Workshop
  - Nursing Informatics Working Group (NIWG)
  - Harriet Werley Award
  - Virginia K. Saba Award
- **Healthcare Information and Management and Systems Society (HIMSS) Annual Conference and Exhibition**
  - Nursing Informatics Symposium
  - Nursing Informatics Task Force
  - Nursing Informatics Leadership Award
- **Annual Summer Institute in Nursing Informatics (SINI) at University of Maryland, Baltimore, MD**
- **Annual Rutgers State University of New Jersey College of Nursing: Nursing and Computer Technology Conference**
  - Rutgers "Outstanding Contribution in Field of NI Award"
- **Annual American Academy of Nursing**
  - Panel of Nursing Informatics Experts
- **Sigma Theta Tau International: Bi-Annual Conference**
  - Virginia K. Saba Nursing Informatics Leadership Award (Bi-Annual)
  - Technology Award; Information Resources (Annual)
- **Nursing Informatics Special Interest Group of the International Medical Informatics Association (IMIA/NI-SIG): Tri-Annual Conference**
  - Starting 2014 Bi-Annual Conference
- **International Medical Informatics Association (IMIA): Triennial Congress**
  - Nursing Sessions and Papers

B. Professional Councils and/or Committees

- **American Nurses Association (ANA)**
  - Nursing Informatics Database Steering Committee
- **National League for Nursing (NLN)**
  - Educational Technology and Information Management Advisory Council (ETIMC)
- **American Academy of Nursing (AAN)**
  - Expert Panel of Nursing Informatics

C. Credentialing/Certification/Fellowship

- **American Nurses Association (ANA); American Nurses Credentialing Center (ANCC)**
  - Informatics Nursing Certification
- **Healthcare Information and Management and Systems Society (HIMSS)**
  - Certified Professional in Healthcare Information Management and Systems (CPHIMS)

TABLE 1.2 Landmark Events in Computers and Nursing, and Nursing Informatics

Year(s)	Title/Event	Sponsor(s)	Coordinator/Chair/NI Representative(s)
1973	First Invitational Conference: Management Information Systems (MISs) for Public and Community Health Agencies	National League for Nursing (NLN) and Division of Nursing, Public Health Service (DN/PHS), Arlington, VA	Goldie Levenson (NLN) Virginia K. Saba (DN/PHS)
1974 to 1975	Five Workshops in USA on MISs for Public and Community Health Agencies	NLN and DN/PHS, selected US Cities	Goldie Levenson (NLN) Virginia K. Saba (DN/PHS)
1976	State-of-the-Art Conference on Management for Public and Community Health Agencies	NLN and DN/PHS, Washington, DC	Goldie Levenson (NLN) Virginia K. Saba (DN/PHS)
1977	First Research: State-of-the-Art Conference on Nursing Information Systems	University of Illinois College of Nursing, Chicago, IL	Harriet H. Werley (UIL) Margaret Grier (UIL)
1977	First undergraduate academic course: Computers and Nursing	The State University of New York at Buffalo, Buffalo, NY	Judith Ronald (SUNY, Buffalo)
1979	First Military Conference on: Computers in Nursing	TRIMIS Army Nurse Consultant Team, Walter Reed Hospital, Washington, DC	Dorothy Pocklington (TRIMIS Army) Linda Guttman (ANC)
1980	First Workshop: Computer Usage in Healthcare	University of Akron, School of Nursing, Continuing Education Department, Akron, OH	Virginia Newbern (UA/SON) Dorothy Pocklington (TRIMIS Army) Virginia K. Saba (DN/PHS)
1980	First Computer Textbook: Computers in Nursing	Nursing Resources, Boston, MA	Rita Zielstorff, Editor
1981	First Special Interest Group Meeting on Computers in Nursing at SCAMC	Annual SCAMC Conference Event, Washington, DC	Virginia K. Saba, Chair (DN/PHS)
1981 to 1991	First Nursing Papers Initiated at Fifth Annual Symposium on Computer Applications in Medical Care (SCAMC)	Annual SCAMC Conference Sessions, Washington, DC	Virginia K. Saba (DN/PHS) Coralee Farlee (NCHSR)
1981 to 1984	Four National Conferences: Computer Technology and Nursing	NIH Clinical Center, TRIMIS Army Nurse Consultant Team, and DN/PHS NIH Campus, Bethesda, MD	Virginia K. Saba (DN/PHS) Ruth Carlsen and Carol Romano (CC/NIH) Dorothy Pocklington and Carolyn Tindal (TRIMIS Army)
1981	Early academic course on Computers in Nursing (NIH/CC)	Foundation for Advanced Education in Sciences (FAES) at NIH, Bethesda, MD	Virginia K. Saba (DN/PHS) Kathleen A. McCormick (NIH/PHS)
1982	Study Group on Nursing Information Systems	University Hospitals of Cleveland, Case Western Reserve University, and National Center for Health Services Research (NCHSR/PHS), Cleveland, OH	Mary Kiley (CWS) Gerry Weston (NCHSR)
1982 to Present	Initiated Annual International Nursing Computer Technology Conference	Rutgers, State University of New Jersey, College of Nursing, CE Department, selected cities	Gayle Pearson (Rutgers) Jean Arnold (Rutgers)

Year	Event	Location	People
1982	First International Workshop: *The Impact of Computers on Nursing*	London Hospital, UK and IFIP-IMIA, Harrogate, UK	Maureen Scholes (UK) Barry Barber (UK)
1982	First Newsletter: *Computers in Nursing*	School of Nursing, University of Texas at Austin, Austin, TX	Gary Hales (UT)
1982 and 1984	Two Boston University (BU) Workshops on *Computers and Nursing*	Boston University School of Nursing, Boston, MA	Diane Skiba (BU)
1982	*PLATO IV CAI Educational Network System*	University of Illinois School of Nursing, Chicago, IL	Pat Tymchyshyn (UIL)
1982	Capital Area Roundtable in Informatics in Nursing (CARING) Founded	Greater Washington, DC	Founding Members: Susan McDermott, P. J. Hallberg, Susan Newbold
1983 to Present (Every 3 Years)	Initiated nursing papers at MED-INFO World Congress on Medical Informatics, International Medical Informatics Association (IMIA)	1983—Amsterdam, The Netherlands 1986—Washington, DC, USA 1989—Singapore, Malaysia 1992—Geneva, Switzerland 1995—Vancouver, Canada 1998—Seoul, South Korea 2001—London, UK 2004—San Francisco, CA 2007—Brisbane, AU 2010—Capetown, SA 2013—Copenhagen, DM	Elly Pluyter-Wenting, First Nursing Chair
1983	Second Annual Joint SCAMC Congress and IMIA Conference	SCAMC and IMIA, San Francisco, CA, and Baltimore, MD	Virginia K. Saba, Nursing Chair
1983	Early Workshop: *Computers in Nursing*	University of Texas at Austin, Austin, TX	Susan Grobe (UT—Austin)
1983	First Hospital Workshop: *Computers in Nursing Practice*	St. Agnes Hospital for HEC, Baltimore, MD	Susan Newbold
1983	First: *Nursing Model for Patient Care and Acuity System*	TRIMIS Program Office, Washington, DC	Karen Rieder (NNC) Dena Nortan (NNC)
1983 to 2012	Initiated International Symposium: *Nursing Use of Computers and Information Science*, IMIA Working Group 8 on Nursing Informatics (IMIA/NI-8)	1983—Amsterdam, the Netherlands 1985—Calgary, Canada	1983—Maureen Scholes, First Chair 1985—Kathryn J. Hannah and Evelyn J. Guillemin

(continued)

TABLE 1.2　Landmark Events in Computers and Nursing, and Nursing Informatics *(continued)*

Year(s)	Title/Event	Sponsor(s)	Coordinator/Chair/NI Representative(s)
2014 (New Q-2 Years)	Renamed: IMIA Nursing Informatics, Special Interest Group (IMIA/NI-SIG)	1988—Dublin, Ireland 1991—Melbourne, Australia 1994—San Antonio, TX, USA 1997—Stockholm, Sweden 2000—Auckland, New Zealand 2003—Rio de Janeiro, Brazil 2006—Seoul, Korea 2009—Helsinki, Finland 2012—Montreal, Canada 2014—Taipei, Taiwan	1988—Noel Daley and Maureen Scholes 1991—Evelyn S. Hovenga and Joan Edgecumbe 1994—Susan Grobe and Virginia K. Saba 1997—Ulla Gerdin and Marianne Tallberg 2000—Robyn Carr and Paula Rocha 2003—Heimar Marin and Eduardo Marques 2006—Hyeoun-Ae Park 2009—Anneli Ensio and Kaija Saranto 2012—Patricia Abbott (JHU) 2014—Polun Chang
1984	American Nursing Association (ANA) Initiated First Council Computer Applications in Nursing (CCAN)	ANA	Harriet Werley, Chair First Exec. Board: Ivo Abraham Kathleen A. McCormick Virginia K. Saba Rita Zielstorff
1984	First Seminar: *Microcomputers for Nurses*	University of California at San Francisco, College of Nursing, San Francisco, CA	William Holzemer, Chair
1984 to present	First Nursing Computer Journal: *Computers in Nursing CIN,* Renamed *Computers, Informatics, Nursing*	JB Lippincott, Philadelphia, PA	Gary Hales (UT Austin) First Editorial Board: Patricia Schwirian (OSU) Virginia K. Saba (GT) Susan Grobe (UT Austin) Rita Zielstorff (MGH Lab)
1984 to 1995	First *Directory of Educational Software for Nursing*	Christine Bolwell and National League for Nursing (NLN)	Christine Bolwell
1985	NLN initiated First National Forum: *Computers in Healthcare and Nursing*	National League for Nursing, New York City, NY	Susan Grobe, Chair First Exec. Board: Diane Skiba Judy Ronald Bill Holzemer Roy Simpson Pat Tymchyshyn
1985	First Annual Seminar on Computers and Nursing Practice	NYU Medical Center, New York, NY	Patsy Marr (NYU) Janet Kelly (NYU)
1985	First Invitational *Nursing Minimum Data Set (NMDS) Conference*	University of Illinois School of Nursing, Chicago, IL	Harriet Werley (UIL) Norma Lang (UM)

Year	Event	Location	Person(s)
1985	Early academic course: *Essentials of Computers*, in Undergraduate and Graduate Programs	Georgetown University School of Nursing, Washington, DC	Virginia K. Saba (GU)
1985 to 1990	Early 5-year Project: Continuing Nursing Education: *Computer Technology, Focus: Nursing Faculty*	Southern Regional Education Board (SREB), Atlanta, GA	Eula Aiken (SREB)
1985	First Test Authoring Program (TAP)	Addison-Wesley Publishing, New York, NY	William Holzemer (UCSF)
1986	Two early *Microcomputer Institutes for Nurses*	Georgetown University, School of Nursing, Washington, DC	Virginia K. Saba (GU)
		University of Southwest Louisiana Nursing Department, Lafayette, LA	Dorothy Pocklington (USL) Diane Skiba (BU)
1986	Established first nurse educator's newsletter: *Micro World*	Christine Bolwell and Stewart Publishing, Alexandria, VA	Christine Bolwell, Editor
1986	*CIN* First Indexed in MEDLINE and CINAHL	J. B. Lippincott Publisher, Philadelphia, PA	Gary Hales, Editor
1986	First *NI Pyramid—NI Research Model*	Published in *CIN* Indexed in MEDLINE and CINAHL	Patricia Schwirian (OSU)
1987	Initiated and Created *Interactive Videodisc Software Programs*	*American Journal of Nursing*, New York, NY	Mary Ann Rizzolo (AJN)
1987	*International Working Group Task Force on Education*	IMIA/NI Working Group 8 and Swedish Federation, Stockholm, Sweden	Ulla Gerdin (NI) Kristina Janson Jelger and Hans Peterson (Swedish Federation)
1987	Videodisc for Health Conference: *Interactive Healthcare Conference*	Stewart Publishing, Alexandria, VA	Scott Stewart, Publisher
1988	Recommendation #3: *Support Automated Information Systems.*	National Commission on Nursing Implementation Project (NCNIP), Secretary's Commission on Nursing Shortage	Vivian DeBack, Chair
1988	Priority Expert Panel E: *Nursing Informatics Task Force*	National Center for Nursing Research, NIH, Bethesda, MD	Judy Ozbolt, Chair
1989	Invitational Conference: *Nursing Information Systems*, Washington, DC	National Commission on Nursing Implementation Project (NCNIP), ANA, NLN, and NIS Industry	Vivian DeBack, Chair
1989 and 1991 to Present	Initiated First Graduate Programs with Specialty in Nursing Informatics, Master's and Doctorate	University of Maryland School of Nursing, Baltimore, MD	Barbara Heller, Dean Program Chairs: Carol Gassert, Patricia Abbott, Kathleen Charters, Judy Ozbolt, and Eun-Shim Nahm

(continued)

TABLE 1.2	Landmark Events in Computers and Nursing, and Nursing Informatics *(continued)*		
Year(s)	**Title/Event**	**Sponsor(s)**	**Coordinator/Chair/NI Representative(s)**
1989	ICN Resolution Initiated Project: *International Classification of Nursing Practice (ICNP)*	International Council of Nurses Conference, Seoul, Korea	Fadwa Affra (ICN)
1990 to 1995	*Annual Nurse Scholars Program*	HBO and HealthQuest Corporation	Roy Simpson (HBO) Diane Skiba (BU) Judith Ronald (SUNY Buffalo)
1990	ANA House of Delegates endorsed: *Nursing Minimum Data Set (NMDS)* to define costs and quality of care	ANA House of Delegates	Harriet Werley (UM)
1990	Invitational Conference: *State-of-the-Art of Information Systems*	NCNIP, Orlando, FL	Vivian DeBack, Chair
1990	Renamed ANA: Steering Committee on Databases to Support Nursing Practice	ANA, Washington, DC	Norma Lang, Chair Kathy Milholland Hunter (ANA) Carol Bickford
1990	Task Force: *Nursing Information Systems*	NCNIP, ANA, NLN, NIS Industry Task Force, Project Hope, VA	Vivian DeBack, Chair
1991 to 2001	First Annual *European Summer Institute*	International Nursing Informatics Experts	Jos Aarts and Diane Skiba (USA)
1991	First *Nursing Informatics Listserv*	University of Massachusetts, Amherst, MA	Gordon Larrivee
1991	Formation of Combined Annual SCAMC *Special Nursing Informatics Working Group* and AMIA NIWG	AMIA/SCAMC Sponsors, Washington, DC	Judy Ozbolt, First Chair
1991 and 1992	Two WHO Workshops: *Nursing Informatics*	World Health Organization and US PHS, Washington, DC, and Geneva, Switzerland	Marian Hirschfield (WHO) Carol Romano (PHS)
1991 to Present	Initiated Annual *Summer Institute in Nursing and Healthcare Informatics (SINI)*	University of Maryland School of Nursing (SON), Baltimore, MD	Program Chairs: Carol Gassert, Mary Etta Mills, Judy Ozbolt, and Marissa Wilson
1992	ANA-approved Nursing Informatics as a new Nursing Specialty	ANA Database Steering Committee, Washington, DC	Norma Lang, Chair
1992	Formation of *Virginia Henderson International Nursing Library (INL)*	Sigma Theta Tau International Honor Society, Indianapolis, IN	Judith Graves, Director
1992	ANA "recognized" four Nursing Terminologies: *CCC System (HHCC), OMAHA System, NANDA, and NIC*	ANA Database Steering Committee, Washington, DC	Norma Lang, Chair
1992	*Read Clinical Thesaurus* added Nursing Terms in UMLS	Read Codes Clinical Terms, Version 3	Ann Casey (UK)
1992	Canadian Nurses Assoc.: *Nursing Minimum Data Set Conference*	Canadian Nurses Association, Edmonton, Alberta, Canada	Phyllis Giovannetti, Chair
1992	American Nursing Informatics Association (ANIA) Founded	Southern, CA	Melodie Kaltenbaugh

Year	Event	Organization/Location	People
1993	Four ANA "Recognized" Nursing Terminologies Integrated into UMLS	ANA Database Steering Committee and NLM	Norma Lang, Chair; Betsy Humphreys (NLM)
1993	Initiated *Virginia Henderson Electronic Library Online* via Internet	Sigma Theta Tau International Honor Society, Indianapolis, IN	Carol Hudgings, Director
1993	Initiated *AJN Network Online* via Internet	American Journal of Nursing Company, New York, NY	Mary Ann Rizzolo, Director
1993	ANC Postgraduate course: *Computer Applications for Nursing*	Army Nurse Corps, Washington, DC	Army Nurse Corps (ANC)
1993	Formation: Nursing Informatics Fellowship Program	Partners Healthcare Systems, Wellesley, MA	Rita Zielstorff, Director
1993	Alpha Version: Working Paper of ICNP	International Council of Nurses, Geneva, Switzerland	Fadwa Affara (ICN)
1993	Formed: *Denver Free-Net*	University of Colorado Health Sciences Center, Denver, CO	Diane Skiba (UC)
1993	Priority Expert Panel E: *Nursing Informatics Report: Nursing Informatics: Enhancing Patient Care*	National Center for Nursing Research (NCNR/NIH), Bethesda, MD	Judy Ozbolt, Chair
1994	*ANA-NET Online*	American Nurses Association, Washington, DC	Kathy Milholland (ANA)
1994	Four Nursing Educators *Workshops on Computers in Education*	Southern Council on Collegiate Regional Education and University of Maryland, Washington, DC; Baltimore, MD; Atlanta, GA; Augusta, GA	Eula Aiken (SREB), Mary Etta Mills (UMD)
1994	*Next Generation: Clinical Information Systems Conference*	Tri-Council for Nursing and Kellogg Foundation, Washington, DC	Sheila Ryan, Chair
1994, 2008, and 2014	First *Nursing: Scope and Standards of Nursing Informatics Practice*	ANA Database Steering Committee	Kathy Milholland (ANA)
1995	First International NI Teleconference: Three Countries Linked Together	International NI Experts: NI, USA; HIS, Australia; NI, New Zealand	Sue Sparks (USA), Evelyn Hovenga (AU), Robyn Carr (NZ)
1995	First Combined NYU Hospital and NYU SON: *Programs on Nursing Informatics and Patient Care: A New Era*	NYU School of Nursing and NYU Medical Center, New York, NY	Barbara Carty, Chair; Janet Kelly, Co-Chair
1995	First *Weekend Immersion in NI (WINI)*	CARING Group, Warrenton, VA	Susan Newbold (CARING), Carol Bickford (ANA), Kathleen Smith (USN Retired)

(continued)

TABLE 1.2 Landmark Events in Computers and Nursing, and Nursing Informatics *(continued)*

Year(s)	Title/Event	Sponsor(s)	Coordinator/Chair/NI Representative(s)
1995	First *CPRI Davies Recognition Awards of Excellence Symposium*	Computer-Based Patient Record Institute, Los Angeles, CA	Intermountain Healthcare, Salt Lake City, UT; Columbia Presbyterian MC, New York, NY; Department of Veterans Affairs, Washington, DC
1995	First ANA Certification in Nursing Informatics	ANA Credentialing Center (ANCC)	Rita Zielstorff, Chair
1996	ANA established *Nursing Information and Data Set Evaluation Center (NIDSEC)*	ANA Database Steering Committee, Washington, DC	Rita Zielstorff, Chair; Connie Delaney, Co-Chair
1996 to 1999	*Nightingale Project—Health Telematics Education*, three Workshops, and two International Conferences	University of Athens, Greece, and European Union	John Mantas, Chair (Greece); Arie Hasman, Co-Chair (the Netherlands); Consultants: Virginia K. Saba (USA); Evelyn Hovenga (AU)
1996	Initiated *TELENURSE Project*	Danish Institute for Health and Nursing Research and European Union	Randi Mortensen, Director; Gunnar Nielsen, Co-Director
1996	First Harriet Werley Award for Best Nursing Informatics Paper at AMIA	AMIA-NI Working Group (NIWG), Washington, DC	Rita Zielstorff (MGH Computer Lab)
1997	Invitational *National Nursing Informatics Workgroup*	National Advisory Council on Nurse Education and Practice and DN/PHS	Carol Gassert, Chair
1997	ANA published *NIDSEC Standards and Scoring Guidelines*	ANA Database Steering Committee	Rita Zielstorff, Chair; Connie Delaney, Co-Chair
1997	National Database of Nursing Quality Indicators (NDNQI®)	American Nurses Association	Nancy Dunton, PI
1997	Initiated *Nursing Informatics Archival Collection*	NLM—History Collection	Virginia K. Saba, Chair (GT)
1998	Initiated NursingCenter.com Web site	JB Lippincott, New York, NY	Maryanne Rizzalo, Director
1999	Beta Version: *ICNP published*	International Council of Nurses, Geneva, Switzerland	Fadwa Affara (ICN)
1999 to 2008	Annual *Summer Nursing Terminology Summit*	Vanderbilt University, Nashville, TN	Judy Ozbolt, Chair
1999	*Convergent Terminology Group for Nursing*	SNOMED/RT International, Northbrook, IL	Suzanne Bakken, Chair (NYU) and Debra Konicek (CAP)
1999 and 2004	*United States Health Information Knowledgebase (USHIK)* Integrated Nursing Data	Department of Defence (Health Affairs), CMS, CDC, AHRQ	M.D. Johnson (OASD/HA); Glenn Sperle (CMS); M. Fitzmaurice (AHRQ); Luann Whittenburg (OASD/HA)
1999	Inaugural Virtual Graduation: Online Post-Masters: *ANP Certificate Program*	GSN, Uniformed Services University VA TeleConference Network, Bethesda, MD Eight Nationwide VA MCs	Faye Abdellah (USU); Virginia K. Saba (USU); Charlotte Beason (VA)

Year	Event	Organization/Location	People
1999	First meeting: *Nursing Data Standards Project for Central Organization (PAHO) and Brazil*	Pan American Health Organization (PAHO), Washington, DC	Roberto Rodriquez (PAHO) Heimar Marin (Brazil)
2000	ICNP Programme Office established	International Council of Nurses, Geneva, Switzerland	Amy Coenen, Director
2000	*Computer-Based Patient Record Institute (CPRI) 2000 Conference*	CPRI, Los Angeles, CA	Virginia K. Saba, Nursing Chair
2001	AMIA Nursing Informatics Leaders	University of Wisconsin, Madison, WI Columbia University, New York, NY	Pattie Brennan, President Suzanne Bakken, Program Chair
2002	ICNP Strategic Advisory Group Established	ICN, Geneva, Switzerland	Amy Coenen, Director
2002	Conference: *Strategy for Health IT and eHealth Vendors*	Medical Records Institute (MRI), Boston, MA	Peter Waegemann, President
2002	AAN Conference: *Using Innovative Technology*	American Academy of Nursing, Washington, DC	Margaret McClure, Chair Linda Bolton, Co-Chair Nellie O'Gara, Co-Chair
2002 to 2006	Initiated AAN Expert Panel on Nursing Informatics	American Academy of Nursing Annual Conference, Naples, FL	Virginia K. Saba, Co-Chair Ida Androwich, Co-Chair
2003	*Finnish Nursing Informatics Symposium*	Finnish Nurses Association (FNA) and Siemens Medical Solutions, Helsinki, Finland	Kaija Saranto (FN) Anneli Ensio (FN) Rosemary Kennedy (Siemens)
2003	First ISO-Approved Nursing Standard: *Integrated Reference Terminology Model for Nursing*	IMIA/NI-SIG and ICN, Oslo, Norway	Virginia K. Saba, Chair (NI/SIG) Kathleen McCormick, Co-Chair (NIWG) Amy Coenen, Co-Chair (ICN) Evelyn Hovenga, Co-Chair (NI/SIG) Susanne Bakken, Chair, Tech. Group
2004	First ICN Research and Development Centre	Deutschsprachige ICNP, Freiburg, Germany	Peter Koenig, Director
2004 to Present	Initiated *Annual Nursing Informatics Symposium* at HIMSS Conference and Exhibition	HIMSS Annual Conference, Orlando, FL	Joyce Sensmeier, Chair
2004	Initial Formation of Alliance for Nursing Informatics (ANI)	AMIA/HIMSS	Connie Delaney, Chair Joyce Sensmeier, Co-Chair
2004 to 2012	First nurse on NCVHS Standards Subcommittee	NCVHS, Washington, DC	Judy Warren, KUMC

(continued)

TABLE 1.2	Landmark Events in Computers and Nursing, and Nursing Informatics *(continued)*		
Year(s)	**Title/Event**	**Sponsor(s)**	**Coordinator/Chair/NI Representative(s)**
2004	Office of the National Coordinator for Health Information Technology (ONC) established	National Coordinators	First Coordinator: Dr. David Brailer Dr. Robert Kolodner Dr. David Blumenthal Dr. Farzad Mostashari Dr. Karen DeSalvo
2004	*Technology Informatics Guiding Education Reform (TIGER)*—Phase I	National Members Online Teleconferences	Marion Ball, Chair Diane Skiba, Co-Chair
2006	First TIGER Summit	100 Invited Representatives from 70 Healthcare Organizations; Summit held at USU, Bethesda, MD	Marion Ball, Chair Diane Skiba, Co-Chair
2006	Revitalized *NI Archival Collection*—Initiated Solicitation of Pioneer NI Documents	AMIA/NIWG Executive Committee	Kathleen McCormick, Chair Bonnie Westra, Co-Chair
2005, 2008, and 2009	*ICNP Version 1.0, Version 1.1, and Version 2*	ICN, Geneva, Switzerland	Amy Coenen, Director
2006 and 2008	*Symposium on Nursing Informatics*	Brazil Medical Informatics Society	Heimar Marin, Chair
2007/2008	First National Nursing Terminology Standard: *Clinical Care Classification (CCC) System*	ANSI-HITSP: Bio-surveillance Committee HITSP Recommended and HHS Secretary Approved	Virginia K. Saba and Colleagues, HITSP Committee Developers
2007 to Present	ANIA/CARING Joint Conferences	Las Vegas, Washington, DC	Victoria Bradley, Chair
2009 to Present	*American Recovery and Reinvestment Act of 2009—Health Information Technology for Economic and Clinical Health (HITECH Act of 2009)*; ONC formed two National Committees, each with one nurse	ONC National Health Information Technology Committee: Health Policy Committee Health Standards Committee	Focus on Hospital HIT/EHR Systems Integrated and Interoperable Terminology Standards Judy Murphy (Aurora Health Systems) Connie Delaney (UMN):
2009	ICNP recognized by WHO as First International Nursing Terminology	ICN and WHO, Geneva, Switzerland	Amy Coenen, Director
2010	Formed Doctor of Nursing Practice Specialty in Informatics	University of Minnesota, Minneapolis, MN	Connie Delaney, Dean Bonnie Westra, Chair
2010	American Nursing Informatics Association (ANIA and CARING) merged	ANIA and CARING	Victoria Bradley, First President
2011	Tiger Initiative Foundation Incorporated	TIGER Initiative	Patricia Hinton Walker, Chair
2012 to Present	ANIA New Re-Named and *First Annual ANIA Conference*	ANIA	Victoria Bradley, President Patricia Sengstack, President (2013/2014)
2013	First NI Nurse to be President of IMIA	IMIA	Hyeoun-Ae Park, PhD, RN, FAAN Seoul National University, Seoul, Korea
2013/2014/2015	*Big Data for Better Health Care:* Invitational Conference	University of Minnesota School of Nursing	Connie Delaney, Chair Bonnie Westra, Co-Chair

the conferences and the appearance of nursing articles, journals, books, and other literature on this topic demonstrated the intense interest nurses had in learning more about computers and information technologies. These advances confirmed the status of NI as a new ANA specialty in nursing and provided the stimulus to transform nursing in the twenty-first century.

ACKNOWLEDGMENTS

The authors wish to acknowledge Patricia B. Wise for her authorship of the original fifth edition Chapter 3 "Electronic Health Records from a Historical Perspective" from which content has been integrated into this chapter.

REFERENCES

American Association of Colleges of Nursing. (2006, October). *The essentials of doctoral education for advanced nursing practice*. Retrieved from http://www.aacn.nche.edu/education/essentials.htm

American Association of Colleges of Nursing. (2011). *The essentials of master's education for professional nursing practice*. Retrieved from http://www.aacn.nche.edu/education-resources/MastersEssentials11.pdf

American Nurses Association. (1997). *NIDSEC standards and scoring guidelines*. Silver Springs, MD: ANA. A high-level summary can be found at http://ana.nursingworld.org/DocumentVault/NursingPractice/NCNQ/meeting/ANA-and-NIDSEC.aspx

American Nurses Association. (2010). *Nursing: Scope and standards of practice*. Washington, DC: ANA.

American Nurses Association. (2008; 2010). *Nursing informatics: Scope & standards of practice*. Washington, DC: ANA.

Bakken, S. (2006). Informatics for patient safety: A nursing research perspective. *Annual Review of Nursing Research, 24*, 219–254.

Bakken, S., Stone, P. W., & Larson, E. L. (2012). A nursing informatics research agenda for 2008–2018: Contextual influence and key components. *Nursing Outlook, 60*, 28–290.

Bitzer, M. (1966). Clinical nursing instruction via the Plato simulated laboratory. *Nursing Research, 15*(2), 144–150.

Blackmon, P. W., Mario, C. A., Aukward, R. K., Bresnahan, R. E., Carlisle, R. G., Goldenberg, R. G., & Patterson, J. T. (1982). *Evaluation of the medical information system at the NIH clinical center. Vol 1, Summary of findings and recommendations* (Publication No. 82-190083). Springfield, VA: NTIS.

Blum, B. I. (1990). Medical informatics in the United States, 1950–1975. In B. Blum & K. Duncan (Eds.), *A history of medical informatics* (pp. xvii–xxx). Reading, MA: Addison-Wesley.

Branchini, A. Z. (2012). *Leadership of the pioneers of nursing informatics: A multiple case study analysis*. Doctoral Dissertations. Paper AAI3529472. Retrieved from http://digitalcommons.uconn.edu/dissertations/AAI3529472

Collen, M. F. (1994). The origins of informatics. *Journal of the American Medical Informatics Association, 1*(2), 91–107.

Collen, M. F. (1995). *A history of medical informatics in the United States, 1950 to 1990*. Bethesda, MD: American Medical Informatics Association.

Dick, R. S., & Steen, E. B. (Eds.). (1991). *The computer-based patient record: An essential technology for healthcare*. Washington, DC: National Academy Press.

Gallagher, L. A. (2010). Revising HIPAA. *Nursing Management, 41*(4), 34–40.

Hammond, W. E. (1994). The role of standards in creating a health information infrastructure. *International Journal of Bio-Medical Computing, 34*, 29–44.

Hobbs, J. (2011). Political dreams, practical boundaries: The case of the Nursing Minimum Data Set, 1983–1990. *Nursing History Review, 19*, 127–155.

Humphreys, B. L., & Lindberg, D. A. B. (1992). The unified medical language system project: A distributed experiment in improving access to biomedical information. In K. C. Lun, P. DeGoulet, T. E. Piemme, & O. Reinhoff (Eds.), *MEDINFO 92: Proceedings of Seventh World Congress of Medical Informatics* (pp. 1496–1500). Amsterdam: North-Holland.

Kemeny, J. G. (1972). *Man and the computer*. New York, NY: Charles Scribner.

Nelson, R. (2013). Introduction: The evolution of health informatics. In R. Nelson & N. Staggers (Eds.), *Health informatics: An interprofessional approach* (pp. 2–17). New York, NY: Mosby Publishing.

Newbold, S., & Westra, B. (2009). American Medical Informatics Nursing Informatics History Committee update. *CIN: Computers, Informatics, Nursing, 27*, 263–265.

Newbold, S. K., Berg, C., McCormick, K. A., Saba, V. K., & Skiba, D. J. (2012). Twenty five years in nursing informatics: A SILVER pioneer panel. In P. A. Abbott, C. Hullin, S. Bandara, L. Nagle, & S. K. Newbold (Eds.), *Proceedings of the 11th International Congress on Nursing Informatics, Montreal, QC, Canada*. Retrieved from http://knowledge.amia.org/amia-55142-cni2012-1.129368?qr=1

Nicoll, L. H. (1998). *Computers in nursing: Nurses' guide to the internet* (2nd ed.). New York, NY: Lippincott.

NINR Priority Expert Panel on Nursing Informatics. (1993). *Nursing informatics: Enhancing patient care*. Bethesda, MD: U.S. Department of Health and Human Services, U.S. Public Health Services, and National Institutes of Health.

Ozbolt, J. G., & Bakken, S. (2003). Patient-care systems. In E. H. Shortliffe, L. E. Perreault, G. Wiederhold, & L. M. Pagan (Eds.), *Medical informatics computer applications in healthcare and biomedicine series: Health informatics* (2nd ed., pp. 421–442). New York, NY: Springer.

Parker, M., Ausman, R. K., & Ovedovitz, I. (1965). Automation of public health nurse reports. *Public Health Reports, 80*, 526–528.

Public Health Service. (1976). *State of the Art in Management Information Systems for Public Health/Community Health Agencies*. Report of the conference. New York, NY: National League of Nursing.

Rajecki, R. (2008). eICU: Big brother, great friend: Remote monitoring of patients is a boon for nurses, patients, and families. *RN, 71*(11), 36–39.

Romano, C., McCormick, K., & McNeely, L. D. (1982). Nursing documentation: A model for a computerized data base. *Advances in Nursing Science, 4*(2), 43–56.

Saba, V. K. (1995). A new nursing vision: The information highway. *Nursing Leadership Forum, 1*(2), 44–51.

Saba, V. K. (1996). Developing a home page for the World Wide Web. *American Journal of Infection Control, 24*, 468–470.

Saba, V. K. (1998). Nursing information technology: Classifications and management. In J. Mantas (Ed.), *Advances in health education: A Nightingale perspective*. Amsterdam: IOS Press.

Saba, V. K., & McCormick, K. A. (2011). *Essentials of nursing informatics* (5th ed). New York, NY: McGraw-Hill.

Saba, V. K., & Westra, B. L. (2011). Historical perspectives of nursing and the computer. In V. K. Saba & K. A. McCormick (Eds.), *Essentials of nursing informatics*, (5th ed., pp. 11–29). New York, NY: McGraw-Hill.

Sackett, K. M., & Erdley, W. S. (2002). The history of healthcare informatics. In S. Englebardt & R. Nelson (Eds.), *Healthcare informatics: An interdisciplinary approach* (pp. 453–476). St. Louis, MO: Mosby.

Sherman, R. (1965). Computer system clears up errors, lets nurses get back to nursing. *Hospital Topics, 43*(10), 44–46.

Shortliffe, E. H., Perreault, L. E., Wiederhold, G., & Pagan, L. M. (Eds.). (2003). *Medical informatics computer applications in healthcare and biomedicine* (2nd ed.). New York, NY: Springer.

Sparks, S. (1996). Use of the Internet for infection control and epidemiology. *American Journal of Infection Control, 24*, 435–439.

Van Bemmel, J. H., & Musen, M. A. (Eds.). (1997). *Handbook of medical informatics*. Germany: Springer-Verlag.

Wang, A. Y., Sable, J. H., & Spackman, K. A. (2002). The SNOMED Clinical Terms development process: Refinement and analysis of content. *Proceedings of American Medical Informatics Association, 2002* (pp. 845–849). Washington, DC: AMIA.

Westra, B. L. (2009). Radio frequency identification—Will it reach a tipping point in healthcare? *American Journal of Nursing, 109*(3), 34–36.

Westra, B. L., Delaney, C. W., Konicek, D., & Keenan, G. (2008). Nursing standards to support the electronic health record. *Nursing Outlook, 56*, 258.e1–266.e1

Westra, B. L., & Newbold, S. K. (2006). American Medical Informatics Association Nursing Informatics History Committee. *CIN: Computers, Informatics, Nursing, 24*:113–116.

Wolkodoff, P. E. (1963). A central electronic computer speeds patient information. *Hospital Management, 96*, 82–84.

World Health Organization. (1992). *ICD-10: International statistical classification of diseases and health related problems*. Geneva: WHO.

Computer Hardware

Mary L. McHugh

• OBJECTIVES

1. Identify the essential hardware components of a computer.
2. List key peripherals attached to most computers.
3. Describe the four basic operations of the central processing unit (CPU).
4. Explain how power is measured for computers.
5. Describe common computer input, output, and storage devices.
6. List the names for six types of computers and describe how they are different.
7. Describe computer network hardware devices and their functions.

• KEY WORDS

CPU (central processing unit)
Motherboard
Memory
Peripherals
Hardware

INTRODUCTION

Computer **hardware** is defined as all of the physical components of a computer. A computer is a machine that uses electronic components and instructions to the components to perform calculations, repetitive and complex procedures, process text, and manipulate data and signals. Computer technology has evolved from huge, room-sized electronic calculators developed with military funding during World War II to palm-sized machines available to virtually everybody. Today, computers are encountered in most areas of people's lives. From the grocery store and the movie theater to the power grid, from the bedside alarm clock to the automobile accelerator, and from infusion pumps to heart monitors, patient record systems, radiology machines, diagnostic devices, order processing systems, and all kinds of machines in the operating room, computer processors are employed so widely that today's society could not function without them.

The basic hardware of a computer composes the computer's architecture, and includes the electronic circuits, microchips, processors, random access memory (RAM), read-only memory (ROM), and graphic and sound cards. These are attached to a component called a motherboard. The motherboard is a square or rectangular board with circuits into which are plugged the main electronics of the computer. Devices that may be inside the computer case but are not part of the architecture include the main storage device, which is usually an internal hard drive, the cooling system, a modem, Ethernet connectors, optical drives, universal serial bus (USB) connectors, and multiformat media card readers. In addition, devices attached or linked to a computer that are peripheral to the main computer box are part of the system's hardware. These include input and output devices including the keyboard, touch screen, mouse, printer, and fax. The storage components are external hard drives, thumb drives, floppy drives, tape drives, sound systems (earphones, microphones, speakers, subwoofers), and the computer monitor. Typically, computer systems are composed of many different components that enable the user to communicate with the computer, and with other computers to produce work. The group of required and optional hardware items that are linked together to make up a computer system is called its configuration. When computers are sold, many of the key components are placed inside a rigid plastic housing or case, which is called the box. What can typically be seen from outside is the box (Fig. 2.1) containing the internal components, and the peripherals such as a keyboard, mouse, speakers, monitor, and printer.

Computer hardware advances during the late 1900s and into the 2000s have made possible many changes to the healthcare industry. The first work to be modified consisted of special administrative functions such as finance, payroll, billing, and nurse staffing and scheduling support. Later, the computer allowed fantastic changes in the practice of radiology and imaging, allowing noninvasive visualization not only of internal structures, but even of metabolic and movement functioning (Falke et al., 2013; Gropler, 2013; Hess, Ofori, Akbar, Okun, & Vaillancourt, 2013; Ishii, Fujimori, Kaneko, & Kikuta, 2013). Computer-enhanced surgical instruments enabled surgeons to insert endoscopy tools that allow for both visualization and precise removal of diseased tissues, leaving healthy tissues minimally damaged and the patient unscarred (Botta et al., 2013; Gumbs et al., 2009). Virtual reality programs in surgery have greatly enhanced the scope and complexity of surgeries that are now amenable to much less invasive surgeries (Volante et al., 2014). As a result, massive damage to skin, subcutaneous tissues, muscles, and organs have been eliminated from many procedures. Today, millions of patients who formerly

would have needed weeks in the hospital for recovery are now released from the hospital the same day as of their surgery or in a day or two at most.

Computers are now pervasive throughout the healthcare industry. Their applications are expected to continue to expand and thereby improve the quality of healthcare while at the same time reducing some costs. Most important, the applications of computers to healthcare will greatly expand the diagnostic and therapeutic abilities of practitioners and broaden the diagnostic and treatment options available to recipients of healthcare. Computers allow for distance visualization and communication with patients in remote areas. Telemedicine is now being used to reduce the impact of distance and location on accessibility and availability of healthcare (Coakley, Hough, Dwyer, & Parra, 2013; Davidson, Simpson, Demiris, Sheikh, & McKinstry, 2013; Russell, 2013; Saleh, Larsen, Bergsåker-Aspøy, & Grundt, 2014; Vowden & Vowden, 2013). None of these changes could have happened without tremendous advances in the machinery, the hardware, of computers.

This chapter covers various aspects of computer hardware: components and their functions and classes of computers and their characteristics and types. It also highlights the functional components of the computer and describes the devices and media used to communicate, store, and process data. Major topics addressed include basic computer concepts and classes and types of computers, components, and computer communications. To understand how a computer processes data, it is necessary to examine the component parts and devices that comprise computer hardware.

REQUIRED HARDWARE COMPONENTS OF A COMPUTER

The box of any computer contains a **motherboard** (Fig. 2.2). The motherboard is a thin, flat sheet made of

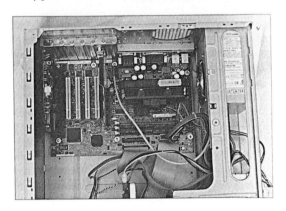

• **FIGURE 2.1.** Computer Box with Components Loaded. (Reproduced, with Permission, from Rosenthal M. (1999). *Build Your Own PC* (p. 82). New York, NY: McGraw-Hill.)

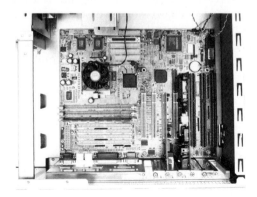

• **FIGURE 2.2.** Motherboard with CPU, Chips, and Slots. (Reproduced, with Permission, from Michael Alan Baxter)

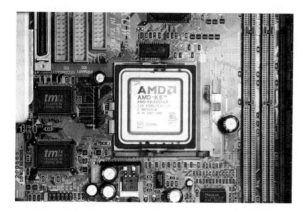

• **FIGURE 2.3.** CPU Chip Attached to Motherboard. (Reproduced, with Permission, from Michael Alan Baxter)

a firm, nonconducting material on which the internal components—printed circuits, chips, slots, and so on—of the computer are mounted. The motherboard is made of a **dielectric** or nonconducting plastic material. Electric conducting lines are etched or soldered onto the bottom of the board. The motherboard has holes or perforations through which components can be affixed so they can transmit data across the circuits on the motherboard (Fig. 2.3). Typically, one side looks like a maze of soldered metal trails with sharp projections (which are the attachments for the chips and other components affixed to the motherboard). The motherboard contains the microchips (including the central processing unit [CPU]), and the wiring, and slots for adding components. The specific design of the components on the motherboard—especially the CPU and other microprocessors—composes the foundation of the computer's architecture.

A computer has four basic components, although most have many more add-on components. At its most basic, a computer must consist of a CPU, input and output controllers, and storage media. The motherboard's storage media is called **memory**. Memory includes the locations of the computer's internal or main working storage. Memory consists of registers (a small number of very high speed memory locations), RAM, which is the main storage area in which the computer places the programs and data it is working on, and cache (a small memory storage area holding recently accessed data).

Memory

Memory refers to the electronic storage devices or chips on the motherboard of a computer. There are three key types of memory in a computer. They are read-only memory (ROM), the main memory known as random access memory (RAM), and cache.

Read-Only Memory. Read-only memory (ROM) is a form of permanent storage in the computer. It carries instructions that allow the computer to be booted (started), and other essential machine instructions. Its programming is stored by the manufacturer and cannot be changed by the user. This means that data and programs in ROM can only be read by the computer, and cannot be erased or altered by users. Theoretically, ROM can be changed by the factory, but effectively, the programs are permanently wired into the memory. ROM generally contains the programs, called firmware, used by the control unit of the CPU to oversee computer functions. In microcomputers, this may also include the software programs used to translate the computer's high-level programming languages into machine language (binary code). ROM storage is not erased when the computer is turned off.

Random Access Memory. Random access memory (RAM) refers to working memory used for primary storage. It is used as temporary storage. Also known as main memory, RAM can be accessed, used, changed, and written on repeatedly. RAM is the work area available to the CPU for all processing applications. When a user clicks on a program icon, such as a word processing program, the computer loads all or part of the program into RAM where it can be accessed very quickly. It saves work done through the programs until the user formally saves the work on the hard drive or other permanent storage. RAM is a permanent part of the computer. Because everything in RAM unloads (is lost) when the computer is turned off, RAM is called volatile memory. The computer programs that users install on their computers to do work or play games are stored on media such as the hard drive. They are not permanent parts of the computer itself. Running programs from the hard drive would be a very slow process, so parts of the programs are loaded and unloaded from the much faster RAM as needed. They are unloaded when the user shuts the program down or turns off the computer. The contents of RAM are erased whenever the power to the computer is turned off. Thus, RAM is made ready for new programs when the computer is turned on again.

Cache. Cache is a smaller form of RAM. Its purpose is to speed up processing by storing frequently called items in a small, rapid access memory location. To understand how cache works, think of a surgical nursing unit. Prior to the 1980s, many hospitals did not have many volumetric pumps, and all were kept in the central supply (CS) department—usually far away in the basement. Whenever a nurse needed a pump (which at that time were used only for especially dangerous intravenous [IV] medication infusions), the nurse had to go to CS and fetch it. When the pump was no longer needed for that patient, it was returned to CS. This is analogous to a system with no cache. This was a good system when pumps were seldom used on any unit as storage space is always limited in nursing units. Now, however, consider changes in practice that have led to the need for one or more volumetric pumps used for every patient. The new plan is to have a storage area in the nursing unit so that when needed the machines are always available nearby. This system is much more efficient for the nurses. Having a space to store the pumps nearby greatly reduces the time needed to access a pump. Rarely used equipment is still often kept in the CS department, but frequently needed items are kept in a nearby storeroom so they can be retrieved more quickly and efficiently. This is similar to cache. Prior to the development of cache, all information had to be fetched from the hard drive, and then stored in RAM. To handle all the work, the processor had to move information into and out of RAM (and back to the hard drive) in order to manage all the data from programs and their output. Given that RAM is large, it takes a bit of searching to find just the pieces needed and is relatively slow. Cache is much smaller than RAM, and thus fetching from cache takes much less time than from RAM. Keeping information that will be used frequently in cache greatly reduces the amount of time needed to move data around among the memory locations. It is a relatively inexpensive way to increase the speed of the computer.

Input and Output

To do work, the computer must have a way of receiving commands and data from outside and a way of reporting out its work. The motherboard itself cannot communicate with users. However, it has slots and circuit boards that allow the CPU to communicate with the outside world. Input and output devices are wired to a **controller** that is plugged into the slots or circuit boards of the computer. Some devices can serve as both input and output devices—for example, the hard drive in which most of the programs are stored receive and store information as well as send their programs to the computer.

Input Devices. These devices allow the computer to receive information from the outside world. The most common input devices are the keyboard and mouse. Others commonly seen on nursing workstations include the touch screen, light pen, voice, and scanner. A touch screen is actually both an input and output device combined. Electronics allow the computer to "sense" when a

particular part of the screen is pressed or touched. In this way, users input information into the computer. The touch screen displays information back to the user, just as does any computer monitor. A light pen is a device attached to the computer that has special software that allows the computer to sense when the light pen is focused on a particular part of the screen. It allows smaller screen location discriminations than does a touch screen. For both the touch screen and light pen, software interprets the meaning of the user-identified screen location to the program. Many other input devices exist. Some devices are used for security and can detect users' fingerprints, retinal prints, voiceprints, or other personally unique physical characteristics that identify users who have clearance to use the system.

In healthcare computing, many medical devices serve as input devices. For example, the electrodes placed on a patient's body provide input to the computerized physiologic monitors. The oximetry device placed on a patient's finger uses light waves to detect impulses that are sent to a computer and then interpreted as oxygen levels in the blood. Voice systems allow the nurse to speak into a microphone (which is the input device) to record data, submit laboratory orders, or request information from the computer. In radiology, most machines today input images from the X-Ray machines to a computer rather than storing them on film. In fact, the most advanced imaging machines could not exist without computer technology. Computerized axial tomography (CAT) scans and medical resonance imaging (MRI) machines are the best-known computerized imaging devices, but most of the radiology applications today are computerized.

Output Devices. These devices allow the computer to report its results to the external world. Output devices are defined as any equipment that translates the computer information into something readable by people or other machines. Output can be in the form of text, data files, sound, graphics, or signals to other devices. The most obvious output devices are the monitor (display screen) and printer. Other commonly used output devices include storage devices such as the USB drive (also known as flash or thumb drive) and optical media. In healthcare settings, a variety of medical devices serve as output devices. Heart monitors are output devices recording and displaying heart rhythm patterns, and initiating alarms when certain conditions are met. Volumetric infusion pump output includes both images on a screen and fluids infused into the patient's body. The pump delivers a specific volume of IV fluids based on commands that the nurse inputs so the ordered fluid volume will be infused in the correct time period.

Storage Media

Storage includes the main memory but also external devices on which programs and data are stored. The most common storage device is the computer's hard drive. Other common media include external hard drives, flash drives, and read/write digital versatile disks (DVDs) and compact disks (CDs). The hard drive and diskettes are magnetic storage media. DVDs and CD-ROMs are a form of optical storage. Optical media are read by a laser "eye" rather than a magnet.

Hard Drive. The hard drive is a peripheral device that has very high speed and high density (Fig. 2.4). That is, it is a very fast means of storing and retrieving data as well as having a large storage capacity compared with other types of storage. The hard drive is the main storage device of a computer. In small computers, typically the inside of the case or box houses the CPR and other internal hardware. Internal hard drives are not portable; they are plugged directly into the motherboard. The storage capacity of hard drives has and continues to increase exponentially every few years. In 2014, most personal computers (PCs) are sold with about a terabyte of storage; in 1990 PCs had about 500 megabytes (MB) of storage capacity (Table 2.1). That is approximately a 2100% increase. On the biggest computers, storage is measured in petabytes (see Table 2.1), which is an almost unimaginably huge number.

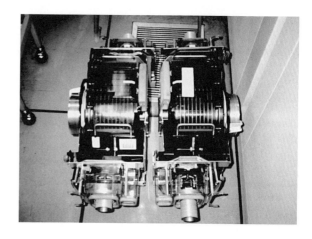

• **FIGURE 2.4.** Hard Disk Platters from an IBM Mainframe Computer. (Reproduced, with Permission, from Ákos Varga.)

USB Flash Drive. With the rise in demands for higher and higher density transportable storage, the popularity of the USB disk has also risen. A USB flash drive is actually a form of a small, removable hard drive that is inserted into the USB port of the computer. The USB drive is also known as pen drive, jump drive, thistle drive, pocket drive, and so forth. This is a device that can store 4 gigabytes (GB) of data for about $10. Flash drives can be very tiny—only

TABLE 2.1	Meaning of Storage Size Terms		
Number of Bytes	**Term**	**Formula ($\approx$ Means "Approximately")**	**Approximate Size in Typed Pages or Other Comparison**
1,024	1 kilobyte (K)	$2^{10} \approx 1,000$	One-third of a single-spaced typed page
1,048,567	1 megabyte (M or MB)	$2^{20} \approx 1,024^2$	600-page paperback book or 30 s of low-definition video
1,073,741,824	1 gigabyte (G or GB)	$2^{30} \approx 1,024^3$	An encyclopedia or 90 min of low-definition video
1,099,511,627,776	1 terabyte (T or TB)	$2^{40} \approx 1,024^4$	200,000 photos or Mp3 songs, 10 TB equals Library of Congress body of print material
1,125,899,906,842,624	1 petabyte (PB)	$2^{50} \approx 1,024^5$	Approximately 1 quadrillion bytes
1,152,921,504,606,846,976	1 exabyte (EB)	$2^{60} \approx 1,024^6$	Approximately 1 quintillion bytes
1,180,591,620,717,411,303,424	1 zettabyte (ZB)	$2^{70} \approx 1,024^7$	Approximately 1 sextillion bytes or 1 billion terabytes
1,000,000,000,000,000,000,000,000	1 yottabyte (YB)	$2^{80} \approx 1,027^8$	Approximately 1 septillion bytes or 1,000 zettabytes or 1 trillion terabytes
1 followed by 27 zeros	1 xenottabyte (XB)	$2^{90} \approx 1,027^9$	So big it feels like infinity

about ½ in. by 1 in. in some cases. They can also be much bigger and can store 128 GB or more data.

The flash drive is highly reliable and small enough to carry comfortably in a pants pocket or on a lanyard as a necklace, or on one's keychain. The device plugs into one of the computer box's USB ports and instead of saving to hard drive or CD-ROM or disk, the user simply saves to the flash drive. Since the flash drive can store so much data in a package so much smaller than a CD or DVD, the convenience makes it worth of a slightly higher price to many users. Of course, as its popularity increases, prices drop.

It should be noted that flash drives are not really used in clinical settings, at least not for business or patient care purposes. However, they are often carried by personnel who may plug them into the hospital's computer to do personal work. There is a danger that they can end up compromising patient's or company's confidentiality. Nurses should not save confidential patient information onto their personal flash drive (or any other personal storage devices). It is too easy to lose the drive itself, and then confidential information could end up anywhere! While working with hard copy medical records, a person had to laboriously copy confidential information manually onto a piece of paper, which creates a risk to confidentiality. With electronic media, it is perilously easy to copy confidential information; since the information becomes so easily accessible, there is a little security for that information. As nurses are responsible for protecting confidential information, as both a personal and company policy, confidential patient or company information should not be downloaded onto personal storage devices without a very good reason and legal permission to do so.

Optical Media. Optical media include CDs, DVDs, and Blu-ray. CD-ROMs and DVDs are rigid disks that hold a higher density of information and have higher speed. Until the late 1990s, CD-ROMs were strictly input devices. They were designed to store sound and data, and held about 737 MB of information (see Table 2.1), and large laser writers were required to store data on them. Thus, they were read-only media. However, technology developed in the 1980s by Philips Corporation permitted the development of a new type of CD that could be written on by the user. It is called CD-RW for compact disc read–write. As technology advanced and people wanted to store motion pictures on computer-readable media, DVDs were developed and held approximately 4.3 GB of information, which handled a regular 2 h movie. These DVDs were too limited to handle high-definition

movies and movies longer than 2 h, and thus media moved to the even higher storage capacity of Blu-ray discs that store approximately 27 GB of information or the equivalent of a 2 h high-definition movie. Double-layer Blu-ray discs can store 54 GB or 4.5 h of high-definition motion picture media. The name is derived from the blue color of the laser that writes on the media and ray for the optical ray that reads the media.

Other Storage Devices. As computers became more standard in offices during the 1990s, more and more corporate and individual information was stored solely on computers. Even when hard copy backups were kept, loss of information on the hard drive was usually inconvenient at the least and a disaster at worst. Diskettes could not store large amounts of data, so people began to search for economical and speedy ways to back up the information on their hard drive. Zip drives, which were mini magnetic tape devices, were a form of relatively fast (in their time) backup storage for people's data. Thumb (USB) and external hard drives were faster than tape media and replaced it as the backup media of choice. Today, many people purchase services that allow them to back up their data online, which means it gets stored on commercial computers that themselves have backup facilities.

Cloud Storage. An extension of the online storage service offered by individual vendors is cloud storage. Data stored "in the cloud" are still stored on commercial computers called servers. However, "cloud" refers to a distributed system of many commercial, networked servers that communicate through the Internet, and work together so closely that they can essentially function as one large system. Physically, enormous numbers of servers that store data are located in buildings, many warehouse sized. These data storage sites are called **data centers**. Multiple data centers are linked together to create cloud storage. The advantage to the customer is safety of the stored data.

A key factor in cloud storage is redundancy. The storage vendors must maintain multiple copies of the data they store. If one server in a data center becomes inoperable, copies of the data on that server are stored elsewhere and thus the data are not lost. They can be retrieved from another server. There are quite a few vendors who offer individuals free cloud storage space for their personal files, such as photos, music, and the like. They may also offer storage for a modest monthly or yearly fee. Some continuously back up data, others back up data at specified times, and typically the user can order files to be backed up whenever he or she wishes. Cloud storage is far more secure and reliable than a personal hard drive or backup drives.

Most users of smartphones, tablet computers, and other portable devices store their data in the cloud not only because of the security of the data, but also because storage in small devices is somewhat limited and the cloud allows more data storage than most individuals need for personal use.

MAJOR TYPES OF COMPUTERS

The computers discussed so far are **general purpose** machines, because the user can program them to process all types of problems and can solve any problem that can be broken down into a set of logical sequential instructions. Special purpose machines designed to do only a very few different types of tasks have also been developed. A category of special purpose computers includes the tablet computers, personal digital assistants (PDAs), and smartphones.

Today, five basic types of computers are generally recognized. Each type of computer was developed as the computer industry evolved, and each was developed for a different purpose. The basic types of computers include the supercomputer, the mainframe, the microcomputer, the handheld, and PDAs. They differ in size, composition, memory and storage capacity, processing time, and cost. They generally have had different applications and are found in many different locations in the healthcare industry.

Supercomputers

The largest type of computer is the supercomputer. First developed by Seymour Cray in 1972, the early supercomputer research, development, and production were carried out by Cray Corporation or one of its affiliates (Cray Corp, 2014). A supercomputer is a computational-oriented computer specially designed for scientific applications requiring a gigantic amount of calculations that, to be useful, must be processed at superfast speeds. The supercomputer is truly a world class "number cruncher." Designed primarily for analysis of scientific and engineering problems and for tasks requiring millions or billions of computational operations and calculations, they are huge and expensive. Supercomputers are used primarily in such work as defense and weaponry, weather forecasting, advanced engineering and physics, and other mathematically intensive scientific research applications. The supercomputer also provides computing power for

the high-performance computing and communication (HPCC) environment.

Mainframes

The mainframe computer is the most common fast, large, and expensive type of computer used in large businesses (including hospitals and other large healthcare facilities) for processing, storing, and retrieving data. It is a large multiuser central computer that meets the computing needs of large- and medium-sized public and private organizations. Virtually, all large- and medium-sized hospitals (300 beds and up) have a mainframe computer to handle their business office operations. They may have the hospital's electronic medical record (EMR) on that computer as well, or they may subcontract mainframe computing from a professional computer system support vendor.

Mainframes are used for processing the large amount of repetitive calculations involved in handling billing, payroll, inventory control, and business operations computing. For example, large volume sales businesses like grocery store chains and the "big box" stores have mainframe computers tracking all sales transactions. In fact, the machines and software that process transactions in high-volume businesses are known as **transaction processing systems** (TPS). The information nurses chart on patients in inpatient care facilities can be viewed as transactions. For example, every time a nurse charts a medication, that charting records use of one or more drugs. That charting in turn is transmitted to the pharmacy so that one item of that drug in inventory can be decreased. Typically, when the count of remaining inventory drops to a certain level, the TPS automatically initiates an order to a pharmacy supply house for more of the drug. Operations like charting a patient's vital signs goes into that person's medical record, and might trigger a warning to the nurse should any of the vital signs be out of range for that patient. For example, if the blood pressure is too high or too low, the system might be programmed to signal a warning so the nurse is advised to assess the patient and take appropriate action. Given the number of these kinds of "transactions" in clinical facilities, a powerful computer is needed to handle them all, and therefore, the hospital's EMR and other clinical applications are often handled through a mainframe computer.

Mainframes always have very high processing speeds (calculated in millions of processes per second, or MIPS, or in floating point operations per second, or FLOPS). In earlier times (prior to the year 2000), mainframes were often defined almost entirely by their high processing speed. However, computer processing speed changes so rapidly that today's mainframes are more defined by the following characteristics than merely processing speed:

1. Their extensive input and output capabilities to support their multiuser environment

2. Complex engineering to support long-term stability with high reliability, allowing these machines to run uninterrupted for decades

3. Their ability to process the massive throughput needed for high-volume business transactions and business office operations

In hospitals, mainframe computers are often used to support the entire Hospital Information Technology (HIT) system, also known as the Hospital Information System (HIS), purchased from one of the 30 or so large HIT vendors. The HIT includes not only business and nursing operations, but also supports many clinical systems. As previously mentioned, the applications nurses use in hospitals and other large healthcare facilities to document patient care, obtain laboratory and radiology results, record medication orders and administration records, and perform many other nursing record-keeping and information retrieval tasks typically involve use of a hospital mainframe computer.

Virtually all inpatient healthcare facility departments need large amounts of computer support. A partial listing of departments that typically have their systems on the hospital's mainframe computer includes the laboratory and radiology systems, the dietary department, the admissions department and its patient location system, the pharmacy department, and the CS department's inventory control system. Sometimes clinical monitoring systems, such as cardiac and fetal monitors, and surgery information systems may be housed on the mainframe, although these systems often reside on their own separate computer hardware.

Today the average sized or large acute care hospital has a HIT system implemented by one of the 30 or so large HIT vendors. It has a hardware configuration of a mainframe that may be located on-site (physically located at the hospital) or it might be located somewhere else. In some cases, the mainframe is not owned by the hospital but by a computer service vendor who provides mainframe computing power to multiple customers. In that case, the hospital's information is processed and stored on the vendor's computer systems.

A mainframe is capable of processing and accessing billions (GB) of characters of data or mathematical calculations per second. Mainframes can serve a large number (thousands) of users at the same time. In some settings, hundreds of workstations (input and output devices that

may or may not have any processing power of their own) are wired directly to the mainframe for processing and communication speeds faster than can be achieved with wireless communications. Typically, there are also wireless and telephone linkages into the computer so that remote users can gain access to the mainframe. As compared with a desktop PC, a mainframe has an extremely large memory capacity, fast operating and processing time, and it can process a large number of functions (multiprocessing) at one time.

Microcomputers (Personal Computers or PCs)

Although mainframe computers provide critical service to the healthcare industry, much smaller computers are also an essential part of healthcare computing systems. Computers designed to support a single user are called microcomputers or personal computers (PCs). Much smaller and less powerful than a mainframe, PCs were designed to be used by one person at a time.

In hospitals, they are used for an increasing number of independent applications as well as serving as an intelligent link to the programs of the mainframe. Hospital nursing departments use PCs to process specific applications such as patient classification, nurse staffing and scheduling, and personnel management applications. Microcomputers are also found in educational and research settings, where they are used to conduct a multitude of special educational and scientific functions. Desktops are replacing many of the mainframe attributes. Desktops can serve as stand-alone workstations and can be linked to a network system to increase their capabilities. This is advantageous, since software multiuser licensing fees are usually less expensive per user than having each user purchase his or her own copy. Computer size has steadily decreased since their invention, while at the same time power has grown exponentially. The components of desktop computer are typically housed in a hard case. Although the size of the case can vary considerably, one common size is 2 ft long by 6 to 10 in. wide. The case is most typically connected via wire or wireless technology to a keyboard, monitor, mouse, and printer.

Microcomputers are also available as portable or laptop computers, and as notebook, tablet, and handheld computers. Laptop computers are highly portable because they are much smaller than the standard desktop microcomputers. Many are less than 2 in. deep. There is huge variation in the length and width, but if a 15 in. viewing screen is used, the case is usually about 16 in. by 12 in. Notebook computers are even smaller; one size marketed in 2014 is 8.5 in. × 11 in. Tablet computers such as the Apple iPad and Samsung Galaxy are smaller with

---

BOX 2.1   HOME COMPUTER SUGGESTIONS

Today, most people need to have a PC in their homes, and need advice on what to buy for a home system to meet their needs. A good rule of thumb is to think of the home computer as a system because much more than the basic hardware is needed by most users. In addition to the CPU, memory, hard drive, and graphics cards, computers in the home should have the following components to meet most people's needs: a printer, monitor screen, keyboard, and mouse. The multifunction printer should be able to print in both black and white and color at the very least. A better machine can also allow the user to scan pictures and documents, make copies in black and white or color, and provide fax capability. These multifunction printers are called "four-in-one" printers that can print-fax-scan-copy. They often come with a price tag not much more than a simple black and white printer. Of course the user must have a mouse, keyboard, and monitor screen for basic input and output. While many laptops come with a built-in video camera and microphone, desktop computers often do not. Fortunately, a basic video camera with microphone can be bought for as little as $30, and that device allows the user to have video-linked conversations with family, friends, and business partners. The user must also budget for purchasing essential software such as an operating system and security software. Most people will also need software for writing documents, which may come bundled with the operating system. The operating system is the most basic software that must be purchased. Most come with a Web browser, which is a program that allows the user to access the Internet. There are several excellent free Web browsers that can be downloaded from the Internet if the one that comes with the operating system is not preferred. In addition to Microsoft's Internet Explorer that comes with the Windows operating system, and the Mac browser that comes with the Mac's operating system, some very popular free Web browsers include Google Chrome, Mozilla Firefox, and Opera. Many users use their home computer to do work at home, and need office productivity software packages that include powerful word processors, a spreadsheet, and a presentation graphics program; the productivity package may also include a database management system.

Once the buyer has budgeted for the essential peripherals and software, then the rest of the budget should buy the most powerful processor and biggest memory and cache the buyer can afford. The processor and cache size are what are going to become obsolete, because program updates will have to be made every few months (many are automatic with the software) and they always consume more processor power and memory storage. Within about 5 years, an average computer will become very slow because its processor, memory, and cache will no longer be big enough to handle the programs the buyer wants to run.

---

a width of about 7 in. and length of about 9 in., but are super thin as compared with the laptop and notebook computers. Less than an inch deep, they end up widened due to the addition of a protective case that usually also serves as a stand.

Desktop and laptop computer systems with wireless connectivity to the hospital's computer are often placed on a rolling cart for use of the nursing staff in recording nursing notes, ordering tests and treatments, looking up medications, and other computer work in inpatient settings. These computers on carts are often referred to as "WOWs" for workstation on wheels, or "COWs" for computer on wheels. Many nurses find these rolling workstations to be much more useful than fixed computers at patient bedsides for a variety of reasons. Additionally, one workstation can be assigned to a nurse to use with his or her assigned patients, thus eliminating the need for a separate computer for every bed. This solution allows nurses to adjust screen height and location of the mouse on the COW for their physical comfort that day rather than having to readjust a separate computer at every bedside (Box 2.1).

Handheld Computers/Personal Digital Assistants

Handheld computers are small, special function computers, although a few "full function" handheld computers were introduced in the late 1990s. Even though of smaller size than the laptop and notebook microcomputers, some have claimed to have almost the same functionality and processing capabilities. However, they are limited in their expansion possibilities, their ability to serve as full participants in the office network, and the peripherals they can support. More popular are the palm-sized computers, including personal digital assistants (PDAs), which are the smallest of the handheld computers. The PDA is a very small special function handheld computer that provides calendar, contacts, and note-taking functions, and may provide word processing, spread sheet, and a variety of other functions (Computer Hope, 2014).

Originally sold as isolated devices, today virtually all PDAs are combined with telephone functionality and sold as **smartphones**. Smartphones are ubiquitous and owned by a huge number of people worldwide, from the slums of South Africa to business people in the most developed countries. Smartphones have replaced wristwatches, pocket calendars, and other personal items people used to keep their lives organized. They feel indispensable to many people who might be more comfortable leaving home without a coat in winter than without their smartphone. These devices provide constant connectivity and access to Internet and telephone functions. They are particularly useful in that they can synchronize with other technology and provide automatic support for such things as the user's calendar.

The processors for most smartphones, tablet computers, and other small but powerful devices are made by Advanced RISC Machines Ltd. (ARM). An RISC processor is a "Reduced Instruction Set Computer," which means it is a special purpose processor. As of 2014, these processors are 32-bit microprocessors that use the RISC architecture.

There are a variety of hardware platforms and operating systems for smartphones and tablet computers. The three most common are the Apple Corporation's iPhone and iPad using the iOS operating system, smartphones and tablets using the Android operating system (owned by Google Corporation), and the Windows operating system for smartphones and tablets from Microsoft Corporation. The Android system is an open source operating system, the other two operating systems are closed and proprietary.

There are thousands of software applications (called **apps**) developed for all these platforms, many of them are free or sold at a very low price. In general, the apps work on only the platform for which they were developed, but quite a few will work on both smartphones and tablets using that platform. For example, many apps that work on the iPad tablet will also work on the iPhone. Clinical applications can allow the nurse to obtain assessments such as electrocardiograms, heart and respiratory rate, hearing acuity, oxygenation, and blood pressure using a smartphone. There are calculators that can make drug dosage calculations safer. There are programs that can help identify drug facts such as actions and dosages, and drug interactions, and remind the nurse of potential complications to watch for as well as special nursing actions to take with various medications. Reminders can help the nurse avoid forgetting to perform a treatment or give a medication on time. Wisely used, tablet computers, smartphones,

and other PDA technologies have the potential to support patient care safety and quality in all settings of care.

As wonderful as these handheld devices can be, there are pitfalls for nurses in their use in clinical areas. They come with both still photo and video capabilities. It can be very easy to forget the legal requirement for permission to photograph anything on a patient, much less make a photo of a patient's face when the technology is so available. It is quite a simple matter to upload information stored on a smartphone onto the Internet. A few nurses have found themselves in serious trouble when they forgot that social media such as Facebook, Twitter, and Linkedin are not private spaces and they uploaded photographs of patients or confidential patient information on social media. Smartphones are incredibly easy media on which to store information. Nurses must remember that most information in their workplace has confidentiality requirements that can be protected only with sophisticated technical barriers to unauthorized access. Those barriers are typically not available in an individual's smartphone.

CONNECTIVITY, COMPATIBILITY, AND INCOMPATIBILITY ISSUES

Communication among various hardware devices cannot be assumed. Given that departments within a single organization have often bought small systems designed to support their work, a single hospital may have literally hundreds of different computers and applications on those computers. Simply wiring incompatible machines so that power can flow between them accomplishes nothing. Often, computers cannot transfer data meaningfully among themselves. This makes it difficult to create a comprehensive medical record for individual patients. Thus, information stored somewhere in the facility may not be available when needed to the providers who need the information to make good patient care decisions.

As greater attention is placed on patient safety and quality improvement, and on analysis of performance data for planning and evaluation, there is a need to acquire and combine data from multiple patient care operations' computers and systems. Unfortunately, different computers have different architectures, hardware configurations, and storage schemes. Software must be specifically designed to communicate with another program for the two to communicate. Therefore, systems not designed specifically to work together cannot communicate information and processes to each other without the addition of complex translation programs (that usually do not exist); that is, they are not **interoperable**.

As a result of the interoperability problems, it can be economically infeasible to move data across different computers and programs. The interoperability problem limits nurses' ability to obtain, combine, and analyze data they need to provide for high quality, safe patient care. Organizationally, progress and performance are hampered when data and information are not available to perform the analysis required to identify problems, for opportunities for improvement, for safety risks, and to make projections about future needs.

Interoperability is necessary to meet the requirements of the Medicare and Medicaid EHR Incentive Programs (which provide financial incentives for the "meaningful use" of certified EHR technology) as part of the HITECH Act of 2009. Interoperability usually requires interoperable software programs such as SNOMED CT, LOINC, and so on (see Chapter 4 "Computer Software").

COMPUTER POWER

The terms **bits** and **bytes** refer to how the machine stores information at the lowest, or "closest to machine registers and memory," level. Computers do not process information as words or numbers. They handle information in bytes. A byte is made up of 8 bits.

Bits and Bytes

A bit (**b**inary dig**it**) is a unit of data in the binary numbering system. Binary means two, so a bit can assume one of two positions. Effectively, a bit is an ON/OFF switch—ON equals the value of 1 and OFF equals 0. Bits are grouped into collections of 8, which then function as a unit. That unit describes a single character in the computer, such as the letter A or the number 3, and is called a byte. A byte looks something like this:

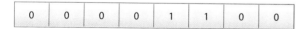

There are 255 different combinations of 0 and 1 in an 8-character (or 1-byte) unit. That forms the basic limit to the number of characters that can be directly expressed in the computer. Thus, the basic character set hardwired into most PCs contains 255 characters. In the early days of PCs, this was a problem because it severely limited the images that could be produced. However, with the advent of graphics cards and the additional character sets and graphics that graphics cards allow, virtually any character can be produced on a computer screen or printed on a printer. Even without graphics cards, additional character

sets can be created by means of programming techniques. The size of a variety of computer functions and components is measured by how many bytes they can handle or store at one time (Table 2.1).

Main memory, which includes the ROM on the motherboard in today's computers, is very large as compared with that of just a few years ago, and continues to increase every year with new computers. Since the size of memory is an important factor in the amount of work a computer can handle, large main memory is another key measure in the power of a computer. In the mid-1970s, the PCs on the market were typically sold with a main memory of between 48 K and 64 K. By 2014, the size of main memory in computers sold to the public had risen exponentially and most computers in 2014 are advertised with between 5 and 16 GB of main memory and computers with 20 GB or more of main memory are available. Cache has also become an important variable in computer power and thus in advertising the power of computers.

Another important selling point of a computer is the size of the hard drive that is installed in the box. The first hard drives sold for microcomputers in the 1970s were external devices that stored about 1500 kilobytes (KB). At that time, home computers were not sold with internal hard drives. When the user turned on the computer, they had to be sure the operating system diskette was in the disk drive, or the computer could not work. This architecture severely limited the size and functionality of programs. Therefore, consumer demand for hard drives was such that their size grew exponentially, while at the same time the cost of hard drive storage decreased exponentially. By late 1999, home computers typically sold had between 6 and 20 GB of space on the hard drive, and in 2010, the typical laptop computer was sold with a 300 to 500 GB hard drive, and desktops often came with hard drives that offered a terabyte or more of storage. By 2014, most home and laptop computers were advertised with 1- to 2-terabyte hard drives, and hard drive space will undoubtedly continue to increase. Applications programs have become so large that both the main memory and the hard drive storage space have had to increase exponentially as well.

COMPUTER SPEED

The basic operations of the CPU are called cycles, and the four types of cycles, or operations of a CPU, include fetch, decode, execute, and store. It takes time for the computer to perform each of these functions or cycles. The CPU speed is measured in cycles per second, which are called the clock speed of the computer. One million cycles per second is called 1 megahertz (MHz) and a billion cycles per second is called 1 gigahertz (GHz). CPU speeds are very fast, but because computers perform many billions of cycles per second, they can be slow if their processors have insufficient speed for the work they are required to process. Clock speeds, like most other components, have greatly improved over time. For example, the original IBM PC introduced in 1981 had a clock speed of 4.77 MHz (4.77 million cycles per second). In 2010, home computers commonly had from 1.8 to 3 GHz speeds. In 2014, advertised computers in the $1000 range have clock speeds of 2.5 to 3 GHz.

In general, the higher the clock speed possessed by the CPU, the faster and (in one dimension) the more powerful the computer. However, clock rate can be misleading, since different kinds of processors may perform a different amount of work in one cycle. For example, general-purpose computers are known as complex instruction set computers (CISCs) and their processors are prepared to perform a large number of different instruction sets. Therefore, a cycle in a CISC computer may take longer than that for a specialized type of computer called a reduced instruction set computer (RISC). Nonetheless, clock speed is one important measure of the power of a computer.

NETWORK HARDWARE

A network is a set of cooperative interconnected computers for the purpose of information interchange. The networks of greatest interest include local area networks (LANs), wide area networks (WANs), and the Internet, which is a network of networks. A LAN usually supports the interconnected computer needs of a single company or agency. The computers are physically located close to each other, and generally, only members of the company or agency have legitimate access to the information on the network. WANs support geographically dispersed facilities, such as the individual grocery stores in a national chain. A subset of WANs include the metropolitan area networks (MANs) that support and connect many buildings of local governmental agencies or university campuses.

The most important components of network hardware are the **adapter or interface card**, **cabling**, and **servers**. The role of hardware in a network is to provide an interconnection between computers. For a computer to participate on a network, it must have at least two pieces of hardware:

1. *Network adapter or network interface card*.
   A network interface card (NIC) is a computer circuit board or card that is installed in a computer so that it can be connected to a network. PCs and workstations on LANs typically contain an NIC specifically designed for the LAN transmission technology, such as Ethernet. NICs provide a dedicated, full-time connection to a network. Most home and portable computers connect to the Internet through modems on an as-needed dial-up connection. The modem provides the connection interface to the Internet service provider.

   The oldest network interface (or "adapter card") is an Ethernet card. But wireless network modems are used more often today. There exist other options such as arcnet, serial-port boards, and so on. Most of the time, the choice of NIC depends on the communication medium.

2. *Communication medium (cabling)*. The "communication medium" is the means by which actual transfer of data from one site to another takes place. Commonly used communication media include twisted pair cable, coaxial cable, fiber-optics, telephone lines, satellites, and compressed video. Most of the time, the choice of a communication medium is based on the following:

   (a) *Distance*. Relatively short distances are required for wireless, compressed video, and coaxial cable systems. For much longer distances, fiber-optics, telephone lines, and satellite transmission are used.

   (b) *Amount of data transfer*. Large amounts of data (especially video) are best handled with coaxial cables and compressed video and through satellite communications (satellite and compressed video are very expensive). Smaller amounts of data or serial (nonvideo) streams are best handled through the other wire types, such as twisted pair copper wire and optical fiber, and are less expensive.

   (c) *How often the transfer is needed*. Coaxial works best for locally wired networks that are used constantly by a very limited number of users. Telephone wires work well for the relatively high-usage public networks (like the Internet) but are more likely to get overloaded when many users try to use the system at the same time. Consider, for example, the busy Internet or phone lines getting clogged up when a tornado or hurricane has struck a community.

   (d) *Availability*. Availability depends on cost, transmission speed, number of users (who might clog up the system), weather conditions (satellites), and so on.

CONCLUSION

The computer is generally described in terms of several major characteristics of its hardware. The speed is determined by how many cycles per second can be processed, the size of its main memory, its cache, and its hard drive. All these factors combine to determine how many programs and data can be permanently stored on the hard drive and how fast the computer can run programs. In turn, these factors determine what kinds of work the user can do with the computer. Playing online games is one activity that takes a large amount of computing power. As a result, "gaming computers" are known to have a lot of computer power. The physical components of the computer itself and its peripheral hardware constitute the architecture of the computer, and these factors determine how it can be used. A great deal of work and playing on computers today involves interactions with other people and machines. Thus, multiple computers must be able to be connected or networked with each other. All the work performed and games played with computers require essential components, including a motherboard, printed circuits, a CPU, other processors, memory chips, controllers, and peripheral devices. This chapter introduced the fundamental hardware of computers and networks.

REFERENCES

Botta, L., Cannata, A., Fratto, P., Bruschi, G., Trunfio, S., Maneggia, C., & Martinelli, L. (2013). The role of the minimally invasive beating heart technique in reoperative valve surgery. *Journal of Cardiac Surgery, 27*(1), 24–28.

Coakley, C., Hough, A., Dwyer, D., & Parra, D. (2013). Clinical video telehealth in a cardiology pharmacotherapy clinic. *American Journal of Health-System Pharmacy, 70,* 1974–1975.

Computer Hope. (2014). *PDA.* Computer Hope website. Retrieved from http://www.computerhope.com/jargon/p/pda.htm. Accessed on April 3, 2014.

Cray Corp. (2014). *Cray History.* Retrieved from http://www.cray.com/About/History.aspx. Accessed on March 20, 2014.

Davidson, E., Simpson, C., Demiris, G., Sheikh, A., & McKinstry, B. (2013). Integrating telehealth care-generated data with the family practice electronic medical record: Qualitative exploration of the views of primary care staff. *Interactive Journal of Medical Research, 2*(2), e29.

Falke, K., Krüger, P., Hosten, N., Zimpfer, A., Guthoff, R., Langner, S., & Stachs, O. (2013). Experimental differentiation of intraocular masses using ultra high-field magnetic resonance imaging. *PLoS ONE, 8*(12), e81284. doi:10.1371/journal.pone.0081284. Retrieved from http://www.plosone.org/article/info%3Adoi%2F10.1371%2Fjournal.pone.0081284. Accessed on December 12, 2013.

Gropler, R. (2013). Recent advances in metabolic imaging. *Journal of Nuclear Cardiology, 20*(6), 1147–1172.

Gumbs, A., Fowler, D., Milone, L., Evanko, J., Ude, A., Stevens, P., & Bessler, M. (2009). Transvaginal natural orifice translumenal endoscopic surgery. *Annals of Surgery, 249*(6), 908–12.

Hess, C., Ofori, E., Akbar, U., Okun, M., & Vaillancourt, D. (2013). The evolving role of diffusion magnetic resonance imaging in movement disorders. *Current Neurology and Neuroscience Reports, 13*(11), 400–416.

Ishii, M., Fujimori, S., Kaneko, T., & Kikuta, J. (2013). Dynamic live imaging of bone: Opening a new era of 'bone histodynametry'. *Journal of Bone and Mineral Metabolism, 31*(5), 507–511.

Russell, T. (2013). Internet-based physical assessment of people with Parkinson disease is accurate and reliable: A pilot study. *Journal of Rehabilitation Research & Development, 50*(5), 643–650.

Saleh, S., Larsen, J., Bergsåker-Aspøy, J., & Grundt, H. (2014). Re-admissions to hospital and patient satisfaction among patients with chronic obstructive pulmonary disease after telemedicine video consultation—a retrospective pilot study. *Multidisciplinary Respiratory Medicine.* Retrieved from http://www.mrmjournal.com/content/9/1/6. Accessed on February 3, 2014.

Volante, F., Buchs, F., Pugin, J., Spaltenstein, B., Schiltz, M., Jung, M., … Ratib, P. (2014). New robotics study findings have been reported by investigators at University Hospital. *Medical Devices and Surgical Technology Week,* February 9, 294.

Vowden, K., & Vowden, P. (2013). A pilot study on the potential of remote support to enhance wound care for nursing-home patients. *Journal of Wound Care, 22*(9), 481–488.

3

Advanced Hardware and mHealth

Kathleen G. Charters / Patricia B. Wise

• OBJECTIVES

1. Identify standards that provide the framework for communication.
2. Identify Internet protocols.
3. Identify standards that provide the framework for interoperability.
4. Describe the enabling technologies for collaborative care.
5. List two examples of the use of collaborative tools.

• KEY WORDS

Advanced hardware
Bluetooth
mHealth
Mobile device
Wi-Fi

INTRODUCTION

Hardware—the silicon, metal, and plastic portion of the hardware–software–human triangle—exists to support the activities in which we engage. New care models are driving a change in the way people think about the use of advanced hardware in healthcare. One activity that is pushing the development of and leveraging the existing advanced hardware is eHealth—the use of information and communication technology for health services and information by both healthcare professionals and the public. At the leading edge of eHealth is the practice of healthcare and public health supported by mobile devices.

The three key synergistic advanced hardware elements enabling mobile health (mHealth) are (1) physical device size, (2) wireless network access, and (3) battery life. mHealth is accelerating due to the convergence of the infrastructure of adequate processing power and storage available on mobile devices (e.g., smartphones, advanced tablets, and wearable/implantable/injectable devices); large capacity redundant storage typically

available through cloud computing services; and long-life batteries.

Hardware

Advances in computer hardware continue two trends: (1) more powerful processing in ever-smaller packages and (2) more power distributed across many, many machines, most commonly seen in cloud services. For example, tablets used to be a bridge between a desktop and a smartphone, allowing mobility but lacking the range of computing capability that a laptop provided. This distinction is disappearing as tablets evolve to provide the same capability as a laptop. A smartphone is a powerful hand-held computer with an operating system and the ability to access the Internet. Wearable devices, the size of a piece of jewelry, collect physiological measures and wirelessly send that data to smartphones or cloud services via the Internet. Implantable devices, such as an implantable cardioverter-defibrillator, not only monitor physiological responses, they also provide interventions. Research on injectable microchips continues, and raises many security, privacy, and ethical issues.

Advances in large capacity redundant storage allows rapid access to massive amounts of data with steadily improving fault tolerance. Redundant arrays of independent disks (RAIDs) for replicating and sharing data among disks make it possible to store larger chunks of information than a single storage device can handle. The combination of accessibility and capacity can be used in healthcare for storage of large data sets such as genomics data. Making this storage accessible through the Internet allows mobile devices to overcome local storage limitations. The ability of a mobile device to access a large number of computers connected through a communication network and run a program or application on many connected computers at the same time is known as cloud computing. A common example of mobile device access to cloud services is when the user of a smartphone takes photos, edits the photos, and shares them, all without having to go back to a desktop machine in order to edit and share.

The length of time a mobile device can work powered by a rechargeable battery is the limiting factor for mobile computing. The most common complaint about the limitation of a mobile device is battery life, which becomes problematic when there is a high level of background activity. For example, running multiple interactive mobile applications (apps) in the background, each of which drains power, shortens the amount of time the device can be used before having to recharge the battery. Use of mobile data and video is rapidly expanding (Moore, 2011), driving research on ways to deliver vastly improved power density (Williams, 2013).

Wireless Communication

The ability of a mobile device to connect with networks in multiple ways is the foundation of mobile computing and mHealth. Technology used to wirelessly communicate with a mobile device includes mobile telecommunications technology, Wi-Fi, Bluetooth, and Radio-Frequency IDentification (RFID). Mobile telecommunications technology continues to evolve (Federal Communications Commission, 2012). Fourth-generation (4G) networks that provide faster performance and more capabilities are replacing third-generation (3G) networks. A 4G network supports all Internet Protocol (IP) communication and uses new technology to transfer data at very high bit rates, significantly improving both the speed of transfer and volume of data over that possible with a 3G network. The International Telecommunications Union-Radio (ITU-R) communications sector sets the standards for International Mobile Telecommunications Advanced

(IMT-Advanced) technology. The peak speed requirements for 4G service are 100 megabits per second for high mobility communication (e.g., communications while traveling by car or train) and 1 gigabit per second for low mobility communication (e.g., communications while walking or standing still). Technologies that do not fulfill 4G requirements but represent the forerunners to that level of service by providing wireless broadband access include Worldwide Interoperability for Microwave Access (Mobile WiMAX) and Long-Term Evolution (LTE), a standard for wireless communication of high-speed data for mobile phones. (Although the standards-setting body is international, due to different frequencies and bands used by different countries, only multi-band phones will be able to use LTE in all countries where LTE is supported.)

Wi-Fi is intended for general local network access, called a wireless local area network (WLAN). Bluetooth is intended for a wireless personal area network (WPAN). Wi-Fi and Bluetooth are complementary. Wi-Fi is access point-centered, with all traffic routed through the access point (typically, several computers, tablets, and other devices share a single access point). Bluetooth is used for symmetrical communication between Bluetooth devices, transferring information between two and seven devices that are near each other in low-bandwidth situations (typically, several devices are paired with a single device, such as Bluetooth keyboards, mice, activity monitors, and cameras paired to a single desktop, tablet, or smartphone). Protocols covering wireless devices include Wireless Application Environment (WAE), which specifies an application framework, and Wireless Application Protocol (WAP), which is an open standard providing mobile devices access to telephony and information services.

Wi-Fi is a technology that allows an electronic device to exchange data or connect to the Internet wirelessly using (in the United States) 2.4 GHz Ultra High Frequency (UHF) waves and 5 GHz Super High Frequency (SHF) waves. Advanced hardware makes this connection through a wireless network access point, or hotspot. Wi-Fi is based on the Institute of Electrical and Electronics Engineers (IEEE) 802.11 standards. To provide a level of security for the wireless connection, various encryption technologies are used, such as Wi-Fi Protected Access (WPA) and Wi-Fi Protected Access II (WPA2) security protocols. To ensure that devices can interoperate with one another, a type of Extensible Authentication Protocol (EAP) is used. Wi-Fi security concerns are covered in the National Institute of Standards and Technology (NIST) *Guidelines for Securing Wireless Local Area Networks* (NIST Special Publication 800-153) (2012b).

Bluetooth is a wireless technology standard for control of and communication between devices, allowing exchange of data over short distances. Bluetooth is used for wirelessly connecting keyboards, mice, light-pens, pedometers, sleep monitors, pulse oximeters, etc. The range is application specific. Bluetooth uses 2.4 to 2.485 GHz UHF radio waves, and can connect several devices. The Bluetooth Special Interest Group (SIG) is responsible for Bluetooth standards. Bluetooth security concerns are addressed in the NIST *Guide to Bluetooth Security* (NIST Special Publication 800-121) (2012a).

Radio-Frequency Identification (RFID) is a technology that uses radio-frequency electromagnetic fields to transfer data, using tags that contain electronically stored information. Typically, RFID is used for equipment tracking and inventory control. For example, in an Operating Room, RFID is used to automatically poll equipment in the suite and cross-reference that equipment with inventories showing the equipment is certified, and the date of the most recent service. Tags contain an integrated circuit for storing and processing information, and modulating and demodulating a radio frequency. Tags also contain an antenna for receiving and transmitting the signal. The tag does not need to be in the line of sight of the reader, and may be embedded in the object to be identified. The reader is a two-way radio transmitter-receiver that sends a signal to the tag and reads its response. Advanced hardware uses increasingly miniaturized RFIDs; some chips are dust-sized. The International Organization for Standardization (ISO) and the International Electrotechnical Commission (IEC), among others, set standards for RFID. The standards for information technology telecommunications and information exchange between systems are ISO/IEC 18092 and ISO/IEC 21481. (Although the standard-setting bodies are international, frequencies used for UHF RFID in the United States are currently incompatible with those of Europe or Japan.) Security concerns are addressed by using cryptography. RFID security concerns are addressed in the NIST *Guidelines for Securing Radio Frequency Identification (RFID) Systems* (NIST Special Publication SP 800-98) (2007).

Standards and Protocols

Use of well-established standards and best practices allows global and easy access to networks and networked information in a standardized way. The networking model and communications protocols used for the Internet are commonly known as Transmission Control Protocol (TCP) and the Internet Protocol (IP) or TCP/IP. This suite of standards provides end-to-end connectivity specifying how data are formatted, addressed, transmitted, routed, and received at the destination. The Internet Engineering Task Force (IETF) maintains the standards for the TCP/IP suite. Some of the most commonly used

protocols for Internet user-interface services and support services include Simple Mail Transfer Protocol (SMTP), File Transfer Protocol (FTP), and HyperText Transfer Protocol (HTTP). Encryption provides confidentiality and integrity for data sent over the Internet. Cryptographic network protocols to protect data in transport are Secure Sockets Layer (SSL) and Transport Layer Security (TLS). Protocols for encrypting data at rest include Pretty Good Privacy (PGP) and GNU Privacy Guard (GPG).

Building on top of network standards, there are standards that ensure health information is properly identified, transmitted correctly, and complete. Health Level Seven International (HL7) maintains the framework and standards for the exchange, integration, sharing, and retrieval of electronic health information. These standards are the most commonly used in the world for packaging and communicating health information from one party to another using language, structure, and data types that allow seamless integration between systems. The HL7 standards support management, delivery, and evaluation of health services and clinical practice (Health Level Seven International, 2014). Clinical Content Object Workgroup (CCOW) is an HL7 standard protocol that enables different applications to synchronize at the user-interface level in real time. This standard allows applications to present information in a unified way. For example, with CCOW enabled, a provider could bring up a patient record in the inpatient electronic record application, and then open the outpatient electronic record in a different application, and CCOW would bring up the same patient in the outpatient application.

Evolution and adoption of existing technologies and standards allow users to benefit from advanced hardware without the need for deep knowledge or expertise. For example, you can watch a feature film on a smartphone without knowing how the underlying hardware and software work. These advances in hardware along with virtualization support new care models.

Drivers of Mobile Healthcare

The 2012 documentary *Escape Fire: The Fight to Rescue Healthcare* is an urgent call to think differently about healthcare. Clinicians shifting from a focus on disease management to a focus on ending lifestyle disease may leverage the use of mobile platforms. For example, during an outpatient visit, Dr. Natalie Hodge prescribes an app for health self-management in the same way that medicine or any other intervention would be prescribed (Wicklund, 2014 February 13). According to the mHIMSS Roadmap, "patients and providers are leveraging mobile devices to seek care, participate in, and deliver care. Mobile devices represent the opportunity to interact and provide this care beyond the office walls" (Healthcare Information and Management Systems Society [HIMSS], 2012b).

Advancements in technology, federal healthcare policy, and commitment to deliver high-quality care in a cost-efficient manner have led to new approaches (mHIMSS, 2014b, 2014c). The Affordable Care Act (ACA) leverages innovative technology to bring about "a stronger, better integrated, and more accessible healthcare system" (HIMSS, 2012b). For example, mobile apps allow expansion of telemedicine and telehealth services. The current healthcare focus is on preventive and primary care to reduce hospital admissions and emergency department utilization. Engaging patients in management of their chronic diseases helps them maintain their independence and achieve a high quality of life. Patients may make use of collaborative tools such as Secure Messaging to communicate with their healthcare team, and may find support through social interactions on a blog.

Technology in Mobile Healthcare

Under the ACA, innovative technology is seen as an integral component of an integrated, accessible, outcome-driven healthcare system. Mobile technology may be key to providing more effective preventative care, improving patient outcomes, improving access to specialized medical services, and driving system-wide cost reduction. Services to patients and families at home will be personalized and delivered by providers equipped with apps for smartphones, tablets, and laptops (Powell, Landman, & Bates, 2014).

The National Institutes of Health defines mHealth as "the use of mobile and wireless devices to improve health outcomes, healthcare services, and health research" (HIMSS, 2012a). A major component of mHealth includes timely access to clinical information such as the data contained in electronic health records (EHRs), personal health records (PHRs), and patient portals. This information should be securely accessible by clinicians, patients, and consumers over various wireless mediums both inside and outside the traditional boundaries of a hospital, clinic, or practice (HIMSS, 2012b). The iPhone and Android operating systems have accelerated the proliferation of mobile data use. By 2015, mobile data traffic will be some 20 times the 2010 level (Moore, 2011).

The concept of mHealth can be traced to the early 1990s when the first 2G cellular networks and devices were being introduced to the market. The bulky handset designs and limited bandwidth deterred growth, lack of communication standards impeded interoperability, and batteries lasted less than 6 hours. A major standards breakthrough occurred in 1997, enabling Wi-Fi capable barcode scanners to be used in hospital inventory management. Shortly thereafter, clinicians began to take an increasing interest in adopting technologies. At this time, nurses began to use personal digital assistants (PDAs) to run applications like general nursing and medical reference, drug interactions, and synchronization of schedules and tasks. This quick rate of adoption was quite notable for clinicians often considered technology adverse. Increased processing capabilities and onboard memory created an appetite for more advanced applications. Network manufacturers were beginning to offer Personal Computer Memory Card International Association (PCMCIA) wireless devices, creating an environment where retrofitted hospital computers or new laptops allowed nurses to access the Internet without adding network cabling.

In 2000, the Federal Communications Commission (FCC) dedicated a portion of the radio spectrum to wireless medical telemetry systems (WMTS), which was widely adopted for remote monitoring of a patient's health. As data transmission rates increased, it became feasible for hospitals to run video or voice applications over the wireless networks. Application-Specific Devices (ASDs) are often integrated with nurse call systems and medical telemetry so that nurses can receive alerts, alarms, and text messages. Many vendors are now beginning to offer the same type of nurse call integration and voice-over Wi-Fi capabilities on popular smartphones (HIMSS, 2012b).

Nurses soon became familiar with Computers on Wheels (COWs), which evolved to workstations on wheels (WOWs). More wireless devices were integrated into networks and a greater emphasis was placed on error detection and prevention, medication administration safety, and computerized provider order entry (CPOE). Parallel to Wi-Fi technology evolution has been the growth in cellular technology. In many healthcare organizations, seamless roaming between the two systems is a reality. Nurses now have immediate access to patient data at the bedside.

Infrastructure. mHealth is a broad, expanding universe that encompasses a wide variety of user stories (use cases) that range from continuous clinical data access to remote diagnosis and even guest Internet access. The role of video in healthcare is evolving as quickly as the standards themselves. Telemedicine carts outfitted with high-resolution cameras include remote translation and interpretation services for non-native speakers as well as the hearing impaired. In the past, WOWs were mainly used to access clinical data, but these carts have gained such wide acceptance that they are often found in use by clinicians on rounds or at change of shift. Hospital systems and ambulatory practices have also started using products like FaceTime, Skype, Google Hangouts, and other consumer-oriented video-telephony and voice-over Internet

Protocol (VOIP) software applications for patient consults, follow-up, and care coordination (mHIMSS, 2014a).

Overlay networks for medical devices are becoming obsolete as hospitals seek economies of scale by utilizing their existing Wi-Fi infrastructure. This places a heavy dependency on the Information Technology department (IT) to ensure that the hospital, clinic, or practice wireless network is secure, designed properly, and robust enough to support various types of medical devices such as infusion pumps, mobile EKG devices, mobile X-ray devices, ultrasounds, and blood gas analyzers on a single infrastructure.

An important and often overlooked aspect of mHealth is patient or guest access to the wireless system. Care must be taken to segregate the guest access wireless network from the health professional networks. Wireless guest access provides a way for patients and their families to access the Internet; it can be a valuable tool for hospitals to engage with patients and guests. In a healthcare setting, organizations generally opt to provide free unencrypted access with a splash page that outlines terms and conditions. This allows the hospital to address liability for the patient's Internet traffic and allows guests and patients to access the network quickly.

Real-time location services (RTLS), a concept dating back to the 1990s, has evolved rapidly over the years. RTLS can be used for asset location tracking using RFID beacons, temperature/humidity monitoring, distress alert badges, and hand washing tracking (mHIMSS, 2014e). A properly configured RTLS system can minimize the task of tracking down medical equipment and show the nurse the status of the equipment. The wide range of options includes using RFID technology. Biomedical, pharmacy, security, and other departments in the hospital are using this technology (see Table 3.1).

Mobile Devices

Smartphones and tablets are ubiquitous in the healthcare setting. What started out as consumer devices are now in the hands of almost all clinicians. In a short period, mobile device performance has improved radically, putting them closer and closer in capability to general computing devices such as laptops and desktops. Battery technology has also improved significantly, with most devices able to go a shift between charging. Within the palm of a nurse's hand is a fully capable computing device able to perform complex and powerful operations. Many mobile devices are using high-resolution touch screens. When clinical information systems are designed to display well on smartphones and tablets, these devices will emerge as the primary computing device for all users. These devices already support text messaging, voice, and video.

Telehealth

One of the latest trends in healthcare IT is the concept of Bring Your Own Device (BYOD). Products in the marketplace today, such as the iPhone, iPad, and similar devices

TABLE 3.1	Major Technology Trends (HIMSS, 2012b)
Trend	**Explanation/Example**
Wireless Patient Monitoring	Technologies that enable remote surveillance of patient vital functions through the use of internally and externally located patient devices.
	Examples: Wirelessly monitored pacemakers and automatic defibrillators
Mobile System Access	Mobile technologies that enable remote/virtual access to current clinical systems such as Electronic Health Records (EHRs) and Picture Archiving and Communication System (PACS).
	Examples: Web sites, portals, mobile apps
Medical Devices	Mobile and/or wireless-enabled technologies that capture and track key care compliance and disease management data.
	Examples: Digital glucometers, blood pressure devices, pedometers
Virtual Consultation	Remote connectivity and multimedia solutions that enable virtual care consultation, education, and therapy.
	Examples: Tele-consultations, mobile video solutions
Aging in Place	Remote technologies that enable clinically monitored independent living for aging populations.
	Examples: Personal Emergency Response Systems (PERS), video consultations, motion/activity monitoring, fall detection, aggregation, transport

from other vendors, have produced loyal customers who do not want to have multiple communication devices attached to their waistband or filling the pockets of their lab coat. They prefer one device, the device that they own. In many hospitals the IT department has already ensured that their devices are secure and able to meet government regulations. Back-end IT systems are required to ensure that a given device does not introduce vulnerabilities into the system. Mobile Device Management products provide policy enforcement on end-user devices, remote wipe capability, and endpoint integrity. To implement BYOD, owners of the devices must be willing to abide by the hospital's mobile device policy and allow their devices to be managed. As the concept of unified communications continues to grow, fed by the challenge to attain work-life balance, BYOD is becoming increasingly attractive in many organizations.

Future of mHealth Inside Healthcare Facilities

The nation's healthcare model is on the path toward consolidated, coordinated, value-based care. Information Technology tools, mobile applications, and clinical information systems provide an evolving platform for the effective delivery of clinical services, increased operational excellence, and cost containment. Wireless networking, specifically Wi-Fi, began to be widely adopted in hospitals about 10 years ago. In the beginning, few organizations had 100% Wi-Fi coverage, but steadily increasing demand resulted in the deployment of wall-to-wall Wi-Fi coverage in hospitals and often in adjacent outside areas. Cellular network coverage in hospitals has also grown. Initially, owners of mobile devices were accustomed to spotty coverage and dropped calls or even policies banning mobile phones. In recent years, thanks to investments by cellular carriers, coverage areas have grown, along with the user's expectation of a quality signal. Distributed Antenna Systems (DAS) are commonly used for providing cellular wireless signals while also providing for two-way radio, paging, and first responder communication systems (HIMSS, 2012b).

Still, unified communications (a combination of messaging, video, and voice) has not yet realized full potential in healthcare facilities. The value of an emergency room nurse being able to instantly create a video session with a remote patient is not in doubt. However, the infrastructure to accomplish this is still fledgling. Enterprise communication platform vendors have provided these capabilities with devices that integrate with their vendor-specific devices. Broader integration with common devices such as smartphones and tablets is an ongoing effort.

Considerations for mHealth Planning

The role of cellular networks in video and voice applications is expanding rapidly. Advances in 4G technologies are beginning to provide the bandwidth necessary for video conferencing and Video Remote Interpreting (VRI). Patients newly discharged from the hospital will be followed by nurses with devices that allow nurses to see and hear the patient, monitor wound healing, and address family concerns. Early intervention for patients with chronic diseases such as asthma, chronic obstructive pulmonary disease (COPD), heart failure, and diabetes will alert caregivers and prevent hospitalizations. Remote monitoring of patients is increasingly viewed as essential for mHealth planning.

It is widely believed that, by 2020, the majority of computing will be edge computing, defined by a constantly changing mix of corporate and privately owned mobile and wireless devices talking to a corporate or enterprise cloud. As a result, healthcare will become more patient-centered, and mobile and health visits will occur in the home, school, and office (mHIMSS, 2014d). Data from home monitoring devices to fitness apps raise questions about which kinds of data will be aggregated, and conventions for meta-tagging the source of that data. Ethical, legal, privacy, and security questions must be addressed. How is the data protected? Who is authorized to use it and for what purposes? How will the data be processed to discover patterns (data mining)?

Setting the Stage for mHealth Adoption

Smartphones and tablets offer a new engagement model for patients, their family members, and healthcare providers. These devices move with their owners from hospital, to home, and beyond. An Internet search for healthcare applications will yield thousands of results and the list constantly grows larger. With the public's increasing interest in wellness, and a large fitness industry attempting to grow their business, peripheral devices are becoming smartphone-ready. Sensors can now measure heart rate, pulse, oxygen saturation levels, speed, and distance for exercise regimens. Devices are emerging for daily blood tests, automated weight tracking, and sleep monitoring. EKGs can be registered and transmitted through a device no larger than a Band-Aid. The concept of home health has been a driving factor in the proliferation of remote monitoring devices (HIMSS, 2012b). Thanks to advances in machine-to-machine (M2M) technology, patients no longer have to travel to the clinic or hospital for routine monitoring. Patients can check their blood sugar, blood pressure, oxygen levels, and other vital signs at home with their results wirelessly transmitted to their healthcare providers. Providing cellular or Wi-Fi communications to the ambulatory practice and the patient's home is a technology trend that has seen affiliate physician offices partnering with larger hospital systems for access to the EHR and to leverage corporate IT services to provide Wi-Fi for their offices.

Privacy and Security

The cornerstone of trust in healthcare is privacy and security. mHealth data present a greater challenge to security and data integrity because this data is in a mobile environment and not collected in stored access facilities and stored behind firewalls. However, many of the same rules apply to mHealth as well as the physical hospital environment. mHealth must comply with all Health Insurance Portability and Accountability Act (HIPAA) mandates, Food and Drug Administration (FDA) regulations, Office of Civil Rights (OCR) enforcements, and requirements from other governing agencies. The only difference between a smartphone, a personal computer, and an enterprise server is size. In a large number of security breaches, the thief simply carried the equipment out the door or removed it from a car. Size does not play a role in protecting the data.

An organization is responsible for securing and verifying security, and testing to locate vulnerabilities in systems. The goal of privacy and security is to provide as much effort as needed to protect patient's personal health information (PHI) from being compromised. The benchmark for privacy must be 100% secure PHI.

Legal and Policy

State and national policy and regulations have not kept pace with the rate of technology innovation. The proliferation of mHealth technology creates several fundamental issues related to the custody of medical information: who owns it, who can access it, and under what circumstances? As information becomes more portable, the question raised is to what extent records of other providers should be incorporated into clinical records of the practice, hospital, or specialist. Consider the transmission of digital radiology images from a hospital or freestanding diagnostic center to a provider's smartphone. Consumers and patients use a multitude of devices to collect wellness data. Should all data be incorporated into the EHR, or just portions of the data? Should data from all devices be incorporated into the record, or data from just one or a few devices? Does having too much data obscure potentially critical information? Under what circumstances is the healthcare provider required to maintain records of these transmissions? If the transmissions are received, must all data be reviewed? What does the record look like for legal purposes? Must the source of the data (e.g., patient-provided, wearable device, etc.) be transparent?

Clinical significance is the central consideration in the determination of whether wellness, monitoring, and other data transmitted by consumers to their providers should be incorporated into the patient's EHR. Incorporating vast amounts of routine data might detract from clinically relevant findings. When data is shared between patient and clinician from such devices, it is desirable to have a thorough understanding between the treatment team and the patient about how the data is going to be reviewed, incorporated (or not) into the record, and used in patient care.

Historically, there has been reluctance to accept any data other than the information collected within the physical boundaries of the hospital or practice, with the exception of routine consultations. Hesitancy to accept outside data is based on the receiving provider's inability to verify the accuracy of the data. Today, however, that paradigm is changing. Healthcare professionals must be engaged in care coordination across the care continuum. Excluding data from other sources may provide an incomplete picture of the patient's care, resulting in inappropriate or substandard treatment.

The term "social media" immediately brings to mind Facebook, LinkedIn, and Twitter, which are accessible at all times, and in all locations via smartphones. Indeed, the world often learns of breaking news through a tweet. User content is developed and shared through platforms such as YouTube, and video is shared through services such as Skype and FaceTime. As pleasant as it is to receive a new picture of a loved one, social media also presents several types of legal and regulatory concerns:

- Professionalism: Because social media is so ubiquitous, healthcare professionals may face new questions such as whether or not it is appropriate to "friend" a patient.

- Privacy: There have been several widely reported incidents of healthcare professionals posting data related to patients on social media sites. Even if the patient's name is not revealed, releasing data that is not completely de-identified violates the HIPAA Privacy Standards.

- Who owns health-related data posted to a social media site? Is ownership relevant?

There is no question that great change is happening in healthcare and among healthcare professionals. The new technology is mobile. The new face of healthcare will be mHealth.

REFERENCES

Federal Communications Commission. (2012). *mHealth Task Force: Findings and recommendations*. Retrieved from http://transition.fcc.gov/cgb/mhealth/mHealthRecommendations.pdf. Accessed on April 13, 2014.

Healthcare Information and Management Systems Society. (2012a). *Definitions of mHealth*. Retrieved from http://www.himss.org/ResourceLibrary/GenResourceDetail.aspx?ItemNumber=20221. Accessed on April 13, 2014.

Healthcare Information and Management Systems Society. (2012b). *mHIMSS roadmap*. Retrieved from http://www.himss.org/files/mHIMSS%20Roadmap-all%20pages.pdf. Accessed on March 2, 2014.

Health Level Seven International. (2014). *Introduction to HL7 standards*. Retrieved from https://www.hl7.org/implement/standards/. Accessed on April 13, 2014.

mHIMSS. (2014a, February). *Case study: Decreasing costs and improving outcomes through community-based care transitions and care coordination technology*. Retrieved from http://himss.files.cms-plus.com/FileDownloads/User%20Case%20Study%20Decreasing%20Costs%20and%20Improving%20Outcomes%20through%20Community-Based%20Care%20Transitions%20and%20Care%20Coordination%20Technology.pdf. Accessed on March 2, 2014.

mHIMSS. (2014b, February). *Case study: Geisinger Health System: Weight management text program*. Retrieved from http://himss.files.cms-plus.com/FileDownloads/Use%20Case%20Study%20Geisinger%20Health%20System%20Weight%20Management%20Text%20Program.pdf. Accessed on March 2, 2014.

mHIMSS. (2014c, February). *Case study: Improving quality of care for the underserved*. Retrieved from http://himss.files.cms-plus.com/FileDownloads/User%20Case%20Study%20Improving%20Quality%20of%20Care%20for%20the%20Underserved.pdf. Accessed on March 2, 2014.

mHIMSS. (2014d, February). *Case study: Reducing patient no-shows*. Retrieved from http://himss.files.cms-plus.com/FileDownloads/Use%20Case%20Study%20Geisinger%20Health%20System%20Reducing%20Patient%20No-Shows.pdf. Accessed on March 2, 2014.

mHIMSS. (2014e, February). *Case study: Vanderbilt University Medical Center: Hand hygiene monitoring app*. Retrieved from http://himss.files.cms-plus.com/FileDownloads/Case%20Study%20Vanderbilt%20University%20Medical%20Center%20Hand%20Hygiene%20Monitoring%20App.pdf. Accessed on March 2, 2014.

Moore, T. (2011, July 27). Spectrum squeeze: The battle for bandwidth. *Fortune*. Retrieved from http://tech.fortune.cnn.com/2011/07/27/spectrum-squeeze-battle-for-bandwidth/. Accessed on April 9, 2014.

National Institute of Standards and Technology. (2007, April). *Guidelines for Securing radio frequency identification (RFID) systems* (NIST Special Publication SP 800-98). Retrieved from http://csrc.nist.gov/publications/nistpubs/800-98/SP800-98_RFID-2007.pdf. Accessed on April 9, 2014.

National Institute of Standards and Technology. (2012a, June). *Guide to bluetooth security* (NIST Special Publication 800-121 revision 1). Retrieved from http://csrc.nist.gov/publications/nistpubs/800-121-rev1/sp800-121_rev1.pdf. Accessed on April 9, 2014.

National Institute of Standards and Technology. (2012b, February). *Guidelines for securing wireless local area networks* (NIST Special Publication 800-153). Retrieved from http://csrc.nist.gov/publications/nistpubs/800-153/sp800-153.pdf. Accessed on April 9, 2014.

Powell, A. C., Landman, A. B., & Bates, D. W. (2014, March 24). In search of a few good apps. *Journal of the American Medical Association*. Retrieved from https://jama.jamanetwork.com/article.aspx?articleid=1852662. Accessed on April 9, 2014.

Wicklund, E. (Ed.). (2014, February 13). A doc's-eye view of mHealth. *mHealth News*. Retrieved from http://www.mhealthnews.com/news/docs-eye-view-mhealth?singlepage=true. Accessed on March 2, 2014.

Williams, M. (2013, October 1). Battery life hasn't kept pace with advances in mobile computing—but that could change soon. *Techradar*. Retrieved from http://www.techradar.com/us/news/phone-and-communications/mobile-phones/why-are-mobile-phone-batteries-still-so-crap--1162779/2#articleContent. Accessed on April 9, 2014.

Computer Software

Mary L. McHugh

• OBJECTIVES

1. Identify the three categories of software and their functions.
2. Describe four important analytic themes in Information Science.
3. Explain five types of programming languages and their general capabilities.
4. Discuss PDA applications that can be used as part of physical assessment.
5. Explain the differences among LANs, WANs, and MANs.

• KEY WORDS

Software
Information science
Programming languages
PDAs
Networks: LANs, WANs, MANs

INTRODUCTION

Software is the general term applied to the instructions that direct the computer's hardware to perform work. It is distinguished from hardware by its conceptual rather than physical nature. Hardware consists of physical components, whereas software consists of instructions communicated electronically to the hardware. Software is needed for two purposes. First, computers do not directly understand human language, and software is needed to translate instructions created in human language into machine language. At the machine level, computers can understand only binary numbers, not English or any other human language.

Second, packaged or stored software is needed to make the computer an economical work tool. Theoretically, users could create their own software to use the computer. However, writing software instructions (programming) is extremely difficult, time-consuming, and, for most people, tedious. It is much more practical and economical for one highly skilled person or programming team to develop programs that many other people can buy and use to do common tasks. Software is supplied as organized instruction sets called programs, or more typically as a set of related programs called a package.

For example, several prominent software companies sell their own version of a package of programs that are typically needed to support an office computer, including a word processing program, a spreadsheet program, a presentation graphics program, and sometimes a database manager. Programs translate operations the user needs into language and instructions that the computer can understand. By itself, computer hardware is merely a collection of printed circuits, plastic, metal, and wires. Without software, hardware performs no functions.

CATEGORIES OF SOFTWARE

There are three basic types of software: system software, utility programs, and applications software. System software "boots up" (starts up and initializes) the computer system; controls input, output, and storage; and controls the operations of the application software. Utility software consists of programs designed to support and optimize the functioning of the computer system itself.

Applications software includes the various programs that users require to perform day-to-day tasks. They are the programs that support the actual work of the user. Some users claim a third type of software called utility programs. These are programs that are used to help maintain the system, clean up unwanted programs, protect the system against virus attacks, access the World Wide Web (WWW), and the like. Sometimes it can get confusing as to whether programs are utility programs or system software because system software packages today usually include a variety of utility programs with the basic system software packages.

System Software

System software consists of a variety of programs that control the individual computer and make the user's application programs work well with the hardware. System software consists of a variety of programs that initialize, or boot up, the computer when it is first turned on and thereafter control all the functions of the computer hardware and applications software. System software helps speed up the computer's processing, expands the power of the computer by creating cache memory, reduces the amount of confusion when multiple programs are running together, "cleans up" the hard drive so that storage is managed efficiently, and performs other such system management tasks.

Basic Input/Output System. The first level of system control is handled by the basic input/output system (BIOS) stored on a ROM chip on the motherboard. The software on the BIOS chip is the first part of the computer to function when the system is turned on. It first searches for an Operating System (OS) and loads it into the RAM. Given that the BIOS consists of a set of instructions permanently burned onto a computer chip, it is truly a combination of hardware and software. Programs on chips are often called firmware, because they straddle the line between hardware and software. For this reason, many computer engineers make a distinction between firmware and software. From that perspective, the OS is actually the first level of system software (Koushanfar & Markov, 2011).

Operating System. An OS is the overall controller of the work of the computer. The OS is software loaded from the hard drive into RAM as soon as the computer is turned on. While the firmware cannot be upgraded without changing the hardware chip, the OS can be upgraded or entirely changed through software. The user can simply delete one system of OS files from the hard drive and installs a new OS. Most users purchase a computer with the OS already installed on the hard drive. However, the OS can be purchased separately and installed by the user. OSs handle the connection between the CPU and peripherals. The connection between the CPU and a peripheral or a user is called an interface. The OS manages the interfaces to all peripheral hardware, schedules tasks, allocates storage in memory and on disks, retrieves programs and data from storage, and provides an interface between the machine and the user.

One of the most critical tasks (from the user's perspective) performed by the OS involves the management of storage. In the early computers, there were no OSs. Every programmer had to include explicit instructions in every program to tell the CPU exactly where-in RAM to locate the lines of program code and data to be used during processing. That meant the user had to keep track of thousands of memory locations, and be sure to avoid writing one line of code over another active line of code. Also, the programmer had to be careful that output of one part of processing did not accidentally get written over output from another part of processing. As can be imagined, the need for management of storage consumed a great deal of time and programming code, and it produced many errors in programs. Since those errors had to be discovered and corrected before the program would run correctly, the lack of an OS made programming enormously time-consuming and tedious. In comparison, programming today—while still a difficult and time-consuming task—is much more efficient. In fact, with the size of programs, memory and storage media today, no programmer could realistically manage all the storage. OSs allowed not only more complex programs and systems, but without them, there could be no home computers, except for skilled programmers.

Utility Software

Utility programs include programs designed to keep the computer system operating efficiently. They do this by adding power to the functioning of the system software or supporting the OS or applications software programs. As such, utility programs are sort of between system software and applications software, although many writers identify this software as part of the system software category. Six types of utility software can describe the majority of utility programs, although there is no formal categorization system for such programs. The categories include at least Security programs, disk management utilities, backup for the user's data, screen savers, archival assistance software, and programming environment support programs.

Security software, including primarily anti-virus, firewall, and encryption programs, protect the computer and its data from attacks that can destroy programs and data. Anti-virus utilities serve primarily to guard against malicious programs inadvertently accessed, usually through e-mail or downloads from the Internet. Firewalls are a type of security program that makes it much harder for unauthorized persons or systems to enter the computer and hijack or damage programs or data on the computer. Firewalls can include both additional hardware and utility software. Encryption software encodes the data so that it cannot be read until it is decoded. The HTTPS letters on a Web page address indicate that the site encrypts data sent through that site. The encryption is sufficiently high level that it cannot be decoded without a program at the receiver site. This encryption makes buying and selling via the Internet much safer. Without such encryption, credit card and other very private data would not be safe to use to purchase anything via the Internet. Security is also a hardware issue and is addressed in chapter 2 "Computer Hardware" (Markov, 2014).

Disk management utilities are designed to help the user keep hard disk space clean and efficient. They do this by analyzing use of disk space, **defragmenting** the drive, and deleting duplicate files if the user so commands. Over time as users store and delete data and programs, information on the disk may become scattered across the disk in an inefficient or fragmented way. The defragmenter moves data around on the disk so that small empty spaces are eliminated and data and programs are relocated to better use the available space. These programs can also compress data to free up disk space, partition a disk so that the user has more control on where different types of information are stored, and clean up disks by eliminating unnecessary data and information. Specifically, many programs and Internet sites temporarily store information on the hard drive as part of their operations, but when those operations are finished, they don't clean the temporary files. Such files can consume quite a bit of disk space over time, and disk cleaners can sometimes free up large amounts of disk space just by eliminating obsolete information. Other disk management utilities include diagnostic programs designed to find problems with programs or the OS so that they can be fixed.

Backup utilities serve to help the users back up their data. Applications programs may be backed up, but usually that is not necessary because legal copies of programs can be reloaded by the person who bought the license. Illegal (or *pirate*) programs are a different issue. The computer owner may not have a backup copy of illegally downloaded

programs. Given that any computer component can fail, it is very important for users to back up any data they have saved that they do not want to lose permanently. When a hard drive fails (or crashes), the user who has not backed up that drive is at risk of permanently losing photos, information, songs, videos, and anything else stored on the computer. Of course, backing up data on the same hard drive is not necessarily much protection. A better choice is to back up one's data to an external (removable) hard drive or an online backup location.

Screen savers are computer programs that either blank the monitor screen or fill it with constantly moving images when the user is away from the computer but does not turn it (and the monitor) completely off. They were originally developed for old technology screens (cathode ray tube [CRT] screens or plasma screens) that would be damaged by having the same image on the screen for a long period of time. Modern computer screen have different technology and so do not suffer that risk. However, screen savers are often entertaining or beautiful to look at, and do provide a small measure of privacy because they hide whatever the user is working on when the user steps away from the computer. Unless also linked with a program that requires the user to sign back in to access the regular screen, they do not provide security because a passing person could also tap a key to get back to the regular screen. However, most people have the good manners to keep their hands off other people's computers, and the screen saver hides what might be personal or confidential data from casual roaming eyes. Screen savers sometimes do require users to log back into their computer to turn off the screen saver, and those do have a security function. Typically, screen savers activate automatically if the computer does not receive any input from the user for a preset time period.

Archival Software usually performs at least two functions. First, it compresses information in files to be archived, and then stores them in a compressed form in some long-term storage device. For Windows, programs such as WinZip and WinRar are well-known archival utilities. When the files are retrieved, software must be used to unpack (or decompress) the data so that it can be read. Terms used to describe the data compression performed by archival software include packing, zipping, compressing, and archiving as well as unpacking, unzipping, de-archiving, and extraction. The compression can sharply reduce the size of a large file such that it can be made small enough to e-mail to another person or location.

Programming environment support programs are used by program developers to support their programming work or to run their programs. Computers cannot read or understand English or any other human language.

Ultimately, programs must change the language in which developers write programs (the source code) into a machine language the computer can understand (assembly or machine language). The program that performs this translation is called a compiler. If a programmer wishes to translate a machine language program into a higher level language a human can understand the programmer uses a decompiler program. Programming is difficult because not only does the programmer have to detail complex logic, but the commands that comprise the program must be written in a specific syntax. Syntax in this usage refers to a set of very specific rules about words, word usage, and word order in order of a computer language. Syntax must be exactly correct for a computer to correctly interpret the code and run the program. Problems with either the logic or syntax will cause the program to fail, or perform incorrectly. These kinds of problems are called "bugs" and correcting them is called "debugging" a program. Utility programs designed to help a programmer debug a program are called debugging programs. The most commonly used utility programs for programmers include the various types of compilers and debuggers.

Applications Software

Applications software includes all the various programs people use to do work, process data, play games, communicate with others, and watch videos and multimedia programs on a computer. Unlike system and utility programs, they are written for system users to make use of the computer. When the user orders the OS to run an application program, the OS transfers the program from the hard drive, or removable media, and executes it.

Application programs are written in a particular programming language. Then the program is "compiled" (or translated) into machine language so the computer can understand the instructions and execute the program. Originally, programs were written for a specific computer and could only run on that model machine. However, the science of programming languages and their translation eventually advanced to the point that programs today can generally be "ported" (or translated) across many machines. This advancement permitted programmers to develop programs that could be used on a class of machines, such as the Windows type or Mac type computers (the two are still generally incompatible). This advance opened a whole new industry, since programs could be mass marketed as off-the-shelf software packages. By far the most commonly used set of programs are the programs in an office package, such as Microsoft Office, ApacheOpen Office, or LibreOffice, or any of the many other office suites. The most useful program in these

packages is, of course, the word processing program. But spreadsheets and presentation graphics are also widely used, as are the Database Management System software packages such as Microsoft Access. Many of these products also offer e-mail systems, publisher programs, flowchart software, and various other application programs.

INFORMATION SCIENCE

Information science is an interdisciplinary field primarily concerned with the analysis, collection, classification, manipulation, storage, retrieval, movement, dissemination, and use of information (Stock & Stock, 2013). It is concerned with technologies, strategies, and methodologies for getting the right information to people when it is needed without people getting overwhelmed with irrelevant and unwanted information. All science is concerned with measurement and analysis, and information science is no different.

Key themes in information science analysis include optimality, performance, complexity, and structure (Luenberger, 2006). Optimality varies with the situation, but generally refers to achieving an optimum value for some desired outcome. For example, when a nurse wants to obtain information on outcomes of patients who suffered a complication for the purpose of determining whether they were rescued or not, the optimal outcome is that the search facility in the information system finds all patient records for patients who were truly at risk, and does not miss any. Additionally, the system retrieves few if any records of patients who did not suffer a high-risk complication. Optimality may refer to almost any variable that is measured on a numerical scale, such as cost, time (e.g., time to answer patient call lights), workload, etc.

Performance is typically considered in the context of average performance of the information system over a series of communication instances. Averages are better representations of performance than long lists of single instance performance. For example, the average time it takes an e-mail to reach the intended recipient is much more useful than a long list of each e-mail and its transmission time.

Complexity is a reality with the enormous masses of data and information generated, collected, stored, and retrieved. A typical measure of complexity in informatics is the amount of time it takes to complete a task. The time required is most often a function of the amount of information that must be dealt with to complete the task, but can also be greatly affected by how well the database was structured.

Structure means developing a system for ordering and cataloging the data and information, particularly in a database. Excellent structure serves to reduce the amount of time required to perform operations on the database, such as search, retrieve, update, sort, and so forth. When data are well structured and cataloged in a database, complexity can actually be reduced because the system will not have to review all the data to find particular items. Rather, it will have to search only the sectors in which the data are going to be found, and the structure tells the programs that operate on the database which sectors to search.

Information science is a rapidly growing field, and much of the progress is based on development and testing of mathematical algorithms related to information management tasks, such as storage and retrieval, database structure, measuring the value of information, and other works involved in increasing the efficiency of using information to make better decisions. In nursing, some key issues include ways nurses use information to make better nursing diagnoses and care decisions. Nursing information science is very concerned with measuring patient care outcomes and what nursing protocols produce the best outcomes. As a relatively new field, information science is only beginning to help people put the vast amount of data stored in multiple databases to work in efforts to improve health. In the future, data mining and other technologies designed to harvest information from very large databases is likely to become a major focus of health research, and holds great promise for improving healthcare by providing accurate information to decision-makers.

Programming Languages

A programming language is a means of communicating with the computer. Actually, of course, the only language a CPU can understand is binary or machine language. While it is certainly possible for programmers to learn to use binary language—some highly sensitive defense applications are still written in machine language—the language is painfully tedious and inefficient use of human resources, and its programs are virtually impossible to update and debug. Since the invention of computers, users have longed for a machine that could accept instructions in everyday human language. Although that goal largely eludes programmers, applications such as office support programs (i.e., word processors, spread sheets, presentation graphics applications, and the like) have become much easier to use with graphical user interface based commands.

Generations and Levels of Programming Languages

Programming languages are divided into five generations, or sometimes into three levels. The term level refers to how close the language is to the actual machine. The first level includes the first two generations of programming languages: machine language and assembly language. The second level includes the next two generations: high-level procedural and nonprocedural languages. The third level (and fifth generation) is natural language.

The low-level languages are machinelike. Machine language is, of course, binary. It consists of strings of 0s and 1s and can be directly understood by the computer. However, it is difficult to use and to edit.

Machine Language. Machine language is the true language of the computer. Any program must be translated into machine language before the computer can execute it. The machine language consists only of the binary numbers 1 and 0, representing the **ON** and **OFF** electrical impulses. All data—numbers, letters, and symbols—are represented by combinations of binary digits. For example, the number 3 is represented by 8 binary numbers (00000011), and 6 is represented by 00000110. Traditionally, machine languages are machine dependent, which means that each model of computer has its own unique machine language.

Assembler Language. Assembler language is far more like the English language, but it is still very close to machine language. One command in machine language is a single instruction to the processor. Assembler language instructions have a one-to-one correspondence with a machine language instruction. Assembler language is still used a great deal by system programmers and whenever application programmers wish to manipulate functions at the machine level. As can be seen from Fig. 4.1, assembly language, while more English-like than machine language, is extremely obscure to the nonprogrammer.

Third-Generation Languages. Third-generation languages include the procedural languages and were the beginning of the second level in programming languages. Procedural

```
PRINT_ASCII PROC
        MOV DL, 00h
        DL MOV CX, 255
PRINT_LOOP:
        CALL WRITE_CHAR
        INC DL
        LOOP PRINT_LOOP
        MOV AH, 4Ch
        INT 21h ;21h
PRINT ASCII       ENDP
```

• **FIGURE 4.1.** Assembler Language Lines of Code.

languages require the programmer to specify both what the computer is to do and the procedure for how to do it. These languages are far more English-like than assembler and machine languages. However, a great deal of study is required to learn to use these languages. The programmer must learn the words the language recognizes, and must use those words in a rigid style and sequence. A single comma or letter out of place will cause the program to fail or crash. The style and sequence of a language are called its syntax. FORTRAN and COBOL are examples of early third-generation languages.

A third-generation language written specifically for use in healthcare settings was MUMPS (**M**assachusetts **G**eneral **H**ospital **U**tility **M**ulti-**P**rogramming **S**ystem). MUMPS was originally developed to support medical record applications at Massachusetts General Hospital. MUMPS offers powerful tools to support database management systems; this is particularly useful in any setting in which many users have to access the same databases at the same time. Therefore, MUMPS is now found in many different industries such as banks, travel agencies, stock exchanges, and, of course, other hospitals. Originally, MUMPS was both a language and a full OS; however, today most installations load MUMPS on top of their own computer's OS.

Today, the most popular computer language for writing new OSs and other system programs is called C. (It was named after an earlier prototype program called simply B.)

Two important late third-generation languages are increasing in importance as the importance of the Internet grows. They include the visual programming languages and Java. Java was developed by Sun Microsystems to be a relatively simple language that would provide the portability across differing computer platforms and the security needed for use on a huge, public network like the Internet. The world community of software developers and Internet content providers has warmly received Java. Java programming skills are critical for any serious Web developer.

Visual Programming Languages. As the popularity of GUI technology grew, several languages were developed to facilitate program development in graphics-based environments. Microsoft Corporation has marketed two very popular such programs: Visual BASIC (**B**eginners' **A**ll-purpose **S**ymbolic **I**nstruction **C**ode) and Visual C++. These programs and their cousins marketed by other companies have been used for a variety of applications, especially those that allow users to interact with electronic companies through the Internet.

Concurrent and Distributed Languages. Another way to categorize programs is whether they were designed to work sequentially or concurrently. Originally, all programming languages were strictly sequential. That is, the CPU processed one line of code at a time, and the next line was not read until the prior line command had been executed. A lot of calculation work and operations such as payroll and invoice processing do require each part of the process to be completed before the next is started. Mathematical and statistical calculations often must be sequential because the results of each calculation is used by the next calculation to complete the work. One way computer speed was increased was to support the CPU with very specialized processors that handled mathematical functions. However, the CPU would wait for the math processor results to continue with the program. As programming addressed much more complex processes, many parts of programs were not dependent on prior processes. That meant different parts of the program could, at least theoretically, be processed simultaneously. However, a single processor can only process one command at a time. Clock speed improvements have been somewhat limited by the heat produced by faster processing.

Originally, computers had only one CPU so they had only one core processor. As programs became more complex, and especially as the Internet advanced into a multimedia environment, the clock speed of a single processor could not keep up. It is extremely slow to wait to load text while pictures are loading, but a single processor cannot do two of those actions at the same time. Those who used computers in the early 1990s may remember that Web pages with lots of images could be impossibly slow to load, and this was at least partly due to personal computers having only a single processor. Even though CPU clock speeds increased steadily, a single processor could not keep up with the video, graphs, and sound demands of Internet pages. According to Igor Markov, "Computer speed is not increasing anymore" (Markov, 2014). Another strategy was needed to improve speed. The solution has been to add more CPU processors, and this solution is called **multiprocessing** which involves multiple processors working in parallel (parallelism).

Around the year 2000, dual core processors became available (Varela, 2013). Although they were expensive, they were essential for people who needed to run complex engineering and scientific programs, and people who liked to play complex online games with sophisticated graphics (these people are called "gamers" and their high power computers are called "gaming computers"). The advantages of multiprocessing were such that by 2014, all personal computers advertised for the home and business had two or more processors to speed up the operation of complex and graphics intensive programs. A high-speed, sophisticated graphics card is also necessary to handle the volume of graphics in today's programs and Web pages. The Intel i7 product had six microprocessors in addition to its graphics card. Program languages designed to take advantage of multiple processors are called **concurrent** languages. Concurrent languages are designed for programs that use multiple processors in parallel, rather than running the program sequentially on a single processor. C++ is an example of a programming language designed as a concurrent language.

Closely associated with the need to run multiple parts of a program at the same time is the need to accommodate multiple users at the same time. This is called ***multithreading*** (Intel, 2003). While multithreading is more of an implementation problem than strictly a programming issue, modern, high-level languages handle multiprocessing and multithreading more easily than older languages. Programming languages like Java, from Sun Microsystems, and Haskell were designed expressly to handle both multiprocessing and multithreading at the same time. However, C11 and C++11 as well as other languages were designed to be used in multiprocessing and multithreading environments. The importance of excellent multithreading programming products was well illustrated when the Affordable Care Act government Web site could not handle the volume of users trying to access the site at the same time.

Fourth-Generation Languages. Fourth-generation languages are specialized application programs that require more involvement of the user in directing the program to do the necessary work. Some people in the computer industry do not consider these to be programming languages. Procedural languages include programs such as spreadsheets, statistical analysis programs, and database query languages. These programs may also be thought of as applications programs for special work functions. The difference between these languages and the earlier generation languages is that the user specifies *what* the program is to do, but not *how* the program is to perform the task. The "how" is already programmed by the manufacturer of the language/applications program. For example, to perform a chi-square calculation in FORTRAN, the user must specify each step involved in carrying out the formula for a chi-square and also must enter into the FORTRAN program all the data on which the operations are to be performed. In Statistical Package for Social Sciences (SPSS), a statistical analysis program, the user enters a command (from a menu of commands) that tells the computer to compute a chi-square statistic on a particular set of numbers provided to the program. That is, the user provides SPSS with a data file and selects the command that

executes a Chi-Square on the selected data. But the user does not have to write code telling the computer which mathematical processes (add, subtract, multiply, divide) to perform on the data in order to calculate the statistic. The formula for chi-square is already part of the SPSS program.

An important Fourth-Generation language is SQL (Structured Query Language). SQL is a language designed for management and query operations on a relational database. It does far more than simply allow users to query a database. It also supports data insert, data definition, database schema creation, update and delete, and data modification. It is not particularly user friendly for non-programmers, but it is an extremely powerful language for information retrieval.

Fifth-Generation Languages. Fifth-generation or third-level languages are called natural languages. In these types of programs, the user tells the machine what to do in the user's own natural language or through use of a set of very English-like commands. Ideally, voice recognition technology is integrated with the language so that voice commands are recognized and executed. True fifth-generation languages are still emerging. Natural language recognition, in which any user could give understandable commands to the computer in his or her own word style and accent, is being performed at the beginning of the twenty-first century. However, natural language systems are clearly in the future of personal computing. The great difficulty is, of course, how to reliably translate natural, spoken human language into a language the computer can understand.

To prepare a translation program for a natural language requires several levels of analysis. First, the sentences need to be broken down to identify the subject's words and relate them to the underlying constituents of speech (i.e., parsed). The next level is called semantic analysis, whereby the grammar of each word in the sentence is analyzed. It attempts to recognize the action described and the object of the action. There are several computer programs that translate natural languages based on basic rules of English. They generally are specially written programs designed to interact with databases on a specific topic. By limiting the programs to querying the database, it is possible to process the natural language terms.

An exciting application of natural language processing (NLP) is called biomedical text mining (BioNLP). The purpose is to assist users to find information about a specific topic in biomedical literature. This method of searching professional literature articles in PubMed or another database increases the likelihood that a relevant mention of the topic will be discovered and extracted, thus increasing the probability of a comprehensive information extraction process. One example is a program called **DNorm.** DNorm detects specific disease names (entered by the searcher) in journal articles or other text documents. It also associates them with search terms in MeSH terms in PubMed and terms in SNOMED-CT[1] (Leaman, Dogan, & Zhivong, 2014).

Text Formatting Languages. Strictly speaking, text formatters are not true programming languages. They are used to format content, originally text, for visual display in a system. However, the skills required to learn to format text are similar to the skills required to learn a programming language, and informally they are called programming languages.

The most famous is HyperText Markup Language (HTML). HTML is used to format text for the World Wide Web and is one of the older formatting languages. These languages specify to the computer how text and graphics are to be displayed on the computer screen. There are many other formatting languages, such as Extensible Markup Language (XML) which is a restricted version of SGML and used in most word processing programs. The original markup language is Standardized General Markup Language (SGML) which is actually a meta-language and the standard for markup languages. HTML and XML adhere to the SGML pattern.

COMMON SOFTWARE PACKAGES FOR MICROCOMPUTERS

The most common package sold with computers is a standard office package. The standard office package includes a word processing program, a spreadsheet program, and a presentation graphics program. The upgraded or professional versions usually add some form of database management system, an e-mail system, a "publisher" program for preparing flyers, brochures, and other column-format documents. The two most commonly used programs are the e-mail system and the word processor. In fact, some people purchase a computer with only an OS, word processor, and an Internet browser, and sign up for their e-mail account and use little else. Another very common product is a desktop publisher. Most of these common programs

---

[1]SNOMED CT is a database containing a comprehensive list of clinical terms. Nursing terms from all the major nursing terminologies have been listed in SNOMED CT. It is owned, maintained, and distributed by the International Health Terminology Standards Development Organisation (IHTSDO).

have to be written in two versions: one for the IBM PC platform and one for the Mac. Typically, software packages are sold on DVDs, although some are available on flash drives and many software companies are now marketing their products through the Internet and customers download the software directly through the Internet from the vendor's Web site.

Security programs are also an important market product. Given the large number of people seeking to steal identities and otherwise use the computer for criminal or malicious activity, every user who accesses the Internet should have security software.

SOFTWARE PACKAGE OWNERSHIP RIGHTS

Protecting ownership rights in software has presented a challenge to the computer software industry. A program sold to one customer can be installed on a very large number of machines. This practice obviously seriously harms the profitability of software development. If programs were sold outright, users would have every right to distribute them as they wished; however, the industry could not survive in such market conditions. As a result, the software industry has followed an ownership model more similar to that of the book publishing industry than to the model used by vendors of most commercial products.

When most commercial products like furniture or appliances are sold, the buyer can use the product or resell it or loan it to a friend if so desired. The product sold is a physical product that can be used only by one customer at a time. Copying the product is not feasible. However, intellectual property is quite a different proposition: what is sold is the idea. The medium on which the idea is stored is not the product. However, when the PC industry was new, people buying software viewed their purchase as the physical diskette on which the intellectual property was stored. Software was expensive, but the diskettes were cheap. Therefore, groups of friends would often pool money to purchase one copy of the software and make copies for everyone in the group. This, of course, enraged the software vendors.

As a result, copyright laws were extended to software so that only the original purchaser was legally empowered to install the program on his or her computer. Any other installations were considered illegal copies, and such copies were called pirate copies. Purchasers of software do not buy full rights to the software. They purchase only a license to use the software. Individually purchased software is licensed to one and only one computer. An exception can be made if the individual has both a desktop and a laptop. Fair use allows the purchaser to install the software on all the machines he or she personally owns—provided the computers are for that user's personal use only. Companies that have multiple computers that are used by many employees must purchase a separate copy for each machine, or more typically, they purchase a "site license." A site license is a way of buying in bulk, so to speak. The company and software vendor agree on how many machines the software may be used on, and a special fee is paid for the number of copies to be used. Additional machines over the number agreed on require an increase in the allowable sites—and payment of the higher site-license fee—or separate copies of the software may be purchased. What is not permitted, and is, in fact, a form of theft is to install more copies of the software than were paid for.

COMMON SOFTWARE USEFUL TO NURSES

In most hospitals, most software systems used by nurses are based in a Hospital Information System (HIS). The HIS is a multipurpose program, designed to support many applications in hospitals and their associated clinics. The components nurses use most include the electronic medical record for charting patient care, admission-discharge-transfer (ADT) systems that help with patient tracking, medication administration record (MAR) software, supplies inventory systems through which nurses charge IVs, dressings, and other supplies used in patient care, and laboratory systems that are used to order laboratory tests and report the results. There are systems for physicians to document their medical orders; quality and safety groups such as the Leapfrog group consider a computer physician order entry (CPOE) system to be so important that they list it as a separate item on their quality checklist. Additionally, nurses may have the support of computer-based systems for radiology orders and results reporting, a computerized patient acuity system used to help with nurse staff allocation, and perhaps there may be a hospital e-mail system used for at least some hospital communications. Increasingly, nurses are finding that they are able to build regional, national, and international networks with their nursing colleagues with the use of chat rooms, bulletin boards, conferencing systems, and listservs on the Internet.

Given that many people have personal digital assistants (PDAs) as part of their cellular phones, nurses may download any of thousands of software applications (apps) onto their PDAs to assist them with patient care. Most are very low cost and some are free. Such programs include drug guides, medical dictionaries, and consult guides for a variety of patient populations and clinical problems (e.g., pediatric pocket consultation, toxicology guide, guide to clinical procedures, and laboratory results guides). Software can now be downloaded onto a PDA to measure heart and respiratory rate, perform ultrasounds on various organs, test hearing, perform a simple EKG, and many other physical assessments can be obtained via a PDA.

As so many items of healthcare equipment have computer processers today, the nurse may not always realize that software is being used. For example, volumetric pumps control IV flow through computer processors. Heart monitors and EKG and EEG machines all have internal computers that detect patterns and provide interpretations of the patterns. Hospital beds may have processors to detect wetness, heat, weight, and other measures. Most radiology equipment today is computer based. Many items of surgery equipment exist only because computer processors are available to make them operate.

Some nursing applications include a handy "**dashboard**," which is an application that provides a sort of a menu of options from which the nurse can choose. Typically, dashboards provide the nurse a quick way to order common output from certain (or all) screens, or may provide some kind of alert that a task is due to be performed.

COMPUTER SYSTEMS

Every functioning computer is a system; that is, it is a complex entity, consisting of an organized set of interconnected components or factors that function together as a unit to accomplish results that one part alone could not. Computer system may refer to a single machine (and its peripherals and software) that is unconnected to any other computer. However, most healthcare professionals use computer systems consisting of multiple, interconnected computers that function to facilitate the work of groups of providers and their support people in a system called a **network**. The greatest range of functionality is realized when computers are connected to other computers in a network or, as with the Internet, a system of networks in which any computer can communicate with any other computer.

Common types of computer networks are point-to-point, local area network (LAN), wide area network (WAN), and metropolitan area network (MAN). A point-to-point network is a very small network in which all parts of the system are directly connected via wires or wireless (typically provided by a router in a single building). LANs, WANs, and MANs are sequentially larger and given the number of users they require communications architecture to ensure all users on the network are served. If the network capacity is too small, some users will experience very long waits or perhaps the system will crash from overload (i.e., stop working and have to be restarted).

Computer networks must allocate time and memory space to many users, and so must have a way to organize usage of the network resources so that all users are served. There are a variety of allocation strategies for high-level communication in networks. The most common are token ring (developed by IBM), star (also called multipoint; all communications go through a single hub computer), bus (in which all computers are connected to a single line), and tree. For very large networks, backbone communication technology is increasingly used.

The use of systems in computer technology is based on system theory. System theory and its subset, network theory, provide the basis for understanding how the power of individual computers has been greatly enhanced through the process of linking multiple computers into a single system and multiple computer systems into networks.

REFERENCES

Intel. (2003). *Intel hyperthreading users technology manual.* Retrieved from http://cache-www.intel.com/cd/00/00/01/77/17705_htt_user_guide.pdf. Accessed on April 2, 2014.

Koushanfar, R., & Markov, I. (2011). *Designing chips that protect themselves.* ACM DAC Knowledge Center. Retrieved from http://web.eecs.umich.edu/~imarkov/pubs/jour/DAC.COM-TrustedICs.pdf. Accessed on March 10, 2014.

Leaman, R., Dogan, R., & Zhivong, L. (2014). *DNorm: Disease name normalization with pairwise learning to rank.* National Center for Biotechnology Information (NCBI), National Library of Medicine. Retrieved from http://www.ncbi.nlm.nih.gov/CBBresearch/Lu/Demo/DNorm/. Accessed on February 15, 2014.

Luenberger, D. (2006). *Information science.* Princeton, NJ: Princeton University Press.

Markov, I. (2014). *Next-generation chips and computing with atoms. Igor Markov: Material for graduate students.* Retrieved from http://web.eecs.umich.edu/~imarkov/. Accessed on February 14, 2014.

Stock, W. G., & Stock, M. (2013). *Handbook of information science.* Berlin: De Gruyter Saur.

Varela, C. (2013). *Programming distributed computer systems.* Cambridge, MA: MIT Press.

5

Open Source and Free Software

David J. Whitten

• OBJECTIVES

1. Describe the basic concepts of open source software (OSS) and free software (FS).
2. Describe the differences between open source software, free software, and proprietary software, particularly in respect of licensing.
3. Discuss why an understanding of open source and free software is important in a healthcare context, in particular where a choice between proprietary and open source software or free software is being considered.
4. Describe some of the open source and free software applications currently available, both healthcare-specific and for general office/productivity use.
5. Introduce some of the organizations and resources available to assist the nurse interested in exploring the potential of open source software.
6. Create and develop an example of OSS.
7. Describe the organization of health databases.
8. Use Boolean Logic to form query conditions.
9. Understand methods for querying and reporting from databases (VistA FileMan, SQL).

• KEY WORDS

Querying databases
Boolean Logic
Open source software
Free software
Linux

INTRODUCTION

It is estimated that, worldwide, over 350 million people use open source software products and thousands of enterprises and organizations use open source code (Anderson & Dare, 2009); free and open source software are increasingly recognized as a reliable alternative to proprietary products. Most nurses use open source and free software (OSS/FS) (Table 5.1) on a daily basis, often without even realizing it. Everybody who sends an e-mail or uses the Web uses OSS/FS most of the time, as the majority of the hardware and software that allows the Internet to function (Web servers, file transmission protocol [FTP] servers, and mail systems) are OSS/FS. As Vint Cerf, Google's "Chief Internet Evangelist" who is seen by many as the "father of the Internet," has stated, the Internet "is fundamentally based on the existence of open, nonproprietary standards" (Openforum Europe, 2008). Many popular Web sites are hosted on Apache (OSS/FS) servers, and increasingly people are using OSS/FS Web browsers

TABLE 5.1	Common Acronyms and Terms

A number of acronyms are used to denote a combination of free software and open source software. OSS/FS is the term that is used for preference in this chapter; others include the following:

OSS: Open source software

OSS/FS: Open source software/free software

FOSS: Free and open source software

FLOSS: Free/libre/open source software

GNU: GNU is Not Unix Project (a recursive acronym). This is a project started by Richard Stallman, which turned into the Free Software Foundation (FSF, www.fsf.org), to develop and promote alternatives to proprietary Unix implementations.

GNU/Linux or Linux: The complete operating system includes the Linux kernel, the GNU components, and many other programs. GNU/Linux is the more accurate term because it makes a distinction between the kernel—Linux—and much of the software that was developed by the GNU Project in association with the FSF.

such as Firefox. While in the early days of computing software was often free, free software (as defined by the Free Software Foundation [FSF]; Table 5.1) has existed since the mid-1980s, the 'GNU is Not Unix' Project (GNU)/Linux operating system (Table 5.1) has been developing since the early 1990s, and the open source initiative (OSI) (Table 5.2) definition of open source software has existed since the late 1990s. It is only more recently that widespread interest has begun to develop in the possibilities of OSS/FS within health, healthcare, and nursing, and within nursing informatics (NI) and health informatics.

In healthcare facilities in many countries, in both hospital and community settings, healthcare information technology (IT) initially evolved as a set of facility-centric tools to manage patient data. This was often primarily for administrative purposes, such that there now exists, in many facilities, a multitude of different, often disconnected, systems, with modern hospitals often using more than 100 different software applications. One of the major problems that nurses and all other health professionals currently face is that many of these applications and systems do not interface well for data and information exchange to benefit patient care. A major challenge in all countries is to move to a more patient-centric system, integrating facilities such as hospitals, physicians' offices, and community or home healthcare providers, so that they can easily share and exchange patient data and allow collaborative care around the patient. Supporters of OSS/FS approaches believe that only through openness,

in respect to open standards and access to applications' source codes, is the user in control of the software and able to adapt the application to local needs, and prevent problems associated with vendor lock-in (Murray, Wright, Karopka, Betts, & Orel, 2009).

However, many nurses have only a vague understanding of what OSS/FS are and their possible applications and relevance to nursing and NI. This chapter aims to provide a basic understanding of the issues, as it is only through being fully informed about the relative merits, and potential limitations, of the range of proprietary software and OSS/FS, that nurses can make informed choices, whether they are selecting software for their own personal needs or involved in procurements for large healthcare organizations. This chapter will provide an overview of the background to OSS/FS, explaining the differences and similarities between open source and free software, and introducing some particular applications such as the GNU/Linux operating system. Licensing will be addressed, as it is one of the major issues that exercises the minds of those with responsibility for decision-making, as issues such as the interface of OSS/FS and proprietary software, or use of OSS/FS components are not fully resolved. Some commonly available and healthcare-specific applications will be introduced, with a few examples being discussed. Some of the organizations working to explore the use of OSS/FS within healthcare and nursing, and some additional resources, will be introduced.

The chapter will conclude with a case study of what many consider the potential "mother of OSS/FS healthcare applications," Veterans Health Information System and Technology Architecture (VistA) (Tiemann, 2004), and recent moves to develop fully OSS/FS versions.

OSS/FS—THE THEORY

Background

While we use the term *open source* (and the acronym OSS/FS) in this chapter, we do so loosely (and, some would argue, incorrectly) to cover several concepts, including OSS, FS, and GNU/Linux. Each of these concepts and applications has its own definition and attributes (Table 5.2). While the two major philosophies in the OSS/FS world, i.e., the free software foundation (FSF) philosophy and the open source initiative (OSI) philosophy, are today often seen as separate movements with different views and goals, their adherents frequently work together on specific practical projects (FSF, 2010a).

The key commonality between FSF and OSI philosophies is that the source code is made available to the users by the programmer. Where FSF and OSI differ in the

TABLE 5.2	Free Software and Open Source Definitions

Free Software

The term *free software* is defined as follows by the Free Software Foundation (FSF) (Version 1.122, 2013, www.gnu.org/philosophy/free-sw.html, emphasis added):

Free software is seen in terms of liberty, rather than price, and to understand the concept, you need to think of "free" as in free speech, not as in free beer. The differences are easier to understand in some languages other than English, where there is less ambiguity in the use of the word *free*. For example, in French, the use of the terms *libre* (freedom) software versus gratis (zero price) software. Free software is described in terms of the users' freedom to run, copy, distribute, study, change, and improve the software. More precisely, it refers to four kinds of freedom for the users of the software:

- The freedom to run the program for any purpose (freedom 0).
- The freedom to study how the program works, and change it to make it do what you wish (freedom 1). Access to the source code is a precondition for this.
- The freedom to redistribute copies so you can help your neighbor (freedom 2).
- The freedom to distribute copies of your modified versions to others (freedom 3). By doing this you can give the whole community a chance to benefit from your changes. Access to the source code is a precondition for this.

A program is free software if users have all of these freedoms.

Open Source Software

The term *open source* is defined exactly as follows by the open source initiative (OSI) (www.opensource.org/docs/osd):

Introduction

Open source does not just mean access to the source code. The distribution terms of open source software must comply with the following criteria:

1. **Free Redistribution**
   The license shall not restrict any party from selling or giving away the software as a component of an aggregate software distribution containing programs from several different sources. The license shall not require a royalty or other fee for such sale.
   Rationale: By constraining the license to require free redistribution, we eliminate the temptation to throw away many long-term gains in order to make a few short-term sales dollars. If we did not do this, there would be lots of pressure for cooperators to defect.

2. **Source Code**
   The program must include source code, and must allow distribution in source code as well as compiled form. Where some form of a product is not distributed with source code, there must be a well-publicized means of obtaining the source code for no more than a reasonable reproduction cost preferably, downloading via the Internet without charge. The source code must be the preferred form in which a programmer would modify the program. Deliberately obfuscated source code is not allowed. Intermediate forms such as the output of a preprocessor or translator are not allowed.
   Rationale: We require access to unobfuscated source code because you cannot evolve programs without modifying them. Since our purpose is to make evolution easy, we require that modification be made easy.

3. **Derived Works**
   The license must allow modifications and derived works, and must allow them to be distributed under the same terms as the license of the original software.
   Rationale: The mere ability to read source is not enough to support independent peer review and rapid evolutionary selection. For rapid evolution to happen, people need to be able to experiment with and redistribute modifications.

4. **Integrity of the Author's Source Code**
   The license may restrict source code from being distributed in modified form only if the license allows the distribution of "patch files" with the source code for the purpose of modifying the program at build time. The license must explicitly permit distribution of software built from modified source code. The license may require derived works to carry a different name or version number from the original software.
   Rationale: Encouraging lots of improvement is a good thing, but users have a right to know who is responsible for the software they are using. Authors and maintainers have reciprocal right to know what they are being asked to support and protect their reputations.

(continued)

TABLE 5.2	Free Software and Open Source Definitions *(continued)*

Open Source Software

Accordingly, an open source license must guarantee that source be readily available, but may require that it be distributed as pristine base sources plus patches. In this way, "unofficial" changes can be made available but readily distinguished from the base source.

5. **No Discrimination Against Persons or Groups**
   The license must not discriminate against any person or group of persons.
   Rationale: In order to get the maximum benefit from the process, the maximum diversity of persons and groups should be equally eligible to contribute to open sources. Therefore, we forbid any open source license from locking anybody out of the process.
   Some countries, including the United States, have export restrictions for certain types of software. An OSD-conformant license may warn licensees of applicable restrictions and remind them that they are obliged to obey the law; however, it may not incorporate such restrictions itself.

6. **No Discrimination Against Fields of Endeavor**
   The license must not restrict anyone from making use of the program in a specific field of endeavor. For example, it may not restrict the program from being used in a business, or from being used for genetic research.
   Rationale: The major intention of this clause is to prohibit license traps that prevent open source from being used commercially. We want commercial users to join our community, not feel excluded from it.

7. **Distribution of License**
   The rights attached to the program must apply to all to whom the program is redistributed without the need for execution of an additional license by those parties.
   Rationale: This clause is intended to forbid closing up software by indirect means such as requiring a nondisclosure agreement.

8. **License Must Not Be Specific to a Product**
   The rights attached to the program must not depend on the program's being part of a particular software distribution. If the program is extracted from that distribution and used or distributed within the terms of the program's license, all parties to whom the program is redistributed should have the same rights as those that are granted in conjunction with the original software distribution.
   Rationale: This clause forecloses yet another class of license traps.

9. **License Must Not Restrict Other Software**
   The license must not place restrictions on other software that is distributed along with the licensed software. For example, the license must not insist that all other programs distributed on the same medium must be open source software.
   Rationale: Distributors of open source software have the right to make their own choices about their own software.

10. **License Must Be Technology-Neutral**
    No provision of the license may be predicated on any individual technology or style of interface.
    Rationale: This provision is aimed specifically at licenses which require an explicit gesture of assent in order to establish a contract between licensor and licensee. Provisions mandating so-called "click-wrap" may conflict with important methods of software distribution such as FTP download, CD-ROM anthologies, and Web mirroring; such provisions may also hinder code reuse. Conformant licenses must allow for the possibility that (a) redistribution of the software will take place over non-Web channels that do not support click-wrapping of the download, and that (b) the covered code (or reused portions of covered code) may run in a non-GUI environment that cannot support pop-up dialogs.

restrictions placed on redistributed source code. FSF is committed to no restrictions, so that if you modify and redistribute free software, as a part or as a whole of aggregated software, you are not allowed to place any restrictions on the openness of the resultant source code (Wong & Sayo, 2004). The difference between the two movements is said to be that the free software movement's fundamental issues are ethical and philosophical, while for the open source movement the issues are more practical than ethical ones; thus, the FSF asserts that open source is a development methodology, while free software is a social movement (FSF, 2010a).

OSS/FS is contrasted with proprietary or commercial software, again the two terms often being conflated but strictly needing separation. Proprietary software is that on which an individual or company holds the exclusive copyright, at the same time restricting other people's access to the software's source code and/or the right to copy, modify, and study the software (Sfakianakis, Chronaki, Chiarugi, Conforti, & Katehakis, 2007). Commercial software is software developed by businesses or individuals with the aim of making money from its licensing and use. Most commercial software is proprietary, but there is commercial free software, and there is noncommercial nonfree software.

OSS/FS should also not be confused with freeware or shareware. Freeware is software offered free of charge, but without the freedom to modify the source code and redistribute the changes, so it is not free software (as defined by the FSF). Shareware is another form of commercial software, which is offered on a "try before you buy" basis. If the customer continues to use the product after a short trial period, or wishes to use additional features, they are required to pay a specified, usually nominal, license fee.

Free Software Definition

Free software is defined by the FSF in terms of four freedoms for software users: to have the freedom to use, study, redistribute, and improve the software in any way they wish. A program is only free software, in terms of the FSF definition, if users have all of these freedoms (see Table 5.2). The FSF believes that users should be free to redistribute copies, either with or without modifications, either gratis or through charging a fee for distribution, to anyone, anywhere without a need to ask or pay for permission to do so (FSF, 2010a).

Confusion around the use and meaning of the term *free software* arises from the multiple meanings of the word *free* in the English language. In other languages, there is less of a problem, with different words being used for the "freedom" versus "no cost" meanings of *free*, for example, the French terms *libre* (freedom) software versus *gratis* (zero price) software. The "free" of free software is defined in terms of liberty, not price, thus to understand the concept, the common distinction is in thinking of free as in free speech, not as in free beer (FSF, 2010b). Acronyms such as FLOSS (free/libre/OSS—a combination of the above two terms emphasizing the "libre" meaning of the word *free*) or OSS/FS are increasingly used, particularly in Europe, to overcome this issue (International Institute of Infonomics, 2005).

Open Source Software Definition

Open source software is any software satisfying the open software initiative's definition (OSI, n.d.). The open source concept is said to promote software reliability and quality by supporting independent peer review and rapid evolution of source code as well as making the source code

of software freely available. In addition to providing free access to the programmer's instructions to the computer in the programming language in which they were written, many versions of open source licenses allow anyone to modify and redistribute the software.

The open source initiative (OSI) has created a certification mark, "OSI certified." In order to be OSI certified, the software must be distributed under a license that guarantees the right to read, redistribute, modify, and use the software freely (OSI, n.d.). Not only must the source code be accessible to all, but also the distribution terms must comply with 10 criteria defined by the OSI (see Table 5.2 for full text and rationale).

OSS/FS Development Models and Systems

OSS/FS has existed as a model for developing computer applications and software since the 1950s (Waring & Maddocks, 2005); at that time, software was often provided free (gratis), and freely, when buying hardware (Murray et al., 2009). The freedoms embodied within OSS/FS were understood as routine until the early 1980s with the rise of proprietary software. However, it was only in the 1980s that the term free software (Stallman, 2002) and in the 1990s that the term open source software, as we recognize them today, came into existence to distinguish them from the proprietary models.

The development models of OSS/FS are said to contribute to their distinctions from proprietary software. Shaw et al. (2002) state that as OSS/FS is "developed and disseminated in an open forum," it "revolutionizes the way in which software has historically been developed and distributed." A similar description, in a UK government report, emphasizes the open publishing of source code and that development is often largely through voluntary efforts (Peeling & Satchell, 2001).

While OSS/FS is often described as being developed by voluntary efforts, this description may belie the professional skills and expertise of many of the developers. Many of those providing the volunteer efforts are highly skilled programmers who contribute time and efforts freely to the development of OSS/FS. In addition, many OSS/FS applications are coordinated through formal groups. For example, the Apache Software Foundation (www.apache.org) coordinates development of the Apache hypertext transfer protocol (HTTP) server and many other products.

OSS/FS draws much of its strength from the collaborative efforts of people who work to improve, modify, or customize programs, believing they must give back to the OSS/FS community so others can benefit from their work. The OSS/FS development model is unique, although it bears strong similarities to the openness of the scientific method, and is facilitated by the communication capabilities of the Internet that allow collaboration and rapid sharing of developments, such that new versions of software can often be made available on a daily basis.

The most well-known description of the distinction between OSS/FS and proprietary models of software development lies in Eric Raymond's famous essay, "The Cathedral and the Bazaar" (Raymond, 2001). Cathedrals, Raymond says, were built by small groups of skilled workers and craftsmen to carefully worked out designs. The work was often done in isolation, and with everything built in a single effort with little subsequent modification. Much software, in particular proprietary software, has traditionally been built in a similar fashion, with groups of programmers working to strictly controlled planning and management, until their work was completed and the program released to the world. In contrast, OSS/FS development is likened to a bazaar, growing organically from an initial small group of traders or enthusiasts establishing their structures and beginning businesses. The bazaar grows in a seemingly chaotic fashion, from a minimally functional structure, with later additions or modifications as circumstances dictate. Likewise, most OSS/FS development starts off highly unstructured, with developers releasing early, minimally functional code and then modifying their programs based on feedback. Other developers may then join, and modify or build on the existing code; over time, an entire operating system and suite of applications develops, evolves, and improves continuously.

The bazaar method of development is said to have been proven over time to have several advantages, including the following:

- Reduced duplication of efforts through being able to examine the work of others and through the potential for large numbers of contributors to use their skills. As Moody (2001) describes it, there is no need to reinvent the wheel every time as there would be with commercial products whose codes cannot be used in these ways
- Building on the work of others, often by the use of open standards or components from other applications
- Better quality control; with many developers working on a project, code errors (bugs) are uncovered quickly and may be fixed even more rapidly (often termed Linus' Law, "given enough eyeballs, all bugs are shallow" [Raymond, 2001])
- Reduction in maintenance costs; costs, as well as effort, can be shared among potentially thousands of developers (Wong & Sayo, 2004).

CHOOSING OSS/FS OR NOT

Proposed Benefits of OSS/FS

OSS/FS has been described as the electronic equivalent of generic drugs (Bruggink, 2003; Goetz, 2003; Surman & Diceman, 2004). In the same way as the formulas for generic drugs are made public, so OSS/FS source code is accessible to the user. Any person can see how the software works and can make changes to the functionality. It is also suggested by many that there are significant similarities between the open source ethos and the traditional scientific method approach (supported by most scientists and philosophers of science), as this latter method is based on openness, free sharing of information, and improvement of the end result. As OSS/FS can be obtained royalty free, it is less expensive to acquire than proprietary alternatives. This means that OSS/FS can transform healthcare in developing countries just as the availability of generic drugs have.

This is only one of several benefits proposed for OSS/FS, with further benefits including lack of the proprietary lock-in that can often freeze out innovation, and with OSS/FS projects supporting open standards and providing a level playing field, expanding the market by giving software consumers greater choice (Dravis, 2003).

Besides the low cost of OSS/FS, there are many other reasons why public and private organizations are adopting OSS/FS, including security, reliability, and stability, and developing local software capacity. Many of these proposed benefits have yet to be demonstrated or tested extensively, but there is growing evidence for many of them, and we will address some of them in the next section.

Issues in OSS/FS

There are many issues in the use of OSS/FS that we cannot address here in detail. However, by providing nurses who are exploring, using, or intending to use OSS/FS with a basic introduction and pointers to additional resources, we facilitate their awareness of the issues and support them in their decision-making. The issues that we introduce include, not necessarily in any order of importance:

- Licensing
- Copyright and intellectual property
- Total cost of ownership (TCO)
- Support and migration
- Business models
- Security and stability

Licensing and copyright will be addressed in the next section, but the other issues will be covered briefly here, before concluding the section with a short description of one possible strategy for choosing OSS/FS (or other software, as the issues are pertinent to any properly considered purchase and implementation strategy).

Total Cost of Ownership. Total cost of ownership (TCO) is the sum of all the expenses directly related to the ownership and use of a product over a given period of time. The popular myth surrounding OSS/FS is that it is always free as in free of charge. This is true to an extent, as most OSS/FS distributions (e.g., Ubuntu [www.ubuntu.com], Red Hat [www.redhat.com], SuSE [www.opensuse.org], and Debian [www.debian.org]) can be obtained at no charge from the Internet; however, copies can also be sold.

No true OSS/FS application charges a licensing fee for usage, thus on a licensing cost basis OSS/FS applications are almost always cheaper than proprietary software. However, licensing costs are not the only costs of a software package or infrastructure. It is also necessary to consider personnel costs, hardware requirements, migration time, changes in staff efficiency, and training costs, among others. Without all of this information, it is impossible to really know which software solutions are going to be the most cost-effective. There are still real costs with OSS/FS, specifically around configuration and support (examples are provided in Wheeler, 2007 and Wong & Sayo, 2004).

Wheeler (2007) lists the main reasons why OSS/FS is generally less expensive, including the following:

- OSS/FS costs less to initially acquire, because there are no license fees.

- Upgrade and maintenance costs are typically far less due to improved stability and security.

- OSS/FS can often use older hardware more efficiently than proprietary systems, yielding smaller hardware costs and sometimes eliminating the need for new hardware.

- Increasing numbers of case studies using OSS/FS show it to be especially cheaper in server environments.

Support and Migration. Making an organization-wide change from proprietary software can be costly, and sometimes the costs will outweigh the benefits. Some OSS/FS packages do not have the same level of documentation, training, and support resources as their common proprietary equivalents, and may not fully interface with other proprietary software being used by other organizations with which an organization may work (e.g., patient data exchange between different healthcare provider systems).

Migration from one platform to another should be handled using a careful and phased approach. The European Commission has published a document entitled the "IDA Open Source Migration Guidelines" (European Communities, 2003) that provides detailed suggestions on how to approach migration. These include the need for a clear understanding of the reasons to migrate, ensuring that there is active support for the change from IT staff and users, building up expertise and relationships with the open source movement, starting with noncritical systems, and ensuring that each step in the migration is manageable.

Security and Stability. While there is no perfectly secure operating system or platform, factors such as development method, program architecture, and target market can greatly affect the security of a system and consequently make it easier or more difficult to breach. There are some indications that OSS/FS systems are superior to proprietary systems in this respect, and the security aspect has already encouraged many public organizations to switch or to consider switching to OSS/FS solutions. The French Customs and Indirect Taxation authority, for example, migrated to Red Hat Linux largely because of security concerns with proprietary software (International Institute of Infonomics, 2005).

Among reasons often cited for the better security record in OSS/FS is the availability of the source code (making it easier for vulnerabilities to be discovered and fixed). Many OSS/FS have a proactive security focus, so that before features are added the security considerations are accounted for and a feature is added only if it is determined not to compromise system security. In addition, the strong security and permission structure inherent in OSS/FS applications that are based on the Unix model are designed to minimize the possibility of users being able to compromise systems (Wong & Sayo, 2004). OSS/FS systems are well known for their stability and reliability, and many anecdotal stories exist of OSS/FS servers functioning for years without requiring maintenance. However, quantitative studies are more difficult to come by (Wong & Sayo, 2004).

Security of information is vitally important in the health domain, particularly in relation to access, storage, and transmission of patient records. The advocates of OSS/FS suggest that it can provide increased security over proprietary software, and a report to the UK government saw no security disadvantage in the use of OSS/FS products (Peeling & Satchell, 2001). Even the US government's National Security Agency (NSA), according to the same report, supports a number of OSS/FS security-related projects. Stanco (2001) considers that the reason the NSA thinks that free software can be more secure is that when anyone and everyone can inspect source code, hiding backdoors into the code can be very difficult.

In considering a migration to OSS/FS, whether it is for everyday office and productivity uses, or for health-specific applications, there are some commonly encountered challenges that one may face. These challenges have traditionally been seen as including the following:

- There is a relative lack of mature OSS/FS desktop applications.

- Many OSS/FS tools are not user-friendly and have a steep learning curve.

- File sharing between OSS/FS and proprietary applications can be difficult.

As OSS/FS applications have matured in recent years, and the user community grown, many of these challenges have been largely overcome, such that today many OSS/FA applications are indistinguishable from proprietary equivalents for many users in terms of functionality, ease of use, and general user-friendliness.

Choosing the Right Software: The Three-Step Method for OSS/FS Decision-Making. Whether one is working with OSS/FS or commercial/proprietary tools, choosing the right software can be a difficult process, and a thorough review process is needed before making a choice. A simple three-step method for OSS/FS decision-making can guide organizations through the process and works well for all kinds of software, including server, desktop, and Web applications (Surman & Diceman, 2004).

Step 1. **Define the needs and constraints**. Needs must be clearly defined, including those of the organization and of individual users. Other specific issues to consider include range of features, languages, budget (e.g., for training or integration with other systems), the implementation time frame, compatibility with existing systems, and the skills existing within the organization.

Step 2. **Identify the options**. A short list of three to five software packages that are likely to meet the needs can be developed from comparing software packages with the needs and constraints listed in the previous phase. There are numerous sources of information on OSS/FS packages, including recommendations of existing users, reviews, and directories (e.g., OSDir.com and OpenSourceCMS.com.) and software package sites that contain promotional information, documentation, and often demonstration versions that will help with the review process.

Step 3. **Undertake a detailed review**. Once the options have been identified, the final step is to review and choose a software package from the short list. The aim here is to assess which of the possible options will be best for the organization. This assessment can be done by rating each package against a list of criteria, including quality, ease of use, ease of migration, software stability, compatibility with other systems being used, flexibility and customizability, user response, organizational buy-in, evidence of widespread use of the software, and the existence of support mechanisms for the software's use. Hands-on testing is key and each piece of software should be installed and tested for quality, stability, and compatibility, including by a group of key users so as to assess factors such as ease of use, ease of migration, and user response.

Making a Decision. Once the review has been completed, if two packages are close in score, intuition about the right package is probably more important than the actual numbers in reaching a final decision.

Examples of Adoption or Policy Regarding OSS/FS

OSS/FS has moved beyond the closed world of programmers and enthusiasts. Governments around the world have begun to take notice of OSS/FS and have launched initiatives to explore the proposed benefits. There is a significant trend toward incorporating OSS/FS into procurement and development policies, and there are increasing numbers of cases of OSS/FS recognition, explicit policy statements, and procurement decisions. Many countries, regions, and authorities now have existing or proposed laws mandating or encouraging the use of OSS/FS (Wong & Sayo, 2004).

A survey from The MITRE Corporation (2003) showed that the US Department of Defense (DoD) at that time used over 100 different OSS/FS applications. The main conclusion of their study (The MITRE Corporation, 2003) was that OSS/FS software was used in critical roles, including infrastructure support, software development, and research, and that the degree of dependence on OSS/FS for security was unexpected. In 2000, the (US) President's Information Technology Advisory Committee (PITAC, 2000) recommended that the US federal government should encourage OSS/FS use for software development for high-end computing. In 2002, the UK government published a policy (Office of the e-Envoy, 2002), since updated, that it would "consider OSS solutions alongside proprietary ones in IT procurements" (p. 4), "only use products for interoperability that support open standards and specifications in all future IT developments" (p. 4) and explore the possibility of using OSS/FS as the default exploitation route for government-funded research and development (R&D) software. Similar policies have been developed in Denmark, Sweden, and The Netherlands (Wong & Sayo, 2004).

European policy encouraging the exploration and use of OSS/FS has been consequent on the European Commission's *eEurope2005—An Information Society for All* initiative (European Communities, 2004) and its predecessors, such as the i2010 strategy (European Communities, 2005) with their associated action plans. These have encouraged the exchange of experiences and best practice examples so as to promote the use of OSS/FS in the public sector and e-government across the European Commission and member states of the European Union (EU). In addition, the EU has funded R&D on health-related OSS/FS applications as well as encouraged open standards and OSS/FS where appropriate in wider policy initiatives.

In other parts of world, Brazil and Peru are among countries whose governments are actively moving toward OSS/FS solutions, for a variety of reasons, including ensuring long-term access to data through the use of open standards (i.e., not being reliant on proprietary software that may not, in the future, be interoperable) and cost reduction. The South African government has a policy favoring OSS/FS, Japan is considering moving e-government projects to OSS/FS, and pro-OSS/FS initiatives are in operation or being seriously considered in Taiwan, Malaysia, South Korea, and other Asia-Pacific countries.

OPEN SOURCE LICENSING

While OSS/FS is seen by many as a philosophy and a development model, it is also important to consider it a licensing model (Leong, Kaiser, & Miksch, 2007; Sfakianakis et al., 2007). In this section, we can only briefly introduce some of the issues of software licensing as they apply to OSS/FS, and will include definitions of licensing, some of the types of licenses that exist, and how licenses are different from copyright. While we will cover some of the legal concepts, this section cannot take the place of proper legal counsel, which should be sought when reviewing the impact of licenses or contracts. Licensing plays a crucial role in the OSS/FS community, as it is "the operative tool to convey rights and redistribution conditions" (Anderson & Dare 2009, p. 101).

Licensing is defined by Merriam-Webster (2010) as giving the user of something permission to use it; in the case

here, that something is software. Most software comes with some type of licensing, commonly known as the end-user licensing agreement (EULA). The license may have specific restrictions related to the use, modification, or duplication of the software. The Microsoft EULA, for example, specifically prohibits any kind of disassembly, inspection, or reverse engineering of software (Zymaris, 2003). Most licenses also have statements limiting the liability of the software manufacturer toward the user in case of possible problems arising in the use of the software.

From this working definition of licensing, and some examples of what can be found in a EULA, we can examine copyright. While licensing gives a person the right to use software, with restrictions in some cases, copyright is described as the exclusively granted or owned legal right to publish, reproduce, and/or sell a work (Merriam-Webster, 2010). The distinctions between ownership of the original work and rights to use it are important, and there are differences in the way these issues are approached for proprietary software and OSS/FS. For software, the *work* means the source code or statements made in a programming language. In general, the person who creates a work owns the copyright to it and has the right to allow others to copy it or deny that right. In some cases the copyright is owned by a company with software developers working for that company, usually having statements in their employment contracts that assign copyright of their works to the company. In the case of OSS/FS, contributors to a project will often assign copyright to the managers of the project.

While in the case of proprietary software, licensing is generally dealt with in terms of restrictions (i.e., what the user is not allowed to do; for OSS/FS, licensing is seen in terms of permissions, rights, and encouraging users to do things). Most software manufacturing companies hold the copyright for software created by their employees. In financial terms, these works are considered intellectual property, meaning that they have some value. For large software companies, such as Oracle or Microsoft, intellectual property may be a large part of their capital assets. The open source community values software differently, and OSS/FS licenses are designed to facilitate the sharing of software and to prevent an individual or organization from controlling ownership of the software. The individuals who participate in OSS/FS projects generally do realize the monetary value of what they create; however, they feel it is more valuable if the community at large has open access to it and is able to contribute back to the project.

A common misconception is that if a piece of software, or any other product, is made freely available and open to inspection and modification, then the intellectual property rights (IPR) of the originators cannot be protected, and the material cannot be subject to copyright. The open source community, and in particular the FSF, have adopted a number of conventions, some built into the licenses, to protect the IPR of authors and developers. One form of copyright, termed *copyleft* to distinguish it from commercial copyright terms, works by stating that the software is copyrighted and then adding distribution terms. These are a legal instrument giving everyone the rights to use, modify, and redistribute the program's code or any program derived from it but only if the distribution terms are unchanged. The code and the freedoms become legally inseparable, and strengthen the rights of the originators and contributors (Cox, 1999; FSF, 2010c).

Types of OSS/FS Licenses

A large and growing number of OSS/FS licenses exist. Table 5.3 lists some of the more common ones, while fuller lists of various licenses and terms can be found in Wong and Sayo (2004). The OSI Web site currently lists over 60 (www.opensource.org/licenses), while the FSF Web site lists over 40 general public license (GPL)-compatible free software licenses (www.gnu.org/licenses/license-list.html). The two main licenses are the GNU GPL and the Berkeley system distribution (BSD)-style licenses. It is estimated that about 75% of OSS/FS products use the GNU GPL (Wheeler, 2010), and this license is designed to ensure that user freedoms under the license are protected in perpetuity, with users being allowed to do almost anything they want to a GPL program. The conditions of the license primarily affect the user when it is distributed to

another user (Wong & Sayo, 2004). BSD-style licenses are so named because they are identical in spirit to the original license issued by the University of California, Berkeley. These are among the most permissive licenses possible, and essentially permit users to do anything they wish with the software, provided the original licensor is acknowledged by including the original copyright notice in source code files and no attempt is made to sue or hold the original licensor liable for damages (Wong & Sayo, 2004).

Here is an example from the GNU GPL that talks about limitations:

> 16. Limitation of Liability. In no event unless required by applicable law or agreed to in writing will any copyright holder, or any other party who may modify and/or redistribute the program as permitted above, be liable to you for damages, including any general, special, incidental, or consequential damages arising out of the use or inability to use the program (including but not limited to loss of data or data being rendered inaccurate or losses sustained by you or third parties or a failure of the program to operate with any other programs), even if such holder or other party has been advised of the possibility of such damages. (FSF, 2007, para. 16)

Like the Microsoft EULA, there are limitations relating to liability in the use of the software and damage that may be caused, but unlike the Microsoft EULA, the GPL makes it clear what you can do with the software. In general, you can copy and redistribute it, sell or modify it. The restriction is that you must comply with the parts of the

---

TABLE 5.3	Common OSS/FS Licenses

GNU GPL: A free software license and a copyleft license. Recommended by FSF for most software packages (www.gnu.org/licenses/gpl.html).
GNU Lesser General Public License (GNU LGPL): A free software license, but not a strong copyleft license, because it permits linking with nonfree modules (www.gnu.org/copyleft/lesser.html).
Modified BSD License: The original BSD license, modified by removal of the advertising clause. It is a simple, permissive noncopyleft free software license, compatible with the GNU GPL (www.oss-watch.ac.uk/resources/modbsd.xml).
W3C Software Notice and License: A free software license and GPL compatible (www.w3.org/Consortium/Legal/2002/copyright-software-20021231).
MySQL Database License: (www.mysql.com/about/legal).
Apache License, Version 2.0: A simple, permissive noncopyleft free software license that is incompatible with the GNU GPL (www.apache.org/licenses/LICENSE-2.0).
GNU Free Documentation License: A license intended for use on copylefted free documentation. It is also suitable for textbooks and dictionaries, and its applicability is not limited to textual works (e.g., books) (www.gnu.org/copyleft/fdl.html).
Public Domain: Being in the public domain is not a license, but means the material is not copyrighted and no license is needed. Public domain status is compatible with all other licenses, including GNU GPL.

Further information on licenses is available at www.gnu.org/licenses/licenses.html and www.opensource.org/licenses.

license requiring the source code to be distributed as well. One of the primary motivations behind usage of the GPL in OSS/FS is to ensure that once a program is released as OSS/FS, it will remain so permanently. A commercial software company cannot legally modify a GPL program and then sell it under a different proprietary license (Wong & Sayo, 2004).

In relation to using OSS/FS within a healthcare environment, as with use of any software, legal counsel should be consulted to review any license agreement made; however, in general terms, when using OSS/FS there are no obligations that would not apply to using any copyrighted work. Someone cannot legally take a body of work, the source code, and claim it as their own. The licensing terms must be followed as with any other software.

Perhaps the most difficult issue comes when integrating OSS/FS components into a larger infrastructure, especially where it may have to interface with proprietary software. Much has been said about the "viral" nature of the open source license, which comes from the requirement of making source code available if the software is redistributed. Care must be taken that components utilized in creating proprietary software either utilize OSS/FS components in such a way as to facilitate distribution of the code or avoid their use. If the component cannot be made available without all of the source code being made available, then the developer has the choice of not using the component or making the entire application open source. Some projects have created separate licensing schemes to maintain the OSS/FS license and provide those vendors that wish to integrate components without making their product open source. MySQL, a popular open source database server, offers such an option (Table 5.3).

Licensing is a complex issue; we have only touched on some of the points, but in conclusion, the best advice is always to read the license agreement and understand it. In the case of a business decision on software purchase or use, one should always consult legal counsel; however, one should remember that OSS/FS licenses are more about providing freedom than about restricting use.

OSS/FS APPLICATIONS

Many OSS/FS alternatives exist to more commonly known applications. Not all can be covered here, but if one thinks of the common applications that most nurses use on a daily basis, these are likely to include the following:

- Operating system
- Web browser
- E-mail client

- Word processing or integrated office suite
- Presentation tools

For each of these, OSS/FS applications exist. Using OSS/FS does not require an all or nothing approach (Dravis, 2003) and much OSS/FS can be mixed with proprietary software and a gradual migration to OSS/FS is an option for many organizations or individuals. However, when using a mixture of OSS/FS and proprietary or commercial software, incompatibilities can be uncovered and cause problems whose severity must be assessed. Many OSS/FS applications have versions that will run on non-OSS/FS operating systems, so that a change of operating system, for example, to one of the many distributions of Linux, is not necessarily needed. Most OSS/FS operating systems now have graphical interfaces that look very similar to Windows or Apple interfaces.

Operating Systems: GNU/Linux

A GNU/Linux distribution (named in recognition of the GNU Project's significant contribution, but often just called Linux) contains the Linux kernel at its heart and all the OSS/FS components required to produce full operating system functionality. *GNU/Linux* is a term that is increasingly used by many people to cover a distribution of operating systems and other associated software components. However, Linux was originally the name of the kernel created by Linus Torvalds, which has grown from a one-man operation to now having over 200 maintainers representing over 300 organizations.

A kernel is the critical center point of an operating system that controls central processing unit (CPU) usage, memory management, and hardware devices. It also mediates communication between the different programs running within the operating system. The kernel influences performance and the hardware platforms that the OSS/FS system can run on, and the Linux kernel has been ported to run on almost any hardware, from mainframes and supercomputers, through desktop, laptop, and tablet machines, to mobile phones and other mobile devices. The Linux kernel is OSS/FS, licensed under the GNU GPL.

Over time, individuals and companies began distributing Linux with their own choice of OSS/FS packages bound around the Linux kernel; the concept of the *distribution* was born, which contains much more than the kernel (usually only about 0.25% in binary file size of the distribution). There is no single Linux distribution, and many commercial distributions and freely available variants exist, with numerous customized distributions that are targeted to the unique needs of different users (Table 5.4). Although all

TABLE 5.4	Some Common Linux Distributions

Ubuntu: Ubuntu is a Linux-based operating system for desktop, server, netbook, and cloud computing environments. First released in 2004, it is loosely based on Debian OS. Ubuntu now releases updates on a six-month cycle. There are increasing numbers of customized variants of Ubuntu, aimed at, for example, educational use (Edubuntu), professional video and audio editing (Ubuntu Studio), and server editions (www.ubuntu.com).

Debian: Debian GNU/Linux is a free distribution of the Linux-based operating system. It includes a large selection of prepackaged application software, plus advanced package management tools to allow for easy installation and maintenance on individual systems and workstation clusters (www.debian.org).

Mandriva (formerly Mandrakelinux): Available in multiple language versions (including English, Swedish, Spanish, Chinese, Japanese, French, German, Italian, and Russian). Mandrakelinux was first created in 1998 and is designed for ease of use on servers and on home and office systems (www2.mandriva.com).

Red Hat (Enterprise): Red Hat Enterprise Linux is a high-end Linux distribution geared toward businesses with mission-critical needs (www.redhat.com).

Fedora: The Fedora Project was created in late 2003, when Red Hat Linux was discontinued. Fedora is a community distribution (fedoraproject.org).

SuSE: SuSE was first developed in 1992. It is a popular mainstream Linux distribution and is the only Linux recommended by VMware, Microsoft, and SAP (www.suse.com and www.opensuse.org).

KNOPPIX: KNOPPIX is a bootable Live system on CD-ROM or DVD, consisting of a representative collection of GNU/Linux software, automatic hardware detection, and support for many graphics cards, sound cards, and peripheral devices. KNOPPIX can be used for the desktop, educational CD-ROM, as a rescue system, or adapted and used as a platform for commercial software product demos. As it is not necessary to install anything on a hard disk, but can be run entirely from CD-ROM or DVD, it is ideal for demonstrations of Linux (www.knoppix.net or www.knoppix.org).

Centos: The CentOS Linux distribution is a stable, predictable, manageable, and reproducible platform derived from the sources of Red Hat Enterprise Linux (RHEL) (centos.org).

There are many Web sites and organizations that maintain lists of the most used Linux distributions: distrowatch.com/dwres.php?resource=major and en.wikipedia.org/wiki/Comparison_of_Linux_distributions as well as www.linux.com/directory/Distributions.

distributions contain the Linux kernel, some contain only OSS/FS materials, while others additionally contain non-OSS/FS components, and the mix of OSS/FS and other applications included and the configurations supported vary. The Debian GNU/Linux distribution is one of the few distributions that is committed to including only OSS/FS components (as defined by the open source initiative) in its core distribution.

Ubuntu, Linux Mint, and PCLinuxOS are generally viewed as the easiest distributions for new users who wish to simply test or gain a general familiarity with Linux. Slackware Linux, Gentoo Linux, and FreeBSD are distributions that require a degree of expertise and familiarity with Linux if they are to be used effectively and productively. openSUSE, Fedora, Debian GNU/Linux, and Mandriva Linux are mid-range distributions in terms of both complexity and ease of use. Recently, Google has released their version of an open source operating system called Android. It is suited for a wide range of devices from personal computer to mobile device. In particular, there is a smartphone now running Android. There are rumors of tablet computers running Android soon to come to market.

Web Browser and Server: Firefox and Apache

While for most people the focus may be on their client-end use of applications, many rely on other, server-side applications, to function. Web browsing is a prime example where both server and client-side applications are needed. Web servers, such as Apache, are responsible for receiving and fulfilling requests from Web browsers. An OSS/FS application, the Apache HTTP server, developed for Unix, Windows NT, and other platforms, is currently the top Web server with 55% of the market share (over twice that of its next-ranked competitor), and serving 67% of the million busiest Web sites. Apache has dominated the public Internet Web server market ever since it grew to become the number one Web server in 1996 (NetCraft Ltd., 2010; Wheeler, 2007). Apache began development in early 1995 and is an example of an OSS/FS project that is maintained by a formal structure, the Apache Software Foundation.

Firefox (technically Mozilla Firefox) is an OSS/FS graphical Web browser, designed for standards compliance, and with a large number of browser features. It derives from the Mozilla Application Suite, and aims to continue Netscape Communicator as an open project and is maintained by the Mozilla Organization and employees of several other companies, as well as contributors from the community. Firefox source code is OSS/FS, and is tri-licensed, under the Mozilla Public License (MPL), the GNU GPL, and the GNU Lesser General Public License (LGPL), which permit anyone to view, modify, and/or redistribute the source code, and several publicly released applications have been built on it. As of May 2010, Firefox had over 24% worldwide usage share of Web browsers, making it the second most used browser, after Internet Explorer (Netmarketshare, 2010), although reports show higher market shares, up to 30%, in some European countries (AT Internet, 2010).

Word Processing or Integrated Office Suite: Open Office (Office Productivity Suite)

While OSS/FS products have been strong on the server side, OSS/FS desktop applications are relatively new and few. Open Office (strictly OpenOffice.org), which is based on the source code of the formerly proprietary StarOffice, is an OSS/FS equivalent of Microsoft Office, with most of its features. It supports the ISO/IEC standard OpenDocument Format (ODF) for data interchange as its default file format, as well as Microsoft Office formats among others. As of November 2009, Open Office supports over 110 languages. It includes a fully featured word processor, spreadsheet, and presentation software. One of the advantages for considering a shift from a Windows desktop environment to Open Office is that Open Office reads most Microsoft Office documents without problems and will save documents to many formats, including Microsoft Word (but not vice versa). This makes the transition relatively painless and Open Office has been used in recent high-profile switches from Windows to Linux. Open Office has versions that will run on Windows, Linux, and other operating systems. (Note that the text for this chapter was originally written using OpenOffice.org Writer, the word processing package within the OpenOffice.org suite.)

The word *PowerPoint* has become almost synonymous with software for making presentations, and is even commonly used as a teaching tool. The OpenOffice.org suite contains a presentation component, called Impress, which produces presentations very similar to PowerPoint; they can be saved and run in OpenOffice format on Windows or Linux desktop environments, or exported as PowerPoint versions.

Some Other OSS/FS Applications

BIND. The Berkeley Internet Name Domain (BIND) is a domain name system (DNS) server, or in other words, an Internet naming system. Internet addresses, such as www.google.com or www.openoffice.org, would not function without DNS. These servers take these human-friendly names and convert them into computer-friendly numeric Internet protocol (IP) addresses and vice versa. Without these servers, users would have to memorize numbers such as 74.125.19.104 in order to use a Web site, instead of simply typing www.google.com.

The BIND server is an OSS/FS program developed and distributed by the University of California at Berkeley. It is licensed under a BSD-style license by the Internet Software Consortium. It runs 95% of all DNS servers including most of the DNS root servers. These servers hold the master record of all domain names on the Internet.

Perl. Practical Extraction and Reporting Language (Perl) is a high-level programming language that is frequently used for creating common gateway interface (CGI) programs. Started in 1987, and now developed as an OSS/FS project, it was designed for processing text and derives from the C programming language and many other tools and languages. It was originally developed for Unix and is now available for many platforms. Perl modules and add-ons are available to do almost anything, leading some to call it the "Swiss Army chain-saw" of programming languages (Raymond, 2003).

PHP. PHP stands for PHP Hypertext Preprocessor. The name is an example of a recursive acronym (the first word of the acronym is also the acronym), a common practice in the OSS/FS community for naming applications. PHP is a server-side, HTML-embedded scripting language used to quickly create dynamically generated Web pages. In an HTML document, PHP script (similar syntax to that of Perl or C) is enclosed within special PHP tags. PHP can perform any task any CGI program can, but its strength lies in its compatibility with many types of relational databases. PHP runs on every major operating system, including Unix, Linux, Windows, and Mac OS X and can interact with all major Web servers.

GT.M is a database engine with scalability proven in the largest real-time core processing systems in production at financial institutions worldwide, as well as in large, well-known healthcare institutions, but with a small footprint that scales down to use in small clinics, virtual machines, and software appliances. The GT.M data model is an NOSQL hierarchical associative memory (i.e., multidimensional array) that imposes no restrictions on the data types of the indexes and the content—the application logic can impose any schema, dictionary, or data organization suited to its problem domain. GT.M's compiler for the standard M (also known as MUMPS) language is the basis for an open source stack for implementation of the VistA Hospital Information System.

LAMP. The Linux, Apache, MySQL, PHP/Perl/Python (LAMP) architecture has become very popular as a way of affordably deploying reliable, scalable, and secure Web applications (the "P" in LAMP can also stand for either PHP or Perl or Python). MySQL is a multithreaded, multiuser, SQL (Structured Query Language) relational database server, using the GNU GPL. The PHP–MySQL combination is also a cross-platform (i.e., it will run on Windows as well as Linux servers) (Murray & Oyri, 2005).

Content Management Systems. Many OSS/FS applications, especially modern content management systems (CMS) that are the basis of many of today's interactive Web sites, use LAMP. A CMS has a flexible, modular framework that separates the content of a Web site (the text, images, and other content) from the framework of linking the pages together and controlling how the pages appear. In most cases, this is done to make a site easier to maintain than would be the case if it was built exclusively out of flat HTML pages. There are now over 200 OSS/FS FLOSS content management systems (see php.opensourcecms.com for an extensive list) designed for developing portals and Web sites with dynamic, fully searchable content. Drupal (drupal.org), for example, is one of the most well-known and widely used CMS and is currently used for the official site of the White House (www.whitehouse.gov), the United Nations World Food Programme (www.wfp.org), and the South African Government for their official 2010 FIFA World Cup Web site (www.sa2010.gov.za). MyOpenSourcematrix, a CMS designed for large organizations, has been used by the UK's Royal College of Nursing to provide a content and communications portal for its 400,000 members (Squiz UK, 2007).

A CMS can be easily administrated and moderated at several levels by members of an online community, which gives complete control of compliance with the organization's policy for published material and provides for greater interactivity and sense of ownership by online community members. In addition, the workload relating to publication of material and overall maintenance of the Web site can be spread among many members, rather than having only one Web spinner. This secures frequent updates of content and reduces individual workloads, making the likelihood of member participation greater. The initial user registration and redistribution of passwords and access can be carried out automatically by user requests, while assignment to user groups is made manually by the site administrators or moderators.

FLOSS applications are gaining widespread use within education sectors, with one example of a widely used e-learning application being Moodle (www.moodle.org). Moodle is a complete e-learning course management system, or virtual learning environment (VLE), with a modular structure designed to help educators create high-quality, multimedia-based online courses. Moodle is translated into more than 30 languages, and handles thematic or topic-based classes and courses. As Moodle is based in social constructivist pedagogy (moodle.org/doc/?frame=philosophy.html), it also allows the construction of e-learning materials that are based around discussion and interaction, rather than static content (Kaminski, 2005).

OSS/FS HEALTHCARE APPLICATIONS

It is suggested that in healthcare, as in many other areas, the development of OSS/FS may provide much-needed competition to the relatively closed market of commercial, proprietary software (Smith, 2002), and thus encourage innovation. This could lead to lower cost and higher quality systems that are more responsive to changing clinical needs. OSS/FS could also solve many of the problems health information systems (HISs) currently face including lack of interoperability and vendor lock-in, cost, difficulty of record, and system maintenance given the rate of change and size of the information needs of the health domain, and lack of support for security, privacy, and consent. This is because OSS/FS more closely conforms to standards and its source code open to inspection and adaptation. A significant motive for supporting the use of OSS/FS and open standards in healthcare is that interoperability of HISs requires the consistent implementation of open standards (Sfakianakis et al., 2007). Open standards, as described by the International Telecommunications Union (ITU), are made available to the general public and developed, approved, and maintained via a collaborative and consensus-driven process (ITU, 2009; Sfakianakis et al., 2007). A key element of the process is that, by being open, there is less risk of being dominated by any single interest group.

Bowen et al. (2009) summarize a number of advantages that open source software offers when compared with proprietary software, including, but not limited to, the following: (1) ease of modification and or customization, (2) large developer community and its benefits, (3) increased compliance with open standards, (4) enhanced security, (5) increased likelihood of source code availability in the event of the demise of the vendor or company, (6) easier to adapt for use by healthcare students, and (7) flexibility of source code to adapt to research efforts. The cost-effectiveness of open source software also lends well to communities or organizations requiring such an approach (e.g., long-term care facilities, assisted living communities, clinics [public health and educational venue clinics], and home care).

Yellowlees, Marks, Hogarth, and Turner (2008) are among those who suggest that many current EHR systems tend to be expensive, inflexible, difficult to maintain, and rarely interoperable across health systems; this is often due to their being proprietary systems. This makes clinicians reluctant to use them, as they are seen as no better than paper-based systems. OSS/FS has been very successful in other information-intensive industries, and so is seen as having potential to integrate functional EHR systems into, and across, wider health systems. They believe that interoperable open source EHR systems would have the potential to improve healthcare in the United States, and cite examples from other areas around the world.

Currently, there is much interest in interoperability testing of systems, not only between proprietary systems, but also among OSS/FS systems, and between OSS/FS systems and proprietary systems. Integrating the Healthcare Enterprise (IHE) has developed a range of open source interoperability testing tools, called MESA, KUDU, and its next generation tool GAZELLE, to test healthcare interoperability according to the standards profiled by the IHE in its technical frameworks. The Certification Commission for Health Information Technology (CCHIT) has developed an open source program called Laika to test EHR software for compliance with CCHIT (CCHIT, n.d.) interoperability standards.

There are, of course, potential limitations regarding open source EHRs. Technology staff may require education in order to be adept with understanding and supporting open source solutions. Open source efforts are more likely to be underfunded, which impacts not only the ability to upgrade but also support of the software. Another limitation is the perception of open source solutions as the forgotten stepchild of certification (at least in the United States). Only recently (mid-2009) did the CCHIT modify requirements to allow for more than just proprietary EHRs to become certified. Additional barriers include limited interoperability, fuzzy ROI, slower uptake by users than proprietary software, personnel resistance to this change, and, as previously alluded, IT employees unfamiliar with open source software. Other barriers to use of OSS/FS for implementation of EHRs or health information systems (HISs) have been identified, including resistance to change among users and IT departments, lack of documentation associated with some OSS/FS projects, and language barriers in some countries, in particular due to the documentation around many OSS/FS developments being in

English, without translation (Bagayoko, Dufour, Chaacho, Bouhaddou, & Fieschi, 2010).

In the case study, we will look at one project, probably the largest, most sophisticated, and furthest developed—VistA. Here we will provide a brief overview of examples of some of the other projects currently existing, some of which have been in development for over 15 years. Many share commonalities in trying to develop components of EHRs and several have online demonstration versions available for exploration. A useful summary of the known projects and products has been provided by the AMIA-OSWG (Valdes, 2008), while a number of Web sites provide catalogues of known OSS/FS developments in health (www.medfloss.org).

Examples exist of OSS/FS electronic medical records (EMRs), hospital management systems, laboratory information systems, radiology information systems, telemedicine systems, picture archiving and communications systems, and practice management systems (Janamanchi, Katsamakas, Raghupathi, & Gao, 2009). A few examples indicate this range, and more extensive lists and descriptions are available at several Web portals, including www.medfloss.org.

ClearHealth

(www.clear-health.com)

ClearHealth is a Web-based, fully comprehensive medical suite offering a wide range of tools to practices of all sizes. It includes scheduling and registration features; EMR including alerts, patient dashboard, laboratory ordering and results, and barcode generation and uses; SNOMED; access via mobile devices; billing and reporting features; and specialist clinical modules (Goulde & Brown, 2006).

Indivo

(indivohealth.org)

Indivo is the original personal health platform, enabling an individual to own and manage a complete, secure, digital copy of her health and wellness information. Indivo integrates health information across sites of care and over time. Indivo is free and open source, uses open, unencumbered standards, including those from the SMART Platforms project and is actively deployed in diverse settings. Indivo is an OSS/FS personally controlled health record (PCHR) system, using open standards. A PCHR enables individuals to own and manage a complete, secure, digital copy of their health and wellness information. Indivo integrates health information across sites of care and over time, and is actively deployed in diverse settings, for example, in the

Boston Children's Hospital and the Dossia Consortium (Bourgeois, Mandl, Shaw, Flemming, & Nigrin, 2009; Mandl, Simons, Crawford, & Abbett, 2007).

SMART Platforms Project

(smartplatforms.org)

The SMART Platforms project is an open source, developer-friendly application programming interface and its extensible medical data representation and standards-based clinical vocabularies. SMART allows healthcare clients to make their own customizations, and these apps can then be licensed to run across the installed base.

As of 2014, SMART works with Cerner Millennium at Boston Children's Hospital, running the SMART app BP Centiles, with i2b2 (a clinical discovery system used at over 75 US academic hospitals), with Indivo (an advanced personally controlled health record system), with Mirth Results (a clinical data repository system for HIEs), with OpenMRS (a common framework for medical informatics efforts in developing countries), with Think!Med Clinical (an openEHR-based clinical information system), and with WorldVistA (an open source EMR based on the US Department of Veterans Affairs VistA system).

GNUMed

(gnumed.de)

The GNUmed project builds free, liberated open source EMR software in multiple languages to assist and improve longitudinal care (specifically in ambulatory settings, i.e., multiprofessional practices and clinics). It is made available at no charge and is capable of running on GNU/Linux, Windows, and Mac OS X. It is developed by a handful of medical doctors and programmers from all over the world.

OpenMRS

(openmrs.org)

OpenMRS® is a community-developed, open source enterprise EMR system platform (Wolfe et al., 2006). Of particular interest to this project is supporting efforts to actively build and/or manage health systems in the developing world to address AIDS, tuberculosis, and malaria, which afflict the lives of millions. Their mission is to foster self-sustaining health IT implementations in these environments through peer mentorship, proactive collaboration, and a code base equaling or surpassing any proprietary equivalent. OpenMRS is a multi-institution, nonprofit collaborative led by Regenstrief Institute, Inc.

(www.regenstrief.org) and Partners In Health (pih.org), and has been implemented in 20 countries throughout the world ranging from South Africa and Kenya to Haiti, India, and China, as well as in the United States. This effort is supported in part by organizations such as the World Health Organization (WHO), the Centers for Disease Control and Prevention (CDC), The Rockefeller Foundation, and the President's Emergency Plan for AIDS Relief (PEPFAR).

District Health Information System

(sourceforge.net/projects/dhis/)

The District Health Information System (DHIS) provides for data entry, report generation, and analysis. It is part of a larger initiative for healthcare data in developing countries, called the Health Information System Programme (HISP).

OpenEHR

(www.openehr.org)

The openEHR Foundation is an international, not-for-profit organization working toward the development of interoperable, lifelong EHRs. However, it is also looking to reconceptualize the problems of health records, not in narrow IT-implementation terms, but through an understanding of the social, clinical, and technical challenges of electronic records for healthcare in the information society. The openEHR Foundation was created to enable the development of open specifications, software, and knowledge resources for HISs, in particular EHR systems. It publishes all its specifications and builds reference implementations as OSS/FS. It also develops archetypes and a terminology for use with EHRs.

Tolven

(www.tolvenhealth.com)

Tolven is developing a range of electronic personal and clinician health record applications, using open source software and health industry standards, including Unified Medical Language Systems and Health Level 7.

European Projects and Initiatives

The European Union (EU) has funded research and development programs through the European Commission. There have been many projects and initiatives to explore and promote the use of OSS/FS within EU member states and organizations. While many of the earlier initiatives were projects whose outputs were not further developed, or are no longer available, several of them laid the basis for current initiatives, such as the Open Source Observatory and Repository Portal (www.osor.eu). Among the early EU projects are the following:

- SMARTIE sought to offer a comprehensive collection, or suite, of selected medical software decision tools, ranging from clinical calculators (i.e., risk factor scoring) up to advanced medical decision support tools (i.e., acute abdominal pain diagnosis).

- openECG sought to consolidate interoperability efforts in computerized electrocardiography at the European and international levels, encouraging the use of standards. The project aimed to promote the consistent use of format and communications standards for computerized ECGs and to pave the way toward developing similar standards for stress ECG, Holter ECG, and real-time monitoring. The openECG portal still provides information on interoperability in digital electrocardiography, and one of the project's outputs, the Standard Communications Protocol for Computer-Assisted Electrocardiography (SCP-ECG), was approved as an ISO standard, ISO/DIS 11073-91064.

- Open source medical image analysis (OSMIA) at www.tina-vision.net/projects/osmia.php was designed to provide an OSS/FS development environment for medical image analysis research in order to facilitate the free and open exchange of ideas and techniques.

- PICNIC from Minoru Development was designed to help regional healthcare providers to develop and implement the next generation of secure, user-friendly regional healthcare networks to support new ways of providing health and social care.

- Free/Libre/Open Source Software: Policy Support (FLOSSpols) (www.flosspols.org) aims to work on three specific tracks: government policy toward OSS/FS; gender issues in open source; and the efficiency of open source as a system for collaborative problem solving; however, it should be noted that many of these are R&D projects only and not guaranteed to have any lasting effect or uptake beyond the lifespan of the project.

- The Open Source Observatory and Repository for European public administrations (www.osor.eu) is a major portal that supports and encourages the collaborative development and reuse of publicly financed free, libre, and open source software (FLOSS) applications developments for use in European public administrations. It is a platform for exchanging information, experiences, and FLOSS-based code. It also promotes and links to the work of national repositories, encouraging the emergence of a pan-European federation of open source software repositories. OSOR.eu is financed by the European Commission through the initiative Interoperable Delivery of European eGovernment Services to Public Administrations, Businesses and Citizens (IDABC) and is supported by European governments at national, regional, and local levels.

- OSOR.eu indexes and describes a number of health-related initiatives, some directly related to providing healthcare and others with lessons that might be applicable across a number of sectors, including healthcare. Among the health-specific initiatives listed are the following:

  o Health Atlas Ireland (www.hse.ie/eng/about/ Who/clinical/Health_Intelligence/About_us/): An OSS/FS application using geographical information systems (GIS), health-related data sets, and statistical software. It received the Irish Prime Minister Public Service Excellence Award because of its capacity to innovate and to improve the quality and the efficiency health services. Health Atlas Ireland is an open source application developed to use a Web environment to add value to existing health data; it also enables controlled access to maps, data, and analyses for service planning and delivery, major incident response, epidemiology, and research to improve the health of patients and the population.

Many hospitals and healthcare institutions in the EU are increasing their use of open source software (OSOR.eu, n.d.). The University Hospital of Clermont Ferrand began using OSS/FS to consolidate data from multiple computer systems in order to improve its invoicing. The Centre Hospitalier Universitaire Tivoli in Louvière, Belgium, in 2006 estimated that about 25% of its software was OSS/FS, including enterprise resource planning (ERP) software, e-mail applications, VPN software openVPN, and the K-Pacs OSS/FS DICOM viewing software. Additionally, many hospitals are moving their Web sites and portals to OSS/FS content management systems, such as Drupal. The St. Antonius hospital in the cities of Utrecht and Nieuwegein (The Netherlands) is migrating to an almost completely OSS/FS IT environment, with 3000 desktops running Ubuntu GNU/Linux, and using OpenOffice for office productivity tools. Growing numbers of examples of the use of OSS/FS for developing hospital and HISs exist, especially in developing countries.

ORGANIZATIONS AND RESOURCES

Over the past 10 years a number of organizations have sought to explore and, where appropriate, advocate the use of OSS/FS within health, healthcare, and nursing. While some of these are still active, others have struggled to maintain activity due to having to rely primarily on voluntary efforts, which can be difficult to sustain over long periods. As a result, current efforts in promoting and publicizing OSS/FS seem to be based around looser collaborations and less formal groups, often working on developing and maintaining information resources. The American Medical Informatics Association (AMIA), International Medical Informatics Association (IMIA), and the European Federation for Medical Informatics (EFMI) all have working groups dealing with OSS/FS who develop position papers, contribute workshops and other activities to conferences, and undertake a variety of other promotional activities. Each of these groups have nurses actively involved.

National (in all countries) and international health informatics organizations seem to be late in realizing the need to consider the potential impact of OSS/FS. The IMIA established an Open Source Health Informatics Working Group in 2002. It aims to work both within IMIA and through encouraging joint work with other OSS/FS organizations to explore issues around the use of OSS/FS within healthcare and health informatics. The mission of the AMIA-OSWG (www.amia.org/working-group/open-source) is to act as the primary conduit between AMIA and the wider open source community. Its specific activities include providing information regarding the benefits and pitfalls of OSS/FS to other AMIA working groups, identifying useful open source projects, and identifying funding sources, and providing grant application support to open source projects. The AMIA-OSWG produced a White Paper in late 2008 that not only addressed and summarized many of the issues on definitions and licensing addressed in this chapter but also provided a list of the major OSS/FS electronic health and medical record systems in use, primarily in the United States, at the time (Valdes, 2008). The AMIA-OSWG identified 12 systems, in use in over 2500 federal government and almost 900 non-federal government sites, which among them held over 32 million individual patient records (Samuel & Sujansky, 2008; Valdes, 2008).

The IMIA-OSWG, in collaboration with several other organizations, including the AMIA-OSWG, organized a series of think-tank meetings in 2004, in Winchester, UK, and San Francisco, USA. The main purpose of these events was to "identify key issues, opportunities, obstacles, areas of work and research that may be needed, and other relevant aspects, around the potential for using open source software, solutions and approaches within healthcare, and in particular within health informatics, in the UK and Europe" (Murray, 2004, p. 4). Three-quarters of attendees at the first event (UK, February 2004) described their ideal vision for the future use of software in healthcare as containing at least a significant percentage of OSS/FS with nearly one-third of the attendees wanting to see an "entirely open source" use of software in healthcare. Similar findings arose from the US meeting of September 2004, which had broader international participation. The emergence of a situation wherein OSS/FS would interface with proprietary software within the healthcare domain was seen to be achievable and desirable. Such use was also likely if the right drivers were put in place and barriers addressed. Participants felt the strongest drivers included the following:

- Adoption and use of the right standards
- The development of a FLOSS "killer application"
- A political mandate toward the use of FLOSS
- Producing positive case studies comparing financial benefits of FLOSS budget reductions

Participants rated the most important issues why people might use or do use FLOSS within the health domain as quality, stability, and robustness of software and data as well as long-term availability of important health data because of not being "locked up" in proprietary systems that limit interoperability and data migration. They felt the two most important areas for FLOSS activity by IMIA-OSWG and other FLOSS groups were political activity and efforts toward raising awareness among healthcare workers and the wider public. There was a feeling, especially from the US meeting, that lack of interaction between OSS/FS groups was a barrier to adoption in healthcare.

Discussions at meetings in 2008 and 2009, and in particular at the Special Topic Conference of the European Federation for Medical Informatics (EFMI) held in London in September 2008, and at the Medical Informatics Europe (MIE) 2009 conference held in Sarajevo, Bosnia and Herzegovina, reflected back on progress made since 2004 (Murray et al., 2009). It was concluded that many of the issues identified in 2004 remained relevant, and while some progress had been made in raising awareness within health and nursing communities of the possibilities of OSS/FS, the same issues were still relevant.

To date, few nursing or NI organizations have sought to address the implications of OSS/FS from a nursing-focused perspective. The first nursing or NI organization to establish a group dealing with OSS/FS issues was the

Special Interest Group in Nursing Informatics of IMIA (IMIA/NI-SIG). Established in June 2003, the IMIA-NI Open Source Nursing Informatics (OSNI) Working Group has many aims congruent with those of the IMIA-OSWG, but with a focus on identifying and addressing nursing-specific issues and providing a nursing contribution within multiprofessional or multidisciplinary domains. However, it has been difficult to maintain specific nursing-focused

activity and many members now work within other groups to provide nursing input.

Among providers of resources (see Table 5.5), the Medical Free/Libre and Open Source Software Web site (www.medfloss.org) provides a comprehensive and structured overview of OSS/FS projects for the healthcare domain; it also offers an open content platform to foster the exchange of ideas, knowledge, and experiences about projects.

| **TABLE 5.5** | Selected Information and Resource Web Sites |

Linux Medical News: The leading news resource for health and medical applications of OSS/FS. The site provides information on events, conferences and activities, software development, and any other issues that contributors feel are relevant to the use of OSS/FS in healthcare (www.linuxmednews.com).

Medical Free/Libre and Open Source Software: A comprehensive and structured overview of Free/Libre and Open Source Software (FLOSS) projects for the healthcare domain. The Web-based resource also offers an open content platform to foster the exchange of ideas, knowledge, and experiences about the projects (www.medfloss.org).

SourceForge: SourceForge is the largest repository and development site for open source software. Many healthcare applications and other OSS/FS applications use it as the official repository of their latest versions (sourceforge.net).

Free and Open Source Software (FOSS) for Health Web Portal: The FOSS for Health Web portal aims to be a dynamic, evolving repository and venue for interaction, sharing, and supporting those who are interested in using OSS/FS in health and e-Health. It is part of the Open Source and Standards PCTA (PANACeA Common Thematic Activities) of the PAN Asian Collaboration for Evidence-based eHealth Adoption and Application (PANACeA) (www.foss-for-health.org/portal).

FOSS Primers: The IOSN is producing a series of primers on FOSS. The primers serve as introductory documents to FOSS in general, as well as covering particular topic areas in greater detail. Their purpose is to raise FOSS awareness, particularly among policy-makers, practitioners, and educators. The following Web site contains summaries of the primers that have been published or are currently being produced (www.iosn.net/publications/foss-primers).

OSS Watch: OSS Watch is an advisory service that provides unbiased advice and guidance on the use, development, and licensing of free and open source software. OSS Watch is funded by the JISC and its services are available free-of-charge for higher and further education within the United Kingdom (www.oss-watch.ac.uk).

The Open Source Observatory and Repository (OSOR): OSOR is a platform for exchanging information, experiences, and FLOSS-based code for use in public administrations (www.osor.eu).

FOSS Open Standards/Government National Open Standards Policies and Initiatives: Many governments all over the world have developed policies and/or initiatives that advocate and favor open source and open standards in order to bring about increased independence from specific vendors and technologies, and at the same time accommodate both FOSS and proprietary software (en.wikibooks.org/wiki/FOSS_Open_Standards/Government_National_Open_Standards_Policies_and_Initiatives).

Free and Open Source Software Portal: A gateway to resources related to free software and the open source technology movement (UNESCO, www.unesco.org/new/en/communication-and-information/access-to-knowledge/free-and-open-source-software-foss).

The Top 100 Open Source Software Tools for Medical Professionals: www.ondd.org/the-top-100-open-source-software-tools-for-medical-professionals

Open Source Methods, Tools, and Applications; Open Source Downloads: www.openclinical.org/opensourceDLD.html

Medsphere OpenVista Project: sourceforge.net/projects/openvista

Open Source Software for Public Health: www.ibiblio.org/pjones/wiki/index.php/Open_Source_Software_for_Public_Health

Clearhealth: www.clear-health.com

VistA Resources

VistA Monograph: www.ehealth.va.gov/VistA_Monograph.asp

VistA CPRS Demo: www.ehealth.va.gov/EHEALTH/CPRS_demo.asp

VistA eHealth: www.ehealth.va.gov/EHEALTH/index.asp

VistA Documentation Library: www.va.gov/vdl

Latest Version of WorldVistA: worldvista.org/Software_Download

A Description of the Historical Development of VistA: VistA Monograph, www.ehealth.va.gov/VistA_Monograph.asp; WorldVista, worldvista.org/AboutVistA/VistA_History; Hardhats, www.hardhats.org/history/HSTmain.html

VistApedia—A Wiki about VistA: (vistapedia.net)

The International Open Source Network (IOSN, www. iosn.net), funded by the United Nations Development Programme (UNDP), is a center of excellence for OSS/ FS in the Asia-Pacific region. It is tasked specifically with facilitating and networking OSS/FS advocates in the region, so developing countries in the region can achieve rapid and sustained economic and social development by using affordable, yet effective, OSS/FS solutions to bridge the digital divide. While its work and case studies have a focus on developing countries, and especially those of the Asia-Pacific region, the materials they produce are of wider value. In particular, they publish a series of free and open source software (FOSS) primers, which serve as introductory documents to OSS/FS in general as well as covering particular topic areas in greater detail. Their purpose is to raise FLOSS awareness, particularly among policy-makers, practitioners, and educators. While there is not currently a health offering, the general lessons from the primers on education, open standards, OSS/FS licensing and the general introductory primer to OSS/FS are useful materials for anyone wishing to explore the issues in greater detail (IOSN, n.d.).

Open Health Tools (www.openhealthtools.org) is an open source community, with members including national health agencies from several countries, medical standards organizations, and software product and service companies. Its vision is of enabling a ubiquitous ecosystem where members of the health and informatics professions can collaborate to build interoperable systems.

SUMMARY

OSS/FS has been described as a disruptive paradigm, but one that has the potential to improve not only the delivery of care but also healthcare outcomes (Bagayoko et al., 2010). This chapter provides a necessarily brief introduction to OSS/FS. While we have tried to explain the underlying philosophies of the two major camps, only an in-depth reading of the explanations emanating from each can help to clarify the differences.

Many of the issues we have addressed are in a state of flux, therefore we cannot give definitive answers or solutions to many of them, as debate and understanding will have moved on. As we have already indicated, detailed exploration of licensing issues is best addressed with the aid of legal counsel. Readers wishing to develop a further understanding of OSS/FS are recommended to read the International Open Source Network's (IOSN) FOSS Primer (Wong & Sayo, 2004). Additional resources are identified in Table 5.5.

CASE STUDY 5.1: VistA (VETERANS HEALTH INFORMATION SYSTEM AND TECHNOLOGY ARCHITECTURE)

This case study focuses on the long-standing HIS of the US Department of Veterans Affairs (VA). As outlined above, VistA is an acronym for Veterans Health Information Systems and Technology Architecture (Tiemann, 2004b). Started in the early 1980s with efforts at electronic record keeping via the Decentralized Hospital Computer Program (DHCP) information system, the US Veterans Health Administration (2010), disseminated this system countrywide by the early 1990s. The name *VistA* dates back to 1996, when the project previously known as the DHCP was renamed to VistA (VistA Monograph [US Department of Veteran Affairs, 2008; WorldVistA, n.d.], www.ehealth. va.gov/VistA_Monograph.asp, WorldVista, worldvista. org/AboutVistA/VistA_History, Hardhats, www.hard hats.org/history/HSTmain.html).

VistA is widely believed to be the largest integrated HIS in the world. Because VistA was originally developed and maintained by the US Department of VA for use in veterans' hospitals it is public domain. Its development was based on the systems software architecture and implementation methodology developed by the US Public Health Service jointly with the National Bureau of Standards. VistA is in production today at hundreds of healthcare facilities across the country, from small outpatient clinics to large medical centers. It is currently used by all VA facilities throughout countries where there is a US military presence, as well as in nonmilitary clinics with both military and civilian focuses.

VistA itself is not strictly open source or free software, but because of its origin as government developed software, it was released to, and remains in, the public domain. Because of this free availability it has been promoted by many OSS/FS organizations and individuals with some suggesting it is the "mother of OSS/FS healthcare applications" (Tiemann, 2004b).

Over the years VistA has demonstrated its flexibility by supporting a wide variety of clinical settings and medical delivery systems inside and outside of facilities ranging from small outpatient-oriented clinics to large medical centers with significant inpatient populations and associated specialties, such as surgical care or dermatology. Hospitals and clinics in many countries depend on it to manage such things as patient records, prescriptions, laboratory results, and other medical information. It contains, among other components, integrated hospital management, patient records management, medication administration (via barcoding), and medical imaging systems.

There are many versions of the VistA system in use in the US Department of Defense Military Health System as the Composite Health Care System (CHCS), the US Department of Interior's Indian Health Service as the Resource and Patient Management System (RPMS), and internationally, including, for example, the Berlin Heart Institute of Germany (Deutsches Herzzentrum Berlin, Deutschland), and National Cancer Institute of Cairo University in Egypt. It is also used by Oroville Hospital in California and at Central Region Hospital of the North Carolina Department of Health and Human Services.

The use of VistA helps demonstrate some of the proposed benefits of OSS/FS. The costs associated with the acquisition and support of an HIS can indirectly affect the quality of healthcare provided by limiting the availability of timely and accurate access to electronic patient records. One solution is to lower the cost of acquiring an HIS by using a software stack consisting of open source, free software (OSS/FS). Since VistA is in the public domain and available through the US Freedom of Information Act (FOIA), software license fees are not an issue with regard to deployment.

Several OSS/FS organizations associated with, and deriving from, VistA are WorldVistA (worldvista.org), Medsphere OpenVista (medsphere.com), DSS vxVistA (www.dssinc.com/dss-vxOpenSource.html), the Open Source Electronic Health Record Software Alliance (osehra.org), and the VISTA Expertise Network (www. vistaexpertise.net).

WorldVistA was formed as a US-based nonprofit organization committed to the continued development and deployment of VistA. It aims to develop and support the global VistA community, through helping to make healthcare IT more affordable and more widely available, both within the United States and internationally. WorldVistA extends and improves VistA for use outside its original setting through such activities as developing packages for pediatrics, obstetrics, and other hospital services not used in veterans' hospitals. WorldVistA also helps those who choose to adopt VistA to learn, install, and maintain the software. WorldVistA advises adopters of VistA, but does not implement VistA for adopters. Other organizations do provide these services.

Historically, running VistA has required adopters to pay licensing fees for the systems on which it runs: the programming environment (Massachusetts General Hospital Utility Multi-Programming System [MUMPS]) and the operating system underneath (such as Microsoft Windows or Linux or VMS). WorldVistA eliminated these fees by allowing VistA to run on the GT.M programming environment and the Linux operating system, which are both open source and free. By reducing licensing costs, users may spend their money on medicine, medical professionals, and other resources more likely to directly improve patient care. The WorldVistA project effort also transfers knowledge and expertise and builds long-term relationships between adopters and the rest of the worldwide VistA community.

The complete WorldVistA package comprises the following:

- GNU/Linux operating system GT.M, an implementation of the Standard M programming system (M = MUMPS)VistA.

- Information on VistA, and WorldVistA and software downloads are available at a number of Web sites, including the following:
  - www.va.gov/vdl/—VistA Documentation Library
  - www1.va.gov/vista_monograph/—VistA Monograph
  - sourceforge.net/projects/worldvista/—latest versions of WorldVistA software
  - www.vistapedia.net—community and user-created documentation about VistA.

A description of the historical development of VistA is available at worldvista.org/AboutVistA/VistA_History. A demonstration of VistA as a Web-based application is also available to try out. It is an installable package for Windows OS computers found at www.ehealth.va.gov/EHEALTH/CPRS_demo.asp. Once installed, the application links to a demonstration server hosted by VA Information Services, thereby allowing the user to enter and retrieve data without risk.

The sharing of veterans' health information between the US Department of Defence (DoD) and the VA has been a continuing effort since the initial installation of the DoD's CHCS in the 1980s. A Directorate (VA/DoD Health Information Sharing Directorate) administers this effort between both of the agencies regarding interoperability along with other initiatives related to IT, healthcare, and data sharing. Efforts coordinated and supported by this intermediary organization currently include bidirectional health information interoperability exchange (BHIE), clinical and health information repository efforts (Clinical Data Repository/Health Data Repository [CHDR]) initiated in 2006, transition of active personnel to veteran status via the Federal Health Information Exchange (FHIE) initiative between the DoD and the VA, laboratory data sharing (Laboratory Data Sharing Interoperability [LDSI]) not only between the DoD and the VA but also among commercial laboratory vendors, and increased quality of care for polytrauma patients due to data exchange. The Directorate also coordinates report generation for the VA, the DoD, and the Office of Management and Budget (OMB). In April 2010, the VA and DoD expanded their Virtual Lifetime Electronic Record (VLER) program to exchange more types of clinical data. In 2013, the iEHR effort between the VA and DoD was initiated by Congress to promote sharing between the agencies.

The VA also provides Web access for its veterans through VistA. These include the HealthyVet project, which provides 24 × 7 Web-based access to VA health services and information, and the Compensation and Pension Records Interchange (CAPRI) which enables veterans service organizations (VSOs) to view only a member's EHR if necessary to assist the individual with benefit claims and drug refills.

Future Direction of VistA

The VistA software is constantly being updated with current technologies and enhancements as the practice of medicine changes. New ways of accessing VistA using data and programming languages are always changing. Of great importance is the current shift to an open source, open standards environment along with development efforts to support and advance VistA.

CASE STUDY 5.2: ORGANIZING DATA IN A HEALTH DATABASE

A database is a part of the computer software that performs the function of a paper record's filing room. In paper files, the information about a patient are stored using standard forms, and in notes. In a health database, a similar model is used.

In the place of a paper form, a database will have records. In the place of questions that may be answered on the form, the database records will have fields. Just as a patient's paper records may have multiple forms that specify standard information, the computer database may have multiple kinds of records that are all tied together with a common reference to a particular patient.

A common way to visualize the various information about a health record is to think of it as a spreadsheet, whether one on paper or on a computer. This model has columns for different kinds of information that may be stored usually with a description at the top of the column. Each successive row or entry in the spreadsheet corresponds to information about a particular event or person.

The database model identifies the various forms in the paper record with various kinds of spreadsheets. These spreadsheets are called Tables in SQL and Files in VistA FileMan. The questions of each kind of paper form are identified with the descriptions at the top of the columns in the spreadsheet. The various rows of the spreadsheet correspond to people, and the answers put into the form are the cells where the rows and columns intersect.

This row and column organization is easy to visualize and corresponds to the simple database model of SQL. VistA FileMan builds upon this simple model by allowing cells to be further subdivided into sub-columns and sub rows. The cells inside these sub-spreadsheets can be further subdivided if needed to accurately reflect the organization of the data. VistA FileMan includes the simple model of SQL, but enhances it to allow more complex medical data to be stored in a more natural way.

Medical Data normally has a many to one and relational nature. Any given patient might have multiple appointments, with each appointment having multiple diagnoses. An appointment for a patient would have a single start time for a particular clinic and a particular clinician. Viewed from the perspective of the clinic, it might have multiple appointments occurring at the same time, with multiple clinicians involved. There may be multiple diagnoses for a particular patient and date time interval, but they would all be from a standard list of diagnoses. Each diagnosis may have multiple treatment options, including particular medications and procedures performed.

Datatypes for Fields

Just as an electronic spreadsheet may have a format for each of the cells, a database will have requirements for what can be stored in the database elements. Usually this kind of information is called the datatype of the element. Generally SQL datatypes are described with a word like INTEGER or TIMESTAMP. VistA FileMan datatypes are described as FREE TEXT or NUMERIC or SET OF CODES. Each of these datatypes correspond to some restrictions because it makes the organization of the database more predictable and efficient. When information that is put into a database has no limits, such as when typing Progress Notes or Discharge Summaries, there are usually very few ways to organize it.

Indexes and Cross-References

To help find particular entries (or rows) in a database record, it is common to index part of the entry in a special cross-reference where some fields (or columns) are stored in a sorted order. When retrieving the record, the database will be searched along this cross-reference for the indexed information, and group together all the records which have the same index. When paper records are stored, the tabs on a folder provide the same function. When a field is cross-referenced, the information can be retrieved faster, and any print processes using that field will work faster.

EXAMPLE DATABASE

Let us use a simple database that has several fields in each PATIENT record. This example database purposely does not have the relational aspects of a true health database as these complicate things, while gaining little in making the process of creating an example report which might have a software license.

The name of the Table in SQL and the name of the File in VistA FileMan for our example database would be simply PATIENT.

The first field named PATNAME has a datatype as a VARCHAR(60) in SQL or a FREETEXT field in VistA FileMan. This field would hold the name of the patient, with no extra padding. The PATNAME field will be indexed.

The second field named DATEOFBIRTH has a datatype of DATE in SQL or DATE/TIME in VistA FileMan. This field will hold the day that the patient was born.

The third field will be AGE which has a datatype of SMALLINT in SQL or NUMBER in VistA FileMan. In SQL, the datatype always has the same lower bound such as between 0 and 255, whereas in VistA FileMan, the number range is defined specifically for each field, such as from 0 to 120. This field will hold the number of years since the patient was born. In VistA FileMan, this field normally will be a COMPUTED field.

The fourth field named GENDER would be a CHARACTER value of 'M' or 'F' or 'U' in SQL, and be a SET OF CODES in VistA FileMan using a mapping of 'M' to MALE, 'F' to FEMALE, and 'U' to UNKNOWN.

Comparison Operations Form Simple Conditions

Each datatype has particular ways of comparing values. How you compare values depends upon what is needed for a particular report. A value may be the name of a field such as AGE or PATIENT NAME from our example database. A value might be a constant like 70 or "SMITH". Comparison operators use two or more values together to produce a Condition. Conditions can be used to include or to filter out rows or entries from the database, again, depending on what the report needs.

A numeric datatype will have operators that allow one to test if the field is larger or smaller than another field or a particular number. A listing of some numeric comparison operators is listed in Table 5.6 for an example. All of these comparison operators do not work on all system. You must test them on the software system you are using to see which apply.

A character-based datatype might be a VARCHAR or a CHARACTER or a MEMO field in SQL. The FREE TEXT datatype or the SET OF CODES datatype in VistA FileMan is also a character-based datatype. Character datatypes will have operators that look for particular text. The CONTAINS operator is to check if a particular field has some text within it. The LIKE operator and the MATCHES operator both look for patterns, such as wildcards in text or unchanging text in a particular order.

TABLE 5.6	(Case Study 5.2) Numeric Comparison Operators Combining to Make Condition
FirstValue > SecondValue	Condition where first value is greater than second value
FirstValue < SecondValue	Condition where first value is less than second value
FirstValue = SecondValue	Condition where first value is equal to second value
FirstValue <> SecondValue	Condition where first value is not equal to second value
FirstValue != SecondValue	Condition where first value is not equal to second value
FirstValue '= SecondValue	Condition where first value is not equal to second value
FirstValue <= SecondValue	Condition where first value is less than or equal to second value
FirstValue !> SecondValue	Condition where first value is less than or equal to second value
FirstValue '> SecondValue	Condition where first value is less than or equal to second value
FirstValue >= SecondValue	Condition where first value is greater than or equal to second value
FirstValue !< SecondValue	Condition where first value is greater than or equal to second value
FirstValue '< SecondValue	Condition where first value is greater than or equal to second value
BETWEEN (FirstValue, SecondValue, ThirdValue)	Condition where the first value is less than the second value and the second value is less than the third value

Most datatypes allow the NULL operator to be used to check if a field is empty.

Boolean Operators Make Complex Conditions

Finally, these conditions can then be combined together using Boolean logic to make a more complex Condition. This logic allows a report writer enough flexibility to include and exclude conditions made up of more than one field and value.

Boolean Logic is named after George Boole who worked on it in the 1800s. He started with just two values, such as TRUE and FALSE, and showed a logical system that combined them together in all 16 possible ways. Later in the century, Charles Pierce was able to prove that using only one of the ways, either using NAND or NOR, comprised a sole sufficient operator. Electronic engineers took advantage of this to simplify the process of creating computer circuits.

If there are two conditions, there are 16 ways to combine them together. With three conditions, there are 32 ways to do so. As you add more conditions, the number of possible ways double each time. This is why some people feel Boolean Logic can be so complex. The following discussion will try to make this simpler.

The two simplest ways to combine values together is to ignore the conditions completely and always produce the same answer. Since there are two possible answers, one operator named Contradiction always gives the value of FALSE, and the other named Tautology always gives the value of TRUE. No one purposely will use these operators, but may accidentally do so. The most common way to use the Contradiction Operator is when you use two conditions, each using a comparison operator, but no value can satisfy both of the comparisons at the same time. Such as checking for a field value like greater than 70 and less than 10 or getting the order wrong on BETWEEN so you test if it is greater than your highest value and lower than your lowest value. Similarly the Tautology Operator may be accidentally used if you look for Conditions that are always TRUE. Some of the ways to combine Conditions can do this and produce a useless search because nothing is excluded from your search, or everything is included.

The AND operator is used when you have a list of conditions that must all be TRUE to include an entry or row. Usually each of the conditions will test different fields, such as testing GENDER = 'M' and at the same time looking for AGE > 70. Since AND requires that both of these succeed for the same entry, it effectively filters out any entries where it fails. You can combine multiple conditions together with AND to create easily understandable search conditions that are targeting very specific subsets of the database.

The OR operator is used when you have a list of conditions where any of them may be true for a particular entry or row. It is common to have multiple conditions which include the same field name, as you are trying to include as many possible entries as you can. Few conditions try to exclude entries, such as GENDER = 'M' or alternately GENDER = 'U'. When you combine multiple conditions together with an OR, it creates a superset of all of the conditions and increases the size of the subset of the database.

The NOT operator is used on a condition to negate its meaning. If the condition originally would include particular entries, then using NOT will exclude them. If the condition pares down the results, the negated condition will increase the results. For example the NAND operator is simply the NOT operator applied to the results of an AND operation. The NOR operator is simply NOT applied to the results of an OR operation. If a particular operation yields a larger subset, NOT will produce the dual smaller subset, and vice versa.

Using Boolean Operators to Form a Query

In SQL, queries are created using a specific language. Every query will use the SELECT syntax with various optional parts. Every SELECT query has to include the fields (columns) and the table name of the database and possibly some extra syntax to limit which entries (rows) are included. Finally, the results are ordered so the output fits the desired report.

In VistA FileMan, queries involve three parts: the SEARCH conditions, the SORT ranges, and the PRINT output. Individual SEARCH comparisons are first stated, then the conditions are combined together to make a total condition. Then entries are organized by specifying what fields are used to group together, allowing for subtotals, or special sorting orders. After this, the data that needs to be output for the report is specified in the PRINT output.

First Example

The simplest SQL query just states what columns are needed from a particular table.

```
i.e.:  SELECT  column1,  column2....columnN
FROM   table_name ;
```

Using our example database this would be

```
SELECT PATNAME, DATEOFBIRTH, AGE, GENDER
FROM PATIENT;
```

Since there are no filtering conditions, every patient in the database will be output.

The VistA FileMan query would just use `PRINT FILE ENTRIES`

```
OUTPUT FROM WHAT FILE: PATIENT//
SORT BY: NAME//
START WITH NAME: FIRST//
FIRST PRINT FIELD: PATNAME
THEN PRINT FIELD: DATEOFBIRTH
THEN PRINT FIELD: AGE
THEN PRINT FIELD: GENDER
THEN PRINT FIELD: ]
Heading (S/C): PATIENT LIST//
STORE PRINT LOGIC IN TEMPLATE:EXAMPLE
   Are you adding 'EXAMPLE' as a new PRINT
TEMPLATE? No// YES  (Yes)
```

For VistA FileMan, every patient in the database will be output, but this also adds the list of output fields as a PRINT Template, so we do not have to tell VistA FileMan every time what list to use. This saves effort, but also makes the process simpler.

Second Example

The next example is to print out the subset of the patients that happen to satisfy a condition that we specify.

This will use a more complex SQL syntax:

```
SELECT column1, column2....columnN
FROM    table
WHERE CONDITION;
```

If our Condition is both the AGE must be greater than 70 and that the PATNAME must equal SMITH, we would write that Condition in SQL as

```
SELECT PATNAME, DATEOFBIRTH, AGE, GENDER
FROM PATIENT
WHERE (AGE > 70) AND (PATNAME = 'SMITH') ;
```

The same query in VistA FileMan would use

```
Select OPTION: SEARCH FILE ENTRIES
OUTPUT FROM WHAT FILE: PATIENT//
   -A- SEARCH FOR PATIENT FIELD: NAME
   -A- CONDITION: = EQUALS
   -A- EQUALS: SMITH

   -B- SEARCH FOR PATIENT FIELD: AGE
   -B- CONDITION: > GREATER THAN
   -B- GREATER THAN: 70

   -C- SEARCH FOR PATIENT FIELD:
```

```
IF: A&B      NAME EQUALS (case-insensitive)
"SMITH"      and AGE GREATER THAN "70"
OR:

STORE RESULTS OF SEARCH IN TEMPLATE:
EXAMPLE2
   Are you adding 'EXAMPLE2' as a new SORT
TEMPLATE? No// Y  (Yes)
DESCRIPTION:
   1>

SORT BY: NAME//
START WITH NAME: FIRST//
FIRST PRINT FIELD: [EXAMPLE]
```

Notice that the VistA FileMan uses a dialog to set up the condition and uses the character & to mean AND. It also automatically asks about OR conditions, but SQL requires you to type the word OR as part of the condition. If you wish to use an OR inside the condition in VistA FileMan, you must use the exclamation point ! to do so.

Each software system will have differences like this. This section is using two different systems as examples, but you must learn the specific way of writing queries for the system you end up using. Just as the Comparison Table 5.6 shows different ways to say the same comparison, each system you use will require specific study.

SUMMARY OF REPORT WRITING

Nursing Informatics involves understanding the information in a computer system and how it is organized. Each clinical information system must be learned independently. A flexible attitude when creating reports is the most successful. Formulating queries using Boolean Logic also is useful beyond reporting results as most Clinical Decision Support systems also require this formal way of specifying rules about patient data. With attention to details and persistence, using formal Boolean Logic is actually the simplest way to organize comparisons and conditions.

ACKNOWLEDGEMENTS

The author wishes to acknowledge Peter J. Murray and W. Scott Erdley for their authorship of the original fifth edition Chapter 9 "Open Source and Free Software" from which content has been integrated into this chapter.

REFERENCES

Anderson, H., & Dare, T. (2009). Passport without a visa: Open source software licensing and trademarks. *International Free and Open Source Software Law Review, 1*(2), 99–110. Retrieved from http://www.ifosslr.org/ifosslr/article/view/11.

AT Internet. (2010). *Web visit distribution by browser family (graphic).* Retrieved from http://www.atinternet-institute.com/en-us/browsers-barometer/browser-barometer-march-2010/index-1-2-3-195.html.

Bagayoko, C-O., Dufour, J-C., Chaacho, S., Bouhaddou, O., & Fieschi, M. (2010). Open source challenges for hospital information system (HIS) in developing countries: A pilot project in Mali. *BMC Medical Informatics and Decision Making, 10*(22). doi:10.1186/1472-6947-10-22.

Bourgeois, F. C., Mandl, K. D., Shaw, D., Flemming, D., & Nigrin, D. J. (2009). Mychildren's: Integration of a personally controlled health record with a tethered patient portal for a pediatric and adolescent population. *AMIA Annual Symposium Proceedings,* 65–69. Retrieved from http://www.ncbi.nlm.nih.gov/pmc/articles/PMC2815447.

Bowen, S., Valdes, I., Hoyt, R., Glenn, L., McCormick, D., & Gonzalez, X. (2009). Open-source electronic Health records: Policy implications. *Open Source EHR Public Policy Wiki.* Retrieved from http://www.openmedsoftware.org/wiki/Open_Source_EHR_Public_Policy.

Bruggink, M. (2003). *Open source in Africa: Towards informed decision-making.* The Hague, The Netherlands: International Institute for Communication and Development (IICD). Retrieved from http://www.iicd.org/files/Brief7.pdf.

Certification Commission for Health Information Technology (CCHIT). (n.d.). *Project Laika.* Retrieved from http://laika.sourceforge.net/

Cox, A. (1999). *The risks of closed source computing.* Retrieved from http://www.ibiblio.org/oswg/oswg-nightly/oswg/en_US.ISO_8859-1/articles/alan-cox/risks/risks-closed-source/index.html.

Dravis, P. (2003). *Open source software: Perspectives for development.* Washington, DC: Global Information and Communication Technologies Department, The World Bank. Retrieved from http://www.infodev.org/en/Publication.21.html.

European Communities. (2003). *The IDA open source migration guidelines.* Morden, Surrey: Netproject Ltd. and Interchange of Data between Administrations, European Commission. Retrieved from http://ec.europa.eu/idabc/en/document/2623/5585.

European Communities. (2004). *e-Europe action plan 2005.* Brussels: European Commission, Directorate-General Information Society. Retrieved from http://europa.eu/legislation_summaries/information_society/l24226_en.htm.

European Communities. (2005). *i2010—A European information society for growth and employment.* Brussels: European Commission, Directorate-General Information

Society. Retrieved from http://www.epractice.eu/node/281014.

Free Software Foundation (FSF). (2007). *GNU general public license. Version 3, 29 June 2007.* Retrieved from http://www.gnu.org/licenses/gpl.html.

Free Software Foundation (FSF). (2010a). *Why 'free software' is better than 'open source'.* Boston, MA: Free Software Foundation. Retrieved from http://www.gnu.org/philosophy/free-software-for-freedom.html.

Free Software Foundation (FSF). (2010b). *The free software definition. Version 1.92.* Boston, MA: Free Software Foundation. Retrieved from http://www.gnu.org/philosophy/free-sw.html.

Free Software Foundation (FSF). (2010c). *What is copyleft?* Retrieved from http://www.gnu.org/copyleft/copyleft.html.

Goetz, T. (2003). Open source everywhere. *WIRED, 11*(11), 158–167, 208–211. Retrieved from http://www.wired.com/wired/archive/11.11/opensource.html.

Goulde, M., & Brown, E. (2006). *Open source software: A primer for healthcare leaders.* California Healthcare Foundation/Forrester Research. Retrieved from http://www.chcf.org/publications/2006/03/open-source-software-a-primer-for-health-care-leaders.

International Institute of Infonomics. (2005). *Free/libre and open source software: Survey and study: FLOSS final report.* University of Maastricht, The Netherlands: International Institute of Infonomics. Retrieved from http://flossproject.org/report/index.htm.

International Open Source Network (IOSN). (n.d.). *FOSS primers.* Retrieved from http://www.iosn.net/publications/foss-primers.

International Telecommunications Union (ITU). (2009). *Definition of "open standards."* Retrieved from http://www.itu.int/ITU-T/othergroups/ipr-adhoc/openstandards.html.

Janamanchi, B., Katsamakas, E., Raghupathi, W., & Gao, W. (2009). The state and profile of open source software projects in health and medical informatics. *International Journal of Medical Informatics, 78*(7), 457–472.

Kaminski, J. (2005). *Moodle: A user-friendly, open source course management system.* Retrieved from http://www.nursing-informatics.com/moodle_article.pdf.

Leong, T. Y., Kaiser, K., & Miksch, S. (2007). Free and open source enabling technologies for patient-centric, guideline-based clinical decision support: A survey. In A. Geissbuhler, R. Haux, & C. Kulikowski (Eds.), *IMIA yearbook of medical informatics 2007.* Retrieved from http://www.schattauer.de/de/magazine/uebersicht/zeitschriften-a-z/imia-yearbook/imia-yearbook-2007/issue/special/manuscript/8416/show.html.

Mandl, K. D., Simons, W. W., Crawford, W. C. R., & Abbett, J. M. (2007). Indivo: A personally controlled health record for health information exchange and communication. *BMC Medical Informatics and Decision Making, 7*(25). doi:10.1186/1472-6947-7-25.

Merriam-Webster. (2010). *Merriam-Webster online.* Retrieved from http://www.merriam-webster.com/netdict/license.

Moody, G. (2001). *Rebel code: Inside Linux and the open source revolution.* Cambridge, MA: Perseus.

Murray, P. J. (2004). *Open steps, release 1.0. Report of a think-tank meeting on free/libre/open source software in the health and health informatics domains.* Retrieved from http://www.peter-murray.net/chiradinfo/marwell04/marwell%20release%201.0.pdf.

Murray, P. J., & Oyri, K. (2005). Developing online communities with LAMP (Linux, Apache, MySQL, PHP)—The IMIA OSNI and CHIRAD experiences. In R. Englebrecht, A. Geissbuhler, C. Lovis, & G. Mihalas (Eds.), *Connecting Medical Informatics and Bio-informatics: Proceedings of MIE2005—The XIXth International Congress of the European Federation for Medical Informatics* (pp. 361–366). Amsterdam: IOS Press.

Murray P. J., Wright G., Karopka T., Betts H., & Orel A. (2009). Open source and healthcare in Europe—Time to put leading edge ideas into practice. In K. P. Adlassnig, B. Blobel, J. Mantas, & I. Masic (Eds.), *Medical Informatics in a United and Healthy Europe: Proceedings of MIE2009* (pp. 963–967). Amsterdam: IOS Press. Retrieved from http://person.hst.aau.dk/ska/MIE2009/papers/MIE2009p0963.pdf.

Netcraft Ltd. (2010). *May 2010 web server survey.* Retrieved from http://news.netcraft.com/archives/2010/05/14/may_2010_web_server_survey.html.

Netmarketshare. (2010). *Browser market share.* Retrieved from http://marketshare.hitslink.com/browser-market-share.aspx?qprid=0&qptimeframe=M&qpsp=136&qpnp=2.

Office of the e-Envoy. (2002). *Open source software: Use within UK government, version 1.* London: Office of the e-Envoy, e-Government Unit. Retrieved from http://archive.cabinetoffice.gov.uk/e-envoy/frameworks-oss-policy/$file/oss-policy.pdf.

Openforum Europe Ltd. (2008). *The importance of open standards in interoperability (OFE one-page brief no. 1 (31.10.08.)).* Retrieved from http://www.openforumeurope.org/library/onepage-briefs/ofe-open-standards-onepage-2008.pdf.

Open Source Initiative (OSI). (n.d.). *The open source definition, version 1.9.* Retrieved from http://www.opensource.org/docs/osd.

Peeling, N., & Satchell, J. (2001). *Analysis of the impact of open source software.* Farnborough: QinetiQ Ltd. Retrieved from http://citeseerx.ist.psu.edu/viewdoc/download?doi=10.1.1.115.8510&rep=rep1&type=pdf.

President's Information Technology Advisory Panel (PITAC). (2000). *Developing open source software to advance high end computing.* Arlington, VA: National Coordination Office for Computing, Information, and Communications. Retrieved from http://www.itrd.gov/pubs/pitac/pres-oss-11sep00.pdf.

Raymond, E. S. (2001). *The Cathedral and the bazaar: Musings on Linux and open source by an accidental revolutionary* (Rev. ed.). Sebastopol, CA: O'Reilly and Associates.

Raymond, E. S. (2003). *The jargon file, version 4.4.7.* Retrieved from http://www.catb.org/~esr/jargon/html/S/Swiss-Army-chainsaw.html.

Samuel, F., & Sujansky, W. (2008). *Open-source EHR systems for ambulatory care: A market assessment.* California Healthcare Foundation. Retrieved from http://www.chcf.org/~/media/Files/PDF/O/OpenSourceEHRSystemsExecSummary.pdf.

Sfakianakis, S., Chronaki, C. E., Chiarugi, F., Conforti, F., & Katehakis, D. G. (2007). Reflections on the role of open source in health information system interoperability. In A. Geissbuhler, R. Haux, & C. Kulikowski (Eds.), *IMIA yearbook of medical informatics 2007.* Retrieved from http://www.schattauer.de/de/magazine/uebersicht/zeitschriften-a-z/imia-yearbook/imia-yearbook-2007/issue/special/manuscript/8412/download.html.

Shaw, N. T., Pepper, D. R., Cook, T., Houwink, P., Jain, N., & Bainbridge, M. (2002). Open source and international health informatics: Placebo or panacea? *Informatics in Primary Care, 10*(1), 39–44.

Smith, C. (2002). *Open source software and the NHS: A white paper.* Leeds, UK: NHSIA.

Squiz UK Ltd. (2007). *Royal College of Nursing case study.* Retrieved from http://www.squiz.co.uk/clients/case-studies/royal-college-of-nursing.

Stallman, R. M. (2002). *Free software free society: Selected essays of Richard M. Stallman.* Boston, MA: GNU Press/Free Software Foundation.

Stanco, T. (2001). *World Bank: InfoDev presentation.* Retrieved from http://lwn.net/2002/0117/a/stanco-world-bank.php3.

Surman, M., & Diceman, J. (2004). *Choosing open source: A guide for civil society organizations.* Toronto, Canada: Commons Group. Retrieved from http://commons.ca/articles/fulltext.shtml?x=335.

The MITRE Corporation. (2003). *Use of free and open-source software (FOSS) in the US Department of Defense, version 1.2.04.* Retrieved from http://www.microcross.com/dodfoss.pdf.

Tiemann, M. (2004a). *Open source: The solution in many countries.* Presentation at HIMSS Annual Conference and Exhibition 2004, Orlando, FL.

Tiemann, M. (2004b). Veterans Health Information System architecture (VistA). Presentation at HIMSS Annual Conference and Exhibition, 2004, Orlando, FL.

US Department of Veterans Affairs. (2008). *VistA monograph.* Retrieved from http://www4.va.gov/VistA_MONOGRAPH/index.asp.

US Department of Veterans Affairs. (2010). *VA HealthIT sharing.* Retrieved from http://www1.va.gov/vadodhealthitsharing.

Valdes, I. (2008). *Free and open source software in healthcare 1.0.* American Medical Informatics Association Open Source Working Group white paper. Retrieved from https://www.amia.org/files/Final-OS-WG%20White%20Paper_11_19_08.pdf.

Waring, T., & Maddocks, P. (2005). Open source software implementation in the UK public sector: Evidence from the field and implications for the future. *International Journal of Information Management, 25*(5), 411–442.

Wheeler, D. A. (2007). *Why open source software/free software (OSS/FS, FLOSS or FOSS)? Look at the numbers!* Retrieved from http://www.dwheeler.com/oss_fs_why.html.

Wheeler, D. A. (2010). *Make your open source software GPL-compatible. or else.* Retrieved from http://www.dwheeler.com/essays/gpl-compatible.html.

Wolfe, B. A., Mamlin, B. W., Biondich, P. G., Fraser, H. S. F., Jazayeri, D., Allen, C., … Tierney, W. M. (2006). The OpenMRS system: Collaborating toward an open source EMR for developing countries. *Proceedings of the AMIA Annual Symposium, 2006,* 1146.

Wong, K., & Sayo, P. (2004). *Free/open source software: A general introduction.* Kuala Lumpur, Malaysia: International Open Source Network (IOSN). Retrieved from http://www.iosn.net/downloads/foss_primer_current.pdf.

WorldVistA. (n.d.). *VistA history.* Retrieved from http://worldvista.org/AboutVistA/VistA_History.

Yellowlees, P. M., Marks, S. L., Hogarth, M., & Turner, S. (2008). Standards-based, open-source electronic health record systems: A desirable future for the US health industry. *Telemedicine and e-Health, 14*(3), 284–288. doi:10.1089/tmj.2007.0052.

Zymaris, C. (2003). *A comparison of the GPL and the Microsoft EULA.* Retrieved from http://www.cyber.com.au/cyber/about/comparing_the_gpl_to_eula.pdf.

6

Data and Data Processing

Irene Joos / Ramona Nelson

• OBJECTIVES

1. Describe the data-related implications for data and database systems within the data to wisdom continuum.
2. Explain file structures and database models.
3. Describe the purpose, structures, and functions of database management systems (DBMSs).
4. Outline the life cycle of a database system.
5. Explore concepts and issues related to data warehouses, big data, and dashboards.
6. Explain knowledge discovery in databases (KDD) including data mining, data analytics, and benchmarking.

• KEY WORDS

Big data
Dashboard
Data
Database
Data analytics
Data mining
Data warehouse
Information
Knowledge
Knowledge discovery in databases (KDD)
Wisdom

The Executive Office of the President produced a document titled *Big Data Across the Federal Government* providing a listing of projects undertaken by the Federal Government (Executive Office of the President, 2012, March 29). This document describes initiatives in a wide range of government agencies including the following health-related agencies:

- Department of Veterans Administration's projects such as Protecting Warfighters using

Algorithms for Text Processing to Capture Health Events (ProWatch), Consortium for Healthcare Informatics Research (CHIR), Corporate Data Warehouse (CDW), Genomic Information System for Integrated Science (GenISIS) to name a few

- Department of Health and Human Services' projects such as BioSense 2.0 (public health surveillance through collaboration), Special Bacteriology Reference Laboratory (SBRL), Virtual Laboratory

Environment (VLE), and a data warehouse based on Hadoop for big data analytics and reporting to name a few

- National Institutes of Health's projects such as The Cancer Imaging Archive (TCIA), The Cancer Genome Atlas (TCGA), and Patient Reported Outcomes Measurement Information System (PROMIS), as examples.

In addition there are a number of other government agencies such as the Department of Defense, Department of Homeland Security, and the Office of Basic Energy Sciences with big data projects that directly or indirectly impact the healthcare community. As these projects demonstrate the Federal Government is using data and especially the big data revolution to advance scientific discovery and innovation in a number of areas including the delivery of quality healthcare and personalized healthcare.

In modern healthcare, the process of moving from data collection to implementing and evaluating the care provided to individuals, families, and communities is highly dependent on automated database systems. The goal of healthcare and the movement to big data and data analytics is to drive quality care at lower costs through reducing overutilization of services, improve coding and billing practices, empowering patients, measuring trends, predicting outcomes, and examining how improved workflow and productivity can influence quality outcomes (Barlow, 2013). This chapter introduces the nurse to basic concepts, theories, models, and issues necessary to understand the effective use of automated database systems and to engage in dialog regarding data analytics, benchmarks, and outcomes.

THE NELSON DATA TO WISDOM CONTINUUM

The Nelson data to wisdom continuum moves from data to information to knowledge to wisdom with constant interaction within and across these concepts as well as the environment (Joos, Nelson, & Smith, 2014). As shown in Fig. 6.1 data are raw, uninterrupted facts without meaning. For example, the following series of numbers are data, with no meaning: 98, 116, 58, 68, 18. Reordered and labeled as vital signs they have meaning

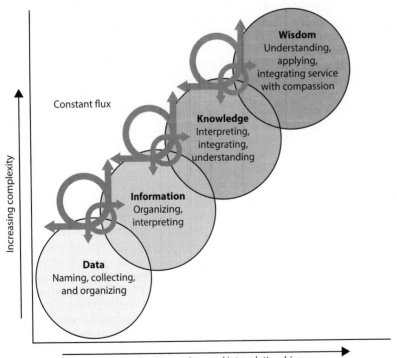

• **FIGURE 6.1.** The Nelson Data to Wisdom Continuum. Revised Data Information Knowledge Wisdom (DIKW) Model-2013 Version (Copyright © 2013 Ramona Nelson, Ramona Nelson Consulting. All rights reserved. Reprinted with permission.)

and now represent information: temperature 98.0, pulse 58, respirations 18, and blood pressure 106/68. These data provide information on a person's basic condition. Using the nurse's knowledge this information is then interpreted. The nurse fits these data into a *pattern* of prior knowledge about vital signs. For example, if these vital signs were recorded as part of a physical for a high school athlete they are in the normal range; however, if these same numbers were part of an assessment on an elderly patient with congestive heart failure, the low pulse and blood pressure could suggest a problem. Context and pattern knowledge allow the nurse to understand the meaning and importance of those data and to make decisions about nursing actions with regard to the information. While data by themselves are meaningless, information and knowledge, by definition, are meaningful. When the nurse uses knowledge to make appropriate decisions and acts on those decisions he or she exhibits wisdom. In other words the nurse demonstrates wisdom when the nurse synthesizes and appropriately uses a variety of knowledge types within nursing actions to meet human needs.

For data to be placed in context so that information is produced, the data must be processed. This means that the data are organized so that patterns and relationships between the data can be identified, thereby producing information. When the user understands and interprets the patterns and relationships in the data, knowledge results. Finally, the user applies the knowledge as the basis for making clinical judgments and decisions and choosing nursing actions for implementation. The "data to information to knowledge to wisdom" progression is predicated on the existence of accurate, pertinent, and properly collected and organized data. There are several approaches to organizing and naming data.

Some common approaches to organizing data include sorting, classifying, summarizing, and calculating. For example, students will often take their notes and handouts from their nursing classes and organize them into folders. The folders can be on a personal computer or other automated device. They may be in a box, in a file cabinet, or on some other storage media. Each folder represents a different topic. Students may organize the data in the folders by nursing problems, interventions, medical diseases, cell biology, or drugs, to name but a few classifications for the information. Sometimes it is difficult to decide which folder is the appropriate one to use to store specific notes. Students may make a copy of the notes and store them in both folders or may put the notes in one folder and use a link or a cross-reference note in the other folder. In the process of organizing the data/information students have created a database.

DEFINING DATA AND DATABASES

Data States

When discussing digital data it is important to discuss the three states of data—data at rest, data in motion, and data in use (Cisco, 2013; Quillin, 2013; and Barney, 2013). Data at rest generally refer to data on storage devices such as a removable one like a USB thumb drive, a hard drive, tape, and a cloud sever. This is archived data that rarely change. You could consider patient's past medical records data at rest. In today's cybercrime world, it is important to protect these data from unauthorized access and use. These data are subject to security protocols to protect the confidential nature of these data. Data in use refer to data that a database program is currently reading or writing; it resides in the computer's temporary memory. This is its most vulnerable state as it becomes open to access or change by others. Some of these data may contain sensitive data-like social security numbers, birth dates, health insurance numbers, results of diagnostic tests, and so forth. One can attempt to secure these data in use through passwords and user IDs, but these are only as secure as the person's ability to keep that information private, and the nature of the encryption technology used. Data in motion are data moving between applications, over the network, or over the Internet. Data in motion are an increasing concern in healthcare because streaming data are now available from sensors, monitoring devices, mobile devices, and so forth. Monitoring activities of patients in their homes places these data at risk as the data move from the source to the destination database. Increasingly healthcare providers require access to data at the point of care through mobile devices. While data in motion entail security risks, they also provides opportunities that we never imagined. For example, monitoring patients in real time in their homes can lead to improved patient care and compliance.

Databases

A database is an organized collection of related data. Placing notes in folders and folders in file cabinets is one example of creating a paper database; however, you can organize and store data in many different formats in a database. Electronic databases like the WhitePages application (app) and electronic library catalogs are replacing paper databases like a phone book or card catalog. Healthcare professionals may store patient medical records in either paper or digital format but more and more healthcare organizations are converting to digital records. They can use each of these databases to store data and to search for information. The possibility of finding information in these databases depends on several factors. Four of the most important are the following:

1. The data naming (indexing) and organizational schemes
2. The size and complexity of the database
3. The type of data within the database
4. The database search methodology

The systematic approach used to name, organize, and store data in a database has a major impact on how easy it is to find information in the database. Electronic phone books permit searching by name, address, or phone number unlike paper ones that permit searching by last name in alphabetical order. A large database can be more difficult to search than a small database. The size of a database is a function of not only the amount of data in the database but also the number and complexity of the relationships between the data. The patient's chart may reflect an overnight observational visit at the hospital. One can organize data in the patient's chart in an infinite number of ways. A wide range of caregivers will see different relationships and reach different conclusions from reading the same chart.

Organizations use information systems to process data and produce information. The term information system traditionally refers to computer systems, but this is only one type of information system. There are manual information systems as well as human information systems. The most effective and complex information system is the human brain. People are constantly taking in data and processing that data to produce meaning.

Types of Data

When developing automated database systems, the designer defines each data element. As part of this process, the designer classifies the data. There are two primary approaches to classifying data in a database system. First, they are classified in terms of how the users will use these data. This is the conceptual view of the data. Conceptual data classifications may include financial data, patient data, or human resource data. The conceptual view of the data has a major impact on how the designer indexes the data. Second, data are classified by their computerized data type. For example, data can be numbers or letters or a combination of both. The designer uses this classification to build the physical database within the computer system. It identifies the number of spaces necessary to capture each data element and the specific functions that the system can perform on these data.

Conceptual Data Types. Conceptual data types reflect how users view the data. The source of the data may be the basis of conceptual data types. For example, the lab produces lab data, and the X-ray department produces image data. Conceptual data can also have its basis on the event that the data are attempting to capture. Assessment data, intervention data, and outcome data are examples of data that reflect event capturing.

Computer-Based Data Types. Alphanumeric data include letters and numbers in any combination; however, you cannot perform numeric calculations on the numbers in an alphanumeric field. For example, an address is alphanumeric data that may include both numbers and letters. A social security number is an example of alphanumeric data compressing numbers and sometimes dashes. It makes no logical sense to add or perform any other numerical functions on either addresses or social security numbers. The designer must identify for the computer system the number of spaces for an alphanumeric field. In the database program this is generally called a text field.

Numeric data can be used to perform numeric functions including addition, subtraction, multiplication, and division. There are several different formats as well as types of numeric data. For example, numeric data types include general number, currency, Euro, fixed, standard, percent, and scientific formats.

Date and time are special types of numeric data with which certain specific numeric functions are appropriate. For example, you could subtract two dates to determine how many days, months, and/or years are between the two dates. However, it would not make sense to add together several different dates, but one might use today's date and date of last mammogram to determine how long it has been since the first one was completed.

Logic data are data limited to two options. Some examples include YES or NO, TRUE or FALSE, 1 or 2, and ON or OFF. In addition there are other data types like rich text, hyperlink, memo, attachments, and lookup which you will learn when you create or use a database. Attachments can take the format of a file or image.

One of the major advantages of an automated information system is that you can capture each of these data elements once and different users can use them many times for different purposes. For example, a patient with diabetes mellitus has an elevated blood sugar level. The physician may use this datum to adjust the patient's insulin dose and the nurse may use it in a patient education program. You can also aggregate and summarize these basic data elements to produce new data and information that a different set of users may use. This attribute of data is referred to as "data collected once, used many times."

Database Management Systems (DBMSs)

DBMSs are computer programs that are used to input, store, modify, process, and access data in a database. Before you can use a DBMS, you must first create the structure for the database using the data elements necessary to manage the data specific to the project. This process of configuring the database software is called database system design. Once you configure the database for the project, you use the database software to enter the project data into the computer. A functioning DBMS consists of three interacting parts. These are the data, the designed database, and the query language that you use to access the data. Some examples of databases in everyday life include computerized library systems, automated teller machines, and flight reservation systems. When you use these systems, the data, the structured database, and the query language interact together.

Earlier in this chapter, the example of creating a database for class notes was introduced. The notes and handouts are the data. The folders and file cabinet demonstrate the design or organization of the database in the DBMS. The labels on the folders and the file cabinet are the fields in the database. With these labels the user is able to understand how the data are organized and how to look for specific pieces of information. This makes it possible for the user to find information in the files. With a manual system, the index and query language are usually in the user's head; however, there are problems storing and finding data with a manual system. One can use different terms for the same concept such as liver or hepatic and the user can forget how specific data was classified or how it was stored. As you add new data, the classification and storage of data can become inconsistent. If there are two or more users the classification system becomes ever more inconsistent. Putting the data in sometimes requires duplicate copies. Once you store the data, it is not unusual to forget where it is stored or to forget about the data completely. Automated DBMSs deal with many of these problems.

Advantages of Automated Database Management Systems. Automated DBMSs decrease data redundancy, increase data consistency, and improve access to all data. These advantages result from the fact that in a well-designed automated system all data exist in only one place. The datum is never repeated.

Data redundancy occurs when one stores the same data in the database more than once or stores it in more than one interrelated database. Making a copy of class notes to store the same notes in two different folders is an example of data redundancy. In healthcare, there are many examples of data redundancy. Patients, as different

healthcare providers assess them, will complain that they have answered the same questions over and over. Often nurses will need to chart the same data on different forms or on different screens in a patient's medical record. The same data may be stored in two different health-related databases. For example, the patient's active medication list may be in both the electronic medical record that the primary provider maintains and in the electronic health record (EHR) at a healthcare instruction. A well-designed automated database links these data and records it once and accesses it from this single location each time they are necessary.

When the same data are in different manuals or automated databases, a second problem emerges. The data become inconsistent. As different users working with different databases update or change data, they do not always consistently record it in the same format. Once the data are inconsistent, it can be impossible to know the correct data. Two examples from education and healthcare may make this clearer. Many departments within a university maintain their own database with student information (i.e., address, phone number). Some of the databases are manual, and some are automated in stand-alone systems while others are in systems that interface with other systems. When a student changes his or her address, it is not unusual for that student to receive mail from the university at both addresses. Current student information systems resolve this problem by storing the address in one database that all with permissions access.

When a doctor admits a patient to a hospital, different caregivers will ask the patient to identify medications he or she is taking at home. Sometimes the patient will list only prescription medications; other times the patient will include over-the-counter drugs taken on a routine basis. Sometimes the patient will forget to include a medication. If caregivers record these different lists in different sections of the medical record, inconsistency occurs. In a well-designed integrated automated database, each caregiver is working with the same list each time data are reviewed. An additional problem occurs if one uses different terms for the same data. For example, sometimes one might use a generic name while other times one might use the brand name for that drug. This is why standards such as standard languages (i.e., SNOMED) are key to the design of EHRs. An automated database design that uses recognized standards as well as consistent input and access to data is imperative to creating databases necessary for the efficient and effective delivery of quality healthcare.

The database management software program uses a structured approach to organize and store data. The same software uses a query language, making it possible for the computer to do the work of searching for the data.

Structure—Fields, Records, and Files. Fields describe the type of data expected in the related field. For example, LName refers to last name and FName the first name. Each row represents a record of the data in each of the fields of the database. For example, row 2 might be the record for Betty Smith. Each record is assigned a primary identifier (also known as primary key or unique identifier). No other record in the database will have that identifier. Needless to say in healthcare institutions where there can be several different interrelated databases or where the institution's databases link to databases outside the institution such as the private office of a Primary Care Provider (PCP), it is imperative that there be a master patient index with a unique identifier for each patient. This is a critical piece for the safe and effective exchange of electronic health information. The Office of the National Coordinator for Health Information Technology (ONC) initiated a collaborative patient matching initiative and three months later some preliminary findings to include standardized patient identifying attributes (Perna, 2013; PMC, 2013; ONC, 2013; Morris, Farnum, Afzal, Robinson, Greene, & Choughlin, 2014). All the records together in a table constitute a file.

In a DBMS, there may be several files. A file is defined as a set of related records that have the same data fields. A database consists of several files. The DBMS can then search across the tables or files to find data related to any one entity in the database as long as they share a common identifier.

Function—Store, Update, Retrieve, Report. The functions of a DBMS are to store the data, update the records, provide easy retrieval of the data, and permit report generation. The first function was addressed above. The next function is the ability to update the data in the database. This means to add a record, delete a record, or change the data in a record. The next function relates to the query language that permits one to retrieve the data. One can search one table or multiple tables depending on the structure of the database. The last function is report generation. Most DBMS permit you to create custom reports based on selections of retrieved data.

Models

A database model is the basis or foundation that determines how one stores, organizes, and accesses or manipulates the data. The American National Standards Institute (ANSI) and the Standards Planning and Requirements Committee (SPARC) identified these views or models in 1975 (IBM, 2013; 1Keydata, 2014). According to these documents, there are three main phases to database design: conceptual design, logical design, and physical design.

In 1987, John Zachman described database models through the framework of information architecture

TABLE 6.1	Database Views
View	**Description**
Ballpark	This includes the scope and/or description of the database listing items of importance to the business.
Owner	This view models the business entities of interest to the business.
Designer	This is the entity or actual record on the computer from the designer's view.
Builder	This describes the actual physical implementation or database design from the conception view.
Out-of-Context	This would include the data definition language for the database.
Actual System	This describes what is actually built.

(Zachman, 2008). Hay (2010) identified six views: ballpark, owner's, designer's, builder's, out-of-context, and the actual system. See Table 6.1 for a definition of these views. These views are helpful in understanding how different groups from information technology (IT) professionals to caregivers will interact with the design and use of a database. It is always important to remember that creating a database that meets the needs of the organization and end users is a complex process. The models and the process of developing them are critical to the success of the database endeavor. The following text describes three primary views or models.

Conceptual Models. A conceptual model identifies the entities and the relationship between those entities. It does not identify the attributes or primary keys or attempt to call out the major details of the database. Figure 6.2

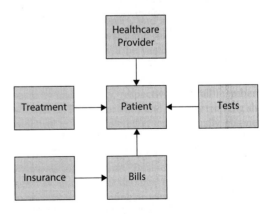

• **FIGURE 6.2.** Conceptual Data Model.

shows a Conceptual Data Model. This phase focuses on constructing a model that accurately reflects the information that organizations or businesses use. It describes the scope of the information of interest. The question here is what are those items of interest to the organization or business and how do they relate to one another?

Logical Models. This model describes the data in more detail without paying attention to the actual physical implementation or design of the database. It defines the structure of the whole database in terms of the attributes of the entities (data elements), their relationships, a primary key for each entity, and so forth. For example, there may be a database system to manage patient medication orders. With each individual order, there will be several entities—patient, medication, pharmacy, physician, and administration as examples. The medication entity attributes would include the specific medication, the dose, the time and frequency of administration, the route of administration, and any specific directions for administering the medication. Each medication order is a written individual order for one patient. This facilitates the normalization process which is the process of reducing the database structure to its lowest form by organizing the fields and tables to minimize redundancy and dependency.

When complete, the logical data model will include a diagram of data entities, the definition and attributes of each entity, and relationships between data. One uses the definitions and the description of each data attribute to create the data dictionary. For nursing, this has been a major challenge. Many of the data elements including nursing diagnosis, interventions, and outcomes have not been included in the data dictionaries of DBMSs used in healthcare. Nursing has had difficulty identifying and defining data elements in a format that an automated system can use. This challenge has been the basis for the development of standard languages within nursing.

When planning a small database for personal use, developing the conceptual and logical model is an important step. There are several questions that can be helpful in thinking through this process.

1. How end users use the database? What kind of information or output does one expect from the system? This includes both online data queries and written reports.

2. What data entities need to be in the database to produce the desired output? What are the attributes of each entity? What type of data are the attributes and how much space does each attribute require? For example, a first name is an alphanumeric data type. The largest name in the database may require

25 character spaces; therefore, this field will require a minimum of 25 spaces.

3. What are easy to remember logical names for each of the data fields or attributes?

4. What approach will be used to create a unique identifier for each record in the database? Will each table have a unique identifier for each record?

5. Does each of the table designs have no unnecessary overlapping data, but does have common data fields so that searches can include several tables?

Once developed, the logical data model provides the foundation for the physical data model.

Physical Data Model. The physical data model includes each of the data elements and the relationship between the data elements, as they will be actually physically stored on the computer. There are four primary approaches to the development of a physical data model. These are hierarchical, network, relational, and object oriented. The initial database models were hierarchical and network. The relational and object oriented are more common today than the hierarchical or network models. With the concern for big data and data analytics, new models such as Massively Parallel Processing (MPP), Column-oriented database, Stream processing (ESP or CEP), and Key-value storage (MapReduce) are popular for overcoming the limitations of traditional models when dealing with large-scale data (Rodrigues, 2012).

Hierarchical Databases. Hierarchical databases have been compared to inverted trees. Access to data starts at the top of the hierarchy or at the root. The table at the root has pointers that point to tables with data that relate hierarchically to the root. Each table is a node. For example, a master patient index might include pointers to each patient's record node. Each of the patient record nodes could include pointers to lab data, radiology data, and medication data for that patient. The patient record nodes are called parent nodes, while the lab, medication, and radiology nodes are called child nodes. In a hierarchical model, a parent node may have several children nodes, but each child node can only have one parent node. Figure 6.3 demonstrates a hierarchical model and the related terminology.

Hierarchical models are very effective at representing one-to-many relationships; however, they have some disadvantages. Many data relationships do not fit the one-to-many model. Remember the class notes that were in two folders? In addition, if the data relationships change, this can require significant redesign of the database.

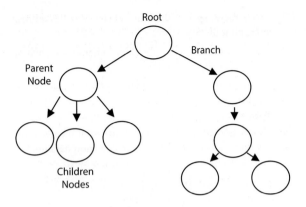

• **FIGURE 6.3.** Hierarchical Database Model.

Network Model. Network models developed from hierarchical models. In a network model, the child node is not limited to one parent. This makes it possible for a network model to represent many-to-many relationships; however, the presence of multiple links between data does make it more difficult if data relationships change and redesign is necessary.

Relational Database Models (RDM). RDM consist of a series of files set up as tables. Each column represents an attribute, and each row is a record. Another name for a row is tuple. The intersection of the row and the column

is a cell. The datum in the cell is the manifestation of the attribute for that record. Each cell may contain only one piece of datum. The datum must be atomic or broken down into its smallest format. For example, a blood pressure reading would be broken into the systolic and the diastolic reading. Because of this limitation, the relationships represented are linear and only relate one data element to another.

A relational database joins any two or more files and generates a new file from the records that meet the matching search criteria. Figure 6.4 includes two related tables: Table A and Table B. Both tables include the patient's ID or master index number. This is the common field by which the relational database joins the tables. By joining these two tables, it is possible to create a new table that identifies by name all patients who have a diagnosis of cerebral vascular accident (CVA). For example, Table C is created by the DBMS in response to the query, "List all patients with a diagnosis of CVA."

While a relational database consists of multiple tables, it is possible to build a simple database with one table. This type of database is a flat file. An Excel spreadsheet is an example of a flat file. This approach is good if you have a relativity small amount of data and simple questions. Excel has a table feature that permits one to delete and add fields, add records, remove duplicate rows, sort data, filter data, and create aggregate subsets of data. For example, asking how many nurses needed recertification on CPR would create a data subset of nurses needing this update.

Table A

ID	L-NAME	F-NAME	SEX	B-DATE
12	Smith	Tom	M	01-23-73
14	Brown	Robert	M	02-01-77
13	Jones	Mary Lou	F	12-12-54
15	Yurick	Edward	M	04-04-38

Table B

ID	DX-1	DX-2	DX-3	DX-4
12	MI	CVA	GLACOMA	PVD
14	CVA	HEPATITIS C	COLITIS	UTI
13	DIABETES M	ANGINA	CVA	GOUT
15	CERF	AMENIA	GLACOMA	PEPTIC ULCER

Table C

ID	L-NAME	F-NAME	DX-1	DX-2	DX-3
12	Smith	Tom		CVA	
14	Brown	Robert	CVA		
13	Jones	Mary Lou			CVA

• **FIGURE 6.4.** Relational Database Model.

Object-Oriented Model. An object-oriented database has evolved because the relational model has limited ability to deal with binary large objects or BLOBs. BLOBs are complex data types such as images, sounds, spreadsheets, or text messages. They are large nonatomic data with parts and subparts that a relational database cannot easily represent. In object-oriented databases the entity as well as attributes of the entity is stored with the object. An object can store other objects as well. In the object-oriented model, the data definition includes both the object and its attributes. For example, amoxicillin is an antibiotic. All antibiotics have certain attributes or actions. Because amoxicillin is an antibiotic, it can be stored in the object antibiotic and inherit the attributes that are true of all antibiotics. For example, all antibiotics can cause diarrhea; therefore, diarrhea can be a side effect of amoxicillin. The ability to handle nonatomic complex data and inheritance attributes are major advantages in healthcare computing.

Database Life Cycle

The development and use of a DBMS follow a systematic process called the life cycle of a database system. The number of steps used to describe this process can vary from one author to another. In this chapter, we use a five-step approach in the life cycle process. While the process of developing a DBMS moves forward through these steps, there is a recursive pattern to the development. Each step in the process provides the developer(s) with new insights. As these new insights occur, it is sometimes necessary to make modifications in previously completed steps of the process.

Initiation. Initiation occurs when one identifies a need or problem and sees the development of a DBMS as a potential solution. This initial assessment looks at what is the need, what do we want to accomplish, what are the current approaches, and what are the potential options for dealing with the need are. For example, the Staff Development Department in a home health agency may want to automate their staff education records. The current approach is to maintain an index card for each staff member. The index card lists all the programs that individual staff members have attended. When the card gets full, the department staples a second card to the first card. When the department needed to know how many total hours of staff development education it had provided monthly by each branch office for the last year, the department had to pay staff several hours of overtime to review the cards and collect these data.

The department made a decision to request assistance from the Information Services Department. Initially the IT department reviewed commercial or "off-the-shelf"

education database management applications developed especially for staff development departments. These programs offered much more functionality than necessary and in addition required a significant investment to purchase the software. The IT department made a decision to design an in-house database using currently owned software. The department had a computer with a generic DBMS software program; however, no one in the department knew how to use the program or how to structure the data for a database program. The nurse who organized most of the reports for the department attended in-service classes and worked with the database administrator from the Information Services Department. Now the Staff Development Department was ready to start planning for their automated DBMS.

Planning and Analysis. This step begins with an assessment of the user's view and the development of the conceptual model and ends with the logical model. What are the information needs of the department and how does the department use the information? This includes the internal and external uses of information. External needs for information come from outside the department. What are the reports that the department produces? What are the requests for information that the department is unable to fill? What information would the department like to report but has not because it is too difficult or time-consuming to collect the data? In the future, what data and in what format—print or electronic—are we anticipating? Internally what information does the department use in planning and/or developing educational programs? How does the department evaluate the quality of individual programs or its overall performance? How does the department evaluate the performance of its staff? By understanding the external and internal informational needs of the department, it is possible to identify data and the data relationships that will need to be captured in the DBMS. IT will use diagrams and narrative reports to describe the data elements, their attributes, and the overall ideal information flow in the conceptual model. A well-developed conceptual and logical model in accordance with a careful assessment of the user's needs will be a major advantage for the database administrator. The logical model provides the framework for the physical model developed by the database administrator.

Detailed Systems Design and Development. The detailed systems design begins with the selection of the physical model: hierarchical, network, relational, or object-oriented. Using the physical model, IT develops each table and the relationships between the tables. At this point, IT will carefully design the data entry screens and the format for all output reports. The users in the department must validate the data entry screens and output formats. It is often helpful to use prototypes and screen shoots to get user input during this stage. Revisions are the norm. Development of the database also involves the development of field naming conventions as well as writing initial drafts of policies and procedures for using the database.

Implementation. Implementation includes training the users, testing the system, finalizing the procedure manual for use of the system, piloting the DBMS, and finally "going live." Training users can take the form of online tutorials or live training as well as access to a help desk and/or super users who can provide help 24/7. Testing the system is generally done in a development environment with simulated data. The procedure manual outlines the "rules" for how one uses the system in day-to-day operations. For example, what is the procedure for recording attendance at individual classes, and when do you provide the attendance data to the data entry clerk? Is the attendance data automatically entered when registering for a class? In going live with a database system, one of the difficult decisions is how much previous data must you load into the DBMS. The initial request that stimulated the development of the DBMS would have required that you load at least one year of previous data into the automated database system.

Evaluation and Maintenance. When IT installs a new database system, the developers and the users can be too anxious to immediately evaluate the system. Initial or early evaluations may have limited value. It will take a few weeks or even months for users to adjust their work routines to this new approach to information management. It is not unusual for there to be adjustments to the database as well as revisions in the procedure manual during this initial period of use. The first evaluations should be informal and focus more on troubleshooting specific problems. Once the system is up and running and users have adjusted to the new information processing procedure, they will have a whole new appreciation of the value of a DBMS. At this point, one can expect a number of requests for new options and capabilities. Maintenance also includes backup of the database on a regular basis. IT in consultation with nursing will need to make a decision as to how often and when to complete the backup of the database.

DATA TO INFORMATION

Common Database Operations

DBMSs vary from small programs running on a personal computer to massive programs that manage the data for large international enterprises. No matter what size or

how a DBMS is used, there are common operations that DBMSs perform. There are three basic types of data processing operations. These include data input, data processing, and data output.

Data Input Operations. One uses data input operations to enter new data, update data in the system, or change/modify data in the DBMS. One usually enters data through a set of screens that the designers have designed for data entry. A well-designed screen will discourage data entry errors. In addition, one can design the program to alert the user to potential errors or to prevent obvious data entry errors. It may not accept data that are out of range. For example, if someone tried to enter a blood pressure of 60/180, the system would issue an error message. The error message can be in the form of a sound or a text message on the screen. It is important that text messages are clear and help the user correct the error. With today's mobile devices, web 2.0 tools, cameras, wearables, dissolvables, and sensors, we are collecting increasing amounts of data without human input (Frost & Sullivan, 2011; Hamilton, 2013). Data coming from automated input technologies decreases data input errors by eliminating the human element. The input of automated data is also contributing to the vast amount of data now available to healthcare organizations for improvement of quality care and cost reductions.

Sometimes one enters data that are unusual but could be correct. For example, a drug dose could be higher than the normal recommendation for that drug. In these cases, one may design the system to offer an alert and request that the user re-enter the data to confirm its accuracy. It is important to evaluate how the alert should function. For example, if this is a clerical office dealing with numerical data, there may be no problem with having the clerk re-enter the data; however, if this is an intensive care unit, where drug doses are often higher than the recommended dose in textbooks, requiring busy caregivers to repeatedly reenter data may not be a good idea.

Database systems also let the user update, modify, or change data that the user has previously entered into the system. Depending on the design of the DBMS, you may overwrite or lose the original data, or you may save the original data to a separate file. With patient data, it is important to be able to track data modifications. This should include who changed the data, what were the original data, and what modifications were made to the data. It may also include why the data were changed.

Data Processing Processes. Data processing processes are DBMS-directed actions that the computer performs on entered data. The purpose is to extract information, discover new meanings, reorder data, and so forth. It is these processes that one uses to convert raw data into meaningful information. These include common database functions discussed previously in this chapter. In large databases these are processes referred to as online transaction processing (OLTP). OLTP is defined as real-time processing of transactions to support the day-to-day operation of the institution.

Data Output Operations. These operations include online and written reports. Output can also include presentation of the processed data in charts and graphs for easier understanding. The approach to designing these reports will have a major impact on what information the reader actually gains from the report. Reports that are clear and concise help the reader see the information in the data. On the other hand, poorly designed reports can mislead and confuse the reader.

The development of a database system within a department serves two important purposes. First, both the developers and the users create a new level of knowledge and skill. Second, as individual departments develop databases, they create institutional data; however, if each department develops its individual database system, in isolation, the institution develops islands of automation.

Data Warehouses

In the late 1980s and early 1990s, a number of changes stimulated the development of the data warehouse concept. Computer systems became more powerful. Database theory and products were more sophisticated. Users were becoming computer literate and developing more requirements. A core of healthcare informatics leaders had developed. The move away from fee-for-service to managed care created a new set of information needs. While systems were still used to track charges for services, it was also necessary to assist analysts to calculate the actual cost of providing health services. Historical data within the computer systems took on a new value. Analyzing historical data for the institution meant the institution must collect and store that data from each of the systems in a common storage system called a data warehouse.

A data warehouse is a large collection of data imported from several different systems into one database. The source of the data includes not only internal data from the institution but can also include data from external sources. For example, one can import standards of practice-related data into data warehouse and use it to analyze how the institution achieved a variety of standard related goals. Smaller collections of data are data marts. One might develop a data mart with the historical data of a department or a small group of departments or one might also develop a data mart by exporting a subset of the data from the data warehouse.

Purposes of a Data Warehouse. The development of a data warehouse requires a great deal of time, energy, and money. An organization's decision to develop a data warehouse is based on several goals and purposes. Because of its integrated nature a data warehouse spares users from the need to learn several different applications. For example, a warehouse no longer requires healthcare providers to access the lab reporting system to see lab work and use a different application with a different interface to view radiology results. When users are viewing several different applications there are several different "versions of the truth." These can result from looking at the database at different times as well as the use of different definitions. For example, the payroll database may show a different number of nurses on staff than the automated staffing system. That is because the payroll database would include nurses in administrative positions; however, the staffing system may only include the nurses that you assign to patient care.

The developer makes these types of decisions in building the warehouse to provide a more consistent approach to making decisions based on the data. A data warehouse makes it possible to separate the analytical and operational processing. With this separation one provides an architectural design for the data warehouse that supports decisional information needs. The user can slice and dice the data from different angles and at different levels of detail.

Functions of a Data Warehouse. The management of a data warehouse requires three types of programs. First the data warehouse must be able to extract data from the various computer systems and import those data into the data warehouse. This is a key point for nursing. If nursing data such as the nursing diagnoses are not in the various computer systems or do not exist in any standardized format, one cannot extract and import it into the data warehouse. Nursing data are not limited to the data that nurses generate but include the data that nurses use for client care, administration, research, and education.

Furthermore, the data definitions that were established in the original computer systems must now be revised so that the data from the different systems can be integrated. For example, does the data definition for patient problem(s) include problems identified by all professional caregivers, or is it limited to the medical diagnosis?

Second, the data warehouse must function as a database able to store and process the data in the database. This includes the ability to aggregate the data and process the aggregated data. For example, the operational database systems used to manage the institution on a day-to-day basis do not usually offer the opportunity to look at data over time, yet a data warehouse supports integration of data and the analysis of trends over time. The individual data elements imported into the warehouse are referred to as primary data. The aggregate data produced by the warehouse database system are referred to as secondary data or derived data.

Third, the data warehouse must be able to deliver the data in the warehouse back to the users in the form of information. They can use information from a data warehouse for decision support systems for both managers and direct care givers. This information can support clinical and administrative research, education, quality improvement, infection control, and a myriad of other decision-making activities in healthcare institutions. The data hospitals collect are already used to support planning, marketing, and project management as well as reporting to accreditation and regulatory agencies. Having it in a data warehouse would greatly improve the efficiency of developing reports. The development of data warehouses promises to convert clinical information from a wasted resource, available only for an individual patient, into a resource that can be used for clinical effectiveness review, clinical research, and serves as a source of new discovery. In these ways, clinical data will ultimately benefit people through improvement in clinical care.

Data from a data warehouse can support a number of activities and provide these benefits:

- End user self-service of their data needs freeing IT for other tasks

- Access to clinical and financial data in one repository

- Creation of standardized reports of core measures, quality indicators, pay-for-performance results, and so forth

- Identification of casual relationships of diseases, symptoms, and treatments

- Focus on common goals regarding data management

- Negotiating with insurance companies

- Reporting on EMR user log data for tracking policy compliance (Doyle, 2013; Enterprise Information Systems Steering Committee, 2009; Inmon, 2007)

Data Analysis and Presentation

With the ability to collect increasing amounts of data, the ability to obtain new information and insights is growing exponentially. In turn the tools that one uses for data analytics and information presentation such as dashboards take on new importance.

Analytics. While there are many definitions of analytics, it is defined here as the process one uses to make realistic,

quality decisions using the available data. This means that data and their analysis guide the decision-making process. Analysis involves a systematic examination and evaluation of data to uncover interrelationships within the data, thereby producing new insights and information. The process usually involves breaking the data into smaller parts to better understand the area of concern. For example, the area of concern might be progress toward meeting the Institute of Medicine's recommendation for nursing education, improving medication safety practices, improving clinical care quality for some group of patients, providing cost-effective care, and so forth. We use the term business intelligence (BI) when the data include administrative data that relates to the day-to-day operation of the institution, as well as strategic or long-range planning data. Analysis in this case includes a host of statistics that one uses for analyzing the wealth of business data. These statistical tests can include simple descriptive statistics like means, averages, frequencies, and so forth to more complex operations such as regression analysis, correlations, and predictions.

Depending on the size of the database, one can use simple tools like spreadsheets or other tools designed for larger data sets. Data tools can be free or must be acquired for a fee. Examples of some available tools include the R Project (http://www.r-project.org/), which is an environment for data analysis and visualization; DataWrangler (http://vis.stanford.edu/wrangler/) for cleaning and rearranging data; and CSVKit (http://csvkit.readthedocs.org/en/latest/index.html) for working with .csv files. An example of a tool for a large data set is Hadoop (http://hadoop.apache.org/).

Dashboards. This concept for dashboards comes from the automobile and airline industry and involves the synthesis and presentation of data in a visual format. Systems process data and then present it in a visual layout so that one can easily visualize the information and the interrelationships in that information for the purpose of decision-making and benchmarking (covered later in this chapter). A dashboard "…is a visual display of the most important information needed to achieve one or more objectives, consolidated and arranged on a single screen so the information can be monitored at-a-glance" (iDashboard, 2013, p. 3). Dashboards are available for clinical performance indicators such as unit census, length of stay, and so forth; for hospital performance indicators such as admissions, income, and utilization; for patient performance indicators such as average length of stay and drug error rates; for physician performance indicators such as number of patients seen; and for nursing performance indicators such as pain assessment, staff turnover rates, educational levels, and pressure ulcer prevalence. For examples of dashboards and related visuals refer to Table 6.2.

TABLE 6.2	Examples of Dashboards
Name	**Location**
Dashboard Data and Measuring Nurse Education	http://campaignforaction.org/webinar/how-do-you-measure-your-progress-dashboard-data-and-measuring-nurse-education
Nursing Dashboard in Excel	http://www.qimacros.com/store/nursing-dashboard/
Health Care Clinical Quality and Safety Dashboard—Using enterprise dashboards for hospital performance improvement	http://dashboardspy.wordpress.com/2006/07/19/health-care-clinical-quality-and-safety-dashboard-using-enterprise-dashboards-for-performance-improvement/
Datasets and Documentation	http://dashboard.healthit.gov/
Adopting Real-Time Surveillance Dashboards as a Component of an Enterprisewide Medication Safety Strategy	http://psnet.ahrq.gov/resource.aspx?resourceID=22476
Beyond Nursing Quality Measurement: The Nation's First Regional Nursing Virtual Dashboard	http://www.ahrq.gov/professionals/quality-patient-safety/patient-safety-resources/resources/advances-in-patient-safety-2/vol1/Advances-Aydin_2.pdf

Data Quality

In a data warehouse, data are entered once but can be used many times by many users for a number of different purposes. As a result, the quality of the data on entry takes on a whole new level of importance. In this situation, the concept of data ownership changes. When dealing with a department information system, the department is usually seen as owning the data and being responsible for the quality of that data. For example, one might expect nurses to be responsible for the quality of data in an application capturing nursing documentation.

However, when thinking about who is responsible for the data in a data warehouse, the concept of a data steward is more appropriate. "Data stewardship is the aspect of data governance that focuses on providing the appropriate access to users, helping users to understand the data, and taking ownership of data quality. Without appropriate stewardship, even the best infrastructures become underutilized and poorly understood by knowledge workers who could be generating value with the data every day" (Just, 2013, p. 4). A data steward does not own the data but ensures its quality. The data steward is the "keeper of the data," not the "owner of the data." See Box 6.1 for implications for nursing.

The National Committee on Vital and Health Statistics (NCVHS) under the authorship of Kanaan and Carr (2009)

BOX 6.1   WHY HEALTHCARE DATA STEWARDSHIP IS SO IMPORTANT IN NURSING*

1. Good data warehouse architecture promotes good data stewardship. In nursing this means standard nursing languages that are consistent with and integrated into other standard languages in healthcare as well as standard nurse-sensitive quality indicators.

2. Good data warehouse tools promote good data stewardship. In nursing, access to data is usually based on who has clinical responsibility for the delivery of care. As a result a top nursing administrator may have access to all patient data. But this may not be the person who can best interpret the implications of the data for meeting specific patient needs. Not only do we need good data warehouse tools but we also need clinical nurse leaders who can access these data and the skills to use the tools for analyzing nursing data and meeting patient needs.

3. Good data stewardship creates a well-informed and thriving user base. Nurses are knowledge workers but only if they have access to the data and the information in that data can they apply that knowledge in meeting the needs of patients, families, and the community of patients with similar needs.

---

* Data from Just (2013).

issued a primer titled "Health Data Stewardship: What, Why, Who, How: An NCVHS Primer." In this primer four key principles were identified with implications for nurses:

- Individual rights to access and to correct their own data. This includes building trust by making the data transparent and by requiring consent for this data use.
- A data steward with responsibilities for data quality, for identifying the purpose in using specific data, application of good statistical practices, and so forth.
- Appropriate safeguards and controls to ensure confidentiality, integrity, and protection of the data from unauthorized access, use, or disclosure.
- Policies for appropriate use and accountability for those using the data.

Given the potential for both benefits and risks from the sharing and reuse of health data, consensus is building in the United States and beyond that everyone who touches individual health data for any purpose—health care, research, quality assessment, population health monitoring, payment, and more—must understand and practice data stewardship (Kanaan & Carr, 2009, p. 5).

The Development of Big Data

Big data is the term used to describe the amount of data generated from digital sources such as sensors, social media, and monitoring devices in addition to traditional digital data from EMRs, diagnostic tests, images, and so forth. The 3 Vs—volume, velocity, and variety—describe big data (Fernandes, O'Connor, & Weaver, 2012). Volume relates to the amount of data that are generated with increasing use of technology. While there is no one source that is quantifying the size of healthcare data, general estimates by McKinsey's Global Institute group place it in the several hundred exabyte (1 000 000 000 000 000 000 bytes) range (Manyika, Chui, Brown, Bughin, Dobbs, Roxburgh, & Byers, 2011). Velocity means the frequency of data delivery; technology is influencing velocity through the use of monitoring and sensing devices, embedded chips, and so forth. Variety means the forms in which data exist. In healthcare this means data in unstructured text format, data from monitoring devices, images, and so forth. These data are more unstructured than one typically finds in a database. The biggest issue in healthcare is how to tap the potential value of these data. Big data present new challenges related to how healthcare data are organized, retrieved, and used to personalize patient care. McKinsey & Company published a report titled "The

'big data' revolution in healthcare: Accelerating value and innovation" that outlines new value pathways to assist in decision-making regarding issues of the correct care for patients while also addressing what is right for the healthcare system (Groves, Kayyali, Knott, & Kuiken, 2013). These five values are right living, right care, right provider, right value, and right innovation. The questions for nursing are: How does nursing tap into big data for benchmarking and outcomes measurements and how do we add value? Is value now the fourth V in big data?

DATA/INFORMATION TO KNOWLEDGE (KDD)

Data Mining

Traditional methods of retrieving information from databases no longer work with the sheer amount of data that the healthcare industry is producing. One can generate and store data far faster than one can analyze and understand it. We can refer to the process of extracting information and knowledge from large-scale databases as knowledge discovery and data mining (KDD). The purpose of data mining is to find previously unknown patterns and trends that will assist in providing quality care, predicting best treatment choices, and utilizing health resources in a cost-effective manner.

A traditional approach to the KDD development includes a seven-step process. These steps are task analysis, data selection, data cleaning, data transformation, data mining, pattern interpretation and evaluation, and deployment. Bagga and Singh (2011) propose a three-step process: pre-processing, data mining, and post-processing. Regardless of the approach, the first task is to define the goal of the process. What is the problem specification? Once this task is complete, one must identify the appropriate data needs, and prepare (clean) and process the appropriate data. This will result in the appropriate data set that is complete and accurate.

The next task is data mining. This means to apply computational techniques to find the patterns and trends. Some examples of data mining techniques include rule set classifiers like IF conditions, THEN conclusion, decision tree algorithms, logistic regression analysis, neuro-fuzzy techniques, and memory-based reasoning (Srinivas, Rani, & Govrdhan, 2010; Zurada & Lonial, 2005).

Once you mine the data, you visualize the results. The question here is how to present the results to decision-makers. What does this mean? How can we use this "new" knowledge? Some questions depending on the goal of the data mining could be: What does this mean for evaluating treatment effectiveness? How might we use this knowledge to impact the management of healthcare? How might this help with detection of fraud and abuse? How might this help predict who is at risk for a certain health problem? How might we provide personalized care and treatment? (Kob & Tan, 2005).

Benchmarking

Benchmarking is a process where one compares outcome measures with industry averages. Sower (2007) proposes that it be expanded to be more than industry averages but a comparison against the best of the best. Healthcare organization should not be content with being average, but should be analyzing what they can do to be the best of the best. The question to ask is, What is x and y doing that makes them stand out in whatever indicators they are assessing? To achieve excellence in x, y, and z, you must analyze what the best are doing in x, y, and z.

The process of benchmarking means to determine the goal or objectives, define appropriate indicators, collect data, and determine results (Nolte, 2010). One of the first items to address in benchmarking is what are you benchmarking and how will you use that to improve performance? Will the benchmark indicators be internal or external? Will you measure structure, process, and outcomes? Structure measures examine the organization and whether a structure is in place that will facilitate quality, cost-effective care. Process measures such things as screening, diagnosing, and managing patient care, addressing how things are done. Outcomes track the results.

Outcome Probabilities

The concept of outcome probability is built on the statistical concept of probability. If one would toss a fair coin in the air 100 times, one would expect that 50% of the time the coin would come up heads. In this example, there are a number of possibilities ranging from 0% heads to 100% heads; however, the farther the actual results are from the 50%, the more probable it is that something is affecting these results besides the random toss of a fair coin. With a slight variation from 50% the variation is likely due to chance. In fact if this experiment is repeated many times 68% of the time the scores will range between 16% and 84% heads.

If this concept is transferred to nursing, the question becomes, What is the probability that a certain intervention will result in a certain outcome? For example, if using alcohol swabs to clean the skin before inserting an IV, will the probability of an infection at the site decrease from the probability if you use nothing? This example represents a simple straightforward question that traditional research approaches can answer. However, with nursing care, as is true in healthcare in general, many of the outcomes are

long-term and influenced by a variety of factors. In the past traditional research has been too slow and too expensive to answer many of these important questions. For example, what is the probability that a home health visit to all new mothers will impact the health status of children at the point they graduate from grade school? Certainly there will be a wide range of outcomes across this population of children, but is there a difference in that pattern of outcomes—are more children experiencing good health? With the advent of EHRs and information exchange networks nurses must now move forward with developing real-time data mining skills in answering these key nursing questions and thereby generating outcome probabilities that are based on big data and not small samples.

WISDOM

The continuum begins with data, the raw facts. As the data are named, collected, and organized, data become information. By discovering the meaningful facts in the information and the relationships between the facts, a knowledge base is built. By understanding the knowledge and the implications of that knowledge nurses are able to manage a wide range of human health problems. The appropriate and ethical use of knowledge to manage human problems is termed wisdom. Certainly this continuum can and does exist without the use of automated systems. But over the last 50 years nursing has experienced the introduction of the computer and the automation of this process. As early as the 1980s, Blum (1986) demonstrated that automated systems could be used to process data, information, and knowledge. Figure 6.5 presents the relationship between automated systems and this continuum. Over the years as computers have become increasingly powerful and able to manage larger and larger data sets a controversial question is, "Can any aspect of wisdom be automated?" A related and equally important question is, "How can we design and implement automated systems especially decision support and expert systems to best support the wisdom of expert nurses while maintaining clear guidelines and standards of practice?"

Knowledge Application

While decision support systems produce knowledge from information, expert systems use that knowledge base and transform it to produce wisdom. With the emergence of supercomputers in the 1990s nursing had a unique opportunity to further nursing's knowledge and practice. A proposed theory of nursing knowledge/wisdom uses the formula NKW(IB) = P, where NK is nursing knowledge, W is wisdom, "IB is the individual nurse's integration

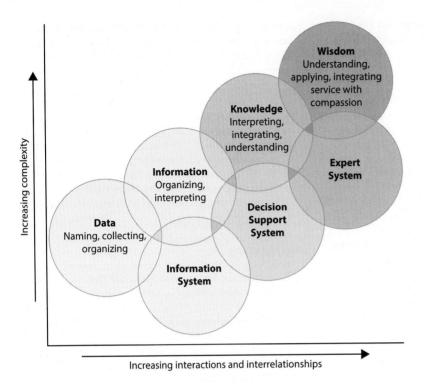

and synthesis of nursing knowledge through cognitive, psychomotor, and affective/spiritual domain of self" (Kalofissudis, 2007, para. 9), and P represents the breadth and depth of practice. Expert systems require a sound knowledge base as one of its components.

Expert Support/Systems

Expert systems represent the present and future vanguard of nursing informatics. These systems aim to help make the nurse "more intelligent" in providing quality care based on evidence. Expert systems use artificial intelligence (AI) to model the decisions an expert nurse would make. They provide the "best decision" recommendation based on what an expert nurse would do unlike decision support systems that provide several options from which the nurse selects.

Some of the advantages of expert systems include the following:

- Provide a solution more quickly than humans
- Reduce waste and cut costs
- Improve patient care by sharing the knowledge and wisdom of human experts

As early as the mid-1980s and early 1990s articles were published describing the components of expert systems and uses in nursing (Darlington, 1997; Turley, 1993). Expert systems have four main components: natural language, knowledge base, a database, and an inference engine as well as a means of capturing expert knowledge and an explanation to the end user as to the rationale behind the recommendation. See Table 6.3 for definitions of these terms.

TABLE 6.3	Definitions of Components of Expert System
Component	**Definition**
Natural Language	Used to interface and interact with the end user
Knowledge Base	Contains rules for decision-making
Database	Facts specific to the domain focus, i.e., nursing
Inference Engine	Links the knowledge base rules with the database

A current example today is IBM's Watson that understands natural language and can process large amounts of data quickly using rules and machine learning. In the medical field Watson can diagnose and suggest a treatment option, search the Internet for new information in real time, and diagnose conditions in some cases with more accuracy than an expert doctor (IBM, n.d.).

Evidence-Based Practice

The concept of evidence-based practice is widely accepted across each of the healthcare disciplines; however, the reality of providing evidence-based care at the point of care is often an elusive goal. With the advent of Big Data and data analytics techniques capable of analyzing Big Data along with expert systems capable of analyzing unstructured data and using natural language to present the resulting conclusions, real-time evidence-based practice is a potential reality. But for nursing to achieve this potential reality nursing data, information, knowledge, and wisdom must consistently be included in building automated healthcare information systems.

SUMMARY

This chapter describes data processing. The focus of the chapter is on understanding concepts and issues necessary to effectively use database systems in healthcare. The chapter begins by discussing the difference between data and information. It describes the process of using an information system to produce information from data. The chapter explains data structures and models and reviews the purpose(s), structures, and functions of automated database systems. The chapter outlines the life cycle of an automated database system. Building on an understanding of databases, the chapter explores concepts and issues that relate to data warehouses and knowledge discovery within large data sets. The chapter concludes by describing how an understanding of databases is key to understanding the data to wisdom continuum in nursing.

REFERENCES

1Keydata. (2014). *Data warehousing>concepts>conceptual data model.* Retrieved from http://www.1keydata.com/datawarehousing/datawarehouse.html

Bagga, S., & Singh, G. (2011). Three phase iterative model of KDD. *International Journal of Information Technology and Knowledge Management, 4*(2):695–697.

Barlow, R. (2013). Making clinical data analytics count: Does size, volume really matter? *Health Management Technology, 43*(12), 8–11.

Barney, K. (2013, April). *Data in motion: An opportunity for healthcare providers.* Retrieved from http://blogs.cisco.com/ioe/data-in-motion-an-opportunity-for-healthcare-providers/

Blum, B. (1986). *Clinical information systems.* New York, NY: Springer-Verlag.

Cisco Public Information. (2013). *White paper: Increase the value and relevance of data in motion.* Retrieved from http://share.cisco.com/DiM/

Darlington, K. (1997). Expert systems in nursing. Retrieved from http://www.bcs.org/upload/pdf/nsg-itin-vol9-darlington1.pdf

Doyle, M. (2013). *6 Surprising benefits of healthcare data warehouse: Getting more than you expected.* Retrieved from http://www.healthcatalyst.com/healthcare-data-warehouse-questions

Enterprise Information Systems Steering Committee, Data Warehousing Work Group. (2009). *Data warehousing: A new focus in healthcare data management.* Retrieved from http://www.himss.org/ResourceLibrary/ResourceDetail.aspx?ItemNumber=7913

Executive Office of the President. (2012, March 29). *Big data across the federal government.* Retrieved from http://www.whitehouse.gov/sites/default/files/microsites/ostp/big_data_fact_sheet_final.pdf

Fernandes, L., O'Connor, M., & Weaver, V. (2012). Big data, bigger outcomes. *Journal of AHIMA, 83*(10), 38–43.

Frost & Sullivan. (2011). *Drowning in big data? Reducing information technology complexities and costs for healthcare organizations.* Retrieved from http://www.emc.com/collateral/analyst-reports/frost-sullivan-reducing-information-technology-complexities-ar.pdf

Groves, P., Kayyali, B., Knott, D., & Kuiken, S. (2013). *The 'big data' revolution in healthcare: Accelerating value and innovation.* Retrieved from http://www.mckinsey.com/insights/health_systems_and_services/the_big-data_revolution_in_us_health_care

Hamilton, B. (2013). Impacts of big data. *Health Management Technology, 34*(8), 12–13.

Hay, D. (2010). *Different kinds of data models: History and a suggestion.* Retrieved from http://www.tdan.com/print/14400

IBM. (n.d.). *Watson in healthcare.* Retrieved from http://www-03.ibm.com/innovation/us/watson/watson_in_healthcare.shtml

IBM. (2013, June). *Introduction to DB2 for z/OS.* Retrieved from http://publib.boulder.ibm.com/iepubs/pdf/dsnitm06.pdf

iDashboards. (2013). *iDashboards for healthcare: Providing insight for operational success.* Retrieved from www.iDashboards.com

Inmon, B. (2007, January). Data warehousing in a healthcare environment. *TDWI World Conference. The Data Administration Newsletter-TDAN.com.* Retrieved from http://inmoncif.com/registration/whitepapers/DATA%20WAREHOUSING%20IN%20THE%20HEALTHCARE%20ENVIRONMENTR1.pdf.

Joos, I., Nelson, R., & Smith, M. (2014). *Introduction to computers for healthcare professionals*. Burlington, MA: Jones & Barlett Learning.

Just, E. (2013, June). *3 reasons why healthcare data stewardship is so important*. Retrieved from http://www.healthcatalyst.com/healthcare_data_stewardship_data_rich_information_rich/

Kalofissudis, I. (2007). The theory of nursing knowledge (editorial). *Health Science Journal, 1*(4). Retrieved from http://www.hsj.gr/volume1/issue4/editorialkalof.pdf

Kanaan, S., & Carr, J. (2009, September). *Health data stewardship: What, why, who, how: An NCVHS Primer*. Retrieved from http://www.ncvhs.hhs.gov/090930lt.pdf

Kob, H., & Tan, G. (2005). Data mining applications in healthcare. *Journal of Healthcare Information Management, 19*(2), 64–72.

Manyika, J., Chui, M., Brown, B., Bughin, J., Dobbs, R., Roxburgh, C., & Byers, A. (2011, May). *Big data: The next frontier for innovation, competition, and productivity*. Retrieved from http://www.mckinsey.com/insights/business_technology/big_data_the_next_frontier_for_innovation

Morris, G., Farnum, G., Afzal, S., Robinson, C., Greene, J., & Coughlin, C. (2014). Patient identification and matching initial findings. *Prepared for the Office of the National Coordinator for Health Information Technology by Aduaciaous, Inquiry, LLC*. Retrieved from http://www.healthit.gov/sites/default/files/patient_Identification_Matching_Final_Report.pdf

Nolte, E. (2010). *International benchmarking of healthcare quality: A review of the literature*. Retrieved from http://www.rand.org/content/dam/rand/pubs/technical_reports/2010/RAND_TR738.pdf

ONC. (2013, December). *ONC releases findings from patient data matching study*. Retreived from http://www.ihealthbeat.org/articles/2013/12/17/onc-releases-findings-from-patient-data-matching-study

Perna, G. (2013, September). *ONC announces patient matching initiative*. Retrieved from http://www.healthcare-informatics.com/news-item/onc-announces-patient-matching-initiative

Quillin, T. (2013, November). *Lock these three doors to help protect your data*. Retrieved from http://blogs.intel.com/technology/2013/11/lock-these-three-doors-to-help-protect-your-data/

Rodrigues, T. (2012). *10 emerging technologies for big data*. Retrieved from http://www.techrepublic.com/blog/big-data-analytics/10-emerging-technologies-for-big-data/

Sower, V. (2007, August). *Benchmarking in hospitals: More than a scorecard*. Retreieved from http://www.shsu.edu/~mgt_ves/BenchmarkingArticle.pdf

Srinivas, K., Rani, B., & Govrdhan, A. (2010). Applications of data mining techniques in healthcare and prediction of heart attacks. *International Journal on Computer Science and Engineering, 2*(2), 250–255.

Turley, J. (1993). *The use of artificial intelligence in nursing information systems*. Retrieved from http://project.net.au/hisavic/hisa/mag/may93/the.htm

Zachman, J. (2008). *John Zachman's concise definition of the Zachman framework*. Retrieved from http://www.zachman.com/about-the-zachman-framework

Zurada, J., & Lonial, S. (2005). Comparison of the performance of several data mining methods for bad debt recovery in the healthcare industry. *The Journal of Applied Business Research, 21*(2), 37–53.

7

Health Data Standards: Development, Harmonization, and Interoperability

Joyce Sensmeier

• OBJECTIVES

1. Discuss the need for health data standards.
2. Describe the standards development process and related organizations.
3. Delineate the importance of health information exchange and interoperability.
4. Describe current health data standards initiatives.
5. Explore the business value of health data standards.

• KEY WORDS

Standards
Health information exchange
Knowledge representation
Interoperability
Clinical integration
Terminology

INTRODUCTION

Standards are foundational to the development, implementation, and exchange of electronic health records (EHRs). The effectiveness of healthcare delivery is dependent on the ability of clinicians to securely access health information when and where it is needed. The capability of exchanging health information across organizational and system boundaries, whether between multiple departments within a single institution or among a varied cast of providers, payers, regulators, and others, is essential. A harmonized set of rules and definitions, both at the level of data meaning as well as at the technical level of data exchange, is needed to make this possible. Additionally, there must be a sociopolitical structure in place that recognizes the benefits of shared information and incentivizes the adoption and implementation of such standards to improve population health management.

This chapter examines health data standards in terms of the following topic areas:

Need for health data standards

Standards development process, organizations, and categories

Knowledge representation

Standards coordination and harmonization

Health information exchange and interoperability

Health data standards initiatives

Business value of health data standards

INTRODUCTION TO HEALTH DATA STANDARDS

The ability to communicate in a way that ensures the message is received and the content is understood is dependent on standards. Data standards are intended to reduce ambiguity in communication so that the actions taken based on data are consistent with the actual meaning of that data. The Health Information Technology for Economic and Clinical Health (HITECH) Act is driving U.S. efforts to transform healthcare through the meaningful use of health data. This goal will be advanced through a phased-in series of improved clinical data capture processes that support more rigorous quality measures and improvements. This transformation requires data capture and sharing and advanced clinical processes, which will enable improved health outcomes. This ultimate end state can only be achieved through the organized structuring and effective use of information to support better decision-making and more effective care processes, thus improving health outcomes and reducing costs.

While current information technology (IT) is able to move and manipulate large amounts of data, it is not as proficient in dealing with ambiguity in the structure and semantic content of that data. The term *health data standards* is generally used to describe those standards having to do with the structure and content of health information. However, it may be useful to differentiate data from information and knowledge. Data are the fundamental building blocks on which healthcare decisions are based. Data are collections of unstructured, discrete entities (facts) that exist outside of any particular context. When data are interpreted within a given context and given meaningful structure within that context, they become information. The term *interoperability* describes the extent to which systems and devices can exchange data, and interpret that shared data. For two systems to be interoperable, they must be able to exchange data and subsequently present that data such that it can be understood by a user (HIMSS, 2013). When information from various contexts is aggregated following a defined set of rules, it becomes knowledge and provides the basis for informed action (Nelson, 2006). Data standards represent both data and their transformation into information. Data analysis generates knowledge, which is the foundation of professional practice standards.

Standards are created by several methods (Hammond, 2005): (1) a group of interested parties comes together and agrees upon a standard; (2) the government sanctions a process for standards to be developed; (3) marketplace competition and technology adoption introduces a de facto standard; (4) a formal consensus process is used by a standards development organization (SDO). The standards development process typically begins with a use case or business need that describes a system's behavior as it responds to a request that originates from outside of that system. Technical experts then consider what methods, protocols, terminologies, or specifications are needed to address the requirements of the use case. An open acceptance or balloting process is desirable to ensure that the developed standards have representative stakeholder input, which minimizes bias and encourages marketplace adoption and implementation.

Legislated, government-developed standards are able to gain widespread acceptance by virtue of their being required by either regulation or in order to participate in large, government-funded programs, such as Medicare. Because government-developed standards are in the public domain, they are available at little or no cost and can be incorporated into any information system; however, they are often developed to support particular government initiatives and may not be as suitable for general, private sector use. Also, given the amount of bureaucratic overhead attached to the legislative and regulatory process, it is likely that they will lag behind changes in technology and the general business environment.

Standards developed by SDOs are typically consensus-based and reflect the perspectives of a wide variety of interested stakeholders. They are generally not tied to specific systems. For this reason, they tend to be robust and adaptable across a range of implementations; however, most SDOs are non-profit organizations that rely on the commitment of dedicated volunteers to develop and maintain standards. This often limits the amount of work that can be undertaken. In addition, the consensus process can be time consuming and result in a slow development process, which does not always keep pace with technological change. Perhaps the most problematic aspect of consensus-based standards is that there is no mechanism to ensure that they are adopted by the industry, since there is usually little infrastructure in place for SDOs to actively and aggressively market them. This has resulted in the development of many technically competent standards that are never implemented. The U.S. Standards Strategy (ANSI, 2005) states, "The goal of all international standards forums should be to achieve globally relevant and internationally recognized and accepted standards that support trade and commerce while protecting the environment, health, safety, and security."

There are a number of drivers in the current standards landscape that are working to accelerate health data standards adoption and implementation through innovative efforts and incentives that address this charge.

STANDARDS CATEGORIES

Four broad areas are identified to categorize health data standards (Department of Health and Human Services, 2010). Transport standards are used to establish a common, predictable, secure communication protocol between systems. Vocabulary standards consist of nomenclatures and code sets used to describe clinical problems and procedures, medications, and allergies. Content exchange standards and value sets are used to share clinical information such as clinical summaries, prescriptions, and structured electronic documents. Security standards are used to safeguard the transmission of health data through authentication and access control.

Transport Standards

Transport standards primarily address the format of messages that are exchanged between computer systems, document architecture, clinical templates, the user interface, and patient data linkage (Committee on Data Standards for Patient Safety, 2004). To achieve data compatibility between systems, it is necessary to have prior agreement on the syntax of the messages to be exchanged. The receiving system must be able to divide the incoming message into discrete data elements that reflect what the sending system wishes to communicate. The following section describes some of the major SDOs involved in the development of transport standards.

Accredited Standards Committee X12N/Insurance. Accredited Standards Committee (ASC) X12N has developed a broad range of electronic data interchange (EDI) standards to facilitate electronic business transactions. In the healthcare arena, X12N standards have been adopted as national standards for such administrative transactions as claims, enrollment, and eligibility in health plans, and first report of injury under the requirements of the Health Insurance Portability and Accountability Act (HIPAA). Due to the uniqueness of health insurance and the varying policies for protection of personal health information from country to country, these standards are primarily used in the United States. HIPAA directed the Secretary of the Department of Health and Human Services (HHS) to adopt standards for transactions to enable health information to be exchanged electronically, and the Administrative Simplification Act (ASA), one of the HIPAA provisions, requires standard formats to be used for electronically submitted healthcare transactions. The American National Standards Institute (ANSI) developed these, and the ANSI X12N 837 Implementation Guide has been established as the standard of compliance for claims transactions.

Institute of Electrical and Electronic Engineers. The Institute of Electrical and Electronic Engineers (IEEE) has developed a series of standards known collectively as P1073 Medical Information Bus (MIB), which support real-time, continuous, and comprehensive capture and communication of data from bedside medical devices such as those found in intensive care units, operating rooms, and emergency departments. These data include physiological parameter measurements and device settings. IEEE standards for IT focus on telecommunications and information exchange between systems including local and metropolitan area networks. The IEEE 802.xx suite of wireless networking standards, supporting local and metropolitan area networks, has advanced developments in the communications market. The most widely known standard, 802.11, commonly referred to as Wi-Fi, allows anyone with a "smart" mobile device or a computer to connect to the Internet wirelessly through myriad access points. IEEE 11073 standards are designed to help healthcare product vendors and integrators create interoperable devices and systems for disease management, health, and fitness. The growing IEEE 11073 family of standards is intended to enable interoperable communication for traditional medical devices, as well as personal health devices.

National Electrical Manufacturers Association. The National Electrical Manufacturers Association (NEMA), in collaboration with the American College of Radiologists (ACR) and others, formed DICOM (Digital Imaging and Communications in Medicine) to develop a generic digital format and a transfer protocol for biomedical images and image-related information. DICOM enables the transfer of medical images in a multi-vendor environment and facilitates the development and expansion of picture archiving and communication systems (PACS). The specification is usable on any type of computer system and supports transfer over the Internet. The DICOM standard is the dominant international data interchange message format in biomedical imaging. The Joint NEMA/The European Coordination Committee of the Radiological and Electromedical Industry/Japan Industries Association of Radiological Systems (COCIR/JIRA) Security and Privacy Committee (SPC) issued a white paper that provides a guide for vendors and users on how to protect health information systems against viruses, Trojan horses, denial of service attacks, Internet worms, and related forms of so-called malicious software.

World Wide Web Consortium. The World Wide Web Consortium (W3C) is the main international standards organization for development of the World Wide Web (abbreviated WWW or W3). W3C also publishes XML

(Extensible Markup Language), which is a set of rules for encoding documents in machine-readable format. XML is most commonly used in exchanging data over the Internet. It is defined in the XML 1.0 Specification produced by the W3C and several other related specifications, all of which are available in the public domain. XML's design goals emphasize simplicity, generality, and usability over the Internet, which also makes it desirable for use in cross-enterprise health information exchange. It is a textual data format, with strong support for the languages of the world. Although XML's design focuses on documents, it is widely used for the representation of arbitrary data structures such as Web Services. Web Services use XML messages that follow the Simple Object Access Protocol (SOAP) standard and have been popular with traditional enterprises. Other transport protocols include the Representational State Transfer (REST) architectural style, which was developed in parallel with the Hypertext Transfer Protocol (HTTP) used in Web browsers. The largest known implementation of a system conforming to the REST architectural style is the World Wide Web.

Communication Protocols. In telecommunications, a protocol is a system of digital rules for data exchange within or between computers. When data are exchanged through a computer network, the rules system is called a network protocol. Communication systems use well-defined formats for exchanging messages. A protocol must define the syntax, semantics, and synchronization of the communication. Examples of communication protocols include the Transmission Control Protocol/Internet Protocol (TCP/IP) which is the suite of communication protocols used to connect hosts on the Internet. TCP/IP is built into the UNIX operating system and is used by the Internet, making it the de facto standard for transmitting data over networks. File Transfer Protocol (FTP) is a standard network protocol used to transfer files from one host to another host over a TCP-based network, such as the Internet. Simple Mail Transfer Protocol (SMTP) is an Internet standard for electronic mail (e-mail) transmission.

Vocabulary Standards

A fundamental requirement for effective communication is the ability to represent concepts in an unambiguous fashion between both the sender and the receiver of the message. Natural human languages are incredibly rich in their ability to communicate subtle differences in the semantic content, or meaning, of messages. While there have been great advances in the ability of computers to process natural language, most communication between health information systems relies on the use of structured vocabularies, terminologies, code sets, and classification systems to represent health concepts. Standardized terminologies enable data collection at the point of care, and retrieval of data, information, and knowledge in support of clinical practice. The following examples describe several of the major systems.

Current Procedural Terminology. The Current Procedural Terminology (CPT) code set, maintained by the American Medical Association (AMA), accurately describes medical, surgical, and diagnostic services. It is designed to communicate uniform information about medical services and procedures among physicians, coders, patients, accreditation organizations, and payers for administrative, financial, and analytical purposes. The current version is the CPT 2013. In addition to descriptive terms and codes, it contains modifiers, notes, and guidelines to facilitate correct usage. While primarily used in the United States for reimbursement purposes, it has also been adopted for other data purposes.

International Statistical Classification of Diseases and Related Health Problems: *Ninth Revision and Clinical Modifications.* The *International Statistical Classification of Diseases and Related Health Problems*: Ninth Revision and Clinical Modifications (ICD-9-CM) (World Health Organization, 1980) is a version of a mortality and morbidity classification used since 1979 for reporting in the United States. It is widely accepted and used in the healthcare industry and has been adopted for a number of purposes including data collection, quality-of-care analysis, resource utilization, and statistical reporting. While ICD-9 procedure codes are the acceptable HIPAA code set for inpatient claims, Healthcare Common Procedure Coding System/Current Procedural Terminology (HCPCS/CPT) codes are the valid set for outpatient claims.

International Statistical Classification of Diseases and Related Health Problems: *Tenth Revision.* The *International Statistical Classification of Diseases and Related Health Problems*: Tenth Revision (ICD-10) is the most recent revision of the ICD classification system for mortality and morbidity, which is used worldwide. In addition to diagnostic labels, the ICD-10 also encompasses nomenclature structures. On October 1, 2014, the ICD-9 code sets used to report medical diagnoses and inpatient procedures will be replaced by ICD-10 code sets. The transition to ICD-10 is required for everyone covered by HIPAA; however, the change to ICD-10 does not affect CPT coding for outpatient procedures and physician services. The transition to ICD-10-CM and ICD-10 Procedural Coding System (ICD-10-PCS) is anticipated to improve the capture of health information and bring the United States in step with coding systems worldwide. For those who prepare appropriately, leveraging the ICD-10 investment will allow organizations to move beyond compliance to achieve competitive advantage (Bowman, 2008). Moving to the new code sets will also improve efficiencies and lower administrative costs due to replacement of a dysfunctional classification system.

Nursing and Other Domain-Specific Terminologies. The American Nurses Association (ANA) has spearheaded efforts to coordinate the various minimum data sets and standardized nursing terminologies. The ANA has recognized the following nursing terminologies that support nursing practice: ABC Codes, Clinical Care Classification, International Classification of Nursing Practice, Logical Observation Identifiers Names and Codes (LOINC), North American Nursing Diagnosis Association, Nursing Interventions Classification (NIC), Nursing Outcome Classification (NOC), Nursing Management Minimum Data Set, Nursing Minimum Data Set, Omaha System, Patient Care Data Set (retired), Perioperative Nursing Data Set, and SNOMED-CT (Rutherford, 2008). These standard terminologies enable knowledge representation of nursing content. Nurses use assessment data and nursing judgment to determine nursing diagnoses, interventions, and outcomes. These elements can be linked together using standards to represent nursing knowledge.

RxNorm. RxNorm is a standardized nomenclature for clinical drugs and drug delivery devices produced by the National Library of Medicine (NLM). Because every drug information system follows somewhat different naming conventions, a standardized nomenclature is needed for the consistent exchange of information, not only between organizations but even within the same organization. For example, a hospital may use one system for ordering and another for inventory management. Still another system might be used to record dose adjustments or to check drug interactions. The goal of RxNorm is to allow various systems using different drug nomenclatures to share data efficiently at the appropriate level of abstraction. RxNorm contains the names of prescription and many nonprescription formulations that exist in the United States, including the devices that administer the medications.

Unified Medical Language System. Currently, the Unified Medical Language System (UMLS) consists of a metathesaurus of terms and concepts from dozens of vocabularies, a semantic network of relationships among the concepts recognized in the metathesaurus, and an information sources map of the various biomedical databases referenced. There are specialized vocabularies, code sets, and classification systems for almost every practice domain in healthcare. Most of these are not compatible with one another, and much work needs to be done to achieve usable mapping and linkages between them. There have been a number of efforts to develop mapping and linkages among various code sets, classification systems, and vocabularies. One of the most successful is the UMLS project undertaken by the NLM.

The NLM supports the development, enhancement, and distribution of clinically specific vocabularies to facilitate the exchange of clinical data to improve retrieval of health information. In 1986, the NLM began an ambitious long-term project to map and link a large number of vocabularies from a number of knowledge sources to allow retrieval and integration of relevant machine-readable information. The NLM is the central coordinating body for clinical terminology standards within HHS (National Library of Medicine, 2010). The NLM works closely with the Office of the National Coordinator for Health Information Technology (ONC) to ensure NLM's efforts are aligned with the goal of the President and HHS Secretary to achieve nationwide implementation of an interoperable health IT infrastructure to improve the quality and efficiency of healthcare.

Other domain-specific terminologies include Current Dental Terminology (CDT), International Medical Terminology (IMT), and *Diagnostic and Statistical Manual of Mental Disorders* (DSM-IV-TR) to name just a few.

Content Standards

Content Standards are related to the data content within information exchanges. Information content standards define the structure and content organization of the electronic message's or document's information content. They can also define a "package" of content standards (messages or documents). In addition to standardizing the format of health data messages and the lexicons and value sets used in those messages, there is widespread interest in defining common sets of data for specific message types. The concept of a *minimum data set* is defined as "a minimum set of items with uniform definitions and categories concerning a specific aspect or dimension of the healthcare system which meets the essential needs of multiple users" (Health Information Policy Council, 1983).

A related concept is that of a *core data element*. It has been defined as "a standard data element with a uniform definition and coding convention to collect data on persons and on events or encounters" (National Committee on Vital and Health Statistics, 1996). Core data elements are seen as serving as the building blocks for well-formed minimum data sets and may appear in several minimum data sets. The following are some examples of minimum, or core, data sets currently in use. As with code sets, professional specialty groups are often the best source for current information on minimum data set development efforts. A number of SDOs have been increasingly interested in incorporating domain-specific data sets into their messaging standards.

American Society for Testing and Materials. The American Society for Testing and Materials (ASTM) is one of the largest SDOs in the world and publishes standards covering all sectors in the economy. More than 13,000 ASTM standards are used worldwide to improve product quality, enhance safety, and facilitate trade. The ASTM Committee E31 on Healthcare Informatics has developed a wide range of standards supporting the electronic management of health information.

Clinical Data Interchange Standards Consortium. The Clinical Data Interchange Standards Consortium (CDISC) is a global, multidisciplinary consortium that has established standards to support the acquisition, exchange, submission, and archive of clinical research data and metadata. CDISC develops and supports global, platform-independent data standards that enable information system interoperability to improve medical research and related areas of healthcare. One example is the Biomedical Research Integrated Domain Group (BRIDG) Model, which is a domain analysis model representing protocol-driven biomedical and clinical research. The BRIDG model emerged from an unprecedented collaborative effort among clinical trial experts from CDISC, the National Institutes of Health (NIH)/National Cancer Institute (NCI), the Food and Drug Administration (FDA), HL7, and other volunteers. This structured information model is being used to support development of data interchange standards and technology solutions that will enable harmonization between the biomedical and clinical research and healthcare arenas.

Health Level Seven. Health Level Seven (HL7) is an SDO that develops standards in multiple categories including transport and content. HL7 standards focus on facilitating the exchange of data to support clinical practice both within and across institutions. HL7 standards cover a broad spectrum of areas for information exchange including medical orders, clinical observations, test results, admission/transfer/discharge, document architecture, clinical templates, user interface, EHR, and charge and billing information. A primary example of an HL7 standard is Clinical Document Architecture (CDA) which is

an XML-based document markup standard that specifies the structure and semantics of clinical documents for the purpose of exchange. HL7 standards are widely implemented by healthcare provider organizations worldwide, many of which have adapted the basic standards for use in their particular settings.

International Health Terminology Standards Development Organisation. The International Health Terminology Standards Development Organisation (IHTSDO) is a not-for-profit association in Denmark that develops and promotes use of SNOMED-CT to support safe and effective health information exchange. It was formed in 2006 with the purpose of developing and maintaining international health terminology systems. SNOMED-CT is a comprehensive clinical terminology, originally created by the College of American Pathologists (CAP) and, as of April 2007, owned, maintained, and distributed by the IHTSDO. The CAP continues to support SNOMED-CT operations under contract to the IHTSDO and provides SNOMED-related products and services as a licensee of the terminology. The NLM is the U.S. member of the IHTSDO and, as such, distributes SNOMED-CT at no cost in accordance with the member rights and responsibilities outlined in the IHTSDO's Articles of Association. SNOMED-CT is one of a suite of designated standards for use in U.S. federal government systems for the electronic exchange of clinical health information and is specified as a required standard for the creation and exchange of patient medical record information within the HHS Electronic Health Record Incentive Program.

LOINC. Logical Observation Identifiers Names and Codes (LOINC) is a database and universal standard for identifying medical laboratory observations. It was developed and is maintained by the Regenstrief Institute in 1994. The purpose of LOINC is to assist in the electronic exchange and gathering of clinical results (such as laboratory tests, clinical observations, and outcomes management and research). Since its inception, the database has expanded to include not just medical and laboratory code names but also nursing diagnosis, nursing interventions, outcomes classification, and patient care data set.

National Council for Prescription Drug Programs. The National Council for Prescription Drug Programs (NCPDP) develops both content and transport standards for information processing in the pharmacy services sector of the healthcare industry. This is a very successful example of how standards can enable significant improvements in service delivery. Since the introduction of this standard in 1992, the retail pharmacy industry has moved to 100% electronic claims processing in real time. NCPDP standards are forming the basis for electronic prescription transactions. Electronic prescription transactions are defined as EDI messages flowing between healthcare providers (i.e., pharmacy software systems and prescriber software systems) that are concerned with prescription orders. NCPDP's Telecommunication Standard Version 5.1 was named the official standard for pharmacy claims within HIPAA, and NCPDP is also named in other U.S. federal legislation titled the Medicare Prescription Drug, Improvement, and Modernization Act. Other NCPDP standards include the SCRIPT Standard for Electronic Prescribing, and the Manufacturers Rebate Standard.

National Uniform Claim Committee Recommended Data Set for a Noninstitutional Claim. Organized in 1995, the scope of the National Uniform Claim Committee (NUCC) was to develop, promote, and maintain a standard data set for use in noninstitutional claims and encounter information. The committee is chaired by the AMA, and its member organizations represent a number of the major public and private sector payers. The NUCC was formally named in the administrative simplification section of HIPAA as one of the organizations to be consulted by ANSI-accredited SDOs and the Secretary of HHS as they develop, adopt, or modify national standards for healthcare transactions. As such, the NUCC has authoritative voice regarding national standard content and data definitions for noninstitutional healthcare claims in the United States.

Security Standards

HIPAA Security Standards for the Protection of Electronic Health Information at 45 CFR Part 160 and Part 164, Subparts A and C. The HIPAA Security Rule was developed to protect electronic health information and implement reasonable and appropriate administrative safeguards that establish the foundation for a covered entity's security program (CMS, 2007). Prior to HIPAA, no generally accepted set of security standards or general requirements for protecting health information existed in the healthcare industry. Congress passed the Administrative Simplification provisions of HIPAA to protect the privacy and security of certain health information, and promote efficiency in the healthcare industry through the use of standardized electronic transactions.

ISO IEC 27002:2005 Standard. The ISO IEC 27002:2005 Standard consists of recommended information security practices. It establishes guidelines and general principles for initiating, implementing, maintaining, and improving information security management in an organization. The objectives outlined provide general guidance on the commonly accepted goals and best practices for control objectives and controls for information security management. ISO/IEC 27002:2005 is intended as a common basis and practical guideline for developing organizational security standards and effective security management practices, and to help build confidence in interorganizational activities.

Implementation Guides

Implementation guides combine one or more standards into a specific guidance set to address focused use cases or user stories. Using implementation guides resolves the issues and challenges of unique and inconsistent standards implementations and enables the integration of base standards in an industry-wide, uniform manner. In order to test and implement the standards in real-life settings, they must be specified to a higher degree of detail. An implementation guide becomes an explicit description of the standards, services, and policies that then conform to the adopted standards and have sufficient detail to be implemented.

Figure 7.1 highlights the distinction between standards and implementation guides.

STANDARDS COORDINATION AND HARMONIZATION

It has become clear to both public and private sector standards development efforts that no one entity has the resources to create an exhaustive set of health data standards that will meet all needs. New emphasis is being placed on leveraging and harmonizing existing standards to eliminate the redundant and siloed efforts that have contributed to a complex, difficult to navigate health data standards environment. Advances are being made in the area of standards harmonization through the coming together of industry groups to accelerate and streamline the standards development and adoption process.

In addition to the various SDOs described above, the following organizations are working at national and international levels to create synergistic relationships between and across organizations. These emerging organizations are involved in standards development, coordination, and harmonization in all sectors of the economy. Since many of the health data standards issues, such as security, are not unique to the healthcare sector, this breadth of scope offers the potential for technology transfer and advancement across multiple sectors. The following is a brief description of some of the major national and international organizations involved in broad-based standards development, coordination, and harmonization.

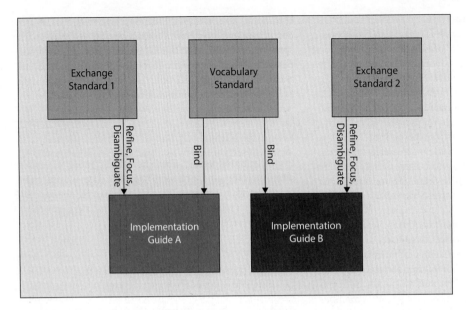

• **FIGURE 7.1.** HIMSS Health Information Standards Work Group, 2013. (Reproduced, with permission, from HIMSS Health Information Standards Work Group. (2013). Evaluating HIT Standards (p. 3). Chicago, IL: HIMSS. Copyright © 2013 Healthcare Information and Management Systems Society (HIMSS).

American National Standards Institute

The American National Standards Institute (ANSI) serves as the U.S. coordinating body for voluntary standards activity. Standards are submitted to ANSI by member SDOs and are approved as American National Standards through a consensus methodology developed by ANSI. ANSI is the U.S. representative to the International Organization for Standardization (ISO), and as such, is responsible for bringing forward U.S. standards to that organization for approval.

European Technical Committee for Standardization

In 1990, TC 251 on medical informatics was established by the European Committee for Standardization (CEN). CEN/TC 251 works to develop a wide variety of standards in the area of healthcare data management and interchange. CEN standards are adopted by its member countries in Europe and are also submitted for harmonization with ISO standards.

Health IT Standards Committee

The American Recovery and Reinvestment Act (ARRA) provided for the creation of the Health IT Standards Committee under the auspices of the Federal Advisory

Committee Act (FACA). The Committee is charged with making recommendations to the US Office of the National Coordinator for Health Information Technology on standards, implementation specifications, and certification criteria for the electronic exchange and use of health information. In developing, harmonizing, or recognizing standards and implementation specifications, the Committee also provides for the testing of the same by the National Institute for Standards and Technology (NIST). The Committee has formed several workgroups to further the work of the FACA. These workgroups are composed of stakeholder representatives and subject matter experts focused on the following topic areas: Clinical Operations, Clinical Quality, Privacy and Security, and Implementation.

Integrating the Healthcare Enterprise

Standards, while a necessary part of the interoperability ecosystem, are not sufficient alone to fulfill the needs. Simply using a standard does not necessarily guarantee health information exchange within or among organizations and systems. Standards can be implemented in various ways, so implementation specifications or guides are critical to make interoperability a reality (Sensmeier, 2010). Standard implementation specifications are designed to provide specific configuration instructions or constraints for implementation of a particular standard or set of standards.

Integrating the Healthcare Enterprise (IHE) is an international organization that provides a detailed framework for implementing standards, filling the gaps between standards and their implementations. While IHE is not a standards body and does not create standards, it offers a common framework, available in the public domain, to understand and address critical integration needs. IHE has published a large body of detailed specifications called integration profiles that are being implemented globally by healthcare providers and regional entities to enable standards-based safe, secure, and efficient health information exchange. Vendors publish IHE integration statements to document the IHE integration profiles supported by their products that were successfully tested at an IHE Connectathon. Users can reference the appropriate integration profiles in requests for proposals, thus simplifying the systems acquisition process.

To better differentiate those products that can deliver robust integration capabilities in production systems, IHE USA (a national deployment committee of IHE International) and ICSA Labs (an HIT testing laboratory and certification body) have implemented a testing program with formalized, rigorous, and independent examination of IHE profiles and specifications in specific versions of products going to market (Morrissey, 2014). This certification testing program is based on industry best practices and international ISO standards. Products that pass this testing and receive the IHE USA's mark of certification will operate as they should in meeting IHE functionality to achieve interoperability.

International Organization for Standardization

The International Organization for Standardization (ISO) develops, harmonizes, and publishes standards internationally. ISO standards are developed, in large part, from standards brought forth by member countries and through liaison activities with other SDOs. Often, these standards are further broadened to reflect the greater diversity of the international community. In 1998, the ISO Technical Committee (TC) 215 on Health Informatics was formed to coordinate the development of international health information standards, including data standards. This Committee published the first international standard for nursing content titled *Integration of a Reference Terminology Model for Nursing.* This standard includes the development of reference terminology models for nursing diagnoses and nursing actions with relevant terminology and definitions for implementation.

In order to address the need for global standards harmonization, the Joint Initiative Council (JIC) was founded as a liaison group under ISO/TC 215. Its goal is to enable common timely health informatics standards by addressing and resolving issues of gaps, overlaps, and counterproductive standardization efforts. Membership in JIC is restricted to international SDOs with a formal relationship to ISO and includes CEN/TC 251, ISO/TC 215, HL7, CDISC, IHTSDO, GS1, and IHE.

Object Management Group

While the organizations described thus far are made up of volunteer-based SDOs, the Object Management Group (OMG) is representative of a different approach to standards development. OMG is an international consortium of primarily for-profit vendors of information systems technology that are interested in the development of standards based on object-oriented technologies. While its standards are developed by private organizations, it has developed a process to lessen the potential problems noted previously with proprietary standards. Standards developed in OMG are required to be implemented in a commercially available product by their developers within one year of the standard being accepted; however, the specifications for the standard are made publicly available. The OMG CORBAMed working group is responsible for development of object-based standards in the health information arena.

Public Health Data Standards Consortium

The Public Health Data Standards Consortium (PHDSC) is a national non-profit membership–based organization of federal, state, and local health agencies; professional associations and academia; public and private sector organizations; international members; and individuals. Its goal is to empower the healthcare and public health communities with health IT standards that improve individual and community health. PHDSC represents a common voice from the public health community about the national effort toward standardization of health information for healthcare and population health by identifying priorities for new standards, promoting integration of health data systems, and educating the public health community about health data standards.

It is increasingly recognized that combining the strengths of these efforts and their approaches tends to minimize individual weaknesses and can lead to significant gains for the healthcare sector as a whole. As we have discussed, this melding of approaches is being achieved both at the organizational and international levels by the development of coordinating bodies and consortia as well as through national, government-directed laws, regulations, committees, and initiatives.

STANDARDS AND INTEROPERABILITY

ONC Standards and Interoperability Framework

The ONC Standards and Interoperability (S&I) Framework is a collaborative community of participants from the public and private sectors who are focused on providing the tools, services, and guidance to facilitate the functional exchange of health information. The S&I Framework, launched in 2011, uses a set of integrated functions, processes, and tools that enable execution of specific value-creating initiatives. Each S&I Initiative tackles a critical interoperability challenge through a rigorous process that typically includes the following:

- Development of clinically oriented user stories and robust use cases
- Harmonization of interoperability specifications and implementation guidance
- Provision of real-world experience and implementer support through new initiatives, workgroups, and pilot projects
- Mechanisms for feedback and testing of implementations, often in conjunction with ONC partners such as NIST

Testing and Certification

To accelerate the development, use, maintenance, and adoption of interoperability standards across the industry, and to spur innovation, the ONC has developed tools to facilitate the entire standards life cycle and maximize reuse of concepts and components, including tools and repositories for browsing, selecting, and implementing appropriate standards. The ONC is working with NIST to provide testing tools to validate that a particular implementation conforms to a set of standards and implementation specifications. The ONC also supports the development of an integration testing "harness" that tests how a particular component that has satisfied conformance testing requirements integrates into the reference implementation (Fridsma, 2010).

A certification process has been established so that organizations can be approved as certifying entities to which vendors may submit their EHR systems for review and certification. *The Health Information Technology: Initial Set of Standards, Implementation Specifications, and Certification Criteria for Electronic Health Record Technology (45 CFR Part 170) Final Rule*, published in 2010 by HHS, identifies the technical standards that must be met in the certification process, and coordinates those requirements with the meaningful use objectives.

CURRENT INITIATIVES

Health Information Exchange and Interoperability

Formal entities are emerging to provide both the structure and the function for health information exchange efforts at independent and governmental or regional/state levels. These organizations, called health information exchanges (HIEs), are geographically defined entities that develop and manage a set of contractual conventions and terms, and arrange for the governance and means of electronic exchange of information.

The HITECH Act authorized the establishment of the State Health Information Exchange Cooperative Agreement Program in the United States to advance appropriate and secure health information exchange across the healthcare system. The purpose of this program was to continuously improve and expand these services to reach all healthcare providers in an effort to improve the quality and efficiency of healthcare. Cooperative agreement recipients were funded, and many are now independently advancing the necessary governance, policies, technical services, business operations, and financing mechanisms for HIE. This program was intended to advance regional and state-level HIEs, while moving toward nationwide interoperability.

Nationwide Health Information Network and the eHealth Exchange

In 2007, ONC provided funding for the Nationwide Health Information Network (NwHIN), which is a set of standards, services, and policies that enable secure health information exchange over the Internet (Office of the National Coordinator for Health IT, 2013). The U.S. intent for the NwHIN was to provide a foundation for the exchange of health IT across diverse entities, within communities and across the country, to achieve the goals of the HITECH Act. This component of the national health IT agenda has enabled health information to follow the consumer, be available for clinical decision-making, and support appropriate use of health information beyond direct patient care so as to improve population health. The NwHIN architecture is a specific network architecture that implements health information exchange specifications based on open standards.

In 2009, the first production exchange began between the Social Security Administration and MedVirginia, followed by the Veterans Health Administration and Kaiser Permanente. This was the beginning of what is now known as the eHealth Exchange. In 2012, the eHealth

Exchange transitioned from operating as an ONC initiative to become a public–private partnership supported by Healtheway, Inc., a non-profit organization established to advance HIE implementation. Today, the eHealth Exchange has become a rapidly growing community of exchange partners, representing thousands of providers and millions of patients in support of treatment, care coordination, and public health purposes.

Clinical Integration and Accountable Care

As implementation of the 2010 Affordable Care Act advances, more organizations will sign on as accountable care organizations (ACOs), thus agreeing to provide care for a particular group of patients and to be paid on how well they do at keeping their patients healthy and lowering the costs of care. This model of care, which is based on clinical integration and focuses on increasing quality and care coordination, requires the use of health IT to enable earlier detection of conditions, preventing them from becoming advanced chronic diseases (Flareau, Yale, Bohn, & Konschak, 2011). Adopting standards-based information systems across the nation will enable wider sharing of patient health data and information with all members of the care team. Legislative and regulatory reforms that are accelerating ACO and clinical integration program development among hospitals and physician practices will support accurate and timely health information exchanged among hospital and office-based electronic medical records. Interoperability in turn will enable the efficient coordination and continuity of care offered by the ACO.

THE BUSINESS VALUE OF HEALTH DATA STANDARDS

The importance of data standards to enhancing the quality and efficiency of healthcare delivery and improving health outcomes is being recognized by national and international leadership. Reviewing the business value of defining and using health data standards is critical for driving the implementation of these standards into applications and real-world systems. Having data standards for data exchange and information modeling will provide a mechanism against which deployed systems can be validated (Loshin, 2004). Reducing manual intervention will increase worker productivity and streamline operations. Defining information exchange requirements will enhance the ability to automate interaction with external partners, which in turn will improve efficiency and decrease costs.

A standardized nursing language is necessary so that nursing knowledge can be represented and communicated consistently among nurses and other healthcare providers. Identifying key data elements, defining them consistently, and capturing them in a database will build a library of evidenced-based care that can be measured and validated (Rutherford, 2008). Enhanced data collection will contribute to greater adherence to standards of care, assessment of nursing competencies, and evaluation of nursing outcomes, thus increasing the visibility of nursing interventions and improving patient care.

By using data standards to develop their emergency department data collection system, New York State demonstrated that it is good business practice (Davis, 2004). Their project was completed on time without additional resources and generated a positive return on investment. The use of standards provided the basis for consensus between the hospital industry and the state, a robust pool of information that satisfied the users, and the structure necessary to create unambiguous data requirements and specifications.

The complex and highly fragmented healthcare system in the United States makes it difficult to develop a nationwide approach to value-based healthcare, according to a new report published by the Boston Consulting Group that called for better data standards and patient registries. The report looked at efforts to improve health outcomes—while also maintaining or lowering costs—in the health systems of 12 countries: Australia, Austria, Canada, Germany, Hungary, Japan, the Netherlands, New Zealand, Singapore, Sweden, the United Kingdom, and the United States.

The report (Soderlund, Kent, Lawyer, & Larsson, 2012) outlined four key success factors:

1. Clinician engagement: The greatest improvement comes when clinicians are responsible not only for collecting and interpreting data but also leading improvement efforts.

2. National infrastructure: It looked for common standards for tracking diagnoses, treatments, outcomes, and costs at the patient level; a limited number of shared IT platforms; and a common legal framework regulating the use of patient data.

3. High-quality data: The most effective way to collect relevant data is through disease registries to promote more effective and cost-efficient care.

4. Outcome-based incentives: Data-driven incentive measures should spur changes in the way clinicians practice, payers reimburse, and suppliers of drugs and medical devices develop and deliver products and services.

Other economic stakeholders for health IT include software vendors or suppliers, software implementers who install the software to support end-user requirements, and the users who must use the software to do their work. The balance of interests among these stakeholders is necessary to promote standardization to achieve economic and organizational benefits (Marshall, 2009). Defining clear business measures will help motivate the advancement and adoption of interoperable health IT systems, thus ensuring the desired outcomes can be achieved. Considering the value proposition for incorporating data standards into products, applications, and systems should be a part of every organization's IT strategy.

SUMMARY

This chapter introduces health data standards, the organizations that develop, coordinate, and harmonize them, the process by which they are developed, examples of current standards initiatives, and a discussion of the business value of health data standards. Four broad areas are described to categorize health data standards. Transport standards are used to establish communication protocols between systems. Vocabulary standards are used to describe clinical problems and procedures, medications, and allergies. Content exchange standards and value sets are used to share clinical information such as clinical summaries, prescriptions, and structured electronic documents. And security standards are those used for authentication, access control, and transmission of health data. Organizations involved in the development, harmonization, and coordination of health data standards are described.

A discussion of the standards development process highlights the international and sociopolitical context in which standards are developed and the potential impact they have on improving the health of patients and populations. The increasingly significant role of regulation, legislation, and the federal government in furthering the development, adoption, and value of health data standards is discussed. Several key initiatives including the ONC S&I Framework, HIEs, and the eHealth Exchange are described, and their potential impacts are highlighted. The influence of the emerging ACO model of care's focus on increasing quality and care coordination is explored. Finally, the business value and importance of health data standards to improving the quality and efficiency of healthcare delivery and the role their adoption plays in improving health outcomes are emphasized.

REFERENCES

ANSI. (2005). *The United States standards strategy*. New York, NY: American National Standards Institute.

Bowman, S. (2008). Why ICD-10 is worth the trouble. *Journal of AHIMA, 79*(3), 24–29.

Centers for Medicare and Medicaid Services (CMS). (2007). *HIPAA security series: Security 101 for covered entities* (Vol. 2, paper 1, pp. 1–11). Washington, DC: Centers for Medicare and Medicaid Services.

Committee on Data Standards for Patient Safety. (2004). *Patient safety: Achieving a new standard for care*. Washington, DC: Institute of Medicine.

Davis, B. (2004). *Return-on-investment for using data standards: A case study of New York State's data system*. Public Health Data Standards Consortium. Retrieved from http://www.phdsc.org/standards/pdfs/ROI4UDS.pdf

Department of Health and Human Services. (2010). *Health information technology: Initial set of standards, implementation specifications, and certification criteria for electronic health record technology*. (45 CFR Part 170). Washington, DC: Office of the Secretary.

Flareau, B., Yale, K., Bohn, J. M., Konschak, C. (2011). *Clinical integration: A roadmap to accountable care* (2nd ed.). Virginia Beach, VA: Convurgent.

Fridsma, D. (2010). *Interoperability framework overview*. Presentation to the HIT Standards Committee, March 24, 2010. Washington, DC.

Hammond, W. E. (2005). The making and adoption of health data standards. *Health Affairs, 23*(5), 1205–1213.

Health Information Policy Council. (1983). *Background paper: Uniform minimum health data sets*. Washington, DC: Department of Health and Human Services.

HIMSS. (2013). *The definition of interoperability*. Retrieved from http://www.himss.org/files/FileDownloads/HIMSS_Interoperability_Definition_FINAL.pdf

HIMSS Health Information Standards Work Group. (2013). *Evaluating HIT standards*. Chicago, IL: HIMSS.

Loshin, D. (2004). The business value of data standards. *DM Review. 14*(6), 20.

Marshall, G. (2009). The standards value chain. *Journal of AHIMA, 10*, 58–65.

Morrissey, J. (2014). *IHE profiles and certification drive interoperability*. ICSA Labs.

National Committee on Vital and Health Statistics. (1996). *Report of the National Committee on Vital and Health Statistics: Core Health Data Elements*. Washington, DC: Government Printing Office.

National Library of Medicine. (2010). *Health information technology and health data standards at NLM*. Retrieved from http://www.nlm.nih.gov/healthit.html

Nelson, R. (2006). Data processing. In V. K. Saba & K. A. McCormick (Eds.), *Essentials of nursing informatics* (4th ed.). New York, NY: McGraw-Hill.

Office of the National Coordinator for Health IT. (2013). *Nationwide Health Information Network (NwHIN)*. Retrieved from http://www.healthit.gov/policy-researchers-implementers/nationwide-health-information-network-nwhin

Rutherford, M. A. (2008). Standardized nursing language: What does it mean for nursing practice? *The Online Journal of Issues in Nursing, 13*(1).

Sensmeier, J. (2010). *The impact of standards and certification on EHR Systems*. Foundations of Nursing Informatics. Atlanta, GA: HIMSS10.

Soderlund, N., Kent, J., Lawyer, P., Larsson, S. (2012). *Progress toward value-based health care: Lessons from 12 countries*. Retrieved at https://www.bcgperspectives.com/content/articles/health_care_public_sector_progress_toward_value_based_health_care/

WEB SITES

The field of data standards is a very dynamic one with existing standards undergoing revision and new standards being developed. The best way to learn about specific standards activities is to get involved in the process. All of the organizations discussed in this chapter provide opportunities to be involved with activities that support standards development, coordination, harmonization, and implementation. Listed below are the World Wide Web addresses for each organization. Most sites describe current activities and publications available, and many have links to other related sites.

Accredited Standards Committee (ASC) X12. www.wpc-edi.com

American Medical Association (AMA). www.ama-assn.org

American National Standards Institute (ANSI). www.ansi.org

American Nurses Association (ANA). www.nursingworld.org

American Society for Testing and Materials (ASTM). www.astm.org

Clinical Data Interchange Standards Consortium (CDISC). www.cdisc.org

Digital Imaging Communication in Medicine Standards Committee (DICOM). www.nema.org

European Committee for Standardization Technical Committee 251 Health Informatics (CEN/TC 251). www.cen.eu/cen

Healtheway. http://healthewayinc.org

Health Level Seven (HL7). www.hl7.org

Institute of Electrical and Electronic Engineers (IEEE). www.ieee.org

Integrating the Healthcare Enterprise (IHE). www.iheusa.org

International Health Terminology Standards Development Organisation (IHTSDO). www.ihtsdo.org

International Organization for Standardization (ISO). www.iso.org

International Statistical Classification of Diseases and Related Health Problems (ICD-9, ICD-9CM, ICD-10). www.cdc.gov/nchs

Logical Observation Identifiers Names and Codes (LOINC). loinc.org

National Committee on Vital and Health Statistics (NCVHS). http://www.aspe.os.dhhs.gov/ncvhs

National Council for Prescription Drug Programs (NCPDP). www.ncpdp.org

National Electrical Manufacturers Association (NEMA). www.nema.org

National Library of Medicine (NLM). www.nlm.nih.gov/healthit.html

National Uniform Claims Committee (NUCC). www.nucc.org

Object Management Group (OMG). www.omg.org

Office of the National Coordinator for Health Information Technology (ONC). www.hhs.gov/healthit

Public Health Data Standards Consortium (PHDSC). www.phdsc.org

RxNorm. www.nlm.nih.gov/research/umls/rxnorm

Standards & Interoperability Framework. http://wiki.siframework.org/Introduction+and+Overview

Unified Medical Language System (UMLS). www.nlm.nih.gov/research/umls

World Wide Web Consortium (W3C). www.w3.org

8

Standardized Nursing Terminologies

Nicholas R. Hardiker / Virginia K. Saba / Tae Youn Kim

- ## OBJECTIVES

  1. Define "standardized nursing terminology."
  2. Describe the impact of terminologies on nursing.
  3. Describe the features of advanced nursing terminology systems.

- ## KEY WORDS

  Advanced nursing terminology
  Concepts
  Concept-Oriented
  Classification
  Data
  Data element
  Nursing terminology
  Vocabulary

INTRODUCTION

In the present technological environment, the need for nursing to become visible through the documentation of nursing practice in emerging Healthcare Information Technology (HIT) and Electronic Health Record (EHR) Systems is critical. Nursing can no longer rely on the intuition of senior nurses or on the trial-and-error of tradition-oriented nursing practice but rather the profession needs to conduct research and generate measures and evidence to prove that their nursing care improves quality, safety, and healthcare outcomes. To become visible nursing needs to electronically document nursing practice using a standardized nursing terminology with coded concepts in order to measure the effectiveness of their care delivery and thus generate the evidence (Elfrink, Bakken, Coenen, McNeil, & Bickford, 2001; Saba & Taylor, 2007; Whittenburg, 2011).

A standardized nursing terminology consists of nursing concepts that represent the domain of nursing. A nursing terminology must include standardized nursing data that represent the essential building blocks for nursing practice. Such nursing data are critical to the development of data sets that can be used for analysis and integrated with the data of other healthcare disciplines. The standardized nursing data sets might also serve as research data to advance the science of nursing practice.

The U.S. Institute of Medicine in a 2012 report recommended that the capture of clinical care data is needed for better patient care coordination and management. It stated that our patient care data is poorly captured and managed, and our evidence poorly used. The report focused on the need recommended by the U.S. National Coordinator for Healthcare Information Technology (ONC) to improve interoperability across systems to support better care. The report also recommended that to be usable the standardized data must be captured in real time and at the point of care (IOM, 2012).

Standardized nursing terminologies are needed to (a) provide valid clinical care data, (b) allow data sharing across today's HIT and EHR systems, (c) support evidenced-based decision making, (d) facilitate evaluation of nursing processes, and (e) permit the measurement of outcomes. Standardized concepts and data elements are also needed to facilitate **aggregation** and **comparison** for clinical, translational, and comparative effectiveness research, as well as for the development of practice-based nursing protocols and evidence-based knowledge, including the generation of healthcare policy (Hardiker, Bakken, Casey, & Hoy, 2002). Lastly, to support continuity of care and the exchange of data, for example, to implement in the United States the federal regulations for "meaningful use" (MU), the standardized nursing concepts must be **interoperable** between HIT and EHR systems, across healthcare settings and population groups. Such demands require that the initial standardized nursing terminology concepts be coded in a structure that is suitable for computer-based processing.

This chapter focuses on providing the background necessary to understand standardized nursing terminologies, standardized nursing concepts and data elements, and their impact on nursing practice. The chapter provides an overview of the characteristics of nursing terminologies and how they are used in today's HIT and EHR systems. It further provides an overview of advanced nursing terminologies and describes how they can contribute to today's informatics infrastructure (Coenen, McNeil, Bakken, Bickford, & Warren, 2001).

Note that the word "terminology" is used throughout the chapter to refer also to "classification," "vocabulary," "taxonomy," or "nomenclature." Concepts and terms that are coded for computer processing are referred to as "data" or "data elements."

BACKGROUND

Historical Events

Terminological work within the nursing professions has been ongoing for many years. As early as 1859, Florence Nightingale named her six canons of care as "what nurses do" in her text *Notes on Nursing* (1859). She considered the six canons to be measures of "good standards" essential for the practice of nursing. It took another 80 years for her work to be expanded in the United States when Virginia Henderson published her *Textbook of the Principles and Practices of Nursing* (1939) in which she delineated her "14 patterns of daily living." Her works were followed by the works of several nurse-theorists who presented their theories and standards of nursing practice such as Peplau's "Four Major Life Tasks," Orem's "Universal Self-Care Deficits," King's "Process of Nursing," Roger's "Four Building Blocks," Abdellah's "21 Problems," etc. (Fordyce,

1984). These models were all developed as approaches to patient care; however, none referred to or predicted the use of computers to support the implementation of nursing practice standards (Englebright, 2014).

In 1970 the American Nurses Association (ANA) approved the **nursing process** as the standard of professional nursing practice (ANA, 2008; Mannino & Feeg, 2011). Yura and Walsh identified the nursing process as representing an orderly, systematic orientation to addressing a client's condition. Yura and Walsh described the Nursing Process as providing the framework for gathering patient care data, beginning with the assessment phase which also identified the client's conditions, which they referred to as, nursing diagnoses, through goal designations and the planning of nursing activities, and ending with evaluation. Yura and Walsh also identified their "34 Human Needs Assessment" which they outlined with the "Proposed Nursing Diagnoses" (Yura & Walsh, 1983, pp. 152–155).

Health Terminologies

During this same time period in the United States computer technology was being introduced in hospitals, albeit primarily for administrative applications. It was relatively easy for vendors to computerize hospital billing applications since hospitals were already using an established terminology for payment for disease conditions and/or services. The International Classification of Diseases (ICD), which was being used internationally for the reporting of mortality and morbidity statistics, was also being used by the U.S. federal government for payment of healthcare services. Subsequently, other hospital specialty departments initiated different terminologies for payment of their specific services such as *Physician's Current Procedural Terminology* (CPT) for surgical procedures (AMA, 2014), *Logical Observation Identifiers Names and Codes* (LOINC) for laboratory tests (Regenstrief Institute, 2014), etc.

During this period, however, nursing did not have any recognized terminologies to characterize their patients, describe nursing interventions, or support documentation. Subsequent nursing terminology development was motivated by a number of factors: (1) the need to quantify nursing resources, (2) the introduction of the electronic health record in healthcare facilities, and (3) the development of knowledge bases and growth of evidence-based nursing practice (Saranto, Moss, & Jylha, 2010).

Nursing and Computers

In 1985, the American Nurses Association (ANA) initiated the Council on Computer Applications in Nursing (CCAN) which promoted the nursing profession to become involved in the integration of computer-based applications in nursing practice, education, and research (Zielstorff, 1998). The CCAN Executive Board, which consisted of several nursing informatics pioneers, was responsible for numerous initiatives and served as a moving force for this new nursing specialty. For example, the CCAN supported the conduct of several conferences on computers in nursing practice such as Werley and her development of the Nursing Minimum Data Set (NMDS) discussed elsewhere in this chapter, or Saba and McCormick who initiated their first book *Essentials of Computers for Nurses* (1986) (see Chapter 1: NI History). This activity was mirrored in a number of countries worldwide.

It was during this time that Graves and Corcoran adapted Blum's concepts of data (discrete entities), information (interpreted data), and knowledge (formalized information) as a framework for understanding the impact of computer-based systems on healthcare (ANA, 2008; Simpson, 2003). They also supported the need for computer-based nursing terminologies by their definition of Nursing Informatics:

> Nursing Informatics combines nursing science, information science, and computer science to manage and process nursing data, information and knowledge to facilitate the delivery of healthcare. (ANA, 2008, p. 7)

In 1992, the CCAN's name was changed to the Database Steering Committee and continued its involvement by approving Nursing Informatics as a new nursing specialty. Also in 1992, the Council developed the criteria for a nursing terminology (see Table 8.1 for proposed updated criteria) as well as "recognizing" the first nursing terminologies as appropriate for the documentation of nursing practice (see Table 8.2 for listing). They included NANDA's Classification of Nursing Diagnoses, Home Health Care Classification (HHCC) (now Clinical Care Classification [CCC] System), Nursing Intervention Classification (NIC), and the Omaha System. The remaining "recognized" terminologies that exist today are Nursing Outcome Classification (NOC), Perioperative Nursing Data Set (PNDS), International Classification for Nursing Practice (ICNP), ABC Codes, Logical Observation Identifiers Names and Codes (LOINC), and Systematic Nomenclature of Medicine—Clinical Terms (SNOMED-CT) (Thede & Schwirian, 2013). Two data sets are also recognized: the Nursing Minimum Data Set (NMDS) and the Nursing Management Minimum Data Set (NMMDS) (http://www.nursingworld.org/MainMenuCategories/ThePracticeofProfessionalNursing/NursingStandards/Recognized-Nursing-Practice-Terminologies.pdf).

TABLE 8.1 Terminology Recognition Criteria Approved by ANA's Congress on Nursing Practice and Economics (2008)

In 2008 the American Nurses Association's Congress on Nursing Practice and Economics approved the following criteria as the framework for the evaluation process for recognition of a terminology supporting nursing practice:

1. The terminology supports one or more components of the nursing process.
2. The rationale for development supports this terminology as a new terminology itself or with a unique contribution to nursing/healthcare.
3. Characteristics of the terminology include:
   - Support of one or more of the nursing domains
   - Description of the data elements
   - Internal consistency
   - Testing of reliability, validity, sensitivity, and specificity
   - Utility in practice showing scope of use and user population
   - Coding using context-free unique identifier
4. Characteristics of the terminology development and maintenance process include:
   - The intended use of the terminology
   - The centricity of the content (patient, community, etc.)
   - Research-based framework used for development
   - Open call for participation for initial and ongoing development
   - Systematic, defined ongoing process for development
   - Relevance to nursing care and nursing science
   - Collaborative partnerships
   - Documentation of history of decisions
   - Defined revision and version control mechanisms
   - Defined maintenance program
   - Long-term plan for sustainability
5. Access and distribution mechanisms are defined.
6. Plans and strategies for future development are defined.

ANA elected to retire its terminology recognition program in 2012 because of the National Committee on Vital and Health Statistics (NCVHS) recommendations for selection of standardized languages for health information technology solutions, the federal government's actions related to the National Library of Medicine's procurement of SNOMED-CT licenses, establishment of the Office of the National Coordinator for the Health Information Technology (ONC) and its various departments and committees, and the resultant decisions identifying standardized terminologies requisite for interoperability and data and information reporting and exchange (see http://www.healthit.gov/policy-researchers-implementers/meaningful-use-stage-2-0/standards-hub for additional details).

Reproduced, with permission, from Westra B.L. (2010). *Testimony Vocabulary Task Force, Standards Committee, Office of the National Coordinator. CIN: Computers, Informatics, Nursing, 28*(6), 380–385.

TABLE 8.2	Current American Nurses Association (ANA)–Recognized Terminologies and Data Sets	
Category	**Setting**	**Content**
Data Element Sets		
1. NMDS Nursing Minimum Data Set www.nursing.umn.edu/ICNP/USANMDS/home.html	All nursing	Clinical data elements
2. NMMDS Nursing Management Minimum Data Set www.nursing.umn.edu/ICNP/USANMMDS/home.html	All settings	Nursing administrative data elements
Interface Terminologies		
3. CCC System Clinical Care Classification (CCC) System www.sabacare.com and www.clinicalcareclassification.com	All settings	Diagnoses, Interventions, and Outcomes

4. ICNP®
International Classification of Nursing Practice
    www.icn.ch/pillarsprograms/international-classification-
    for-nursing-practicer/
	All Nursing	Diagnoses, Interventions, and Outcomes

5. NANDA NANDA International www.nanda.org	All nursing	Diagnoses

6. NIC
Nursing Intervention Classification
    www.nursing.uiowa.edu/excellence/nursing_knowledge/
    clinical_effectiveness/index.htm
	All nursing	Interventions

7. NOC
Nursing Outcome Classification
    www.nursing.uiowa.edu/excellence/nursing_knowledge/
    clinical_effectiveness/index.htm
	All nursing	Outcomes

8. Omaha System Omaha System www.omahasystem.org	Home care, public health, and community	Diagnoses, Interventions, and Outcomes

9. PNDS
Perioperative Nursing Data Set
    www.aorn.org/PracticeResources/PNDSAndStandardized
    PerioperativeRecord/
	Perioperative	Diagnoses, Interventions, and Outcomes

Multidisciplinary Terminologies		
10. ABC Codes ABC Codes www.abccodes.com	Nursing and other	Interventions
11. LOINC Logical Observation Identifiers Names and Codes www.loinc.org	Nursing and other	Outcome and Assessments
12. SNOMED-CT Systematic Nomenclature of Medicine-Clinical Terms www.ihtsdo.org/snomed-ct/	Nursing and other	Diagnoses, Interventions, and Outcomes

The majority of these terminologies are considered to be "interface terminologies," "user terminologies," or "point-of-care" terminologies, using common terms that nurses use and understand in daily practice. ICNP and SNOMED-CT also have reference properties. A reference terminology acts as a common reference point that can for example facilitate cross-mapping between interface terminologies.

Several nursing terminologies have been integrated into the Metathesaurus of the Unified Medical Language System (UMLS), developed by the U.S. National Library of Medicine (NLM). The Metathesaurus in the UMLS is a large, multipurpose, and multilingual thesaurus that contains millions of biomedical and health-related concepts, their synonymous names, and their relationship (http://uts.nlm.nih.gov//home.html/).

Nursing terminologies vary in scope, structure, and content. They were developed by different organizations, with different funding sources, for different purposes, with different foci, and with different copyright privileges. Most of the early terminologies were initially developed for paper-based documentation of nursing care; the CCC System was designed specifically for computer-based documentation and processing (Saba, 2012) see *Appendix A: Overview of Clinical Care Classification (CCC) System* (http://www.sabacare.com/About). However, over time and with the advancement of technology, all of the nursing terminologies have now been adapted for computer processing.

Coding Structure and Terminology

A standardized nursing terminology with nursing concepts and data requires a tree structure that allows for the data to be aggregated upward and parsed downward to the atomic level data elements. The coded data might also be organized using a nursing terminology framework to document and link the nursing process phases together (assessment, diagnosis, expected outcome, planning, implementation, and evaluation of the actual outcomes). The framework should allow for the collection of data to be in real time at the point of care, with ongoing processing that allows for feedback loops (reuse of the data concepts) based on the patient's responses to their interventions/actions (care), and then be able to generate outcomes for comparison.

Nursing Terminology Challenges

Currently, there is a movement to harmonize nursing and multidisciplinary terminologies. However, there are two major challenges. Firstly, the existence of multiple, specialized terminologies has resulted in areas of overlapping content, areas for which there was no content, and large numbers of different codes and terms (Chute, Cohn, & Campbell, 1998; Cimino, 1998a). Secondly, existing terminologies most often were developed to provide sets of terms and definitions of concepts for human interpretation, with computer interpretation only as a secondary goal (Rossi Mori, Consorti, & Galeazzi, 1998). The latter is particularly true for nursing terminologies that have been designed primarily for direct use by nurses in the course of clinical care (Association of Operating Room Nurses [AORN], 2007; Johnson et al., 2006; Martin, 2005; Saba & Taylor, 2007). It is unfortunate that knowledge eminently understandable by nurses is often confusing, ambiguous, or opaque to computers, and, consequently, previous efforts often resulted in terminologies that in some ways were inadequate in meeting the data needs of nursing practice in today's HIT and EHR systems.

ADVANCED TERMINOLOGY SYSTEMS IN NURSING

Nursing Requirements

The HIT and EHR systems that support functionality such as decision support may require more granular (i.e., less abstract) data than may be found in today's interface terminologies (Campbell et al., 1997; Chute, Cohn, Campbell, Oliver, & Campbell, 1996; Cimino, 1998b; Cimino, Hripcsak, Johnson, & Clayton, 1989). More advanced terminology systems are needed that allow for much greater granularity through controlled composition, while avoiding a combinatorial explosion of pre-coordinated terms.

Formal Terminologies

Advanced terminology systems such as ICNP and SNOMED-CT are a focus of today's harmonizing efforts. Both terminologies facilitate two important facets of knowledge representation for HIT and EHR systems that support clinical care: (1) **describing concepts** and (2) **manipulating and reasoning** about those concepts using computer-based tools. Advantages resulting from the first facet—describing concepts—include (a) non-ambiguous representation of concepts, (b) facilitation of data abstraction or de-abstraction without loss of original meaning (i.e., "loss-less" data transformation), (c) non-ambiguous mapping among terminologies, (d) data reuse in different contexts, and (e) data interoperability across settings. These advantages are particularly important for clinical uses of the terminology. Advantages gained from the second facet—manipulating and reasoning—include (a) auditing the terminology system, (b) automated classification of new concepts, and (c) an ability to support multiple inheritance of defining characteristics (e.g., "acute postoperative pain" is both a "pain" and a "postoperative symptom"). Both facets are vital to the maintenance of the terminology itself as well as to the ability to subsequently support the clinical utility of the terminology (Campbell, Cohn, Chute, Shortliffe, & Rennels, 1998; Rector et al., 1997).

Characteristics of Advanced Terminologies

Healthcare terminologies suitable for implementation in HIT systems have been studied by numerous experts who have provided an evolving framework that enumerates the recommended criteria. The characteristics apply to any terminology being used in the healthcare industry as well as for a nursing terminology. It is clear that such terminologies must be concept-oriented (with explicit semantics), rather than based on surface linguistics (Chute et al., 1998; Cimino, 1998b; Cimino et al., 1989). Other recommended criteria for terminologies include domain completeness and a polyhierarchical organization. Additional criteria applying to concepts themselves include being atomic-level (single concept coded as a single data element), non-redundancy (unique identifier), nonambiguity (explicit definition), concept permanence (cannot be duplicated), compositionality (ability to combine concepts to form new unique concepts), and synonymy (a single concept supports multiple terms or synonyms) (Henry & Mead, 1997; de Keizer & Abu Hanna, 2000; Zielstorff, 1998).

Concept Orientation

In order to appreciate the significance of concept-oriented approaches, it is important to first understand the definitions of and relationships among things in the world (objects), our thoughts about things in the world (concepts), the labels we use to represent and communicate our thoughts about things in the world (terms), and the coded data elements needed to represent and be processed by computer (Bakken et al., 2000; Moss, Damrongsak, & Gallichio, 2005). The terminology relationships are depicted by a descriptive model commonly called the semiotic triangle (Fig. 8.1) (Ingenerf, 1995; Ogden & Richards, 1923). The International Organization for Standardization (ISO) International Standard ISO 1087-1:2000 provides definitions for elements that correspond to each vertex of the triangle:

> **Concept** (i.e., thought or reference): Unit of knowledge created by a unique combination of characteristics—a characteristic is an abstraction of a property of an object or of a set of objects.

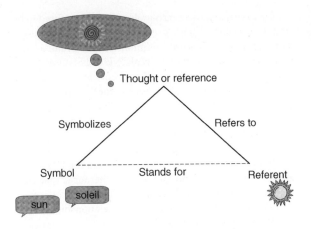

• **FIGURE 8.1.** The Semiotic Triangle Depicts the Relationships among Objects in the Perceivable or Conceivable World (Referent), Thoughts about Things in the World, and the Labels (Symbols or Terms) Used to Represent Thoughts about Things in the World.

> **Object** (i.e., referent): Anything perceivable or conceivable.
>
> **Term** (i.e., symbol): Verbal designation of a general concept in a specific subject field—a general concept corresponds to two or more objects which form a group by reason of common properties (ISO, 1990).

As specified by the criteria in Table 8.3 and illustrated in Fig. 8.2, a single concept may be associated with multiple terms (synonym).

Model Structures

A terminology model is a concept-based representation of a collection of domain-specific terms (data elements) that is optimized for the management of terminological definitions. It encompasses both "schemata" and "type definitions" (Campbell et al., 1998; Sowa, 1984). Schemata incorporate domain-specific knowledge about the typical constellations of entities, attributes, and events in the real world and, as such, reflect plausible combinations of concepts for naming a nursing diagnosis or problem, for example, "pain" may be combined with "acute" or "chronic" to make "acute pain" or "chronic pain" or for naming clinical nursing intervention, for example, "vital signs" may be combined with "teach" to form "teach vital signs."

Schemata may be supported by either formal or informal composition rules (i.e., grammar). Type definitions address obligatory conditions that state only the essential properties of a concept (Sowa, 1984), for example, a

TABLE 8.3	Evaluation Criteria Related to Concept-Oriented Approaches

Atomic-based—concepts must be separable into constituent components (Chute et al., 1998)

Compositionality—ability to combine simple concepts into composed concepts, e.g., "pain" *and* "acute" = "acute pain" (Chute et al., 1998)

Concept permanence—once a concept is defined it should not be deleted from a terminology (Cimino, 1998b)

Language independence—support for multiple linguistic expressions (Chute et al., 1998)

Multiple hierarchy—accessibility of concepts through all reasonable hierarchical paths with consistency of views (Chute et al., 1998; Cimino, 1998b; Cimino et al., 1989)

Nonambiguity—explicit definition for each term, e.g., "patient teaching related to medication adherence" defined as an *action* of "teaching," *recipient* of "patient," and *target* of "medication adherence" (Chute et al., 1998; Cimino, 1998b; Cimino et al., 1989)

Nonredundancy—one preferred way of representing a concept or idea (Chute et al., 1998; Cimino, 1998b; Cimino et al., 1989)

Synonymy—support for synonyms and consistent mapping of synonyms within and among terminologies (Chute et al., 1998; Cimino, 1998b; Cimino et al., 1989)

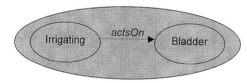

• **FIGURE 8.2.** A simple Graphical Example of a Formal Representation of the Nursing Activity Concept "Bladder Irrigation."

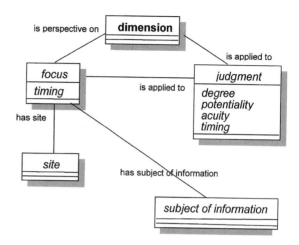

• **FIGURE 8.3.** Reference Terminology Model for Nursing Diagnoses. (This excerpt is from ISO 18104:2014, Figure 1 on page 9, with the permission of ANSI on behalf of ISO. © ISO 2015 - All rights reserved.)

Reference Terminology Models for Nursing

In 2003, the ISO which is responsible for identifying international standards for Health Informatics passed ISO 18104:2003, *Integration of a Reference Terminology Model for Nursing*, which covers two Reference Terminology Models: one for Nursing Diagnoses (Fig. 8.3) and one for Nursing Actions (Fig. 8.4) (ISO, 2003). The standard was developed by a group of experts within ISO Technical Committee 215 (Health Informatics) Working Group 3 (Semantic Content), including representatives of the International Medical Informatics Association–Nursing Informatics Working Group (IMIA-NI) and the International Council of Nurses (ICN). The model built on work originating within the European Committee for Standardization (CEN) (European Committee for Standardization, 2000).

Development of ISO 18104:2003

The development of ISO 18104:2003 was motivated in part by a desire to harmonize the plethora of nursing terminologies in use around the world (Hardiker, 2004). Another major incentive was to integrate with other evolving terminology and information model standards—the development of ISO 18104:2003 was intended to be "consistent with the goals and objectives of other specific health terminology models in order to provide a more unified reference health model" (ISO, 2003, p. 1). Potential uses identified for

nursing activity must have a *recipient*, an *action*, and a *target*. Examples of terminology models that can be used to guide or underpin nursing terminologies are embedded within the international technical standard *ISO 18104:2003 Integration of a reference terminology model for nursing*, described below (Bakken, Cashen, & O'Brien, 1999; Hardiker & Rector, 1998; ICN, 2001; ISO, 2003; Saba, Hovenga, Coenen, & McCormick, 2003).

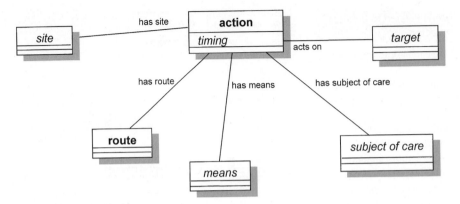

the terminology models included to (1) facilitate the representation of nursing diagnosis and nursing action concepts and their relationships in a manner suitable for computer processing; (2) provide a framework for the generation of compositional expressions from atomic concepts within a reference terminology; (3) facilitate the mapping among nursing diagnosis and nursing action concepts from various terminologies; (4) enable the systematic evaluation of terminologies and associated terminology models for purposes of harmonization; and (5) provide a language to describe the structure of nursing diagnosis and nursing action concepts in order to enable appropriate integration with information models (ISO, 2003).

The standard is not intended to be of direct benefit to practicing nurses. It is intended to be of use to those who develop coding systems, terminologies, terminology models for other domains, health information models, information systems, software for natural language processing, and markup standards for representation of healthcare documents. The ISO 18104:2003 models have undergone substantial bench testing, both during their development and through independent research (Hwang, Cimino, & Bakken, 2003; Moss, Coenen, & Mills, 2003; Saba et al., 2003). The standard was under revision at the time of writing this text.

Ontologies

Terminology models may be formulated and elucidated in an ontology language that represents classes (also referred to as concepts, categories, or types) and their properties

(also referred to as relations, slots, roles, or attributes) such as Web Ontology Language (OWL) (Rector, 2004). In this way, ontology languages or terminologies are able to support, through explicit semantics, the formal definition of concepts in terms of their relationships with other concepts (Fig. 8.2); they also facilitate reasoning about those concepts, for example, whether two concepts are equivalent or whether one concept, such as "vital sign," subsumes (is a generalization of) another, such as "temperature, pulse, and respirations (TPR)" (Hardiker, Hoy, & Casey, 2000). Ontology languages are often used to support advanced terminologies. One example is the use of OWL to represent ICNP.

OWL Representation of ICNP

Outside the health domain, work in relation to the Semantic Web has resulted in the recognition of OWL as an emerging standard (i.e., a W3C recommendation) (McGuiness & van Harmelen, 2004). OWL is intended for use where applications, rather than humans, process information. As such, it should be able to meet the requirements of advanced terminology systems that support contemporary healthcare. OWL builds on existing recommendations such as Extensible Markup Language (XML) (surface syntax for structured documents), Resource Description Framework (RDF) (a data model for resources), and RDF Schema (a vocabulary for describing the properties and classes of resources) by providing additional vocabulary and a formal semantics. Software, both proprietary and open source, is available for (a) managing

TABLE 8.4	Possible OWL Representation (in XML) of the Nursing Activity Concept "Bladder Irrigation"

```
<owl:Class rdf:ID="BladderIrrigation">
 <owl:equivalentClass>
  <owl:Class>
   <owl:intersectionOf rdf:parseType="Collection">
   <owl:Class rdf:about="#Irrigating"/>
   <owl:Restriction>
    <owl:onProperty>
     <owl:FunctionalProperty rdf:about="#actsOn"/>
    </owl:onProperty>
    <owl:someValuesFrom>
     <owl:Class rdf:about="#Bladder"/>
    </owl:someValuesFrom>
   </owl:Restriction>
   </owl:intersectionOf>
  </owl:Class>
 </owl:equivalentClass>
</owl:Class>
```

terminology models or ontologies developed in OWL (e.g., Protégé, 2010) and (b) reasoning on the model (e.g., FaCT++ (Tsarkov, 2009). Work within nursing is now well-established. For example, ICNP is maintained in OWL—it is a compositional standards-based terminology for nursing practice (Hardiker & Coenen, 2007). The compositionality of ICNP further facilitates the development of and the cross-mapping among local terminologies and existing classification systems (ICN, 2009).

An OWL representation (in XML) of the nursing activity concept "Bladder Irrigation" is provided in Table 8.4.

ICNP as a Terminology

The ICNP is a major product of the International Council of Nurses (ICN), Geneva, Switzerland. It is a formal terminology for nursing practice and is used to represent nursing diagnosis, outcomes, and interventions. The primary motivation for an international nursing terminology involves sharing and comparing nursing data across settings, countries, and languages. These data can be used to support clinical decision making, evaluate nursing care and patient outcomes, develop health policy, and generate knowledge through research (Coenen, Marin, Park, & Bakken, 2001; Moen, 1999). Using a formal ontological approach, ICNP can complement existing terminologies, such as the CCC System and SNOMED-CT.

The CCC has been demonstrated to support the electronic capture of discrete patient care data for documenting and coding the "essence of care" and measuring the relationship of nursing care to patient outcomes. The CCC, an "interface terminology," is being mapped to ICNP which will benefit both terminologies and their users, for example, by enabling ICNP users to code their terminologies using the CCC or to allow the comparison of CCC data with data recorded using other terminologies (ICN, 2012).

SNOMED-CT

SNOMED-CT is another advanced terminology system being used within a wider healthcare context (including within nursing). SNOMED-CT, which was developed collaboratively by the College of American Pathologists and the UK National Health Service (Wang, Sable, & Spackman, 2002), now falls under the responsibility of the International Health Terminology Standards Development Organization (IHTSDO). In common with ICNP, SNOMED-CT possesses both reference properties and user interface terms. SNOMED-CT is considered to be the most comprehensive, multilingual clinical healthcare terminology in the world and integrates, through external mappings, concepts from many nursing terminologies.

In the United States, SNOMED-CT is distributed at no cost by the NLM. Licensees of the UMLS Metathesaurus are granted free access to SNOMED-CT. SNOMED-CT is one of a suite of designated standards for use for the electronic exchange of health information and also is a required standard in interoperability specifications of the U.S. Health Information Technology Standards Panel (HITSP) (http://www.nlm.nih.gov/research/umls/SNOMED.snomed_main.html).

A harmonization agreement exists between IHTSDO and ICN (http://www.icn.ch/images/stories/documents/news/press_releases/2010_PR_04_AC-ICNP_IHTSDO.pdf). Joint work between IHTSDO and ICN has resulted in a table of equivalents for concepts within SNOMED-CT and ICNP (http://www.icn.ch/images/stories/documents/news/press_releases/2014_PR_02_ICNP_SNOMED.pdf). These equivalencies are important as they mean that those who choose to use ICNP are able to play a full part in any broader health informatics infrastructure.

Nursing Minimum Data Set (NMDS)

Terminologies obviously rely on structures and processes that guide the collection of data. A Nursing Minimum Data Set (NMDS) identifies essential, common, and core data elements to be collected for all patients/clients receiving nursing care (Werley & Lang, 1988). An NMDS generally

TABLE 8.5	The U.S. Nursing Minimum Data Set (NMDS) Data Elements

Nursing Care Elements

Nursing diagnosis

Nursing intervention

Nursing outcome

Intensity of nursing care

Patient or Client Demographic Elements

Personal identification[a]

Date of birth[a]

Sex[a]

Race and ethnicity[a]

Residence[a]

Service Elements

Unique facility or service agency number[a]

Unique health record number of patient or client[a]

Unique number of principal registered nurse provider

Episode admission or encounter date[a]

Discharge or termination date[a]

Disposition of patient or client[a]

Expected payer for most of this bill (anticipated financial guarantor for services)[a]

[a]Elements of the Uniform Hospital Discharge Data Set (UHDDS).

TABLE 8.6	Nursing Minimum Management Data Set (NMMDS) Data Elements

Environment

Facility unique identifiers

Nursing delivery unit or service

Patient/client population

Volume

Method of care delivery

Patient/client accessibility

Clinical decision-making complexity

Environmental complexity

Autonomy

Accreditation

Nursing Care

Management demographic profile

Staff demographic profile

Staffing

Staff satisfaction

Financial Resources

Payer type

Reimbursement

Budget

Expense

includes three broad categories of elements: (a) nursing care, (b) patient or client demographics, and (c) service elements (see Table 8.5). Many of the NMDS elements are consistently collected in the majority of patient/client records across healthcare settings in especially the patient and service elements. The aim of the NMDS is not to be redundant with respect to other data sets, but rather to identify what minimal data are needed to be collected from records of patients receiving nursing care.

Nursing Minimum Management Data Set (NMMDS)

NMDSs such as the U.S. NMDS often address "intensity"; however, no current NMDS addresses the essential breadth of contextual variables. The development within the United States of the NMMDS addresses this void. The 18 NMMDS elements are organized into three categories: environment, nursing care resources, and financial resources (see Table 8.6). The NMMDS is the minimum set of items of information with uniform definitions and categories concerning the specific dimension of the context of patient/client care delivery. It represents the essential data used to support the management and administration of nursing care delivery across all types of settings. The NMMDS most appropriately focuses on the nursing delivery unit/service/center of excellence level across these settings. The NMMDS supports numerous constructed variables as well as aggregation of data, for example, unit level, institution, network, system. This NMMDS provides the structure for the collection of uniform information that influences quality of patient care, directly and indirectly. These data, in combination with actual patient data identified in the NMDS, support clinical decision making; management decisions regarding the quantity, quality, and satisfaction of personnel; costs of patient care; clinical outcomes; and internal and external benchmarking. The Environment and Nursing Care categories for the NMMDS have been reviewed, normalized to national data definition standards, and incorporated into LOINC (Regenstrief Institute, 2014). Consequently, most elements of the NMMDS are available through implementation of the LOINC standard, making collection of these contextual variables and inclusion in outcomes analysis more efficient.

International Nursing Minimum Data Set

The International Nursing Minimum Data Set (i-NMDS) project is intended to build on and support data set work already underway in individual countries. Data collected in the i-NMDS pilot project will be cross-mapped and normalized to ICNP. This i-NMDS work will assist in testing the utility of i-NMDS and also advancing the ICNP as a unifying framework. Overall, the i-NMDS project focuses on coordinating ongoing national-level efforts (Kunkle et al., 2012; Westra, Matney, Subramanian, Hart, & Delaney, 2010a, 2010b).

The i-NMDS includes the core, internationally relevant, essential, minimum data elements to be collected in the course of providing nursing care (Clark & Delaney, 2000). These data can provide information to describe, compare, and examine nursing practice around the globe. Work toward the i-NMDS is intended to build on the efforts already underway in individual countries.

SUMMARY AND IMPLICATIONS FOR NURSING

The majority of nursing terminologies that exist today were developed originally many years ago and were primarily designed for the manual documentation of nursing practice. However, with the heavy emphasis on automation, the emergence of HIT and EHR systems, and the entrance of the federal government mandating technological regulations, the configuration of hospitals' HIT and EHR systems have changed to a more business model. For example in the United States, with the passage of the HITECH Act of 2009, and the implementation of "MU" Stages regulating technological processing of all patient services for federal payment, the documentation of patient care and the development of nursing plans of care have become secondary to the revenue generating departments' processing of their services.

The developers of nursing and healthcare terminologies and informatics scientists have made significant progress. From decades of nursing language research, there exists an extensive set of terms describing patient problems, nursing interventions and actions, and nursing-sensitive patient outcomes (AORN, 2007; Dochterman & Bulechek, 2004; ICN, 2009; Martin, 2005; Moorhead, Johnson, & Maas, 2004; NANDA, 2008; Ozbolt, 1998; Saba, 2006; Coenen, 2003) and robust information models, such as the

NMDS, to guide the collection of those terms. Through the efforts of nursing professionals, new terms which are useful for representing nursing-relevant concepts have been integrated into or linked into large healthcare terminologies (Bakken et al., 2000; Bakken et al., 2002; Henry, Holzemer, Reilly, & Campbell, 1994; Lange, 1996; Matney, Bakken, & Huff, 2003).

A number of efforts within nursing (e.g., ICNP) and the larger healthcare arena (e.g., SNOMED-CT) are aimed toward the achievement of advanced terminology systems that support semantic interoperability across healthcare information systems; collaborative working is facilitating this process. Ontology languages supported by suites of software tools have been developed within the context of terminologies with broad coverage of the healthcare domain (Campbell et al., 1998). Applicability of these tools to the nursing domain has been demonstrated (Hardiker & Rector, 1998; Zingo, 1997). A major ongoing challenge is the development of granular nursing content. However, existing standardized nursing terminologies continue to be an excellent source.

Today, advanced concept-oriented terminology systems are emerging as essential infrastructure for clinical practice. They now (a) provide for nonambiguous concept definitions, (b) facilitate composition of complex concepts from more primitive concepts, and (c) support mapping among terminologies (Campbell et al., 1997; Chute et al., 1996; Cimino, Clayton, Hripcsak, & Johnson, 1994; Henry et al., 1994). A number of benefits are being realized through the use of advanced terminology systems such as (a) the facilitation of evidence-based practice (e.g., linking of clinical practice guidelines to appropriate patients during the patient-provider encounter); (b) the matching of potential research subjects to research protocols for which they are potentially eligible; (c) the detection and prevention of potential adverse outcomes; (d) the linking online information resources; (e) the increased reliability and validity of data for quality evaluation; and (f) the data mining of concepts for purposes such as clinical research, health services research, or knowledge discovery.

In addition, other research is focusing on examining how terminology models and advanced terminology systems relate to other types of models that support semantic interoperability, such as (a) the Health Level 7 Reference Information Model (RIM) (Goossen et al., 2004), (b) the open EHR Archetypes (Beale, 2003), (c) the Detailed Clinical Models (Goossen, 2008), and (d) the ontology for document naming (Hyun et al., 2009; Dykes, Dadamio, & Kim, 2012). Such interoperability is a prerequisite to meeting the information demands of today's complex healthcare, management, and nursing environments.

ACKNOWLEDGMENTS

The authors wish to acknowledge Connie White Delaney for summarizing content from the 5th Ed. Chapter 13: Connie White Delaney and Bonnie Westra, "Nursing Minimum Data Sets Systems," and Suzanne Bakken for her contribution to the original 5th Ed. Chapter 12: Nicholas Hardiker, Suzanne Bakken, and Tae Youn Kim, "Advanced Terminological Approaches in Nursing" and Amy Coenen for her review of this update.

REFERENCES

American Medical Association. (2014). *CPT-2014: Current procedural terminology*. Chicago, IL: AMA.

American Nurses Association. (2008). *Nursing informatics: Scope and standards of practice*. Silver Spring, MD: ANA.

Association of Operating Room Nurses. (2007). *PNDS— Perioperative nursing data set* (2nd ed., rev.). Denver, CO: AORN Inc.

Bakken, S., Cashen, M., & O'Brien, A. (1999). Evaluation of a type definition for representing nursing activities within a concept-based terminologic system. In N. Lorenzi (Ed.), *1999 American Medical Informatics Association Fall Symposium* (pp. 17–21). Philadelphia, PA: Hanley & Belfus.

Bakken, S., Cimino, J. J., Haskell, R., Kukafka, R., Matsumoto, C., Chan, G. K., & Huff, S. M. (2000). Evaluation of the clinical LOINC (Logical Observation Identifiers, Names, and Codes) semantic structure as a terminology model for standardized assessment measures. *Journal of the American Medical Informatics Association, 7*(6), 529–538.

Bakken, S., Warren, J. J., Lundberg, C., Casey, A., Correia, C., Konicek, D., & Zingo, C. (2002). An evaluation of the usefulness of two terminology models for integrating nursing diagnosis concepts into SNOMED clinical terms. *International Journal of Medical Informatics, 68*(1–3), 71–77.

Beale, T. (2003). Archetypes and the EHR. *Studies in Health Technology and Informatics, 96*, 238–244.

Campbell, J., Carpenter, P., Sneiderman, C., Cohn, S., Chute, C., & Warren, J. (1997). Phase II evaluation of clinical coding schemes: Completeness, taxonomy, mapping, definitions, and clarity. *Journal of the American Medical Informatics Association, 4*(3), 238–251.

Campbell, K., Cohn, S., Chute, C., Shortliffe, E., & Rennels, G. (1998). Scalable methodologies for distributed development of logic-based convergent medical terminology. *Methods of Information in Medicine, 37*(4–5), 426–439.

Chute, C., Cohn, S., & Campbell, J. (1998). A framework for comprehensive terminology systems in the United States: Development guidelines, criteria for selection, and public policy implications. ANSI Healthcare Informatics Standards Board Vocabulary Working Group and the Computer-based Patient Records Institute Working Group on Codes and Structures. *Journal of the American Medical Informatics Association, 5*(6), 503–510.

Chute, C. G., Cohn, S. P., Campbell, K. E., Oliver, D. E., & Campbell, J. R. (1996). The content coverage of clinical classifications. *Journal of the American Medical Informatics Association, 3*(3), 224–233.

Cimino, J. (1998a). The concepts of language and the language of concepts. *Methods of Information in Medicine, 37*(4–5), 311.

Cimino, J. (1998b). Desiderata for controlled medical vocabularies in the twenty-first century. *Methods of Information in Medicine, 37*(4–5), 394–403.

Cimino, J., Hripcsak, G., Johnson, S., & Clayton, P. (1989). Designing an introspective, multi-purpose, controlled medical vocabulary. In L. C. Kingsland, III (Ed.), *Symposium on Computer Applications in Medical Care* (pp. 513–518). Washington, DC: IEEE Computer Society Press.

Cimino, J. J., Clayton, P. D., Hripcsak, G., & Johnson, S. B. (1994). Knowledge-based approaches to the maintenance of a large controlled medical terminology. *Journal of the American Medical Informatics Association, 1*(1), 35–50.

Clark, E., & Delaney, C. (2000). Conceptualizing and feasibility of an International Nursing Minimum Data Set (i-NMDS). (Abstract). In V. Saba, R. Carr, W. Sermeus, & P. Rocha (Eds.), *One Step Beyond: The Evolution of Technology and Nursing: Proceedings of the 7th Congress on Nursing Informatics* (p. 865). Aukland, New Zealand: Adis International.

Coenen, A. (2003). Building a unified nursing language: The ICNP. *International Nursing Review, 50*(2), 65–66.

Coenen, A., Marin, A. F., Park, H. A., & Bakken, S. (2001). Collaborative efforts for representing nursing concepts in computer-based systems. *Journal of American Medical Informatics Association, 8*, 202–211.

Coenen, A., McNeil, B., Bakken, S., Bickford, C., & Warren, J. J. (2001). Toward comparable nursing data: American Nurses Association criteria for datasets, classification systems, and nomenclatures. *Computers in Nursing, 19*(6), 240–246.

deKeizer, N. F., & Abu-Hanna, A. (2000). Understanding terminology systems II: Experience with conceptual & formal representation of structure. *Methods of Information in Medicine, 39*, 22–29.

Dochterman, J., & Bulechek, G. M. (2004). *Nursing interventions classification* (4th ed.). St. Louis, MO: C. V. Mosby.

Dykes, P. C., Dadamio, R. R., Kim, H. E. (2012, June 23). A framework for harmonizing terminologies to support representation of nursing practice in electronic records. *Nursing informatics: Proceedings of the International Congress on Nursing Informatics. 2012*, (p. 103). Montreal, Canada.

Elfrink, V., Bakken, S., Coenen, A., McNeil, B., & Bickford, C. (2001). Standardization of nursing vocabularies:

A foundation for quality care. *Seminars in Oncology Nursing, 17*(1), 18–23.

Englebright, J. (2014). Defining and incorporating basic nursing actions into the electronic health record. *Journal of Nursing Scholarship, 46,* 50–57.

European Committee for Standardization. (2000). *CEN ENV health informatics: Systems of concepts to support nursing.* Brussels, Belgium: CEN.

Fordyce, E. M. (1984). Theorists in nursing. In J. M Fynn & P. B. Heffron (Eds.), *Nursing from concept to practice* (pp. 237–258). Bowie, MD: Brady.

Goossen, W., Ozbolt, J., Coenen, A., Park, H., Mead, C., Ehnfors, M., & Marin, H. (2004). Development of a provisional domain model for the nursing process for use within the Health Level 7 reference information model. *Journal of the American Medical Informatics Association, 11*(3), 186–194.

Goossen, W. T. F. (2008). Using detailed clinical models to bridge the gap between clinicians and HIT. In E. de Clercq, G. De Moor, J. Bellon, M. Foulon, & J. Van der Lei (Eds.), *Collaborative patient centered ehealth* (pp. 3–10). Brussels, Belgium: IOS Press.

Hardiker, N. (2004). An international standard for nursing terminologies. In J. Bryant (Ed.), *Current perspectives in healthcare computing* (pp. 212–219). Swindon, UK: Health Informatics Committee of the British Computer Society.

Hardiker, N. R., Bakken, S., Casey, A., & Hoy, D. (2002). Formal nursing terminology systems: A means to an end. *Journal of Biomedical Informatics, 35*(5–6), 298–305.

Hardiker, N. R., Hoy, D., & Casey, A. (2000). Standards for nursing terminology. *Journal of American Medical Association, 7*(6), 523–528.

Hardiker, N. R., & Rector, A. (1998). Modeling nursing terminology using the GRAIL representation language. *Journal of the American Medical Informatics Association, 5*(1), 120–128.

Hardiker, N. R., & Coenen, A. (2007). Interpretation of an international terminology standard in the development of a logic-based compositional terminology. *International Journal of Medical Informatics, 76S2,* S274–S280.

Henry, S. B., Holzemer, W. L., Reilly, C. A., & Campbell, K. E. (1994). Terms used by nurses to describe patient problems: Can SNOMED III represent nursing concepts in the patient record? *Journal of the American Medical Informatics Association, 1*(1), 61–74.

Henry, S. B., & Mead, C. N. (1997). Nursing classification systems: Necessary but not sufficient for representing "what nurses do" for inclusion in computer-based patient record systems. *Journal of the American Medical Informatics Association, 4*(3), 222–232.

Hwang, J. I., Cimino, J. J., & Bakken, S. (2003). Integrating nursing diagnostic concepts into the medical entities dictionary using the ISO Reference Terminology Model for Nursing Diagnosis. *Journal of the American Medical Informatics Association, 10*(4), 382–388.

Hyun, S., Shapiro, J., Melton, G. B., Schlegel, C., Stetson, P., Johnson, J. B., & Bakken, S. (2009). Iterative evaluation of the Health Level 7—LOINC clinical document ontology for representing clinical document names: A case report. *Journal of the American Medical Informatics Association,* (3), 395–399.

Ingenerf, J. (1995). Taxonomic vocabularies in medicine: The intention of usage determines different established structures. In R. A. Greenes, H. E. Peterson, & D. J. Protti (Eds.). *Proceedings: MedInfo 95'* (pp. 136–139). Vancouver, BC: HealthCare Computing and Communications, Canada.

Institute of Medicine. (2012). *Best care at low cost: The path to continuously learning healthcare in America.* Washington, DC: IOM.

International Council of Nurses. (2001). *International Classification for Nursing Practice* (beta 2 version). Geneva, Switzerland: International Council of Nurses.

International Council of Nurses. (2009). *International Classification for Nursing Practice* (version 2). Geneva, Switzerland: International Council of Nurses. Retrieved from http://www.Icn.ch/PillarsPrograms/International-classification-for-nursing-practice-icnpr/. Accessed on June 1, 2014.

International Council of Nurses. (2012, June). *Press release: Harmonizing nursing terminology internationally: Collaboration between the International Council of Nurses and SabaCare.* Geneva, Switzerland: ICN.

International Organization for Standardization. (1990). *International Standard ISO 1087 1:2000 terminology: Vocabulary: Part 1: Theory and application.* Geneva, Switzerland: International Organization for Standardization.

International Organization for Standardization. (2003). *International Standard ISO 18104:2003 Health Informatics—Integration of a reference terminology model for nursing.* Geneva, Switzerland: International Organization for Standardization.

Johnson, M., Bulechek, G., Butcher, H., Dochterman, J. M., Maas, M., Moorhead, S., & Swanson, E. (2006). *NANDA, NOC, and NIC linkages: Nursing diagnoses, outcomes, & interventions.* St. Louis, MO: Mosby.

Kunkle, D., Westra, B. L., Hart, C. A., Subramanian, A., Kenny, S., & Delaney, C. W. (2012). Updating and normalization of the nursing management. Minimum data set: Element 6: Patient/Client accessibility. *Computers in Nursing, 30*(3), 134–141.

Lange, L. (1996). Representation of everyday clinical nursing language in UMLS and SNOMED. In J. Cimino (Ed.), *1996 American Medical Informatics Association Fall Symposium* (pp. 140–144). Philadelphia, PA: Hanley & Belfus.

Mannino, J. E., & Feeg, V. D. (2011). Field-testing a PC electronic documentation system using the Clinical Care Classification (CCC) System work with nursing students. *Journal of Healthcare Engineering, 2*(2), 223–240.

Martin, K. S. (2005). *The Omaha System: A key to practice, documentation, and information management.* St. Louis, MO: Elsevier.

Matney, S., Bakken, S., & Huff, S. M. (2003). Representing nursing assessments in clinical information systems using the logical observation identifiers, names, and codes database. *Journal of Biomedical Informatics, 36*(4–5), 287–293.

McGuiness, D. L., & van Harmelen, F. (Eds.), (2004). *OWL Web Ontology Language overview.* World Wide Web consortium. Retrieved from www.w3.org/TR/owl-features/. Accessed on July 27, 2010.

Moen, A. (1999). Representing nursing judgements in the electronic health record. *Journal of Advanced Nursing, 30*(4), 990–997.

Moorhead, S., Johnson, M., & Maas, M. (Eds.), (2004). *Nursing outcomes classification* (3rd ed.). St. Louis, MO: C. V. Mosby.

Moss, J., Coenen, A., & Mills, M. (2003). Evaluation of the draft international standard for a reference terminology model for nursing actions. *Journal of Biomedical Informatics, 36*(4–5), 271–278.

Moss, J. A., Damtongsak, M., & Gallichio, K. (2005). *Proceedings of 2005 AMIA Annual Symposium* (pp. 545–549). Washington, DC: AMIA.

Nightingale, F. (1859). *Notes on nursing.* Commemorative edition. Philadelphia, PA: J. B. Lippincott.

North American Nursing Diagnosis Association. (2008). *NANDA nursing diagnoses 2009–20011: Definitions and classification 2009–2011.* Philadelphia, PA: North American Nursing Diagnosis Association.

Ogden, C., & Richards, I. (1923). *The meaning of meaning.* New York, NY: Harcourt, Brace & World.

Ozbolt, J. G. (1998). *Ozbolt's Patient Care Data Set (Version 4.0).* Nashville, TN: Vanderbilt University.

Protégé. (2010). *What is Protégé-OWL?* Retrieved from http://protege.stanford.edu/overview/protege-owl.html. Accessed on July 27, 2010.

Rector, A. L. (2004). Defaults, context, and knowledge: Alternatives for OWL-indexed knowledge bases. *Pacific Symposium on Biocomputing* (pp. 226–237), January 6–10, 2004, Hawaii.

Rector, A. L., Bechhofer, S., Goble, C. A., Horrocks, I., Nowlan, W. A., & Solomon, W. D. (1997). The GRAIL concept modelling language for medical terminology. *Artificial Intelligence in Medicine, 9,* 139–171.

Regenstrief Institute. (2014). *Logical Observation Identifiers Names and Codes (LOINC).* Indianapolis, IN: Regenstrief Institute Inc.

Rossi Mori, A., Consorti, F., & Galeazzi, E. (1998). Standards to support development of terminological systems for healthcare telematics. *Methods of Information in Medicine, 37*(4–5), 551–563.

Saba, V. (2006). *Clinical Care Classification System.* Retrieved from www.sabacare.com. Accessed on July 27, 2010.

Saba, V., Hovenga, E., Coenen, A., & McCormick, K. A. (2003, September). *Nursing language: Terminology models for nurses.* Geneva, Switzerland: ISO Bulletin.

Saba, V. K. (2012). *Clinical Care Classification (CCC) System, Version 2.5: User's guide.* New York, NY: Springer.

Saba, V. K., & McCormick, K. A. (1986). *Essentials of computers for nurses.* Philadelphia, PA: J. B. Lippincott.

Saba, V. K., & Taylor, S. L. (2007). Moving past theory: Use of a standardized, coded nursing terminology to enhance nursing visibility. *CIN: Computers, Informatics, Nursing, 25*(6), 324–331.

Saranto, K. A., Moss, J., & Jylha, V. (2010). Medication counselling: Analysis of electronic documentation using the Clinical Care Classification System. In C. Safran, H. Marin, & S. Reti. (Eds.), *Proceedings of the MEDINFO 2010.* The Netherlands: IOS Press.

Simpson, R. L. (2003). Information technology. What's in a name? The taxonomy and nomenclature puzzle, Part 1. *Nursing Management, 34*(6), 14–18.

Sowa, J. (1984). *Conceptual structures.* Reading, MA: Addison-Wesley.

Thede, L. O., & Schwirian, P. M. (2013). Informatics: The standardization nursing terminologies: A national survey of nurses' experience and attitudes—Survey II: Participants' documentation use of standardized nursing terminologies. *The Online Journal of Issues in Nursing, 19*(1). doi:10.3912/OJIN.Vol19No01InfoCol01

Tsarkov, D. (2009). *factplusplus.* Retrieved from http://code.google.com/p/factplusplus/. Accessed on July 27, 2010.

Wang, A., Sable, J. H., & Spackman, K. (2002). The SNOMED clinical terms development process: Refinement and analysis of content. In I. Kohane (Ed.), *2002 American Medical Informatics Association Fall Symposium* (pp. 845–849). Philadelphia, PA: Hanley & Belfus.

Werley, H. H., & Lang, N. M. (Eds.), (1988). *Identification of the Nursing Minimum Data Set.* New York, NY: Springer.

Westra, B., Matney, S., Subramanian, A., Hart, C., & Delaney, C. (2010a). Update of the NMMDS & mapping to LOINC®. In C. Weaver, C. Delaney, P. Weber, & R. Carr (Eds.), *Nursing and Informatics for the 21st Century: An International Look at Practice, Education, and EHR Trends* (2nd ed.). *Healthcare Information and Management Systems Society (HIMSS) & American Medical Informatics Association* (AMIA) (pp. 269–275). Chicago, IL: HIMSS.

Westra, B. L., Subramanian, A., Hart, C. M., Matney, S. A., Wilson, P. S., Huff, S. M., Huber, D. L., & Delaney, C. W. (2010b). Achieving "meaningful use" of electronic health records through the integration of the Nursing Management Minimum Data Set. *Journal of Nursing Administration, 40*(7/8), 336–343.

Whittenburg, L. (2011). *Postpartum nursing records: Utility of the Clinical Care Classification System.* Doctoral dissertation. George Mason University, Fairfax, VA.

Yura, H., & Walsh, M. B. (1983). *The Nursing Process* (4th ed.). Norwalk, CT: Appleton-Century-Crofts Publishing.

Zielstorff, R. D. (1998, September 30). Characteristics of a good nursing nomenclature from an informatics perspective. *Online Journal of Issues in Nursing, 3*(2). Manuscript 4. Retrieved from www.nursingworld. org/MainMenuCategories/ANAMarketplace/ANAPeriodicals/OJIN/TableofContents/Vol31998/No2Sept1998/CharacteristicsofNomenclaturefromInformaticsPerspective.aspx

Zingo, C. A. (1997). Strategies and tools for creating a common nursing terminology within a large health maintenance organization. In U. Gerdin, M. Tallberg, & P. Wainwright (Eds.), *Proceedings: Nursing Information 1997* (pp. 27–31). Stockholm, Sweden: IOS Press.

9

Human–Computer Interaction

Gregory L. Alexander

- OBJECTIVES
  1. Recognize theoretical underpinnings for Human–Computer Interaction.
  2. Discuss Human–Computer Interaction principles.
  3. Apply the use of Human–Computer Interaction principles to a healthcare model called Aging in Place.
  4. Propose how the application of Human–Computer Interaction principles can improve nurse and patient outcomes in healthcare.

- KEY WORDS

  Human–Computer Interaction
  Patient care
  Information technology
  Patient safety
  System design

INTRODUCTION

Human–Computer Interaction (HCI) is broadly defined as an intellectually rich and highly impactful phenomenon influenced by four disciplines: (1) Human Factors/Ergonomics, (2) Information Systems, (3) Computer Science, and (4) Library and Information Science (Grudin, 2012). Aspirations of fledgling HCI researchers and practitioners, over the past 30 years, were to develop better menus, enhance use of graphical user interfaces, advance input devices, construct effective control panels, and improve information comprehension (Shneiderman, 2012). There are few fields, like HCI, which can claim such a rapid expansion and strong influence on the design of ubiquitous technologies including desktops, Web, and mobile devices used by at least 5 billion users around the world (Shneiderman, 2012). This chapter provides important information for nurses engaged in HCI efforts to improve healthcare systems and processes. The purpose of this chapter is to elevate nurses' understanding of theoretical underpinnings for HCI

approaches used to evaluate clinical technologies; to infuse HCI concepts by identifying important HCI approaches, during this time of rapid and continuous change; and finally, to describe how HCI evaluation can lead to improved performance and outcomes in nurse-led systems.

HUMAN FACTORS: A BUILDING BLOCK FOR HUMAN–COMPUTER INTERACTION

Human factors is a discipline that optimizes relationships between technology and humans (Kantowitz & Sorkin, 1983; McCormick & Sanders, 1982). Human factors has been defined in a number of ways by a number of experts (see Table 9.1). In healthcare, human factors experts attempt to understand relationships between humans, tools they use (i.e., computers), living and work environments, and tasks they perform (Staggers, 1991; Staggers, 2003; Weinger, Pantiskas, Wiklund, & Carstensen, 1998). Human factors

TABLE 9.1		Human Factors Definitions
Author	**Year**	**Human Factors Definition**
McCormick, E. J. and Sanders, M. S.	1982	The systematic application of relevant information about human abilities, characteristics, behaviors, and motivations to the execution of functions.
Kantowitz, B. H. and Sorkin, R. D.	1983	The discipline that tries to optimize the relationship between technology and the human.
Meister, D.	1989	HF is the study of how humans accomplish work-related tasks in the context of human machine-system operation and how behavioral and nonbehavioral variables affect that accomplishment. HF is also the application of behavioral principles to the design, development, testing, and operation of equipment and systems.
Weinger, M. B. and Englund, C. E.	1990	Refers to the designing of equipment, machines, or systems to accommodate the characteristics, expectations, and behaviors of the humans who use them in their everyday working and living environments.
Staggers, N.	1991	Optimal match between humans, their environments, technology, and the task at hand.
Traub, P.	1996	The application of scientific information about human beings (and scientific methods of acquiring such information) to the problems of design. Human factors is not (1) just applying checklists and guidelines, (2) using oneself as the model for designing things, (3) just common sense, or (4) a styling exercise.
Sawyer, D.	1996	Is a discipline that seeks to improve human performance in the use of equipment by means of hardware and software design that is compatible with the abilities of the user population.
Hasler, R. A.	1996	• An applied science focused on minimizing human errors and optimizing performance where human beings interface with a device. • HF engineering…also known as ergonomics…is the study of the physical characteristics and limitations of humans, which can be further subdivided into physical and anatomical characteristics.
Weinger, M., Pantiskas, C., Wiklund, M. E., and Carstensen, P.	1998	Human factors is the study of the interrelationships between humans, the tools they use, and the environments in which they live and work.
Welch, D. L.	1998	Improvement in efficiency, safety, and user satisfaction.
Rogers, W. A., Lamson, N., and Rousseau, G. K.	2000	A general tenet of human factors design is that safety should be ensured through design of the system. If potential hazard cannot be designed out, then it should be guarded against. If guarding against the hazard is not possible, then an adequate warning system should be developed.
Lin, L., Vicente, K., and Doyle, D. J.	2001	This discipline focuses on the interaction between technology, people, and their work context. HF has sometimes been narrowly associated with HCI design guidelines.
Weinger, M. B. and Slagle, J.	2002	Techniques to extract detailed information about system performance and risks to safety.
Wears, R. L. and Perry, S. J.	2002	The study of how human beings interact with their environment for useful purposes. The study of factors that make work easy or hard.
Gosbee, J.	2002	• The discipline that uses methods and concepts to understand and build systems that are more efficient, comfortable, and safe. • A discipline concerned with the design of tools, machines, and systems that take into account human capabilities, limitations, and characteristics. • Ergonomics, usability engineering, and user-centered design are considered synonymous.

(continued)

TABLE 9.1	Human Factors Definitions *(continued)*	
Author	**Year**	**Human Factors Definition**
Bates, D. W. and Gawande, A. A.	2003	Principles of design using HF suggest it is important to make warnings that are more serious and look different than those that are less serious.
Nemeth, C.	2004	The development and application of knowledge about human physiology and behavior in the operational environment.
Potter, P., Boxerman, S., Wolf, L., Marshall, J., Grayson, D., Sledge, J., and Evanoff, B.	2004	The study of human beings and their interactions with products, environments, and equipment in performing tasks and activities.
Boston-Fleischhauer, C.	2008	The discipline that studies human capabilities and limitations and applies that knowledge to the design of safe, effective, and comfortable products, processes, and systems for the human beings involved.
Sharples, S., Martin, J., Lang, A., Craven, M., O'Neill, S., and Barnett, J.	2012	The discipline of human factors has demonstrated that if a device is well designed then this will have positive implications for usability, defined as "the extent to which a product can be used by specified users to achieve specified goals with effectiveness, efficiency, and satisfaction in a specified context of use." (ISO 9241-11)
Vincent, C. J., Li, Y., and Blandford, A.	2013	The application of theory, principles, data, and methods to design in order to optimize human well-being and overall system performance.

Bates, D. W., & Gawande, A. A. (2003). Improving safety with information technology. *New England Journal of Medicine, 348*, 2526–2534.

Boston-Fleischhauer, C. (2008). Enhancing healthcare process design with human factors engineering and reliability science, Part 1: Setting the context. *Journal of Nursing Administration, 38*, 27–32.

Gosbee, J. (2002). Human factors in engineering and patient safety. *Quality and Safety in Health Care, 11*, 352–354.

Kantowitz, B. H., & Sorkin, R. D. (1983). *Human factors: Understanding people—System relationships.* New York, NY: Wiley.

Lin, L., Vicente, K. J., & Doyle, D. J. (2001). Patient safety, potential adverse drug events, and medical device design: A human factors engineering approach. *Journal of Biomedical Informatics, 34*, 274–284.

McCormick, E., & Sanders, M. S. (1982). *Human factors in engineering and design* (5th ed.). New York, NY: McGraw-Hill.

Meister, D. (1989). *Conceptual aspects of human factors.* Baltimore, MD: The Johns Hopkins University Press.

Rogers, W. A., Lamson, N., & Rousseau, G. K. (2000). Warning research: An integrative perspective. *Human Factors, 42*, 102–139.

Sawyer, D. (1996). *Do it by design: An introduction to human factors in medical devices.* Retrieved from http://www.fda.gov/cdrh/humfac/doitpdf.pdf

Sharples, S., Martin, J., Lang, A., Craven, M., O'Neill, S., & Barnett, J. (2012). Medical device design in context: A model of user-device interaction and consequences. *Displays, 33*, 221–232.

Traub, P. (1996, April). Optimising human factors integration in system design. *Engineering Management Journal*, 93–98.

Vincent, C.J., Li, Y., & Blandford, A. (2014). Integration of human factors and ergonomics during medical device design and development: It's all about communication. *Applied Ergonomics, 45*(3), 413–419. Available online June 15, 2013.

Wears, R. L., & Perry, S. J. (2002). Human factors and ergonomics in the emergency department. *Annals of Emergency Medicine, 40*, 206–212.

Weinger, M. B., & Slagle, J. (2002). Human factors research in anesthesia patient safety: Techniques to elucidate factors affecting clinical task performance and decision making. *Journal of the American Medical Informatics Association, 9*, S58–S63.

Welch, D. L. (1998, May–June). Human factors engineering. Human factors in the health care facility. *Biomedical Instrumentation & Technology, 32*(3), 311–316.

Wickens, C. D., Lee, J. D., Liu, Y., & Gordon-Becker, S. E. (2004). *An introduction to human factors engineering* (2nd ed.). Upper Saddle River, NJ: Pearson Prentice Hall.

experts apply information about human characteristics and behavior to determine optimal design specifications for tools people use in their daily life (Johnson & Barach, 2007). The goal of a human factors approach in nurse-led systems is to optimize the interactions between nurses and the tools they use to perform their jobs, minimize error, and maximize efficiency, optimize well-being, and improve quality of life.

HCI, concerned with interactions between people and computers, is an area of study concentrated on by human factors experts (Staggers, 2002). HCI is defined as the study of how people design, implement, and evaluate interactive computer systems in the context of users' tasks and work (Nelson & Staggers, 2014). HCI emerged in the 1980s as an interdisciplinary field incorporating ideals of computer science, cognitive science, and human factors engineering professionals, but since has grown into a science incorporating concepts and approaches from many other disciplines. An excellent history of HCI written by Grudin can be found in *Human Computer Interaction*

Handbook (Grudin, 2012). Some critics believe current descriptions of HCI require broader definitions. Critics suggest that current definitions do not reflect ubiquitous, pervasive, social, embedded, and invisible user-oriented technologies (Shneiderman, 2012). Further, some HCI critics want to move beyond computer use to emphasize other components of HCI including "…user experience, interaction design, emotional impact, aesthetics, social engagement, empathetic interactions, trust building, and human responsibility" (Shneiderman, 2012).

FRAMEWORKS FOR HCI IN NURSING

Early pioneers in nursing informatics set the stage for development of nursing information systems and their use in storing information, knowledge development, and development of technology in caregiving activities (Graves & Corcoran, 1989; Schwirian, 1986; Turley, 1996; Werley & Grier, 1981). These early models had several limitations including a lack of environmental and task-oriented elements, conceptual differences across frameworks, and a lack of time dimensions; subsequently, nursing frameworks were proposed to illustrate dynamic interactions occurring between nurses, computers, and enabling elements that optimize a user's ability to process information via computers (Staggers & Parks, 1993). These became the early foundations for incorporating human factors approaches into the design of information technologies used by nurses. However, there were still limitations identified in these early models because they did not explicitly make the patient part of the model and they didn't define the context or include all elements of nursing's metaparadigm (Effken, 2003). Effken (2003) proposed the Informatics Research Organizing Model, which emphasized all elements of nursing's metaparadigm including the system, nurse, patient, and health. Later, Alexander's Nurse—Patient Trajectory Framework was proposed (Alexander, 2007, 2011). Alexander's framework utilizes nursing process theory, human factors, and nursing and patient trajectories as components of a framework that can be used to evaluate patient care systems. The midrange framework specifically emphasizes the use of human factors approaches to link patient care processes, nurse and patient trajectories, and nursing and patient outcomes. In this discussion, the framework (see Fig. 9.1) has been modified to explore HCI in the context of nurse and patient trajectories as technology is integrated into nurse-led systems. Examples of HCI design and research using this model will be used to achieve the objectives.

DESIGNING FOR HCI

The discipline of HCI incorporates proponents of interaction design. Interaction designers are concerned with shaping digital things for people's use (Lowgren, 2013). Concepts proposed by interaction designers in healthcare have significant implications for design of pervasive technologies that are being developed and adopted by healthcare providers and patients. Interaction designers are characterized as shaping and transforming processes through the use of digital devices; they consider all possible futures for a digital design space; designers frame a problem at the same time they are creating a solution; and finally, designers address instrumental and technical aspects of digital media, but also recognize aesthetical and ethical aspects of designs (Lowgren, 2013).

AGING IN PLACE: AN EXAMPLE OF INTERACTION DESIGN

One problem for the millions of older adults who have multiple chronic illnesses is that they want to remain at home as long as possible. However, at the end of life, these chronic illnesses result in greater frailty, decline in independent daily activities, and greater safety concerns such as falls. Furthermore, as these conditions progress often older adults experience reduced mobility with greater isolation from their peers. Solutions to problems faced by these frail individuals are needed to help them age in place and to have better experiences at the end of their life.

Solutions for these problems are being developed by an interdisciplinary team of software designers at the University of Missouri in an independent living facility called TigerPlace (Rantz et al., 2013). To maximize efforts, the formation of an interdisciplinary interaction design team was critical in initial and ongoing stages of developing solutions for these age-old problems. The multidisciplinary team included nurses, physicians, sociologists, computer engineers, architectural designers, and informatics specialists. Rich dialog was produced from multiple perspectives that enhanced our ability to produce a wide variety of solutions, including embedded sensor systems that assisted in early detection of declining health experienced by older adults living in TigerPlace. While developing these solutions the design team concurrently considered crucial aspects of HCI design such as aesthetics, ethics, usability, and user experience (Alexander et al., 2011a). Examples are drawn from these experiences to demonstrate principles of HCI design.

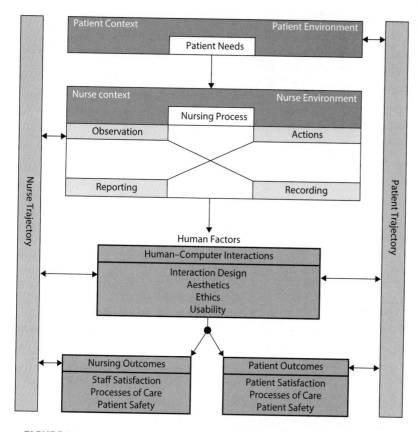

Patient Context

Patient Environment

Patient Needs

Nurse context

Nurse Environment

Nursing Process

Observation

Actions

Reporting

Recording

Human Factors

Human–Computer Interactions

Interaction Design
Aesthetics
Ethics
Usability

Nursing Outcomes

Staff Satisfaction
Processes of Care
Patient Safety

Patient Outcomes

Patient Satisfaction
Processes of Care
Patient Safety

Nurse Trajectory

Patient Trajectory

· **FIGURE 9.1.** Trajectory HCI. (Reproduced, with Permission, from Gregory L. Alexander, PhD.)

AESTHETICS IN HCI

Aesthetics has been defined as, "of or relating to beauty", and "pleasing in appearance: ATTRACTIVE easy to use keyboards, clear graphics, and other ergonomic and aesthetic features" (Merriam Webster, 2014). Aesthetics influences cognitive and emotional processes of people who interact with technology and is a strong determinate of user satisfaction and pleasure, which are important HCI outcome metrics (Tractinsky, 2013). Traditionally, HCI researchers have emphasized objective performance criteria, such as time to learn, error rates, and task completion times; other aspects such as aesthetics have been neglected (Lavie & Tractinsky, 2004). In the current context, aesthetics refers to the beauty and pleasing appearance of technological artifacts designed to solve complex health-related problems.

Aesthetics for Aging in Place Technologies

Referring back to our Aging in Place HCI model, our team has found that aesthetic design features influence

the adoption of technologies by patients who want to age in place; additionally, aesthetics are important to healthcare providers whose healthcare decisions are influenced during interactions with the technology (Demiris et al., 2004). As an example of aesthetic appeal, we will use descriptions of the functional components of our IT system used by patients and providers who live and work, respectively, with our sensor system. Aesthetic design has important ramifications for patient and provider trajectories in Alexander's framework illustrated in Fig. 9.1. The influence of aesthetic appeal for our users has important implications for technology acceptance in the lived environments of our patients and for providers (Venkatesh, Morris, Davis, & Davis, 2003).

Information about how the TigerPlace sensor system operates can be found in past publications (Rantz et al., 2013). We will provide a brief description here. TigerPlace residents who consent to have sensor systems have the option of having motion sensors placed throughout their apartment that detect motion, location, and functional activity levels in each room and in certain places, such as opening the refrigerator or turning on the stove. Another option, for TigerPlace residents, is to have a water-filled sensor installed under their mattress on their bed that detects bed restlessness, breathing patterns, and heart rate, while they are lying on the bed. Another option, for residents, is technology that captures gait parameters including most used walking paths and fall detection images. All of these data are collected in a secure server, accessed only by research staff with proper authorization. The data can be viewed via a computer interface which we have developed with HCI methods (Alexander et al., 2011a).

Residents, who live at TigerPlace, have expressed aesthetic concerns about the technology, which have influenced our product design and implementation in residents' apartments. In the initial stages of product development, the design team made a conscious decision to make all the technologies as noninvasive to the users as possible, including deploying technologies that are not worn by end users. The design team decided that technologies that are worn may infringe on the independence of the older adults, and furthermore, could contribute to the stigma of frailty that older adults may

experience. Older adults at TigerPlace expressed that they felt safer living with the technology, but they did not want the technology to stand out (Demiris, 2009). The invisibility of the technology was an important aesthetic design factor the team had to consider as we developed the product. HCI metrics that help us understand the perceptions of noninvasiveness and invisibility have been rarely measured, but are important considerations for prevailing IT systems that will be embedded where people live.

TigerPlace providers, nurse care coordinators who care for TigerPlace residents, want a system that can contribute to earlier detection of health decline for residents who are aging in place. However, a sensor system that captures activity data around the clock, 24/7, can be daunting to search through in order to make appropriate decisions about care coordination. One problem that designers faced was how to develop an interface that supports proper data visualization, of this big data, with good aesthetic appeal for end users. Using an interactive, iterative HCI process, the design team worked together with care coordinators to discuss concerns about the early illness warning system and suggest solutions (Alexander et al., 2011a). Figure 9.2

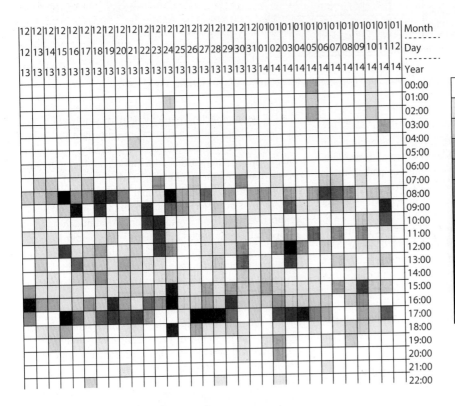

• **FIGURE 9.2.** Sensor–System Interface.

illustrates the outcome of this critical work engaging end users and software developers in the design process of an interface for our sensor system.

The design teams worked to incorporate colors along a longitudinal graph for each hour of each day, which we call a motion density map, to help providers easily detect resident activity level change. More vivid blues and yellows on the motion density map indicate greater activity levels, which are easily detectable, compared to the duller hues. Additionally, the design layout expedited the ability to detect important activity changes at different times of the day, such as during the nighttime when residents should be sleeping (yellow and gray hues between midnight and 6:00 AM). Design aesthetics incorporated into longitudinal data, as illustrated in Fig. 9.2, is being used by healthcare providers to detect patient decline. The aesthetic design of these interfaces is crucial to facilitate proper use and detection of early illness decline experienced by residents and observed for by providers.

ETHICS IN HCI

For a long while, perceptions have been that information technology can help improve diagnostic accuracy, make information more accessible, and can improve the representation of facts in medical records (Miller, Schaffner, & Meisel, 1985; Staggers, Thompson, & Snyder-Halpern, 2001). However, with the everywhereness of technology embedded throughout our world and the robust forms of technology being used, ethical considerations for HCI are becoming paramount. For instance, consider the example of designing for mobile platforms, three main problem areas of design have been proposed for these types of devices including use of screen space, interaction mechanisms, and design of mobile user interfaces (Nilsson, 2009). Designers assume great responsibility to address these problems by designing in solutions that optimize use of these platforms, while minimizing potential pitfalls of HCI design problems (Association for Computing Machinery, 2014). Mobile healthcare platforms, such as telemonitoring equipment, Web-based support systems, or bedside clinical decision support systems to help frontline nurses manage critical symptom changes are a few examples (van der Krieke, Emerencia, Aiello, & Syteme, 2012; Winkler et al., 2011; Yuan, Finley, Long, Mills, & Johnson, 2013). Designers assume an ethical responsibility to test these platforms using HCI methods not only in controlled settings during early stages of development life cycles but also at periods of implementation in the field where unintended consequences can occur (Ash, Berg, & Coiera, 2004).

Ethics for Aging in Place Technologies

The sensor technologies being used at TigerPlace have been incorporated into the living environments of residents choosing to age in place at this facility. Future use of these sensors includes possible interactions with other types of users, such as families, physicians, nurses. So, their input into the development of this technology is critical during all stages of development and implementation.

In order to meet ethical obligations to the public who will eventually use these sensor systems, the design team incorporated multiple HCI methodologies to examine user's perceptions of the interface and to examine the functionality of the interface. For instance, our team conducted many key informant interviews with residents living with sensors to explore their lived experiences with the sensor systems (Demiris et al., 2004). Finally, we conducted task-oriented usability assessments that were electronically documented with usability software, called Morae, with each type of end user (residents, families, nurses, physicians) (Alexander et al., 2011b). Through these usability assessments the design team identified potential problem areas encountered during interactions for each user type. Again, these findings were used by software designers to improve the functionality, aesthetics, and appearance of the sensor interface. Usability methodologies are important to meet ethical obligations of software design.

USABILITY IN HCI

Usability evaluation determines the extent that a technology is easy and pleasurable to use by determining if it is well adapted to users, their tasks, and that negative outcomes are minimized as a result of use (Bastien, 2010). Usability evaluation has been a staple of HCI researchers for the past 30 years and continues to grow in prominence as technology advances have been made around the world. HCI designers have proposed that usability is inherently measureable in all electronic technologies, that usability evaluation determines if an interactive system is usable, and if a system is usable, then usability evaluation can determine the extent of usability using hardy usability metrics, and finally, that usability evaluation is an accessible form of analysis and easy enough to learn about in HCI literature (Cockton, 2013). There are a large number of methods available for designers to use to assess the usefulness of a piece of medical technology. Table 9.2 provides a comparison of HCI methods for capturing user requirements to help interested readers in selecting some appropriate HCI methods.

TABLE 9.2	Comparison of Methods for Capturing User Requirements						
Method	**Contextual Inquiry**	**Cognitive Task Analysis**	**Usability Tests**	**Heuristics**	**Cognitive Walkthrough**	**Focus Groups**	**Delphi Technique**
Relative costs	Moderate/ high	Moderate	Moderate	Low	Low	Low	Low
Time	Moderate/ high	Moderate	Moderate	Low	Low	Moderate	Moderate
Setting	Field	Field/lab	Field/lab	Lab	Lab	Conference room	Office
Stage of product develop- ment	Pre-concept/ concept	Evaluation	Concept through to evaluation	Evaluation	Evaluation	All	Pre-concept/ concept
Type of data	Qualitative	Qualitative	Qualitative and Quantitative	Quantitative	Qualitative and Quantitative	Qualitative	Quantitative
Type of user	"Real" users	"Real" users	"Real" users and proxies	Proxies	Proxies	"Real" users and proxies	"Real" users
Level of inves- tigator expertise required	Moderate/ high	Moderate/ high	Moderate	Moderate	Moderate	Moderate	Moderate
Information yield	Moderate/ high	Moderate/ high	Moderate/ high	Low/ moderate	Low/moderate	Low/ moderate	Moderate

Reprinted with permission from Martin, J. L., Norris, B. J., Murphy, E., & Crose, J. A. (2008). Medical device development: The challenge for ergonomics. *Applied Ergonomics, 39*, 271–283. Copyright Elsevier.

Contextual Inquiry

Contextual inquiry is qualitative in nature. This methodology is derived from ethnography, which focuses on scientific descriptions and illustrations of social groups and systems. Contextual inquiry is usually conducted in the field using extensive, well-designed, systematic observations to capture how people interact with technology in real-world settings. Through this method the researcher becomes immersed in the group or system to understand how interactions take place. This method provides rich data that can be voluminous depending on number of settings involved, time spent in the settings, and the number of observations captured in the setting. Typically, sample subjects are key informants who have specialized knowledge, status, or skills which are of interest to the researcher. Oftentimes one, two, or more subjects can be observed individually or in dyads over periods of time to understand how interactions take place or how technology may influence interactions. Decisions about the sample

and settings also have impacts on costs of conducting contextual inquiry research, which can be high. Researchers using contextual inquiry methods use their interpretations of observations as a source to answer important questions about social groups or systems. In many studies, other methods are used concurrently with contextual inquiry, such as focus groups in order to validate researchers' interpretations of phenomenon observed in the field.

Cognitive Task Analysis

Cognitive research is used to describe psychological processes associated with the acquisition, organization, and use of knowledge (Hollnagel, 2003). Cognitive processes in human–machine interactions are complex and involve continuous exchanges of information between operators and the machines they use, which is a type of shared cognition. For example, nurses and physicians work in tandem to deliver optimal care for each patient. The design of human–machine interfaces such as nursing and physician interfaces used for documentation and medical record review must consider the nature of interdisciplinary work. Unfortunately, studies typical of evaluating nursing workflow disruption have not been a focus in similar studies assessing physician workflow; for instance, investigating how nursing roles and activities are affected by physician orders when implementing a clinical information system would provide valuable design input for electronic medical record designs (Lee & McElmurry, 2010). Medical devices are also an important human–machine interface which are sometimes shared and need to be tested collaboratively by interdisciplinary healthcare teams, but these evaluations are limited, such as evaluations including both nurses and pharmacists should provide important design considerations for computerized provider order entry for pharmacy and medication administration systems to ensure safe execution of orders and delivery of medications (Alexander & Staggers, 2009).

Cognitive processes in human–machine systems involve the operator providing input to the machine, the machine acting on the input, and displaying information back to the operator; the operator processes information through sensing mechanisms such as visual, auditory, somatosensory, and vestibular systems; and finally, the operator determines if the information from the machine is accurate, providing correct communication, decides what actions to take, and provides new input to the machine (Proctor & Proctor, 2006). Attempts to understand and exploit human capabilities and strengths within the area of human cognitive ability are critical to the safe design of technology. Safe design includes responses to human stress and is an important variable in HCI research. For example, the ability of a nurse to make timely and accurate decisions and to be vigilant of machine alarms during periods of sleep deprivation while working several 12-h night shifts in a row is a common work scenario that is worthy of attention in HCI research. Furthermore, human factors experts in nursing have begun using mapping techniques called link analysis to map the cognitive processes of nursing work to understand what stresses or interruptions nurses encounter during work, which contribute to cognitive delay. For example, nonlinearity of nursing work, which requires frequent shifts in the process of delivering care results in interruptions and delays in care that contribute to unsafe environments (Potter et al., 2004). Understanding cognitive abilities of operators in the healthcare sector provides better understanding of physical and operational structures that affect clinical decision-making and clinical reasoning that may lead to potential system failures.

Cognitive task analysis used to evaluate task load has been used in healthcare settings. These type of analyses are typically qualitative in nature and involve interactions with "real" users to inform the design of new devices, which have usability outcomes already established (Martin, Norris, Murphy, & Crowe, 2008). Examples of CTA, in health care research, include the identification of potential errors performed with computer-based infusion devices used for terbutaline administration in preterm labor; to evaluate cognitive and physical burdens during period of high workload and stress while using computer-based physiological monitoring systems in cardiac anesthesia; and to gain new perspectives in the work of nursing processes to understand how disruptions can contribute to nursing error in acute care environments (Cook & Woods, 1996; Obradovich & Woods, 1996; Potter et al., 2004).

Usability Tests

The International Organization for Standardization's definition of usability is "The extent to which a product can be used by specified users to achieve specified goals with effectiveness, efficiency, and satisfaction in a specified context of use" (ISO/IEC, 1998). Usability evaluations are viewed as a critical component to inform all stages of medical device product development from initial concepts through evaluation. The potential impacts of well-designed usability studies for medical devices are reduced user errors and intensification of patient safety efforts. For example, the National Institute of Standards and Technology in the U.S. Department of Commerce issued a report describing why usability of electronic medical records is critical (Lowry et al., 2012). In the report, the authors outline a three-step process for electronic health record evaluation and human user performance testing including the following: (1) During the electronic health record design stage, users, work settings, and workflows are documented to determine possible system usability problems and to develop a working model that minimizes potential safety risks; (2) conduct an expert analysis comparing the prototype interface designs to rigorously established design standards, such as heuristics discussed next in order to establish estimates of effectiveness, efficiency, and potential risks; and finally (3) examine critical tasks to be performed with real users documenting objective performance measures, such as task completion times, number of errors, and failures. Additionally, subjective measures are important to identify, such as mismatches between user expectations identified during periods when users are encouraged to think aloud about their experiences. Subject measures can be measured with simple usability scales, as the System Usability Scale, which is freely available for researchers. These processes, if conducted in a rigorous way, could be applied to any medical device usability evaluation, not just electronic health records.

Usability studies are often conducted in labs during early conceptual and prototype stages of a project. However, usability studies should also be conducted through to final evaluation stages in the field. This is important because field experiments can bring about unintended consequences due to workflows and processes encountered by users during interactions with devices. There is evidence in the literature that field studies are not conducted as often as they should be for crucial medical devices being implemented in patient care settings (Alexander & Staggers, 2009). Reasons for a lack of usability studies in the field could be increased costs and disruptions to services from excessive time commitments required for these types of assessments.

Heuristics

This type of HCI evaluation involves a small group of experts, who evaluate quantitatively how well a device meets established design standards, called heuristics (Sharp, Rogers, & Preece, 2008). Procedures for a heuristic evaluation are part of an iterative design process that enables identification and, hopefully, elimination of potential risks that may cause dangerous outcomes. For example, designers of the Aging in Place sensor system, discussed throughout this chapter, supported an extensive heuristic analysis of the sensor data display using three outside experts who were trained in HCI methods. The sensor data display was evaluated against 16 heuristics, which included 96 heuristic criteria in total, during the conceptual phase, before it was deployed in the clinical setting where care coordinators use the sensor interface to coordinate care. The assessment was conducted in a usability lab where the expert reviewers could interact with the sensor interface. Many recommendations were made by reviewers to the design team to improve the sensor data interface, which were incorporated into the subsequent interface designs.

The heuristic evaluation resulted in 26 recommendations for design change. Findings were classified according to their importance, the most important being heuristic criteria that were not met. The most important design changes that were not met included flexibility and efficiency of use of the interface due to lack of functional descriptions of interface components provided, help and frequently asked question (FAQ) documentation that were provided to users, lack of the interface to support all skill levels of users, and poor navigational issues related to lack of feedback about where users were located in the system during interactions. Positive ratings were given heuristic

criteria related to aesthetic appeal of the interface and minimalist design (Alexander et al., 2008). Through this process the design team was able to identify weaknesses in system design prior to implementation, responded by redesigning the interface to strengthen support of these established criteria, and reducing the risk of potential negative outcomes of use of the system.

Cognitive Walkthrough

Similar to heuristic evaluation, cognitive walkthrough is conducted using expert evaluators who are not necessarily part of the population of end users of a technological device (Martin et al., 2008). Cognitive walkthrough evaluations are task-specific, as compared to heuristic evaluation, which provides a holistic view of the interface and system features. To be successful an investigator conducting a cognitive walkthrough must be aware of who are the systems users, what tasks are to be analyzed, and sequences of tasks to be conducted, and that evaluators must know how the interface functions (Unknown, 2014). This means that evaluators must be familiar with tasks, their composition, how tasks are allocated, and feedback given in response to tasks.

Tasks. Tasks involve interplay between physical and cognitive activities and may be considered to follow a continuum between nearly pure physical tasks, such as transporting a patient to an X-ray to nearly pure cognitive tasks such as assessing hemodynamic status. Tasks tend to describe discrete, detailed behaviors needed to carry out functions and functions tend to describe continuous, macro-level behaviors, such as analyzing or detecting (Sharit, 1997).

Task Composition. A task or action sequence starts with a goal, then steps are initiated based upon user intentions, followed by the sequence of actions to be performed or intended to be performed, and the steps in the execution of the task. After tasks are executed they are evaluated based on user perception, interpretation, and evaluation of the interpretations of the actions. Task structures may be shallow, narrow, wide, and deep. Most everyday tasks, which occupy most of a human's time, are considered shallow, narrow structures that are opportunistic in nature, requiring little complexity in analysis and minimal conscious activity. In shallow and narrow structures, humans need only examine alternative actions and act; alternatively, wide and deep structures require a considerable amount of conscious planning and thought, and usually require deliberate trial-and-error functions (Norman, 2002).

Feedback. Conditions that have been found to hinder feedback in healthcare environments include incomplete awareness that system failures have occurred, time and work pressures, delays in action or outcome sequences, case infrequence, deficient follow-up, failed communication, deficient reporting systems, case review biases, shift work and handoffs (Croskerry, 2000). Feedback is an important element that may be derived from display information in human–computer interactions and is important in the perception, implementation, and evaluation of tasks. Not all system feedback mechanisms are technical in nature, sometimes feedback mechanisms are created through human quality audits, peer reviews, and data mining. Emotional risks associated with the failure to provide feedback include loss of confidence, uncertainty about performance, and increased stress.

Feedback mechanisms have been recognized as important components in nurse–computer interactions. Improvements have been recognized in the visibility and standardization of coordination of care mechanisms in wireless computerized information systems in nursing home information systems. In these settings, improved feedback mechanisms positively affected staff documentation and communication patterns in automated wireless nursing home environments where mobile devices were used by nurse assistants to document activities of daily living as they occurred; simultaneously, nurses were able to see what cares had been completed and outcomes related to the care. This seamless transition resulted in better quality and efficiency of patient care (Rantz et al., 2010). In other reports evaluations of response times to critical laboratory results using automated feedback mechanisms resulted in decreased response times following an appropriate treatment order (Kuperman et al., 1999). Information technologies that facilitate transmission of important patient data can improve the quality of care.

Focus Groups

Focus groups are an excellent method to cumulate rich qualitative descriptions of how people interact with technological systems. These are low costs methodologies that require little overhead to conduct, but can provide a significant amount of information about usefulness of technologies, system processes, and satisfaction of people using technology. Focus groups methodologies can be used throughout all product design stages and usually involve small groups of users being interviewed by researcher who is interested in a specified phenomenon familiar to the users (Krueger, 1994). Focus groups are usually conducted in a controlled environment to avoid distraction, such as a conference room, where people can feel free to share openly about their experiences. Typically, focus groups are conducted using well-thought-out questions, which are used by researchers to maintain some methodological consistency. Taking time to think about these questions ahead of time will enhance reliability and reduce bias that could be introduced by randomly questioning participants. Data from multiple focus groups are usually analyzed for emerging themes that help support the research question. Data are analyzed until data saturation is reached and all themes are realized from the data.

Delphi Technique

The Delphi technique is used to gain consensus from experts on a subject. This method uses multiple rounds of data collection from experts, with each round using data from previous rounds. The questions posed focus on the opinions, forecasts, and judgments of experts on a specific topic. Each round of questions completed is analyzed, summarized, and returned to the experts with a new questionnaire. With each round of questions experts look over previous information provided by the group and formulate opinions based on the whole group's feedback until a consensus is reached. This process of response, feedback, and response is usually repeated at least three times, or until a general group consensus is obtained. Benefits of this methodology is acquiring input from multiple experts who may be geographically dispersed, further, overhead and costs are generally low to conduct the method. Some limitations to this method is that it can be time consuming and cooperation of consensus panel members might be reduced over the length of the study.

OUTCOMES IN HCI

Traditional outcomes associated with HCI methods are efficiency, effectiveness, and satisfaction, which, as stated, are highly related to how usable a piece of technology is. These outcomes have been a long-standing, central feature of HCI for many years. With current emphasis by national institutes, such as National Institute of Standards and Technology, on incorporating HCI methodologies into the life cycle of developing technologies, HCI principles and methods will continue to grow in importance. Theoretical frameworks or models of clinical care using any form of technology should incorporate HCI outcomes related to both the clinician and the patient. For example, satisfaction with particular technologies will differ depending on whether the interaction being evaluated is between a patient and a computer or a nurse and a computer. In the examples used throughout this chapter, the patients who are aging in place, living with sensor systems have a very different set of expectations, compared to nurses who are using the sensor system for early detection of health decline and care coordination. Patients claim they feel safer living with the technology, but they are not necessarily interested in seeing or using the data being collected by the sensors. Nurses have shown that the sensor data are useful in helping to predict early illness decline, but tracking big data longitudinally presents some unique challenges in data visualization and prediction of health events. As new forms of technologies evolve, traditional HCI outcomes may require updating to keep pace with development.

REFERENCES

Alexander, G. L. (2007). The nurse-patient trajectory framework. *Studies in Health Technology and Informatics, 129,* 910–914.

Alexander, G. L. (2011). Human factors. In V. K. Saba & K. A. McCormick (Eds.), *Essentials of nursing informatics* (5th ed., pp. 119–132). New York, NY: McGraw-Hill.

Alexander, G. L., Rantz, M. J., Skubic, M., Aud, M., Wakefield, B., Florea, E., & Paul, A. (2008). Sensor systems for monitoring functional status in assisted living facility residents. *Research in Gerontological Nursing, 1,* 238–244.

Alexander, G. L., Rantz, M. J., Skubic, M., Koopman, R., Phillips, L. J., Guevara, R. D., & Miller, S. J. (2011a). Evolution of an early illness warning system to monitor frail elders in independent living. *Journal of Healthcare Engineering, 2,* 259–286.

Alexander, G. L., & Staggers, N. (2009). A systematic review on the designs of clinical technology: Findings and recommendations for future research. *Advances in Nursing Science, 32,* 252–279.

Alexander, G. L., Wakefield, B. J., Rantz, M. J., Aud, M. A., Skubic, M., & Erdelez, S. (2011b). Evaluation of a passive sensor technology interface to assess elder activity in independent living. *Nursing Research, 60,* 318–325.

Ash, J. S., Berg, M., & Coiera, E. (2004). Some unintended consequences of information technology in health care: The nature of patient care information system-related errors. *Journal of the American Medical Informatics Association, 11,* 104–112.

Association for Computing Machinery. (2014). *Software engineering code of ethics and professional practice.* Retrieved from http://www.acm.org/about/se-code

Bastien, J. M. (2010). Usability testing: A review of some methodological and technical aspects of the method. *International Journal of Medical Informatics, 79,* e18–e23.

Cockton, G. (2013). *Usability evaluation. "The encyclopedia of human-computer interaction."* Retrieved from http://www.interaction-design.org/encyclopedia/interaction_design.html

Cook, R. I., & Woods, D. D. (1996). Adapting to new technology in the operating room. *Human Factors, 38,* 593–613.

Croskerry, P. (2000). The feedback sanction. *Academic Emergency Medicine., 7,* 1232–1238.

Demiris, G. (2009). Privacy and social implications of distinct sensing approaches to implementing smart homes for older adults. In IEEE (Ed.), *Engineering in Medicine and Biology Society (EMBC), 2009. Annual International Conference of the IEEE* (pp. 4311–4314). New York, NY: IEEE.

Demiris, G., Rantz, M. J., Aud, M. A., Marek, K. D., Tyrer, H. W., Skubic, M. et al. (2004). Older adults' attitudes towards and perceptions of 'smart home' technologies: A pilot study. *Medical Informatics, 29,* 87–94.

Effken, E. (2003). An organizing framework for nursing informatics research. *Computers Informatics Nursing, 21,* 316–325.

Graves, J. R., & Corcoran, S. (1989). The study of nursing informatics. *Image Journal of Nursing Scholarship, 21,* 227–231.

Grudin, J. (2012). A moving target: The evolution of human–computer interaction. In J. Jacko (Ed.), *Human–computer interaction handbook* (3rd ed.). London: CRC Press.

Hollnagel, E. (2003). Prolegomenon to cognitive task design. In E. Hollnagel (Ed.), *Handbook of cognitive task design* (pp. 3–15). Mahwah, NJ: Lawrence Erlbaum.

ISO/IEC. (1998). *Ergonomic requirements for office work with visual display terminals (VDTs)—Part 14 Menu dialogue* (Rep. No. (ISO/IEC 9241-14)).

Johnson, J. K., & Barach, P. (2007). Clinical microsystems in health care: The role of human factors in shaping the microsystem. In P. Carayon (Ed.), *Handbook of human factors and ergonomics in health care and patient safety* (pp. 95–107). Mahwah, NJ: Lawrence Erlbaum.

Kantowitz, B. H., & Sorkin, R. D. (1983). *Human factors: Understanding people—System relationships.* New York, NY: Wiley.

Krueger, R. A. (1994). *Focus groups: A practical guide for applied research* (2nd ed.). Thousand Oaks, CA: Sage.

Kuperman, G. J., Teich, J. M., Tanasijevic, M. J., Ma'Luf, N., Rittenberg, E., Jha, A., … Bates, B. W. (1999). Improving response to critical laboratory results with automation. *Journal of the American Medical Informatics Association, 6,* 512–522.

Lavie, T., & Tractinsky, N. (2004). Assessing dimensions of perceived visual aesthetics of web sites. *International Journal of Human Computer Interaction, 60,* 269–298.

Lee, S., & McElmurry, B. (2010). Capturing nursing care workflow disruptions: Comparison between nursing and physician workflows. *CIN: Computers, Informatics, Nursing, 28,* 151–159.

Lowgren, J. (2013). *Interaction design-brief intro. "The encyclopedia of human–computer interaction."* Retrieved from http://www.interaction-design.org/encyclopedia/interaction_design.html

Lowry, S. Z., Quinn, M. T., Mala, R., Shumacher, R. M., Patterson, E. S., North, R., … Abbott, P. A. (2012).

Technical Evaluation, Testing, and Validation of the Usability of Electronic Health Records (Rep. No. NIST Interagency/Internal Report (NISTIR)—7804). National Institute of Standards and Technology.

Martin, J. L., Norris, B. J., Murphy, E., & Crowe, J. A. (2008). Medical device development: The challenge for ergonomics. *Applied Ergonomics, 39*, 271–283.

McCormick, E. J., & Sanders, M. S. (1982). *Human factors in engineering and design* (5th ed.). New York, NY: McGraw-Hill.

Merriam Webster. (2014). *Merriam Webster online dictionary*. Retrieved from http://www.merriam-webster.com/dictionary/aesthetic

Miller, R. A., Schaffner, K. F., & Meisel, A. (1985). Ethical and legal issues related to the use of computer programs in clinical medicine. *Annals of Internal Medicine, 102*, 529–536.

Nelson, R., & Staggers, N. (2014). *Health informatics*. St. Louis, MO: Mosby.

Nilsson, E. G. (2009). Design patterns for user interface for mobile applications. *Advances in Engineering Software, 40*, 1318–1328.

Obradovich, J. H., & Woods, D. D. (1996). Users as designers: How people cope with poor HCI design in computer-based medical devices. *Human Factors, 38*, 574–592.

Potter, P., Boxerman, S., Wolf, L., Marshall, J., Grayson, D., Sledge, J., & Evanoff, B. (2004). Mapping the nursing process: A new approach for understanding the work of nursing. *Journal of Nursing Administration, 34*, 101–109.

Proctor, R. W., & Proctor, J. D. (2006). Sensation and perception. In G. Salvendy (Ed.), *Handbook of human factors and ergonomics* (3rd ed., pp. 53–88). Hoboken, NJ: Wiley.

Rantz, M. J., Alexander, G. L., Galambos, C., Flesner, M. K., Vogelsmeier, A., Hicks, ... Greenwood, L. (2011). The use of bedside electronic medical record to improve quality of care in nursing facilities: A qualitative analysis, *CIN: Computers, Informatics, Nursing, 29*(3), 149–156.

Rantz, M. J., Skubic, M., Miller, S., Galambos, C., Alexander, G. L., Keller, J., & Popescu, M. (2013). Sensor technology to support Aging in Place. *Journal of the American Medical Informatics Association, 14*, 386–391.

Schwirian, P. M. (1986). The NI pyramid: A model for research in nursing informatics. *Computers in Nursing, 4*, 134–136.

Sharit, J. (1997). Allocation of functions. In G. Salvendy (Ed.), *Handbook of human factors and ergonomics* (2nd ed., pp. 302–337). New York, NY: Wiley.

Sharp, H., Rogers, Y., & Preece, J. (2008). Interaction heuristic evaluation toolkit. The interaction design: Beyond human–computer interaction. Retrieved from http://www.id-book.com/catherb/index.htm

Shneiderman, B. (2012). Expanding the impact of human–computer interaction. In J. Jacko (Ed.), *Human–computer interaction handbook* (3rd ed., pp. xv-xvi). London: CRC Press.

Staggers, N. (1991). Human factors. The missing element in computer technology. *Computers in Nursing, 9*, 47–49.

Staggers, N. (2002). Human–computer interaction. In S. Englebardt & R. Nelson (Eds.), *Information technology in health care: An interdisciplinary approach* (pp. 321–345). San Diego, CA: Harcourt Health Science Company.

Staggers, N. (2003). Human factors: Imperative concepts for information systems in critical care. [Review] [24 refs]. *AACN Clinical Issues, 14*, 310–319.

Staggers, N., & Parks, P. L. (1993). Description and initial applications of the Staggers & Parks nurse–computer interaction framework. *Computers in Nursing, 11*, 282–290.

Staggers, N., Thompson, C. B., & Snyder-Halpern, R. (2001). History and trends in clinical information systems in the United States. *Journal of Nursing Scholarship, 33*, 75–81.

Tractinsky, N. (2013). *Visual aesthetics. "The encyclopedia of human–computer interaction."* Retrieved from http://www.interaction-design.org/encyclopedia/interaction_design.html

Turley, J. (1996). Toward a model for nursing informatics. *Image Journal of Nursing Scholarship, 28*, 309–313.

Unknown. (2014). *Cognitive walkthrough*. Retrieved from http://www.pages.drexel.edu/~zwz22/CognWalk.htm

van der Krieke, L., Emerencia, A. C., Aiello, M., & Syteme, S. (2012). Usability evaluation of a web-based support system for people with a schizophrenia diagnosis. *Journal of Medical Internet Research, 14*, e24.

Venkatesh, V., Morris, M. G., Davis, G. B., & Davis, F. D. (2003). User acceptance of information technology: Toward a unified view. *MIS Quarterly, 27*, 425–478.

Weinger, M., Pantiskas, C., Wiklund, M. E., & Carstensen, P. (1998). Incorporating human factors into the design of medical devices. *Journal of the American Medical Association., 280*, 1484.

Werley, H. H., & Grier, M. R. (1981). *Nursing information systems*. New York, NY: Springer.

Winkler, S., Axmann, C., Schannor, B., Kim, S., Leuthold, T., Scherf, M., ... Koehler, F. (2011). Diagnostic accuracy of a new detection algorithm for atrial fibrillation in cardiac telemonitoring with portable electrocardiogram devices. *Journal of Electrocardiology, 44*, 460–464.

Yuan, M. J., Finley, G. M., Long, J., Mills, C., & Johnson, R. K. (2013). Evaluation of user interface and workflow design of a bedside nursing clinical decision support system. *Interactive Journal of Medical Research, 2*, e4.

10

Trustworthy Systems for Safe and Private Healthcare

Dixie B. Baker

• OBJECTIVES

1. To explain the critical role that "trustworthiness" plays in healthcare quality and safety.
2. To explain the relationship among security, privacy, and trust.
3. To propose adherence to fair information practices principles as essential to privacy and trust.
4. To introduce and describe a trust framework comprising seven layers of protection essential for protecting sensitive and safety-critical health information and services.

• KEY WORDS

Health information technology
Trustworthy systems
Security
Privacy
Fair Information Practices Principles

INTRODUCTION

The healthcare industry is in the midst of a dramatic transformation that is changing everything from frustrating and costly administrative inefficiencies to how conditions are diagnosed and treated, to how biomedical science advances. This transformation is driven by a number of factors, most prominently the skyrocketing cost of healthcare in the United States; the exposure of care-related, patient-safety problems; advances in genomics and "big data" analytics; and an aging, socially networked population that expects the healthcare industry to effectively leverage information technology to manage costs, improve health outcomes, advance medical science, and engage consumers as active participants in their own health.

The U.S. Health Information Technology for Economic and Clinical Health (HITECH) Act in 2009 was enacted as part of the American Recovery and Reinvestment Act (USC, 2009) and provided major structural changes; funding for research, technical support, and training; and financial incentives designed to significantly expedite and accelerate this transformation. The HITECH Act codified the Office of National Coordinator (ONC) for Health Information Technology (HIT) and assigned it responsibility for developing a nationwide infrastructure that would facilitate the use and exchange of electronic health information, including policy, standards, implementation specifications, and certification criteria. In enacting the HITECH Act, Congress recognized that the meaningful use and exchange of electronic health information was key to improving the quality, safety, and efficiency of the U.S. healthcare system.

At the same time, the HITECH Act recognized that as more health information was recorded and exchanged electronically to coordinate care, monitor quality, measure outcomes, and report public health threats, the risks to personal privacy and patient safety would be heightened. This recognition is reflected in the fact that four of the eight areas the HITECH Act identified as priorities for the ONC specifically address risks to individual privacy and information security:

1. Technologies that *protect the privacy* of health information and *promote security* in a qualified electronic health record (EHR), including for the *segmentation and protection from disclosure* of specific and sensitive individually identifiable health information, with the goal of minimizing the reluctance of patients to seek care (or disclose information about a condition) because of privacy concerns, in accordance with applicable law, and for the use and disclosure of *limited data sets* of such information.

2. A nationwide HIT infrastructure that allows for the electronic use and *accurate exchange* of health information.

3. Technologies that as a part of a qualified EHR allow for an *accounting of disclosures* made by a covered entity (as defined by the Health Insurance Portability and Accountability Act [HIPAA] of 1996) for purposes of treatment, payment, and healthcare operations.

4. Technologies that allow individually identifiable health information to be *rendered unusable, unreadable, or indecipherable to unauthorized individuals* when such information is transmitted in the nationwide health information network or physically transported outside the secured, physical perimeter of a healthcare provider, health plan, or healthcare clearinghouse (ARRA, 2009, pp. 120, 121).

The HITECH Act resulted in most significant amendments to the Health Insurance Portability and Accountability Act (HIPAA) Security and Privacy Rules since the rules became law (USC, 2013).

Maintaining Trust, Despite Increasing Risk

As noted by former National Coordinator David Blumenthal, MD, MPP, "Information is the lifeblood of modern medicine. Health information technology is destined to be its circulatory system. Without that system, neither individual physicians nor healthcare institutions can perform at their best or deliver the highest-quality care" (Blumenthal, 2009, p. 382). To carry Dr. Blumenthal's analogy one step further, at the heart of modern medicine lies "trust." Caregivers must trust that the technology and information they need will be available when they are needed at the point of care. They must trust that the information in a patient's EHR is accurate and complete and that it has not been accidentally or intentionally corrupted, modified, or destroyed. Consumers must trust that their caregivers will keep their most private health information confidential and will disclose and use it only to the extent necessary and in ways that are legal, ethical, and authorized consistent with individuals' personal expectations and preferences. Above all else, consumers must trust that their caregivers and the technology they use will "do no harm."

The nursing profession is firmly grounded in a tradition of ethics, patient advocacy, care quality, and human safety. The registered nurse is well indoctrinated on clinical practice that respects personal privacy and that protects confidential information and life-critical information services. The American Nurses Association's (ANA's) *Code of Ethics for Nurses with Interpretive Statements* includes a commitment to "promote, advocate for, and strive to protect the health, safety, and rights of the patient" (ANA, 2001, Provision 3). The International Council of Nurses (ICN) Code of Ethics for Nurses affirms that the nurse "holds in confidence personal information" and "ensures that use of technology…[is] compatible with the safety, dignity, and rights of people" (ICN, 2000, p. 2). Fulfilling these ethical obligations is the individual responsibility of each nurse, who must trust that the information technology she relies upon will help and not harm patients and will protect their private information.

Recording, storing, using, and exchanging information electronically do indeed introduce new risks. As anyone who has used e-mail or texting knows, very little effort is required to instantaneously send information to millions of people throughout the world. Try doing that with a paper record and a fax machine! We also know that nefarious "spyware," "viruses," and "Trojan horses" skulk around the Internet and insert themselves into our laptops, tablets, and smartphones, eager to capture our passwords, identities, and credit card numbers. At the same time, the capability to receive laboratory results within seconds after a test is performed; to continuously monitor a patient's condition remotely, without requiring him to leave his home; or to align treatments with outcomes-based protocols and decision-support rules personalized according to the patient's condition, family history, and genetics, all are enabled through HIT.

As HIT assumes a greater role in the provision of care and in healthcare decision-making, the nurse increasingly must trust HIT to provide timely access to accurate and complete health information and support for decision-making, while assuring that individual privacy is continuously protected. Legal and ethical obligations, as well as consumer expectations, drive requirements for assurance that data and applications will be available when they are needed; that private and confidential information will be protected; that data will not be modified or destroyed other than as authorized; that systems will be responsive and usable; and that systems designed to perform health-critical functions will do so safely. These are the attributes of trustworthy HIT—technology that is worthy of our trust. The Markle Foundation's Connecting for Health collaboration identified privacy and security as a technology principle fundamental to trust: "All health information exchange, including in support of the delivery of care and the conduct of research and public health reporting, must be conducted in an *environment of trust,* based on conformance with appropriate requirements for patient privacy, security, confidentiality, integrity, audit, and informed consent" (Markle, 2006, Privacy and Security).

Security and Privacy

Many people think of "security" and "privacy" as synonymous. These concepts are indeed related in that security mechanisms can help protect personal privacy by assuring that confidential personal information is accessible only by authorized individuals and entities. However, privacy is more than security, and security is more than privacy. Healthcare privacy principles were first articulated in 1973 in a U.S. Department of Health, Education, and Welfare report entitled *Records, Computers, and the Rights of Citizens* as "fair information practice principles" (DHEW, 1973). The Markle Foundation's Connecting for Health collaboration updated these principles to incorporate new risks created by a networked environment in which health information routinely is electronically captured, used, and exchanged (Markle, 2006). Based on these works, as well as other national and international privacy and security principles focusing on individually identifiable information in an electronic environment (including but not limited to health), the ONC developed a *Nationwide Privacy and Security Framework for Electronic Exchange of Individually Identifiable Health Information* that identified eight principles intended to guide the actions of all people and entities that participate in networked, electronic exchange of individually identifiable health information (ONC, 2008). These principles, described in Table 10.1, essentially articulate the "rights" of individuals to openness, transparency, fairness, and choice in the collection and use of their health information (Table 10.1). Whereas privacy has to do with individual rights, security deals with protection. Security mechanisms and assurance methods are used to protect

TABLE 10.1	The Nationwide Privacy and Security Framework Defines Eight Privacy Principles
Principle	**Description**
Individual access	Individuals should be provided simple and timely means to access and obtain their individually identifiable health information in a readable form and format.
Correction	Individuals should be provided a timely means to dispute the accuracy or integrity of their individually identifiable health information and to have erroneous information corrected or the dispute documented.
Openness and transparency	Policies, procedures, and technologies that directly affect individuals and their individually identifiable health information should be open and transparent.
Individual choice	Individuals should be provided a reasonable opportunity and capability to make informed decisions about the collection, use, and disclosure of their individually identifiable health information.
Collection and use	Individually identifiable health information should be collected, used, and/or disclosed only to the extent necessary to accomplish a specified purpose(s) and never to discriminate inappropriately.
Data quality and integrity	People and entities should take reasonable steps to ensure that individually identifiable health information is complete, accurate, and up-to-date to the extent necessary for intended purposes and that it has not been altered or destroyed in an unauthorized manner.
Safeguards	Individually identifiable health information should be protected with reasonable administrative, technical, and physical safeguards to ensure its confidentiality, integrity, and availability and to prevent unauthorized or inappropriate access, use, or disclosure.
Accountability	These principles should be implemented—and adherence assured—through appropriate monitoring and other means, and methods should be in place to report and mitigate nonadherence and breaches.

Reproduced from ONC (2008).

the confidentiality and authenticity of information, the integrity of data, and the availability of information and services, as well as to provide an accurate record of activities and accesses to information. While these mechanisms and methods are critical to protecting personal privacy, they are also essential in protecting patient safety and care quality—and in engendering trust in electronic systems and information. For example, if laboratory results are corrupted during transmission, or data in an EHR are overwritten, or if an electronic message claiming to have been sent by another health professional proves to be fraudulent, the nurse is likely to lose confidence that the HIT can be trusted to help her provide quality care. If a miscreant alters a clinical decision-support rule or launches a denial-of-service attack on a sensor system for tracking wandering Alzheimer's patients, individuals' lives are put at risk.

Trustworthiness is an attribute of each system component and of integrated enterprise systems as a whole—including those components that may exist in "clouds" or in coat pockets. Trustworthiness is very difficult to retrofit, as it must be designed and integrated into the system and conscientiously preserved as the system evolves. Discovering that an operational system cannot be trusted generally indicates that extensive—and expensive—changes to the system are needed. In this chapter, we introduce a framework for achieving and maintaining trustworthiness in HIT.

WHEN THINGS GO WRONG

Although we would like to be able to assume that computers, networks, and software are as trustworthy as our toasters and refrigerators, unfortunately that is not the case, and when computers, networks, and software fail in such a way that critical services and data are not available when they are needed, or confidential information is disclosed, or health data are corrupted, personal privacy and safety are imperiled. One of the more dramatic examples was reported in the cover story for the February 2003 issue of *CIO Magazine*, which relates in detail the occurrence and recovery from "one of the worst healthcare IT crises in history"—a catastrophic failure in the network infrastructure that supported CareGroup, one of the most prestigious healthcare organizations in the United States. The source of the problem ultimately was traced to network switches that directed network traffic over a highly overburdened and fragile network that was further taxed when a researcher uploaded a multigigabyte file into the picture archiving and communication system (PACS). The failure resulted in a four-hour closure of the emergency room,

a complete shutdown of the network, and two days of paper-based clinical operations—a true "retro" experience for many of the physicians who had never practiced without computers. Network services were not fully recovered until six days after the onset of the disaster (Berinato, 2003). Through this experience, CareGroup learned a valuable lesson about the importance of assessing and mitigating risk to the confidentiality, integrity, and availability of critical systems and information—and what to do when disaster strikes.

One might surmise that today the risk of overloading networks might be mitigated by migrating systems to the cloud, where storage and infrastructure resources are made available upon demand, and services are provided in accordance with negotiated service-level agreements (SLAs). However, today's cloud environments are equally susceptible to outages. Even the largest global cloud computing infrastructures can be brought down by seemingly minor factors—in some cases factors intended to provide security. One such example is a major crash of Microsoft's Azure Cloud that occurred in February 2013, when a secure socket layer (SSL) certificate used to authenticate the identity of a server was allowed to expire. The outage brought down cloud storage for 12 hours and affected secure Web traffic worldwide. Over 50 different Microsoft services reported performance problems during the outage (Microsoft, 2013).

Identity theft is a felonious and seriously disruptive invasion of personal privacy that also can cause physical harm. In 2006, a 27-year-old mother of four children in Salt Lake City received a phone call from a Utah social worker notifying her that her newborn had tested positive for methamphetamines and that the state planned to remove all of her children from her home. The young mother had not been pregnant in more than two years, but her stolen driver's license had ended up in the hands of a methamphetamine user who gave birth using the stolen identity. After a few tense days of urgent phone calls with child protective services, the victim was allowed to keep her children. She hired an attorney to sort out the damages to her legal and medical records. Months later, when she needed treatment for a kidney infection, she carefully avoided the hospital where her stolen identity had been used. But her caution did no good—her electronic record, with the identity thief's medical information intermingled, had circulated to hospitals throughout the community. The hospital worked with the victim to correct her charts to avoid making life-critical decisions based on erroneous information. The data corruption damage could have been far worse had the thief's baby not tested positive for methamphetamines, bringing the theft to the victim's attention (Rys, 2008).

One's personal genome is the most uniquely identifying of health information, and it contains information not only about the individual but also about their parents and siblings. One determined and industrious 15-year-old used his own personal genome to find his mother's anonymous sperm donor (Stein, 2005). Even whole genome sequences that claim to be "anonymized" can disclose an individual's identity, as demonstrated by a research team at Whitehead Institute for Biomedical Research (Gymrek, McGuire, Golan, Halperin, & Erlich, 2013). As genomic data are integrated into EHRs and routinely used in clinical care, the potential for damage from unauthorized disclosure and identity theft significantly increases.

In July 2009, after noting several instances of computer malware affecting the United Kingdom's National Health Service (NHS) hospitals, a British news broadcasting station conducted a survey of the NHS trusts throughout England to determine how many of their systems had been infected by malware. Seventy-five percent replied, reporting that over 8000 viruses had penetrated their security systems, with 12 incidents affecting clinical departments, putting patient care at risk, and exposing personal information. One Scottish trust was attacked by the Conficker virus, which shut down computers for two days. Some attacks were used to steal personal information, and at a cancer center, 51 appointments and radiotherapy sessions had to be rescheduled (Cohen, 2009). The survey seemed to have little effect in reducing the threat—less than a year later, NHS systems were victimized by the Qakbot data-stealing worm, which infected over a thousand computers and stole massive amounts of information (Goodin, 2010).

For decades, organizations and individuals have known that they need to fortify their desktop computers and laptops to counter the threat of computer malware. However, as medical device manufacturers have integrated personal computer technology into medical devices, they have neglected to protect against malware threats. The Department of Veterans Affairs (VA) reported that between 2009 and 2013, malware infected at least 327 medical devices in VA hospitals, including X-ray machines, lab equipment, equipment used to open blocked arteries, and cameras used in nuclear medicine studies. In one reported outbreak, the Conficker virus was detected in 104 devices in a single VA hospital. A VA security technologist surmised that the malware most likely was brought into the hospital on infected thumb drives used by vendor support technicians to install software updates. Infections from malware commonly seen in the wild are most likely to cause a degradation of system performance or to expose patients' private data. However, malware written to target a specific medical device could

result in even more dire consequences. Recognizing the safety risk posed by malware, the Food and Drug Administration (FDA) in 2013 began warning device manufacturers that their devices were at risk of being infected by malware that could endanger patients. The FDA recommended that manufacturers seeking approval for their devices submit security plans to counter the malware threat, and that hospitals vigilantly report cybersecurity attacks (WSJ, 2013).

Since 2009, entities covered under the HIPAA have been required to notify individuals whose unsecured protected health information may have been exposed due to a security breach, and to report to the Department of Health and Human Services (HHS) breaches affecting 500 or more individuals. HHS maintains a public Web site, frequently referred to as the "wall of shame," listing the breaches reported. Between September 22, 2009 and January, 2014, a total of 804 breaches, affecting 29.3 million individuals, were reported (HHS, 2014). Seven breaches, each of which affected over a million individuals, accounted for over half of the individuals affected, and all were attributed to the loss or theft of equipment or media—the most visible and easily detected types of breaches. Thus, one might surmise that this accounting may be just the tip of the iceberg of electronic breaches of health information.

The bottom line is that systems, networks, and software applications, as well as the enterprises within which they are used, are highly complex, and the only safe assumption is that "things will go wrong." Trustworthiness is an essential attribute for the systems, software, services, processes, and people used to manage individuals' personal health information and to help provide safe, high-quality healthcare.

HIT TRUST FRAMEWORK

Trustworthiness can never be achieved by implementing a few policies and procedures, and some security technology. Protecting sensitive and safety-critical health information and assuring that the systems, services, and information that nurses rely upon to deliver quality care are available when they are needed require a complete HIT trust framework that starts with an objective assessment of risk, and that is conscientiously applied throughout the development and implementation of policies, operational procedures, and security safeguards built on a solid system architecture. This trust framework is depicted in Fig. 10.1 and comprises seven layers of protection, each of which is dependent upon the layers below it (indicated by the arrows in the figure), and all of which must work together to provide a trustworthy HIT environment for

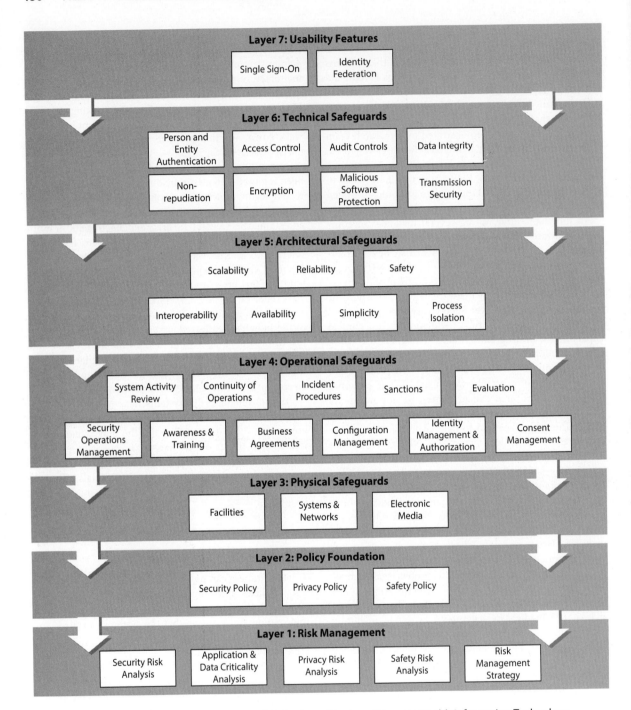

• **FIGURE 10.1.** A Framework for Achieving and Maintaining Trustworthiness in Health Information Technology Comprises Multiple Layers of Trust, Beginning with Objective Risk Assessment that Serves as the Foundation for Information Assurance Policy, and Operational, Architectural, and Technological Safeguards.

healthcare delivery. This trust framework does not dictate a physical architecture; it may be implemented within a single or across multiple sites, and may comprise enterprise, mobile, and cloud components.

Layer 1: Risk Management

Risk management is the foundation of the HIT trust framework. Objective risk assessment informs decision-making and positions the organization to correct those physical, operational, and technical deficiencies that pose the highest risk to the information assets within the enterprise. Objective risk assessment also puts into place protections that will enable the organization to manage the residual risk and liability. Patient safety, individual privacy, and information security all relate to *risk*, which is simply the probability that some "bad thing" will happen. Risk is always with respect to a given context comprising relevant threats, vulnerabilities, and valued assets. Threats can be natural occurrences (e.g., earthquake, hurricane), accidents, or malicious people and software programs. Vulnerabilities are present in facilities, hardware, software, communication systems, business processes, workforces, and electronic data. Valued assets can be anything from reputation to business infrastructure to information to human lives.

A security risk is the probability that a threat will exploit a vulnerability to expose confidential information, corrupt or destroy data, or interrupt or deny essential information services. If that risk could result in the unauthorized disclosure of an individual's private health information or the compromise of an individual's identity, it also represents a privacy risk. If the risk could result in the corruption of clinical data or an interruption in the availability of a safety-critical system, causing human harm or the loss of life, it is a safety risk as well.

Information security is widely viewed as the protection of information confidentiality, data integrity, and service availability. Indeed, these are the three areas directly addressed by the technical safeguards addressed in the HIPAA Security Rule (CFR, 2013). Generally, safety is most closely associated with protective measures for data integrity and the availability of life-critical information and services, while privacy is more often linked to confidentiality protection. However, the unauthorized exposure of private health information, or corruption of one's personal EHR as a result of an identity theft, also can put an individual's health and safety at risk.

Risk management is an ongoing, individualized discipline wherein each individual or each organization examines its own threats, vulnerabilities, and valued assets and decides for itself how to deal with identified risks—whether to reduce or eliminate them, counter them with protective measures, or tolerate them and prepare for the consequences. Risks to personal privacy, patient safety, care quality, financial stability, and public trust all must be considered in developing an overall strategy for managing risks both internal and external to an organization. In bygone times, risk assessment focused on resources within a well-defined physical and electronic boundary that comprised the "enterprise." In today's environment, where resources may include cloud components, bring-your-own devices (BYOD), and any Wi-Fi device within signal range of a wireless network, risk assessment is far more complex and will require careful analysis of potential data flows and close examination of SLAs for enterprise and cloud services and data-sharing agreements with trading partners.

Layer 2: Information Assurance Policy

The risk management strategy will identify what risks need to be addressed through an information assurance policy that governs operations, information technology, and individual behavior. The information assurance policy comprises rules that guide organizational decision-making and that define behavioral expectations and sanctions for unacceptable actions. The policy defines rules for protecting individuals' private information, for securing all confidential information, and for providing choice and transparency with respect to how individuals' health information is used and shared. It includes rules that protect human beings, including patients, employees, family members, and visitors, from physical harm that could result from data corruption or service interruption. Overall, the information assurance policy defines the rules enforced to protect the organization's valued information assets from identified risks to confidentiality, data integrity, and service availability.

Some policy rules are mandated by applicable state and federal laws and regulations. For example, the HIPAA Security Rule requires compliance with a set of administrative, physical, and technical standards, and the HIPAA Privacy Rule (CFR, 2013) sets forth privacy policies to be implemented. However, although the HIPAA regulations establish uniform minimum privacy and security standards, state health privacy laws are quite diverse. Because the HIPAA regulations apply only to "covered entities" and their "business associates" and not to everyone who may hold health information, and because the HIPAA regulations preempt only those state laws that are less stringent, the privacy protections of individuals and security protections of health information vary depending on who is holding the information and the state in which they are located (Pritts, Choy, Emmart, & Hustead, 2002).

The policy that codifies the nurse's obligation to protect patients' privacy and safety is embodied in the ICN Code of Ethics for Nurses (ICN, 2000):

- The nurse holds in confidence personal information and uses judgment in sharing this information.
- The nurse takes appropriate action to safeguard individuals whose care is endangered by a co-worker or any other person.

HIT information assurance policy provides the foundation for the development and implementation of physical, operational, architectural, and security technology safeguards. Nursing professionals can provide valuable insights, recommendations, and advocacy in the formulation of information assurance policy within the organizations where they practice, as well as within their professional organizations and with state and federal governments.

Layer 3: Physical Safeguards

Physically safeguarding health information, and the information technology used to collect, store, retrieve, analyze, and exchange health data, is essential to assuring that information needed at the point and time of care is available, trustworthy, and usable in providing quality healthcare. Although the electronic signals that represent health information are not themselves "physical," the facilities within which data are generated, stored, displayed, and used; the media on which data are recorded; the information system hardware used to process, access, and display the data; and the communications equipment used to transmit and route the data are. So are the people who generate, access, and use the information the data represent. Physical safeguards are essential to protecting these assets in accordance with the information assurance policy.

The HIPAA Security Rule prescribes four standards for physically safeguarding electronic health information protected under HIPAA: facility-access controls, workstation-use policies and procedures, workstation-security measures, and device and media controls. Physically safeguarding the lives and well-being of patients is central to the roles and responsibilities of nurses. Protecting patients requires the physical protection of the media on which their health data are recorded, as well as the devices, systems, networks, and facilities involved in data collection, use, storage, and disposal.

Healthcare organizations are increasingly choosing to purchase services from third parties, rather than hosting and maintaining these services within their own facilities. Third-party services include EHR software-as-a-service (SaaS) applications, outsourced hosting services, and cloud storage and infrastructure offerings. The HIPAA Security Rule requires that the providers of these services sign a business associate agreement in which they agree to meet all of the HIPAA security standards. However, if a breach occurs, the covered entity retains primary responsibility for reporting and responding to the breach. So it is essential that healthcare entities perform due diligence to assure that their business associates understand and are capable of providing the required levels of physical protection and data isolation.

Layer 4: Operational Safeguards

Operational safeguards are processes, procedures, and practices that govern the creation, handling, usage, and sharing of health information in accordance with the information assurance policy. The HIT trust framework shown in Fig. 10.1 includes the following operational safeguards.

Security Operations Management. HIPAA regulations require that each healthcare organization designate a "security official" and a "privacy official" to be responsible for developing and implementing security and privacy policies and procedures. The management of services relating to the protection of health information and patient privacy touches every function within a healthcare organization.

Awareness and Training. One of the most valuable actions a healthcare organization can take to maintain public trust is to inculcate a culture of safety, privacy, and security. If every person employed by, or associated with, an organization feels individually responsible for protecting the confidentiality, integrity, and availability of health information, and the privacy and safety of patients, the risk for that organization will be vastly reduced. Recognition of the value of workforce training is reflected in the fact that the HIPAA Security and Privacy Rules require training in security and privacy, respectively, for all members of the workforce. Formal privacy and security training should be required to be completed at least annually, augmented by simple and frequent reminders.

Business Agreements. Business agreements help manage risk and bound liability, clarify responsibilities and expectations, and define processes for addressing disputes among parties. The HIPAA Privacy and Security Rules require that each person or organization that provides to a covered entity services involving individually identifiable health information must sign a "business associate" contract obligating the service provider to comply with HIPAA requirements, subject to the same enforcement and sanctions as covered entities. Business associates include entities that provide services delivered within the covered entity's own premises, entities that provide health-information-exchange services, and entities that provide services in the "cloud." The HIPAA Privacy Rule also requires "data use agreements" defining how "limited data sets" will be used. Organizations wishing to exchange health information as part of the National eHealth Collaborative must sign a Data Use and Reciprocal Support Agreement (DURSA) in which they agree to exchange and use message content only in accordance with the agreed upon provisions (HHS, 2011). Agreements are only as trustworthy as the entities that sign them. Organizations should exercise due diligence in deciding with whom they will enter into business agreements.

Configuration Management. Configuration management refers to processes and procedures for maintaining an accurate and consistent accounting of the physical and functional attributes of a system throughout its life cycle. From an information assurance perspective, configuration management is the process of controlling and documenting modifications to the hardware, firmware, software, and documentation involved in the protection of information assets.

Identity Management and Authorization. Arguably the operational processes most critical to the effectiveness of technical safeguards are the process used to positively establish the identity of the individuals and entities to whom rights and privileges are being assigned, and the process used to assign authorizations to those identities. Many of the technical safeguards (e.g., authentication, access control, audit, digital signature) rely upon and assume the accuracy of an identity that is established when an account is created.

Identity management begins with verification of the identity of each individual before creating a system account for him. This process, called "identity proofing," may require the person to present one or more government-issued documents containing the individual's photograph, such as a driver license or passport. Once identity has been positively established, one or more system accounts are created, giving the individual the access rights and privileges essential to performing his assigned duties, and a means of "authenticating" this identity when the individual attempts to access resources is assigned. (See Security Technology Safeguards section below.) The

life cycle of identity management includes the prompt termination of identities and authorizations when the individual leaves the organization or otherwise no longer needs the resources and privileges assigned to him, as well as ongoing maintenance of the governance processes that support this life cycle.

Consent Management. Obtaining an individual's consent prior to taking any actions that involve her physical body or personal information is fundamental to respecting her right to privacy, and a profusion of state and federal laws set forth requirements for protecting and enforcing this right. Medical ethics and state laws require that providers obtain a patient's "informed consent" before delivering medical care, or administering diagnostic tests or treatment. The Common Rule, designed to protect human research subjects, requires informed consent before using an individual or her biological materials in research (HHS, 2009). The HIPAA Privacy Rule specifies conditions under which an individual's personal health information may be used and exchanged, including uses and exchanges that require the individual's express "authorization." Certain types of information, such as psychotherapy notes and substance abuse records, have special restrictions and authorization requirements. Managing an individual's consents and authorizations and assuring consistent adherence to the individual's privacy preferences is a complex process, but essential to protecting personal privacy.

Today, consent management is primarily a manual process, and consents are collected and managed within a single institution. However, as access to health information and biological specimens is shared among multiple institutions, consent management becomes much more complex. At the same time, the risk to personal privacy is heightened. New standards and models for electronically capturing and exchanging individual permissions, and for "segmenting" data for special protection, are beginning to emerge.

System Activity Review. One of the most effective means of detecting potential misuse and abuse of privileges is by regularly reviewing records of information system activity, such as audit logs, facility access reports, security incident tracking reports, and accountings of disclosures. The HIPAA Privacy Rule requires that covered entities provide to patients, upon request, an accounting of all disclosures (i.e., outside the entity holding the information) of their protected health information except for those disclosures for purposes of treatment, payment, and healthcare operations (TPO). The HITECH Act dropped the TPO exception; as of this writing, regulation to implement this requirement is still in development. Although technology to automate system-activity review exists, many health-care organizations still rely on manual review of audit logs to detect potential intrusions and misuse. As more clinical data are generated and exchanged, the sheer volume will overpower system-activity review as a manual operation. Further, the HITECH Act's requirement to include TPO in an accounting of disclosures will necessitate the use of automated review.

Continuity of Operations. Unexpected events, both natural and human-produced, do happen, and when they do, it is important that critical health services can continue to be provided. As healthcare organizations become increasingly dependent on electronic health information and information systems, the need to plan for unexpected events, and to develop operational procedures that will enable the organization to continue to function, becomes more urgent. The HIPAA Security Rule requires that organizations establish and implement policies and procedures for responding to an emergency. Contingency planning is part of an organization's risk-management strategy, and the first step is performed as part of a risk assessment—identifying those software applications and data that are essential for enabling operations to continue under emergency conditions and for returning to full operations. These business-critical systems are those to which architectural safeguards such as fail-safe design, redundancy and failover, and availability engineering should be applied.

Incident Procedures. Awareness and training should include a clear explanation of what an individual should do if she suspects a security incident, such as a malicious code infiltration or denial-of-service attack or a breach of confidential information. Organizations need to plan their response to an incident report, including procedures for investigating and resolving the incident, notifying individuals whose health information may have been exposed as a result of the incident, and penalizing parties responsible for the incident. Individuals whose information may have been exposed as a result of a breach must be notified, and breaches affecting 500 or more individuals must be reported to the HHS.

Not all security incidents are major or require enterprise-wide response. Some incidents may be as simple as a user accidentally including PHI in a request sent to the help desk. Incident procedures should not require a user or help-desk operator to make a judgment call on the seriousness of a disclosure; procedures should clearly specify what an individual should do when he or she notices a potential security incident.

Sanctions. The HIPAA law (USC, 1996), as amended by the HITECH Act (USC, 2009), prescribes severe civil and criminal penalties for sanctioning entities that fail to comply with the privacy and security provisions. Organizations must implement appropriate sanctions to penalize workforce members who fail to comply with privacy and security policies and procedures.

Evaluation. Periodic, objective evaluation of the operational and technical safeguards in place helps measure the effectiveness, or "outcomes," of the security management program. A formal evaluation should be conducted at least annually and should involve independent participants who are not responsible for the program. Security evaluation should include resources and services maintained within the enterprise, as well as resources and services provided by business associates—including SaaS and cloud-services providers. Independent evaluators can be from either within or outside an organization, so long as they can be objective. In addition to the annual programmed evaluation, security technology safeguards should be evaluated whenever changes in circumstances or events occur that affect the risk profile of the organization.

Layer 5: Architectural Safeguards

A system's architecture comprises its individual hardware and software components, the relationships among them, their relationship with the environment, and the principles that govern the system's design and evolution over time. As shown in Fig. 10.1, specific architectural design principles, and the hardware and software components that support those principles, work together to establish the technical foundation for security technology safeguards. In simpler times, the hardware and software components that comprised an enterprise's architecture were under the physical and logical control of the enterprise itself, but in an era when an enterprise may depend upon external providers of enterprises services (e.g., a health exchange service, hosting service, backup service), and virtualized services (e.g., SaaS, cloud resources), this may not be the case. Still, the design principles discussed below apply whether an enterprise's architecture is centralized or distributed, physical or virtual.

Scalability. As more health information is recorded, stored, used, and exchanged electronically, systems and networks must be able to deal with that growth. The catastrophic failure at CareGroup (mentioned earlier in this chapter) resulted from the network's inability to scale to the capacity required. The most recent stage in the evolution of the Internet specifically addresses the scalability issue by virtualizing computing resources into services, including software as a service (SaaS), platforms as a service (PaaS), and infrastructure as a service (IaaS)—collectively referred to as "cloud" services. Indeed, the Internet itself was created on the same principle as cloud computing—the creation of a virtual, ubiquitous, continuously expanding network through the sharing of resources (servers) owned by different entities. Whenever one sends information over the Internet, the information is broken into small packets that are then sent ("hop") from server to server from source to destination, with all of the servers in between being "public"—in the sense that they probably belong to someone other than the sender or the receiver. Cloud computing, a model for providing "on demand" computing services accessible over the Internet, pushes virtualization to a new level by sharing applications, storage, and computing power to offer scalability beyond what would be economically possible otherwise.

Reliability. Reliability is the ability of a system or component to perform its specified functions consistently, over a specified period of time—an essential attribute of trustworthiness. Security- and safety-critical system components should be engaged and integrated so that no single point of failure exists. If a given component fails, the system should engage a second, backup component with no breach of sensitive information, interruption of operations, or corruption of data.

Safety. Safety-critical components, software, and systems should be designed so that if they fail, the failure will not cause people to be physically harmed. Note that fail-safe design may indicate that, under certain circumstances, a component should be shut down, or forced to violate its functional specification, to avoid harming someone. So the interrelationships among redundancy and failover, reliability, and fail-safe design are complex, yet critical to patient safety. The "break-the-glass" feature that enables an unauthorized user to gain access to patient information in an emergency situation is an example of fail-safe design. If, in an emergency, an EHR system "fails" to provide a nurse access to the clinical information he or she needs to deliver care, the "break-the-glass" feature will enable the system to "fail safely." Fail-safe methods are particularly important in research where new treatment protocols and devices are being tested for safety.

Interoperability. Interoperability is the ability of systems and system components to work together. To exchange health information effectively, healthcare systems must interoperate not only at the technical level, but also at the syntactic and semantic levels. The Internet and its

protocols, which have been adopted for use both within and between enterprises, package and transmit data in small packets (electronic bits) over a network in such a way that upon arrival at their destination the data appear the same as when they were sent. If the data are encrypted, the receiving system must be able to decrypt the data, and if the data are wrapped in an electronic envelope (e.g., electronic mail message, HL7 message), the system must open the envelope and extract the content. Finally, the system must translate the electronic data into health information that the system's applications and users will understand. Open standards, including encryption and messaging standards, and standard vocabulary for coding and exchanging security attributes and patient permissions—e.g., Security Assertion Markup Language [SAML], eXtensible Access Control Markup Language [XACML]—are fundamental to implementing interoperable healthcare systems.

Availability. Required services and information must be available and usable when they are needed. Availability is measured as the proportion of time a system is in a functioning condition. A reciprocal dependency exists between security technology safeguards and high-availability design—security safeguards depend upon the availability of systems, networks, and information, which in turn enable those safeguards to protect enterprise assets against threats to availability, such as denial-of-service attacks. Resource virtualization and "cloud" computing are important technologies for helping assure availability.

Simplicity. Safe, secure architectures are designed to minimize complexity. The simplest design and integration strategy will be the easiest to understand, to maintain, and to recover in the case of a failure or disaster.

Process Isolation. Process isolation refers to the extent to which processes running on the same system at different trust levels, virtual machines (VMs) running on the same hardware, or applications running on the same computer or tablet are kept separate. Isolation is important to ensuring that if one process, VM, or application misbehaves or is compromised, other processes, VMs, or applications can continue to operate safely and securely. Process isolation is particularly important to preserve the integrity of the operating system itself. The operating system is the most critical component in a system because it is responsible for managing, protecting, and provisioning all system resources (e.g., data files, directories, memory, application processes, network ports). Within today's operating systems, processes critical to the security and reliability of the system execute within a protected hardware state, while untrusted applications execute within a separate state.

However, this hardware architectural isolation is undermined if the system is configured so that untrusted applications are allowed to run with privilege, which puts the operating system itself at risk. For example, if a user logs into an account with administrative privileges and then runs an application that has been infected by a virus (or opens an infected e-mail attachment), the entire operating system may become infected.

Within a cloud environment, the hypervisor is assigned responsibility for assuring that VMs are kept separate so that processes running on one subscriber's VM cannot interfere with those running on another subscriber's VM. In general, the same security safeguards used to protect an enterprise system are equally effective in a cloud environment—but only if the hypervisor is able to maintain isolation among virtual environments. Another example of isolation is seen in the Apple iOS environment. Apps running on an iPad or iPhone are isolated such that not only are they unable to view or modify each other's data, but also one app does not even know whether another app is installed on the device. (Apple calls this architectural feature "sandboxing.")

Layer 6: Security Technology Safeguards

Security technology safeguards are software and hardware services specifically designed to perform security-related functions. Essential technical safeguards are depicted in Fig. 10.1; Table 10.2 provides a sampling of standards that are useful in implementing these safeguards.

Person and Entity Authentication. The identity of each entity, whether it be a person or a software entity, must be clearly established before that entity is allowed to access

protected systems, applications, and data. Identity management and authorization processes are used to validate identities and to assign them system rights and privileges. (See Identity Management and Authorization above.) Then, whenever the person or application requires access, it asserts an identity (userID) and authenticates that identity by providing some "proof" in the form of something it has (e.g., smartcard), something it knows (e.g., password, private encryption key), or something it is (e.g., fingerprint). The system then checks to verify that the userID represents someone who has been authorized to access the system, and then verifies that the "proof" provided provides the evidence required. While only people can authenticate themselves using biometrics, both people and software applications can authenticate themselves using public–private key exchanges.

Individuals who work for federal agencies, such as the Department of Veterans Affairs (VA), are issued Personal Identity Verification (PIV) cards containing a digital certificate that uniquely identifies the individual and the rights assigned to him. The National Strategy for Trusted Identities in Cyberspace (NSTIC) program is working toward an "identity ecosystem" in which each individual possesses trusted credentials for proving her identity (NIST, 2014).

Access Control. Access-control services help assure that people, computer systems, and software applications are able to use all of and only the resources (e.g., computers, networks, applications, services, data files, information) that they are authorized to use and only within the constraints of the authorization. Access controls protect against unauthorized use, disclosure, modification, and destruction of resources, and unauthorized execution of

TABLE 10.2	Many Open Standards Address Security Technology Safeguards	
Safeguard	**Standard**	**Description**
Person and Entity Authentication	ITU-T X.509: Information technology— open systems interconnection—the directory: public-key and attribute-certificate frameworks	Standard for public-key infrastructure (PKI), single sign-on, and privilege-management infrastructure (PMI); includes standard formats for public-key certificates, certificate revocation lists, attribute certificates, and a certification path-validation algorithm
	OASIS security assertion markup language (SAML)	XML-based protocol for exchanging authentication and authorization data ("assertions") between an identity provider and a service provider; used to enable single sign-on
	OpenID Foundation OpenID Connect	Standard for a simple identity layer that lies on top of the OAuth 2.0 protocol

(continued)

TABLE 10.2	Many Open Standards Address Security Technology Safeguards *(continued)*	
Safeguard	**Standard**	**Description**
Access Control	IETF OAuth 2.0 Authorization Framework; RFC 6749	Standard for enabling a third-party application (or mobile app) to obtain limited access to a Web service, either on behalf of a resource owner by orchestrating an approval interaction between the resource owner and the Web service or by allowing the third-party application to obtain access on its own behalf
	ANSI/INCITS 359-2004: Information technology—role-based access control (RBAC)	Specifies RBAC elements (users, roles, permissions, operations, objects) and features required by an RBAC system
	HL7 Version 3 confidentiality code system	HL7 V3 value set for coding confidentiality attributes
	HL7 Version 3 role-based access control (RBAC) healthcare permission catalog	Permission vocabulary to support RBAC, consistent with OASIS XACML and ANSI INCITS RBAC standards
	OASIS extensible access control markup language (XACML)	XML-based language for expressing information technology security policy
Audit Controls	ASTM E-2147-01: Standard specification for audit and disclosure logs for use in health information systems	Specifies how to design audit logs to record accesses within a computer system and disclosure logs to document disclosures to external users
Data Integrity	FIPS PUB 180-3 secure hash standard (SHS)	Specifies five hash algorithms that can be used to generate message digests used to detect whether messages have been changed since the digests were generated
Nonrepudiation	ASTM E-1762-95(2003): Standard guide for electronic authentication of healthcare information	Standard on the design, implementation, and use of electronic signatures to authenticate healthcare data
	ETSI TS 101 903: XML advanced electronic signatures (XadES)	Defines XML formats for advanced electronic signatures, based on the use of public-key cryptography supported by public-key certificates
Encryption (confidentiality)	FIPS 197, advanced encryption standard, November 2001	Specifies a symmetric cryptographic algorithm that can be used to protect electronic data
Transmission Security	IETF transport layer security (TLS) protocol: RFC 2246, RFC 3546	Standard for establishing secured channel at layer 4 (transport) of the open systems interconnection (OSI) model; includes authentication of sender and receiver and encryption and integrity protection of the communication channel
	IETF IP security protocol (IPsec): RFCs listed at http://datatracker.ietf.org/wg/ipsec/	Standard for establishing virtual private network (VPN) at layer 3 (network) of the OSI model; includes authentication of sender and receiver and encryption and integrity protection of the communication channel
	IETF secure/multipurpose internet mail extensions (S/MIME): RFC 2633	Internet mail protocol for providing authentication, message integrity and nonrepudiation of origin (digital signatures), and confidentiality protection (encryption)
	OASIS WS-security (WSS)	Extension to the simple object access protocol (SOAP) transport protocol used to access Web services; includes encryption and digital signing of messages and exchange of security tokens, including SAML assertions

ANSI, American National Standards Institute; ASTM, ASTM International (originally American Society for Testing and Materials); ETSI, European Telecommunications Standards Institute; FIPS, National Institute of Standards and Technology (NIST) Federal Information Processing Standard; HL7, Health Level Seven; IETF, Internet Engineering Task Force; INCITS, InterNational Committee for Information Technology Standards; ITU-T, International Telecommunication Union—Telecommunication Standardization Sector; OASIS, Organization for the Advancement of Structured Information Standards.

system functions. Access-control rules are based on federal and state laws and regulations, the enterprise's information assurance policy, as well as consumer-elected preferences. These rules may be based on the user's identity, the user's role, the context of the request (e.g., location, time of day), and/or a combination of the sensitivity attributes of the data and the user's authorizations.

Audit Controls. Security audit controls collect and record information about security-relevant events within a system component or across a network. Audit logs are generated by multiple software components within a system, including operating systems, servers, firewalls, applications, and database management systems. Many healthcare organizations manually review these logs to detect potential intrusions and misuse. Automated intrusion and misuse detection tools are increasingly being used to normalize and analyze data from network monitoring logs, system audit logs, application audit logs, and database audit logs to detect potential intrusions originating from outside the enterprise, and potential misuse by authorized users within an organization.

Data Integrity. Data integrity services provide assurance that electronic data have not been modified or destroyed except as authorized. Cryptographic hash functions are commonly used for this purpose. A cryptographic hash function is a mathematical algorithm that uses a block of data as input to generate a "hash value" such that any change to the data will change the hash value that represents it—thus detecting an integrity breach.

Non-Repudiation. Sometimes the need arises to assure not only that data have not been modified inappropriately, but also that the data are in fact from an authentic source. This proof of the authenticity of data is often referred to as "non-repudiation" and can be met through the use of digital signatures. Digital signatures use public-key (assymetric) encryption (see Encryption below) to encrypt a block of data using the signer's private key. To authenticate that the data block was signed by the entity claimed, one only needs to try decrypting the data using the signer's public key; if the data block decrypts successfully, its authenticity is assured.

Encryption. Encryption is simply the process of obfuscating information by running the data representing that information through an algorithm (sometimes called a "cipher") to make it unreadable until the data are decrypted by someone possessing the proper encryption "key." "Symmetric" encryption uses the same key to both encrypt and decrypt data, while "asymmetric" encryption

(also known as "public-key encryption") uses two keys that are mathematically related such that one key is used for encryption and the other for decryption. One key is called a "private" key and is held secret; the other is called a "public key" and is openly published. Which key is used for encryption and which for decryption depends upon the assurance objective. For example, secure e-mail encrypts the message contents using the recipient's public key so that only a recipient holding the private key can decrypt and view it, then digitally signs the message using the sender's own private key so that if the recipient can use the sender's public key to decrypt the signature, thus being assured that the sender actually sent it. Encryption technology can be used to encrypt both data at rest and data in motion. So it is used both to protect electronic transmissions over networks and to protect sensitive data in storage.

Malicious Software Protection. Malicious software, also called "malware," is any software program designed to infiltrate a system without the user's permission, with the intent to damage or disrupt operations, or to use resources to which the miscreant is not authorized access. Malicious software includes programs commonly called viruses, worms, Trojan horses, and spyware. Protecting against malicious software requires not only technical solutions to prevent, detect, and remove these invasive pests, but also policies and procedures for reporting suspected attacks.

Transmission Security. Sensitive and safety-critical electronic data that are transmitted over vulnerable networks, such as the Internet, must be protected against unauthorized disclosure and modification. The Internet protocol provides no protection against the disclosure or modification of any transmissions, and no assurance of the identity of any transmitters or receivers (or eavesdroppers). Protecting network transmissions between two entities (people, organizations, or software programs) requires that the communicating entities authenticate themselves to each other, confirm data integrity using something like a cryptographic hash function, and encrypt the channel over which data are to be exchanged.

Both the Transport Layer Security (TLS) protocol (IETF, 2008) and Internet Protocol security (IPsec) protocol suite (IETF, 1998) support these functions, but at different layers in the Open System Interconnection (OSI) model (ISO, 1996). TLS establishes protected channels at the OSI transport layer (layer 4), allowing software applications to exchange information securely. For example, TLS might be used to establish a secure link between a user's browser and a merchant's check-out application on the Web. IPsec establishes protected channels at the

OSI network layer (layer 3), allowing Internet gateways to exchange information securely. For example, IPsec might be used to establish a virtual private network (VPN) that allows all hospitals within an integrated delivery system to openly yet securely exchange information. Because IPsec is implemented at the network layer, it is less vulnerable to malicious software applications than TLS and also less visible to users (e.g., IPsec does not display an icon in a browser).

Layer 7: Usability Features

The top layer of the trust framework includes services that make life easier for users. "Single sign-on" often is referred to as a security "service," but in fact it is a usability service that makes authentication services more palatable. Both single sign-on and identity federation enable a user to authenticate himself or herself once and then to access multiple applications, multiple databases, and even multiple enterprises for which he or she is authorized, without having to reauthenticate himself or herself. Single sign-on enables a user to navigate among authorized applications and resources within a single organization. Identity federation enables a user to navigate between services managed by different organizations. Both single sign-on and identity federation require the exchange of "security assertions." Once the user has logged into a system, that system can pass the user's identity, along with other attributes, such as role, method of authentication, and time of login, to another entity using a security assertion. The receiving entity then enforces its own access-control rules, based on the identity passed to it.

Neither single sign-on nor identity federation actually adds security protections (other than to reduce the need for users to post their passwords to their computer monitors). In fact, if the original identity-proofing process or authentication method is weak, the risk associated with that weakness will be propagated to any other entities to which the identity is passed. Therefore, whenever single sign-on or federated identity is implemented, a key consideration is the level-of-assurance provided by the methods used to identity-proof and authenticate the individual.

SUMMARY AND CONCLUSIONS

Healthcare is in the midst of a dramatic and exciting transformation that will enable individual health information to be captured, used, and exchanged electronically using interoperable HIT. The potential impacts on individuals' health and on the health of entire populations are dramatic. Outcomes-based decision support will help improve the safety and quality of healthcare. The availability of huge quantities of de-identified health information will help scientists discover the underlying genetic bases for diseases, leading to earlier and more accurate detection and diagnoses, more targeted and effective treatments, and ultimately personalized medicine.

In this chapter we have explained the critical role that trustworthiness plays in HIT adoption and in providing safe, private, high-quality care. We have introduced and described a trust framework comprising seven layers of protection essential for establishing and maintaining trust in a healthcare enterprise. Many of the safeguards included in the trust framework have been codified in HIPAA standards and implementation specifications. Building trustworthiness in HIT always begins with objective risk assessment, a continuous process that serves as the basis for developing and implementing a sound information assurance policy and physical, operational, architectural, and technological safeguards to mitigate and manage risks to patient safety, individual privacy, care quality, financial stability, and public trust.

REFERENCES

American Nurses Association (ANA). (2001). *Code of ethics for nurses with interpretive statements*. Silver Spring, MD: Nursesbooks.org. Retrieved from http://www.nursingworld.org/MainMenuCategories/EthicsStandards/CodeofEthicsforNurses/Code-of-Ethics.pdf. Accessed on February 19, 2014.

American Recovery and Reinvestment Act of 2009 (ARRA). (2009). H.R. 111-5, 111th Cong. Retrieved from http://frwebgate.access.gpo.gov/cgi-bin/getdoc.cgi?dbname=111_cong_bills&docid=f:h1enr.pdf. Accessed on January 31, 2014.

Berinato, S. (2003). All systems down. *CIO* (pp. 46–53). Retrieved from http://www.cio.com.au/article/65115/all_systems_down/. Accessed on January 31, 2014.

Blumenthal, D. (2009). Launching HITECH. *New England Journal of Medicine*. December 31, 2009. Retrieved from http://www.nejm.org/doi/full/10.1056/NEJMp0912825. Accessed on January 31, 2014.

Cohen, B (2009). NHS hit by a different sort of virus. *Channel 4 News*. July 9, 2009. Retrieved from http://www.channel4.com/news/articles/science_technology/nhs+hit+by+a+different+sort+of+virus/3256957. Accessed on January 31, 2014.

Code of Federal Regulations (CFR). (2013). *Health Insurance Portability and Accountability Act (HIPAA) Privacy, Security, and Enforcement Rules*. 45 CFR Parts 160, 162 and 164. Most recently amended January 25, 2013. Retrieved from http://www.ecfr.gov/. Accessed on January 31, 2014.

Department of Health, Education, and Welfare (DHEW). (1973). *Records, Computers and the Rights of Citizens: Report of the Secretary's Advisory Committee on Automated Personal Data Systems.* July 1973. Retrieved from http://epic.org/privacy/hew1973report/. Accessed on January 31, 2014.

Department of Health and Human Services (HHS). (2009). *Protection of human subjects.* 45 CFR Part 46. January 15, 2009. Retrieved from http://www.hhs.gov/ohrp/policy/ohrpregulations.pdf. Accessed on January 29, 2014.

Department of Health and Human Services (HHS). (2011). *Restatement I of the data use and reciprocal support agreement (DURSA).* May 3, 2011. Retrieved from http://www.nationalehealth.org/ckfinder/userfiles/files/Restatement%20I__DURSA_5_3_11_FINAL_for%20PARTICIPANT%20SIGNATURE.pdf. Accessed on January 27, 2014.

Department of Health and Human Services (HHS). (2014). *Health information privacy: Breaches affecting 500 or more individuals.* Retrieved from http://www.hhs.gov/ocr/privacy/hipaa/administrative/breachnotificationrule/breachtool.html. Accessed on January 23, 2014.

Goodin, D. (2010). NHS computers hit by voracious, data-stealing worm. *The Register.* April 23, 2010. Retrieved from http://www.theregister.co.uk/2010/04/23/nhs_worm_infection/. Accessed on January 31, 2014.

Gymrek, M., McGuire, A. L., Golan, D., Halperin, E., Erlich, Y. (2013). Identifying personal genomes by surname inference. *Science, 339,* 321. Retrieved from http://data2discovery.org/dev/wp-content/uploads/2013/05/Gymrek-et-al.-2013-Genome-Hacking-Science-2013-Gymrek-321-4.pdf. Accessed January 23, 2014.

International Council of Nurses (ICN). (2000). *The ICN code of ethics for nurses.* Geneva, Switzerland. ISBN: 92-95005-16-3. Retrieved from http://www.icn.ch/images/stories/documents/about/icncode_english.pdf. Accessed on February 19, 2014.

International Organization for Standardization (ISO). (1996). *Information technology—Open systems interconnection—Basic reference model: The basic model* (2nd ed.). ISO/IEC 7498-1.1994-11-15. Corrected and reprinted, 1996-06-15. Retrieved from http://standards.iso.org/ittf/licence.html. Accessed on January 31, 2014.

Internet Engineering Task Force (IETF). (1998). *Security architecture for the internet protocol. RFC 2401.* November 1998. Retrieved from http://www.ietf.org/rfc/rfc2401.txt. Accessed on January 31, 2014.

Internet Engineering Task Force (IETF). (2008). *The transport layer security (TLS) protocol.* Version 1.2. RFC 5246. August 2008. Retrieved from http://tools.ietf.org/html/rfc5246. Accessed on January 31, 2014.

Markle Foundation Connecting for Health (Markle). (2006). *The common framework. Connection professionals: Overview and principles. Markle connecting for health's technology principles.* Retrieved from http://www.markle.org/health/markle-common-framework/connecting-professionals/overview. Accessed on February 19, 2014.

Microsoft Corporation (Microsoft). (2013). *Windows Azure team blog. Windows Azure service disruption from expired certificate.* Retrieved from http://blogs.msdn.com/b/windowsazure/archive/2013/02/24/windows-azure-service-disruption-from-expired-certificate.aspx. Accessed on January 21, 2014.

National Institute of Standards and Technology (NIST). *National strategy for trusted identities in cyberspace.* Available at http://www.nist.gov/nstic/. Accessed on January 30, 2014.

Office of the National Coordinator for Health Information Technology, U.S. Department of Health and Human Services (ONC). (2008). *Nationwide privacy and security framework for electronic exchange of individually identifiable health information.* December 15, 2008. Retrieved from http://www.healthit.gov/policy-researchers-implementers/nationwide-privacy-and-security-framework-electronic-exchange. Accessed on January 31, 2014.

Pritts, J., A. Choy, L. Emmart, & J. Hustead. (2002, June 1). *The state of health privacy: A survey of state health privacy statutes* (2nd ed.). Available at http://ihcrp.georgetown.edu/privacy/pdfs/statereport2.pdf. Accessed on January 27, 2014.

Rys, R. (2008). *The imposter in the ER: Medical identity theft can leave you with hazardous errors in health records.* March 13, 2008. Retrieved from http://www.msnbc.msn.com/id/23392229/ns/health-health_care. Accessed on January 31, 2014.

Stein, R. (2005). Found on the Web, with DNA: A boy's father. *Washington Post.* November 13, 2005. Retrieved from http://www.washingtonpost.com/wp-dyn/content/article/2005/11/12/AR2005111200958.html. Accessed on January 23, 2014.

United States Congress, 104th Session (USC). (1996). Health Insurance Portability and Accountability Act of 1996. *Public Law,* 104–191. August 21, 1996. Retrieved from http://aspe.hhs.gov/admnsimp/pl104191.htm. Accessed on January 31, 2014.

United States Congress, 111th Session (USC). (2009). *American Recovery and Reinvestment Act of 2009 (ARRA).* January 6, 2009. Retrieved from http://www.healthit.gov/sites/default/files/hitech_act_excerpt_from_arra_with_index.pdf. Accessed on February 19, 2014.

Weaver, C. (2013, June 13) Patients put at risk by computer viruses. Wall Street Journal Online. Retrieved from http://online.wsj.com/news/articles/SB10001424127887324188604578543162744943762. Assessed on October 29, 2014.

PART 2

System Life Cycle

Virginia K. Saba

11

System Life Cycle: A Framework

Marina Douglas / Marian Celli

• OBJECTIVES

1. Describe a methodology and checklist for the phases of a system implementation life cycle.
2. Describe barriers and critical success factors related to implementation.
3. Describe the Nursing Informaticist role in a clinical system's implementation life cycle.
4. Discuss the heightened impact of regulatory and financial requirements on the Electronic Health Record (EHR).

• KEY WORDS

Project Scope
Request for Proposal (RFP)
Request for Information (RFI)
Workflow Analysis
Workplan
Feasibility Study
Go Live Plan
Communication Plan
Issue's List

OVERVIEW

In the past, clinical systems implementation projects were considered successful when implemented on time and within budget. Later, the concepts of end-user perceptions determining project success in conjunction with streamlining clinician workflow layered clinical systems projects with additional success criteria. In the past five years, the focus for clinical systems implementations has been on systems improving patient safety through evidence-based medicine while meeting the federal requirements set forth in the Health Information and Technology for Economic and Clinical Health (HITECH) Act of 2009 (Trotter & Ulman, 2013).

As part of the HITECH Act, the Centers for Medicare & Medicaid Services (CMS), set forth a program providing organizations who demonstrate the meaningful use of an EHR to improve patient safety significant financial incentives. Today, the successful system implementation project must be completed on time, within budget, and offer end users streamlined workflow, with added safety in the delivery of healthcare and qualifying the organization for the financial benefits of meeting the meaningful use requirements.

The System Life Cycle (SLC) outlined in this chapter discusses the tasks multiple disciplines must accomplish to produce a technically sound, regulatory compliant and user-friendly EHR supporting safe, effective, and efficient patient care delivery. The SLC framework described by the American Nurses Credentialing Center's Nursing Informatics, (2012) (Available from http://www.nurse credentialing.org/Informatics-TCO2012) consists of four major phases. The chapter further defines these phases into the key tasks of a practical clinical systems implementation checklist and high-level workplan used successfully for real-world implementations in the acute care setting. Many examples in this chapter refer to the implementation of an EHR; however, the framework, phases, and tasks discussed can and should be applied to any clinical system or application implementation.

ELECTRONIC HEALTH RECORD

The Electronic Health Record (EHR) is a longitudinal electronic record of patient health information generated by one or more encounters in any care delivery setting. Included in this information are patient demographics, progress notes, problems, medications, vital signs, past medical history, immunizations, laboratory data, and radiology reports. The EHR automates and streamlines the clinician's workflow. The EHR has the ability to generate a complete record of a clinical patient encounter—as well as support other care-related activities directly or indirectly via interface (Anderson, 2011; Rouse, 2010).

The skills required to deliver direct patient care include the ability to understand and coordinate the work of multiple disciplines and departments. As multiple departments work in concert for optimum and safe patient care delivery, the components of an EHR integrate data in a coordinated fashion to provide an organization's administration and clinicians demographic, financial, and clinical information. The SLC provides a framework to attain a successful implementation.

CURRENT LANDSCAPE

The U.S. government has become one of the largest payers of healthcare. As the costs of healthcare increase, both the U.S. population as well as the US government have become more critical of a payer-based health system. Four factors impacting healthcare payments and hospital information systems implementations are the evolution of evidence-based healthcare/medicine, the Federal Meaningful Use requirements set forth in the HITECH Act of 2009, the cost of technology, and the use of Project Management principles.

Evidence-Based Medicine (EBM)

Both the Cochrane Collaboration and the Centre for Evidence Based Medicine have adopted the definition of EBM as "...the conscientious, explicit, and judicious use of current best evidence in making decisions about the care of individual patients" (Sachett, Rosenberg, Gray, Haynes, & Richardson, 1996). The purpose of EBM is to utilize scientific studies to determine the best course of treatment. Functionality within the EHR provides access to the studies to understand the recommended treatment while reviewing a patient's data in real time (Timmermans & Mauch, 2005).

Federal Initiative—HITECH Act 2009. This act seeks to promote the meaningful use of information technology to improve patient safety in healthcare delivery. The initiative requires an organization or provider to demonstrate consistent and appropriate use of information technology. Adoption of the technology is required in stages, with increasing numbers of requirements in each stage. Federal financial incentives are awarded to those meeting each stage. Financial penalties will be levied against organization failing to meet the requirements by 2016 (Trotter & Ulman, 2013).

The Meaningful Use requirements leverage the results published in studies indicating a marked increase in patient safety when specified functions of an information system are utilized. In addition, standardized terminology criteria permitting comparison of healthcare treatments and outcomes across healthcare facilities are incorporated into the later HITECH Act's stages. Legislative and legal aspects of informatics are discussed in another chapter.

Technology: Cost, Benefit, and Risk. Technology costs are high, increasing the risk of significant financial losses from a poor implementation. Vendors deliver the same software to clients; the success of an information system project often rests on a well-planned and well-executed implementation. A well-planned implementation dovetails an organization's strategic goals and culture, with the introduction of and ability to assimilate technology and workflow changes into the daily practice of healthcare delivery. The SLC provides a structured implementation approach to accomplish this.

Healthcare information systems implementation time lines are often long, spanning 10 to 16 months for a full hospital information system implementation.

Increasing a project's risk level, a technology generation, now only 6 to 8 months in length, can render partial obsolescence of a system by one technology generation before the first productive use of a system is sometimes obtained. A well-planned and executed implementation, on the other hand, provides a high level of risk mitigation and cost containment. It is important to remember that technology is not the best solution to every problem; failure to recognize problems caused inefficient processes from an information system problem contributes to the risk and potential costs of a system.

Project Management

With roots in the construction industry, a significant body of knowledge in the area of planning and tracking large-scale projects has evolved. The Project Management Institute (PMI) has become the central and certifying organization for project management professionals. The Project Management Plan (PMP) developed through their efforts has migrated to the Information Technology (IT) area and is commonly called a project workplan (PMI, 2014). It is the main planning document for an IT project and describes how major aspects of the project will be executed and managed. The workplan is a living document, updated continually throughout the project. Nurses have the ability to coordinate and manage multiple diverse care situations; this affords them strong skills to manage complex projects using a Project Workplan as a primary tool (Wilson, 2012). See also Chapter 14 which is devoted to Project Management.

A second essential tool for clinical implementations is the project's "issues list." As concerns, unusual situations, special education/training needs, programming errors, sequencing concerns impacting workflow, and new regulations are uncovered, they are placed on the issue's list. Issues are added to the list and prioritized in relation to other issues and to the project goals and given a status. Examples of issue statuses are open, in progress, testing, and closed. The progress of an issue is tracked by the team on a regular basis with short progress notes added to the issue. When a resolution is reached, the resolution is documented in the issue's list and the status is updated. The resolution documentation detail helps eliminate the need for the team to revisit the decision.

Suggested data elements in an issue's list are as follows:

- Issue number
- Status
- Date added to the list
- Person identifying the problem/adding it to the list
- Module/application involved
- Description of the problem/issue
- Type of problem (e.g., programmatic, training, process, hardware, network)

- Note date
- Notes (e.g., work/efforts to resolve issue)
- Responsible party
- Resolution date
- Resolution description

SYSTEM LIFE CYCLE

The System Life Cycle is defined by the major components of (a) Planning, (b) Analysis, (c) Design/Develop/Customize, and (d) Implement/Evaluate/Maintain/Support. While this chapter discusses phases of the SLC related to an EHR implementation in an acute care setting, it is applicable to many healthcare settings and projects. To continue to meet new regulatory and professional standards, EHRs and software applications must be continuously updated and upgraded in the Maintenance Phase (Wilson, 2012).

Regardless of the size or type of the system, any EHR, single application implementation, or upgrade project, should address each of the items on the clinical system implementation checklist in Fig. 11.1. Though not every

System Life Cycle Phases	Clinical Software Implementation Major Tasks
Planning	Governance Structure Project Purpose Project Scope Document Resource Planning
Analysis	Technical Requirements Functional Design Document System Proposal Document

Design, Develop, and Customize	Design
	  Functional Specifications
	  Technical Specifications
	Develop
	  Focused Plans
	Customize
	  System Dictionary Data and Profiles
	  Policies and Procedures

Implement, Evaluate, Support, and Maintain	Implement
	  Plans
	  Policies and Procedures
	  Live Operations
	    Cut Over and Go Live Plans
	Evaluate—post-live
	Daily support operations
	Ongoing maintenance

• **FIGURE 11.1.** SLC Stages in Relation to Clinical Software Implementation Checklist.

project will require interfacing or data conversion or the addition of new devices, review of the checklist's steps will assure essential considerations are not overlooked (Fig. 11.1).

The SLC phases use a problem-solving, scientific approach. Problem solving begins with observation and understanding of the operations of the current systems or processes, sometimes referred to as the "Current State." The second phase requires an in-depth assessment and definition of the new system's requirements: defining the "Future State." Designing, developing, and customizing a plan to meet requirements are addressed in the third phase. The last phase, implementing, evaluating, supporting, and ongoing maintenance, assures the system is sustainable after implementation.

Nurses' daily use of the Nursing Process, a problem-solving methodology, underlies the successes nurses have achieved in clinical informatics. Countless iterations of the problem-solving methodology are used during the implementation and updating/upgrading of software.

Inherent in the implementation process is the need to recognize and manage change and its impact on patient care delivery and clinician work patterns/workflow. "The ability to manage change often marks the difference between the success and failure of implementing a change initiative and moving an organization forward" (Ritter & Glaser, 1994, p. 168). Often, finding a balance between the technical data capture criteria and the daily workflow of clinicians is required. Details are discussed in Chapter 13, System Life Cycle Tools.

As noted, vendors supply essentially the same software to clients at the time of purchase. The abilities of the project team members and organization to introduce and assimilate changes into daily practice can determine the success of a project. Literature focusing on the workflow impact of an EHR and the cultural impact to an organization are well documented by the Project Management Institute (PMI) and the Healthcare Information Management Systems Society (HIMSS). Ash et al. (2000), Augustine (2004), Kaplan (1997), Lorenzi and Riley (2000) all stress the need to manage the change process foundational to an EHR implementation if success is to be attained.

Attempting to implement or upgrade a system without reviewing each of the checklist items within the SLC framework generally results in failure in one or more of the following areas:

- EHR or application does not meet the stated goal of the project.
- There is failure to gain end-user acceptance.
- Expenditures exceed budget.
- Anticipated benefits are unrealized.

In recent years the quality and abundance of online resources specific to clinical systems implementation have grown significantly. Due in large part to the Federal HITECH meaningful-use requirements, the PMI and HIMSS both offer training and certification processes specific to healthcare-related projects.

The following online sites provide additional and supporting information:

www.pmi.org

www.himss.org

www.cms.gov/EHRincentivePrograms

www.hhs.gov/ocio/eplc/Enterprise%20
Performance%20Lifecycle%20Artifacts/eplc_
artifacts.html

www.hitechacthelp.com/2010/05/25/
understanding-the-state-hie-toolkit/

www.ahima.org/advocacy/rec/default.aspx

www.healthit.hhs.gov/portal/server.pt/community/
healthit_hhs_gov_home/1204

PLANNING PHASE

The planning phase of the project begins once an organization has determined an existing requirement may be filled or solved by the development or implementation of an EHR or application. Establishing the committee framework to research and making recommendations for the project are an important first step.

The key documents created in the Planning Phase are the following:

- Project Governance Structure
- Gap Analysis
- Feasibility Study
- Project Scope Document
- Development of a high-level workplan and resource requirements

Governance Structure and Project Staff

The clinical leadership of an organization is highly involved in the establishment of an EHR committee structure. The organization's strategic goals and priorities must be reviewed and considered. The informatics nurse and information systems management team provide oversight; however, committees work to develop the structure and participate to best guarantee the success of the project. Assigning the appropriate resources, whether financial or personnel, is a critical success factor (McCormick & Gugerty, 2013; Protti & Peel, 1998; Schooler & Dotson, 2004; Trotter & Ulman, 2013).

Recent evaluations of both successful and less than successful implementations have stressed the need to anticipate the impact of the new system on the culture of the organization and to take active steps to mitigate the effects of change on the organization (Lorenzi & Riley, 2000; Peitzman, 2004). Transition management is a series of "…deliberate, planned interventions undertaken to assure successful adaptation/assimilation of a desired outcome into an organization" (Douglas & Wright, 2003). The nursing informaticist often leads the assessment and documentation of the "Current State" and development of the desired "Future State." Cognizance of the new system's impact serves as a visible leader in the transition management efforts.

Steering Committee

Before an EHR is developed or selected, the organization must appoint an EHR steering committee. The EHR steering committee, composed of internal and external stakeholders, is charged with providing oversight guidance to the selection and integration of the organization's strategic goals relative to the EHR requirements. During the planning phase, the projected return on investment (ROI) is established. The Steering Committee members' collective knowledge of the organization's daily operations provides global insight and administrative authority to resolve issues. In most facilities, the Steering Committee has the ultimate authority for decision-making (Fig. 11.2).

Project Team

The project team is led by an appointed project manager (often the Nurse Informaticist) and includes a designated team leader for each of the major departments affected by the system selection, implementation, or upgrade proposed. The objectives of the project team are to (1) understand the technology and technology restrictions of the proposed system, (2) understand the impact of intradepartmental EHR decisions, (3) make EHR decisions at the interdepartmental level, and (4) become the key resource for their application. A stated goal for the selection, implementation, or upgrading of an EHR is to improve

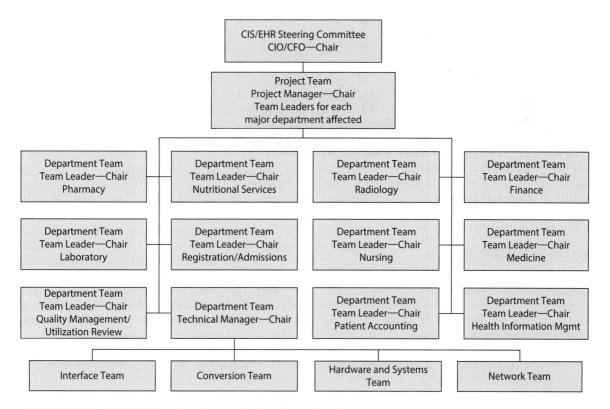

• **FIGURE 11.2.** Clinical Information System Steering Committee Structure.

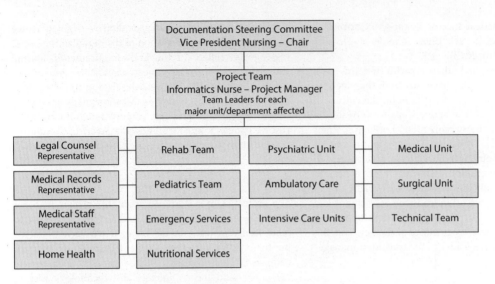

• **FIGURE 11.3.** Application Implementation Committee Structure.

patient safety and care; gains made by one department at the expense of another department rarely work to improve overall patient safety and care delivery. The project team's ability to evaluate multiple departments' information requirements in light of the capabilities of the proposed system is integral to overall success. Issues unable to be resolved by the Project Team are presented to the Steering Committee for resolution (Fig. 11.3).

The project manager is responsible for managing all aspects of the project; this includes software application development, hardware, and network acquisition/readiness, as well as oversight of the interface and conversion tasks. The project manager must possess good communication, facilitation, organizational, and motivational skills when leading a successful implementation. A sound knowledge of healthcare delivery, regulatory requirements, and hospital culture, processes, and politics is essential. .

Departmental Teams

The charge of the departmental teams is (1) to thoroughly understand the department's information requirements and workflow, (2) to gain a full understanding of the software's features and functions, (3) to complete a gap analysis for the new system's capabilities with the department's requirements, (4) to assist in the system testing effort, (5) to participate in developing and conducting end-user education, and (6) to provide a high level of support during the initial activation period of the new system. The team leaders must possess a sound knowledge of the

hospital and departmental policies and procedures (both formal and informal), and good organizational and communication skills, and must be adept at gaining consensus and resolving conflict.

Team members may well change during the course of a 10- to 16-month implementation. Hospital leaders, visionaries, and change agents' participation must balance the pragmatic, bottom line dictated by organizational needs (e.g., meaningful use incentives vs. patient outcomes). Shabot (2004) notes, "…both excellent leaders and excellent followers will be needed to make the new clinical information system a success" (p. 269).

DEVELOP PROJECT SCOPE

During the planning phase, the problem statement and goals of the implementation are defined, committee structures established, and the organization's requirements are defined for selecting, implementing, or upgrading an EHR or application, including the implications for regulatory compliance for safe and quality clinical practice. Commercial software developers and consultants rank this phase as the most critical factor in the selection of a system, even more important than the system itself (Zinn, 1989). Excellent planning takes time and thoughtful consideration. Time spent in developing a sound plan that encompasses all the checklist steps will reduce the amount of time spent in reworking areas not reviewed during the planning phase. Plan the work and then work the plan.

The planning phase involves the following tasks:

- Definition of committee structure
- Definition of requirements and/or stated goal
- Feasibility study
- Gap analysis
- Documentation and negotiation of project scope document
- Development of a high-level workplan
- Allocation of resources

Definition of the Project's Purpose

Definition of the project's purpose/stated goal is essential and often not readily apparent. Not until the information requirements of the project and/or stated goal and outcomes are precisely defined will the real characteristics of the requirements be revealed (Fitzgerald, Fitzgerald, & Satllings, 1981).

The project definition includes a description of how the system will be evaluated. Establishing the evaluation criteria early in the process supports the successful management philosophy of beginning with the end in mind (Convey, 1992). The results and improvements expected from implementing the system are described by realistic goals for the system. They might include increased functionality, decreased costs, increased personnel productivity, and meeting Federal Meaningful Use requirements. When updating or expanding the EHR or application, the project definition includes the identification of equipment currently available, its age, the degree of amortization, and the need for hardware or operating system software upgrades prior to undertaking an upgrade project.

Feasibility Study

A feasibility study is a preliminary analysis to determine if the proposed problem can be solved by the implementation of an EHR or component application. The feasibility study not only clarifies the problem and/or stated goal but also helps identify the information needs, objectives, and scope of the project. The feasibility study helps the EHR steering committee understand the real problem and/or goal by analyzing multiple parameters and by presenting possible solutions. It highlights whether the proposed solution will produce usable products and whether the proposed system's benefits more than justify the costs. Operational issues are reviewed to determine if the proposed solution will work in the intended environment. Technical issues are reviewed to ensure the proposed system can be built and/or will be compatible with the proposed and/or current technology. Legal and statutory regulations are reviewed to ensure

compliance with local and federal law. The feasibility study includes a high-level description of the human resources required and how the selected system will be developed, utilized, and implemented. The feasibility study describes the management controls to be established for obtaining administrative, financial, and technical approvals to proceed with each phase of the project. The feasibility study seeks to answer the following questions:

- What is the real problem to be solved and/or stated goal to be met?
- Where does the project fit into the overall strategic plan of the organization?
- What specific outcomes are expected from the project?
- What are the measurable criteria for determining project success from the above outcomes?
- What research and assumptions support the implementation project?
- What are the known limitations and risks to the project?
- What is the timing of the remaining phases of the project?
- Who will be committed to implementing the project?
- What are the estimated costs in both dollars and personnel time?
- What is the justification for the project, including the relationship between costs and benefits?

A feasibility study includes the following topic areas.

Statement of the Objective

The first step in conducting a feasibility study is to state the objectives for the proposed system. These objectives constitute the purpose(s) of the system. All objectives are outcome-oriented and are stated in measurable terms. The objectives identify the "end product" by defining what the EHR will do for the end users.

Environmental Assessment

The project is defined in terms of the support it provides to both the mission and the strategic plans of the organization. The project is evaluated relative to the organization's competition. The impact of legal, regulatory, and ethical considerations is reviewed. The regulatory impact of the Meaningful Use criteria is far reaching. Often one resource is assigned to assure each Meaningful Use criteria will meet the HITECH requirements. Individual software vendors often provide "best practice" guidelines demonstrating their software's intended functionality relative to Meaningful Use criteria.

Scope

The scope of the proposed system establishes system constraints and outlines what the proposed system will and will not produce. Included in the scope are the criteria by which the success of the project will be judged. The Scope Document outlines the boundaries of the project, establishes responsibilities for each team members, and sets up procedures as to how completed work will be verified and approved (Rouse, 2012).

Timeline

A project timeline is developed providing an overview of the key milestone events of the project. The projected length of time for each major phase of the project is established. Often called a project workplan, the major steps required for project are outlined in sufficient detail to provide the steering committee background on the proposed development or implementation process.

Recommendations

Committees may lose sight of the fact that not all projects are beneficial to the strategic mission of the organization. A decision can be made not only to proceed but also not to proceed with a project. The viability of the project is based on the review of the multiple factors researched in the feasibility study. It is critical to consider whether more personnel or equipment is necessary rather than more computerization. In addition to identifying potential hardware and software improvements, the costs and proposed benefits are factored into the project's viability decision. In upgrading or considering expansion of a system, a concerted effort to maximize use of the current system and to make process improvements in the current management and coordination of existing systems should be undertaken before deciding to procure a new system(s). If, based on the findings of the feasibility study, the project steering committee determines to continue with the project, a project scope agreement is prepared.

Documentation and Negotiation of a Project Scope Document

A project scope document is drafted by the project team and submitted to the project's steering committee for acceptance. The project scope document includes the scope of the project, the application level management requirements, the proposed activation strategy for implementing the EHR or application, and the technical management and personnel who will implement and maintain the equipment and programs. The Scope Document is based on the findings of the feasibility study.

The project scope document becomes the internal organizational contract for the project. It defines the short- and long-term goals, establishes the criteria for evaluating the success of the project, and expands the workplan to include further detail regarding the steps to be accomplished in the development or implementation of a system or application.

Resource Planning

An important step in the planning phase is to determine what resources are required to successfully carry out the agreed upon project scope. A firm commitment of resources for development of the entire EHR project includes all phases of implementation and is for the system to fulfill its stated objectives. The following points should be considered when planning for resources:

- Present staffing workload
- Human resources (i.e., number of personnel, experience and abilities, and percentage of dedicated time to the project)
- Present cost of operation
- Relationship of implementation events with non-project events (e.g., The Joint Commission accreditation process, state certification inspections, peak vacation and census times, union negotiations, and house staff turnover)
- Anticipated training costs
- Space availability
- Current and anticipated equipment requirements for the project team

Highly successful projects have spent the requisite amount of time to thoroughly complete the planning phase. Further, successful organizations have communicated senior management and administration's project expectations through dissemination of the project scope document to all departments in the organization.

ANALYSIS PHASE

The system analysis phase, the second SLC phase of developing an EHR, is the fact-finding phase. All data needs related to the requirements are defined in the project scope agreement developed in the Analysis Phase.

Key documents created in this phase are the following:

- Gap Analysis
- Technical requirements for hardware, software, networks
- Functional Design Document
- System Proposal Document

Data Collection

The collection of data reflecting the existing problem or goal is the first step in the system analysis phase. As a result of thorough data collection, refinements to the project scope agreement may occur. Added benefits to the organization may be realized through the small refinements. Larger project scope refinements should be carefully researched and evaluated (using the steps outlined in the feasibility study methodology) prior to requesting a major project scope change. Large or small, all changes must continue to support the goal(s) of the project and the strategic plan of the organization.

Two important documents are created as a result of data collection. The first is the creation of a workflow document for each major goal or problem to be resolved by the implementation of the new software or system; the second is a functional design document outlining how the new system will resolve the identified goals/problem.

Gap Analysis

Drawing on the work completed in the Planning phase, the workflow document, and the system proposal document from the analysis phase, a comparison of what is available in the current processes and what is desired in the new system is completed. Often referred to as a Gap Analysis, the comparison provides the project team with a list of features and functions desired but not immediately available in the new system/application. The departmental teams review the features/functions and estimated costs, evaluate alternatives to achieving them, and make recommendations to the Steering Committee. Features/functions may be delayed to a subsequent activation phase of the project, lobbied for inclusion in the current activation plan, or eliminated from the project.

Data are collected and analyzed to gain a sound understanding of the current system, "Current State," how it is used, and what is needed from the new system. Process analysis is foundational to the actual system design, since it examines the objectives and project scope in terms of the end-user requirements, the flow of information in daily operation, and the processing of required data elements.

Through the analysis effort, the individual data elements, interfaces, and EHR decision points of the project are identified (www.pmi.org). The "Future State"—how the system will look and function upon completion of the implementation begins to take shape. The review of requirements of the Americans with Disability Act (www.ada.gov/) is done to assure compliance with special needs of staff. Stakeholders review the document to assist in the prioritization of problems/issues to be resolved. Current costs and resources required for processing the organization's volume of data are compared with estimates for the cost of processing with the new system. If a system is being upgraded or expanded, the current equipment and functions are described. Careful evaluation is undertaken to ensure compatibility with the new system's requirements and to maximize the use of available equipment as long as possible. Depreciation costs of available equipment and projected budget expenditures are reviewed.

The importance of this phase should not be underestimated. Design changes made during the analysis stage often add minimal costs to the project; as the project progresses to the development and implementation phases, the cost of programmatic or design changes increases dramatically. According to one source, when a project is in the planning phase, the relative cost to make a design change or fix an error is one; in the analysis phase, the relative cost to fix the error/design change is three to six times that of the planning phase. The relative cost to fix an error or change a system design jumps to 40 to 1000 times once the system is operational.

Technical Analysis

A review of the project's technical requirements is conducted in the Analysis Phase. Trained/certified technical personnel review the requirements for EHR software to run efficiently. This may include programs to run the EHR software, hardware, and networks. Physical requirements for space, electrical needs, and air conditioning/cooling are considered. A technical architecture is developed to assure the speed of data transmissions, and sufficient storage capability to meet clinical and financial requirements over time. These requirements in conjunction with costs are evaluated and compiled into technical recommendations for the project.

Determination of Information Needs

A needs assessment outlines the high-level information required by multidisciplinary users. Standard terminology use as defined by the Centers for Medicare & Medicaid Services (CMS) and the Office of the National Coordinator for Health Care Information Technology (ONC) is critical to meeting Federal Meaningful Use requirements. The numbers of federally mandated data elements are significant, and increase with each Meaningful Use stage. Planning for the data collection across an organization's multiple departments and clinician workflow is imperative to successfully meeting the requirements of the HITECH Act. Workflow review and identification of the information needed clarify what users will expect from the system and how it can be collected in the course of daily operations. Such knowledge is essential in designing the system's output, input, and processing requirements constituting the basis for the new "Future State."

Workflow Document

The workflow document assimilates the data collected into logical sequencing of functions/tasks performed by the end users for each goal or problem area. Departmental standards of care, ordering patterns, procedures, operating manuals, reports (routine, regulatory, and year-end), and forms used in day-to-day operations are collected. Individual data elements required by clinicians in each department are identified and analyzed for continuity, duplication, and cross-referenced to the required HITECH data elements. The workflow document includes the following:

- A list of assumptions about the process or work effort
- A list of the major tasks performed by the user
- A list of the subtasks and steps the user accomplishes and outlines
- The determination of optional or required status for each task
- The frequency of the task being performed
- The criticality and important factors of the tasks/ subtasks
- The order of the subtasks
- The number and frequency of alternate scenarios available to the end user to accomplish a particular task

There are multiple sources of data for completing a workflow document. These include the following:

- Written documents, forms, and flow sheets
- Policy and procedure manuals
- Questionnaires
- Interviews
- Observations

- Development of workflow diagrams utilizing available software is most helpful in documenting the flow of information, people, and processes involved in the "Current State." The graphic representation provided by workflow diagrams allows a clear visualization of the gains proposed in the "Future State."

Functional Design Document

The functional design document is the overview statement of how the new system will work. It uses the workflow documents as its base, adding the critical documentation of the integration of each of the workflow documents to create a new system, implement a commercial software application, or upgrade a system. The functional design document, in this phase, outlines the human and machine procedures, the input points, the processing requirements, the output from the data entry, and the major reports to be generated from the new system. The functional design is a description of the functions required from the proposed EHR system or component and describes how tasks will be accomplished. From the functional design document, database structure will be determined.

Two data types are often used in databases—free text data (allowing the user to describe a response in their own words) and discrete data (structured data presented in application via check boxes or drop-down lists). Discrete data elements with links to standard terminology are the preferred data type. They increase the ability to report on and compare data. Meaningful Use 2014 requirements include the use of structured data linked to standard terminologies such as SNOMED-CT (Structured Nomenclature of Medicine—Clinical Terminology) and LOINC (Logical Observation Identifiers Names and Codes) used for laboratory tests. See also Chapter 8, Standardized Nursing Terminologies.

When new software is being created, the functional design document provides the programmers with a view of screens, linkages, and alternate scenarios to accomplish a task. Initial programming efforts can begin once the functional design is accepted. In the instance where a commercially available system or application is being implemented, the functional design outlines how the end users will use the system's programs to accomplish their tasks. In some cases, commercial software provides multiple pathways to accomplish a single task; the functional specification may suggest deploying a limited number of available pathways.

Data Analysis

The analysis of the collected data is the second step in the analysis phase. The analysis provides the data for development of an overview of the clinical requirements and/or stated goal defined in the project scope agreement.

Several software tools can be used in the development of the workflow and functional design documents and are discussed in Chapter 12, System and Functional Testing.

Data Review

The third step in the analysis phase is to review the data collected in the feasibility study, the workflow documents, and the functional specification and provide recommendations to the project steering committee for the new system. The review focuses on system requirements and/or attaining the project goals outlined in the feasibility study based on the best methods or pathways derived from the workflow documents and the functional design. Recommendations for streamlining workflow are suggested. The success of an EHR implementation project rests on the ability of the departmental and project teams to analyze the data and propose solutions benefiting the total organization without favoring certain departments at the expense of others. The benefits of a thorough structured analysis provide objective data to support the EHR. The careful analysis of end-user requirements and potential solutions has been proved to reduce the cost of design and implementation (Gause & Weinburg, 1989).

Benefits Identification

The overall anticipated benefits from the system are documented in the fourth step in the system analysis process. The benefits are stated in quantifiable terms and become the criteria for measuring the ROI and success of the project.

System Proposal Development

The final document created in the system analysis stage is a system proposal document. The proposal is submitted to the project's steering committee for review and approval. It sets forth the problems and/or goals and the requirements for the new system's overall design. It outlines the standards, documentation, and procedures for management control of the project, and it defines the information required, the necessary resources, anticipated benefits, a detailed workplan, and projected costs for the new system. The system proposal furnishes the project steering committee with recommendations concerning the proposed EHR or application. The system proposal document answers four questions:

1. What are the major problems and/or goals under consideration?

2. How will the proposed EHR solution correct or eliminate the problems and/or accomplish the stated goals?

3. What are the anticipated costs?

4. How long will it take?

The system proposal describes the project in sufficient detail to provide a management level understanding of the system or application without miring in minutiae. Much of the information required in the system proposal is collected in the earlier phases of the analysis. It has been suggested this proposal is best accepted when presented as a business proposal and championed by a member of the project's steering committee. The format of the final system proposal includes the following information:

- A concise statement of the problem(s) and/or goal(s)
- Background information related to the problem
- Environmental factors related to the problem
- Competition
- Economics
- Politics
- Ethics
- Anticipated benefits
- Proposed solutions
- Budgetary and resource requirements
- Project timetable

Acceptance of the system proposal by the project steering committee provides the project senior management support. Following acceptance by the project steering committee, it is not unusual for major EHR proposals to be presented to the institution's governing board for their acceptance and approval and to receive funding. Often the requirement for board approval is dependent on the final cost estimates of the system. Acceptance of the proposal by the project steering committee and the governing board assures not only funding for the project but critical top-down management and administrative support for the project. The final system proposal is an internal contract between the EHR committees/teams (steering, project, and departmental) and the institution.

As noted earlier, the active support and involvement of all senior executives in the development of the feasibility study are essential. The championing of the final system proposal greatly enhances the chances of acceptance of the system proposal.

SYSTEM DESIGN, DEVELOPMENT, AND CUSTOMIZATION PHASE

In this phase, the design details to develop the system and the detailed plans for implementing and evaluating the system evolve for both the functional and the technical components. Data dictionaries are populated with entries and project team's work to assure the functional design supports the clinician and departmental workflows. Policies and procedures are reviewed and updated to reflect the use of the new application/system in the delivery of care. Thorough testing of the new system occurs and detailed plans, developed in this, as well as previous phases, are executed.

There are multiple project documents created in this phase:

- Gap Analysis
- Functional specifications
- Technical specifications
- Implementation Workplan containing detailed plans specific to
  - Hardware and Peripheral Devices
  - Interfaces
  - Conversions
  - Testing
  - End-User Training
  - Cut Over Plan
  - Go Live Plan
- Post-Live Evaluation Reports

System Design

The project teams receive application training often directly from the vendor. In some cases a limited number of team members attend training with the expectation they will train other team members. The Project Teams determine the best utilization of functionality based upon the identified elements of project goals, scope, software functionality, and the organization's workflow. The definition of current workflow, documented in the analysis phase, serves as the bases for changes, both programmatic and process-oriented, required to support the new system's workflow.

Functional Specifications. The functional specifications use the functional design document developed in the system analysis phase of an EHR and builds on the design by formulating a detailed description of ALL system inputs, outputs, and processing logic required to complete the scope of the project. It further refines what the proposed system will encompass and provides the framework for its operation.

Commercial software vendors generally provide a detailed functional specification document for their system or application in the form of manuals. The manuals, usually application-specific, include an introduction, a section for each workflow, and a technical section. From the provided documentation, the hospital's departmental and project teams produce the organization's functional specification by evaluating the available commercial software's functions with the organization's workflow documents and making decisions on the functionality to be used by the institution.

The detailed functional specifications are critical to the system's acceptance; each screen, data flow, and report the user can expect to see is analyzed. The examples incorporate real data into the explanations and drawings. The technical aspects of the HITECH Act and Meaningful Use criteria must be fully understood and followed carefully including the use of both evidence-based medicine links and clinical decision support rules for patient safety within clinical workflows. Additional information can be found at http://www.healthit.gov/providers-professionals/ehr-implementation-steps/step-5-achieve-meaningful-use.

During this step, the departmental teams and users determine what the actual data will look like in its output form, and they gain consensus from the departmental teams for the proposed workflow design. Requirements for meeting the HITECH Meaningful Use data collection are integral to completing the functional specifications. In-depth understanding of the federal criteria, layered with thoughtful implementation planning and execution, will lead to staff's universal adoption of new data collection and data sharing procedures.

There is fluidity between the functional specification and initial programming prototype efforts. The design team creating the new application often works closely with the programmers, making adjustments in the design and specification based on federal requirements, programming logic, newly identified information needs, and/or technologies. As the functional specification matures and major design decisions (e.g., selection of the underlying application technology and database structure) have occurred, a design freeze point is established. This indicates the functional specification is complete and full programming efforts can begin.

Once completed, the functional specification provides not only the road map for programming efforts but also the starting point for developing testing and training plans. The advantages of establishing testing plans in concert with the development of the functional specification include a more thorough test plan (workflows are not missed), and "what if" questions often spark the need to develop or allow alternate workflow.

Technical Specifications

In the system design phase, technical personnel work closely with the project and departmental teams to ensure the components of the proposed system work in concert with technology and end-user needs and to assist in the development of the implementation plan. A dedicated technical manager is required. He or she is responsible for the coordination of efforts in five major areas: hardware, networks, software, interface application, and legacy system data conversion. Detailed technical specifications are developed for each area. The project's technical manager and team leaders ensure all of the components/applications of the EHR work in concert with all the other components.

Hardware

In the case of new software development, the technical project manager ensures the new software uses the best technology platform available. The ability to operate the new application on multiple hardware platforms is often desired. Technical specifications describing the recommended equipment are developed and tested in the development laboratory.

When commercial software is being implemented or upgraded, the technical project manager ensures the physical environment for the new system conforms to the new system's technical specifications. This may include the need to build a new computer room, establish or upgrade a network, and procure the correct devices for the new system. The types of devices to be used (mobile PCs vs. handheld vs. bedside devices) require dialog and testing with team leaders and department team members. The testing and deployment of the new equipment (terminals, multiple types of printers [e.g. card, label, prescription], Internet output [e.g. electronic prescription systems], and/or wireless devices) are the responsibility of the technical manager. Ongoing maintenance requirements for the new system's processing unit, operating systems, and network are coordinated by the project's technical manager.

Selecting the correct hardware for the system depends on its design, application, and software requirements. Technical conditions may dictate selection of a mainframe, a minicomputer, a microcomputer, or a combination of the above. Computer hardware is obtained in several different ways. Central processing may be purchased or leased from a hardware vendor for in-house use; however, when cost is a significant factor, timesharing computer processing with other facilities may be considered. Many Internet Web-hosted medical applications are now available. The technical manager must evaluate such offerings in light of interoperability with the main hospital information system as well as data security during transmissions to and from the Web. Input, output, and processing media, including secondary storage, are selected.

Peripheral Device Plan

Knowledge of the many clinical workflows is an important component of the Peripheral Device Plan. There are now many types of devices available to clinicians to support their daily workflow. For some data collection, wireless tablets may work well when full features and functions are needed (e.g., provider/nursing/ancillary rounding). For other data collection, smaller handheld devices may provide connectivity for limited data collection needs. Nurse Informaticists are integral in reviewing the primary needs of each stakeholder, suggesting a limited number of companies/devices to trial, and providing the compilation of the trial evaluation data. Nursing Informaticians and the technical team work together to assure all hardware is installed and tested at the appropriate time.

Networks

Proliferation of Web-based applications and reference/search engines in addition to the locally based EHR necessitates a thorough review of the current and anticipated volume of transactions (financial and clinical) and high utilization times for accessing the EHR. The EHR no longer resides simply within the walls of a hospital. Health systems composed of inpatient, outpatient, long-term care, home health, and patient access are variables to be considered when determining the size and types of networks. "During day to day utilization, what users want is sub-second screen flip response time" (Shabot, 2004, p. 265).

Application Software

The project's technical manager is responsible for establishing the technical specifications outlining the operational requirements for the new system. The specifications detail the procedures required to maintain the application software on a daily, weekly, and monthly basis. The specifications are compiled as the starting point for determining the operations schedule for the system and/or the institution. The operations plan includes detailed information related to when the system will be scheduled for routine maintenance, plans for operations during system failures, and acceptable periods, if needed, during the week/month for the system to be unavailable to the users. Additional requirements for assuring data reliability and availability following planned and unplanned system downtime as well as procedures outlining data recovery following a downtime are developed. Change control policies and procedures for identifying, tracking, testing, and applying software fixes are established. Mark Anderson, the healthcare IT futurist, acknowledges prevailing requirements from panel of physicians stating "…if the system was not available a minimum of 99% of the time, they (physicians) would not consider the application reliable enough to use…" (Anderson, 2011, p. 2).

With the popularity of Web-based systems, Web design, maintenance, and security have added a level of complexity to maintaining a system within a healthcare environment's security regulations (e.g. HIPAA, Meaningful Use). Often niche software (e.g., patient portal, secure texting software, e-prescribing, appointment scheduling, preventative healthcare alerts) complements the central hospital information system. Requirements of each must be reviewed and outlined in the technical specifications.

Interface Applications

An interface system defines those programs and processes required to transmit data between disparate systems. The project's technical manager coordinates all interfacing activities for the new application. While utilization of the industry's Health Level Seven (HL7) interface standards has greatly reduced the effort required to establish clinical interfaces by providing a standard specification for the transmission of data, the number of clinical interfaces in an EHR has dramatically increased. It is not unusual for an EHR to interface with separate registration, patient billing, ancillary departmental systems (e.g., lab, radiology, pharmacy, ICU systems), as well as multiple types of wireless devices. With the advent of Health Information Exchanges (HIEs), patient data will be sent via interfaces outside a healthcare systems domain. Interface developments advocate the use of an interface engine decreasing the number of individual interfaces to be managed. System security is detailed Chapter 10, Trustworthy Systems for Safe and Private Health Care.

Meaningful Use Stage 2 requirements encompass the ability to share data electronically with Federal and local agencies as well as with the patient. Implementation and use of an Internet portal by patients is a Meaningful Use Stage 2 requirement. Adherence to the Federal Meaningful Use data and transmission criteria is, therefore, essential.

More complex environments may include interfaces to physiological monitors and wireless portable devices, and provide remote access into the healthcare network's clinical system for physicians and their staff.

The interface specification details whether the interface will be one-way or bidirectional. A bidirectional interface implies data are flowing both to and from a system. Conversely, a one-way interface may either send data to or receive data from a separate system but does not do both.

An important process in development of the interface specification is the comparison of data elements in each system in order to determine the data elements and their technical format be included in the interface.

LEGACY SYSTEMS DATA CONVERSIONS

The conversion of data from legacy systems to a new system is a major area of coordination for the project's technical manager. Most hospitals currently use automated registration and billing systems; determining the conversion requirements and developing and testing the conversion programs are critical steps in implementing a new system or application.

While all steps are important in the implementation of a new system, the interface and conversion design and testing tasks are frequent areas causing project delays. The importance of oversight and communication by the project technical manager to keep the technical tasks on the established timetable should not be underestimated.

Development

Multiple plans are developed during this portion of the Design, Develop, Implement, and Evaluate Phase. The detailed implementation workplan encompasses the multiple plans targeting specific aspects of the EHR. Often the appropriate departmental teams are responsible for creating the details for a focused plan. Together with the Project Manager and Team Leaders, the focused plans are incorporated into the implementation workplan. At a minimum the following focused plans are required:

- Communications Plan
- Hardware and Peripheral Devices plan
- Interface plan
- Conversion plan
- Testing plan
- End-User Training plan

The developed functional and technical specifications define a significant amount of form and substance for the new EHR. The next step is to assess the timeframes established in the final scope document with the development timeframes established during the system design and the interface and conversion requirements to establish a detailed workplan. The workplan identifies a responsible party and a beginning date and end date for each phase, step, task, and subtask. This plan coordinates all tasks necessary to complete the development of new software, implement a new system, and/or upgrade a current system. Many software vendors and consultants provide an implementation workplan for their system or applications. The supplied workplans must be reviewed and revised to meet the individual needs and timetables of the organization's project. Automated workplan software is available to create and monitor a project/implementation plan. The implementation checklist describes the high-level tasks to be included in clinical implementation workplans. It is advisable to take advantage of automated software and existing plans. Figure 11.4 provides an example of detailed workplan based on the checklist.

Whether the project is software development or the implementation or upgrading of a system, the implementation workplan details the following:

- Personnel
- Timeframes

Clinical Implementation Workplan Sample

- **PROJECT ADMINISTRATION**
  - Identify Initial Project Team
  - Project Coordination Meeting
  - Initiate Target Hardware/Software Delivery Dates
  - Establish Project Control
  - **Project Supervision/Order Management**
    - **Project Status Meetings**
    - **Project Steering Committee Meeting**
  - **REQUIREMENTS AND PLANNING**
    - Network Kickoff / Review Application Network Overview
    - Project Definition -
      - Project Definition Planning Session
      - Complete Project Definition Document
      - Complete Workplan for
      - **Develop Project Charter**
        - Determine 3 indicators for quantified benchmarking
        - Develop plan for collection of pre-system indicator data
        - Execute plan for collection of pre-system indicator data
    - Finalize/Approve Project Scope/Workplan
    - **Project Organization -**
      - Organize Implementation Project Team -
      - Organize Workflow Design and Project Task Force(s) -
      - Organize Data Standardization Task Force

• **FIGURE 11.4.** Sample Clinical Implementation Workplan.

- Costs and budgets
- Facilities and equipment required
- Operational considerations

A successful implementation ensures all checklist items are planned, executed, and tracked by the project manager and project team leaders.

System Selection

In the instance where commercially available software is being considered, the key documents completed in earlier phases assist in beginning the system selection process. The task of selecting a new system becomes more objective as a result of the thoughtful evaluation for the functional specification and design document. The process and documents provide the steering committee and project team with information to objectively evaluate commercial system offerings. The system proposal document also assists the institution's legal team in formulating a contract with the software vendor as well as providing the basis for the development of a formal request for proposal (RFP) or request for information (RFI) to potential vendors.

Request for Proposal (RFP)/Request for Information (RFI)

The creation of a Request for Information (RFI) document is sent to selected vendors indicating the organization's interest in gaining knowledge about the vendor's products. At a high level, the key features desired for the new system are listed. Vendors respond to the RFI with their product's likely ability to meet the high-level requirements. Additional knowledge about available technical solutions not considered is often gained from the RFI responses. The project team reviews the responses and selects two to four vendors meeting the majority of the high-level requirements. A Request for Proposal (RFP) document is created by the project team and sent to the selected vendors outlining in greater detail the features and functions desired for the new system. Clinical and financial workflow scenarios as well as the desired functions developed by the project team can be included in the RFP. The vendor RFP responses are equally detailed; they are closely evaluated both from the written responses and during subsequent in-person or webinar style demonstrations of their product.

A number of system evaluation tools (Nielsen, 1992; Shneiderman, 1998) have been published. A heuristic method relies on information common to the evaluators in assessing the usability of a system. The 14-point tool, termed the Nielsen–Shneiderman Tool (Zhang, Johnson, Patel, Paige, & Kubose, 2003, p. 25), provides a list of areas

Information System Application			Vendor A Costs			Vendor B Costs			Vendor C Costs		
			Year 1	Year 2	Year 3	Year 1	Year 2	Year 3	Year 1	Year 2	Year 3
Nursing Documentation											
	Implementation										
	License										
	Hardware										
	Training										
	Support										
	Interfaces										
	Conversions										
Order Entry											
	Implementation										
	License										
	Hardware										
	Training										
	Support										
	Interfaces										
	Conversions										
	Yearly Total		$	$	$	$	$	$	$	$	$
	3 Year Total		$			$			$		

• **FIGURE 11.5.** Sample Cost Comparison Worksheet.

to be assessed during the review and evaluation of systems or applications. Preparation activities for project team members evaluating demonstrations of systems or applications for purchase should include a discussion of aspects of the evaluation tool to be used and the definition of the criteria to increase objectivity in the selection process.

Figures 11.5 and 11.6 are examples of tools utilized in evaluating the cost and potential usability of prospective vendors' software.

Communications Plan

Healthcare systems or applications often affect more than one department. Results from a laboratory system are reviewed by clinicians; the pharmacy system utilizes creatine results to adjust medication dosages for renal impaired patients. Documented nursing observations (e.g., wounds, catheters, psychosocial assessments) are utilized by case management, providers, and insurance companies. New functionality must be planned and communicated to all stakeholders. A communications plan is often created in conjunction with the organization's public relations department. The plan is developed to promote frequent face-to-face communications among departments, to multiple levels of administration, and to external stakeholders (e.g., regulatory organizations, payers, and the local communities served). Communications to all stakeholders/constituents affected by the project are developed. Segment-targeted communications plans are developed identifying the type, content level, and media for information dissemination to each identified

stakeholder. Rarely have staff complained of receiving too much information about a new process or change. More often the complaint is "…no one told us!" Multiple communication mediums are utilized, including but not limited to the following:

- Verbal updates presented at departmental/staff meetings
- Fact sheets/newsletters/flyers
- Faxes, e-mail, and Web site posting
- Social media/blogs

The communication plan, once developed and executed, must be monitored and modified as the implementation progresses.

Up to this point, thorough planning and thoughtful design discussions have been held. During Development, the decisions are actualized with the entry of elements into the data dictionaries, and comparison of the clinical and departmental workflow to those created in the system. The functional specification indicating how the departments and clinicians want the system to work and the workflow document describing how processes are carried out are established by populating in the data dictionaries. The plans for Interfaces, Conversions, Testing, Communications, and Training are carried out.

Policies and Procedures

Reviews of policies and procedures are conducted, revisions reflecting changes being implemented with

Reviewer Name: _____
Department: _____ Date: _____
Application: _____ Vendor:_____

SYSTEM ATTRIBUTES	CIRCLE SCORE
	POOR (1) AVG (2–3) GOOD (4–5)
Consistency and use of standards	1 2 3 4 5
Visibility of system state	1 2 3 4 5
Match between system and world	1 2 3 4 5
Minimalist—without extra distractions	1 2 3 4 5
Minimize memory load	1 2 3 4 5
Informative feedback	1 2 3 4 5
Flexibility	1 2 3 4 5
Good error messages	1 2 3 4 5
Error prevention	1 2 3 4 5
Clear closure	1 2 3 4 5
Reversible actions	1 2 3 4 5
User's language	1 2 3 4 5
User is in control	1 2 3 4 5
Help and documentation availability	1 2 3 4 5
Overall system desirability	1 2 3 4 5
Total Average Rating	**1 2 3 4 5**

COMMENTS:_____
_____

• **FIGURE 11.6.** Sample Demo Ranking Form. (Data from Zhang, J., et al, 2003.)

the new system/application workflows. It is advisable to complete the policy reviews and complete procedure revisions prior to the start of end-user training.

Workflow, Dictionaries, and Profiles

In this portion of the phase, project team members review data requirements and workflow previously documented. Data dictionaries and profiles are populated with entries to established desired new system workflow. This becomes an iterative process of populating data dictionaries with values supporting the workflow design and functional specification; testing the design with the project team; evaluating options suggested as a result of testing; and refining/reevaluating the functional specification.

As data dictionaries are established, project teams begin to develop clinical decision support functions. Clinical decision support is defined as "…an application that analyzes data to help healthcare providers make clinical decisions" (Rouse, 2010). "Clinical Decision Support Software (CDSS) is software designed to be a direct aid to clinical decision-making in which the characteristics of an individual patient are matched to a computerized

clinical knowledge base and patient-specific assessments or recommendations are then presented to the clinician or the patient for decision" (Sim et al., 2001, p. 528). Two main types of clinical decision support systems exist. One type uses a knowledge base while systems without a knowledge base rely on machine learning to analyze data. The challenge for the project team is to find the correct balance of the number and types of alerts presented to the clinician. Clinical alert fatigue, caused "…by excessive numbers of warnings about items such as potentially dangerous interaction presented to the clinician and as a result the clinician may pay less attention or even ignore some vital alerts…" (Kesselheim, 2011, p. 2310) is a well-documented phenomena (see Chapter 40, Evidenced-Based Practice).

Testing

The system, whether newly developed or commercially available, must be tested to ensure all data are processed correctly and the desired outputs are generated. Testing verifies the computer programs are written correctly and when implemented in the production (live) environment the system will function as planned. System implementation requires three levels of testing. The first level is often called a functional test. During this round of testing, the departmental teams test and verify the databases (files, tables, data dictionaries), ensuring correct data have been entered into the system. The expected departmental reports are reviewed to assure correctness and accuracy. Multiple iterations of the functional test often occur until the departmental team is confident the system setup and profiles support the work of the department. The second level of testing, integrated systems testing, begins when all departments indicate successful completion of their functional testing. During integrated testing, the total system is tested; this includes interfaces between systems as well as the interplay between applications within the same system. The integrated test must mimic the production (live) environment in terms of the volume of transactions, the number of users, the interfaced systems, and the procedures to be followed to carry out all functions of the system. It is at this point, organization-wide procedures to be instituted when the system is unavailable, often called downtime procedures, are thoroughly tested. Downtime procedures must be taught during end-user training.

At the end of integrated testing, the organization makes a formal decision to proceed or postpone activation of the new systems. Often referred to as the "Go-No Go" decision, members of the steering committee, project team, and technical staff review the outstanding issues from both unit and integrated testing to make their decision. The final round of testing occurs during end-user training. As more users interact with the new system, previously unfound problems may surface. Evaluation of the severity of the newly discovered concerns and the corrective action required is an ongoing process during implementation. Significant information on testing processes and tools can be found in Chapter 12, System and Functional Testing.

End-User Training. It is essential to train the end users on how to use the system in their daily workflow. An EHR will function only as well as its users understand its operation and the operations streamline their workflow. Two levels of training take place for the implementation of a system. The project team and selected members of the departmental team receive training from the developers or vendor. This training details the databases (files and tables), processing logic, and outputs of all the system's features and functions. End-user training takes place once the departmental and project teams have finished profiling the system to meet the functional and technical specifications developed and functional testing has been completed. The preparation for end-user training necessitates

a "mini-workplan" often developed and managed by a team led by the Education/Training department. End-user training stresses how the user will complete his or her workflow using the system features and functionality.

All users of the new system or application must receive training. Training on a new system should occur no more than six weeks prior to the activation of the new system. When training occurs for more than six weeks before activation of the system, additional refresher training is often required by the end users.

Training takes place before and during the activation of a new system. After system implementation, refresher courses as well as new employee introductory training on the use of the system are often provided by the institution. The large number of provider, nursing and ancillary staff members to be trained necessitates a significant amount of advance planning.

Training is most effective when hands-on, interactive instruction is provided. Training guides or manuals explain the system; however, retention of information is increased if the learners are able to interact with the new system in a manner simulating their workflow with the system. Computer-assisted instruction (CAI) can be used to provide hands-on experience. Often the Web-based training provides the user opportunities for self-paced, on-demand learning. End-user training is offered with two perspectives. One perspective provides a general overview of the system, and the second perspective explains how the user will interact with the system to complete his or her daily work. While a training manual is developed for the training sessions, most end users express the desire to have a pocket-size reminder ("cheat sheet") outlining the key functions of the new system or application. Both the user's manual and the pocket reminders should be available for departmental use. When possible, a training environment on the computer system should be established for the organization. Establishing a training lab as well as providing access to the training environment from the departments and nursing units prior to the activation of the new system provides end users the opportunity to practice at times convenient to their work requirements and reinforces the training.

IMPLEMENT, EVALUATE, MAINTAIN, AND SUPPORT PHASE

System Documentation

The preparation of documents to describe the system for all users is an ongoing activity, with development of the documentation occurring as the various system phases and steps are completed. Documentation should begin with the final system proposal. Several manuals are prepared: a user's manual, a reference manual, and an operator's maintenance manual. These manuals provide guides to the system components and outline how the entire system has been developed.

Implementation—Go Live

Few if any healthcare organizations have the luxury to stop operations during an implementation (Lorenzi et al., 2008). Implementation encompasses the Cut Over plan (data driven) and the Implementation plan for the facility to continue to operate (people/processes) during this period. Staffing, patient care delivery, and support of the end user during the "Go Live" period are detailed within the "Go Live" plan. The planning includes assuring patient care functions as smoothly as possible during the time between the cutoff of the old system and the start of processing on the new system. Downtime functions/processes and forms are reviewed to assure patient care, and processing of data continues and is able to be accurately reflected in the patient's record. This often includes developing forms streamlining the documentation to be entered when the new system is available (Fig. 11.7).

Sample Cutover Plan

Four activation approaches are possible: (1) parallel, (2) pilot, (3) phased-in, and (4) big bang theory. In the parallel approach, the new system runs parallel with the existing system until users can adjust. In the pilot approach, a few departments or units try out the new system to see how it works and then help other units or departments to use it. In the phased-in approach, the system is implemented by one unit or department at a time. In the big bang approach, a cutover date and time are established for the organization, the old system is stopped, and all units/departments begin processing on the newly installed system.

The timing of conversion activities and the activation of all interfaces require particular coordination between the technical staff and the project teams. The project's technical manager, in conjunction with the project manager, is responsible for assuring the development of thorough go live plans. A command center is established to coordinate all issues, concerns, and go live help desk functions. A sufficient number of phone lines and beepers/cell phones are secured to support the move to the live production environment. Team members and trainers often serve as resources to the end users on a 24-hour basis for a period of time post-implementation. Sometimes called "super users," these team members are available in the departments and on the nursing units to proactively

assist users during the first one to two weeks of productive use of the new system or application.

The coordination of all activities requires a cohesive team effort. Communication among the team members is foundational; end users are informed of the sequence events, the expected time frames for each event, and the channels established for reporting and resolving issues. Daily meetings of key team members to review issues and chart the progress of the new system are held. Decisions affecting the "Go Live" are made in a timely manner and require a thoughtful and thorough approach when changes to procedures and computer programs are contemplated. The executive team and senior management group are kept as up to date as the end users. The goal of most clinical implementations is to improve the delivery of information to the end user. The end-user suggestions and issues, therefore, must be tracked and resolved. Providing timely follow up to issues and suggestions will be critical to the success of the new system. Often, the informatics nurses are responsible for this follow-up.

It is highly recommended to have all end-user logins, passwords, and system devices and printers tested five to seven days before going live. Requests for login and password support comprise the largest number of calls to the Command Center during the first few weeks of a new system's use. Clinical and departmental managers are in the best position to assure all staff have logged into the new system and have the appropriate role for their job requirements. Login issues are followed closely by printer issues (e.g., printer offline, printer settings incorrect, output expected to print at a location doesn't print) during the first weeks of a new system. The Hardware team members can troubleshoot issues best if they have been given a script outlining one or two functions resulting in a printed output. Assuring these two areas are addressed completely prior to "Go Live" will dramatically lessen the anxiety of the end user as well as eliminate a large number of calls to the Command Center during the "Go Live" period.

With an organized and thorough Integrated Testing period, the actual first productive use of the system and subsequent days of the "Go Live" period are likely to be a "boring" nonevent. Feedback from the end users and administrative staff will help determine how long the Command Center will need to be staffed on a 24-hour-a-day basis.

The command center is set up and ready to coordinate all issues, concerns, and "Go Live" Help Desk functions. The Command Center has a sufficient number of phone lines and beepers to support the move to the Live, production environment. For a period of time, this will include 24 hours a day operations. Often, the representatives/consultants of the new software company are on site to

DONE	DATE	START TIME	TARGET END TIME	SEQUENCE	TASK DESCRIPTION	TASK DEPENDENCY	RESP. PERSON	HANDOFF CONTACT	COMMENTS
	2-Nov	8:30	30-Nov	SMS-1	Change profile PRFDT to 29 days. Continue changing this profile (minus one day) on a daily basis until 11/30 when it is set to 1.	none			All areas that enter orders. To prevent future orders to be placed in legacy system with start date greater than conversion date.
	30-Nov	12:00	23:00	CAI-1	Review/Final configuration changes	none			
	30-Nov				*CHECKPOINT CONFERENCE CALL*	*scheduled*	*ALL*		
	30-Nov	14:00	16:00	**MD-1**	Order rewrites by physicians. Nursing staff will hold on to any orders which can be held until 02:00	none			6 a.m. Lab draws should not wait until 2 p.m. Enter when orders are rewritten. **WE ARE NOT REWRITING MEDICATION ORDERS!**
	30-Nov	14:00	16:00	**Nursing-1**	Enter orders for 6 a.m. Lab draw in legacy system	Legacy Lab Up	Nursing Staff		
	30-Nov	18:00	00:00	**Nursing-2**	Validation of Allergies (including food allergies) and patient factors data on Go Live patient factor validation checklist		Nurses Only	Hand off validation checklist	Go Live patient factor validation form checklist created to help with this.

· **FIGURE 11.7.** Sample Cutover Plan.

assist with "Go Live" support and staffing of the Command Center. The advantages of having designated command center include close proximity of clinical, administrative, technical, and vendor team members to quickly assess and prioritize issues. This close proximity also allows rapid communications and trending of problems in near real time during the first days of the new system's use. Team members, trainers, and super users serve as resources to the end users on a 24-hour basis during "Go Live," often a period of one to two weeks.

Evaluation Post-Live. The important tasks of Evaluation are:

- Collection of post-live Success Criteria
- Completion of a System/Project Evaluation including the results of the Success Criteria
- Transitioning end-user support from the Command Center to the Help Desk
- Closure of the project

The system is evaluated to determine whether it has accomplished the Project Scope's stated objectives. It involves a comparison of the working system with its functional requirements to determine how well the requirements are met, to determine possibilities for growth and improvement, and to preserve the lessons learned from the implementation project for future efforts. The Post "Go Live" evaluation describes and assesses, in detail, the new system's performance. Utilizing the criteria established in Planning Phase, the evaluation process summarizes the entire system, identifying both the strengths and weaknesses of the implementation process. Comparison of the pre- and post-implementation Success Criteria data provide quantitative data as to the successes obtained with the new system. The evaluation often leads to system revisions and, ultimately, a better system.

To evaluate an implemented hospital information system, many principles are important. One authority suggests evaluating duplication of efforts and data entry, fragmentation, misplaced work, complexity, bottlenecks, review/approval processes, error reporting via the Issue Tracking mechanism, or the amount of reworking of content, movement, wait time, delays, set up, low importance outputs, and unimportant outputs.

This evaluation component becomes a continuous phase in total quality management. The system is assessed to determine whether it continues to meet the needs of the users. The totally implemented system will require continuous evaluation to determine if upgrading is appropriate and/or what enhancements could be added to the current system. Formal evaluations generally take place no less than every six months and routinely every two to

four years after the systems have been implemented. The formal evaluation can be conducted by an outside evaluation team to increase the objectivity level of the findings. Informal evaluations are done on a weekly basis.

Other approaches to evaluating the functional performance of a system exist. The Clinical Information System Evaluation Scale (Gugerty, Miranda, & Rook, 2006) describes a 37-item measurement tool for assessing staff satisfaction with a CIS. Investigating such functions as administrative control, medical/nursing orders, charting and documentation, and retrieval and management reports are used to assess system benefits. Each of these areas is evaluated through time observations, work sampling, operational audits, and surveys (Nahan, Vaydua, Ho, Scharf, & Seagull, 2007). System functional performance can be assessed by examining nurses' morale and nursing department operations.

Documentation of care must be assessed if patient care benefits are to be evaluated. The following questions should be asked:

- Does the system assist in improving the documentation of patient care in the patient record?
- Does the system reduce patient care costs?
- Does the system prevent errors and save lives?
- To evaluate nurses' morale requires appraising nurses' satisfaction with the system. The following questions may be considered useful:
  - Does the system facilitate nurses' documentation of patient care?
  - Does it reduce the time spent in such documentation?
  - Is it easy to use?
  - Is it readily accessible?
  - Are the display "screens" easy to use?
  - Do the displays capture patient care?
  - Does the system enhance the work situation and contribute to work satisfaction?

To evaluate the departmental benefits requires determining if the CIS helps improve administrative activities. The following questions must be answered:

- Does the new system enhance the goals of the department?
- Does it improve department efficiency?
- Does it help reduce the range of administrative activities?
- Does it reduce clerical work?

Other criteria are necessary to evaluate technical performance; these include reliability, maintainability, use, response time, accessibility, availability, and flexibility to meet changing needs. These areas are examined from several different points—the technical performance of the software as well as hardware performance. The following questions must be answered:

- Is the system accurate and reliable?
- Is it easy to maintain at a reasonable cost?
- Is it flexible?
- Is the information consistent?
- Is the information timely?
- Is it responsive to users' needs?
- Do users find interaction with the system satisfactory?
- Are input devices accessible and generally available to users?

Implementation of a clinical system is a project; by definition a project has a beginning, a middle, and an end (Lewis, 2007; Project Management Institute, 2014). The transitioning of the end-user support functions from the Command Center to the Help Desk and submission of the Post-Live Evaluation to the Steering Committee are particularly important events in determining the end of an implementation project and the beginning of the maintenance and growth phases of the new system.

Daily Support Operations

Daily support operations begin during the Go Live period. "Help Desk" functions for recording and tracking end-user calls/tasks for help are often managed by the Go Live team in the Command Center during the first one to three weeks post-live. Daily meetings/huddles are held with the Go Live team and IT Help Desk staff to review both type and frequency of problems encountered by the end users. The most frequent type of call during the Go Live period are from users unable to log into the system. The proactive recommendation is to include a task in the Cut Over Plan to assign user logins and have all users log into the new system two to seven days before Go Live. The second most frequently received calls stem from the user's lack of knowledge on how to complete a specific task. Reinforcement of training through one-to-one interventions as well as via mass communications (e-mails/flyers/Web site updates) are done. Early resolution of problems and communication back to staff is imperative and fosters confidence that the Project Team and the organization are addressing their needs during this stressful period.

Ongoing Maintenance

The requirement for support resources in the hospital/healthcare environment is a challenge for organizations. Many organizations utilize technical, analyst, and nursing informatics resources to provide the 24/7 support coverage. Strong communication and issue/task resolution procedures assist in responding to user needs.

The technical manager reviews requirements for networks, servers, hardware, and certain software concerns. Commercial software companies continue to provide upgrades and updates to their systems/applications. Ongoing review of new features and functions, federal and state requirements, and insurance and billing requirements occur. Nursing Informatics personnel must bridge the support of the basic system requirements with the fast paced release of new technologies used in patient care. The cost of purchase and implementation is high; maintaining and improving the system's ability to support all aspects of patient care delivery are mandatory.

To upgrade a system, the same phases and activities described for the SLC must occur; however, when upgrading, dovetailing the changes into the current system will require close evaluation and planning.

SUMMARY

This chapter describes the process of designing, implementing, and/or upgrading a clinical information system/EHR in a patient healthcare facility. It outlines and describes the four phases of the SLC process—planning, system analysis, system design, development, implementation, and evaluation and system maintenance and support. The upgrading process reviews all of the components described to assure a technically sound, regulatory complete implementation supporting safe patient care and streamlined workflow. A clinical system/EHR implementation checklist utilizing the SLC process has been developed (Fig. 11.8).

The planning phase determines the problem scope and outlines the entire project to determine if the system is feasible and worth developing and/or implementing. The analysis phase assesses the problem being studied through extensive data gathering and analysis. The design phase produces detailed specifications of the proposed system. Development involves the actual preparation of the system, support of workflow, review of policies and procedures impacted by the new system, and detailed implementation planning. Testing is generally conducted on three levels for both the design and implementation of a commercially available system. Training focuses on the use of the system to improve their everyday workflow. Implementation outlines the detailed

1. **PLANNING PHASE**
   Project Governance Structure
   Project Purpose
      Feasibility Study
   Project Scope Document
   Resource Planning

2. **ANALYSIS PHASE**
   Data Collection
      Determine Information Needs
         Gap Analysis
      Workflow Document
      Functional Design Document
         Data Analysis
         Data Review
         Benefits Identification
   Technical Analysis
      Hardware
      Software
      Networks
   System Proposal Document

3. **DESIGN, DEVELOP, AND CUSTOMIZE PHASE**
   System Design
      Functional Design Document
      Technical Specifications
         Hardware and Peripheral Device Plan
         Networks
         Application Software
          Interface
         Legacy System Data Conversion

3. **DESIGN, DEVELOP, AND CUSTOMIZE PHASE (cont)**
   Develop Detailed Workplan
      Focused Plans
         Communications
         Hardware and Peripheral Devices
         Interface
         Conversion
         Testing
         End-User Training
   Customize
         System Dictionary Data and Profiles
         Policies and Procedures
   Conduct Testing
         Functional
         Integrated
   Conduct End-User Training
   System Documentation

4. **IMPLEMENT, EVALUATE, MAINTAIN, AND SUPPORT PHASE**
   Implement
      Determine Go Live Approach
         Cutover Plan
         Go Live Plan
         Conduct Live Operations
   Evaluate Post-Live
   Daily Support Operations
   Ongoing Maintenance

• **FIGURE 11.8.** Clinical Systems/EHR Implementation Checklist.

plans for moving the new system into the production or live environment. Evaluating the system determines the positive and negative results of the implementation effort and suggests ways to improve the system. Upgrading the system involves expansion or elaboration of initial functions by expanding capability or function or by adding entirely new applications. Upgrading projects requires all implementation phases be reviewed to assure success.

REFERENCES

American Nurses Credentialing Center. (2012). *Informatics nurse test content outline.* Retrieved from http://www.nursecredentialing.org/Informatics-TCO2012

Anderson, M. (2011). *The costs and implications of EHR system downtime on physician practices.* Retrieved from www.stratus.com/extresources/email/corp/effect_of_downtime_on_physician_practices.pdf. Accessed on October 15, 2013.

Ash, J., Anderson, J., Gorman, P., Zielstorff, R., Norcross, N., Pettit, J., & Yao, P. (2000). Managing change: Analysis of a hypothetical case. *Journal of the American Medical Informatics Association, 7*(2), 125–134.

Augustine, J. (2004). System redesign and IT implementation. *Advance for Health Information Executives, 8*(1), 41–43.

Convey, S. (1992). *The seven healthy habits of highly effective people: Restoring the character ethic* (pp. 95–144). New York, NY: Fireside.

Douglas, M., & Wright, B. (2003). *Zoom–Zoom, turbo charging clinical implementations.* Presentation at Toward an Electronic Health Record—Europe, London, 2003.

Fitzgerald, J., Fitzgerald, A., & Satllings, W. (1981). *Fundamentals of systems analysis* (2nd ed.). New York, NY: Wiley.

Gause, D., & Weinberg, G. (1989). *Exploring requirements: Quality before design.* New York, NY: Dorset House Publishing.

Gugerty, B., Miranda, M., & Rook, D. (2006). The Clinical information system implementation evaluation scale. *Student Health Technology Informatics, 122,* 621–625.

Kaplan, B. (1997). Addressing organizational issues into the evaluation of medical systems. *Journal of the American Medical Informatics Association, 4*(2), 94–101.

Kesselheim, A., Cresswell, K., Phansalkar, S., Bates, D., & Sheikh, A. (2011). Clinical decision support systems could be modified to reduce 'alert fatigue' while still minimizing the risk of litigation. *Health Affairs (Millwood), 30*(12), 2310–2317. Pubmed.gov PMID:22147858 [Pubmed-indexed for MEDLINE].

Lewis, J. (2007). *Fundamentals of project management* (p. 11). New York, NY: ADCOM.

Lorenzi, N., & Riley, R. (2000). Managing change. *Journal of the American Medical Informatics Association, 7*(2), 116–124.

Lorenzi, N., Novak, L., Weiss, J., Gadd, C., & Unerti, K. (2008). Crossing the implementation chasm. *Journal of the American Medical Informatics Association, 15*(3), 290–296.

McCormick, K., & Gugerty, B. (2013). *Healthcare information technology exam guide* (p. 906–910). New York, NY: McGraw-Hill.

Nahan, E., Vaydua, V., Ho, D., Scharf, B., & Seagull, J. (2007). Outcomes assessment. *Nursing Outlook, 55*(6), 282–288.

Nielsen, J. (1992). Finding usability problems through heuristic evaluation. *Proceedings of ACM CHI'92*, 372–380.

Peitzman, L. (2004). Addressing physician resistance to technology. *Advance for Health Information Executives, 8*(5), 69–70.

Project Management Institute (2014). *What is Project Management?* Retrieved from http://www.pmi.org/About-Us-What-is-Project-Management.aspx. Accessed on October, 1, 2014.

Protti, D., & Peel, V. (1998). Critical success factors for evolving a hospital toward an electronic patient record system: A case study of two different sites. *Journal of Healthcare Information Management, 12*(4), 29–37.

Ritter, J., & Glaser, J. (1994). Implementing the patient care information system strategy. In E. Drazen, J. Metzger, J. Ritter, & M. Schneider (Eds.), *Patient care information systems: Successful design and implementation* (pp. 163–194). New York, NY: Springer-Verlag.

Rouse, M. (2010). *A definition of Clinical Decision Support System (CDSS).* Retrieved from http://searchhealthit.techtarget.com/definition/clinical-decision-support-system-CDSS; http://HIMSS.org/library/ehr 20140122140737937388062. Accessed on October 18, 2013.

Rouse, M. (2012). *A definition of Project Scope.* Retrieved from http://Searchcio.techtarget.com/definition/project-scope. Accessed on November 10, 2013, posted by M. Rouse, July 2012.

Sachett, D., Rosenberg, W., Gray, J., Haynes, R., & Richardson, W. (1996, Jan. 13). Evidence based medicine: What it is and what it isn't. *British Medical Journal, 312*(7023), 71–2.

Schooler, R., & Dotson, T. (2004). Rolling out the EHR. *Advance for Health Information Executives, 8*(2), 63–70.

Shabot, M. (2004). The 10 commandments of the clinical information system. *BUMC Proceedings, 17*, 265–269.

Shneiderman, B. (1998). *Designing the user interface* (3rd ed.). Reading, MA: Addison-Wesley.

Sim, I., Gorman, P., Greenes, R., Haynes, B., Kaplan, B., Lehmann, H., & Tang, P. (2001). Clinical decision support system for the practice of evidence based medicine. *Journal of American Medical Informatics Association, 8*, 527–534.

Timmermans, S., & Mauch, A. (2005). The promises and pitfalls of evidence-based medicine. *Health Affairs, 24*(1), 18–28.

Trotter, F., & Ulman, D. (2013). *Hacking healthcare: A guide to standards, workflow and meaningful use.* Safari online (pp. 1–2). Retrieved from http://hhs.gov /ocr/privacy/ hippa/administrative/enforcementrule/hitechenforce mentifr.html. Accessed on October 24, 2013.

Wilson, M. (2012). *Clinical informatics: Evaluation, selection, implementation and management of electronic health records.* Presented at QSEN conference 2012, San Francisco, CA. Retrieved from www.aacn.nche.edu/qsen-informatics/2012/workshop/presentation/Wilson/clinical-informatics.pdf. Accessed on November 10, 2013.

Zhang, J., Johnson, T., Patel, V., Paige, D., & Kubose, T. (2003). Using usability heruistics to evalutate patient safety of medical devices. *Journal of Biomedical Informatics, 36*, 23–30.

Zinn, T. K. (1989). Automated systems selection. *Health Care, 10*, 45–46.

SUGGESTED READINGS

American Nurses Association. (2008). *Nursing informatics: Scope and standards of practice.* Silver Spring, MD: American Nurse Publishing.

American Nurses Association. (2010). *Nursing: Scope and standards of practice.* Silver Spring, MD: American Nurse Publishing.

Arnold, J., & Pearson, G. (1992). *Computer applications in nursing education and practice* (Pub. No. 14-2406). New York, NY: National League for Nursing.

Axford, R., & Carter, B. (1996). Impact of clinical information systems on nursing practice: Nurses' perspective. *Computers in Nursing, 14*(3), 156–163.

Aydin, C., Rosen, P., Jewell, S., & Felitti, V. J. (1995). Computers in the examining room: The patient's perspective. *American Medical Informatics Association Proceedings*, pp. 824–828.

Ball, M. J., & Collen, M. F. (Eds.). (1992). *Aspects of the computer-based patient record.* New York, NY: Springer-Verlag.

Burnard, P. (1991). Computing: An aid to studying nursing. *Nursing Standard, 5*(17), 16–22.

Campbell, B. (1990). The clinical director's role in selecting a computer system. *Caring, 9*(6), 36–38.

Center for Healthcare Information Management (CHIM). (1991). *Guide to making effective H.I.S. purchase DeEHRions.* Ann Arbor, MI: Center for Healthcare Information Management.

Freudenheim, M. (2004). Many hospitals resist computerized patient care. *New York Times*, April 6.

Gillis, P. A., Booth, H., Graves, J. R., Fehlauer, C. S., Soller, J. (1994). Translating traditional principles of system development into a process for designing clinical information systems. *International Journal of Technology Assessment in Health Care, 10*(2), 235–248.

Holzemer, W. L., & Henry, S. B. (1992). Computer-supported versus manually-generated nursing care plans: A comparison of patient problems, nursing interventions and AIDS patients outcomes. *Computers in Nursing, 10*(1), 19–24.

Mills, M. (1994). Nurse-computer performance considerations for the nurse administrator. *Journal of Nursing Administration, 24*(11), 30–35.

Mohr, D., Carpenter, P., Claus, P., Hagen, P. T., Karsell, P. R., & Van Scoy, R. E. (1995). Implementing an EMR: Paper's last hurrah. *American Medical Informatics Association Proceedings*, pp. 157–161.

Protti, D., & Peel, V. (1998). Critical success factors for evolving a hospital toward an electronic patient record system: A case study of two different sites. *Journal of Healthcare Information Management, 12*(4), 29–37.

Warnock-Matheron, A., & Plummer, C. (1988). Introducing nursing information systems in the clinical setting. In M. Ball, K. Hannah, U. Gerdin-Jelger, & H. Peterson. (Eds.), *Nursing informatics: Where caring and technology meet* (pp. 115–127). New York, NY: Springer-Verlag.

Zielstorff, R., Grobe, S., & Hudgins, C. (1992*). Nursing information systems: Essential characteristics for professional practice.* Kansas City, MO: American Nurses Association.

12

System and Functional Testing

Theresa J. Settergren

• OBJECTIVES

1. Differentiate testing and quality assurance.
2. Differentiate testing types related to the system life cycle.
3. Describe testing levels, methodologies, and tools.
4. Examine barriers and success factors related to testing.
5. Discuss roles and skillsets of the informatics nurse in system and functional testing.

• KEY WORDS

Commercial-Off-The-Shelf (COTS) System
Unit Testing
Integrated Testing
Usability Testing
Interoperability
Implementation strategy

INTRODUCTION

System and functional testing are critical components of the system life cycle, whether the software or system is under new development or is commercial off-the-shelf (COTS) software that is being configured for a customer's specific needs. Testing definitions and goals have evolved over the past 60 years from the most simplistic "bug detection" process, conducted toward the end of the design and coding phases. The more contemporary definition goes far beyond bug detection to include dimensions of "correctness" (Lewis, 2009) and alignment of the technology to the business goals, with the intent that the software does what it is supposed to do, errors are caught and resolved very early in the development process, and testing includes the business and end-user impacts.

Testing and quality assurance are not synonymous (Beizer, 1984). Testing is composed of activities performed at various intervals during the development process with the overall goal of finding and fixing errors. The system life cycle phase usually drives how testing activities are organized, but the testing plan will normally include coordination of test efforts (scheduling resources, preparing scripts and other materials), test execution (running prepared test scripts with or without automated tools), defect management (tracking and reporting of errors and issues), and a formulation of a test summary. Quality assurance (QA) is a proactive, planned effort to ensure that a defect-free product fulfills the user-defined functional requirements. Testing is an indispensable tool, but it represents the most reactive aspect of the quality assurance process. Testing is all about finding defects. Quality assurance is all about preventing defects. In theory, an exceptional QA process would all but eliminate the need for bug fixing. Although QA is utilized widely in the broader information technology industry to help guarantee that a product being marketed

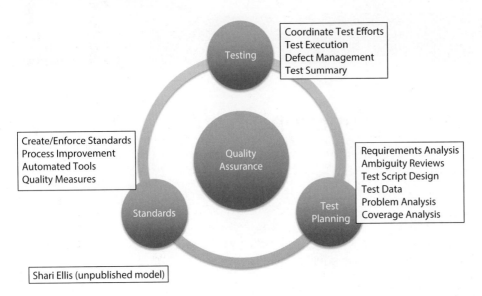

• **FIGURE 12.1.** Testing and Quality Assurance. (Reproduced, with Permission, from Shari Ellis.)

is "fit for use," many—perhaps even most—healthcare organizations rely on testing alone. Quality assurance can be best envisioned as an integrated approach, composed of test planning, testing, and standards (Fig. 12.1; Ellis, 2012). Test planning activities include the following:

- Requirements analysis: User needs are compared to the documented requirements.
- Ambiguity reviews: Identification of flaws, omissions, and inconsistencies in requirements and specifications.
- Nonredundant test script design: All key functions are tested only once in the scripts.
- Creation of test data: The right kinds of test patients and data to test all functions.
- Problem analysis: Defect management includes uncovering underlying issues.
- Coverage analysis: The scripts will test all key functions, and all key nonfunctional components and features.

Standards, the third element of quality assurance, involves the creation and enforcement of testing standards, process improvement activities related to QA, evaluation and appropriate use of automated testing tools, and quality measures (application of effectiveness metrics to the QA function itself). Software quality assurance is a planned effort to ensure that a software product fulfills verification and validation testing criteria and additional

attributes specific to the project, for example, portability, efficiency, reusability, and flexibility. Though this chapter focuses primarily on testing types and levels that are most commonly employed in the implementation and maintenance of COTS clinical systems, it will also review testing and quality assurance in the context of information technology industry standards.

TESTING MODELS AND METHODOLOGIES

Testing models have evolved in tandem with the ever-increasing complexity of healthcare software and systems. Early software development models were derived from Deming's Plan-Do-Check-Act cycle (Graham, Veenendaal, Evans, & Black, 2008; Lewis, 2009). The Waterfall model, for example, was characterized by relatively linear phases of design, development, and testing. Detailed definition of end-user requirements, including any desired process redesign, flowed to logical design (data flow, process decomposition, and entity relationship diagrams), which flowed to physical design (design specifications, database design), then to unit design, and ultimately to coding (writing in a programming language). Testing occurred toward the end of the Waterfall development model—a bit late for any substantive code modifications. This Iterative software development model employed cyclical repeating phases, with incremental enhancements to the software during each define-develop-build-test-implement cycle.

TABLE 12.1	V-Model	
Development Phase	**Interactions**	**Testing Type**
User Requirements	Development Phase Informs Appropriate Testing	User Acceptance
Specifications		System Testing
Design	Testing Types Verify Appropriate Development	Integration Testing
Implementation		Unit Testing

The main advantage of an iterative approach was earlier validation of prototypes, but the costs of multiple cycles were often prohibitive. As software development models evolved, testing levels were correlated with the Waterfall technical development phases (Table 12.1) to demonstrate how development phases should inform the testing plan and how testing should validate the development phases.

Agile software development, in contrast to some of the earlier models, is characterized by nearly simultaneous design, build, and testing (Watkins, 2009). Extreme Programming (XP) is a well-known Agile development life cycle model that emphasizes end-user engagement. Characteristics include the following:

- Generation of business stories to define the functionality.
- On-site customer or end-user presence for continual feedback and acceptance testing.
- Programmer–tester pairs to align coding with testing—and in fact, component test scripts are expected to be written and automated before code is written.
- Integration and testing of code are expected to occur several times a day.
- Simplest solution is implemented to solve today's problems.

Scrum is a project management method that accelerates communication by all team members, including customers or end users, throughout the project. A key principle of Scrum is the recognition that customers are likely to change their minds about their needs (requirements churn). Scrum approaches requirements churn as an opportunity to respond quickly to emerging requirements and to better meet the business needs of the customer. The Agile software development–Scrum project management model encompasses some key quality

assurance principles, is adaptable to healthcare information technology COTS implementation projects, and the intense end-user participation almost guarantees the end product will be "fit for use."

TESTING STRATEGY AND PROCESS

Broad goals for health information technology system and functional testing include building and maintaining a better product, reducing costs by preventing defects, meeting the requirements of and maintaining credibility with end users, and making the product fit for use. Failure costs in system development may be related to fixing the product, to operating a faulty product, and/or to damages caused by using faulty product. Resources required to resolve defects may start with programmer or analyst time at the component level, but in the context of a clinical information system thought to be "ready for use," defect resolution includes multiple human resources: testing analysts, interface analysts, analysts for upstream and downstream applications, analysts for integrated modules, database administrators, change management analysts, technical infrastructure engineers, end users of the new system and upstream and downstream interfaced systems, and others. In addition to the human resource expenses, unplanned fix-validate cycles require significant additional computer resources and may impact project milestones with deleterious cascading effects on critical path activities and the project budget. Operating a faulty software product incurs unnecessary costs in computer resources and operational efficiencies, and potential damages include patient confidentiality violations, medical errors, data loss, misrepresentation of or erroneous patient data, inaccurate aggregated data, and lost revenue. There may be also costs associated with loss of credibility. An inadequately tested system that fails "fit for use" criteria will negatively, perhaps irreparably, influence end-user adoption.

A testing plan is as indispensable to a clinical system project as an architect's drawing is to a building project. You wouldn't try to build a house without a plan—how would you know if it will turn out "right"? Test planning should begin early in the system life cycle (Saba & McCormick, 2011), and should align closely with business and clinical goals. Project definition and scope, feasibility assessments, functional requirements, technical specifications, required interfaces, data flows, workflows and planned process redesign, and other outputs of the planning and analysis phases become the inputs to the testing plan. Technological constraints of the software and hardware, and the ultimate design configuration to support the workflows, represent additional inputs to the testing plan.

Testing predictably takes longer than expected, and the testing timeline is often the first project milestone to be compressed, so it is advisable to plan for contingency testing cycles. Depending on the complexity and magnitude of a COTS system implementation, three or more months should be reserved for testing in the project timeline. Figure 12.2 depicts a testing timeline for multiple concurrent projects, and reflects varying scope and complexity of the projects.

SYSTEM ELEMENTS TO BE TESTED

Commonly tested clinical system elements include software functions or components, software features, interfaces, links, devices, reports, screens, and user security and access (Saba & McCormick, 2011). Components and features include clinical documentation templates and tools, order and results management functions, clinician-to-clinician messaging, care plans, and alerts and reminders based on best care practices. Testing of the documentation features should, at minimum, include the capture of clinical data and how the data are displayed in the system. Are the data elements nonredundant? Are the data captured during a clinical documentation episode displayed correctly, completely, and in the expected sequence in the resulting clinical note? Are discrete data elements captured appropriately for secondary use, such as for building medication, allergy, immunization, and problem lists, driving clinical alerts and reminders, and populating operational and clinical reports? Can clinicians and others, such as ancillary department staff, billing staff, and auditors, easily find recorded data? Can the user add data and modify data in the way expected in that field—structured coded values versus free text, for example. Once accepted, can data be deleted or modified with a version trail that is visible to an end user? Do the entered values show up in the expected displays?

System outputs to test include printing, faxing, and clinical messaging. Do test requisitions, patient education and clinical summaries, and letters print where they are supposed to print? Are prescriptions for scheduled medications printing on watermarked paper, if required? Do the documents print in the right format, and without extra pages? Faxing is important to thoroughly test, to prevent potential violations of patient confidentiality. The physical transmission is tested to ensure that it gets to the correct destination and includes all required data, formatted correctly, and inclusion of contact information in case a fax gets to the wrong recipient. Testing should also include the procedures that ensure fax destinations are periodically verified.

Order entry and transmittal testing occurs at several levels. The simplest level of testing is unit testing: does each orderable procedure have the appropriate billing code associated? Are all orderables available to ordering providers in lists or sets, via searches, and are the orderables named in a clinically identifiable and searchable way, including any abbreviations or mnemonics? Does each order go where it is supposed to go and generate messages, requisitions, labels, or other materials needed to complete the order? For example, an order entered into the electronic health record (EHR) for a laboratory test on a blood specimen collected by the ICU nurse generates an order message that is transmitted into the laboratory information system, and may generate a local paper requisition or an electronic message telling the nurse what kind and how many tubes of blood to collect, as well as generating specimen labels. These outputs for a nurse-collected lab specimen order are tested, as well as the outputs for the same ordered lab specimen collected by a phlebotomist. At the integrated level of testing, the order message and content received in the laboratory information system (LIS) is reviewed for completeness and accuracy of the display—does the test ordered exactly match the test received? Does the result value received from the LIS display correctly, with all expected details, such as the reference ranges and units, collection location, ordering provider, and other requirements?

Interface testing includes system modules, external systems, medical devices, and file transfers. Interfaces are tested for messaging and content, data transformation, and processing time. Interface data flows may be unidirectional or bidirectional. System module interfaces include admission/discharge/transfer (ADT), clinical documentation, order entry and results management, document management, patient and resource scheduling, charge entry and editing, coding, claims generation and edit checking, and other major functions. A data conversion from one system to another system is also a type of interface. Data dictionary testing is vital. In a fully integrated clinical system, the master files for data elements may be shared, so a change to the metadata in a master file needs to be tested for unintended impacts across modules. Other clinical systems may have redundant master files within multiple modules, and testing plans should ensure that the data elements are synchronized across the modules and interfaced systems. Data conversion testing must ensure that the data being converted from one system will populate the new system accurately. This often requires multiple test cycles in nonproduction environments to test each component of each data element being converted, prior to the actual conversion into the live production environment.

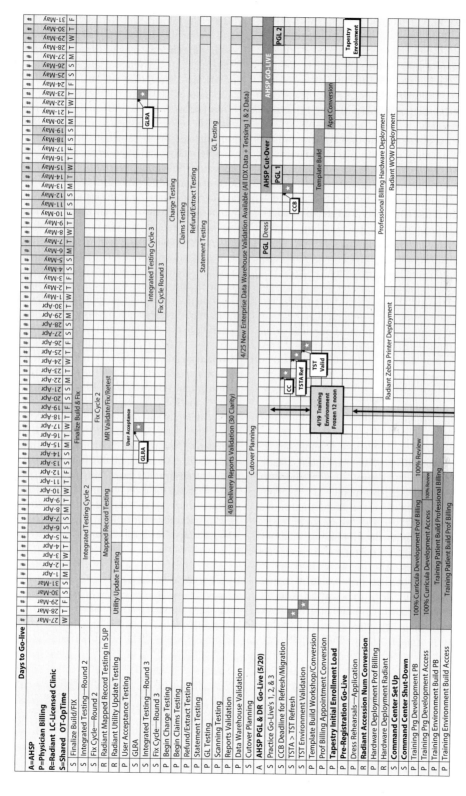

• **FIGURE 12.2.** Testing Timeline Example.

Clinical systems testing include links to third-party content for patient education, clinical references and peer-reviewed evidence, coding support systems, and others. Links to Web content resources for clinicians, including software user support, can be embedded into the software in multiple locations. These links should be tested in every location to ensure that they work properly and bring the user to the right content.

Medical device interfaces include invasive and noninvasive vital signs monitoring, oximetry, wired and wireless cardiac monitoring, hemodynamic monitoring, ventilators, infusion pump integration, urimetry monitoring, and other devices. Middleware can be used to acquire the data and provide the nurse with an interim step of validating data before accepting it into the clinical system. Newer medical devices include wireless continuous vital signs monitoring worn in the hospital or at home, nurse call systems, and bed or chair fall alarm systems. Testing outcomes for medical devices should consider data validation and alert or alarm risk mitigation steps. Data validation refers to the accurate capture of physiological and device data, such as blood pressure and concurrent pump infusion rate, such as the dose of a vasopressor, and requires the nurse to review and accept or reject the data. Alerts and alarms for data captured into the clinical system must be thoroughly tested for relevant settings, such as range and sensitivity. It is critical to minimize false alarms, which may result in alert fatigue, yet still alert nurses and other clinicians to genuine patient status changes.

Reports testing should be performed at multiple levels. Reports may be static or dynamic. Examples of static reports include the formatted display of a documentation episode, specialized displays that pull in data from multiple modules within the clinical system, requisitions that are generated from orders, and the multiple report types that are generated from a data warehouse and may be linked to the clinical system. Data warehouse reports typically contain day-old data. The reports are intended to support individual clinical decision-making as well as provide snapshots of population-level information used for trending, quality improvement, operational assessment, and various external reporting requirements. Dynamic reports (using "real-time" data) provide clinical and operations staff with current information on individual or aggregated patients, and can be updated real time. Examples of dynamic reports include patient lists or registries, appointment no-shows, and queries relevant to a provider ("all of my patients that have a statin prescription") or nurse ("all of my heart failure patients"). Reports testing includes the formatting, accurate inclusion of required data, and also comparing the source data to the data in the reports. For example, a Certification Commission for

Healthcare Information Technology (CCHIT)–certified EHR is capable of producing a CCD document to meet health information exchange standards, but there are differences among the vendors and among data dictionaries, and testing ensures that the data elements are populating values to the CCD document correctly.

User security and access can make or break go live success. User access is designed to be role-based, so that each user role has specific functions and views associated. For example, a physician requires the ability to order tests and procedures including referrals and consults, e-prescribe, document with tools tailored to specialty as well as electronic medication administration and reconciliation, update problem lists and allergy lists, view customized displays of data, query data real time, calculate and submit professional charges, generate health information exchanges, among other functions. The nurse role requires specified documentation activities, some of which may be required, and will usually incorporate a subset of physician functions. Nursing activities generally depend on the location of care. Hospital nurses generally do not have full ordering privileges, but can enter orders under protocol, and some of those orders require physician co-signature. Hospital nurses may or may not be able to update the patient's problem list, as per the organization's policy, but typically can update allergy lists and prior-to-admission medication lists. The security needed for ordering can be different in an ambulatory clinical setting, where physicians may delegate some ordering tasks, and advanced practice nurses practice independently. For an enterprise-wide EHR, practice scope differences must be thoroughly tested to ensure that each clinician has the right access in the right care location. Testing should also include what the person in that role should not be able to perform, such as a hospital registrar ordering medications. This is sometimes termed "negative testing."

TESTING TYPES

Testing types used vary based on where in the system life cycle testing is planned, and the degree of development or programming that is involved. Table 12.2 (Beizer, 1984; Graham et al., 2008; Lewis, 2009; Watkins, 2009) describes common testing types suggested, based on magnitude, for development of the testing plan. The first step in test planning is to define what is to be accomplished (Graham et al., 2008). The goals should include the scope, expectations, critical success factors, and known constraints, which will be used to shape the rest of the plan. Testing approach defines the "how"—the techniques or types of testing, the entrance and exit criteria, defect management

TABLE 12.2	Testing Types Grid			
Test Name	**General Description**	**New Software Development**	**COTS System Configuration**	**Maintenance/ Optimization**
Acceptance	End-user validation testing or final testing based on end-user requirements	X	X	X
Ad hoc	Off-script testing intended to discover issues; "try to break it"	X	X	X (major changes)
Alpha	First customer use of an application nearing development completion	X		
Beta	Customer use when development is complete, to uncover any additional issues before general release	X		
Black Box	Cases developed for functional testing	X		
Comparison	Assessing against competitor products	X	X	
Compatibility	Software performance in different environments (with various software, hardware, network, operating systems)	X	X	X
Coverage	Each branch has true and false outcomes; each condition considers all possible outcomes	X		
Database	Integrity of DB field values	X	X	X
End-to-end	System testing that mimics real-world environment	X	X	X
Exception	Error messages and exceptions—identification and handling processes	X		
Exploratory	Informal testing, often untrained users, to identify unimagined issues	X	X	
Functional	Focused on meeting user-defined requirements; includes unit/component, integration, regression, and acceptance testing	X	X	X
Integration	Testing application parts to ensure they function together correctly; can mean "pieces of code" within a module, or between modules	X	X	X
Interoperability	Disparate systems are able to exchange a defined data set, as in Health Information Exchange	X	X	X (major changes)
Load	High volume testing, often automated, to determine point at which system response time degrades	X	X	
Nonfunctional	Testing outside of the user requirements that define the functions; typically includes interoperability, load/volume, performance/reliability, efficiency, security	X	X	X (Major Changes)
Parallel	Literally "side by side" testing: Same work done in old system and new system to compare results	X	X (less common)	
Performance	Often used interchangeably with stress—may include volume, reliability	X	X	
Recovery	Testing recovery time after a software crash or hardware failure, or other failure	X		
Regression	Testing planned changes for unintended ripple effects	X	X	X

(continued)

TABLE 12.2	Testing Types Grid *(continued)*	New Software Development	COTS System Configuration	Maintenance/ Optimization
Test Name	**General Description**			
Security	How well does system protect against unauthorized use, damage, data loss, etc.	X	X	X
Stress	Similar to load testing: Functional testing for very high loads of users, queries, repeated inputs, etc.	X	X	
System	Includes functional and nonfunctional testing, using both black box and white box techniques	X	X	X
Unit	Lowest level that focuses on a selected function or piece of code to see if it works as designed—usually performed by the programmer or builder	X	X	X
Usability	Focus on ease of use as defined by end users	X	X	
White Box	Testing the logic paths based on the defined specifications	X		

and tracking, feedback loop with development, status and progress reporting, and perhaps most importantly, exceptionally well-defined requirements as the foundational component. The environment for testing defines the physical conditions: end-user hardware to be included in testing (desktops, laptops, wireless workstations, tablets, smartphones, thick client, thin client, scanners, printers, e-signature devices, and other), the interfaces to be included, the test environment for the application and other systems to be tested, automated tools, type of help desk support needed, and any special software or system build required to support testing.

Multiple test user roles are needed for testing to assure appropriate role-based tools, functions, and views. Test patient records are created so that age- and gender-appropriate documentation tools and decision support, including alerts and reminders, are tested. Laboratory values and other diagnostic results for test patients can be manually built into the test system, or copied over from a real patient without identifiers, to allow testing of expected results-driven decision support, flags, displays, and temporal views such as graphs and charts.

Next, testing specifications are developed that define format standards, identify features to be tested, cross-reference features to the functional requirements, and break down the work into manageable pieces. The testing team documents how each feature will be tested, existing interdependencies, and the test workflows, which will be devised to include all of the required test specifications, but in efficient and nonredundant flows that usually will not match end-user workflows. Scripts that emulate end-user workflows are usually utilized for acceptance testing.

Scheduling is a vital test planning component, and involves coordination of multiple human and technical resources. Testing requires scheduling many of the technical participants discussed earlier for integrated testing, plus others from the software, infrastructure, vendor, and clinical and business areas. Ideally, end users have been involved in all system life cycle phases, including testing, but test planning includes scheduled formal user acceptance testing (UAT). Testers should work together in the same location, often requiring equipment set up for workstations, printers, scanners, electronic signature devices, medical devices, and other peripheral equipment needed for end-to-end testing scenarios. Magnitude and complexity of the system as well as testing goals and deadlines are inputs into the number of testing cycles, resources to be scheduled, progress checkpoints, and contingency planning. The final step in test planning is sign-off by stakeholders, a vital checkpoint for review of the goals, requirements, and resources, as well as contingency planning, including "go-no go" decisions.

A typical testing plan for a COTS system requires that all functional modules, features, and interfaces (upstream and downstream) are unit-tested prior to the first integrated test cycle. Three or more integrated test cycles are not uncommon for new implementations or extensive upgrades, though a subset of tests would be conducted for smaller system changes. Two weeks of integrated testing plus two weeks for fixes and unit testing are desirable for each cycle, always ending on a test cycle...never ending on a fix cycle. Daily testing status updates are essential to monitor outcomes and the potential need for plan modifications (Fig. 12.3). During the two weeks of integrated

testing, new software changes should generally not be introduced, and a "code freeze" may be instituted wherein only the highest priority changes are permitted, to reduce unintended ripple effects. The testing team works through expected and unexpected outcomes of all scripts and

documents in the designated tool. Members of the training team and other analysts may also participate, but programmers/builders typically do not test their own work during integrated testing. Builders inherently want their code to work, and they know how to make it work—and they did

From: Tester, Happy
Sent: Monday, April 29, 2013 4:11 PM
To: Group EIS QAT Integrated Test Status
Subject: Status Report PRC - Radiant - AHSP (TST) Cycle 2 Day 3

Script Execution	On Track
Defects	Many normal defects
Resources	Short 3 resources for AMB

Overall Summary
- Day 3 of Cycle 2
- 12 defects were found today.
- 4 scripts are behind due to resource issues.

Defect Summary

Module	Total NON-Script Error Defects	Open NON-Script Error Defects
ADT	2	1
AMB	4	4
Ancillary		
ASAP	1	0
Bridges		
Cadence	1	0
Canto		
CDR		
ClinDoc	6	2
Device Integration		
Epic Rx	1	1
Haiku		
HB	1	0
HID	2	1
Interfaces (SI)		
Orders	5	2
Radiant	3	1
PB		
Security		
Total*	**24**	**12**

Priority (Open)	
High	3
Normal	8
Low	1
Total	**0**

* Total #'s may differ due to defects reported by multiple teams.

- **FIGURE 12.3.** Testing Status Update.

Script Summary

Complete	6
In Progress	8
Behind	0
Fail	0
Not Started	30
Total Scripts	44

Execution Schedule AHSP - PRC - Radiant Cycle 2	Mon 4/29 Day 1	Tue 4/30 Day 2	Wed 5/1 Day 3	Thu 5/2 Day 4	Fri 5/3 Day 5	Status	Comments
Script							
PRC01- Administration of Immunization		1	2	3		In Progress	
PRC02 - Error Encounter				1		Not Started	
PRC03- Insurance Referral		1				Complete	
PRC04- Mental Health			1			Behind	No resource available
PRC05- Mosaic				1		Not Started	
PRC06- Research	1					Complete	
PRC07 - Vision Office Visit		1				Complete	
PRC08 - Reg Employee		1				Fail	Security files not migrated
PRC09 - Reg Dual Insurance Commercial		1	1			Behind	
PRC10 - Reg Deal Insurance Medical			1			Fail	Security files not migrated
PRC11 - Reg Minor						Not Run	
PRC12 - Self Pay						Not Run	
PRC13 - Schuyler				1	2	Not Started	

• **FIGURE 12.3.** Testing Status Update. *(continued)*

that during unit testing. Testers want to test for failures. In their attempts to break the system, defects are uncovered that might otherwise have been missed. Defects may include functions that do not work as designed, workflow issues that were not identified during requirements definition and workflow analysis, or unintended effects. Defects are usually given a priority. The project team should establish definitions for priorities. Priority examples include (Douglas & Celli, 2011) the following:

- Critical: Significant impact to patient safety, regulatory compliance, clinical workflow, or other aspect, for which no workaround is possible.

- High: Significant impact to workflow or training or other aspect, for which the resolution effort or the workaround is in itself a major effort and may be high risk.

- Medium: Impact on workflow or training is noteworthy but a reasonable workaround exists.

- Low: Impact on workflow or training is minimal; workaround is not required.

Defects are communicated back to the programmers/builders, and are followed through to resolution using a defect tracking tool. These cycles repeat until all critical and high defects, at minimum, are resolved. Contingency planning should allow for additional testing cycles.

The testing plan usually culminates in regression and user acceptance testing. Regression testing ensures that fixes implemented during the integration cycles did not break something else. Acceptance testing allows users to validate that the system meets their requirements, and is usually conducted using scripts that reflect redesigned processes from the workflow analysis phase. User acceptance testing ideally occurs after successful integrated and regression testing cycles are completed, and prior to the start of training to avoid the risk of changes that necessitate retraining—since users should have been involved throughout the project, UAT should represent a final validation of "fit for use," but not a "surprise" to end users.

Alpha and/or beta testing may be scheduled when a software or system is newly developed, and both mimic real-world use. Healthcare organizations tend to avoid alpha and beta software because the cost of resources to test immature systems typically outweighs the benefit. Alpha testing is usually conducted in a simulated fashion. Beta testing is more apt to be conducted in a live setting. Both testing strategies can include parallel testing, wherein the users are performing dual data entry—entering data in the new system and in the old system (electronic or paper) to determine whether all required functions exist under

normal conditions of use, and the system outputs are as expected. Parallel testing may be more useful for ensuring appropriate charges are generated or other billing-related functions than for clinician workflow testing, such as "shadow charting."

Usability and safety are valuable barometers for evaluating testing success. The International Organization for Standardization defines usability in terms of a user performing a set of tasks effectively, efficiently, and with satisfaction, and includes learnability, error frequency, and memorability aspects of the user experience (Rose et al., 2005), with special focus on an attractive user interface that is easy to understand and navigate. Usability's broadest definition, "quality in use," includes the user and task dimensions along with the tool and the environment (Yen & Bakken, 2012). Usability testing ideally begins early in the design phase and is conducted throughout the system life cycle, through optimization and maintenance as well as during implementation. An HIMSS Task Force developed a usability testing tool. Figure 12.4 (HIMSS, 2009) demonstrates the tool adapted for an implementation. Iterative usability evaluations by actual users could be expected to enable the clinical system to better meet user efficacy and patient safety goals (Staggers & Troseth, 2011).

Technology-induced errors are on the rise, and usability factors, such as small or very dense displays and lack of data visibility (Borycki, 2013), may be related to higher error rates. Information overload related to the sheer quantity of digital data is compounded by organization and display of data that fails to support pattern recognition and other cognitive tasks (Ahmed, Chandra, Herasevich, Gajic, & Pickering, 2011). User interface design factors contribute to technology-induced errors, and data displays related to a specific user task should be an integral component of testing plans. Data integrity failures in EHRs and other HIT systems are among the top 10 technology hazards for 2014 (ECRI, 2013), citing the following contributing factors:

- Patient/data association errors—patient data associated with another patient's record

- Missing data or delayed data delivery

- Clock synchronization errors

- Inappropriate use of default values

- Use of dual workflows—paper and electronic

- Copying and pasting of older information into a new report

- Basic data entry errors, which now can be propagated much further than could have occurred in paper records

Please rate your experience with the software design by completing the following checklist when you have finished entering the patient scenarios.
Please rate the attribute in the box to the right according to how you feel the task met that principle design. Place a check if it meets the criteria, otherwise, rate 1–4 as defined below.

#	Scenario/ Workflow	Form / process	Simplicity	Visibility	Minimalist	Naturalness	Consistency	Memory	Cognition	Feedback	Flexibility	Language	Presentation	Error Free	Comments—Use back page
1	Admission	Triage Note													
		OB Patient Profile													
2	Labor	OB Patient Care Flowsheet													
3	Delivery	OB Delivery Record													
4	PACU / Recovery	OB Patient Care Flowsheet													
5	Mother/Baby Care	OB Patient Care Flowsheet													
6	Education	Education FS													
7	Plan of Care	Education FS													
8	Discharge	OB Discharge Record													

Usability Attributes

Usability Attributes	Description
Simplicity	Lack of visual clutter; Concise information display
Visibility	Appropriate feedback and display of information
Minimalist	Less is more. Contains only pertinent information and avoids extraneous information
Naturalness	Familiarity and ease of use; Common terminology; Flows with user tasks and expectations
Consistency	Learnability—matches experience with other systems; internal consistency with layout throughout the application
Memory	Minimize requirement for user to memorize a lot of information to carry out tasks
Cognition	Presents the information needed for the task at hand; do not need to seek other places for information; minimal mental interruptions
Feedback	Informative feedback. Prompts and informative feedback given for users actions in the system, Good error messages to direct the user.
Flexibility	Allows users to customize and utilize shortcuts in order to accelerate their performance
Effective use of language	Concise, unambiguous, standard, approved terminology (no use of unapproved abbreviations)
	Density—80% of screen is meaningful
Effective presentation	Color—meaningful to user (red, yellow, green)
	Readability—scan quickly with high comprehension
Error Free	Completion of tasks without errors

Score	Rating	Description
☑	No problem	Not a usability problem
1	Cosmetic problem only	Does not need fixing unless extra time is available
2	Minor usability problem	Fixing-low priority. No impact on patient safety - workaround
3	Major usability problem	Fixing-High priority. Patient safety impact & nurse productivity with difficult workarounds
4	Usability catastrophe	Imperative to fix. Severe patient safety and nurse productivity issues.

Date: _____ Printed Name: _____

Signature: _____

• **FIGURE 12.4.** Usability Tool Exchange.

Safety testing incorporates the people-, process-, technology-, environmental-, and organization-related issues identified in the literature, with a focus on provider order entry, clinical decision support, and closed-loop (bar-coded) medication administration (Harrington, Kennerly, & Johnson, 2011).

CHALLENGES AND BARRIERS

Resources, timeline pressures, and materials comprise the most common barriers to sufficient testing. Liberating end users from their regular work for testing can prove difficult, especially in understaffed nursing environments. Direct care clinicians with varying computer skill levels, not just trainers or nursing "early adopters," are essential to include in testing as they represent a realistic cross-section of users. This approach produces significant budgetary impacts due to the costs of back-filling staff to be "out-of-count," including overtime and/or temporary staffing costs. The staffing crisis may be exacerbated if training is allowed to overlap testing cycles. Costs may be balanced by benefits in going live with a fully tested and well-vetted clinical system that enables nurses and the care team to be efficient and effective in care delivery and satisfied with the system. Timeline pressures constitute a universal barrier to sufficient testing. Extending a project timeline to accommodate additional testing adds cost. Pressure to attain project milestones may tempt even the most seasoned project managers to shorten test cycles or use testing shortcuts, though the costs of failure may outweigh costs of timeline changes.

A third major barrier to testing success is inadequate script development. Testing scripts for integrated testing cycles are typically nonredundant, and do not closely emulate a particular clinical workflow—this is efficient and very appropriate, and an ideal test script could be successfully run by a random person off the street. However, user acceptance testing requires detailed scenario-driven scripts that simulate real workflows. These more detailed scripts will be continually updated throughout the system life cycle, as clinicians provide feedback on nuances of use cases that may have been overlooked. These nuances are valuable findings prior to go live to close safety gaps and avert potentially inefficient or even unsafe workarounds—nurses can be very creative.

Nursing informatics experts can play key roles in the testing process. Informatics nurses can help make the case for sufficient testing by tying testing outcomes back to the original project goals for adoption and care improvements, including quantification of costs of clinical adoption failures, patient safety issues, inability to

meet efficiency, and effectiveness targets. Informatics nurses can help develop and execute testing plans and scripts, ensuring that appropriate use cases are iteratively documented for testing that will continue into the system optimization and maintenance phase. Informatics nurses play a valuable role in ensuring data validation across disparate systems. Evaluation of testing effectiveness, usability, and user acceptance are key skills that informatics nurses bring to testing. Informatics nurses also bring value through research.

The Nursing Informatics International Research Network conducted a recent survey to identify nursing informatics research priorities. Development of systems that provide real-time safety-related feedback to nurses, systems' impact on nursing care, nursing decision support systems, and systems' workflow impacts were the top ranked international research priorities (Dowding et al., 2013). These aspects are very tactical and close to nursing practice, and have implications for various types of system and functional testing. In summary, system and functional testing are critically important to successful implementation and maintenance of clinical information systems, and informatics nurses have a responsibility to inform, champion, and evaluate testing processes and outcomes.

REFERENCES

Ahmed, A., Chandra, S., Herasevich, V., Gajic, O., & Pickering, B. W. (2011). The effect of two different electronic health records user interfaces on intensive care provider task load, errors of cognition, and performance. *Critical Care Medicine, 39*(7), 1626–1634.

Beizer, B. (1984). *Software system testing and quality assurance.* New York, NY: Van Nostrand Reinholt.

Borycki, E. M. (2013). *Technology-induced errors: Where do they come from and what can we do about them?* Retrieved from http://cshi2013.org/files/Elizabeth%20Borycki.pdf

Douglas, M., & Celli, M. (2011). System life cycle: Implementation and evaluation. In V. A. Saba & K. A. McCormick (Eds.), *Essentials of nursing informatics* (5th ed., pp. 93–106). (Kindle Edition). Retrieved from http://www.amazon.com

Dowding, D. W., Currie, L. M., Borycki, E., Clamp, S., Favela, J., Fitzpatrick, G., & Dykes, P. C. (2013). *International priorities for research in nursing informatics for patient care.* Medinfo 2013. Retrieved from http://ebooks.iospress.nl/volumearticle/34021

ECRI Institute. (2013). *Top 10 health technology hazards for 2014: Executive summary report.* Retrieved from http://www.ecri.org/2014hazards.org

Ellis, S. (2012). Unpublished figure depicting a testing-quality assurance model (Personal communication).

Graham, D., Veenendaal, E. V., Evans, I., & Black, R. (2008). *Foundations of software testing: ISTQB certification* (2nd ed.). London: Cengage Learning (EMEA).

Harrington, L., Kennerly, D., & Johnson, C. (2011). Safety issues related to the electronic medical record (EMR): Synthesis of the literature from the last decade, 2000–2009. *Journal of Healthcare Management, 56*(1), 31–43.

HIMSS. (2009). Defining and testing EMR usability (adapted for use at University of Kentucky by C. Page). Retrieved from http://www.himss.org/files/HIMSSorg/content/files/HIMSS_DefiningandTestingEMRUsability.pdf

Lewis, W. E. (2009). *Software testing and continuous quality improvement* (3rd ed.). Boca Raton, FL: Auerback.

Rose, A. F., Schnipper, J. L., Park, E. R., Poon, E. G., Li, Q., & Middleton, B. (2005). Using qualitative studies to improve the usability of an EMR. *Journal of Biomedical Informatics, 35,* 51–60.

Saba, V. A., & McCormick, K. A. (Eds.). (2011). *Essentials of nursing informatics* (5th ed.). (Kindle edition). Retrieved from http://www.amazon.com.

Staggers, N., & Troseth, M. R. (2011). Usability and clinical application design. In M. Ball, K. J. Hannah, D. Dulong, S. Newbold, J. E. Sensmeier, D. J. Skiba, M. R. Troseth, & J. V. Douglas (Eds.), *Nursing informatics: Where technology and caring meet* (4th ed., pp. 219–242). London: Springer-Verlag.

Watkins, J. (2009). *Agile testing: How to succeed in an extreme testing environment.* New York, NY: Cambridge University Press.

Yen, P.-Y., & Bakken, S. (2012). Review of health information technology usability study methodologies. *Journal of the American Medical Informatics Association, 19,* 413–422.

13

System Life Cycle Tools

Denise D. Tyler

• OBJECTIVES

1. Identify two tools to assist with each phase of the System Life Cycle.
2. Describe two pre- and post-implementation metrics.
3. Describe diagrams that can be utilized for clinical workflow and data workflow.
4. Discuss ways to assess the reporting needs of an organization in relationship to all levels of staff.

• KEY WORDS

Business intelligence
Clinical workflow
Data workflow
Failure Modes and Effects Analysis (FMEA)
Lean methodology
Plan Do Study Act (PDSA)
Process diagram
Systems Life Cycle

INTRODUCTION

Like the nursing process, the system life cycle (SLC) is a continuous series of system changes, or evolutions. Even after the system is installed, there is continuous analysis, design, and implementation of new modules, upgrades, and improvements. Nurses are accustomed to leading interdisciplinary team in the patient care environment, so leading interdisciplinary teams to address clinical information systems is a natural progression.

The American Nurses Credentialing Center defines the System Life Cycle as having five phases: System Planning; System Analysis; System Design, Development, and Customization; System Functional Testing; and System Implementation, Evaluation, Maintenance, and Support (American Nurses Credentialing Center, 2012). There are variations of these phases, some experts include the

functional testing in the analysis phase, and some include, for example, the development and customization in the system design phase. No matter how they are broken down, each of these phases has specific elements and tools that can aid in the goal of a successfully installed and maintained system that meets the needs of all stakeholders.

ANALYSIS AND DOCUMENTATION OF THE CURRENT PROCESS AND WORKFLOW

All phases of the SCL may require analyzing the data and workflow. Karsh & Alper (2005) describe system analysis and workflow analysis as a way to understand how a system works, and how the different elements in the system interact. There are many ways to depict a workflow, but the critical part is the analysis of the process or workflow and accurately and completely documenting each step.

Documenting a workflow may be done by walking through the steps via an intensive interview with those intimately familiar with the process by observation or by a combination of the two. Interviewing staff about how a lab or diet order is processed from the time it is entered until it is completed is an example using the interview to document a process. A combination of observation and interviews might be the most effective way to capture all of the nuances for medication administration, and observation alone would be effective for a time and motion study. Analysis provides the data with which you will base decisions that must be made in the design, development, implementation, and evaluation stages of the training project according to Kulhanek (2011, p. 5).

A workflow diagram is generally prepared to document the current state when planning for a system implementation and to identify problems or areas that need improvement. A workflow diagram documents the processes of the users; the data workflow diagram documents the interaction and flow of the information system(s). There are several types of diagrams that can be utilized to document a process, including swim lanes, data flow diagrams (DFDs).

A swim lane diagram represents a process and is usually grouped in lanes (either columns or rows) to help visualize the users or departments involved. Workflow can be documented using a simple list of the steps in the process, a swim lane, or a workflow diagram. No matter what method is used to display the process, it needs to be clear and complete for accurate analysis. A simplified process for a diet order might be documented and displayed in the following manner:

1. Nursing performs the assessment and documents no known allergies or issues related to swallowing or diet intake.
2. The provider reviews assessment data and enters the order.
   a. Nursing reviews the order.
   b. The order prints in the dietary department.
3. The diet aide files the order.
4. The diet prints for the tray line preparation.
5. The diet is delivered to the unit.
6. The tray is delivered to the patient.

Figure 13.1 displays an example of the same simplified process for a diet order in a swim lane format. The swim

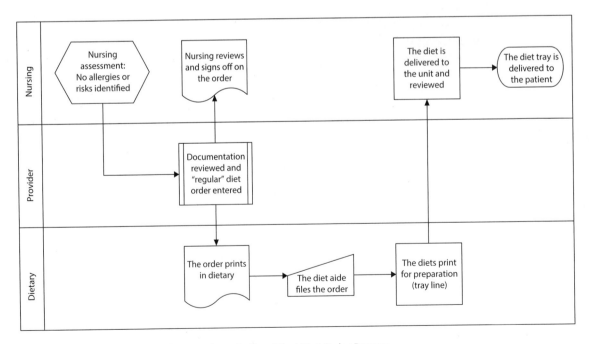

· **FIGURE 13.1.** A Swim Lane Presentation of a Simplified Diet Order Process.

lanes can be displayed in either a vertical or horizontal format. In the example below, each row is a "swimlane." This and other workflow diagrams can be developed using sticky notes rather than a computer program effectively, but transcribing into an electronic display increases the ability to read and share the information. More details on diagrams will be discussed in Chapter 41.

System Selection and Implementation

An information system should support patient care by allowing clinical staff to easily navigate the system to enter information about the system, monitor, and be alerted to changes. Selecting a system that meets the needs of all levels of stakeholders, from bedside staff to the executive team, is a complicated process with multiple factors involved. The TIGER Usability and Clinical Application design team came up with the following attributes of successful implementations (The TIGER Initiative, n.d., p. 20).

- User and key stakeholder involvement began early in the project with system requirements development and system selection.
- Clinicians worked with developers to create definitions, wording, and graphics that represented workflow process.

Systems must be easy to use in relation to entering and obtaining data and information. Today's clinical systems included embedded analytics, clinical decision support (CDS) to prompt clinicians with warnings and evidence-based suggestions, as well as business intelligence to capture financial and operational data. Clinical and Business Intelligence provides historical and predictive perspective of the operations and clinical areas to improve business and clinical decisions (Carr, n.d.).

Understanding how the different parts of the system work together as well as how the system will impact the clinical workflow is key to be considered during the system selection process. While having a system that is easy to learn and use is important, if the data cannot be reported or shared its value decreases significantly. Figure 13.2 is an example of a system diagram, which shows how the Clinical Information System (CIS) relates to other systems required for patient care. For example, the CIS sends reports to the Document Imaging (DI) system, that also stores scanned documents such as a Durable Power of Attorney, which are in turn available in the CIS. The Pharmacy system works with the Bar Code Medication Administration (BCMA) system and Pyxis (Smart pumps thought not displayed here would be another component of medication safety). The financial components that

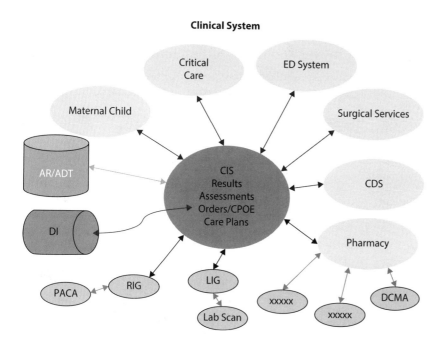

• **FIGURE 13.2.** An Example of How Systems Might Work Together with More Difficult Work and Maintenance.

include Accounts Receivable (AR), Registration functions including Admission, Transfer, and Discharge (ADT) send patient information to the CIS, which can send updates, alerts, and requests back. The Lab Information System (LIS) may work with an application similar to the barcoding used for drug administration to ensure that the correct tests are drawn; some may also be used for blood administration. Orders may be sent from the CIS to the LIS and Radiology Information System (RIS) that in turn send Order Status Updates (OSU) along with results, reports, and images back into the CIS. For more on System Selection see Chapter 41.

System Implementation

System implementation requires system design and building, and testing. System design should involve key

stakeholders, especially end users throughout. Testing involves making sure that each part of the system works, and that the system works correctly with other modules and systems. Table 13.1 is an example of the unit testing required for a lab interface, whether the LIS, the CIS, or both are being replaced or implemented. Each order needs to be tested from start to finish, so ordered, the Order Status Update (OSU) received in the CIS when Lab puts the order in progress, and when the preliminary and final results are posted. Each result associated with the order should display correctly (many lab orders, such as a CBC, have multiple results associated with them). The charge also needs to be verified for each order. Table 13.2 is an example of a tool that can be used when testing Radiology orders. Like Lab, each order needs to be tested from the time it is ordered through the time it is performed and the final report is posted. Also, being able to display the report

TABLE 13.1	A Simple Example of Unit Testing (Lab), Testing Each Test								
				Unit Testing: Lab					
Date	Test	Order Received in Lab	Label Printed in Lab	OSU Received in CIS			Result Received in CIS	Result Displayed Correctly in CIS	Charge Dropped
				In progress	Prelim Result	Final Result			
4/01	CBC	Yes	Yes	Yes	Yes	Yes	Yes	Yes	4/05
4/01	Chem Panel	Yes	Yes	Yes	Yes	Yes	Yes	Yes	4/05
4/01	Urinalysis	Yes	Yes	Yes	Yes	Yes	Yes	Yes	4/05
4/01	Type and Cross	Yes	Yes	Yes	Yes	Yes	Yes	Yes	4/05

Additional testing of orders entered from the ancillary system, as well as order modifications and cancellations should also be tested.

TABLE 13.2	A Simple Example of Unit Testing (Radiology), Testing Each Test								
				Unit Testing: Radiology					
Date	Test	Order Received in Radiology	Transport Method	OSU Received in CIS			Result/Report Received in CIS	Result Displayed Correctly in CIS With Link to PACS Image	Charge Dropped
				In progress	Prelim Result	Final Result			
4/01	Chest X-ray	Yes	Yes	Yes	Yes	Yes	Yes	Yes	4/05
4/01	CT, Head	Yes	Yes	Yes	Yes	Yes	Yes	Yes	4/05
4/01	MRI, Knee	Yes	Yes	Yes	Yes	Yes	Yes	Yes	4/05
4/01	Ultrasound, Abdomen	Yes	Yes	Yes	Yes	Yes	Yes	Yes	4/05

Additional testing of orders entered from the ancillary system, as well as order modifications and cancellations should also be tested.

and the associated image from the picture archiving and communication systems (PACS) needs to be verified for each exam. Verification that the appropriate charges drop is also important.

Integrated testing is done after unit testing has been accomplished and is the last phase of testing, ensuring that all systems that share data are working correctly in real-life scenarios (National Learning Consortium, 2012), similar tools can be used for integrated testing involving interfaced system or conversion verification to ensure that converted information is correct. Table 13.3 is an example of a tool to verify that the fields related to patient information are correct when being converted from one system to another, or when being interfaced from one system

TABLE 13.3	Integrated Testing Day 1: Verify Correct Patient Demographics Online and on Printed Documents

Integrated Testing Day 1

Date	Patient 1 Verify:	Correct	Notes
	Name		
	DOB		
	SSN		
	Marital Status		
	Mother Maiden Name		
	Race		
	Ethnicity		
	Organ Donor		
	Adv Directive		
	Address		
	Phone 1		
	Phone 2		
	Email		
	Contact 1 Name		
	Contact 1 Phone		
	Contact 1 Relationship		
	Contact 2 Name		
	Contact 2 Phone		
	Contact 2 Relationship		
	Employer: Status		
	Employer: Name		
	Employer: Job Title		
	Employer: Address		

(continued)

TABLE 13.3	Integrated Testing Day 1: Verify Correct Patient Demographics Online and on Printed Documents *(continued)*

Integrated Testing Day 1

Date	Patient 1 Verify:	Correct	Notes
	Employer: Phone		
	MRN #		
	Visit/Account #		
	Hospital		
	Nurse Station		
	Room		
	Isolation		
	Visit Type		
	Patient Type		
	Admit date		
	Chief Complaint		
	Guarantor Name		
	Guarantor Relationship		
	Guarantor Phone 1		
	Guarantor Phone 2		
	Guarantor Address		
	Insurance 1 Name		
	Insurance 1 Address		
	Insurance 1 Phone		
	Insurance 1 Group #		
	Insurance 1 Group #		

to another. Attention to each field on both displays and printed documents are required. Doing an analysis of each type of admission to make sure a good sampling is done for integrated testing will help ensure that testing is comprehensive. Testing needs to include all aspects of the patients' experience, from registration to any testing, documentation, and verification that the bill has dropped correctly.

Testing fields that are used by multiple applications such as the height (ht), weight (wt), and allergies (Table 13.4) are also important. If both standard and metric values are allowed, both need to be tested. Even though the interfaces were already tested for ancillary departments during unit testing, they need to be tested again during integrated testing. This testing should include any printed notices that are associated with the orders, along with populating work lists and reports as shown

TABLE 13.4	Verify Interfaces/Integration of Patient Information				
Integrated Testing Day 1: Enter the following information and Verify:					
		Received in:	**Received in:**	**Received in:**	**Received in:**
Date	**Interfaced Field Entered in CIS**	**Pharmacy**	**Radiology**	**Cardiology**	**Dietary**
	Allergies (specify what to enter)				
	Ht/Wt (specify what to enter)				
	Pregnancy/Lactation (specify what to enter)				
	Transportation (specify what to enter)				
Date	**Interfaced Field Entered in Pharmacy**	**CIS**	**Radiology**	**Cardiology**	**Dietary**
	Allergies (specify what to enter)				
	Ht/Wt (specify what to enter)				
	Pregnancy/Lactation (specify what to enter)				
	Transportation (specify what to enter)				
Date	**Interfaced Field Entered in Radiology**	**CIS**	**Pharmacy**	**Cardiology**	**Dietary**
	Allergies (specify what to enter)				
	Ht/Wt (specify what to enter)				
	Pregnancy/Lactation (specify what to enter)				
	Transportation (specify what to enter)				

in Table 13.5. Each field for each assessment needs to be tested and verified for all displays during unit testing and a large, realistic sampling also needs to be included in the integrated testing. Table 13.6 is an example of assessment testing that includes integration of plan of care and alerts based on the assessments. Any printed documents such as discharge instructions should also be included.

Another trend in healthcare is converting not from paper to an electronic record, but from one electronic system to another system. Whether this conversion is due to replacing a legacy system or due to a merger, the complexity of a system conversion brings its own set of requirements in the user expectation, the design and build, testing and the decision of what information to convert, and what to "backload" from the existing system to the new system.

Backloading, or manually entering information into the new system (Ohio KePRO, n.d.), is often done in between two and five days before a new system is live so that important patient information is available. Table 13.7 is an example of a report from the legacy system with the information on it. The report may be very accurate, but the information may be outdated before it is printed and distributed, requiring a second or third report with updated information. The other option is a modification of the report available online, staff doing the backload can either work in pairs, or work off of dual monitors with the

legacy system on one monitor and the new system on the other monitor.

Stakeholder involvement in a project is improved with regular status reporting (Pitagorsky, 2012). Reporting the status of the project from implementation through optimization is critical. Stakeholders, according to Hanson, Stephens, Pangaro, and Gimbel (2012), include clinicians, nurse/ancillary, patients, and administrators. During the implementation, the timeline, progress, teams, and schedule for training can be maintained and updated on the intranet site. Managers and executives might require more detailed report. A general status update can be helpful in visualizing the overall project status. Table 13.8 is an example of a columnar report, and Fig. 13.3 is an example of a chart that depicts the anticipated progress and budget compares it to the actual progress and budget.

System Optimization and Metrics

The system life cycle, like the nursing process, is a fluid process of assessment, diagnosis, planning, implementation, and evaluation. After the system is implemented, the process of system changes does not end. System optimization and support along with changes due to upgrades, regulatory and payer changes, as well as clinical changes due

TABLE 13.5   An Example of Testing Orders to Multiple Departments

Integrated Testing Day 1: Enter orders for:

Date	Lab Order	Order Received in Lab	Label Printed in Lab	OSU Received in CIS			Result Received in CIS	Result Displayed Correctly in CIS
				In Progress	Prelim Result	Final Result		
	CBC							
	Chem Panel							
	Urinalysis							
	Type and Cross							

Integrated Testing Day 1

Date	Radiology Order	Order with Reason for Study Received in Radiology Information System (RIS)	Transport Method	OSU Received in CIS			Result/Report Received in CIS	Result Displayed Correctly in CIS with link to PACS Image
				In Progress	Prelim Result	Final Result		
	y							
	Chest X-ray Daily							

Integrated Testing Day 1

Date	Cardiology Order	Order with Reason for Study Received in Cardiology System	Transport Method	OSU Received in CIS			Result/Report Received in CIS	Result Displayed Correctly in CIS with link to Image
				In Progress	Prelim Result	Final Result		
	Doppler Study							
	EKG							

Integrated Testing Day 1

Date	Dietary Order	Order Received in Dietary System	Order Printed in Department
	Renal Diet, vegetarian, 2000 cc fluid restriction		

Integrated Testing Day 1: Enter orders for:

Date	Telemetry	Wave Form Visible in CIS	Order Printed in Central Monitoring Area
	Telemetry		

Integrated Testing Day 1

Date	Order	Order on Worklist for Department Providing Service	Order Printed in Department
	Discharge Planning		
	Oxygen		
	Wound Nurse Consult		

TABLE 13.6	An Example of a Way to Verify That Charting Pathways Work as Designed, also to Verify That Each Charted Value Displays Correctly and Reports Correctly

Integrated Testing Day 1 Enter Assessments:

Charted (specify what to document)	Pathway Flows (specify)	Yes/No	Kicked Off Care Plan? (specify)	Yes/No	Kicked Off Orders (specify)	Yes/No	Kicked Off Alert (specify)	Yes/No
Risk for skin								
Risk for fall								
Risk for suicide								
Criteria for vaccinations								

TABLE 13.7	An Example of a Report That Can Be Utilized for Backloading Clinically Significant Information into the New System During the System Conversion

Pt. Loc: **4E**   Account #: **12345678**   MR/MPI #: **54121**   Visit Status: **IP**

Pt Name: **John Doe**   Pt DOB: **05/25/1979**   Pt Sex: **M**

HEIGHT and WEIGHT

HtObtained	On	At	Wt		Obtained	On	At	
6/1/	Stated	4/04	1950		210	Standing	4/05	0600

PREGNANCY and LACTATION

ALLERGIES

Alg name	Category	Reaction	Severity
Peanut	Food	Rash	
Peanut	Drug	Rash	
Penicillin	Drug	Rash	

RISK DOCUMENTATION

Fall
Risk for Injury from Fall
Nutrition
Skin

VACCINATION

Influenza
Pneumonia
DPaT

MEDICAL HISTORY

CAD.....................	No	CHF....................	Yes	Stroke....................	Yes
Hypertension.......................	Yes	Dialysis.....................	Yes	Cancer Type..............	Prostate
2001 Arthritis..........................	No	GERD......................	Yes	Ulcer......................	No
Obstructive Sleep Apnea.............	No	Diabetes Type 1............	Yes	Diabetes Type 2..........	No
Surgical History					
Education					
History of MRSA......................	No	History of VRE..............	No		

(continued)

TABLE 13.7	An Example of a Report That Can Be Utilized for Backloading Clinically Significant Information into the New System During the System Conversion *(continued)*

		HOME MEDICATIONS		
Medication	**Dose**	**Route**	**Frequency**	**Indication**
Humera	40 mg	Subcutaneously	Weekly	Arthritis

NON-MEDICATION ORDERS

Lab
CBC daily × 5 days, lab to collect start on 4/04
Radiology
Chest X-ray in the morning, pneumonia transport: Wheelchair
Diets
Regular diet with snacks start 04/04
Nursing
Change dressing to left foot daily
Up in chair for meals
Up to bathroom ad lib
Code Status
Full code

LEGAL	
Durable Power of Attorney	No
Legal Guardian	No

TABLE 13.8	An Example of a Project Status Report

Application	Anticipated % Done	Actual % Done	Reasons
Nursing Assessments	50	40	New regulations
Rehab Therapies Assessments	50	40	Change in resources
Respiratory Assessments	50	60	Decrease in charging components
Care Planning	50	55	
Orders	50	45	Change in resources
Reports	50	40	Dependent on orders and assessments
Budget	35	45	Loss of resources

to new research all lead to constant changes to the system. As stakeholders become more familiar with the system, they will have ideas on improvements and enhancements to make the system more user friendly, as well as improving the ability of the system to prompt staff to improve patient care.

Along with the process improvement strategies listed below, getting pre- and post-implementation metrics will assist. Surveys can be done post-implementation to evaluate staff satisfaction with the system, the education, and/or the support. Examples of pre- and post-implementation metrics include accuracy and completeness of charting, charging, and time studies. The evaluation of charges would include the timeliness, accuracy, and whether the charges were supported by the orders and the documentation. Also included would be the pre and post metrics for charting Core measures such as vaccinations and education on smoking. The time to document specific types of

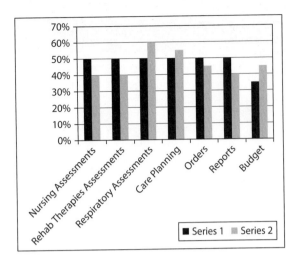

• **FIGURE 13.3.** Table and Graphic Examples of Status Reporting.

charting can be measured and recorded by using a tool similar to that presented in Table 13.9.

MEASURING SUCCESS, CONTINUING TO IMPROVE

Continuous Quality Improvement (CQI) is based on the principle that there is an opportunity for improvement in every process (Wallin, Bostrom, Wikblad, & Ewald, 2003). CQI begins with a culture of change and improvement, and encourages all levels of staff to look for ways to improve the current process, and for variations of the process, which can create errors. There are many philosophies that can be utilized to implement a CQI program; some can be used in combination. Some of these include the following:

- Six Sigma is a "data-driven quality improvement methodology that uses statistical analysis to reduce process variation. Six Sigma has a strong focus on reducing variation, in fact the term, Six Sigma refers to a defect rate of 3.4 defects per million opportunities and represents a statistically high standard of quality" (Anderson-Dean, 2012). Six Sigma utilizes five steps to evaluate metrics, known as DMAIC: **D**efine, **M**easure, **A**nalyze, **I**mprove, and **C**ontrol. Six Sigma focuses on the reduction of variation to improve processes (Nave, 2002); the goal is to permanently resolve errors by focusing on the underlying processes (DMAIC, n.d.).

- Lean Six Sigma has a strong focus on eliminating waste by removing non-value activities including defects, unnecessary, or redundant steps using value stream mapping (VSM). It focuses on the process and works best if all employees are involved (Clancy, 2011). According to Sitterding and Everett (2013), Lean Six Sigma creates a "culture and practices that continually improve all

TABLE 13.9	Example of an Interdisciplinary Time Study Done Pre- and Post-implementation							
Date and Time	**Time Spent Before**			**Category**	**Unit/Area**	**Time Spent After**		
	Admission	**Shift**	**Other**	**RN**	**3S**	**Admission**	**Shift**	**Other**
7/18	19		6	LVN	3S	22		4
7/18			8	LVN	3N			10
7/18	23		10		3S	20		9
7/18			6	RN	3N			5
7/20			2	RT	3W			2
7/20			3	RT	3W			3
7/20			3	RT	3W			3
7/20			2		3W			2
8/10	6		2	RT	3N		9	2
8/10		15	4	FS	3W		12	3
8/11	6		4	RN	3N		6	3
8/11	5		4	RN	3S		7	3
8/11	5		5.5	RN	3S		5	6

TABLE 13.10	An Example of Executive Dashboard With Both Clinical and Non-clinical Measurements			
Strategic Measurement				
Vision—ex. Quality, Vision, Integrity, Care, Respect, Stewardship				
Measurement		**Goal**	**% of Goal**	**On Target**
MeStroke (Venous Thromboembolism [VTE] Prophylaxis, Discharged on Antithrombotic Therapy, Anticoagulation Therapy for Atrial Fibrillation/Flutter, Thrombolytic Therapy, Antithrombotic Therapy By End of Hospital Day 2, Discharged on Statin Medication, Stroke Education, Assessed for Rehabilitation)		100%	99.70%	....
Immunizations (Pneumococcal Immunization, Pneumococcal Immunization—Age 65 and Older, Pneumococcal Immunization—High-Risk Populations [age 6 through 64 years], Influenza Immunization)		100%	95%	....
Tobacco Treatment (Screening, Treatment, Treatment Provided or Offered at Discharge, Treatment at Discharge, Assessing Status After Discharge)		100%	100%	....
Value-Based Purchasing (Consists of weighted components, with targets based on current performance and the goal of reaching the 90th percentile)		90%	99%	....
Readmissions (Composite score of AMI, HF, and PN readmissions back to the same facility in 30 days)		10%	99%	....
Patient Satisfaction (Top priority that hospital staff took patient preference into account; understood the purpose of taking meds, staff do everything to help with pain)		80%	85%	....

functions by all people at all levels in the organization, and also utilizes the DMAIC model."

- Plan Do Study Act (PDSA) is a process for enacting and evaluating change; according to Nakayama et al. (2010) it has been recommended by the Joint Commission and the Institute of Medicine as an effective tool for complex processes. It is a four-step scientific method to enact and evaluate change: **P**lanning, **D**o it—or implement the change, **S**tudy the results, and **A**ct—which may include modifying the change based on the results of the initial test (Quality Tool, 2013).

- Failure Mode and Effects Analysis (FMEA) can be used throughout the system life cycle to evaluate processes for real or potential failure points. The processes are mapped out and each step of the process is documented. Flow charts or Swim Lane Process maps can be used to help visualize the process maps. The process maps or process flows are then used to identify where in the process there are risks for failure (or errors), and the associated risks including the severity and likelihood. The FMEA team, which includes representatives of all affected areas, then identifies solutions and implements them. The implementation is followed by an evaluation, and reevaluation process until no failures can be identified (Mohiuddin, 2011).

How does the CQI process affect the Clinical Information System (CIS)? System design issues can create errors or minimize the risk of errors. By studying and documenting the workflow and processes problems with the current system (paper or electronic) the clinical system can be designed to minimize the risk of errors, and to decrease the risk of errors by both good design and embedding EBP and CDS, using alerts as warnings and suggestions.

One way to visualize the progress of quality improvement initiatives as well as organizational goals is with reports and dashboards. Table 13.10 is an example of an executive dashboard that enables leadership to "visualize strategic metrics to guide decision making grounded in actionable information" (Aydin, Bolton, Donaldson, Brown, & Mukerji, 2008). A more detailed report that is printed, e-mailed, or viewed online each shift can give timely and meaningful feedback to the staff entering the information into the CIS so that any issues can be fixed in a timely manner, improving learning and compliance.

SUMMARY

This chapter reviews the stages of the system life cycle and some of the tools available that can be modified to assist with each phase in almost any scenario. Tools like workflow analysis and documentation can be utilized in multiple phases, and may be displayed in many ways. Like the nursing process of **A**ssessment, **D**iagnosis, **O**utcomes/**P**lanning, **I**mplementation, and **E**valuation (American Nurses Association, n.d.), the system life cycle is a continuous cycle that involves complex teams, and requires involving those affected—the end users and other stakeholders. Design is a continuous cycle based on user requirements and recommendations as well as regulatory changes and new research on best practices which need to be embedded in the CIS. Because of these changes as well as upgrades, testing and evaluation will also be done throughout the system life cycle.

REFERENCES

American Nurses Association. (n.d.). *The nursing process.* Retrieved from http://www.nursingworld.org/EspeciallyForYou/What-is-Nursing/Tools-You-Need/Thenursingprocess.html

American Nurses Credentialing Center. (2012). *Informatics nurse test content outline.* Retrieved from http://www.google.com/url?sa=t&rct=j&q=&esrc=s&source=web&cd=1&cad=rja&ved=0CCYQFjAA&url=http%3A%2F%2Fwww.nursecredentialing.org%2FInformatics-TCO2012.pdf&ei=emYEU8fxEojboATKvYKYBw&usg=AFQjCNG2jZEvVSDg47q0R_xk_ZrKXLhaRw&bvm=bv.61535280,d.cGU.

Anderson-Dean, C. (2012). The benefits of Lean Six Sigma for nursing informatics. *ANIA-CARING Newsletter, 27*(4), 1–7.

Aydin, C., Bolton, L. B., Donaldson, N., Brown, D. S., & Mukerji, A. (2008). *Beyond nursing quality measurement:The nation's first regional nursing virtual dashboard.* Retrieved from http://www.google.com/url?sa=t&rct=j&q=&esrc=s&frm=1&source=web&cd=1&cad=rja&uact=8&ved=0CC8QFjAA&url=http%3A%2F%2Fwww.ahrq.gov%2Fdownloads%2Fpub%2Fadvances2%2Fvol1%2FAdvances-Aydin_2.pdf&ei=nLo7U9-LHMrTsAT4i4HQCA&usg=AFQjCNG04rqFVS-AkKDZTt-5ulSfaRXpsg. Accessed on December 11, 2008.

Carr, D. M. (n.d.). *Clinical and business intelligence.* Retrieved from https://www.himss.org/library/clinical-business-intelligence?navItemNumber=17599

Clancy, T. (2011). The integration of complex systems theory into Six Sigma methods of performance improvement: A case study. In V. A. Saba & K. A. McCormick (Eds.), *Essentials of nursing informatics.* New York, NY: McGraw-Hill Publishing. (5th ed., pp. 373–389).

DMAIC Tools. (n.d.). *Network Diagram Examples: Automate any Network Diagram Professional Quality.* Retrieved from http://www.dmaictools.com/

Hanson, J. L., Stephens, M. B., Pangaro, L. N., & Gimbel, R. W. (2012). Quality of outpatient clinical notes:

A stakeholder definition derived through qualitative research. *BMC Health Services Research, 12*(1), 407-418. doi:10.1186/1472-6963-12-407.

Karsh, B. T., & Alper, S. J. (2005, February). *The key to understanding health care systems.* Agency for Healthcare Research and Quality (US). Retrieved from http://www.ncbi.nlm.nih.gov/books/NBK20518/

Kulhanek, B. (2011). Why reinvent the wheel?. *ANIA-CARING Newsletter, 26*(3), 4–8.

Mohiuddin, N. (2011). FMEA: Uses in informatics projects. *ANIA-CARING Newsletter, 26*(4), 6–7.

Nakayama, D., Bushey, T., Hubbard, I., Cole, D., Brown, A., Grant, T., & Shaker, I. (2010). Using a Plan-Do-Study-Act cycle to introduce a new OR service line. *AORN Journal, 92*(3), 335-343. doi:10.1016/j.aorn.2010.01.018.

National Learning Consortium. (2012). *Electronic health record (EHR) system testing plan.* Retrieved from http://www.google.com/url?sa=t&rct=j&q=&esrc=s&source=web&cd=3&ved=0CDUQFjAC&url=http%3A%2F%2Fwww.healthit.gov%2Fsites%2Fdefault%2Ffiles%2Fehr-system-test-plan.docx&ei=lcZJU_qeM4SL8AHOjYCwAg&usg=AFQjCNHp9vk8TrNPxOeOL_nW6koWyWDa5g&bvm=bv.64542518,d.b2U&cad=rja

Nave, D. (2002). How to compare Six Sigma, Lean and the theory of constraints. *Quality Progress, 35*(3), 73.

Ohio KePRO. (n.d.). Electronic health record implementation in physician offices: Critical success factors. Retrieved from http://www.google.com/url?sa=t&rct=j&q=&esrc=s&source=web&cd=2&ved=0CEUQFjAB&url=http%3A%2F%2Fwww.midwestclinicians.org%2Fsharedchcpolicies%2Fehr%2FPreinstallb.doc&ei=0f5JU4G-JuPS8AGCpIGoCg&usg=AFQjCNG2C3BYUnnmPKVPbMnTDLlXoRlWzA&bvm=bv.64542518,d.b2U&cad=rja

Pitagorsky, G. (2012). *Status reporting, clarity and accountability.* Retrieved from http://www.projecttimes.com/george-pitagorsky/status-reporting-clarity-and-accountability.html

Quality Tool: Plan Do Study Act (PDSA) Cycle. (2013) Retrieved from http://www.innovations.ahrq.gov/content.aspx?id=2398

Sitterding, M., & Everett, L. Q. (2013, February). *Reaching new heights: A hospital system approach maximizing nurse work efficiency.* Symposium conducted at the meeting of the American Organization of Nurse Executives.

The TIGER Initiative. (n.d.). *Designing usable clinical information systems: Recommendations from the TIGER Usability and Clinical Application Design Collaborative Team.* Retrieved from http://www.tigersummit.com/Usability_New.html

Wallin, L., Bostrom, A. M., Wikblad, K., & Ewald, U. (2003). Sustainability in changing clinical practice promotes evidence-based nursing care. *Journal of Advanced Nursing, 41*(5):509–518.

14

Healthcare Project Management

Judy Murphy / Patricia C. Dykes

• OBJECTIVES

1. Describe the five process groups in project management methodology, and identify key inputs and outputs for each.
2. Illustrate the "triple constraint" relationship between scope, cost, and time and how it can impact project quality.
3. Explain how a clinical system project is initiated and the role of the project charter.
4. Identify five techniques that will positively impact the quality, efficiency, and effectiveness of a clinical system implementation.

• KEY WORDS

Project management
Project methodology
Health information technology
Process groups
Triple constraint

INTRODUCTION

It is difficult to read a newspaper, magazine, or Web page today without somehow hearing about the impact of information technology. Information in all forms is traveling faster and being shared by more individuals than ever before. Think of how quickly you can buy just about anything online, make an airline reservation, or book a hotel room anywhere in the world. Consider how fast you can share photos or video clips with your family and friends. This ubiquitous use of technology is permeating the healthcare industry as well, and the future of many organizations may depend on their ability to harness the power of information technology, particularly in the area of electronic health records and health information exchange.

Good project management is needed in order to accomplish the work, facilitate the change, and deliver the improvements facilitated by health information technology implementation. Project management is not a new concept—it has been practiced for hundreds of years, as any large undertaking requires a set of objectives, a plan, coordination, the management of resources, and the ability to manage change. Today, however, project management has become more formal with a specified body of knowledge, and many healthcare organizations have adopted the project-oriented approach as a technique to define and execute on their strategic goals and objectives.

Good project managers for health information technology projects are in high demand. Colleges have responded by establishing courses in project management and making them part of the health informatics' curriculums for continuing education, certificate and degree programs. This chapter provides a high-level look at the methodology behind project management in order to provide a framework for the project manager skills development, structure for the implementation work processes, and organization of the projects' tasks.

CHAPTER OVERVIEW

This chapter augments the Systems Life Cycle chapters, as it outlines the project management phases, called *Process Groups*, used to organize and structure the Systems Life Cycle in order to successfully complete all the implementation steps of a project. The Overview section will provide an introduction to project management and background information on project definitions and project manager skills. Each subsequent section will review one of the five project management process groups. The last section will describe some additional considerations for health information technology projects, such as governance and positioning of project management in the healthcare organization.

What Is a Project?

There are many different definitions of a project, but they all have the same components—a project is temporary, has a defined beginning and end, and is managed to time, budget, and scope. Kerzner defines a project as a temporary endeavor undertaken to create a unique product, service, or result. Distinguishing features of a project are specific objectives, defined start and end dates, defined funding limitations, consumption of resources (human, equipment, materials), and if needed, a multifunctional or cross-organizational structure (Kerzner & Saladis, 2006). The Project Management Institute (PMI) defines a project as "a temporary endeavor undertaken to create a unique product or service with a definite beginning and a definite end. The product or service is different or unique from other products or services" (PMI, 2013, 2014). Schwalbe differentiates a project from operations by defining operations as ongoing work done to sustain the business. Projects are different from operations in that they end when the project objectives are reached or the project is terminated (Schwalbe, 2014).

What Is Project Management?

Project management is facilitation of the planning, scheduling, monitoring, and controlling of all work that must be done to meet the project objectives. PMI states that "project management is the application of knowledge, skills, tools and techniques to project activities to meet project requirements" (PMI, 2013). It is a systematic process for implementing systems on time, within budget, and in line with customer expectations of quality. Project managers must not only strive to meet specific scope, time, cost, and quality project goals, they must also facilitate the entire process to meet the needs and expectations of the people involved in or affected by project activities.

Introduction to the Five Process Groups

The project management process groups progress from initiation activities to planning activities, executing activities, monitoring and controlling activities, and closing activities. Each of these will be described in detail in ensuing sections of this chapter. However, it is important to note here that these groups are integrated and not linear in nature, so that decisions and actions taken in one group can affect another. Figure 14.1 shows the five groups and how they relate to each other in terms of typical level of activity, time, and overlap. Of course, the level of activity and length of each process group varies for each project (Schwalbe, 2014).

Project Management Knowledge Areas

The Project Management Knowledge Areas describe the key competencies that project managers must develop and use during each of the Process Groups. Each of these competencies has specific tools and techniques associated with it, some of which will be elaborated in the following sections of this chapter. Table 14.1 shows the nine knowledge areas of project management. The four core areas of project management (bolded in the table) are project scope, time, cost, and quality management. These are considered core as they lead to specific project objectives. The four facilitating knowledge areas of project management are human resources, communication, risk, and procurement management. These are considered facilitating as they are the processes through which the project objectives are achieved. The ninth knowledge area, project integration management, is an overarching function that affects and is affected by all of the other knowledge areas. Project managers must have knowledge and skills in all of these nine areas.

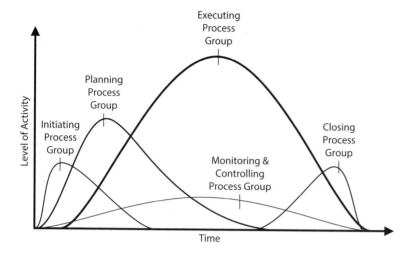

• **FIGURE 14.1.** Level of Activity and Overlap of Process Groups Overtime. (Republished, with permission of Course Technology, Cengage Learning, from Schwalbe K. (2006). *Information Technology Project Management*, 4th ed. (p. 73). Permission conveyed through Copyright Clearance Center, Inc.)

TABLE 14.1	Knowledge Areas Used in Each Process Group				
Knowledge Area	**Project Management Process Group**				
	Initiating	**Planning**	**Executing**	**Monitoring and Controlling**	**Closing**
Project Integration Management	X	X	X	X	X
Project Scope Management		X		X	
Project Time Management		X		X	
Project Cost Management		X		X	
Project Quality Management		X	X	X	
Project Human Resource Management		X	X	X	
Project Communications Management		X	X	X	
Project Risk Management		X		X	
Project Procurement Management		X	X	X	X

Bold indicates the four core knowledge areas.
(Adapted from Schwalbe, 2010, pages 83–84)

INITIATING PROCESS GROUP

The Initiating Process Group (IPG) is defined by the PMI as follows: "those processes performed to authorize and define the scope of a new phase or project or that can result in the continuation of halted project work" (PMI, 2013). The purpose of the IPG is to formally define a project including the business need, key stakeholders, and the project goals. A clear definition of the business case is critical for defining the scope of the project and for identifying the opportunity associated with completing the project. The business case includes the potential risks associated with completing or not completing the project at a given point in time. The work completed throughout the IPG builds a foundation for buy-in and commitment from the project sponsors and establishes understanding of associated challenges. The IPG is characterized by information gathering and research that leads to full disclosure of both the benefits and the costs associated with a given project (Peykari et al., 2013). Historical information is assembled during the IPG to identify related projects or earlier attempts at similar projects. Historical information provides insight into challenges associated with the project and buy-in from stakeholders. The IPG may lead to formal project selection or it may culminate in a decision to forgo or to postpone a project.

The set of work completed in the IPG is often done directly for a business sponsor and may be accomplished without a formal project team in place. During the IPG the goals of the proposed project are analyzed to determine the project scope and associated time, costs, and resource requirements. Key stakeholders are identified and may be engaged in defining the project scope, articulating the business case and developing a shared vision for the project deliverables. The inputs needed to support the work of the IPG include tools and information that support the knowledge area of project integration management. "Project integration management includes the processes and activities needed to identify, define, combine, unify and coordinate the various processes and project management activities within the project management process groups" (PMI, 2013).

Sound integration management contributes to a solid understanding of whether the project is a good match for the organization and if so, how the project fits into the organizational mission and vision. The involvement of stakeholders in the process of project integration management is fundamental to their engagement in the project and involvement in defining and working toward project success. Informational inputs such as the sponsor's description of the project, the organizational strategic plan, the published organizational mission, and historical information on related projects support the integration work of the IPG. Examples of tools and techniques that facilitate completing the information gathering, research,

and related analysis required during the IPG include the SWOT (Strengths, Weaknesses, Opportunities, Threats) analysis, stakeholder analysis, and the value risk assessment (see Table 14.2 and Fig. 14.2).

Tangible outputs of the IPG include the completed project charter (see Table 14.3) that formally defines the project including the business case, key stakeholders, project constraints, and assumptions. The project charter includes signatures of the project sponsors and team members, indicating a shared vision for the project and formal approval to move forward with planning the project. The outputs from the IPG are used to inform project planning and reused during project closure to facilitate evaluation of the project deliverables.

PLANNING PROCESS GROUP

The Planning Process Group (PPG) is often the most difficult and unappreciated process in project management, yet it is one of the most important and should not be rushed. This is the phase where decisions are made on how to complete the project and accomplish the goals and objectives defined in the Initiating Process Group. The *project plan* is created, whose main purpose is to guide the project execution phase. To that end, the plan must be realistic and specific, so a fair amount of time and effort needs to be spent and people knowledgeable about the work need to help plan the work. The project plan also provides structure for the project monitoring and controlling process, as it creates the baseline to which the work is measured against as it is completed.

During the initiating phase, a lot of information was collected to define the project, including the scope document and project charter, which provide validation and approval for the project. During the planning phase, the approach to accomplish the project is defined to an appropriate level of detail. This includes defining the necessary tasks and activities in order to estimate the resources, schedule, and budget. Failure to adequately plan greatly reduces the project's chances of successfully accomplishing its goals (Schwalbe, 2014).

TABLE 14.2	Tools to Support the Initiating Process Group	
SWOT Analysis	**Stakeholder Analysis**	**Value Risk Assessment**
Method for identifying potential Strengths and Weaknesses of the project team/organization relative to a proposed project and the potential Opportunities and Threats inherent in conducting a project	Documents important information about stakeholders that makes explicit their support, level of influence on a project, and strategies for managing relationships to ensure project success (Fig. 14.1)	Tool that supports objective rating of a project using pre-established criteria that are consistent with the mission, vision, and values of an organization

Step 1: List Stakeholders and Assign Code. Classify Stakeholders According to Influence Level

Stakeholder analysis coding key	
Code/Name	Influence level
A.	(H)
B.	(H)
C.	(H)
D.	(H)
E.	(H)
F.	(H)
G.	(H)
H.	(H)
I.	(M)
J.	(H)
K.	(L)
L.	(L)
M.	(H)
N.	(H)

Step 2: Identify Sources and Causes of Resistance and Strategies for Overcoming

Source of resistance	Causes of resistance	Strategies for overcoming resistance
Technical	• Lack of coding skills • Lack of documentation skills • Lack of understanding • Inadequate tools to support skill level	• Education & training • Use of dissemination tool (Marketing w/"on call," mox, e-mail, etc...) • Involve staff in tool development to support new skills
Political	• Job responsibility • Scope • Territoriality • Us vs. We (David vs. Gollith)	• Clarify responsibility • Disseminate "elevator speech" • Involving stakeholders • Past successes
Cultural	• Ingrained departmental • Resistance to change • "If it ain't broke...	• Education & training • Involve staff in tool development to support new skills

Step 3: Plot Strategies for Managing Stakeholders

Stakeholder analysis: *outpatient oncology care: improving the reimbursement process*

Names/influence level	Strongly against (−2)	Moderately against (−1)	Neutral (0)	Moderately supportive (+1)	Strongly supportive (+2)	Strategies for overcoming resistance
A. (H)					X	
B. (H)					X	
C. (H)					X	
D. (H)					X	
E. (H)					X	
F. (H)					X	
G. (H)					X	
H. (H)					X	
I. (M)					X	
J. (H)					X	
K. (L)			X			
L. (L)			X			
M. (H)					X	
N. (H)			X (C) √			(4,8)
O. (M)			X (P)		√	(1,2,7)
P. (M)			X (P)		√	(2,4,7)
Q. (L)		X (C,T)	√			(2,3,4)
R. (H)	X		√			(7)
S. (H)			X			
T. (H)				X		
U. (H)			X			
V. (H)			(P,C,V)		√	(2,3,4)
W. (H)					X	
X. (H)				X		
Y. (L)				X		
Z. (L)				X		
AA. (L)				X		

1. Use of dissemination tool (Marketing w/"on call," mox, e-mail, etc...)	2. Clarify responsibility	3. Education & training
4. Involve staff in tool development to support new skills	5. Disseminate "elevator speech"	6. Past successes
7. Involving stakeholders		

• **FIGURE 14.2.** Stakeholder Analysis.

TABLE 14.3	Sample Table of Contents for Project Charter

Project Charter Table of Contents

Project planning generally consists of the following steps:

- Define project scope.
- Refine project objectives.
- Define all required deliverables.
- Create framework for project scheduled.
- Select the project team.
- Creating the work breakdown structure.
- Identify the activities needed to complete the deliverables.
- Sequence the activities and define the critical path activities.
- Estimating the resource requirements for the activities.
- Identify required skills and resources.
- Estimating work effort, time, and cost for activities.

TABLE 14.4	Planning Process Group Tools and Techniques
Scope Statement	Defines the boundaries of the project work; often developed directly from: • Voice of the customer • Project charter • SWOT analysis (strengths, weaknesses, opportunities, and threats) • Stakeholder analysis • Value Risk Assessment
Project Charter	Describes the high-level scope, time, and cost goals for the project objectives and success criteria, a general approach to accomplishing the project goals, and the roles and responsibilities of project stakeholders.
RACI Chart	Helps define the roles and responsibilities of project teams and team members—shows who is: • **R**esponsible—completes the task • **A**ccountable—signs off on the task • **C**onsulted—has information necessary to complete the task • **I**nformed—needs to be notified of task status or results.
Work Breakdown Structure (WBS)	Displays the project graphically subdivided into manageable work activities, including the relationship of each task to other tasks, the allocation of responsibility, the resources required, and the time allocated.
Risk Register	Prioritizes the list of project risks, often including a plan for risk avoidance and risk mitigation strategies.

- Developing the schedule.
- Developing the budget.
- Complete risk analysis and avoidance.
- Create communication plan.
- Gaining formal approval to begin work.

Some of the tools and techniques employed during the PPG are listed in Table 14.4. One of the most important is the Work Breakdown Structure (WBS). Projects are organized and understood by breaking them into a hierarchy, with progressively smaller pieces until they are a collection of defined "work packages" that include tasks. The WBS is used as the outline to provide a framework for organizing and managing the work. The deliverable of this phase is a comprehensive project plan that is approved by the sponsor(s) and shared with the project team in a project kick-off meeting (Houston & Bove, 2007; Maas, 2013).

EXECUTING PROCESS GROUP

The Executing Process Group (EPG) is defined by the PMI as follows: "Those processes performed to complete the work defined in the project management plan to accomplish the project's objectives defined in the project scope statement" (PMI, 2013). The EPG is characterized by carrying out the work of the project and associated activities defined by the project plan to meet project requirements. During the EPG the project team follows the project plan and each team member contributes to the ongoing progress of the plan. Project deliverables are managed during the EPG by careful tracking of scope, time, and resource

use with ongoing updates made to the project plan and timeline to reflect progress made.

The key responsibilities of the project manager during the EPG are integration of the project team and activities to keep the work of the project moving toward the established milestones set during the project planning phase (e.g., PPG). Clear communication and effective management of project resources are essential. The inputs needed to support the work of the EPG include tools and information that facilitate assimilation of the following knowledge areas into project efforts (PMI, 2013; Schwalbe, 2014):

- Integration management: Coordination of project resources and activities to complete the project on time, within budget, and in accordance with the project scope defined by the customer.

- Quality management: Monitoring of project performance to ensure that the deliverables will satisfy the quality requirements specified by the customer.

- Human resource management: Enhancing and motivating performance of project team members to ensure effective use of human resources to advance project deliverables.

- Communication management: Distribution of information in a complete and timely fashion to ensure all stakeholders are informed and miscommunication channels are minimized.

- Procurement management: Obtaining goods and services from outside an organization including identifying and selecting vendors and managing contracts.

TABLE 14.5	Executing Process Group Tools and Techniques
Project meetings	Gathering of project team for the purpose of advancing the work of the project. All participants have a pre-defined role; action items and decisions are tracked and formally communicated.
Gantt chart	Tracks and communicates project tasks, resources, and milestones against time over the course of a project. (Many of the Web references at the end of the chapter contain links to sample Gantt charts.)
Request for proposal	Used to solicit proposals from prospective vendors.
Issue log	Provides a means to prioritize and track items that represent a degree of risk to meeting project deliverables.
Progress reports	Keep project team informed of project status, milestones to date, and areas of concern.

As noted above, the inputs needed to support the work of the EPG include tools and information that promote clear communication, control the work, and manage project resources. Some common tools employed during the EPG are described in Table 14.5.

The tools and techniques used during the EPG and associated documentation facilitate completion of project work and provide a means to identify and track ongoing activities against the project plan. Variances may arise during project execution and may trigger an evaluation and a re-planning of activities. Deliverables produced through use of the EPG input tools and techniques are then used as outputs to inform the work conducted over subsequent process group phases. For example, during the EPG, the Gantt chart provides a means to monitor whether the project is on schedule and for managing dependencies between tasks. This same tool is useful in the monitoring and controlling process groups (MCPG) where the Gantt chart is used to proactively identify when remedial action is needed and to ensure that project milestones are met in accordance with the project plan.

MONITORING AND CONTROLLING PROCESS GROUP

The purpose of the Monitoring and Controlling Process Group (MCPG) is to observe project execution so that issues and potential problems can be identified in a timely manner and corrective action can be taken when necessary to control execution of the project. It is the process of measuring progress toward project objectives, monitoring deviation from the plan, and taking corrective action to ensure progress matches the plan. The MCPG is performed throughout life of project across all phases, and provides feedback between project phases (PMI, 2013, 2014).

The project manager facilitates project control by measuring actual performance against the planned or estimated performance from the project plan in the areas of scope, resources, budget, and time. The key benefit

of project controls occurs when project performance is observed and measured regularly, variance to the plan can be identified and mitigated quickly to minimize delays and avoid cost overruns. Estimates say that 80% of healthcare projects fail; one-third are never completed; and most are over budget, behind schedule, or go live with reduced scope (Kitzmiller, Hunt, & Sproat, 2006). The reasons for these failures vary, but project control can help improve on-time, on-budget, and in-scope delivery of projects. During the control phase, the project manager needs to support the project team with frequent checks and recognition of the completion of incremental work efforts. This way, the project manager can adapt the work as needed. Project managers also need to work with the project sponsors to identify the risks of keeping on time and on budget versus modifying the schedule or scope to better meet the organizations' need for the project (Houston & Bove, 2007).

The Triple Constraint

Every project is constrained in some way by scope, cost, and time. These limitations are known as the triple constraint. They are often competing constraints that need to be balanced by the project manager throughout the project life cycle (Maas, 2013; Schwalbe, 2014). Scope refers to the work that needs to be done to accomplish the project goals. Cost is the resources required to complete the project. Time is the duration of the project. The concept is that a modification to the project will impact one or more of the three constraints, and often require trade-offs between them. For example, if there is an increase in scope, either cost or time or both will need to be increased as well. Or in another example, if time is decreased when a deadline is moved up, either scope will need to decrease or cost (resources) will need to increase. It is a balancing act.

The tools and techniques employed during the MCPG are described in Table 14.6.

TABLE 14.6	Monitoring and Controlling Process Group Tools and Techniques
Project management methodology	Follows a methodology that describes not only what to do in managing a project, but how to do it.
Project management information systems	Hundreds of project management software products are available on the market today, and many organizations are moving toward powerful enterprise project management systems that are accessible via the Internet.
Time reporting tools	Ability to enter and track project effort by resource and against the project tasks.
Progress reports	Answer the questions: • How are my projects doing overall? • Are my projects on schedule? • Are my estimates accurate? • Are my resources properly utilized?

CLOSING PROCESS GROUP

The Closing Process Group (CPG) is defined by the PMI as follows: "Those processes performed to formally terminate all activities of a project or phase and transfer the completed product to others or close a cancelled project" (PMI, 2013). The goal of CPG is to finalize all project activities and to formally close the project. During the CPG the project goals and objectives set during the IPG are compared with deliverables and analyzed to determine the project success. Key stakeholders are engaged with evaluating the degree to which project deliverables were met. The inputs needed to support the work of the CPG include the outputs from earlier process group phases and the tools and information that support the knowledge areas of project integration and procurement management (PMI, 2013).

• Integration management: Coordination of project closure activities including formal documentation of project deliverables and formal transfer of ongoing activities from the project team to established operational resources.

• Procurement management: Coordination of formal contract closure procedures including resolution of open issues and documentation of archival of information to inform future projects.

Some common tools employed during the CPG are described in Table 14.7.

The tools and techniques used during the CPG and associated documentation facilitate project closure and provide a means to identify lessons learned. Moreover, these tools and techniques are used to document best practices including updates to the organization's project management toolbox (Milosevic, 2003). During the CPG, standard tools available to the project team to support best practices are identified and made available to support application of best practices in future projects. Including a formal step for adapting the project management toolbox during the CPG ensures that the toolbox remains pertinent and continues to support best practices relative to the types of projects typically conducted within an organization.

TABLE 14.7	Closing Process Group Tools and Techniques
Post-implementation survey	Provides an opportunity for project stakeholders to evaluate the project from multiple perspectives including product effectiveness, management of the triple constraint, communication management, and overall performance of the project team.
Post-mortem review document	Provides a means to document the formal project evaluation and summarizes the pluses and deltas associated with a given project. Facilitates discussion related to lessons learned that can be applied to future projects.
Project closeout checklist	Used to ensure that agreed upon features of project closure are completed related to the following: post-implementation review, administrative closeout procedures, and formal acknowledgment of the project team.

OTHER CONSIDERATIONS

Project Governance

There is just no question that successful projects are owned and sponsored by the leaders and staff that will be making the practice change and will be benefiting by the change. So in the ideal scenario, the Governance Committee(s) are led by top business and clinical leaders, with membership built on broad representation from key business and clinical departments. In addition to evaluating and ranking the technology project proposals brought to them, they take responsibility for generating an overall roadmap to use to compare each proposal against. They set guiding principles for concepts like integration versus best-of-breed systems. They consider where the organization needs to be going and what practice and care changes are required, then solicit proposals from the strategic business units who are responsible for making those changes. In other words, they do not just see themselves as "governing" the project selection process, but rather as "driving" the implementation of projects that support strategic initiatives and deliver strategic value. It may be a nuance here, but there is a real argument that these are not Governance Committees that pick IT projects, but rather are Governance Committees that allocate IT resources to strategic projects (PMI, 2013).

Skills Needed for Project Managers

There is general agreement that good project managers need to have both people skills and leadership skills. Here is one skills list that describes the many facets of the project manager role:

- Communication skills: Listens, persuades.
- Organizational skills: Plans, sets goals, analyzes.
- Team-building skills: Shows empathy, motivates, promotes esprit de corps.
- Leadership skills: Sets examples, provides vision (big picture), delegates, positive, energetic.
- Coping skills: Flexible, creative, patient, persistent.
- Technology skills: Experience, project knowledge.

Project Management Office

There are different ways to position project managers in a healthcare organization. Some have them in the information technology department, some have them in the clinical department, others have them in an informatics department, and still others have matrix roles. Many have now created a project management office (PMO) to provide best practices and support for managing all projects in an organization. The office can also provide education, coaching, and mentoring, as well as project management resources. With the federal incentives for health information technology, the industry has begun the challenging task of implementing electronic health record system projects to demonstrate meaningful use. With this increase in projects, there is an increased demand for good project managers and consistent project management methodology for completing projects.

Project Management Institute

The Project Management Institute (PMI) was founded in 1969 by a group of project managers and is considered to be the leading professional organization for project managers worldwide. The primary goal of the PMI is "to advance the practice, science and profession of project management throughout the world in a conscientious and proactive manner so that organizations everywhere will embrace, value and utilize project management and then attribute their successes to it." (PMI, 2014) The PMI publishes the *Guide to the Project Management Body of Knowledge (PMBOK® Guide)*, which is a collection of consensus-based standards and best practices. The *PMBOK® Guide* is currently in its 5th edition and has been adopted as an American National Standard (ANSI) (PMI, 2014).

Project Management Professionals

The Project Management Institute (PMI) offers multiple levels of credentialing to assist project professionals with advancing their careers in project, program, and portfolio management. PMI credentials are available related to many aspects of project management including program management, scheduling, and risk management. PMI membership is not required for credentialing (PMI, 2014). In addition to meeting a set of published pre-requisite requirements, PMI credentialing requires that candidates successfully pass a credentialing exam. Complete information about PMI credentials and the credentialing process can be accessed from the PMI Web site.

Project Management Resources on the Web

Many Web-based resources exist to support project management best practices. A recent search using the key words "project management resources" on a popular search engine returned over 70 million results. A list of validated Web-based resources is included in the Resource List at the end of the chapter.

SUMMARY

Today, as so often in history, healthcare resources are limited. Yet there are many, varied, and complex healthcare technology projects demanding resources. So how does one ensure that healthcare dollars and clinician time are spent wisely on projects that guarantee patient-driven outcomes? In addition to selecting and funding the projects wisely, the authors believe, good project management also minimizes risk and enhances success. We further contend that clinicians, and particularly nurses, are excellent candidates, once trained in PM techniques, to be good project managers. Executive management should support, and maybe even demand, project management training for the organization's clinical IT project team leaders.

Nursing informatics has been evolving since its inception some 25 years ago. More often than ever, project management skills are being included in training and formal education programs. And, increasingly, informatics nurses are stepping up to the plate and taking on key roles in the planning, selection, implementation, and evaluation of the critical clinical systems needed in healthcare today. We hope that we have provided a glimpse as to the skills that will enable this to happen. Good project management holds part of the key to consistent success with electronic health record system implementations in healthcare today.

REFERENCES

Houston, M., & Bove, L. (2007). *Project management for healthcare informatics*. Health Informatics Series 2007. New York, NY: Springer.

Kerzner, H., & Saladis, F. (2006). *Project management workbook and PMP/CAPM exam study guide* (9th ed.). Hoboken, NJ: John Wiley & Sons, Inc.

Kitzmiller, R., Hunt, E., & Sproat, S. (2006). Adopting best practices: "Agility" moves from software development to healthcare project management. *Computers, Informatics, Nursing, 24*(2), 75–83.

Maas, J. (2013). Project management; considerations for success. *Journal of Healthcare Protection Management, 29*(2), 74–82.

Milosevic, D. (2003). *Project management tool box 2003*. Hoboken, NJ: Wiley & Sons.

Peykari, N., Owlia, P., Malekafzali, H., Ghanei, M., Babamahmoodi, A., & Djalalinia, S. (2013). Needs assessment in health research projects: A new approach to project management in Iran. *Iranian Journal of Public Health, 42*(2), 158–163.

PMI. (2013). *A guide to the project management body of knowledge (PMBOK guide)* (5th ed.). Newton Square, PA: Project Management Institute, Inc.

PMI. (2014). The Project Management Institute. (cited 2014, January 15). Retrieved from http://www.pmi.org/

Schwalbe, K. (2006). Course Technology. *Information Technology Project Management* (5th ed.). Independence, KY: Cengage Learning.

Schwalbe, K. (2010). Course Technology. *Information Technology Project Management*. Independence, KY: Cengage Learning.

OTHER RESOURCES

Books

Cleland, D., & Ireland, L. (2007). *Project management strategic design and implementation* (5th ed.). New York, NY: McGraw-Hill.

DeCarlo, D. (2004). *Extreme project management*. Hoboken, NJ: Jossey-Bass.

Kendrick, T. (2000). *The project management tool kit*. Washington, DC: American Management Association.

Kerzner, H. (2006). *Project management: A systems approach to planning, scheduling and controlling* (9th ed.). Hoboken, NJ: John Wiley & Sons, Inc.

Manas, J. (2006). *Napoleon on project management: Timeless lessons in planning, execution and leadership*. Nashville, TN: Thomas Nelson.

Murphy, J., & Gugerty, B. (2006). Nurses in project management roles. In C. A. Weaver, C. W. Delaney, P. Weber, & R. L. Carr (Eds.), *Nursing and informatics for the 21st century: An international look at practice, trends and the future*. Chicago, IL: HIMSS Press.

Project Management Institute. (2013). *A guide to the project management body of knowledge (PMBOK guide)* (5th ed.). Newton Square, PA: Project Management Institute, Inc.

Web Sites

Agile Project Leadership Network. (2014, February 2). *Organization to connect, develop and support great project leaders*. Retrieved from http://www.agileleader shipnetwork.org/

Bright Hub. (2014, February 2). *Free project management forms & templates you can download*. Retrieved from http://www.brighthub.com/office/project-management/articles/26131.aspx#ixzz0rs5TNOvf

Cornell University. (2014, February 2). *Cornell project management methodology (CPMM)*. Retrieved from https://confluence.cornell.edu/display/CITPMO/Cornell+Project+Management+Methodology+%28CPMM%29

Lewis Institute. (2014, February 2). *Lewis project management systems*. Retrieved from http://www.lewisinstitute.com

Musser, J. (2014, February 2). *Project reference*. Retrieved fromhttp://www.projectreference.com/

Project Management.com. (2014, February 2). *The online community for IT project managers*. Retrieved from http://www.projectmanagement.com

State of New York (2014, February 2). *Project management*. Retrieved from http://www.its.ny.gov/pmmp/guidebook2/index.htm

Journal Articles

Becker, J., & Rhodes, H. (2007). Enterprise project management is key to success: Addressing the People, process and technology dimensions of healthcare. *Journal of Healthcare Information Management, 21*(3), 61–66.

Chaiken, P. B., Christian, E. C., & Johnson, L. (2007). Quality and efficiency successes leveraging IT and new processes. *Journal of Healthcare Information Management, 21*(1), 48–53.

Corfield, L. (2008). Project management skills prove invaluable. *Health Estate, 62*(8), 19–20.

James, D., Kretzing, J. E., & Stabile, M. E. (2007). Showing "what right looks like"—How to improve performance through a paradigm shift around implementation thinking. *Journal of Healthcare Information Management, 21*(1), 54–61.

Lang, R. D. (2005). IT project management in healthcare: Improving the odds for success. *Journal of Healthcare Information Management, 19*(1), 2–4.

Loo, R. (2003). Project management: a core competency for professional nurses and nurse managers. *Journal of Nursing Staff Development, 19*(4), 187–193; discussion 194.

Sa Couto, J. (2008). Project management can help to reduce costs and improve quality in healthcare services. *Journal of Evaluation in Clinical Practice, 14*(1), 48–52.

Shellenbarger, T. (2009). Time and project management tips for educators. *Journal of Continuing Education in Nursing, 40*(7), 292–293.

Simpson, R. L. (2013). Chief nurse executives need contemporary informatics competencies. *Nursing Economic$, 31*(6), 277–288.

Wolff, P. (2003). Is your organization project management savvy? *Journal of Healthcare Information Management, 17*(1), 50–54.

PART 3

Informatics Theory Standards—Foundations of Nursing Informatics

Virginia K. Saba

15

The Practice Specialty of Nursing Informatics

Kathleen M. Hunter / Carol J. Bickford

• OBJECTIVES

1. Relate the definition of nursing informatics and its qualifications as a distinct specialty.
2. Discuss models and theories that support nursing informatics.
3. Identify available organizational resources.
4. Describe the relationship of the standards of practice in nursing informatics to the scope of practice statement.

• KEY WORDS

Informatics
Competencies
Models
Theory
Nursing process
Scope of practice
Standards of practice
Standards of professional performance

ABSTRACT

Nursing informatics is an established and growing area of specialization in nursing. All nurses employ information technologies in their practice. Informatics nurses are key persons in the design, development, implementation, and evaluation of these technologies and in the development of the specialty's body of knowledge.

This chapter addresses pertinent concepts, definitions, and interrelationships of nursing, nursing informatics, and healthcare nursing informatics. Evolution of definitions for nursing informatics is presented. The recognition of nursing informatics as a distinct nursing specialty is discussed. Models and theories of nursing informatics and supporting sciences are described. The identification of various sets of nursing-informatics competencies is explained. A collection of international and national organizations of interest to informatics nurses is presented. This chapter also addresses the requisite components of the scope of practice and the standards of practice and professional performance for nursing informatics.

INTRODUCTION

Decision-making is an integral part of daily life. Nurses regularly make frequent, critical, life-impacting decisions. Good decisions require accurate and accessible data as well as skill in processing information. At the heart of nursing informatics is the goal of providing nurses with the data, information, and support for information processing to make effective decisions. This decision-making can encompass any and all of the following areas of nursing practice: client care, research, education, and administration.

INFORMATICS NURSE/INFORMATICS NURSE SPECIALIST

An informatics nurse (IN) is a registered nurse who has experience in nursing informatics. Informatics nurse specialists (INS) are prepared at the graduate level (master's degree) with specialty courses in nursing informatics. An INS functions as a graduate-level-prepared specialty nurse.

Foundational Documents Guide Nursing Informatics Practice

Nursing informatics practice and the development of this specialty has been guided by several foundational documents. These documents are listed in Table 15.1 and described in this section.

In 2001, the American Nurses Association (ANA) published the *Code of Ethics for Nurses with Interpretive Statements*, a complete revision of previous ethics provisions and interpretive statements that guide all nurses in practice, be it in the domains of direct patient care, education, administration, or research. Nurses working in the informatics specialty are professionally bound to follow these provisions. Terms such as decision-making, comprehension, information, knowledge, shared goals, outcomes, privacy, confidentiality, disclosure, policies, protocols, evaluation, judgment, standards, and factual documentation abound throughout the explanatory language of the interpretive statements (American Nurses Association, 2001a). The text of the document is available at the ANA Web site.

In 2003, a second foundational professional document, *Nursing's Social Policy Statement, Second Edition* (American Nurses Association, 2003), provided a new definition of nursing that was reaffirmed in the 2010 *Nursing's*

Social Policy Statement: The Essence of the Profession: "Nursing is the protection, promotion, and optimization of health and abilities, prevention of illness and injury, alleviation of suffering through the diagnosis and treatment of human response, and advocacy in the care of individuals, families, communities, and populations " (p. 3) (American Nurses Association, 2010).

Again, informatics nurses must be cognizant of the statements and direction provided by this document to the nursing profession, its practitioners, and the public.

The ANA's *Nursing: Scope and Standards of Practice, Second Edition,* (2010) further reinforces the recognition of nursing as a cognitive profession. The exemplary competencies accompanying each of the 16 Standards of Professional Nursing Practice, comprised of Standards of Practice and Standards of Professional Performance, reflect the specific knowledge, skills, abilities, and judgment capabilities expected of registered nurses. The standards include data, information, and knowledge management activities as core work for all nurses. This cognitive work begins with the critical-thinking and decision-making components of the nursing process that occur before nursing action can begin (American Nurses Association, 2010).

The nursing process (Figs. 15.1 and 15.2) provides a delineated pathway and process for decision-making. Assessment, or data collection and information processing, begins the nursing process. Diagnosis or problem

TABLE 15.1	Foundational Documents	
Code of Ethics for Nurses With Interpretive Statements	2001
Nursing's Social Policy Statement, Second Edition	2003
Nursing's Social Policy Statement: The Essence of the Profession	2010
Nursing: Scope and Standards of Practice, Second Edition	2010

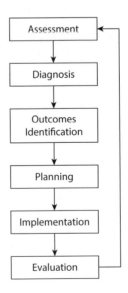

• **FIGURE 15.1.** Nursing Process. (Reproduced, with permission, from American Nurses Association. (2010). Nursing's Social Policy Statement: *The Essence of the Profession*, 3rd ed. (p. 23). Silver Springs, MD: nurses books.org. © 2010 American Nurses Association.)

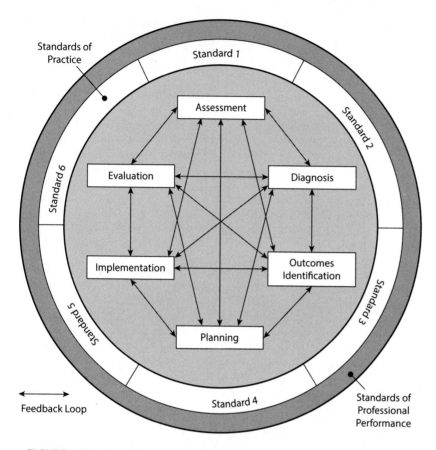

• **FIGURE 15.2.** The Nursing Process Standards. (Reproduced, with permission, from American Nurses Association. (2010). Nursing's Social Policy Statement: *The Essence of the Profession*, 3rd ed. (p. 23). Silver Springs, MD: nurses books.org. © 2010 American Nurses Association.)

definition, the second step, reflects the interpretation of the data and information gathered during assessment. Outcomes identification is the third step, followed by planning as the fourth step. Implementation of a plan is the fifth step. The final component of the nursing process is evaluation. The nursing process is most often presented as a linear process with evaluation listed as the last step. However, the nursing process really is iterative, includes numerous feedback loops, and incorporates evaluation activities throughout the sequencing. For example, evaluation of a plan's implementation may prompt further assessment, a new diagnosis or problem definition, and decision-making about new outcomes and related plans.

The collection of data about a client or about a management, education, or research situation is guided by a nurse's knowledge base built on formal and informal educational preparation, evidence and research, and previous experiences. In healthcare, as in most areas of our lives, data, information, and knowledge are growing at astronomical rates and demand increasing reliance on computer and information systems for collection, storage, organization and management, analysis, and dissemination. For example, in clinical nursing practice, consider the significant expansion in the amount and types of data that *must* be collected for legal, regulatory, quality, and other reasons; the data, information, and knowledge, like genetic profiles, related to specific client health conditions; and the information and knowledge about the healthcare environment, such as that associated with billing and reimbursement, health plan, and available formulary options. Collecting data in a systematic, thoughtful way, organizing data for efficient and accurate transformation into information, and documenting thinking and actions are critical to successful nursing practice. Nursing informatics is the nursing specialty that endeavors to make the collection, management, and dissemination of data, information, and knowledge—to support decision-making—easier for the practitioner, regardless of the domain and setting.

INFORMATICS AND HEALTHCARE INFORMATICS

Informatics is a science that combines a domain science, computer science, information science, and cognitive science. Thus, it is a multidisciplinary science drawing from varied theories and knowledge applications. Healthcare informatics may be defined as the integration of healthcare sciences, computer science, information science, and cognitive science to assist in the management of healthcare information. Healthcare informatics is a subset of informatics. Imagine a large umbrella named informatics and imagine many persons under this umbrella. Each person represents a different domain science, one of which is healthcare informatics.

Because healthcare informatics is a relatively young addition to the informatics umbrella, you may see other terms that seem to be synonyms for this same area, such as health informatics or medical informatics. Medical informatics, historically, was used in Europe and the United States as the preferred term for healthcare informatics. Now, medical informatics is more clearly realized as a subset of healthcare informatics, and health informatics may mean informatics used in educating healthcare clients and/or the general public. As healthcare informatics evolves, so will the clarity in definition of terms and scopes of practice.

Healthcare informatics addresses the study and management of healthcare information. A model of overlapping discrete circles could depict the integrated content most often considered representative of the multiple and diverse aspects of healthcare informatics. Healthcare informatics would be the largest encompassing circle surrounding smaller intersecting circles. These aspects include specific content areas such as information retrieval, ethics, security, decision support, patient care, system life cycle, evaluation, human–computer interaction (HCI), standards, telehealth, healthcare information systems, imaging, knowledge representation, electronic health records (EHRs), education, and information retrieval.

Nursing Informatics

Nursing informatics (NI) is a subset of healthcare informatics. It shares common areas of science with other health professions and, therefore, easily supports interprofessional education, practice, and research focused on healthcare informatics. Nursing informatics also has unique areas that address the special information needs for the nursing profession. Nurses work both collaboratively with other healthcare professionals and independently when engaged in clinical and administrative nursing practice. Nursing informatics reflects this duality as well, moving in and out of integration and separation as situations and needs demand.

In 1985, Kathryn Hannah proposed a definition that nursing informatics is the use of information technologies in relation to any nursing functions and actions of nurses (Hannah, 1985). In their classic article on the science of nursing informatics, Graves and Corcoran presented a more complex definition of nursing informatics. Nursing informatics is a combination of computer science, information science, and nursing science designed to assist in the management and processing of nursing data, information, and knowledge to support the practice of nursing and the delivery of nursing care (Graves & Corcoran, 1989).

The ANA modified the Graves and Corcoran definition with the development of the first scope of practice statement for nursing informatics. The ANA defined nursing informatics as the specialty that integrates nursing science, computer science, and information science in identifying, collecting, processing, and managing data and information to support nursing practice, administration, education, research, and the expansion of nursing knowledge (American Nurses Association, 1994). The explanation of the accompanying standards of practice for nursing informatics followed in 1995 with ANA's publication of the *Standards of Nursing Informatics Practice* (American Nurses Association, 1995).

In 2000, the ANA convened an expert panel to review and revise the scope and standards of nursing informatics practice. That group's work included an extensive examination of the evolving healthcare and nursing environments and culminated in the publication of the *Scope and Standards of Nursing Informatics Practice* (American Nurses Association, 2001b). This professional document includes an expanded definition of nursing informatics that was slightly revised in the 2008 *Nursing Informatics: Scope and Standards of Practice* to include wisdom:

> Nursing informatics (NI) is a specialty that integrates nursing science, computer science, and information science to manage and communicate data, information, knowledge, and wisdom in nursing practice. NI supports consumers, patients, nurses, and other providers in their decision-making in all roles and settings. This support is accomplished through the use of information structures, information processes, and information technology. (American Nurses Association, 2008, p. 1)

Further into the revised 2008 document, a slightly amended definition is provided:

> Nursing informatics is a specialty that integrates nursing science, computer science, and information science to manage and communicate data, information, knowledge, and wisdom in nursing practice. Nursing informatics facilitates the integration of data, information, knowledge, and wisdom to support patients, nurses, and other providers in their decision-making in all roles and settings. This support is accomplished through the use of information structures, information processes, and information technology. (American Nurses Association, 2008)

The Nursing Informatics Special Interest Group of the International Medical Informatics Association (IMIA-NI) adopted the following definition in 2009:

> Nursing informatics science and practice integrates nursing, its information and knowledge and their management with information and communication technologies to promote the health of people, families, and communities worldwide.

Then, in 2014, ANA's second edition of *Nursing Informatics: Scope and Standards of Practice* presented an updated definition:

> Nursing informatics (NI) is a specialty that integrates nursing science with multiple information management and analytical sciences to identify, define, manage, and communicate data, information, knowledge, and wisdom in nursing practice. NI supports consumers, patients, nurses, and other healthcare professionals in their decision-making in all roles and settings to achieve desired outcomes. This support is accomplished through the use of information structures, information processes, and information technology. (American Nurses Association, 2014)

These multiple definitions illustrate the dynamic, developing nature of this still-young nursing specialty. Development of different definitions and a healthy debate on those definitions promotes validation of key elements and concepts. A willingness to continue exploring possible definitions can prevent premature conceptual closure, which may lead to errors in synthesis and knowledge development.

Nursing Informatics as a Specialty

Characteristics of a nursing specialty include differentiated practice, a well-derived knowledge base, a defined research program, organizational representation, educational programs, and a credentialing mechanism.

In early 1992, the ANA recognized nursing informatics as a specialty in nursing with a distinct body of knowledge. Unique among the healthcare professions, this designation as a specialty provides official recognition that nursing informatics is indeed a part of nursing and that it has a distinct scope of practice.

The core phenomena of nursing are the nurse, person, health, and environment. Nursing informatics focuses on the information of nursing needed to address these core phenomena. Within this focus are the metastructures or overarching concepts of nursing informatics: data, information, knowledge, and wisdom. It is this special focus on the information of nursing that differentiates nursing informatics from other nursing specialties.

Research programs in NI are guided by the research priorities set by National Institute for Nursing Research (NINR). These priorities, first identified in 1993, are using data, information, and knowledge to deliver and manage care; defining and describing data and information for patient care; acquiring and delivering knowledge from and for patient care; investigating new technologies to create tools for patient care; applying patient care ergonomics to the patient–nurse–machine interaction; integrating systems for better patient care; and evaluating the effects of nursing informatics solutions. Table 15.2 lists the specific informatics priorities identified by NINR.

Nursing informatics is represented in international, national, regional, and local organizations. For example, there is a nursing informatics working group in the American Medical Informatics Association (AMIA) and in the International Medical Informatics Association (IMIA). Nursing informatics is part of the clinical section of the Healthcare Information and Management Systems Society (HIMSS). The International Council of Nurses regularly addresses NI issues and NI use in nursing practice.

Increasingly, nursing school curricula include content, and sometimes complete courses, on information technologies in healthcare and nursing. In 1989, the University of Maryland established the first graduate program in nursing informatics. The University of Utah followed in 1990. Now, there are several in-person and online programs for graduate work in this specialty. Doctoral programs in nursing informatics have been established.

Following the publication of the first nursing informatics scope of practice and standards documents,

TABLE 15.2	Summary of NI Research Priorities From NINR Expert Panel (1993) and Delphi Survey (1998)

Priority Research Areas

User needs

Identification of users' (nurses, patients, families) information needs

Nature and processes of clinical decision-making and skill development

Match information technologies to nursing work patterns

Capture, representation, and storage of data, information, and knowledge

Develop, validate, and formalize nursing language terms, taxonomies, and classifications

Interdigitate nursing language schemes with larger standards initiatives

Design and management of nursing information databases for use in patient management, clinical records, and research

Develop and test clinical data storage schemes that optimize single-recording, multiple use in nursing

Develop alternative modes of conceptualizing, operationalizing, quantifying, and representing nursing information for incorporation into future information systems

Demonstrate connectivity architecture for capture and storage of patient care information across settings

Informatics support for nursing and healthcare practice

Technology development, including decision support systems to support nursing practice (integrates human–computer interaction)

Use of telecommunications technology for nursing practice

Professional practice issues (e.g., competencies, confidentiality)

Informatics support for patients/families/consumers

Patients' use of information technology

Consumer health informatics

Informatics support for practice-based knowledge generation

Develop systems to build clinical databases to generate and analyze knowledge linkages among resource consumption (structure), care processes (including nursing diagnoses and interventions), and outcomes to guide practice and policy

Design and evaluation methodologies

Develop evaluation methodologies for studying system use and impact on nursing decision-making, nursing practice, and, if possible, patient outcomes

Systems modelling and evaluation

Reproduced, with permission, from Bakken, S., Stone, P.W., & Larson, E.L. (2008). A nursing informatics research agenda for 2008-18: Contextual influences and key components. *Nursing Outlook, 56*(5), 206–214. e3. © Elsevier.

the American Nurses Credentialing Center (ANCC) established a certification process and examination in 1995 to recognize those nurses with basic informatics specialty competencies. The ANCC has used scholarship on nursing-informatics competencies and its own role-delineation studies to develop and maintain the nursing-informatics certification examination. The ANCC-designated NI content-expert panel has oversight responsibility for the content of this examination and considers the current informatics environment and research when defining the test-content outline. The test-content outline is available for free on the ANCC Web site.

The Healthcare Information and Management Systems Society (HIMSS) established a certification program, known as the certified professional in healthcare information and management systems (CPHIMS), which may be of interest to informatics nurses.

Two other informatics-related certification programs are offered by the American Health Information Management Association (AHIMA). The first certification is as a registered health information administrator (RHIA). A RHIA manages patient health information and medical records, administers computer information systems, collects and analyzes patient data, and uses various classification systems and medical terminologies. The second

AHIMA certification is as a registered health information technician (RHIT). In this specialty, professionals ensure the completeness and accuracy of patient data entered into computer systems and focus on coding of diagnoses and patient procedures.

Models for Nursing Informatics

The foundations of nursing informatics are the core phenomena and nursing-informatics models. The core phenomena are data, information, knowledge, and wisdom and the transformations that each of these undergo.

Models are representations of some aspect of the real world. Models show particular perspectives of a selected aspect and may illustrate relationships. Models evolve as knowledge about the selected aspect changes and are dependent on the worldview of those developing the model. It is important to remember that different models reflect different viewpoints and are not necessarily competitive; that is, there is no one, right model.

A clinical-information-system (CIS) model shows how modelling can be used to organize different concepts into a logical whole. The purpose of this model is to depict system components, influencing factors, and relationships that need to be considered when attempting to capture the complexities of professional nursing practice.

Different scholars in nursing informatics have proposed different models. Some of these models are presented here to provide further perspectives on nursing informatics, to demonstrate how differently scholars and practitioners may view what seems to be the same thing, and to show that nursing informatics is an evolutionary, theoretical, and practical science. Again, remember that there is no one, right model nor are any of the models presented here exhaustive of the possible perspectives of nursing informatics.

Graves and Corcoran's seminal work included a model of nursing informatics. Their model placed data, information, and knowledge in sequential boxes with one-way arrows pointing from data to information to knowledge. The management processing box is directly above, with arrows pointing in one direction from management processing to each of the three boxes (Graves & Corcoran, 1989). The model is a direct depiction of their definition of nursing informatics.

In 1986, Patricia Schwirian proposed a model of nursing informatics intended to stimulate and guide systematic research in this discipline. Her concern was over the sparse volume of research literature in nursing informatics. The model provides a framework for identifying significant information needs, which, in turn, can foster research. In this model, there are four primary elements arranged

in a pyramid with a triangular base. The four elements are the raw material (nursing-related information), the technology (a computing system comprised of hardware and software), the users surrounded by context (nurses, students), and the goal (or objective) toward which the preceding elements are directed. Bidirectional arrows connect the three base components of raw material, user, and computer system to form the pyramid's triangular base. The goal element is placed at the apex of the pyramid to show its importance. Similarly, all interactions between the three base elements and the goal are represented by bidirectional arrows (Schwirian, 1986).

Turley, writing in 1996, proposed another model in which the core components of informatics (cognitive science, information science, and computer science) are depicted as intersecting circles. In Turley's model, nursing science is a larger circle that completely encompasses the intersecting circles. Nursing informatics is the intersection between the discipline-specific science (nursing) and the area of informatics (Turley, 1996).

McGonigle and Mastrian (2012) developed the foundation of knowledge model. The base of this model shows data and information distributed randomly. From this base, transparent cones grow upward and intersect. The upward cones represent acquisition, generation, and dissemination of knowledge. Knowledge processing is represented by the intersections of these three cones. Circling and connecting all of the cones is feedback. The cones and feedback circle are dynamic in nature (McGonigle & Mastrian, 2012).

Theories Supporting Nursing Informatics

A theory is a scholarly, organized view of some aspect of the world (reality). Theories can describe, explain, predict, or prescribe selected phenomena within this reality. The concepts within a theory are interrelated. Testing of these relationships through research is how theories gain or lose supporting evidence (Karnick, 2013). A profession needs theories to build evidence for the existence of a unique body of knowledge (Bond et al., 2011).

Theories can be classified as grand, middle-range, and situation-specific or practice theories. Grand theories are broad in scope and the most complex of the three classifications. Practice theories are the most specific of the three. These theories usually provide prescriptions or directions for practitioners. Middle-range theories are somewhere in the middle of these two ends—they are more specific than grand theories but not as prescriptive as practice theories.

Theories are part of an interrelated, circular triad: research, theory, and practice. Entry into this triad can occur at any point. For example, research leads to the development of theory, which can be applied to practice. Alternatively, practitioners can raise questions about clients and/or activities related to clients, which leads to research that generates theory. As pointed out earlier, theory generates research for testing. Validation of a theory can guide practice.

Theories related to and supportive of nursing informatics are numerous. These theories include—but are not limited to—information, cognitive, computer science, systems, change, adult learning, organizational behavior, management, and group dynamics.

Nursing Theories. Nursing theories are about nursing practice—a nurse's interactions or relationships with individuals, groups, or communities (also known as patients or clients) focused on applying the nursing process. Grand nursing theories discuss nursing practice in broad terms, providing different worldviews of how, when, and why nurses relate to clients. Middle-range nursing theories might describe a particular phenomenon of interest to nurses, explain how one phenomenon relates to one or more other phenomena, or predict how a phenomenon impacts nurses and/or clients. A particular approach to breast feeding or a set of specific principles for the care of preterm infants that improves their health outcomes are two examples of practice theories in nursing. Any nursing theory might be useful for an informatics nurse, since informatics nurses work with individuals, groups, and communities. It is beyond the scope of this chapter to examine particular theories and how they can be applied. Informatics nurses are encouraged to consult the numerous texts on nursing theory.

Novice to Expert. In 1989, Dreyfus and Dreyfus published a model on how people in a profession become experts. They proposed five stages: novice, advanced beginner, competent, proficient, and expert (Dreyfus & Dreyfus, 1980). Patricia Benner and other nurse educators adapted this model to explain how nursing students and professional nurses acquired nursing skills. A novice follows rules provided for each situation and is not flexible in real-life situations. As a novice acquires real-life experiences and can appreciate environmental influences on rule sets, he or she moves to the advanced beginner stage. At the competent stage, a learner is able to tell what is important and what is not important in assessing a given situation—a learner has gained perspective. A proficient practitioner is able to see a situation in terms of the larger setting or environmental situation and begins to use intuition in decision-making. Finally, an expert intuitively understands a situation and immediately connects action to this understanding (Ajay, 2003).

Computer Science. Computer science is the study of algorithms for solving computation problems. If an algorithm can be identified for solving a particular problem, an automated solution to the problem can be developed. Once an automated solution is developed, a machine can be built (or a person can be hired) to solve the solution without the person or machine needing to understand the solution. A computer is a tool of this science, not its focus.

Computer science has many subfields. Some emphasize computation of specific results (such as computer graphics), while others relate to properties of computational problems (for example, computational complexity). Others focus on challenges in implementing computations. For example, programming language theory studies ways to describe computations; computer programming applies specific programming languages to solve specific computational problems. Despite its name, computer science rarely involves the study of computers themselves. A computer is a tool of this science, not its focus. Computer science research has often crossed into other disciplines, such as artificial intelligence, cognitive science, physics, information science, and linguistics.

Information Science. Information science focuses on the gathering, manipulation, classification, storage, and retrieval of recorded knowledge. Information science can be socially oriented, focused on humans and machines, and closely linked to communications and human behavior. Information science tries to understand problems from the perspective of the stakeholders and applies information and technology as needed to solve the problems. Three important branches of information science are information retrieval, human–computer interactions—from the perspective of knowledge manipulation, and information handling within a system (human or machine).

For classic information theory, a central problem has been the engineering problem of the transmission of information over a noisy channel. The decisive event that established the discipline of information theory, and brought it to immediate worldwide attention, was the publication of Shannon's classic paper, A Mathematical Theory of Communication, in the *Bell System Technical Journal* in 1948 (Shannon, 1948). Soon after this publication, Weaver coauthored with Shannon a book titled *The Mathematical Theory of Communication* (1949). This work introduced the concept of the communication channel. This communication channel consists of a sender (a source of information), a transmission medium (with noise and distortion), and a receiver (whose goal is to reconstruct the sender's messages).

Another core concept is encoding and decoding. If the amount of information to be transmitted exceeds the channel capacity, there are unavoidable and uncorrectable errors in the transmission. If the amount of information to be sent is below the channel capacity, there is a way to encode the information so that it can be received without errors. Once encoded, the receiver has to decode the message.

These authors, for the first time, introduced the qualitative and quantitative model of communication as a statistical process underlying information theory, opening with the assertion that: "The fundamental problem of communication is that of reproducing at one point, either exactly or approximately, a message selected at another point" (p. 3).

Communication. Communication theory uses these core concepts and additional principles developed since then to analyze information transfer and the effectiveness and efficiency of communications. If the sender's entropy rate is below the channel capacity, there is a way to encode the information so that it can be received without errors. This is true even if the channel distorts the message during transmission.

Within a communication model, Bruce I. Blum presented a taxonomy, with definitions, of the central concepts of data, information, and knowledge. These are the concepts adopted by NI. Blum defined data as discrete entities that are described objectively without interpretation. That is, the facts, without context. Data are sometimes referred to as being "raw." Information is data that are interpreted, organized, or structured. It brings in the idea of processing data so that it can be displayed or presented for human use (Blum, 1985). Knowledge is information that has been synthesized so that interrelationships of data and information are identified and formalized. Many informatics theorists have added the concept of Wisdom to Blum's theory. Think of wisdom as the appropriate use of knowledge in managing and solving problems. As noted earlier, these terms are on a continuum of simple to complex, beginning with data and proceeding toward wisdom.

Cognitive Science. At its most basic, cognitive science is the study of the mind—of how we think. Another way of saying this is that cognitive science looks at mental activities and processes. This science is broad in scope and in the sciences it encompasses. Cognitive technologies, including computers, smart phones, and Web browsers, are media emerging from cognitive science that help in learning, memory, problem solving, and living daily life in modern society. Cognitive enhancements of biological-based

intelligence and so-called artificial intelligence are two significant branches of these technologies (Verdoux, 2011).

Systems. Systems theory relates to the properties of systems as a whole. Systems theory focuses on the organization and interdependence of relationships within a system. A system is any set (group) of interdependent or temporarily interacting parts. Parts are systems themselves and are composed of other parts. The boundary of a system may be open or closed. A closed system has an impermeable boundary and does not interact with the surrounding environment. One example of a closed system is the human circulatory system. The circulatory system is considered closed because the blood never leaves the system of blood vessels.

An open system can be influenced by events outside of the actual or conceptual boundaries. Open systems usually have semipermeable boundaries that restrict the exchange of selective components but allow free exchange of all other components. An open system interacts with the surrounding environment. Information systems and people are usually considered open systems, although there can be closed systems within these open systems (e.g., the circulatory system).

The basic model of a system is one of inputs crossing the boundary, processing of the input through the system (throughput), and the emergence through the system boundary of some kind of output. Along with this basic model, there are other common elements to every open system. These are feedback, control, environment, and goal.

Systems are constantly changing. There are six key concepts related understanding system change: dynamic homeostasis, entropy, negentropy, specialization, reverberation, and equifinality. Dynamic homeostasis preserves the character of a system through its growth. From an organizational perspective, look at this concept by considering that open organizational systems use internal review processes to modify their environmental scanning, input, transformation, and output processes in order to adapt to the changing environment, while still staying focused on their core competency. These modifications lead to quantitative and qualitative growth of an organization's ability to respond to future events. The same processes hold true for organizational programs and projects such as information system implementation.

While there are many definitions of entropy, all seem to point in the same direction—entropy is disorder or breaking down into the smallest parts. In communication theory, entropy is a measure of the loss of information in a transmitted message. Reverberation is the idea that when one part of a system changes, other parts of the system are affected. The effects on other parts of the system can lead to expected and unexpected consequences. Equifinality is the principle by which a system can get to the same end (or goal) from various different routes. That is, the same inputs can result in the same outputs but by different processes. If you (as a subsystem) are required to obtain a book via input from the system (e.g., a course on informatics), you may return to the system with the book (a form of output) that you may have picked up from a friend, a bookstore, or a library.

Behavioral and Social Sciences. The study of behavior—the processes driving actions—is the focus of the behavioral and social sciences. These two terms, behavioral and social, are often combined or used interchangeably when examining how people act alone (as individuals) and with others. Behavior can include emotions, cognition, and motivation. Social processes and acts can be status (demographic, economic, or cultural), levels of social context, and biosocial interactions (Office of Behavioral and Social Sciences, 2010).

Change. Change is disruptive, messy, and complicated. Even with the best laid plans, events rarely occur exactly as they were predicted. In healthcare informatics and nursing informatics, change most often has to be dealt with among groups of people and healthcare organizations. Change processes entail not only structures and ways of doing tasks, but also the performance, expectations, and perceptions of all involved parties.

The informatics nurse specialist (INS) is often the primary change agent in facilitating the implementation of clinical information systems (CIS) in healthcare settings. The INS has a unique understanding of the nursing issues that can affect the change process, and thus, is in a key position to facilitate positive implementation outcomes.

A study of change processes and change theories will show many models and theories of planned change. A planned-change theory is a collection of ideas about modifications to an organization or social system that are explicitly designed and put into place. That is, the changes do not happen by chance. These theories provide overall guidance for change-agent efforts. Two of the most familiar perspectives are Lewin's theory on planned change and the diffusion-of-innovations model developed by Rogers.

Lewin's basic planned-change model has three stages: unfreezing, changing, and refreezing. Unfreezing involves overcoming inertia and dismantling the existing mind-set. Defense mechanisms or resistance patterns have to be bypassed. Measuring the perceptions of those who will experience the change is an important part of this stage. A change agent must uncover reasons or rewards that will be influential in unfreezing or changing a behavior—that

is, what is important to the people? To apply this idea to nursing informatics, consider an information system implementation. In this situation, the identified reasons or rewards can be used to help convert behavioral intent (e.g., people considering adopting the system) to actual behavior (people become active system users) (Wells, Manuel, & Cunning, 2011).

In the second stage, called moving, the behavioral change occurs. Typically, this stage is a period of confusion. People are aware that the old ways are being challenged but do not yet have a clear picture of how to replace the old ways. The third—final—stage is "refreezing." A new mind-set has formed, and the comfort level is returning to previous levels (Wells et al., 2011).

Diffusion of innovation looks at how, why, and at what rate new ideas and technologies spread through cultures. It is examination of the process for communicating an innovation throughout a social system.

Everett Rogers formalized the diffusion-of-innovations theory in a 1962 book called *Diffusion of Innovations.* In his work, Rogers identified five specific groups of innovation adopters. These groups are known as innovators, early adopters, early majority, late majority, and laggards. The distribution (or percentage of each category in a population) approximates a bell curve. Each adopter's willingness and ability to adopt an innovation would depend on their awareness, interest, evaluation, trial, and adoption. Rogers also presented characteristics for each category of adopter (Rogers, 2003).

Along with the concept of different categories of innovation adopters, Rogers proposed a five-stage model for the diffusion of innovation:

- Stage 1 is knowledge—learning about the existence and function of the innovation.
- Stage 2 is persuasion—becoming convinced of the value of the innovation.
- In Stage 3, the adopter makes a decision—committing to the adoption of the innovation.
- Implementation—putting it to use—is Stage 4.
- The final Stage is confirmation—the ultimate acceptance (or rejection) of the innovation (Rogers, 2003).

How does this theory apply to the work of an informatics nurse? Understanding the social forces underlying innovation diffusion is critical for effective management of the process of implementing an informatics innovation, such as a healthcare information system. Because of the investment of time, energy, and economic resources in implementing an information system, organizations—and the people involved in the implementation—must be aware of the human elements influencing successful implementation and subsequent adoption. To be adopted, innovations must appeal to people. People must see something in an innovation that they like or want.

Rogers also identified characteristics of an innovation that most affect the rate of adoption. These characteristics are relative advantage, compatibility, complexity, trialability, and observability.

Relative advantage refers to the degree to which an innovation is perceived as better than the idea it replaces. This is a positive characteristic. Another positive characteristic is compatibility. Compatibility is the degree to which an innovation is perceived as being consistent with existing values, past experiences, and needs of potential adopters. Complexity, as defined by Rogers, is a negative characteristic. It is the degree to which an innovation is perceived as difficult to understand and use. Trialability, another positive characteristic, is the degree to which an innovation may be tried out or experimented with. The last characteristic, observability, is the degree to which the results of an innovation are visible to others. It also is a positive characteristic. In summary, Rogers asserts that innovations perceived by potential adopters as having greater relative advantage, compatibility, trialability, and observability, and less complexity will be adopted more rapidly than other innovations (Rogers, 2003). In other words, the adoption of an innovation by an individual depends on how the individual perceives that innovation.

Learning. Learning is a process of acquiring knowledge, skills, attitudes, or values through study, experience, or teaching. Learning causes a change in behavior that is persistent, measurable, and specified. Learning allows someone to formulate a new mental construct or revise a prior mental construct. There are numerous theories addressing how people learn. Obviously, it is beyond the scope of this chapter to delve into all these theories. A look at categories of these theories will help guide further study. One approach is to categorize learning theories as behavioral, cognitive, adult learning, and learning styles.

Behaviorists believe that learning processes can be studied most objectively when the focus is on stimuli and responses (also known as operant conditioning). At a very simplistic level, think of this learning approach as having two basic elements. First, there is a pairing—a combination of a stimulus and a response. Then, there is reinforcement, which is the stimulus-response element that has two pathways. One is positive reinforcement in which every stimulus is followed by something pleasant or in which the stimulus itself is a good experience. This positive experience encourages continued learning. The other pathway

is negative reinforcement where learners may associate a stimulus with unpleasant or painful experiences.

Cognitive learning theory focuses on internal mental processes, including insight, information processing, memory, and perception. Cognitivists attempt to model how information is received, assimilated, stored, and recalled. Cognitive learning theory divides learning (or to be more precise, it divides information processing) into four steps. These are information input (information is received by the learner), input processing (the information is either remembered only for a short time or is moved to long-term memory where it can be drawn upon as needed), output behaviors (that demonstrate if learning has taken place), and the use of feedback to embed the same information more firmly or to correct errors.

Proponents of learning styles theory assert that individuals have a tendency to both perceive and process information differently. There are concrete and abstract perceivers and active and reflective processors. Concrete perceivers absorb information through direct experience by doing, acting, sensing, and feeling. Abstract perceivers take in information through analysis, observation, and thinking. Active processors make sense of an experience by immediately using the new information. Reflective processors make sense of an experience by reflecting on and thinking about it.

Adult learning theory focuses on understanding how adults learn as opposed to children. Adult learners bring a great deal of experience to the learning environment. Educators can use this experience as a resource. Adults expect to have a high degree of influence on what they are to be educated for and how they are to be educated. The active participation of learners should be encouraged in designing and implementing educational programs. Adults need to be able to see applications for new learning. Adult learners expect to have a high degree of influence on how learning will be evaluated. Adults expect their responses to be acted upon when asked for feedback on the progress of the program.

Organizational Behavior. Organizational behavior is a distinct field focused on organizations. In this field, organizations are examined, using the methods drawn from economics, sociology, political science, anthropology, and psychology. Both individual and group dynamics in an organizational setting are studied, as well as the nature of the organizations themselves. Organizational behavior is becoming more important in the global economy as people with diverse backgrounds and cultural values have to work together effectively and efficiently. A healthy organization has a balance, among the participants, of autonomy, control, and cooperation. Understanding how organizations behave, and how a particular organization behaves, can guide planning for information system implementations.

Management. Management science uses mathematics and other analytical methods to help make better decisions, generally in a business context. While often considered synonymous with operations research (OR), management science is differentiated from OR by a more practical, rather than academic, bent.

The management scientist uses rational, systematic, science-based techniques to inform and improve decisions of all kinds. Naturally, the techniques of management science are not restricted to business applications but may be applied to military situations, clinical decision support, public administration, charitable groups, political groups, or community groups. Some of the methods within management science are decision analysis, optimization, simulation, forecasting, game theory, graph theory, network problems, transportation-forecasting models, mathematical modeling, and queuing theory, as well as many others.

Group Dynamics. Group dynamics is a social science field that focuses on the nature of groups. Urges to belong or to identify may make for distinctly different attitudes (recognized or unrecognized), and the influence of a group may rapidly become strong, influencing or overwhelming individual proclivities and actions.

Within any organization, there are formal and informal groups, each applying pressure on individuals to different degrees. Informal groups have a powerful influence on the effectiveness of an organization, and can even subvert its formal goals. But the informal group's role is not limited to resistance. The impact of the informal group upon the larger formal group depends on the norms that the informal group sets. So the informal group can make the formal organization more effective, too.

Bruce Tuckman (1965) proposed a four-stage model, called Tuckman's stages, for a group. Tuckman's model states that the ideal group decision-making process should occur in four stages:

- Forming (pretending to get on or get along with others)

- Storming (letting down the politeness barrier and trying to get down to the issues even if tempers flare up)

- Norming (getting used to each other and developing trust and productivity)

- Performing (working in a group to a common goal on a highly efficient and cooperative basis)

COMPETENCIES

Benner's work, built on the Dreyfus model of skill acquisition, describes the evolution of novice to expert and merits discussion for nursing informatics. This desired change in skills involves the evolution from a novice level to advanced beginner to competent to proficient to, finally, an expert level. Every nurse must continually exhibit the capability to acquire and then demonstrate specific skills, beginning with the very first student experience. As students, most individuals can be described as novices having no experience with the situations and related content in those situations where they are expected to begin developing competencies by performing tasks that refine their skills. The advanced beginner can marginally demonstrate acceptable performance, having built on lessons learned in an expanding experience base. Individuals at these levels often need oversight by teachers or experienced colleagues to help structure the learning experience and support appropriate and successful workplace decision-making and action (Benner, 2004).

Increased proficiency over time results in enhanced competencies reflecting mastery and the ability to cope with and manage many contingencies. Continued practice, combined with additional professional experience and knowledge, allows the nurse to evolve to the proficient level of appreciating the rules and maxims of practice and the nuances that are reflected in the absence of the normal picture. The expert has the capacity to intuitively understand a situation and immediately target the problem with minimal effort or problem solving (Benner, 2004).

Staggers, Gassert, and Curran are most often cited as the first published research identifying the informatics competencies necessary for all nurses (Staggers, Gassert, & Curran, 2001). Their conceptual framework included computer skills, informatics knowledge, and informatics skills as the informatics competencies. Their research, however, only identified informatics competencies for four levels of nurses: beginning nurse, experienced nurse, informatics specialist, and informatics innovator. The comprehensive list of 304 competencies posed a significant challenge for professional development and academic faculties wishing to address each of the competencies when preparing curricula and then teaching educational programs for all skill levels.

Further competencies-definition work was completed by the workgroup that developed the 2008 NI scope and standards document. Their review of the literature culminated in a two-page matrix that included delineation by computer and information literacy (American Nurses Association, 2008).

The Technology Informatics Guiding Educational Reform (TIGER) initiative moved from an invitational conference to volunteer task forces, also known as collaboratives, to systematically develop key content related to discrete topics, including nursing informatics competencies. The TIGER collaborative on competencies focused on the minimum set of informatics competencies needed by every nurse. These competencies are organized into three categories: basic computer skills, information literacy, and information management (The TIGER Initiative, n.d.).

The National League for Nursing (NLN) has developed a set of competencies for nursing educators. These may be found on the NLN Web site. A recent study presents an updated summary and analysis of other work done on developing nursing-informatics competencies (Carter-Templeton, Patterson, & Russell, 2009). These authors note variation in content, presentation, and audience among the sets of competencies reviewed.

Instruments to assess perceived levels of NI competency are emerging in the scholarly literature. Yoon, Yen, and Bakken (2009) described the validation of an instrument titled the Self-Assessment of Nursing Informatics Competencies Scale. This scale incorporates selected items from the work of Staggers, Gassert, and Curran along with items addressed in a specific NI curriculum (Yoon et al., 2009). In 2013, Hunter, McGonigle, and Hebda published the results of validity and reliability testing on an online self-assessment tool entitled TIGER-based Assessment of Nursing Informatics Competencies (TANIC)©. TANIC uses all of the competencies identified by the TIGER Institute (Hunter, McGonigle, & Hebda, 2013). The level 3 and level 4 competencies identified by Staggers, Gassert, and Curran were organized into an online instrument by McGonigle, Hunter, Hebda, and Hill. This instrument, titled Nursing Informatics Competencies Assessment Level 3 and Level 4 (NICA L3/L4©), has demonstrated reliability and validity (McGonigle, Hunter, Hebda, & Hill, 2013).

ORGANIZATIONS AS RESOURCES

Many organizations have emerged to provide information resources and value-added membership benefits that support those individuals interested in healthcare and nursing informatics. Clinical specialty and other professional organizations have also appreciated the evolving healthcare-information-management focus and have established organizational structures such as informatics sections, divisions, workgroups, or special-interest groups. Some have incorporated informatics and information system technology initiatives in strategic plans with dedicated staffing and ongoing financial support. In many instances, informal networking groups have evolved into international organizations with hundreds of members connected via the Web.

The nature, purposes, and activities of the multiple informatics organizations have sufficient differences that there is bound to be at least one organization, if not more, for everyone interested in nursing informatics. Information about a few of these organizations is provided here. The information for each group was adapted from each group's Web site.

Only national or international informatics-related organizations with nursing groups are included. All of the groups presented here are accessible to individual nurses for more information and/or participation. This content is in no way an exhaustive presentation. To learn more about these organizations and others, consult the Internet, informatics colleagues, and the scholarly literature. A list of these organizations is found in Table 15.3.

American Nurses Association and Specialty Nursing Organizations

The American Nurses Association (ANA) and its affiliates and several nursing-specialty organizations have informatics committees and government affairs offices addressing information technology, EHRs, standards, and other informatics issues. Membership and active participation in such professional organizations demonstrate compliance with Provisions 8 and 9 of the

TABLE 15.3	Resource Organizations
American Nurses Association	
AMIA Nursing Informatics Working Group (NIWG)	
American Nursing Informatics Association (ANIA)	
British Computer Society (BCS) Nursing Specialist Group (NSG)	
HIMSS Nursing Informatics Community	
NLN Educational Technology and Information Management Advisory Council (ETIMAC)	
Nursing Informatics Australia (NIA)	
Nursing Informatics Special Interest Group of the International Medical Informatics Association (IMIA/NI-SIG)	
Alliance for Nursing Informatics (ANI)	
TIGER Initiative Foundation	
Canadian Nursing Informatics Association (CNIA)	
American Academy of Nursing (AAN) Expert Panel on Nursing Informatics and Technology	
Sigma Theta Tau International (STTI)	

Code of Ethics for Nurses with Interpretive Statements (ANA, 2001a) and Standard 12: Leadership, described in *Nursing Informatics: Scope and Standards of Practice*, 2nd ed. (American Nurses Association, 2014).

AMIA Nursing Informatics Working Group

AMIA is a non-profit membership organization of individuals, institutions, and corporations dedicated to developing and using information technologies to improve healthcare. The Nursing Informatics Working Group (NIWG) within AMIA aims to promote and advance nursing informatics within the larger context of health informatics.

The NIWG pursues this mission in many areas, such as professional practice, education, research, governmental and other service, professional organizations, and industry. Member services, outreach functions, official representation to Nursing Informatics Special Interest Group of the International Medical Informatics Association (IMIA-NI), and liaison activities to other national and international groups are some of the activities of this working group.

NIWG has established three awards that recognize excellence in nursing informatics: the Student Award, the Harriet Werley Award, and the Virginia K. Saba Informatics Award.

American Nursing Informatics Association

In January 2010, two nursing-informatics organizations (American Nursing Informatics Association and CARING) merged to form American Nursing Informatics Association (ANIA). The combined organization, with a 3000-plus membership in 50 states and 34 countries, is one of the largest associations of its kind in the United States. The organization is dedicated to advancing the field of nursing informatics through communications, education, research, and professional activities. There is an annual spring conference. A newsletter is published quarterly and is indexed in CINAHL and Thompson. ANIA runs a very active e-mail list and provides access to a large job bank, listing over 800 employer-paid positions.

British Computer Society Nursing Specialist Group

The British Computer Society (BCS) promotes wider social and economic progress through the advancement of information technology science and practice. The Nursing Specialist Group (NSG) is one of five health informatics specialist groups (HISGS) within the BCS. NSG contributes to national and international debates on information management and information technology issues within healthcare. NSG converses and collaborates with other nursing groups within the United Kingdom and with international informatics groups. The NSG contributes to the annual Healthcare Computing (HC) Conferences run by the BCS Health Informatics Committee (HIC), supplemented by special topic meetings organized by the various focus, geographic, and affiliated groups.

HIMSS Nursing Informatics Community

The Healthcare Information and Management Systems Society (HIMSS) provides leadership for the management of healthcare-related technology, information, and change through publications, educational opportunities, and member services. The HIMSS Nursing Informatics Community reflects the increased recognition of the role of the informatics nurse professional in healthcare information and management systems. This community speaks in a unified voice for the HIMSS members who practice in the nursing informatics community and provides nursing informatics expertise, leadership, and guidance internally to HIMSS and externally with the global nursing informatics community. The HIMSS Nursing Informatics Committee serves as the leadership for this community. The Nursing Informatics Community has a membership of more than 2000 nurses, representing nearly 10% of HIMSS members.

NLN Educational Technology and Information Management Advisory Council (ETIMAC)

The mission of the NLN is to advance quality nursing education that prepares the nursing workforce to meet the needs of diverse populations in an ever-changing healthcare environment. This advisory group within NLN functions to promote the use of educational technology as a teaching tool, advance the informatics competencies of faculty, integrate informatics competencies into nursing school curricula, promote development of nursing education information management systems, advise professional organizations and other groups about informatics competencies, and collaborate with other NLN advisory councils and groups.

Nursing Informatics Australia

The Nursing Informatics Australia (NIA) is a special interest group (SIG) of the Health Informatics Society of Australia (HISA). The NIA sees the priorities for nursing informatics in Australia as appropriate language, education, and ongoing research. It aims to encourage nurses to embrace information and communication technologies and establish strong foundations for taking these developments forward. The NIA works to ensure nursing has the data and resources to continue providing evidence-based, quality, cost-effective, and outcome-driven care for patients and clients into the future. The NIA holds an annual conference on nursing informatics.

Nursing Informatics Special Interest Group of the International Medical Informatics Association (IMIA/NI-SIG)

This SIG was originally established by IMIA in 1983 as Working Group 8 of IMIA, dedicated to serving the specific needs of nurses in the field of nursing informatics. IMIA-NI focuses on fostering collaboration among nurses and others who are interested in nursing informatics; exploring the scope of nursing informatics and its implication for information-handling activities associated with the delivery of nursing care, nursing administration, nursing research, and nursing education; supporting the development of nursing informatics in the member countries; providing appropriate informatics meetings, conferences, and post-conferences to provide knowledge-sharing opportunities; encouraging dissemination of nursing-informatics research findings; and developing recommendations, guidelines, and courses related to nursing informatics.

Alliance for Nursing Informatics

The Alliance for Nursing Informatics (ANI) is a collaboration of organizations that provides a unified voice for nursing informatics. NI brings together over 25 nursing-informatics groups, mainly in the United States, that function separately at local, regional, national, and international levels. Each of these organizations has its own established programs, publications, and organizational structures. ANI envisions the transformation of health and healthcare through nursing informatics and innovations. Its mission is advancing nursing-informatics leadership, practice, education, policy, and research through a unified voice.

TIGER Initiative Foundation

TIGER is an acronym, standing for Technology Informatics Guiding Education Reform. The TIGER Initiative, a collaboration of individuals and organizations, was created to better enable practicing nurses and nursing students to use information technology and informatics to improve patient-care delivery. The focus of TIGER is to improve the pre-licensure and post-licensure informatics education of registered nurses. TIGER produced a series of collaborative reports describing the current state of affairs for seven critical areas of informatics education and proposing action plans for improving these areas. The TIGER Initiative Foundation was formed in 2011 to carry on this work.

Canadian Nursing Informatics Association

The Canadian Nursing Informatics Association (CNIA) is organized to help Canadian nurses learn about informatics and share, research, and create informatics-related projects and experiences. The result of these endeavors will be to boost the competencies, theory, and practice of nursing informatics across Canada. The mission of the CNIA is to be the voice for nursing informatics in Canada. Recognizing the importance of the work the CNIA is undertaking, the Canadian Nurses Association has granted associate group status to the CNIA. The CNIA is also affiliated with COACH: Canada's Health Informatics Association and the IMIA/SIG-NI.

AMERICAN ACADEMY OF NURSING EXPERT PANEL ON NURSING INFORMATICS AND TECHNOLOGY

This expert panel gathers and disseminates health policy data and information and advises and represents the American Academy of Nursing (AAN) on issues related to health information management, implementation of informatics and information technology through EHRs and PHRs (electronic and personal health records), HIPAA, patient-safety initiatives, consumer and personal health, workforce issues and training, bioterrorism and biosurveillance, evidence-based practice, clinical-decision support, and other areas of concern related to the use of informatics and information technology in nursing education, practice, administration, and research.

Sigma Theta Tau International

Sigma Theta Tau International's mission is to support the learning, knowledge, and professional development of nurses who are committed to making a difference in health worldwide. It has established the Virginia K. Saba Nursing Informatics Leadership Award, given to an informatics expert whose contributions have the capacity and scope to enhance quality, safety, outcomes, and decision-making in health and nursing care from a national or an international perspective. The Ruth Lilly Nursing Informatics Scholar is a two-year award to an individual to contribute to the vision and plan for the Virginia Henderson International Nursing Library's continued contributions to nursing knowledge. STTI is a collaborator in the work of the TIGER Initiative Foundation.

SCOPE OF PRACTICE AND STANDARDS OF PRACTICE

The ANA provides the definition of nursing and is the steward of the nursing profession's foundational documents: the non-negotiable *Code of Ethics for Nurses With Interpretive Statements* (2001) and *Nursing: Scope and Standards of Practice, Second Edition*. ANA, in its role as the professional organization for all registered nurses (RNs) and advanced practice registered nurses (APRNs), also serves as the convening body to facilitate the development and scheduled revision of select specialty-nursing scope of practice statements and accompanying standards of practice. This section provides the history of such ANA action related to the development and recognition of nursing informatics as a nursing specialty. More detailed descriptions of the nursing informatics scope and standards of practice content follow.

NURSING INFORMATICS SCOPE OF PRACTICE STATEMENT

The current, detailed nursing informatics scope-of-practice statement available in *Nursing Informatics: Scope and Standards of Practice, Second Edition*, (2014) provides the definition of nursing informatics and builds on the content incorporated in ANA's 2001 *Code of Ethics for Nurses With Interpretive Statements* and 2010 *Nursing: Scope and Standards of Practice, Second Edition*. Such a nursing scope of practice statement is expected to adequately answer six questions—who, what, when, where, how, and why—so the readers can close their eyes and easily envision both the informatics nurse and the nursing informatics practice. Thoughtful and precise descriptive answers to the six questions in the narrative scope of practice statement provide clarity to enhance understanding about the demonstrated passion of the informatics nurse and informatics nurse specialist, practice characteristics, and professional expectations. Professional colleagues, educators developing curricula and teaching the requisite nursing informatics content, administrators and employers, researchers, healthcare consumers, regulatory and credentialing authorities, and others find such details helpful.

This specialty's registered nurses who have an interest in nursing informatics, have experience, and have been educationally prepared at a baccalaureate level, are identified as informatics nurses (INs). The informatics nurse specialist (INS) is a registered nurse with additional formal graduate-level education in informatics or related fields. The available nursing informatics board certification credentialing option can be obtained and maintained by qualified individuals who meet defined criteria, pass an initial certification examination, and complete continuing education and work-hour requirements. Certification renewals must be completed every five years and require evidence of continuing education and lifelong learning experiences as well as attestation of the required number of informatics-practice hours.

Informatics nurses assume a plethora of titles in their work environments. The diversity of position titles for informatics nurses encountered within the nursing services sector is equivalent to the multitude of titling conventions present in the healthcare or corporate information systems/services divisions. Informatics nurses who bravely embark on entrepreneurial opportunities often create very distinct titles. Examination of job posting/career opportunities boards and services similarly reflect numerous titles that give little inkling of how an informatics nurse might be a stellar candidate. Therefore, the nursing informatics scope-of-practice authors elected to focus on the characteristics, knowledge, skills, and abilities informatics nurses bring to every setting and role.

Further description of the "who" in nursing informatics addresses the recipient of the informatics nurse's and informatics nurse specialist's actions, decisions, and interactions. Professional colleagues, educators developing curricula and teaching the requisite nursing informatics content, administrators and employers, researchers, healthcare consumers, regulatory and credentialing authorities, and others have occasion to interact with informatics nurses. Such interactions include the expectation that the IN and INS easily transition between leader and member roles within interprofessional teams in all practice settings. Note that the IN and INS are most often the individuals who ensure the interprofessional team includes healthcare consumers and redirect the focus to patient/healthcare-consumer centricity.

Diversity, change, and innovation best characterize the activities, decision-making, concerns, foci, goals, and outcomes of nursing informatics practice. Every day, and sometimes every hour, generates unique challenges and opportunities. Perceived barriers need to be addressed and minimized to "speed bump" levels. The "what" so often includes complex, disparate components of a dysfunctional system or enterprise. Nursing informatics practice also addresses the need for assessment, definition, identification of expected outcomes, planning, implementation, and evaluation of the transformation from an "as is" state, condition, or operation to an envisioned and preferred "to be" level or entity. The data, information, knowledge, and wisdom framework, as well as decision support, analytics, and research, constitute additional components of the scope of nursing informatics.

The description of timing and sequencing, understanding the history of a project or program, and appreciation of project management and a system's life cycle are exemplars of the "when" component of a scope of practice statement for nursing informatics. Strategic planning focused on prevention of errors, problems, and unintended consequences, along with attention to effective change management practices and strategies, provide some hope for success in any nursing informatics initiative. Informatics nurses rely on their rich history of attention to detail to precise timing and sequencing ingrained into practice, beginning in the undergraduate nursing education and practicum experiences related to medication administration, clinical documentation, and care planning.

The evolution of the nursing informatics specialty has seen an explosion in the location and settings or "where" of nursing informatics practice. The academic, professional-development, and continuing-education venues have moved from a discrete physical location to a global virtual presence and increasingly embrace online learning programs, gaming, and simulation experiences. INs and INSs are often key developers and contributors in this space. Similar evolution has occurred in the clinical environment with the proliferation of telehealth, tele-ICUs, patient engagement via mobile applications, home health monitoring, and e-mail and other virtual communications technologies. The informatics nurse is no longer limited to employment in acute-care settings and can be found in post-acute and long-term care facilities, public and private school systems, insurance and data analytics venues, corporate offices, research and development environments, and the exciting world of the entrepreneur. The organizational charts and reporting structures vary significantly, so informatics nurses may find themselves assigned to nursing or patient services, information technology or information services, quality improvement and risk management, legal counsel, clinical informatics, or other departments, divisions, or entities. It is not uncommon for the informatics nurse to be assigned to report to supervisors in two divisions, such as nursing services and information technology services. The knowledge, skills, and abilities of the IN and INS to be the liaison or translator are invaluable enablers wherever they practice.

The "how" of nursing informatics begins with the nurse's reliance on the incorporation of the nursing process into all thinking actions and practice activities. The interrelated and iterative nursing-process steps of assessment; diagnosis, problem, or issue identification; outcomes identification; planning; implementation; and evaluation are reflected in the nursing informatics standards of practice and accompanying competencies described later. The nursing informatics professional-performance standards and accompanying competencies provide more detail about the expected professional role performance of the IN and INS.

Nursing informatics practice encompasses a systems perspective where the whole is greater than the sum of its parts. Proactive and preventive thinking and approaches, like those embraced in the clinical practice realm, are particularly helpful during assessment, diagnosis, outcomes identification, planning, and implementation activities. Definition of outcomes is of key importance in any setting and project. Without such clarity, the IN and INS often must address the ensuing ill-defined plans, floundering implementation activities, and unwanted results. The IN and INS rely on both project and change-management knowledge and skills to facilitate successful implementation actions for large projects or smaller upgrades or changes.

In today's healthcare environment, safe, quality, patient-centric, cost-effective, and team-based care is the focus. The informatics nurse and informatics nurse specialist are the primary and often the only advocates for the patient/healthcare consumer-centric perspective in systems' design, development, testing, implementation, and evaluation environments. The IN/INS advocacy role also extends to calling for and all stakeholders, including healthcare consumers, are engaged members of the team. Each IN and INS also has obligations to protect the employer, organization, or enterprise from untoward outcomes.

The "why" of nursing informatics practice derives from the mandate for all registered nurses to abide by the profession's 2001 *Code of Ethics for Nurses With Interpretive Statements*. Each of the nine provisions is applicable to nursing informatics practice and is included in the detailed scope of practice statement in the 2014 *Nursing Informatics: Scope and Standards of Practice, Second Edition*. Standards and best practices for data and information privacy, security, and confidentiality provide detailed direction and guidance for the IN and INS. Local, state, and federal legislation and regulations provide mandates for compliance and reporting that the informatics nurse and informatics nurse specialist address in daily practice such as reporting morbidity, mortality, and operations details via ICD-10-CM, ICD-10-PCS, CPT4, and DSM-5. Publication of metrics associated with safety, quality, and achievement of expected outcomes has gained increased importance because of the call for openness and transparency in healthcare services delivery and the evolution to reimbursement for quality performance. Often, informatics nurses help develop and maintain the resulting dashboards and reports that provide meaningful details and information to healthcare consumers and healthcare professionals.

Data, information, and knowledge management strategies and capabilities associated with department, facility, and enterprise reporting are also requisite for identifying and detailing the contributions and impact of nursing, registered nurses, and advanced practice registered nurses in the delivery of local, regional, state, national, and global healthcare services. Increased public accountability for evidence-based best-practice nursing care requires standardization of metrics and identification and remediation of variances, key concerns for informatics nurses addressing the viability, and availability of supporting healthcare information system resources. Informatics nurses and informatics nurse specialists are integral partners in the innovative development underway and future implementation and reporting for the first electronic quality measure—pressure ulcer incidence and prevention.

Risk mitigation and concerns about legal issues may prompt informatics nurses to delve more deeply into system security, implementation and monitoring of audit trails, prevention of misuse of data, forensics and e-discovery, corporate or organizational liability, de-identified data and big data analytics, and information governance. The IN and INS seek to prevent unintended consequences and harm resulting from implementation of healthcare information systems and poorly designed workflows. Each informatics nurse also has the responsibility to contribute, as a partner, in emergency preparedness and disaster recovery by thinking and keeping the requisite data, information, and knowledge acquisition, management, communication, and storage processing capabilities and actions intact at all times.

STANDARDS OF NURSING INFORMATICS PRACTICE

The nursing informatics scope of practice statement provides a very brief narrative description of the significant diversity, magnitude, influence, and impact of this specialty nursing practice. The accompanying standards of nursing informatics practice content must be

considered as integral to practice and includes two sections: Standards of Practice and Standards of Professional Performance. Each standard statement and the accompanying competencies reflect the language and influence of the general standards of practice and professional performance delineated in the 2010 *Nursing: Scope and Standards of Practice, Second Edition*. Both informatics nurses and informatics nurse specialists are expected to practice in accordance with the standards and demonstrate competence characterized by the accompanying competency statements. In certain instances, additional competencies are applicable to the informatics nurse specialist and are intended to reflect higher expectations for this role's advanced level of practice. The detailed competency statements are not intended to be a complete listing and can be supplemented with additional delineated competencies associated with setting, role, or organizational policy.

Standards of Practice

The Standards of Practice identify how the informatics nurse and informatics nurse specialist are expected to incorporate the nursing process into all thinking and practice activities.

Standard 1. Assessment addresses the collection of data, information, and emerging evidence as the first step of the nursing process.

Standard 2. Diagnosis, Problems, and Issues Identification calls for the informatics nurse to complete an analysis of the data to identify problems and issues, thus, linking Standard 1 and Standard 2.

Standard 3. Outcomes Identification describes how the informatics nurse identifies expected outcomes that then drive development of an individualized plan to achieve those outcomes.

Standard 4. Planning identifies that the informatics nurse develops a plan with prescribed strategies, alternatives, and recommendations aimed at achieving the delineated expected outcomes.

Standard 5. Implementation addresses that the informatics nurse implements the identified plan. Standard 5a. Coordination of Activities, Standard 5b. Health Teaching and Health Promotion, and Standard 5c. Consultations are specifically delineated implementation activities that describe key nursing activities that merit additional attention.

Standard 6. Evaluation speaks about the expectation that the informatics nurse evaluates progress toward attainment of the outcomes. Accompanying competencies affirm collaboration and partnerships are key components in effectively demonstrating such an evaluation.

Standards of Professional Performance

The Standards of Professional Performance express the role performance requirements for the informatics nurse and informatics nurse specialist.

Standard 7. Ethics identifies the informatics nurse practices ethically, with further detailing of associated competencies, such as the use of the *Code of Ethics for Nurses with Interpretive Statements* to guide practice.

Standard 8. Education addresses the need for the informatics nurse to attain knowledge and competence, including the competency associated with demonstration of a commitment to lifelong learning.

Standard 9. Evidence-based Practice and Research confirms that the informatics nurse integrates evidence and research findings into practice.

Standard 10. Quality of Practice describes the expectation for the informatics nurse's contribution related to the quality and effectiveness of both nursing and informatics practice.

Standard 11. Communication explains that the informatics nurse communicates effectively through a variety of formats, with several accompanying competencies delineating specific requisite knowledge, skills, and abilities for demonstrated success in this area.

Standard 12. Leadership promotes that the informatics nurse leads in the professional practice setting, as well as the profession. Accompanying competencies address such skills as mentoring, problem solving, and promoting the organization's vision, goals, and strategic plan.

Standard 13. Collaboration encompasses the informatics nurse's collaborative efforts with the healthcare consumer, family, and others in the conduct of nursing and informatics practice.

Standard 14. Professional Practice Evaluation identifies that the informatics nurse conducts evaluation of their own nursing practice considering professional practice standards and guidelines, relevant statutes, rules, and regulations.

Standard 15. Resource Utilization addresses that the informatics nurse uses appropriate resources to plan and implement safe, effective, and fiscally responsible informatics and associated services.

Standard 16. Environmental Health closes out the list of professional performance standards by describing that the informatics nurse supports practice in a safe and healthy environment.

Consult the 2014 *Nursing Informatics: Scope and Standards of Practice, Second Edition*, for the precise standards and accompanying competencies language that provides additional details about the nursing informatics specialty and its members.

SUMMARY

Concepts of informatics, healthcare informatics, and nursing informatics were explained and their relationships to each other were discussed. The core concepts of nursing informatics were presented and described. The establishment of the specialty of nursing informatics was explained. Models of nursing informatics were described, and supporting models and theories were summarized. Competency work related to the practice of nursing informatics was presented. International and national resources for informatics nurses were provided. A discussion on how the nursing informatics scope of practice details the "who, what, when, where, how, and why" associated with this specialty was related. The nursing informatics standards of practice and standards of professional performance were briefly described. The 2014 *Nursing Informatics: Scope and Standards of Practice, Second Edition*, contains the official scope of practice statement, standards, and all accompanying competencies, including additional competencies delineated as applicable for the advanced level of practice of the informatics nurse specialist.

REFERENCES

Ajay, B. (2003). Student profiling: the Dreyfus model revisited. *Education for Primary Care, 14*(3), 360.

American Nurses Association. (1994). *The scope of practice for nursing informatics.* Washington, DC: American Nurses Publishing.

American Nurses Association. (1995). *Standards of nursing informatics practice.* Washington, DC: American Nurses Publishing.

American Nurses Association. (2001a). *Code of ethics for nurses with interpretive statements.* Washington, DC: American Nurses Publishing.

American Nurses Association. (2001b). *Scope and standards of nursing informatics practice.* Washington, DC: American Nurses Publishing.

American Nurses Association. (2003). *Nursing's social policy statement. 2nd ed.* Washington, DC: nursesbooks.org.

American Nurses Association. (2008). *Nursing informatics: Scope and standards of practice.* Washington, DC: nursebooks.org.

American Nurses Association. (2010). *Nursing: Scope and standards of practice* (2nd ed.). Washington, DC: nursebooks.org.

American Nurses Association. (2014). *Nursing informatics: Scope and standards of practice.* Silver Spring, MD: American Nurses Association.

Benner, P. (2004). Using the Dreyfus model of skill acquisition to describe and interpret skill acquisition and clinical judgment in nursing practice and education.

Bulletin of Science, Technology and Society, 24(3), 188–199. doi:10.1177/0270467604265061

Blum, B. I. (1985). *Clinical information systems.* New York, NY: Springer.

Bond, A. E., Eshah, N. F., Bani-Khaled, M., Hamad, A. O., Habashneh, S., Kataua, H., ... Maabreh, R. (2011). Who uses nursing theory? A univariate descriptive analysis of five years' research articles. *Scandinavian Journal of Caring Sciences, 25*(2), 404–409. doi:10.1111/j.1471-6712.2010.00835.x

Carter-Templeton, H., Patterson, R., & Russell, C. (2009). An analysis of published nursing informatics competencies. *Studies in Health Technoogy and Informatics, 46,* 540–545.

Dreyfus, S., & Dreyfus, H. (1980). *A five stage model of the mental activities involved in directed skill acquisition.* Berkeley, CA: California University Berkeley Operations Research Center.

Graves, J., & Corcoran, S. (1989). The study of nursing informatics. *Image: Journal of Nursing Scholarship, 21*(4), 227–231.

Hannah, K. (1985). Current trends in nursing informatics: Implications for curriculum planning. In K. Hannah, E. J. Guillemin, & D. N. Conklin (Eds.), *Journal of Nursing Scholarship* (pp. 181). The Netherlands: Elsevier Science.

Hunter, K. M., McGonigle, D., & Hebda, T. (2013). TIGER-based measurement of nursing informatics competencies: The development and implementation of an online tool for self-assessment. *Journal of Nursing Education and Practice, 3*(12), 70–80.

Karnick, P. M. (2013). The importance of defining theory in nursing: Is there a common denominator? *Nursing Science Quarterly, 26*(1), 29–30. doi:10.1177/0894318412466747

McGonigle, D., Hunter, K. M., Hebda, T., & Hill, T. (2013). *Assessment of Level 3 and Level 4 nursing informatics (NI) competencies tool development* Paper presented at the Summer Institute on Nursing Informatics (SINI) Beyond Stage 7 and Meaningful Use: What's Next?, Baltimore, MD.

McGonigle, D., & Mastrian, K. (2012). *Nursing Informatics and the Foundation of Knowledge* (2nd ed.). Burlington, MA: Jones & Bartlett.

Office of Behavioral and Social Sciences. (2010). *Behavioral and social sciences (BSSR) definition.* Retrieved from http://obssr.od.nih.gov/about_obssr/BSSR_CC/BSSR_definition/definition.aspx. Accessed on December 31, 2013.

Rogers, E. M. (2003). *Diffusion of innovations* (5th ed.). New York, NY: Free Press.

Schwirian, P. M. (1986). The NI pyramid—A model for research in nursing informatics. *Computers in Nursing, 43*(3), 1.

Shannon, C. E. (1948). A mathematical theory of communication. *Bell System Technical Journal, 27*(379–423), 623–656.

Shannon, C. E., & Weaver, W. (1949). *The mathematical theory of communication.* Chicago, IL: University of Illinois.

Staggers, N., Gassert, C. A., & Curran, C. (2001). Informatics competencies for nurses at four levels of practice. *Journal of Nursing Education, 40*(7), 303–316.

The TIGER Initiative. (n.d.). Informatics competencies for every practicing nurse: Recommendations from the TIGER Collaborative: Technology Informatics Guiding Education Reform.

Tuckman, B. (1965). Developmental sequence of small groups. *Psychological Bulletin, 63,* 384–399.

Turley, J. (1996). Toward a model for nursing informatics. *Image: Journal of Nursing Scholarship, 28*(4), 309–313.

Verdoux, P. (2011). Emerging technologies and the future of philosophy. *Metaphilosophy, 42*(5), 682–707. doi:10.1111/j.1467-9973.2011.01715.x

Wells, J., Manuel, M., & Cunning, G. (2011). Changing the model of care delivery: nurses' perceptions of job satisfaction and care effectiveness. *Journal of Nursing Management, 19*(6), 777–785. doi:10.1111/j.1365-2834.2011.01292.x

Yoon, S., Yen, P., & Bakken, S. (2009). Psychometric properties of the self-assessment of nursing informatics competencies scale. In K. Saranto, P. Flatley Brennan, H.-A. Park, M. Tallberg, & A. Ensio (Eds.), *Connecting health and humans* (Vol. 146, pp. 546–550). Amsterdam, The Netherlands: IOS Press.

16

Nursing Informatics and Healthcare Policy

Judy Murphy / Elizabeth (Liz) O. Johnson

• OBJECTIVES

1. Discuss the significant impact of federal legislation from 2009 and 2010 on the use of health information technology.
2. Describe the creation of the office of the National Coordinator for Health Information Technology and summarize the major role it plays in the implementation of health information technology.
3. Discuss the implications of policy on nursing informatics as a specialty.
4. Identify the impact that national trends and events focused on information and information technology have on nursing informatics practice.
5. Outline the role of health IT in key emerging payment and clinical practice change initiatives, both in the government and private sectors.

• KEY WORDS

Informatics
Health information technology
Public policy
Health policy
Electronic health record
HITECH

INTRODUCTION AND BACKGROUND

On March 23, 2010, President Barack Obama signed into law the landmark Patient Protection and Affordable Care Act (ACA). As upheld on June 28, 2012, in an historic and landmark decision by the U.S. Supreme Court, ACA was a hard-fought federal statute that represents the sweeping healthcare-reform agenda envisioned by the Democratic 111th Congress and the Obama Administration. Despite legal challenges that sought and to reverse "Obamacare," the law was and is dedicated to replacing a broken system with one that ensures all Americans access to healthcare that is both affordable and driven by quality standards. It includes broad provisions for the improvement of healthcare delivery that, unless declared unconstitutional, will run through the end of the present decade (Obama Care, 2013).

For the Obama administration and the nation, ACA turned a spotlight on the ever-increasing recognition that advanced health information technology (health IT) is and will be essential to support the massive amounts of electronic information exchange foundational to industry reform. In fact, the universal agreement that meaningful healthcare reform cannot be separated from the national— and arguably global—integration of health IT based on accepted, standardized, and interoperable methods of data exchange provided the linchpin for other critically important legislation that created a glide path for ACA.

It was such consensus that resulted in the broad support and passage into law of the American Recovery and Reinvestment Act (ARRA) of 2009 and its key Health Information Technology Act (HITECH) provision in the early weeks of Mr. Obama's presidency. Backed with an allocation of around $22 billion, this legislation authorized the Centers for Medicare & Medicaid Services (CMS) to provide reimbursement incentives for eligible professionals and hospitals that take steps to become "meaningful users" of certified Electronic Health Records (EHRs) technology to improve care quality and better manage care costs (ARRA and HITECH Act Resource Center, 2009).

At the core of the new reform initiatives, the incentivized adoption of EHRs by eligible hospitals and providers across the nation improves care quality and better manages care costs. It also helps meet clinical and business needs, since capturing, storing, and displaying clinical information from EHRs when and where it is needed improves individual patient care while providing aggregated, cross-patient data analysis.

EHRs manage healthcare data and information in ways that are patient centered, secure, and information rich. Improved information access and availability across the continuum of care increasingly enables both the provider and the patient to better manage each patient's health by using capabilities provided through enhanced clinical decision support and customized education materials.

In this massive transformation from disconnected, inefficient, paper-based "islands" of care delivery to a nationwide, interconnected, and interoperable system driven by EHRs and advancing health IT innovation, the importance of nurses and nursing informatics (NI) are difficult to overstate. For decades, nurses have proactively contributed resources to the development, use, and evaluation of information systems. Today, they constitute the largest single group of healthcare professionals and include experts who serve on national committees and participate in interoperability initiatives focused on policy, standards and terminology development, standards harmonization, and EHR adoption. In their front-line roles, nurses continue to have a profound impact on the quality and cost of healthcare and are emerging as leaders in the effective use of HIT to improve the safety, quality, and efficiency of healthcare services (ANI, 2009).

It is informatics nurses who are key contributors to a working knowledge about how evidence-based practices designed in information systems can support and enhance clinical processes and decision-making to improve patient safety and outcomes. Also, as the "glue" of acute care delivery settings who are responsible for care coordination and promotion of wellness, nurses are often the patient's primary contact—and the last defensive line in care delivery where medical errors or other unintended actions can be caught and corrected. In addition, as drivers in organizational planning and process reengineering to improve the healthcare delivery system, informatics nurses are increasingly sought out by nurses and nurse managers for leadership as their profession works to bring IT applications into the mainstream healthcare environment (ANI, 2009).

The importance of nursing in healthcare reform was confirmed in the 2010 landmark report, *The Future of Nursing: Leading Change, Advancing Health* from the Institute of Medicine (IOM) and the Robert Wood Johnson Foundation (RWJF). Based on the report's recommendations, the RWJF began the Initiative on the Future of Nursing. Through the Initiative, RWJF continues to support the research agenda set forth by the report and implement the recommendations in the areas of nurse training, education, professional leadership, and workforce policy (Institute of Medicine, 2013).

Therefore, it will be increasingly essential to the success of today's healthcare-reform movement that nurses are involved in every aspect of selecting, designing, testing, implementing, and developing health information systems. Further, the growing adoption of EHRs must incorporate nursing's unique body of knowledge with the nursing process at its core.

Major forces of reform are fueling sharply increased demand for a larger health IT workforce across the U.S. healthcare landscape. Wrote *The New York Times'* Reed Abelson in late 2011, "… health care in America has changed in ways that will not be easily undone. Provisions already put in place, like tougher oversight of health insurers … are already well cemented and popular" (Abelson, Harris, & Pear, 2011).

In a similar article, *USA Today* concurred, reporting that health IT job growth is being driven by the general restructuring of the healthcare industry. This includes not only ACA, but also 2009 federal stimulus funding, new government regulations, and increasing use of health IT across the industry (Mitchell, 2011). Supporting this viewpoint, the Bureau of Labor Statistics has projected that employment growth in the health IT area will increase overall by 20% through 2020, with some segments like network and computer systems administrators expanding by 28% (Bureau of Labor Statistics, 2012).

Information security concerns are also increasing for many healthcare organizations as managers realize that current security measures are insufficient to protect the privacy of growing volumes of patients' protected healthcare information (PHI). As a direct result, more new opportunities for computer and information management professionals will be driven by organizations upgrading their health IT systems and switching to newer, faster, and more mobile networks.

As a major factor in such dynamics, the growing commitment by health systems and physician practices to the implementation and demonstrated meaningful use of certified EHR systems will also continue to create new opportunities for health IT professionals. Three years into the program to drive the adoption and meaningful use of certified EHRs, 63% of all eligible providers and 86% of all eligible hospitals have received an EHR incentive payment from either Medicare or Medicaid, as of November 2013. Three out of every five Medicare eligible physicians and professionals are meaningful users of EHRs (Centers for Medicare and Medicaid Services, 2011).

As of November 2013, participation in meaningful-use has accounted for well more than $17.8 billion in Medicare and Medicaid incentives payments to nearly 310,000 hospitals and physicians (Golden, 2013). More than half of all doctors and all other eligible providers have received incentive payments for meaningful use, and by May 2013, Health and Human Services (HHS) had exceeded its goal of 50% of doctors and 80 of eligible hospitals using EHRs by the end of 2013 (Centers for Medicare and Medicaid Services, 2014).

All in all, some 50,000 qualified health IT workers will be needed to meet the demands of hospitals and physicians as they move to adopt EHRs and connect to state-wide health information exchanges (HIEs). In fact, the Bureau of Labor Statistics, Department of Education, and independent studies estimate a workforce shortfall over the next five years. One recent study, conducted by PwC's Health Research Institute and released in March 2013, shows that the growing shortage appears greater than previously reported. According to the report, nearly 80% of global healthcare CEOs surveyed expect to increase technology investments in 2013, yet more than half (51%) fear their staff cannot keep up with the pace of technological change. Seventy-seven percent say they are revisiting their hiring and promotion strategies to address gaping holes in health IT (Monegain, 2013).

CHAPTER OVERVIEW

Given the critical importance of nurses and health IT professionals to the future of healthcare transformation, it is important to understand the key components driving change in the industry: the primary influencers, organizations, programs, and processes that have shaped or defined policies for the integration of health IT that will

affect all segments of healthcare. Therefore, the purpose of this chapter is to identify and define the historic and present roles of such influencers, including sections on:

- Forces of Change in Today's National Healthcare System
- Mandate for Reform: ARRA and its HITECH Act Provision
- State and Regional Health IT Programs
- Health IT Federal Advisory Committees and Agencies
- Nursing Informatics and Healthcare Reform
- The Road Ahead

FORCES OF CHANGE IN TODAY'S NATIONAL HEALTHCARE SYSTEM

The long journey to the passage of ACA, ARRA, and HITECH goes back several decades. In 1991, the IOM concluded that computerization could help improve patient records and information management, leading to higher quality of care in its landmark report, *The Computer-Based Patient Record: An Essential Technology for Healthcare* (Dick & Steen, 1997). That was followed nearly a decade later with other groundbreaking reports calling for the use of health IT to improve the efficiency, safety, and quality of the U.S. healthcare system—*To Err Is Human in 1999* (Kohn, Corrigan, & Donaldson, 1999) and *Crossing the Quality Chasm in* 2001 (Institute of Medicine, Committee on Quality of Health Care in America, 2001). These reports were a call to action for a paradigm shift from reliance on paper and verbal communication for managing patient care to a new era where healthcare professionals are supported in their clinical decision-making by technology while providing patient care.

IOM followed up on these reports in 2012 with *Best Care at Lower Cost: The Path to Continuously Learning Health Care in America*, which urged systemic transformation to reduce inefficiencies in the health system (Smith, Saunders, Stuckhardt, & McGinnis, 2013). The report said the complexity and inefficiencies in American's healthcare system are a threat not only to quality healthcare, but to the nation's economic stability and global competitiveness.

Further, the early report on the Computer-Based Patient Record called for an urgent across-the-board commitment to continuous improvement; incremental upgrades by individual hospitals and other providers would no longer suffice. One of the main points of the report was that better data management, including EHRs and mobile technologies would be a key method in upgrading health-care while reducing inefficiency and lowering costs (Dick & Steen, 1997).

In looking back at other significant forces of change, one of the earliest and most influential was PITAC: The President's Information Technology Advisory Committee.

The President's Information Technology Advisory Committee

In 1997, an Executive Order of the President estab-lished the visionary, 24-member President's Information Technology Advisory Committee (PITAC), which was comprised of both corporate and academic leaders from across the United States. Since its inception, the com-mittee has provided the President, Congress, and those federal agencies involved in networking and information technology (IT) research and development with expert, independent advice on maintaining American preemi-nence in advanced information technologies.

In 1999, as part of its seminal work to define how IT could drive progress in the twenty-first Century, PITAC established a panel to provide guidance on how IT could be leveraged to transform healthcare and increase access to care for all citizens. Driving the panel's work was the firm conviction that the Federal government's role in lead-ing the way to healthcare reform through technology was both critical and, at the time, sorely lacking (Computing Research Association, 1999).

A few years later, in a report entitled *Transforming Health Care through Information Technology*, PITAC found that "at present, the U.S. lacks a broadly dissemi-nated and accepted national vision for information tech-nology in healthcare" (President's Information Technology Advisory Committee, 2001). To rectify the situation, the panel strongly recommended that HHS define a clear vision of how IT could improve the U.S. healthcare sys-tem, follow up with resources sufficient to accomplish its objectives, and appoint a senior IT person to provide stra-tegic leadership.

President's Council of Advisors for Science and Technology

After allowing PITAC's charter to expire, President George W. Bush announced that the President's Council of Advisors for Science and Technology (PCAST) would oversee the Networking and Information Technology Research and Development (NITRD) Program. As such, PCAST membership would increase and assume PITAC's responsibilities. The National Coordinating Office for IT called it an elevation of the role of external information

technology advice in the White House, and assigned a broader charter than the former committee's narrow focus on IT (Harsha, 2005). Over next few years, PCAST studied and produced reports on issues ranging from energy and technology to nanotechnology to personalized medicine (Marburger & Kvamme, 2008).

One of the most highly anticipated reports was the 2010 report, *Realizing the Full Potential of Health Information Technology to Improve Healthcare for Americans: The Path Forward* (President's Council of Advisors on Science and Technology, 2010). The report pointed out the necessity of using health technology to increase access to patient infor-mation, streamline patient diagnoses and care, improve monitoring of public health trends, and enhance the abil-ity to conduct clinical trials. With the use of technology, these healthcare goals could be accomplished while lower-ing costs and giving patients "unprecedented" control over who may access their records.

In a letter to the President accompanying the report, PCAST co-chairs John P. Holdren and Eric Lander said it "is crucial that the Federal Government facilitate the nationwide adoption of a universal exchange language for healthcare information and a digital infrastructure for locating patient records while strictly ensuring patient privacy." Moreover, the co-chairs urged the Office of the National Coordinator for Health Information Technology (ONC) and CMS to develop guidelines for the transition from traditional EHRs to the health information exchanges (President's Council of Advisors on Science and Technology, 2010).

President Bush's Executive Order and the Birth of ONC

On January 20, 2004, President George W. Bush in his State of the Union address called for "… an Electronic Health Record for every American by the year 2014 … By com-puterizing health records, we can avoid dangerous medical mistakes, reduce costs, and improve care" (Bush, 2004a). He went on to issue an executive order that same year: "Incentives for the Use of Health Information Technology and Establishing the Position of the National Health Information Technology Coordinator," which has had an impact on every healthcare entity, provider, and informat-ics professional in the United States (Bush, 2004b).

Components of the order were to (1) establish a national health information technology coordinator position; (2) develop a nationwide interoperable health IT infra-structure; and (3) develop, maintain, and direct imple-mentation of a strategic plan to guide implementation of interoperable health IT in both public and private sectors. Dr. David Brailer was appointed as the first national coor-dinator by Tommy Thompson, then Secretary of HHS.

ONC remains today the principal federal entity charged with coordination of nationwide efforts to implement and use the most advanced health IT and the electronic exchange of health information. ONC is a key player in the execution of ARRA and its HITECH Act provision. ARRA authorized the creation of two committees—the Health IT Policy Committee and the Health IT Standards Committee—that make recommendations to the ONC. The Policy Committee works on a policy framework for a nationwide health information infrastructure, including the exchange of patient medical information. The Standards Committee recommends specifications and certification criteria for the electronic exchange and use of health information.

Dr. Farzad Mostashari, who was appointed by HHS Secretary Kathleen Sebelius in May 2011, succeeded Dr. David Blumenthal, as the National Coordinator. Mostashari stepped down in October 2013. The new National Coordinator, Dr. Karen DeSalvo, was appointed by Secretary Sebelius in January 2014.

Health IT Training Programs: An Essential Element of Reform

As discussed in the introduction, today's urgent need for health IT experts is challenged by a shortage of the very professionals who are best positioned to carry transformation forward. With consensus around the essential requirement for advanced health IT and the mounting pressures of shortages in nursing, health IT experts, and other medical professions, the U.S. Government through HHS has enlisted the talent and resources of some of the nation's leading universities, community colleges, and major research centers to advance the widespread adoption and meaningful use of health IT. These schools are offering a wide variety of training programs that are helping build the depth and breadth of the health IT workforce as a critical component in the transformation of American healthcare delivery.

Both on-campus and online programs in health IT are available at the certificate, associate, bachelor's, and master's degree levels. Certificate programs typically consist of between 15 and 30 credit hours and are often designed for working professionals. The American Medical Informatics Association (AMIA) created a revolutionary "10 × 10" Program in 2005, with the goal of training 10,000 healthcare professionals in applied health informatics within 10 years, and became a model for certificate-based programs (AMIA, 2005).

Through an ARRA-funded cooperative agreement program, federal awards and grants totaling some $118 million to 16 universities and 82 community colleges provided incentives for health IT education to speed the growth of a new pool of health IT professionals. These programs supported the training and development of more than 20,000 new health IT professionals. For more information, see *Workforce Training* in the next section on ARRA.

The Health IT Workforce Development workgroup of the Health IT Policy Committee was formed in July 2012 to make recommendations so that within one year, health IT training needs and competencies are identified and tools for implementation are recommended. The workgroup recommended that ONC-funded programs and their core competencies be summarized and publicized along with the many resources available for education and best practices.

The workgroup also recommended new programs and funding to address emerging needs, such as team-based care, population health, and patient engagement, and studies to assess the impact of health IT on the incumbent workforce. Last, health IT needs to be represented in the Standard Occupational Classification (SOC), and the Committee is seeking input to have it included in the next addition, due out in 2018 (Health IT Workforce Development Sub Group, 2013).

The Health Insurance Portability and Accountability Act: Privacy and Security

The Health Insurance Portability and Accountability Act (HIPAA), which passed in 1996, required HHS to develop regulations protecting the privacy and security of electronic health information as well as facilitate its efficient transmission. HIPAA's goals are to allow the flow of health information needed to provide and promote high-quality healthcare while protecting the public's health and well-being. Prior to HIPAA, no generally accepted set of standards or requirements for protecting health information existed in the healthcare industry. At the same time, new technologies were evolving to move the healthcare industry away from paper processes and to increase the reliance on electronic information systems to conduct a host of administrative and clinically based functions, such as providing health information, paying claims, and answering eligibility questions (All Things Medical Billing, 2014).

To comply with the requirements of the Act, HHS published what are commonly known as the HIPAA Privacy Rule and the HIPAA Security Rule. The rules apply to all health plans, healthcare clearinghouses, and any healthcare provider that transmits health information in electronic form.

The HIPAA Privacy Rule. The HIPAA Privacy Rule, which took effect on April 14, 2003, established national standards for the protection of individually identifiable health information. As such, the rule regulates the use and disclosure of an individual's health information, referred to as Protected Health Information (PHI), and sets forth standards for individuals' privacy rights to understand and control how their health information is used. The rule applies to those organizations identified as "covered entities," which include healthcare clearinghouses, employer-sponsored health plans, health insurers, and other medical service providers that engage in the transfer of PHI. PHI is defined broadly and includes any part of an individual's medical record or payment history (Office for Civil Rights, DHHS, 2005).

The final HIPAA/HITECH Act Privacy, Security, Enforcement, Breach Notification Rules were published in the *Federal Register* on January 25, 2013. The final omnibus rule greatly enhances a patient's privacy protections and provides individuals new rights to their health information. While the original HIPAA Privacy and Security Rules focused on healthcare providers, health plans, and other entities that process health insurance claims, the changes expanded many of the privacy requirements to business associates of these entities that receive protected health information, such as contractors and subcontractors. In addition, the rule increased penalties for non-compliance based on the level of negligence with a maximum penalty of $1.5 million per violation (HHS Press Office, 2013).

The HIPAA Security Rule. The HIPAA Security Rule took effect on April 21, 2003, with a compliance date of April 21, 2005, for most covered entities. The Security Rule complements the Privacy Rule; while the Privacy Rule pertains to all PHI including paper and electronic records, the Security Rule deals specifically with Electronic Protected Health Information (ePHI). Still, a major goal of the Security Rule is to protect the privacy of individuals' PHI while allowing covered entities to adopt new technologies to improve the quality and the efficiency of patient care. Given the diversity of the healthcare marketplace, the Security Rule is designed to be flexible and scalable so that a covered entity can implement policies, procedures, and technologies that are appropriate for the entity's particular size, organizational structure, and risks to consumers' electronic ePHI (Office of Civil Rights, DHHS, May, 2005).

In the years following its passage and implementation, HIPAA regulations have had a significant impact on health informatics. For example, under HIPAA, patients must be permitted to review and amend their medical records. Healthcare providers have expressed concern that patients who choose to access their records could experience increased anxiety. Other studies, however, have determined that counter-benefits already include enhanced doctor–patient communications and only minimal risks in increasing patients' access to their records.

The passage of ARRA expanded HIPAA's mandate to impose new privacy and security requirements. One of the greatest changes to HIPAA presently affecting the healthcare community and health IT professionals are the modifications published on January 16, 2009, in the HIPAA Electronic Transaction Standards Final Rule.

As originally framed, the old version of the American National Standards Institute (ANSI) X12 Standards for HIPAA transactions were to be replaced by Version 5010, which regulates the transmission of certain healthcare transactions among hospitals, physician practices, health plans, and claims clearinghouses. In addition, the old version of the National Council for Prescription Drug Program (NCPDP) standard for pharmacy and supplier transactions was to be replaced by Version D.0 (Blue Cross Blue Shield of Michigan, 2009).

As the first major change since HIPAA's implementation, the introductions of these new standards are meant to enhance business functionality, clarify ambiguities, and better define situational and required data elements. The new rules apply to all physicians, providers, and suppliers who bill Medicare carriers, fiscal intermediaries, Medicare administrative contractors (MACs), and durable medical equipment MACs for services provided to Medicare beneficiaries (Centers for Medicare and Medicaid Services, February, 2012).

When first announced, the switch to the 5010 standards was supposed to be in place on January 1, 2012. In November 2011, however, CMS decided that, although it would not change the actual deadline for complying with the standards, it would not initiate enforcement action until March 31. Soon thereafter, in continued reconsideration of what it called "a number of outstanding issues and challenges impeding full implementation," CMS pushed the enforcement date back to July 1, 2012 (Robezniks, 2012). The conversion to the HIPAA 5010 standards is seen as key to the larger switch from the ICD-9 clinical coding system to the vastly more detailed ICD-10 system—ICD-10 conversion is set for October 1, 2014.

More recently, the final rule to HIPAA, as mentioned in the previous section, enhances the HITECH Breach Notification requirements by clarifying when breaches of unsecured health information must be reported to HHS. The changes also strengthen the government's ability to enforce the law.

EHR Certification and Testing

With the passage of ARRA and HITECH, ONC has become the driving force behind the definition of meaningful use of EHRs and the certification of EHR systems. This new reality changed the operating environment for the Certification Commission for Healthcare Information Technology (CCHIT), which until 2009 had been the sole organization to certify EHR systems.

CCHIT was founded in 2004 with support from three industry associations in healthcare information management and technology: the American Health Information Management Association (AHIMA), the Healthcare Information and Management Systems Society (HIMSS), and the National Alliance for Health Information Technology (NAHIT). In September 2005, HHS awarded CCHIT a contract to develop the certification criteria and inspection process for EHRs and the networks through which they interoperate. The certification criteria were developed through a voluntary, consensus-based process engaging diverse stakeholders. Many health IT professionals were involved in this process—helping to define the certification criteria for the hospital and ambulatory environments as well as to outline the testing processes used by CCHIT (Certification Commission for Healthcare Information Technology, 2014).

However, in the months following the 2009 passage of ARRA, questions surfaced about CCHIT's unique role going forward. On March 2, 2010, ONC confirmed the merits of this debate when it issued a new Notice of Proposed Rulemaking, which proposed the establishment of two certification programs for the purposes of testing and certifying EHRs—one temporary and one permanent. These new programs were not limited to CCHIT. Then, on June 24, 2010, ONC published the Final Rule on the Temporary Certification Program for EHRs.

Under the temporary program, ONC authorized approved organizations, called ONC-Authorized Testing and Certification Bodies (ONC-ATCBs), to both test and certify EHRs and EHR Modules, thereby ensuring the availability of Certified EHR Technology prior to the beginning of the reporting period defined under ARRA. After the first year, the permanent certification program replaced the temporary program and now separates the responsibilities for performing testing and certification, now called Authorized Test Labs (ATLs) and Authorized Certification Bodies (ACBs). In addition to EHR and EHR module certification, the permanent program includes the certification of other types of health IT, such as personal health records (PHRs) and health information exchange (HIE) networks. With the launch of the ONC Health IT Certification Program, the Temporary Certification Program sunset on October 4, 2012 (Health IT, 2012).

Standards and the Nationwide Health Information Network

In late 2005, the U.S. Department of Health and Human Services commissioned the Healthcare Information Technology Standards Panel (HITSP) to assist in developing a Nationwide Health Information Network (NwHIN), which would create a nation-wide, interoperable, private, and secure exchange of health information between EHRs (Enrado, 2011).

As envisioned then and now, NwHIN is intended to provide a set of standards that regulate the connections among providers, consumers, and others involved in supporting health and healthcare. The purpose of these standards is to enable normalized health information to follow the consumer; it is intended to make health records, laboratory results, medication information, and related medical data readily available and accessible to providers, pharmacists, and even consumers over the Internet, thereby helping achieve the goals of the HITECH Act. At the same time, NwHIN is also dedicated to ensuring that consumers' health information remains secure and confidential in the electronic environment.

In January 2011, NwHIN began to be referenced as the "Nation*wide* Health Information Network"—or NwHIN. The change emphasizes that NwHIN is a set of standards, services, and policies that enable secure health information exchange over the Internet. These standards are today being used by three Federal initiatives: The Direct Project, NwHIN Exchange, and the CONNECT software project. It also served notice that NwHIN continues to evolve with the government acting as a facilitator—not as an infrastructure builder. In fact, its development depends on an environment of collaboration, transparency, and buy-in from the bottom up, including small as well as large physician groups and health systems who are working to share patient records with other care delivery entities across the continuum of care.

In October, 2012, ONC launched the NwHIN Exchange, which includes federal and non-federal agencies that share patient information for care. Currently the exchange encompasses more than 20 federal and non-federal agencies. They also announced that the NwHIN Exchange had officially been converted into eHealth Exchange, a public–private partnership to increase health information exchange (HIE) innovation in the private sector. It was developed under the auspices of the ONC and is managed by a non-profit industry coalition called HealtheWay.

Interoperability

Interoperability is the ability of health information systems to work together within and across organizational boundaries to advance the effective delivery of healthcare for individuals and communities by sharing data between EHRs. It is not simply the exchange of data between two organizations, but rather the ability of the two organizations to exchange and consume data to and from each other's EHRs. For interoperability to occur, standards are required for data transport, content exchange, and vocabulary management. This is why standards development is so important—it enables the interoperability needed for regional and national health data exchange and is essential to the development of the NwHIN.

Debate exists as to how interoperability should develop relative to EHR adoption in terms of timing. On the one hand, many industry leaders believe that interoperability should precede EHR use. They are convinced that the ability to share information should be designed into EHRs and that the infrastructure and industry capacity for securely networking this information should exist up front. On the other hand, others argue that interoperability will follow widespread EHR adoption. This side of the debate believes that once health information becomes electronic and everyone is using EHRs, interoperability will naturally follow, since it will be easier and cheaper than manual data sharing (Barr, 2008; Connor, 2007).

HIE Governance. In May 2012, ONC released to the public a request for information (RFI) on the governance of the Nationwide Health Information Network, believing this would constitute a critical step toward enabling trusted and interoperable electronic health information exchange nationwide. ONC saw a common set of "rules of the road" for privacy, security, business, and technical requirements as a means of laying the necessary foundation to enable our nation's electronic health information exchange capacity to grow. It could also help achieve the Bush and Obama Administration's vision for an electronically connected health system for the twenty-first Century that delivers efficient and quality healthcare for all Americans.

The RFI asked for public feedback on how a governance mechanism would best provide confidence to patients that their health information is being shared appropriately and securely; reassure providers they are dealing with trusted entities when sending or receiving patient information; promote an open and competitive market for electronic health information exchange; and enable innovation to thrive. The response to the RFI was a desire not to regulate, but to let the market mature and follow a non-regulatory approach. As such, the Governance Framework for Trusted Electronic Health Information Exchange (the Governance Framework) was released in May 2013 and is intended to serve as guiding principles on HIE governance (Office of the National Coordinator

for Health Information Technology, 2013e). It is meant to provide a common conceptual foundation applicable to all types of governance models and express the principles ONC believes are most important for HIE governance. The Governance Framework does not prescribe specific solutions but lays out milestones and outcomes that ONC expects for and from HIE governance entities as they enable electronic HIE (Mostashari, 2013).

The exchange standards were specified by ONC to correspond with the CMS meaningful use measures to promote the use of EHRs to improve healthcare by providing complete and accurate patient information and increased access to information as well as to encourage patients' involvement in their own healthcare. Stage 1 of Meaningful provided incentives to help providers implement EHRs. Now at Stage 2, in effect at the end of 2013, measures focus on health information exchange to improve the flow of information between providers and with patients.

Integrating the Healthcare Enterprise. Integrating the Healthcare Enterprise (IHE) is a global initiative, now in its twelfth year, to create the framework for passing vital health information seamlessly from application to application, system to system, and setting to setting across multiple healthcare enterprises. IHE brings together health IT stakeholders to demonstrate the implementation of standards for communicating patient information efficiently throughout and among healthcare enterprises by developing a framework of interoperability. Because of its proven process of collaboration, demonstration, and real world implementation of interoperable solutions, IHE is in a unique position to significantly accelerate the process for defining, testing, and implementing standards-based interoperability among EHR systems (Health Information and Management Systems Society, 2010).

Non-Profit Organizations Driving Reform

Among the many non-profit organizations today advancing health IT and nursing informatics, few have had such positive impact on the industry than the American Medical Informatics Association (AMIA) and the Healthcare Information and Management Systems Society (HIMSS). Both organizations have significant numbers of health IT professionals who are expert informaticists as well as committees, task forces, and working groups for the health IT community.

AMIA. AMIA is dedicated to promoting the effective organization, analysis, management, and use of information in healthcare to support patient care, public health, teaching, research, administration, and related policy. For more than 30 years, the 4000 some members of AMIA and its honorific college, the American College of Medical Informatics (ACMI), have sponsored meetings, education, policy, and research programs. The federal government frequently calls upon AMIA as a source of informed, unbiased opinions on policy issues relating to the national health information infrastructure, uses and protection of personal health information, and public health considerations, among others.

ONC, for example, requested input from AMIA on the proposed Health IT Patient Safety Action and Surveillance Plan. After review, the AMIA submitted its comments to ONC, which was able to incorporate some of their recommendations in the final plan, published July 2, 2013 (Fickenscher, 2013; Office of the National Coordinator for Health Information Technology, 2013a).

With an overall mission of advancing the informatics profession relating to health and disease, AMIA champions the use of health information and communications technology in clinical care and research, personal health management, public health/population, and transactional science with the ultimate objective of improving health. The association is also dedicated to expanding the size and strengthening the competency of the U.S. health informatics workforce and supporting the continued development of the health informatics profession.

HIMSS. HIMSS, founded in 1961, is a comprehensive healthcare-stakeholder membership organization exclusively focused on providing leadership for the optimal use of IT and management systems for the betterment of healthcare. A global organization with offices in Chicago, Washington, D.C., Brussels, and Singapore, HIMSS represents more than 23,000 members, 73% of whom work in patient care delivery settings. HIMSS also includes corporate members and not-for-profit organizations that share its mission to transform healthcare through the effective use of IT and management systems.

The society was founded on the premise that an organized exchange of experience among members could promote a better understanding of the principles underlying healthcare systems and improve the skills of those who direct health IT programs and the practitioners who analyze, design, or evaluate health IT systems. In today's environment of rapid reform and transformation, HIMSS frames and leads healthcare public policy and industry practices through its educational, professional development, and advocacy initiatives designed to promote information and management systems' contributions to ensuring quality patient care (HIMSS Legacy Workgroup, 2007). HIMSS, like AMIA, often provides input on Health

IT issues and government programs. It also recently provided comments to ONC on the Health IT Patient Safety Action and Surveillance Plan (Fields & Lieber, 2013).

MANDATE FOR REFORM: ARRA AND ITS HITECH ACT PROVISION

ARRA and its important HITECH Act provision were passed into law on February 17, 2009. Commonly referred to as "The Stimulus Bill" or "The Recovery Act," the landmark legislation allocated $787 billion to stimulate the economy, including $147 billion to rescue and reform the nation's seriously ailing healthcare industry. Of these funds, about $22 billion in financial incentives were earmarked for the relatively short period of five years to drive reform through the use of advanced health IT and the adoption of EHRs. As noted in this chapter's introduction, the incentives were intended to help healthcare providers purchase and implement health IT and EHR systems, and the HITECH Act also stipulated that clear penalties would be imposed beyond 2015 for both hospitals and physician providers who failed to adopt use of EHRs in a meaningful way. This section describes some of the key components of ARRA and HITECH.

Incentives for Meaningful Use of EHRs

The majority of the HITECH funding will be used to reward hospitals and eligible providers for "meaningful use" of certified EHRs by "meaningful users" with increased Medicare and Medicaid payments. The law specifies that eligible healthcare professionals and hospitals can qualify for both programs when they adopt certified EHR technology and use it in a meaningful way. Exactly what HITECH, as administered by ONC and CMS, means by the term "meaningful use" is a dynamic, evolutionary process that will involve three stages (Office of the National Coordinator for Health Information Technology, 2013g):

Stage 1: Beginning in 2011 as the incentive program's starting point for all providers; "meaningful use" here consists of transferring data to EHRs and beginning to share information, including electronic copies and visit summaries for patients.

Stage 2: To be implemented in 2014 "meaningful use" includes significant new exchange functionality such as online patient access to their health information and electronic health information exchange during transitions between providers.

Stage 3: Expected to begin in 2017, "meaningful use" in this stage is projected to include measures that demonstrate improvement in the quality of healthcare.

Milestones in Meaningful Use Program

Milestone dates and their significance to the Meaningful Use Program in the United State are summarized in the following paragraphs:

December 31, 2009: CMS, with input from ONC and the HIT Policy and Standards Committees, published a Stage 1 Proposed Rule on Meaningful Use of EHRs and began a 60-day public comment period.

July 28, 2010: After reviewing more than 2000 comments, HHS issued the Stage 1 Final Rule, with final criteria for meeting "Meaningful Use" divided into five initiatives:

1. Improve quality, safety, efficiency, and reduce health disparities.
2. Engage patients and families.
3. Improve care coordination.
4. Improve population and public health.
5. Ensure adequate privacy and security protections for personal health information.

Specific objectives were written to demonstrate that EHR use would have a "meaningful" impact on one of the five initiatives. Under the final rule, participating providers are today working to meet 14 "core" (required) objectives for hospitals and 15 for providers. For both hospitals and providers, the rule sets out 10 other objectives in a "menu set" from which they must choose and comply with five. If the objectives are met during the specified year and the hospital or provider submits the appropriate measurements, then the hospitals or providers will receive the incentive payment. The hospital incentive amount is based on the Medicare and Medicaid patient volumes; the provider incentives are fixed per provider. The incentives are paid over five years, and the hospital or provider must submit measurement results annually during each of the years to continue to qualify.

November 30, 2011: In the launch of an initiative called, "We Can't Wait," HHS and the Obama Administration acknowledged the challenges of meeting Stage 2 timeline requirements. Under the original requirements, eligible doctors and hospitals that begin participating in the Medicare EHR Incentive Programs in 2011 would have to meet new standards for the program in 2013. But if they chose not to participate in the program until 2012, they could wait to meet the same standards until 2014 and still be eligible for identical incentive payments. Therefore, to encourage faster adoption, the HHS' announcement cleared the way for doctors and hospitals to adopt health IT in 2011without formally meeting the new standards until 2014. These policy changes were also accompanied by greater outreach efforts to provide more information to doctors and hospitals about best practices. They also sought to help vendors whose products were straining to keep up with the changing requirements for their technologies, which allow healthcare providers to meaningfully use EHRs (HHS Press Office, 2011).

February 23–24, 2012: CMS and HHS announced Stage 2 meaningful-use steps for providers using EHR technology and receiving Stage 1 incentives payments from Medicare and Medicaid. The proposed rule, which was submitted to the public for a comment period that ended on May 7, 2012, was intended to define more than the Stage 2 criteria that eligible providers must meet to qualify for incentives payments (Monticello, 2012). In addition, the finalized Stage 2 rules define the "payment adjustments" or penalties that, beginning in 2015, providers will face if they fail to demonstrate the meaningful use of certified EHR technology and fail to meet other program participation requirements.

August 23, 2012: The federal government released the final rules for Stage 2 of meaningful use with assurance that the public's voice was heard. The rules, which focus on health information exchange and access to data, will begin January 1, 2014. The final rules outline the certification criteria for the certification of EHR technology, so eligible professionals and hospitals may be assured that the systems they use will work. The rule also helps them meaningfully use health information technology and qualify for incentive payments. In addition, the rules modify the certification program to cut red tape and make the certification process more efficient (Manos & Mosquera, 2012).

What Is New in Stage 2?

With Stage 2, HHS expanded the meaningful use of EHR technology The Stage 2 criteria for meaningful use focuses on increasing the electronic capture of health information in a structured format, as well as increasing the exchange of clinically relevant information between providers of care at care transitions. To accomplish such objectives, the rule maintains the same core and menu structures as were used in Stage 1. The final rule contains 20 measures for physicians, of which 17 are core and 3 of 6 are menu objectives, and 19 measures for hospitals, of which 16 are core and 3 of 6 are menu. The Stage 2 meaningful use final rule includes many measures aimed at improving quality and efficiency, reducing disparities, engaging patients, improving care coordination, safeguarding privacy and more. The Stage 2 rule includes:

- Changes to the denominator of computerized provider order entry (optional in Stage 1; required in Stage 2)

- Elimination of the "exchange of key clinical information" core objective from Stage 1 in favor of a "transitions of care" core objective that requires electronic exchange of summary of care documents in Stage 2 (new in Stage 2)

- Replacing "provide patients with an electronic copy of their health information" objective with a "view online, download and transmit" core objective (new in Stage 2) (News Staff, 2012)

The Stage 2 rule also proposes new objectives that have greater applicability to many specialty providers. The addition of these objectives recognizes the leadership role that many specialty providers have played in the meaningful use of health IT for quality improvement purposes with respect to:

- Imaging results and information accessible through certified EHR technology

- Capability to identify and report cancer cases to a State cancer registry, except where prohibited, and in accordance with applicable law and practice

- Capability to identify and report specific cases to a specialized registry (other than a cancer registry), except where prohibited, and in accordance with applicable law and practice (News Staff, 2012)

Proposed Stage 3

As the goal for Stage 1 was data capture and patient access and information exchange and care coordination for Stage 2, the goal for Stage 3 Meaningful use is improved outcomes. An ONC presentation in July 2013 outlines the adoption of a new model of care that is team based, outcome oriented, and population management driven. In addition, it should address national health priorities and have broad applicability. The hope is that Stage 3 criteria will simplify and reduce reporting requirements and that adherence will rely more on market incentives to promote innovation and reward good behavior (Office of the National Coordinator for Health Information Technology, 2013d). None of these Stage 3 recommendations have been finalized or released at the time of this chapter's publication, since release of the NPRM has been postponed until late 2014.

Quality Measures

One of the "meaningful use" criteria for both hospitals and physicians is the requirement to report clinical quality measures (CQMs) to either CMS (for Medicare) or the States (for Medicaid). Quality measurement is considered one of the most important components of the incentive program under ARRA/HITECH, since the purpose of the health IT incentives is to promote reform in the delivery, cost, and quality of healthcare in the United States. Dr. David Blumenthal, the former national coordinator of health IT, emphasized this point when he said that "health IT is the means, but not the end. Getting an EHR up and running in healthcare is not the main objective behind the incentives provided by the federal government under ARRA. Improving health is. Promoting healthcare reform is" (Blumenthal, 2009).

For providers, the Stage 1 final rule lists 44 quality measures, with a requirement to report on six of them. For hospitals, Stage 1 meaningful use lists 15 measures, with a requirement to report on all of them (Medicare and Medicaid EHR Incentive Program). Because HHS itself was not yet ready to electronically accept quality measure reporting in 2011, the Stage 1 rule specified that hospitals and eligible providers could submit summary information on clinical quality measures to CMS through attestation. For Stage 2, CMS posted its proposed clinical quality measures approximately one month after releasing the proposed rules in late February (CMS, 2014). To comply with Stage 2 meaningful use, physicians will have to measure 12 of the 125 clinical quality measures from various areas, including patient/family engagement, population health, and others. CMS noted on its Web site, "some of these measures are still in development; therefore, the descriptions provided … may change before the final rule is published." Furthermore, some of the measures had not been endorsed by the National Quality Forum (NQF), a nonprofit that HHS brought in to develop healthcare-related benchmarks, at the time of posting (Perna, 2012).

Beginning in 2014, all providers, regardless of whether they are in Stage 1 or Stage 2 of meaningful use, will be required to report on the 2014 CQMs finalized in the Stage 2 rule. CMS has also provided information on what to report in 2013 as well as how to begin the transition for reporting in 2014. In addition, beginning in 2014, all EPs and EHs beyond their first year of meaningful use will be required to submit CQMs electronically (Centers for Medicare and Medicaid Services, 2013–2014).

Looking ahead to Meaningful Use Stage 3, the ONC Health IT Policy Committee is considering both e-clinical quality measures and the data intermediaries and standards to support them. The Policy Committee's Quality Measures Workgroup is tasked with developing recommendations for data intermediaries—and first and foremost to offer ONC leaders a sense of what the healthcare and health IT communities envision for intermediaries' roles. At the same time data intermediaries will be encouraged to develop proprietary measurements—or novel ways of measuring quality, according to *Government Health IT News* (Brino, 2013).

ONC and Establishment of the HIT Policy and Standards Committees

To drive the rapid, health IT-based reform under such an aggressive plan, the HITECH legislation re-energized ONC with specific accountabilities and significant funding. It also created the two new Federal Advisory Committees under its control: the HIT Policy Committee and the HIT Standards Committee, which have already been discussed in this chapter. Members of the two committees are public and private stakeholders who are tasked to provide recommendations on the HIT policy framework, standards, implementation specifications, and certification criteria for the electronic exchange and use of health information Additional information regarding these two committees is provided in the next section: "Health IT Federal Advisory Committees and Agencies."

ONC continues to stress the importance of working with all stakeholders to create workable plans. In the 2013 Federal Health IT Strategic Plan Report, ONC stated that its priorities will center on collaborating with Federal partners and private stakeholders to help providers, hospitals and other facilities, and others in the healthcare system to use tools and processes designed for the Meaningful Use EHR Incentive Program to achieve quality improvement goals in clinical practice and population health; expand health information exchange and interoperability capacity; and increase patient engagement, using health IT to foster consumer confidence and equal partnerships in making health decisions (Office of the National Coordinator for Health Information Technology, 2013b).

Many challenges remain. ONC and Federal partners will continue to engage with the public through open dialog, including the Health IT Policy and Standards Committees, to address existing and emergent policy and market changes. One of the steps ONC took in 2013 to meet these challenges was the formation of three new workgroups: Accountable Care, Consumer Empowerment, and the Food and Drug Administration Safety and Innovation Act (FDASIA), which is a joint workgroup of ONC and the FDA.

Challenges to Achieving Widespread Health Information Exchange

The Information Exchange Workgroup (IEW) makes recommendations to the Health IT Policy Committee on policies, sustainability, and implementation approaches to enhance the flow of health information. However, wide-scale interoperability challenges exist, leaving some primary care physicians and other providers with few options for meeting the health information exchange objectives included in meaningful use Stage 2 (MU2). EHR vendors, along with the federal government and the states, are taking steps to address the interoperability issue and provide doctors and hospitals with the tools to meet the MU2 requirements, but progress is sometimes slow.

The slow progress of EHR interoperability has not gone unnoticed in Congress, either. In October 2012, four powerful Republican members of the U.S. House of Representative Ways and Means Committee wrote to Kathleen Sebelius, secretary of HHS. They expressed "serious concerns that MU2 rules fail to achieve comprehensive interoperability in a timely manner, leaving our healthcare system trapped in information silos. The letter urged Sebelius to suspend incentive payments and delay penalties until HHS promulgates universal interoperable standards" (Bendix, 2013).

The IEW addressed these issues at the April 2013 Health IT Policy Committee Meeting. Micky Tripathi, M.D., chair of the workgroup, said that new payment policies were beginning to create the business case and spur provider demand for information exchange. However, the workgroup recommended that HHS harmonize requirements for all the new payment models for public and private providers and offer supplemental payments to motivate switches to HIE activities (Office of the National Coordinator for Health Information Technology, 2013k).

Gaps in HIE occur when providers are unable to exchange information with pharmacists, commercial labs, and other care settings such as behavioral health and long-term post-acute care facilities that lack compatible exchange systems. The IEW recommended that HHS and CMS simplify and coordinate required documentation as well as provide incentives for HIE activities with these other providers and in these alternate venues.

Another issue addressed by the IEW is the lack of cohesive program requirements across state-level programs, which inhibits seamless exchanges for multi-state providers and technology vendors. Tripathi said that variation may be the result of differences in programs that have federal and state components and/or where states have independent policy authority (e.g., privacy, liability, etc.). The workgroup recommendations included that CMS include HIE requirements in all programs including state waivers. In addition, HHS should create model language for state programs and encourage harmony in state-level HIE policies.

Patient-Centered Outcomes Research

ARRA and HITECH increased funding by more than $1 billion for Comparative Effectiveness Research (CER) and established the Federal Coordinating Council for Comparative Effectiveness Research (FCC-CER). This group is an advisory board comprised of clinical experts responsible for reducing duplication of efforts and encouraging coordination and complementary uses of resources, coordinating related health services research, and making recommendations to the President and Congress on CER infrastructure needs.

As part of this legislation, The Agency for Healthcare Research and Quality (AHRQ) received $1 billion of additional funding for CER. As one of 12 agencies within the Department of Health and Human Services, AHRQ supports research that helps people make more informed decisions and improves the quality of healthcare services. Some of AHRQ's funding must be shared with the National Institutes of Health (NIH) to conduct or support CER (Agency for Healthcare Research and Quality, 2009).

Additional funding was also made available to the Patient-Centered Outcome Research Institute (PCORI), a non-profit, public–private partnership organization created by legislative authority in March 2010 to conduct research that would provide information about the best available evidence to help patients and their healthcare providers make more informed decisions. PCORI's research is intended to give patients a better understanding of the prevention, treatment, and care options available as well as the science that supports those options (Patient-Centered Outcomes Research Institute. March, 2010).

In 2013, Joe Selby, M.D., executive director, PCORI, reported at the June 5 Health IT Policy Committee on two funding announcements for up to $68 million for Clinical Data Research Networks (CDRN) and Patient-Powered Research Networks (PPRN), of which $12 million would support up to 18 new or existing Patient-Powered Research Networks (PPRN) for 18 months. The research should involve patients with a single condition (Selby, 2013).

The remaining $56 million would support up to eight new or existing Clinical Data Research Networks for 18 months. Each network should include at least two healthcare systems that are willing to participate in collaborative studies with data-sharing as part of a national research infrastructure and can enroll at least 1,000,000 patients. Both types of networks must be open to data standardized within network and with other awardees' networks; patients, system, and clinicians engaged in governance and use; and capable of implementing clinical trials.

Currently, PCORI has approved 197 awards totaling more than 27 million to fund patient-centered CER projects (Patient-Centered Outcomes Research Institute. March, 2010).

Workforce Training

As discussed in this chapter's introduction, the rapid advancement toward a more technologically enabled healthcare system is driving a growing demand for health IT professionals—highly skilled health IT experts who can support the provider community in the adoption and meaningful use of electronic health records. To meet this demand, ONC funded the *Health IT Workforce Development Program* (Office of the National Coordinator for Health Information Technology, 2013f). The program's goal was to train a new workforce of health IT professionals who will be ready to help providers implement EHRs to improve healthcare quality, safety, and cost-effectiveness. But now it is even more important to pivot to integrated training of the incumbent workforce, aimed at helping them understand how to use health IT as a tool to enable care delivery and payment reform. This was addressed during a report from the Workforce Workgroup of the Health IT Policy Committee in June 2013.

Patricia Dombrowski, Bellevue College, reported on the adaptation of the curriculum for rural physician practices in rural and migrant clinics and for the VA. A five-hour online class was designed that VA employees could take, but on their own time. Nevertheless, the demand was high. An adaption is being designed for community colleges to use with veterans with funding from the Department of Labor.

Norma Morganti and Rita Horwitz, Cuyahoga Community College, talked about role-based workforce competencies for patient-centered care via HIT and focusing on PCMH, HIE, meaningful use, and population management. The design is based upon input from subject matter experts and was facilitated with a partnership with Better Health Greater Cleveland. The resources were built to be widely distributed and used by educators and healthcare organizations that are ready to move to patient-centered care supported by health IT. For each role, there are competencies, learning objectives, and resources.

Consumer/Patient Engagement and eHealth

"Patient-centered care is considered one pillar of a high-performing, high-quality health care system. It is a key component of many efforts to transform care and achieve better population health. Expansion of health information technology and consumer e-health tools—electronic tools and services such as secure e-mail messaging between patients and providers, or mobile health apps—have created new opportunities for individuals to participate actively in monitoring and directing their health and health care. [ONC] leads the strategy to increase electronic access to health information, support the development of tools that enable people to take action with that information, and shift attitudes related to the traditional roles of patients and providers" (Ricciardi, Mostashari, Murphy, Daniel, & Siminerio, 2013).

In the article quoted above, the ONC authors wrote that patients who use electronic health tools tend to be more engaged in managing their care. Such patients also tend to be better at finding the best quality and most cost-effective care, but often they lack access, despite the increase in mobile technologies. To address this issue, ONC is working to expand access to personal health technologies; promote a more collaborative partnership between patients and their healthcare providers; and boost awareness of patients' ability to request electronic access to their health data.

NIH and NLM Grants to Support Health IT Research

The passage of ARRA and the HITECH Act provision earmarked substantial funding in support of health IT research, in addition to programs supporting health IT training. For its part, the NIH received an infusion of funds for 2009 and 2010 as part of ARRA. NIH had designated more than $200 million in these two years for a new initiative called the NIH Challenge Grants in Health and Science Research. This program supported research on topics that address specific scientific and health research challenges in biomedical and behavioral research that would benefit from significant, two-year jump start funds. NIH funded more than 200 grants, each up to $1 million, depending on the number and quality of applications (National Institutes of Health, DHHS, 2009–2010).

In addition, the National Library of Medicine (NLM) offers Applied Informatics grants to health-related and scientific organizations that wish to optimize use of clinical and research information. These grants help organizations leverage the capabilities of health IT to bring usable, useful biomedical knowledge to end users by translating the findings of informatics and information science research into practice through novel or enhanced systems, incorporating them into real-life systems and service settings. In April 2012, Donald A.B. Lindberg, M.D., Director of the National Library of Medicine (NLM), announced that NLM had awarded 14 five-year grants totaling more than $67 million for research training in biomedical informatics, the discipline that seeks to apply computer and communications technology to improve health (National Library of Medicine, NIH, DHHS. April, 2012).

SHARP Research Grants

Alongside the NIH and NLM focus on incentivizing research, ONC also made available $60 million to support the development of Strategic Health IT Advanced Research Projects (SHARP). The SHARP Program funds research focused on achieving breakthrough advances to address well-documented problems that have impeded adoption of health IT and accelerating progress toward achieving nationwide meaningful use of health IT in support of a high-performing,

continuously learning healthcare system. ONC awarded four cooperative agreements of $15 million, with each awardee implementing a research program addressing a specific research focus area: Health IT Security, Patient-Centered Cognitive Support, Healthcare Application and Network Architectures, and Secondary Use of Health IT Data.

In 2012, ONC shifted the focus of SHARP grants to address the barriers to Meaningful Use in three major areas: EHRs, HIE, and Telemedicine, with Personal Health Records (PHRs) as a major subtopic. Another goal for the shift was to create an integrated security and privacy research IT community that can continue after the SHARP funding expires. The program has worked to automate complex decisions about sharing health records, develop ways to analyze personal health records access logs to catch policy violations, and ensure security and privacy in emerging telemedicine systems (Office of the National Coordinator for Health Information Technology, 2012).

STATE AND REGIONAL HEALTH IT PROGRAMS

With recognition that the regional electronic exchange of health information is essential to the successful implementation of NwHIN and to the success of national healthcare reform in general, the HITECH Act authorized and funded a State HIE Cooperative Program and a Regional HIT Extension Program. Taken together, these grant programs offer much-needed local and regional assistance and technical support to providers while enabling coordination and alignment within and among states. Ultimately, this will allow information to follow patients anywhere they go within the United States healthcare system (Office of the National Coordinator for Health Information Technology, 2013h; Office of the National Coordinator for Health Information Technology, 2013i).

State Health Information Exchange Cooperative Agreement Program

The State HIE Cooperative Agreement Program funds states' efforts to rapidly build capacity for exchanging health information across the healthcare system both within and across states. Awardees are responsible for increasing connectivity and enabling patient-centric information flow to improve the quality and efficiency of care. Key to this is the continual evolution and advancement of necessary governance, policies, technical services, business operations, and financing mechanisms for HIE over each state, territory, and SDE's four-year performance period. This program is building on existing efforts to advance regional and state-level health information exchange while moving toward nationwide interoperability.

On January 27, 2011, an additional $16 million was made available to states through ONC's new Challenge Grants program. This program will provide funding to states to encourage breakthrough innovations for health information exchange that can be leveraged widely to support nation-wide health information exchange and interoperability.

A major challenge for state health information exchanges is the question of sustainability—how will they survive once federal and state grants terminate?

To this end, the National Association of State Chief Information Officers (NASCIO) and HIMSS collaborated on a study of state level health information exchanges, the results of which were released in June 2013. The study showed that most states still rely on federal and state grants; however, some are becoming independent (NASCIO, 2013).

The study surveyed 26 U.S. states and territories about their health IT structures and programs. Most of the responding states, 58%, indicated that they had designated third parties to develop health exchanges in their states. The rest of those survey said the state owned and operated the HIE. Most of the states that reported having active HIEs were those that had a designated third party operating their exchanges.

While state-run HIEs relied heavily on subscription fees, the third-party-managed exchanges had a broader base of revenue, including membership dues and licensing fees as well as subscription fees. The third-party run exchanges sustain funding for operation by meeting the needs of the market, or the needs of hospitals and other providers to share health information.

"So how will state-level HIEs achieve sustainability? The model for success is already in place in some of the more successful HIEs across the country, who understand that the exchange of health information is only one of many services healthcare organizations find valuable" (Murphy, 2013).

Beacon Communities

Also funded by HITECH, ONC's Beacon Community Program will help guide the way to a transformed healthcare system. The program is working to fund more than a dozen demonstration communities that have already made inroads into the adoption of health IT, including EHRs and health information exchange. Beacon Communities are designed to advance new, innovative ways to improve care coordination, improve the quality of care, and slow the growth of healthcare spending. Their goals are to show how health IT tools and resources can contribute to communities' efforts and make breakthrough advancements in healthcare quality, safety, efficiency, and in public health at the community level, demonstrating that these gains are sustainable and replicable (Office of the National Coordinator for Health Information Technology, 2013j).

In 2010, ONC awarded $250 million in grants over three years to 17 selected communities throughout the United States. These communities have already made inroads in the development of secure, private, and accurate systems of EHR adoption and health information exchange. Each of them, with its unique population and regional context, is actively pursuing the following areas of focus:

- Building and strengthening the health IT infra-structure and exchange capabilities within communities, positioning each community to pursue a new level of sustainable healthcare quality and efficiency over the coming years

- Translating investments in health IT in the short run to measureable improvements in cost, quality, and population health

- Developing innovative approaches to performance measurement, technology, and care delivery to accelerate evidence generation for new approaches

In February 2013, the HIT Policy Committee noted that all 17 communities of the Beacon Communities have at least two measures trending positively and the launch of new exchange capabilities in communities like New Orleans and San Diego. The collaboration has enabled 51 primary care practice locations representing 432 providers and 447,000 patients to exchange a consistent patient summary care document to better manage transitions of care and to populate community data repositories or registries (Office of the National Coordinator for Health Information Technology, 2013k).

Health IT Regional Extension Program

The HITECH Act authorized a Health Information Technology Extension Program, which consists of Regional Extension Centers (RECs) and a national Health Information Technology Research Center (HITRC). The regional centers offered technical assistance, guidance, and information on best practices to support and accelerate healthcare providers' efforts to become meaningful users of Electronic Health Records (EHRs). The extension program established 62 regional centers, each serving a defined geographic area. The regional centers supported over 120,000 primary care providers through participating non-profit organizations in achieving meaningful use of EHRs and enabling nationwide health information exchange (Office of the National Coordinator for Health Information Technology, 2013i).

The Extension Program also established an HITRC, funded separately, to gather relevant information on effective practices and help the regional centers collaborate with one another and with relevant stakeholders to identify and share best practices in EHR adoption, effective use, and provider support.

In addition to helping individual and small practice providers, RECs are helping critical-access hospitals and other rural hospitals with targeted technical systems. These hospitals are important, because almost one-fifth of the American population lives in rural areas. However, they face unique challenges because of their remote geographic locations, small sizes and low patient volumes, limited workforces, shortages of clinicians, constrained financial resources, and lack of affordable, adequate connectivity. To help critical access and rural hospitals overcome these obstacles, ONC and the RECs offer a number of tools on the ONC Web site (Office of the National Coordinator for Health Information Technology, 2013l).

As of July 2013, more than 147,000 providers are currently enrolled with a Regional Extension Center. Of these, more than 124,000 are now live on an EHR and more than 70,000 have demonstrated Meaningful Use. Some 41% of PCPs nationwide are enrolled with a REC; 51% of rural PCPs are enrolled. Of these .85% of REC-enrolled providers are live on an EHR vs. 62% live on an EHR in the general provider population (Office of the National Coordinator for Health Information Technology, 2013i).

The RECs participate in eight "Community of Practice" working groups on emerging business lines in support of practice transformation including privacy and security, accountable care organizations, patient-centered medical home, health information exchange, and patient engagement.

HEALTH IT FEDERAL ADVISORY COMMITTEES AND AGENCIES

In 1972, decades before ARRA, HITECH, and ACA, the Federal Advisory Committee Act became law and is still the legal foundation defining how Federal Advisory Committees and Agencies (FACAs) should operate. As then prescribed, characteristics of such groups included openness and inclusiveness, specific authorization by either the President or the head of the overseeing agency, transparency, and clearly defined timelines for operation, termination, and renewal. In 2009, as mandated by ARRA and HITECH, ONC created two new Federal Advisory Committees, the HIT Policy Committee and the HIT Standards Committee, in order to gain broad input on the use of health IT to support healthcare reform. It is these committees, their leaders, and members who are changing the infrastructure of health IT across the nation.

The Health IT Policy Committee

The HIT Policy Committee is charged with making recommendations to ONC on a policy framework for the development and adoption of a nationwide health information infrastructure, including standards for the exchange of patient medical information (Office of the National Coordinator for Health Information Technology, 2013c). Originally serving the Committee were seven workgroups to address and make recommendations to the full committee on key reform issues such as meaningful use of EHRs, certification and adoption of EHRs, information exchange, NwHIN, the strategic plan framework, privacy and security policy, and enrollment in Federal and State health and human services programs. However, as the ONC has taken on a number of issues to expand and protect the future of health IT in America, those seven groups have grown to 14, including new workgroups for accountable care, consumer empowerment, and FDSIA. With the adoption of EHRs a primary concern for health IT, the Meaningful Use workgroup is currently weighing the issues for MU Stages 3 and 4 (Raths, 2013). The ultimate goal is secure, accessible information for providers and patients to aid in quality healthcare.

The Health IT Standards Committee

The HIT Standards Committee is charged with making recommendations to ONC on standards, implementation specifications, and certification criteria for the electronic exchange and use of health information (Office of the National Coordinator for Health Information Technology, 2013m). In harmonizing or recognizing standards and implementation specifications, the HIT Standards Committee is also tasked with providing for all associated testing by the National Institute of Standards and Technology (NIST). Originally serving the Committee are four workgroups addressing clinical operations, clinical quality, privacy and security requirements, and implementation strategies that accelerate the adoption of proposed standards. The Committee has now expanded to eight workgroups, to include ones focused on patient engagement, consumer technology, NwHIN, and vocabulary for this emerging field.

With the increased emphasis on accountable care, a new diagnostic coding system, and Meaningful Use for EHRs, the clinical and health technology sectors are feeling the crunch. In February 2013, members of the HIT Standards Committee felt that rather than operate independently, they needed to coordinate more with the Policy Committee (Halamka, 2013). The Committee decided to work toward a proposal with the HIT Policy Committee that would include these elements:

1. Capability that needs to be broadly adopted to support national goals

2. Programmatic alignment for that capability (e.g., MU3/4, ACO/PCMH, etc.) both at the Federal/state and commercial levels

3. Suggested timeline for adoption of the capability (where the timeline includes stakeholder alignment, standards development, technology development, deployment, and adoption)

Currently both Committees are working on priorities for Meaningful Use Stage 3.

In addition to the HIT Policy and Standards Committees, two other key groups are involved in the national healthcare reform movement, including the National Committee on Vital and Health Statistics and the National Quality Forum.

The National Committee on Vital and Health Statistics

The National Committee on Vital and Health Statistics (NCVHS) was originally established more than 60 years ago by Congress to serve as an advisory body to the HHS on health data, statistics, and national health information policy (National Committee on Vital and Health Statistics, 2009). It fulfills important review and advisory functions relative to health data and statistical problems of national and international interest, stimulates or conducts studies of such problems, and makes proposals for improvement of U.S. health statistics and information systems. In 1996, NCVHS was restructured to meet expanded responsibilities under HIPAA. In 2009, the committee was the first to hear testimony and make recommendations to ONC on meaningful use criteria to measure effective EHR use. Currently, NCVHS is the driving force behind the implementation of ICD-10, a new set of codes for medical diagnoses and inpatient stays. Because other areas of health IT depend on the coding system, NCVHS recommended that HHS not delay ICD-10, which is set to begin October 1, 2014. The Committee also recommends education, outreach, and practical guidance for those who must adopt the new standards (Green, 2013).

The National Quality Forum

The National Quality Forum (NQF) is a non-profit organization that aims to improve the quality of healthcare for all Americans through fulfillment of its three-part mission: to set national priorities and goals for performance improvement; to endorse national consensus standards for measuring and publicly reporting on performance; and to promote the attainment of national goals through education and outreach programs. NQF has taken the lead in defining the quality measures to qualify for the meaningful use incentives under HITECH. Currently, NQF is working

with the HIT Standards Committee to determine specific goals and deliverables for the second revision of Health Level Seven International (HL7), the global authority on standards for interoperability of health information technology with members in more than 55 countries (National Quality Forum, 2014).

NURSING INFORMATICS AND HEALTHCARE REFORM

In 2009, a survey sponsored by HIMSS' Nursing Informatics community entitled *Informatics Nurse Impact Survey* concluded that the passage of the ARRA and its provision of incentives to promote the meaningful use of EHRs created new opportunities for informatics nurses "to apply their ability not only to understand all sides of the IT process, but to act as a translator between those who understand the language of the technology and the language and needs of clinicians and patients" (HIMSS, 2009). HIMSS reinforced this stance in 2011 when it released its Position Statement on Transforming Nursing Practice through Technology and Practice that said in part, "Nurses are key leaders in developing the infrastructure for effective and efficient health information technology that transforms the delivery of care. Nursing informatics professionals are the liaisons to successful interactions with technology in healthcare" (HIMSS, 2011).

For years, informatics nurses have contributed to the work of healthcare reform implementation teams, creating constantly stronger positions from which to help put the new national healthcare infrastructure in place. Given the aggressive timeframes written into the new healthcare reform legislation, however, collaboration between public and private healthcare entities has never been more important. This call to action in the transformation of the healthcare industry has raised the visibility of a number of respected nursing and nursing informatics professional organizations, whose missions seek to advance the practice of informatics nurses and strengthen the profession's collective voice and impact. This section highlights some of the involvement that nurses have had in the work of HIT and healthcare reform.

Nursing Informatics Competencies

Today's informatics nurse combines clinical knowledge with IT to improve the ways nurses diagnose, treat, care for, and manage patients. Essentially, informatics nurses support, change, expand, and transform nursing practice through the design and implementation of information technology. The ANI defines nursing practice as "a specialty that integrates nursing science, computer science, and information science to manage and communicate data, information, knowledge, and wisdom in nursing practice" (RNDegrees, n.d.).

In the transforming healthcare industry environment, informatics nurses help design the automated tools that help clinicians, nurse educators, nursing students, nurse researches, policy-makers, and consumers as they increasingly seek to manage their own health. Therefore, it is essential that a nursing culture that promotes the acceptance and use of information technology is sustained and advanced by establishing informatics nurse competencies and the educational processes that help nurses achieve them.

Many in the profession emphasize the need for every nurse, whether employed in a practice or educational setting, to develop a minimum or "user" level of computer literacy and informatics theory. A second tier includes the intermediate level of literacy, which includes nurses who may work part time on teams to design, modify, or evaluate HIT systems. The third level of competency is the advanced or innovator level where a nurse has begun to specialize. A more complete discussion of competencies and competency development for nurses is provided elsewhere in this book.

Again, it is important to note that the informatics competencies described here are for nurses and nurse leaders, not informatics nurses. Practicing nurses' understanding of the role HIT plays to drive quality care and healthcare reform directly impacts their adoption of HIT and their definition of best practice use of HIT.

The Intersection of HIT Policy and Nursing Informatics

Informatics nurses are poised to play pivotal leadership roles in defining new policies that help make the goals of ARRA and HITECH a reality over coming years. To make such a profound difference in today's constantly changing healthcare environment, informatics professionals must be aware of existing and proposed healthcare policy on an ongoing basis. Policy is defined as a course of action that guides present and future decisions, is based on given conditions, and is selected from among identified alternatives. Healthcare policy is established on local, state, and national levels to guide the implementations of solutions for the population's health needs. Both existing conditions and emerging trends in the healthcare industry influence policy decisions. Policy decisions often establish the direction for future trends that impact informatics. Informatics nurse professionals, therefore, must become more cognizant of events and the healthcare policies that will affect their practices (Gassert, 2006).

As aptly summarized by one of nursing's most active and respected organizations, the ANI, "…'meaningful use' of

HIT, when combined with best practice and evidence-based care delivery, will improve healthcare for all Americans. This is an essential foundation for the future of nursing, and informatics nurses must be engaged as leaders in the effective use of information technology to impact the quality and efficiency of healthcare service" (Sensmeier, 2009).

Influencing Health IT Transformation Through Testimony and Comment

This chapter has discussed the need for health IT competencies, awareness of how health IT is changing the way we diagnose, treat, care for, and manage patients, as well as healthcare policies that affect healthcare practices and the global healthcare landscape. In addition, healthcare informatics professionals should never underestimate the power of communication to bring about meaningful change in our Nation's healthcare delivery system.

In 2005, the World Health Organization's Commission on the Social Determinants of Health asked, "What narrative will capture the imaginations, feelings, intellect and will of political decision-makers and the broader public and inspire them to action?" (World Health Organization Secretariat of the Commission on Social Determinants of Health, 2005) Years later, the question is more important than ever to the health IT professionals who stand in an unprecedented position to effect change. Public comment through the growing number of media outlets—supported by the emergence of the internet and social media—translates theory and knowledge into meaningful activity that can drive and define local, state, and federal policy, addressing key health and social issues and improving the lives of patients affected by them (Kaminski, 2007).

Outlets for communications that can reach pivotal society segments and the ears of key individual influencers in healthcare reform include not only traditional media (newspapers, magazines, books) but also new mass media formats like Web-based video and blogs, Twitter, and other social media sites. Whether commenting over these outlets from organizations like HIMSS or AMIA or as an individual active in healthcare transformation, such communication can change public perceptions of current issues and help form and influence public attitudes and decisions.

Many health IT agencies also collaborate with and testify to federal committees to influence healthcare laws. In July 2013, HIMSS commented on the Senate Finance Committee's hearing on Healthcare Quality. While agreeing with the federal government's desire and plan to move toward quality healthcare, HIMSS urged the Finance Committee to focus on solidifying the Health IT infrastructure before introducing new quality measures (MacLean & Lieber, 2013).

Paul Ginsberg of the Center for Studying Health System Challenges testified before the U.S. Senate Committee on Finance regarding the high price and low transparency of healthcare costs (Ginsburg, 2013). The June 18, 2013, testimony came before the rollout of the Health Insurance Exchange in October and touch on one of the key issues of the new ACA.

THE ROAD AHEAD

Leaders in healthcare agree: the future depends on a system that will continue to innovate using health IT and to rely on informatics to play instrumental roles in patient safety, change management, and quality improvement, as evidenced by quality outcomes, enhanced workflow, and user acceptance. These areas highlight the value of an informatics-trained workforce and their roles in the adoption of health information technologies that deliver higher quality clinical applications across healthcare organizations.

That value can only increase as new directions and priorities emerge in healthcare. In an environment where the roles of all healthcare providers are diversifying, informatics nurses must prepare to guide the profession appropriately from their positions as project managers, consultants, educators, researchers, product developers, decision support and outcomes managers, chief clinical information officers, chief information officers, advocates, policy developers, entrepreneurs, and business owners. This is especially true where informatics nurses can contribute leadership in the effective design and use of EHR systems. To achieve our nation's healthcare reform goals, the healthcare community must leverage the sources of patient-care technologies and information management competence that informatics nurses provide to ensure that the national investment in HIT and EHRs is implemented properly and effectively over coming years.

In fact, in its October 2009 recommendations to the Robert Wood Johnson Foundation (RWJF) on the future of nursing, the ANI argued that nurses will be integral to achieving a vision that will require a nationwide effort to adopt and implement EHR systems in a meaningful way. "This is an incredible opportunity to build upon our understanding of effectiveness research, evidence-based practice, innovation and technology to optimize patient care and health outcomes. *The future of nursing will rely on this transformation, as well as on the important role of nurses in enabling this digital revolution*" (ANI, 2009).

For no professional group does the future hold more excitement and promise from so many productive perspectives than it does for informatics nurses.

SUMMARY

The passage of landmark healthcare reform legislation including ARRA and the HITECH Act in 2009 and ACA in 2010—as upheld by the U.S. Supreme Court on June 28, 2012—have changed the landscape of the U.S. healthcare industry forever, perhaps more than any expert envisioned just scant years ago.

The Obama Administration's hard-fought legislative success is testimony to the growing recognition that advanced health IT is essential to support the enormous amounts of electronic information that will be collected and exchanged will be foundational to industry transformation and healthcare reform. As the massive transformation from disconnected, inefficient, paper-based "islands" of care delivery to a nationwide, interconnected, and interoperable system driven by EHRs and health IT innovation, the importance of nurses and nursing informatics has become increasingly evident. For decades, nurses have proactively contributed resources to the development, use, and evaluation of information systems. Today, they constitute the largest single group of healthcare professionals, and include experts who serve on national committees and initiatives focused on HIT policy, standards and terminology development, standards harmonization, and EHR adoption. Performing their front-line roles, nurses will continue to have a profound impact on the quality and effectiveness of healthcare and are emerging as leaders in the effective use of HIT to improve the quality and efficiency of healthcare services.

REFERENCES

Abelson, R., Harris, G., & Pear, R. (2011). Whatever court rules, major changes in health care likely to last. *The New York Times*. Retrieved from http://www.nytimes.com/2011/11/15/health/policy/health-care-is-changing-despite-federal-uncertainty.html?pagewanted=all

Agency for Healthcare Research and Quality. (2009). What is comparative effectiveness research. *Effective Health Care Program*. Retrieved from http://effectivehealthcare.ahrq.gov/index.cfm/what-is-comparative-effectiveness-research1/

All Things Medical Billing. (2014). *History of HIPAA*. Retrieved from http://www.all-things-medical-billing.com/history of HIPAA.html

AMIA. (2005). AMIA 10x10 courses: Training health care professionals to serve as Informatics leaders. *Virtual Courses*. Retrieved from http:www.amia.org/education/10x10-courses

ANI. (2009). *Testimony to the Robert Wood Johnson Foundation initiative on the future of nursing: acute care, in Los Angeles, California, on October 19, 2009*. Retrieved from http://journals.lww.com/cinjournal/Documents/

ANI%20Response%20to%20RWJ_IOM%20on%20The%20
Future%20of%20Nursing.pdf
ARRA and HITECH Act Resource Center, *First Insight*®.
(2009). Retrieved from http://www.first-insight.com/
News_Events-ARRA-HITECHACT.html
Barr, F. (2008, November 6). *Healthcare interoperability:
the big debate, e Health Insider*. Retrieved from http://
informaticsprofessor.blogspot.com/2014/10/what-are-
realistic-goals-for-ehr.html
Bendix, J. (2013). Meaningful use 2: 2013's interoperability challenge. *Medical Economics*. Retrieved from
http://medicaleconomics.modernmedicine.com/
medical-economics/news/tags/meaningful-use/
meaningful-use-2-2013s-interoperability-challenge
Blue Cross Blue Shield of Michigan. (2009, January 16).
What everyone should know about HIPAA Version 5010.
The Record. Retrieved from
http://www.bcbsm.com/newsletter/therecord/
record_1210/record_1210b.shtml/
Blumenthal, D. (2009, September 16). *National HIPAA
Summit in Washington, D.C.* Retrieved from http://www.
hipaasummit.com/past17/index.html
Brino, A. (2013). ONC crafting e-quality measure
policies for MU3. *Government Health IT News*.
Retrieved from http://www.govhealthit.com/news/
crafting-e-quality-measure-policies-mu3
Bush, G. W. (2004a, January 20). *State of the union address*.
Retrieved from http://www.americanrhetoric.com/
speeches/stateoftheunion2004.htm
Bush, G. W. (2004b). *Executive order, incentives for the use
of health information technology and establishing the
position of the National Health Information Technology
Coordinator*. Retrieved from http://edocket.access.gpo.
gov/cfr_2005/janqtr/pdf/3CFR13335.pdf
Bureau of Labor Statistics, U.S. Department of Labor. (2012).
Medical records and health information technicians.
Occupational Outlook Handbook (2012–2013, ed.).
Retrieved from http://www.bls.gov/ooh/healthcare/
medical-records-and-health-information-
technicians.htm.
Centers for Medicare and Medicaid Services. (2012,
February 22). An introductory overview of the HIPAA
5010, *MLN (Medicare Leadership Network Matters)*.
Retrieved from http://www.cms.gov/Outreach-
and-Education/Medicare-Learning-Network-MLN/
MLNMattersArticles/
downloads//se0904.pdf
Centers for Medicare and Medicaid Services. (2011).
Medicare and Medicaid EHR incentive program basics.
Regulations and Guidance Legislation. Retrieved from
http://www.cms.gov/Regulations-and-Guidance/
Legislation/EHRIncentivePrograms/Downloads/HITPC_
Jan2014_Full_Deck.pdf
Centers for Medicare and Medicaid Services. (2013). *Clinical
quality measures (CQMs)*. Retrieved from http://www.
cms.gov/Regulations-and-Guidance/Legislation/
EHRIncentivePrograms/ClinicalQualityMeasures.html

Centers for Medicare and Medicaid Services (2014).
Proposed clinical quality measures for 2014. Retrieved
from https://www.cms.gov/Medicare/Quality-Initiatives-
Patient-Assessment-Instruments/QualityMeasures/
ProposedClinicalQualityMeasuresfor2014.html
Certification Commission for Healthcare Technology.
(2014). *About CCHIT*. Retrieved from http://www.cchit.
org/about-cchit
Computing Research Association. (1999, February 24). *The
President's Information Technology Advisory Committee
(PITAC) Final Report: Fact Sheet*. Retrieved from http://
www.cra.org/govaffairs/advocacy/pitac_fs.pdf
Connor, D. (2007). Healthcare pros debate interoperability
standards. *Network World*. Retrieved from http://www.
networkworld.com/news/2007/022707-healthcare-pros.
html
Dick, R., & Steen, E. (1997). *The computer-based patient
record: An essential technology for healthcare*. Institute of
Medicine, Committee on Improving the Patient Record.
Washington, DC: National Academy Press. Retrieved
from http://www.iom.edu/Reports/1997/The-Computer-
Based-Patient-Record-An-Essential-Technology-for-
Health-Care-Revised-Edition.aspx
Enrado, P. (2011). NNIN's evolution to NwHIN: From
the ground up. *Healthcare IT News NHIN Watch*.
Retrieved from http://www.nhinwatch.com/perspective/
nhins-evolution-nwhin-ground
Fickenscher, K. (2013). AMIA comments to Farzad
Mostashari, Office of the National Coordinator for
Health Technology. *AMIA*. Retrieved from http://www.
amia.org/sites/amia.org/files/AMIA-ResponseSubmitted-
toONC-HIT-Patient-Safety-Plan.pdf
Fields, W., & Lieber, H. (2013). *Comments to Farzad
Mostashari, national coordinator, ONC*. Retrieved from
http://www.himss.org/files/HIMSSorg/content/files
/2013Feb4HIMSSCommentPatientSafetyAction
Plan.pdf
Gassert, C. A. (2006). Nursing informatics and health-
care policy. In Saba, V., & McCormick, K. (Eds), *Issues
in Informatics* (pp. 183–194). Essentials of Nursing
Informatics, Issues in Informatics, USA, The McGraw Hill
Companies, Inc.
Ginsburg, P. (2013). *High prices, low transparency: The bitter
pill of healthcare costs*. Testimony before the US Senate
Committee on Finance. Retrieved from http://www.
hschange.com/CONTENT/1362/
Golden, P. (2013). *Meaningful use payments top 15.5B*.
Massachusetts eHealth Institute. Retrieved from http://
www.cms.gov/Regulations-and-Guidance/Legislation/
EHRIncentivePrograms/Downloads/September2014_
SummaryReport.pdf
Green, L. (2013). *Findings from the June 2013 NCVHS hear-
ing on current state of administrative simplification
standards, code sets, and operating rules*. Retrieved from
http://www.ncvhs.hhs.gov/130920lt.pdf
Halamka, J. (2013). The February HIT Standards
Committee meeting. *Healthcare IT News*. Retrieved

from http://www.healthcareitnews.com/blog/february-hit-standards-committee-meeting

Harsha, P. (2005). *PCAST to assume PITAC's role.* Computing Research Association. Retrieved from http://cra.org/govaffairs/blog/2005/09/pcast-to-assume-pitacs-role/

Health Information and Management Systems Society. (2010). *Integrating the Healthcare Enterprise (IHE).* Retrieved from http://www.himss.org/ASP/topics_ihe.asp

Health IT (2012, October 4). *Temporary Certification Program.* Retrieved from http://www.healthit.gov/policy-researchers-implementers/temporarycertification-program

Health IT Workforce Development Sub Group. (2013). *Health IT Workforce recommendations.* Health IT Policy Committee. Retrieved from http://www.healthit.gov/archive?dir=HIT%20Policy%20Committee/2013/Certification%20%26%20Adoption/2013-05-16

HHS Press Office. (2011). *We can't wait: Obama administration takes new steps to encourage doctors and hospitals to use health information technology to lower costs, improve quality, create jobs.* U.S. Department of Health & Human Services. Retrieved from http://www.hhs.gov/news/press/2011pres/11/20111130a.html

HHS Press Office. (2013). *New rule protects patient privacy, secures health information.* Retrieved from http://www.hhs.gov/news/press/2013pres/01/20130117b.html

HIMSS (Health Information and Management Systems Society) Legacy Workgroup. (2007). *The history of HIMSS.* Retrieved from http://www.himss.org/content/files/HIMSS_HISTORY.pdf

HIMSS (Health Information and Management Systems Society). (2009, April 2). *Informatics nurse impact survey, sponsored by McKesson. Executive summary.* Retrieved from http://www.himss.org/files/HIMSSorg/content/files/HIMSS2009InformaticsNurseImpactSurvey.pdf

HIMSS (Health Information and Management Systems Society). (2011). *HIMSS position statement on transforming nursing practice through technology and informatics.* Retrieved from http://www.himss.org/files/HIMSSorg/handouts/HIMSSPositionStatementTransformingNursingPracticethroughTechnologyInformatics.pdf

Institute of Medicine, Committee on Quality of Health Care in America. (2001). *Crossing the quality chasm: A new health system for the 21st century.* Washington, DC: National Academy Press. Retrieved from http://www.nap.edu/catalog.php?record_id=10027

Institute of Medicine. (2013, October 25). *Robert Wood Johnson Foundation initiative on the future of nursing.* Retrieved from http://www.iom.edu/Activities/Workforce/Nursing.aspx.

Kaminski, J. (2007). *Activism in education focus: Using communicative and creative technologies to weave social justice and change theory into the tapestry of nursing curriculum.* Retrieved from http://econurse.org/EthelJohns.html

Kohn, L., Corrigan, J., & Donaldson, M., (Eds.). (1999). *To err is human: Building a safer health system.* Institute of Medicine. Washington, DC: National Academy Press. Retrieved from http://www.nap.edu/openbook.php?isbn=0309068371

MacLean, S., & Lieber, S. (2013). *Comments to Senate Committee on finance.* Retrieved from http://himss.files.cms-plus.com/FileDownloads/72013%20Senate%20Finance%20Letter%20on%20Quality%20Measurement%20FINAL%2007-30-13.pdf

Manos, D., & Mosquera, M. (2012). Final rules for Stage 2 meaningful use released. *Healthcare IT News.* Retrieved from http://www.healthcareitnews.com/news/final-rules-stage-2-meaningful-use-released?page=1

Marburger, III, J., & Kvamme, E. (2008). Transition letter to the next PCAST. Office of Science Technology and Policy. Retrieved from http://www.whitehouse.gov/files/documents/ostp/PCAST/PCAST%20Transition%20Letter%202008-2.pdf

Mitchell, R. (2011). Health care jobs grow … in administration. *USA Today.* Retrieved from http://www.usatoday.com/money/industries/health/story/2011-11-30/health-care-creates-jobs/51506244/1

Monegain, B. (2013). Health IT worker shortage looms. *Healthcare IT News.* Retrieved from http://www.healthcareitnews.com/news/health-it-worker-shortage-looms

Monticello, K. (2012). *Public comments for meaningful use Stage 2 NPRM due May 7, legal health information exchange.* Retrieved from http://www.legalhie.com/meaningful-use/public-comments-for-meaningful-use-stage-2-nprm-due-may-7/

Mostashari, F. (2013). Electronic health information exchange governance framework released. *Health IT Buzz.* Retrieved from http://www.healthit.gov/buzz-blog/from-the-onc-desk/electronic-health-information-exchange-governance-framework-released/

Murphy, K. (2013). How will sate HIEs achieve sustainability, success? *EHR intelligence.* Retrieved from http://ehrintelligence.com/2013/06/17/how-will-state-level-hies-achieve-sustainability-success/

National Committee on Vital and Health Statistics. (2009). Introduction to the NCVHS. Retrieved from http://www.ncvhs.hhs.gov/intro.htm

National Institutes of Health (2009–2010). *Challenge grants in health and science research.* Retrieved from http://grants.nih.gov/grants/funding/challenge_award/

National Library of Medicine. NIH, DHHS, (2012, April). *University-based biomedical informatics research training programs.* Retrieved from http://www.nlm.nih.gov/ep/GrantTrainInstitute.html

NASCIO (National Association of State Chief Information Officers). (2013). NASCIO/HIMMS State CIO Survey Collaboration. *The health IT landscape in the States.*

Retrieved from http://www.nascio.org/publications/ documents/The_Health_IT_Landscape_in_the_States_ NASCIO_HIMSS.pdf

National Quality Forum. (2014). *Effective communication and care coordination*. Retrieved from http://www.quality forum.org/About_NQF/About_NQF.aspx

News Staff. (2012). At a glance: Stage 2 final rule. *Healthcare IT News*. Retrieved from http://www.healthcareitnews. com/news/glance-stage-2-final-rule

Obama Care. (2013, October 25). *Obama care explained*. Retrieved from http://Obama-care.org/ obama-care-explained/

Office of Civil Rights DHHS. (2005, May). *Summary of the HIPAA Privacy Rule: HIPAA Compliance Assistance*. Retrieved from http://www.hhs.gov/ ocr/privacy/hipaa/understanding/summary/privacy summary.pdf

Office of the National Coordinator for Health Information Technology. (2012, May 26). *Strategic health IT advanced research projects (SHARPS) presentation*. Retrieved from http://www.healthit.gov/sites/default/files/sharp_final_ report_appendices.pdf

Office of the National Coordinator for Health Information Technology. (2013a). *Health IT patient safety action and surveillance plan*. Retrieved from http://www.healthit. gov/sites/default/files/safety_plan_master.pdf

Office of the National Coordinator for Health Information Technology. (2013b). *Federal health IT strategic plan*. Retrieved from http://www.healthit.gov/sites/default/ files/federal-health-it-strategic-plan-progress-report- 0613.paper_version.v2.pdf

Office of the National Coordinator for Health Information Technology. (2013c, February 6). *Health IT Policy Committee*. Retrieved from http://www.healthit.gov/ FACAS/calendar/2013/03/14/hit-policy-committee.

Office of the National Coordinator for Health Information Technology. (2013d). *Meaningful use Stage 3 recommen- dations power point*. Retrieved from http://www.healthit. gov/facas/calendar/2013/07/16/policy-meaningful-use- workgroup

Office of the National Coordinator for Health Information Technology. (2013e). *Governance framework for trusted electronic health information exchange*. Retrieved from http://www.healthit.gov/sites/default/files/ GovernanceFrameworkTrustedEHIE_Final.pdf

Office of the National Coordinator for Health Information Technology. (2013f, June). *Health IT Workforce Development Programs*. Retrieved from http://www.healthit.gov/providers-professionals/ workforce-development-programs

Office of the National Coordinator for Health Information Technology. (2013g). *HITECH and funding opportunities*. Retrieved from http://www. healthit.gov/policy-researchers-implementers/ meaningful-use-regulations

Office of the National Coordinator for Health Information Technology. (2013h). *State Health Information*

Exchange Cooperative Program. Retrieved from http://www.healthit.gov/providers-professionals/ health-information-exchange/nationwide-hie-strategy

Office of the National Coordinator for Health Information Technology. (2013i). *Regional exten- sion centers (RECs)*. Retrieved from http:// www.healthit.gov/providers-professionals/ regional-extension-centers-recs

Office of the National Coordinator for Health Information Technology. (2013j). *Beacon Community Program: Improving health through health information technology*. Retrieved from http://www.healthit.gov/providers- professionals/faqs/what-beacon-community-cooperative- agreement-program

Office of the National Coordinator for Health Information Technology. (2013k). *Health IT Policy Committee (a Federal Advisory Committee)*. Retrieved from http:// www.healthit.gov/policy-researchers-implementers/ health-it-policy-committee

Office of the National Coordinator for Health Information Technology. (2013l). *REC—Rural health resources*. Retrieved from http://www.healthit.gov/providers- professionals/benefits-critical-access-hospitals-and- other-small-rural-hospitals

Office of the National Coordinator for Health Information Technology. (2013m). *Health IT Standards Committee (a Federal Advisory Committee)*. Retrieved from http:// www.healthit.gov/facas/health-it-standards-committee

Patient-Centered Outcomes Research Institute. (2010). *Funding awards*. Retrieved from http://www.pcori.org/ pfaawards/

Perna, G. (2012). *CMS posts Stage 2 quality measures, healthcare informatics*. Retrieved from http:// www.healthcare-informatics.com/news-item/ cms-posts-stage-2-clinical-quality-measures

President's Council of Advisors on Science and Technology. (2010). *Realizing the full potential of health information technology to improve healthcare for Americans: The path forward*. Retrieved from http://www.whitehouse. gov/sites/default/files/microsites/ostp/pcast-health-it- report.pdf

President's Information Technology Advisory Committee. (2001, February). *Panel on transforming health care, transforming health care through information technology, report to the president*. Retrieved from http://cra.org/ govaffairs/blog/2005/09/pcast-to-assume-pitacs-role/

Raths, D. (2013). Health IT Policy Committee meeting: The year ahead and a glimpse at Stage 4 of meaningful use. *Healthcare Informatics*. Retrieved from http://www. healthcare-informatics.com/article/health-it-policy- committee-meeting-year-ahead-and-glimpse-stage- 4-meaningful-use

Ricciardi, L., Mostashari, F., Murphy, J., Daniel, G. J., & Siminerio, E. P. (2013). A national action plan to support consumer engagement via e-health. *Health Affairs, 32*(2). Retrieved from http://content.healthaffairs.org/ content/32/2/376.abstract

RNDegrees.net. (n.d.). Nursing Informatics Degree Programs: Section on Nursing Informatics. *Nursing Education Guide*. Retrieved from http://rndegrees.net/nursing-informatics-degree-programs.html

Robeznieks, A. (2012). *CMS delays 5010 enforcement, again, modern healthcare*. Retrieved from http://www.modernhealthcare.com/article/20120315/NEWS/303159955

Selby, J. (2013). *PCORI briefing to the ONC Health IT Policy Committee*. Retrieved from http://www.healthit.gov/FACAS/calendar/2013/07/09/hit-policy-committee

Sensmeier, J. (2009, September–October). Don't overlook the role of nurses in the digital revolution. GHIT. Retrieved from http://www.allianceni.org/docs/GHIT_JSensmeier.pdf

Smith, M., Saunders, R., Stuckhardt, L., & McGinnis, J. M. (Eds.). (2013). *Best care at lower cost: The path to continuously learning health care in America*. Institute of Medicine, Committee on the Learning Health Care System in America. Washington, DC: National Academy Press. Retrieved from http://www.iom.edu/Reports/2012/Best-Care-at-Lower-Cost-The-Path-to-Continuously-Learning-Health-Care-in-America.aspx

World Health Organization Secretariat of the Commission on Social Determinants of Health. (2005 Background Report). Action on the social determinants of health: Learning from previous experiences, p. 44.

OTHER RESOURCES

Murphy, J. (2009, Fall). Meaningful use for nursing: Six themes regarding the definition for meaningful use, nursing informatics commentary. *Journal of Healthcare Information Management, 23*(4), 9–11.

Murphy, J. (2010, Winter). This is our time: How ARRA changed the face of health IT, nursing informatics commentary. *Journal of Healthcare Information Management, 24*(1), 8–9.

Patient-Centered Outcomes Research Institute. Retrieved from http://www.pcori.org/

PART 4

Nursing Informatics Leadership

Kathleen Smith

17

The Role of the Nurse Executive in Information Technology Decision-Making

Roy L. Simpson

• OBJECTIVES

1. Discuss why the technology lifecycle virtually ensures perpetual healthcare information technology (HIT) decision-making in healthcare delivery environments.
2. Describe the need for executive nurses to commit to lifelong learning if they are to participate and actively lead HIT decision-making.
3. Identify the two most important HIT processes that demand nurse executive involvement.
4. Discuss where to turn for help in developing and maintaining a nursing-centric, deep HIT competency.
5. Describe the value that only nurse executives, acting as the all-important "voice of the patient," bring to HIT decision-making.

• KEY WORDS

Technology lifecycle
Process mapping
Workflow designs
Nursing-centric HIT expertise
Voice of the patient
Nursing Informatics

To productively contribute and, ultimately, drive technology decisions, nurse executives need to be constantly updating and advancing their hospital information technology (HIT) knowledge. This knowledge needs to go beyond baseline functionality-level information of nursing and clinical information systems, which describes what systems can accomplish, to more a complex understanding of enterprise-wide integration, data and process mapping, and business analytics. Commanding a deep well of HIT expertise helps nurse executives understand the delicate interplay of nursing and outcome data inside the healthcare organization and beyond—to the regulator and payer worlds.

Few industries collect, analyze, and disseminate information with the velocity seen in healthcare and in no industry does the data-driven decision have more importance. In healthcare, every patient care decision can have a life-and-death implication. That is why the timely communication of accurate data plays such a critical role in healthcare delivery.

FLAWED THINKING

Most nurse executives view technology-related decision-making as an episodic responsibility that takes place once every seven to 10 years, the timeframe when major HIT systems are replaced. However, this widely held assumption could not be further from the truth. In the lived experience, technology decision-making happens with regularity throughout the year—every year. From an executive nurse perspective, the complexity of HIT, coupled with the speed of innovation and the rapid adoption of emerging technologies, requires that theoretical and applied knowledge of HIT be up-to-date at all times. As the largest "user group" in most healthcare organizations, nursing feels the impact of technology decisions faster and more often than other user populations in the healthcare organization.

The intricate and interwoven nature of the healthcare technology, especially those systems directly involved in managing, monitoring, and tracking patient care, makes even what appears to be a "small decision" an important one. Technology selections and deployments, with their organizationally transformative potential, come with wide-reaching impacts that can be felt for decades. Consider the decision to upgrade a messaging technology, which would be viewed by many executives as a "small decision." The speed with which nursing data needs to be communicated, and its inherent criticality, can transform the inevitable glitches in new technology introduction into minefields for patient care that reach far beyond the organizational boundaries of nursing.

In addition to the potential impact on patient care the "simplest" technology decision has, consider all the third parties outside the healthcare organization that depend on it for documentation of activities, results, and outcomes. A variety of regulator- and payer-specified formats drive how this documentation must be reported, further complicating results and outcome reporting. Financial reimbursement, the lifeblood of the healthcare organization, literally hangs in the balance for all but the rare privately funded institution.

TECHNOLOGY'S LIFECYCLE

To better understand the incessant nature and far-reaching impact of technology-related decisions, consider the six-stage Technology Life Cycle (Fig. 17.1).

The lifecycle of every technology investment spans six distinct phases, from planning to procurement to deployment to management to support and disposition, only to cycle back to planning. However, various "stops" and "starts," some are internally caused and others are

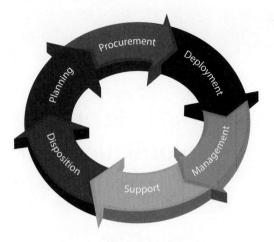

• **FIGURE 17.1.** Technology Life Cycle.

triggered externally. Issues that did not surface during "Planning" or "Procurement" make themselves known during "Deployment," "Management," "Support," or even "Disposition," wreaking havoc on the most well-conceived implementation plan.

Overlaying this lifecycle with an ever-present technology obsolescence complicates technology-related decision-making further. Three key types of obsolescence exist:

- Technology providers' architecture, product, and integration plans
- Third parties' priority shifts
- Regulators' unexpected recalls

The impact of planned obsolescence cannot be overlooked when nurse executives make HIT-related decisions (The Economist, 2009). Technology providers worldwide require engineers to design obsolescence into their systems to ensure ongoing market demand, protect market share, and preserve revenue streams (The Economist, 2009). Technology providers with nurse executives on staff tend to exercise considerable influence over architecture, product, and integration efforts. However, those without such internal nursing advocates may find nursing issues significantly overshadowed by the financial and business pressures public and privately held technology companies face.

In addition to providers' planned obsolescence, systems face being updated or even phased out when the external market landscape changes. Consider the massive overhaul needed to move financial information systems from a cost-plus orientation to a system of capped reimbursement. Virtually overnight, healthcare organizations had to replace large, charge-capture legacy systems with technology that could accurately predict total costs by procedure. Shifts in regulatory- or payer-related priorities can trigger a range of system changes from code revisions all the way up to system replacement. When healthcare organizations face significant penalties, such as funding losses or reductions, fines and legal consequences, and fiscal threats to their very existence, non-compliance is not an option. Complying with these environmental mandates can throw technology lifecycles into free fall as legacy systems struggle to accommodate regulator or payer mandates that were nowhere on the horizon when these systems were built.

A third type of obsolescence, one of an unexpected nature, can derail technology decision-making and implementation in short order as well. This third type pertains to regulators changing the status of a medical device or technology, either narrowing the approved scope of use or even recalling the product, after it has been introduced to the market and is generally available. For example, one hospital selected an FDA-approved monitoring device and conducted extensive staff training only to have the product recalled three months before its formal deployment. In this case, the completed pre-rollout work was of no use as institutional leaders scrambled to vet a replacement device and reconvene round-the-clock training on the new monitoring technology. Obviously, the rollout was delayed but considerable time and money were expended for a second time, which created a previously unpredictable drain on cost and staff.

While each of these types of obsolescence carries an import all its own, it is even more critical for nurse executives to recognize that the healthcare organization controls none of them. In each case, these third-party decisions have enormous impact on when and how nursing uses technology-based products, devices, and systems. Additionally, these third-party decisions occur on a timetable over which healthcare organizations have little to no influence.

Planned obsolescence, shifting environmental mandates from regulators and payers, and changes in regulatory status complicate the already complex landscape of technology-related decision-making. What used to be episodic decision-making has morphed the six-stage lifecycle into a technology model with ever-cycling potential.

MULTI-LAYERED DECISION-MAKING

While the lifecycle seems straightforward, its overlay with content, outcomes, Nursing Informatics, and client intervention makes for a complexity not seen in other types of healthcare decision-making. Nursing-centric technology decisions emerge from a context that includes cultural, economic, social, and physical requirements. Adding an outcome orientation to those decisions layer impacts the cost, quality, safety, and satisfaction. Nursing Informatics staff then views technologies under consideration from the dual perspectives of content structure and information flow. Finally, the client factor encompasses the site-specific political, cultural, and social aspects of embracing technology. The Informatics Research Organizing model (Effken, 2003) captures the intrinsic complexity of the healthcare-centered technology decision-making process.

While the IRO model addresses HIT decision-making from an organizational perspective, a nursing-centric analysis of the process reveals further complexity coming from the dynamics of the physician-dominated HIT discussions (Simpson, 2012). The nursing-centered discussion of HIT decision-making highlights several reasons why medical staff demands often relegate nursing's HIT requirements to a subservient position during technology evaluation and selection (Simpson, 2012).

NURSE INFORMATICIST ROLE

Technologies optimized for the nursing process organize and prioritize patient care data against a complex backdrop of quality and patient safety. Nurse executives' responsibility to evaluate, select, and deploy these advanced technologies requires one of two things: (1) either a deep personal and nursing-centric knowledge of technology or (2) access to that knowledge, which is resident in a technology expert. Considering the organizational and interdisciplinary demands on nurse executives, a direct reporting structure to the technology expert offers the most efficient and effective pathway to this highly specialized knowledge. Often, this direct reporting relationship with the technology-infused individual leads to a Nurse Informaticist (NI). While some confusion over the preferred background of the graduate-prepared NI exists, nursing experts agree that effective NIs command highly specialized knowledge from three distinct disciplines: clinical nursing, information technology, and research. NIs use this rich, interdisciplinary perspective to analyze patient care and outcome data, creating new knowledge that advances the clinical practice of nursing. As a trusted advisor to the nurse executive, the NI serves a "translator" of technology capabilities, options, and alternatives to the nurse executive, who looks to the NI to align technologies and systems under consideration with organizational objectives.

Even with such an expert on staff, the nurse executive must be able to converse, debate, and champion specific technologies and clinical information systems personally. Simply put, there is no one else at the executive decision-making table with the expertise, knowledge, or perspective to advance the requirements and needs of patient care during technology-related discussions and debates.

TWO KEY AREAS OF EXPERTISE

Nurse executives and NIs involved in technology decision-making need to leverage two specific type of IT expertise when they evaluate, select, and implement clinical information systems: process mapping and workflow design. Process mapping delineates the actual steps of clinical practice as they occur during patient care, while workflow design spans the mechanical arrangement of information, forms, and triggers to document nursing practice. The success of every HIT implementation hinges on having a clear understanding of process mapping and workflow design, as well as the ability to chart these activities in a format understandable by computers.

Vendor-resident engineers lack the site-specific and nursing practice-specific knowledge required to add the context of the lived experience to the workflow creation process. While evidence in the standardization of processes and practices is a universal application goal, site-specific modifications are needed to have the software accepted and used by nurses delivering patient care.

From a nursing perspective, leaving this critical foundational work to engineers and technologists who lack the hands-on experience of delivering patient care at the bedside is pure folly. Delegating these two key foundational activities to non-nurses resembles the potential disaster created by allowing individual motorists to build their own roads—with no regard for the needs of their fellow motorists and no knowledge of construction, traffic flow, volume, or local weather conditions.

STANDARDIZATION LACKING

The importance of process mapping and workflow design in the binary world of computers where options are limited to "yes" or "no" collides head-on with the lack of standardization in nursing process, procedure, and operation. Only the nurse executive or an NI working in concert with the nurse executive can design and implement overarching nursing workflows that reflect the organization's nursing process. Even in healthcare organizations where these key tasks can be delegated to an NI, it remains the responsibility of the nurse executive that this foundational work be managed and overseen.

While some aspects of patient care remain resistant to standardization, the vast majority of these processes can be architected into workflows in much the same way that engineering has codified its processes and procedures. The criticality of these two elements and their foundational importance make a working knowledge of process mapping and workflow design knowledge essential to nurse executives' evaluation and selection of clinical information systems (Simpson, 2012).

NURSE EXECUTIVES MARGINALIZED

Nurse executives point to two specific ways they are marginalized in the evaluation and selection of clinical information systems, according to recent research (Simpson, 2012). Most often, the nurse executives found their review responsibilities limited to the functional level; that is, looking at the systems' features, rather than their ability to advance nursing practice. Second, nurse executives explained that CMO-led physician contingents regularly dominated IT decision-making, relegating nurse executives to a "specifier/recommender" role. As a result, nurse executives found their opportunities to advocate effectively for technology needed to support nursing practice during the evaluation and selection of clinical information systems to be limited. With nurse executives relegated to the sideline, no one at the executive decision-making table advocated for the needs of patient care during all-important technology discussions (Simpson, 2012).

In addition to being marginalized during the technology evaluation and selection process, nurse executives found they lacked technology-related competency despite their advanced degrees. Nothing in their traditional business and clinical education prepared them for technology-related decision-making. This lack of foundational knowledge, the nurse executives pointed out, hampered their ability to debate the functions of the clinical information systems with their medical staffs.

What they lacked, the nurse executives said, was the ability to view technology from a strategic and operational perspective. That deficiency hampered their adjustment of the systems' standard architectural design, workflow, and processes for deployment in their specific patient care environments. As a result, nurses, the largest user population in the healthcare organization, often find their technology needs falling in behind physician-championed system requirements.

This same research set out to answer the question, "What is the state of Chief Nurse Executives' HIT-related decision-making as compared to the competencies outlined in AONE's recommended information technology competencies?" Participating nurse executives demonstrated competency in and applied the majority of the AONE-outlined capabilities to their decision-making process related to the evaluation, selection, deployment, and utilization of HIT. However, the majority were not able to demonstrate a competency specific to the AONE's mandate to "demonstrate an awareness of societal and technological trends, issues and new developments as they relate to nursing" (AONE, 2011).

NEW FRONTIER: SOCIAL MEDIA

Although the informant nurse executives demonstrated knowledge of technology-fueled innovation in nursing practice, two substantial gaps exist between their knowledge and AONE's stated competency:

- Nurse executives' awareness of societal and technological trends, issues, and new developments as they relate to the clinical practice of nursing.
- Nurse executives' awareness of legal and ethical issues related to client data, information, and confidentiality.

It is interesting to note that nurses' use of social media lies at the intersection of these two gaps.

In the lived experience, for example, nurses routinely use social media to communicate nurse-to-nurse, nurse-to-patient and nurse-to-patient family, nurse-to-physician, and nurse-to-interdisciplinary team (Black, Light, Paradise, & Thompson, 2013). It is troubling that this pervasive communication violates HIPAA regulations and occurs with regularity in the majority of facilities, even where nurse executives have "banned" social media (U.S. Department of Health and Human Services, 1996).

Recently, researchers from the University of Florida examined 15 days' worth of anonymous network utilization records for 68 workstations located in the Emergency Department (ED) of an academic medical center, comparing data from the ED workstations to work index data from the hospital's information systems. Throughout the 15-day study period, healthcare workers spent 72.5 hours browsing Facebook, visiting the social networking site 9369 times, and spending 12 minutes per hour on the site. The amount of time spent on Facebook, while significant, was overshadowed by a second research finding: that the hospital workers' time on Facebook actually increased as patient volume in the ED rose. As a result, the researchers recommended future studies look at the impact of restricting Facebook use to break rooms and other non-working parts of the hospital (Narsi, 2013).

No matter what their "social media use at work" policies say, nurse executives cannot claim naiveté when it comes to the use of social media in their organizations. This lived experience does not support nurse executives' beliefs that they have protected the confidentiality of vitally important health information. Additionally, the use of social media exposes critically sensitive patient data to another vulnerability when personal communications and computing devices, such as smart phones, tablets, laptops, and notebooks are backed up via cloud computing. As the lines between communication and computing blur, and as handheld devices gain in power, more and more personal data are pushed to "the cloud" automatically. Few users of mobile communications and computing segment the information on their devices, which means that every piece of data on the device is backed up on the cloud.

As a result, sensitive patient data can be duplicated right next to all those family photos, recipes, and blog postings, on the cloud. This backup of the device's data in its totality most often occurs automatically and requires human intervention to be altered, partitioned, or stopped, potentially breaching the confidentiality and privacy that healthcare organizations work so hard to ensure.

QUICKENING PACE OF TECHNOLOGY ADOPTION

This inability to maintain current knowledge, of both technical capabilities and the application of those capabilities to the healthcare organization, presents a particularly troubling scenario when viewed against an emerging trend: the swift pace of technology adoption. While considerable debate surrounds the rate at which technical innovation occurs, with some experts say it is slowing while others point to a quickening, the adoption of new technologies clearly is picking up speed.

Consider the pace of "no phone-to-smart phone" adoption. It took 39 years for American's first landline phones to make their way into 40% of American households and an additional 15 years for the telephone to become prevalent. That is a total of 54 years. Yet, it took only 10 years for the smart phone to reach the 40% penetration rate in 2012 (DeGusta, 2013). That is why the smart phone has been touted as the most rapidly adopted technology in recorded history.

SUMMARY

Nurse executives at healthcare organizations of all sizes need help if they are to acquire and maintain current knowledge of HIT. First, nurse executives need to take seriously their commitment to lifelong learning, especially as it pertains to technology. Second, nurse executives need to lead the process mapping and workflow design of their HIT systems. Third, the profession needs to enlist the help of academic leaders and regulators to build a learning infrastructure capable of creating deep HIT competencies for America's executive nurses. Fourth, this learning infrastructure need not be built "from scratch" as several viable educational options, including but not limited to credentialing organizations and accreditation agencies, such as AONE Certification Center, NLN's credentialing center (National League for Nursing), NLN-AC (National League for Nursing Accrediting Commission), ANCC (American Nurses Credentialing Center), and CCNE (Commission on Collegiate Nursing Education), already exist. These centers would be well served to crystallize educational content to address nurse executives' lack of technology knowledge.

Building and maintaining this deep technology competency across the country's ranks of nurse executives will ensure that the "voice of the patient" is heard when these all-important technology decisions are made. Failing to answer nursing's needs with advanced technologies and systems tailored to their specific clinical environments imperils the quality of patient care as it risks the longevity of nurses and the healthcare organization as well.

REFERENCES

American Organization of Nurse Executives (AONE). (2011). *The AONE nurse executive competencies, information management and technology.* Retrieved from www.aone.org/resources/leadership%20tools/PDFs/AONE_NEC.pdf

Black, E., Light, J., Paradise, B. N., Thompson, L. (2013). Offline social network use by health care providers in a high traffic patient care environment. *Journal of Medical Internet Research, 15*(5):e94. Retrieved from htttp://www.jmir.org/2013/5/e94/?utm_source=feedburner&utm_medium=feed&utm_campaign=Feed%3A+JMedInternetRes+%28Journal+of+Medical+Internet+Research+%28atom%29%29. Accessed on May 20, 2013.

DeGusta, M. (2013). *MIT technology review. Are smart phones spreading faster than any technology in human history?* Retrieved from http://www.technologyreview.com/news/427787/are-smart-phones-spreading-faster-than-any-technology-in-human-history/. Accessed on March 26, 2014.

Effken, J. A. (2003). An organizing framework for nursing informatics research. *Computers, informatics, nursing: CIN, 21*(6), 316–323. Retrieved from http://at.phcc.edu/NUR2820/PDFs/MOD2/Nursing_Informatics.pdf. Accessed on May 28, 2012.

Narsi, S. (2013). *Healthcare business and technology.* Retrieved from http://www.healthcarebusinesstech.com/healthcare-workers-on-facebook/. Accessed on May 22, 2013.

Simpson, R. L. (2012). State of contemporary informatics competencies for chief nurse executives. Capstone requirements for doctorate of nursing practice, American Sentinel University.

The Economist. (2009). *Idea: Planned obsolescence.* Retrieved from http://www.economist.com/node/13354332. Accessed on May 14, 2012.

U.S. Department of Health and Human Services. (1996). *The Health Insurance Portability and Accountability Act of 1996.* Retrieved from http://www.hhs.gov/ocr/privacy/hipaa/understanding/summary. Accessed on May 19, 2013.

18

Establishing Nursing Informatics in Public Policy

Dana Alexander / Elizabeth Casey Halley

• OBJECTIVES

1. Examine the course to navigate public policy as related to healthcare and nursing informatics.
2. Define the public policy process.
3. Analyze the skills and competencies nursing informaticists must possess in order to effectively communicate with policy-makers and those in positions to sway policy-makers.
4. Explore how nursing informaticists are impacting public healthcare policy.
5. Review how education for nurses continues to increasingly leverage technology for learning and supporting nursing practice.
6. Encourage the nursing profession to collaborate, educate, and coordinate efforts in policy formulation to support nursing's roles in quality, safety, and patient advocacy.

• KEY WORDS

Accountable care
Healthcare informatics
Healthcare reform
Health information technology
Nursing informatics
Public health policy
Public healthcare policy
Public policy

INTRODUCTION

Nursing informatics leaders should be engaged in all levels of health IT policy and strategy-setting committees and initiatives. HIMSS Position Paper: Transforming Nursing Practice through Technology & Informatics

Understanding the public policy process and avenues for influence can assist nursing informaticists in engaging in and influencing public healthcare policy to improve healthcare delivery and quality patient care.

Although nursing informatics (NI) has had a role in shaping public health information Technology (IT) policy, it must continue to be engaged in shaping public healthcare policy. In this era of the U.S. Health Information Technology for Economic and Clinical Health (HITECH) Act (GPO, 2009), and the Patient Protection and Affordable Care Act (PPACA) (GPO, 2010), it is especially critical for the NI community to understand public healthcare policy drivers and how to deliver a unified message to those who create public healthcare policy. This will not happen by chance; carefully crafted strategy and collaboration needs to occur now. Those who will lead the efforts to ensure that NI public policy issues are heard require education, competencies, avenues for collaboration, and support.

This chapter explores various components of public policy impacting healthcare, health IT, and NI. It provides a highlight of legislative initiatives, the public policy process, and avenues for engagement of and influence by NI. This chapter also presents considerations relating to healthcare reform now and in the future including bridging settings of care for healthier individuals, communities, and population health, and engaging the patient and family toward better health. This chapter includes a call to collaboration and opportunities for the NI community to engage with public and private stakeholders.

NAVIGATING THE COURSE IN PUBLIC POLICY TO IMPACT HEALTHCARE

Nearly every aspects of the healthcare system including finance and reimbursement; education; facilities, products, and services; professional practice and workforce capacity; and technology, including health IT, are influenced by public policy. It is vital that the NI community understand and acquire skills to navigate the public policy process to ensure that the nurses' voices and their critical positions on healthcare and health IT are heard. This includes understanding the policy process as well as politics.

With an expected 33 million additional Americans to have access to healthcare under PPACA (CBO, 2012), along with initiatives like Medical Homes and Accountable Care Organizations (ACOs), PPACA will have significant impact on our healthcare providers, including nursing's role in providing care. Primary care provider shortfalls may increase up to 46,000 by 2020 (HRSA, 2010), as well as current undersupply of 7550 physicians in primary care Health Professional Shortage Areas (HPSAs) (HRSA, 2013). In addition, by 2020 there is an expected overall physician shortage of over 90,000 and shortage of primary care physicians of over 45,000 (AAMC, 2013) . Positioned to fill some of this need, Nurse Practitioners (NP) and Physician Assistants (PA) are the fastest growing provider segments in primary care (GAO, 2008).

Another critical public policy and health interface was the passage of the HITECH Act, as part of the American Recovery and Reinvestment Act (ARRA) of 2009. This legislation was a culmination of various efforts over the years to recognize and facilitate the adoption of health IT throughout the United States. The HITECH Act included significant incentives for acute care eligible hospitals, critical access hospitals (CAHs), and eligible providers (EP) to acquire and implement electronic health records (EHR) and supporting technology. Also known as the Medicare and Medicaid EHR Incentive Programs, it provides incentive payments to adopt, implement, upgrade, or demonstrate "meaningful use" (MU) of certified EHR technology (CMS, 2013a).

Since the passage of HITECH Act, hospital and providers' implementation and use of EHR technology have dramatically increased. Hospitals' meeting MU objectives grew significantly, with increases ranging from 32% to 167% (ONC Data Brief No.10, 2012a). Also since HITECH Act started, physician adoption of EHR technology meeting MU objectives has increased from 66% to 97% (ONC Data Brief No.7, 2012b).

In addition, since the passage of HITECH Act, four in five NPs in the United States are enrolled with a Regional Extension Center (REC) and are live with an EHR. Operating at the top of their license, NPs and PAs offer treatment, patient education, and care coordination. These providers are fundamental to broad expansions of healthcare and payment reforms facilitated by MU of health IT, EHR, and health information exchange (HIE). (ONC Data Brief No.11, 2013b).

However, it is worth noting while health reform is providing expanded opportunities for NPs, there remain restrictions on practice autonomy by many states and NPs that do practice with independent authority are not eligible to participate in the EHR Eligible Provider incentive for Medicare. According to CMS, to address this oversight in the Medicare MU program to include NPs with independent authority for the Medicare Eligible Provider program would require a congressional legislative modification. Hopefully, with nursing public policy advocacy, this change will occur in the near-term future.

The extent to which nurses contribute to policy development, including the PPACA, is nearly impossible to comprehend. The American Nurses Association (ANA) created *Healthcare Reform: Key Provisions Related to Nursing* and the American Association of Colleges of Nursing (AACN) created *Patient Protection and Affordable Care Act* which provide charts outlining how the law supports continued nurse education and all sectors of the nursing workforce (AACN, 2010; ANA, 2010). These charts also explain how PPACA addresses the nursing shortage (especially as related to skilled nursing), quality improvement, best practices, and public health initiatives. While impressive, nursing's participation to engineer these changes is only one aspect of the role played in creating PPACA. And nurses are involved in numerous other initiatives related to improving the quality and delivery of care.

Legislative initiatives create opportunities for nurses to help shape policies that will drive the implementation of technology to support a cost-effective, accessible, patient-centered, and continuity-of-care model to improve health outcomes in our country and the increasingly important role of nurses in the creation and execution of public health policy cannot be overlooked.

Collaboration at the public healthcare policy level impacts the future of nursing and care delivery while setting expectations for standards of care that nurses are responsible for advancing at the most salient level. With over 3.1 million nurses in the United States alone, nurses are the apparatus for implementation of public healthcare policy (HRSA, 2010).

Exploring the Public Policy Process and NI Influence

This section focuses on navigating the public policy path particularly how it impacts public healthcare policy, health IT, and NI. Understanding and exploring ways to navigate various aspects of the public policy process and identifying avenues for impact in order to influence changes in healthcare delivery, partly through the use of technology, is an essential skill set for nurse informaticists.

Public policy is the action taken by government to address a particular public issue. Local, state, federal, and international government organizations all craft and implement public policy to protect and benefit their populations (JHU, 2013).

Health policy refers to decisions, plans, and actions that are undertaken to achieve specific healthcare goals within a society. An explicit health policy can achieve several things: it defines a vision for the future which in turn helps establish targets and points of reference for the short and medium term. It outlines priorities and the expected roles of different groups, and it builds consensus and informs people (WHO, 2013). Health policy is a course of action that influences healthcare decisions (www.aacn.org).

During the Institute of Medicine's (IOM's) Forum on the Future of Nursing, Selecky noted, "Public health cannot be separated from politics ... as demonstrated by the term 'public'" (IOM, 2010, p. 10).

Nurses have led public health initiatives throughout the United States and beyond that are widely recognized as unquestionable successes. These initiatives include vaccination campaigns (IOM, 2010, p. 7), AIDS prevention

and awareness, infection control, and disaster response mobilization (Robert Wood Johnson Foundation, 2008).

Public healthcare policy is that piece of health policy that deals with the organization, financing, and delivery of healthcare services. This includes training of health professionals, overseeing the safety of drugs and medical devices, administering public programs like Medicare, and regulating private health insurance. The obligation of government to promote and protect the public's health is grounded in the U.S. Constitution. Connected to all of this is a myriad of details concerning the licensing of health professionals and facilities, health information privacy protections, measures of healthcare quality and mistakes, malpractice, electronic medical records, and efforts to control healthcare costs (Acuff, 2010). Figure 18.1 provides an illustration of these various public policy components.

So how do the ideas that originated at the grassroots, clinical practice level make it through the public policy process and become laws?

While the exact process varies from state to state and from state to national levels, if the right people and organizations have been engaged, the nursing informaticist's recommended best practices are sponsored by a legislator and introduced in a bill. From here, the bill goes to committee and experts from various groups that the committee anticipates will be impacted by the bill are asked to provide their reasons for supporting or opposing the bill. The committee may also seek recommendations for modification. Eventually, this bill goes to the floor where the

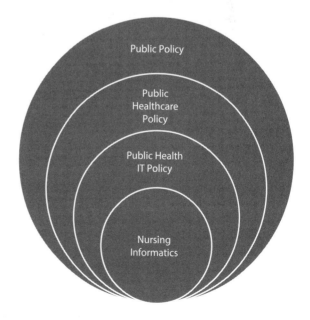

• **FIGURE 18.1.** Policy Component.

House will vote on whether to approve it. If the bill is not passed, it will either be dropped, sent back to the committee for modification, or sit for a time before it is reintroduced. If and when the bill is passed in one House, the bill is sent to the other House where this process is repeated. This is why it is ideal to have both chambers introduce the same bill, known as a companion bill. When both Houses agree on a bill, it is sent to the highest-ranking official (i.e., Governor or President). The President or Governor then either signs the bill into law or employs veto power to prohibit passage of the bill. If the bill is vetoed, it needs to be reintroduced in one of the Houses before any law-making activities resume.

While this process may read easily on paper, there are many factors that impact a federal bill's viability in Congress,

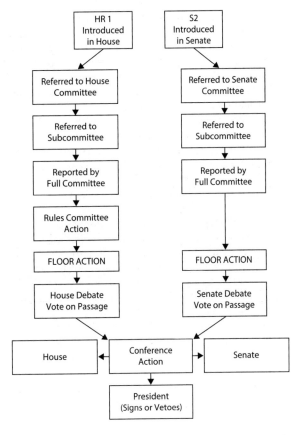

• **FIGURE 18.2.** How a Bill Becomes a Law. (Reproduced, with permission, from How a Bill Becomes a Law. Retrieved on 12 January, 2015 from www.apa.org/about/gr/advocacy/bill.aspx. Copyright © 2015 American Psychological Association)

such as the number of Congressional co-sponsors supporting the bill, the level of support from constituents and national organizations, and the current political agenda. On average, it can take seven to eight years for legislation to pass if it is not on the national agenda. Although there are no guarantees, some bills based on the national agenda are never even reported out of committee. For these reasons, it is important that nurses understand the politics and policy of the issues they are working with to create change. They must work closely with experts in the field, in addition to political strategy and advocacy experts, to move an issue forward. Figure 18.2 provides a simplified graphic outlining how a bill becomes a law.

Examples of public healthcare policy include federal legislation, such as HITECH Act and PPACA, discussed in the previous section, and their associated regulatory rules. These public healthcare policies have produced a significant increase in healthcare technology adoption, as well as new models for healthcare access, reimbursement, and delivery.

The goals of these national healthcare policies include improving access, quality, and safety and reducing costs of healthcare. The National Quality Strategy (NQS), called for under the PPACA, created national aims and priorities to guide local, state, and national efforts to improve the quality of healthcare in the United States. The NQS noted three aims ("Triple Aims") for the healthcare system including Better Care, Healthy People and Communities, and Affordable Care (AHRQ, 2011). These are the goals to which NI should aspire. Being engaged in the national conversation regarding the use of technology and information to improve care and health of our patients while reducing costs is a natural role for NI.

Avenues for Influencing Policy

In addition to the legislative levers, nurse informaticists should understand the roles of and consider participating in other policy development efforts such as advisory committees, policy institutes, professional organizations, technical expert panels, and NI policy advocates.

Federal Advisory Committees. Three important healthcare and health IT–related federal advisory committees are the National Committee on Vital and Health Statistics (NCVHS, 2013) established in 1949 by Congress to serve as an advisory body to the Department of Health and Human Services (HHS) on health data, statistics, and national health information policy and the Health Information Technology Policy Committee (HITPC) and the Health Information Technology Standards Committee

(HITSC) established through ARRA for developing policy recommendation to the National Coordinator for Health IT. These three committees operate under the rules established by the Federal Advisory Committee Act (FACA). The FACA defines *advisory committee* as "any committee, board, commission, council, conference, panel, task force, or other similar group" that dispenses "advice or recommendations" to the President of the United States, and excludes bodies that also exercise operational functions (FACA, 1972).

Policy Institutes. A policy institute (often termed "think tank" by journalists) is an organization that performs research and advocacy concerning topics such as social policy, political strategy, economics, military, technology, and culture (Stone, 2006). There are numerous institutes that conduct research and analysis; develop white papers and policy positions; and provide recommendations specifically on healthcare-related topics, but a prominent voice in healthcare thought leadership is the IOM (IOM, 2013).

Professional Organizations. Another important avenue for influencing health IT and informatics policy is engagement with professional associations. Previously mentioned in this chapter are the ANA and AACN, both actively engaged in healthcare policy issues and deliberations.

Also initially a subsidiary of the ANA and now a nonprofit corporation, the American Academy of Nursing (AAN), serves the public and the nursing profession by advancing health policy and practice through the generation, synthesis, and dissemination of nursing knowledge. The Academy and its member Fellows create and execute knowledge-driving and policy-related initiates to drive reform of America's healthcare system.

In 2013, The Academy released the report, "The Importance of Health Information Technology in Care Coordination and Transitional Care." Based upon the premise that care coordination and transitional care services are strategically important after achieving the National Quality Strategy of the Triple AIMs to improve the health and quality of healthcare, the AAN believes that HIT is essential to enable care and communication across communities of care to include the patient and family. This report "offers a set of recommendations to guide the development of the infrastructure, standards, content and measures for electronically enabled care coordination and transitions in care as well as research needed to build the evidence base to assess outcomes of the associate interventions" (AACN, 2013).

Another professional organization involved in health IT and NI policy deliberations and active contributor to policy comments is the Alliance for Nursing Informatics (ANI). The ANI, in coordination with the American Medical Informatics Association (AMIA) and the Healthcare Information and Management Systems Society (HIMSS), is a collaboration that represents multiple nursing informatics organizations, and responds as one voice to federal health policy initiatives by sharing nursing informatics perspectives for shaping health policy.

The ANI enables a unified voice for the NI community through the American Nursing Informatics Association (ANIA) regional organization members to engage in issues in the public healthcare policy process; information technology standards; information systems design, implementation, and evaluation; and shared communication and networking opportunities (McCormick, Sensmeier, Delaney, & Bickford, 2013).

Another professional organization involved in emerging health technologies is the American Telemedicine Association (ATA) which brings together diverse groups, including nursing associations, for the advancement of telemedicine in healthcare delivery. In January 2014, ATA released draft *ATA Core Guidelines for Telemedicine Operations* to assist practitioners to provide effective and safe medical care. The draft guidelines recognize that safe and effective practices require specific training, skills, and techniques for telemedicine (ATA, 2014).

In many cases, professional organizations like AMIA, ANIA, and HIMSS can legitimize claims made by those in NI leadership positions by accepting their recommendations. These organizations network with other professional organizations, as well as professional lobbyists, to promote the causes of nursing informatics and effective care delivery.

The AMIA Nursing Informatics Working Group (NIWG) and the Public Policy Committee have and continue to influence healthcare public policy and HIT policy. In coordination with its members, AMIA works with key decision-makers, policy-makers, and other health stakeholders to help shape public policies that effectively address today's ongoing biomedical and health informatics issues (AMIA, n.d.).

The American Nursing Informatics Association (ANIA) comprises of more than 3000 nurses and other healthcare professionals in informatics practice and includes roles in: system design and implementation, education, research (analysis and evaluation), standards and policy development, quality improvement, as well as those in management and administration. Their role is to advance the field of nursing informatics through communication, education, research and professional activities. They collaborate with affiliate organizations (ANA, AONE, AMIA, HIMSS, State Nursing Organizations, etc.) to provide informatics education, and develop a collective voice for nursing informatics on relevant issues.

Patricia Sengstack, DNP, RN-BC, CPHIMS, president of ANIA was one of the 10 Influential Women in Health IT in 2014 for her outspoken advocacy on the use of health technology among nurses, according to FierceHealthIT. (https://www.ania.org/)

HIMSS is a global, cause-based organization with a national Government Relations office and engaged NI Community that frames and leads healthcare practices and public policy through its content expertise, professional development, and research initiatives. HIMSS impacts health policy through a variety of avenues including direct legislative outreach, participation in public comments, guidance documents, position statements, and professional tools boxes. Leveraging and incorporating the NI expertise in position papers and deliberations is an important aspect of ensuring the NI voice is heard in policy debates.

Technical Experts Panels. Another avenue for influencing policy are Technical Expert Panels (TEPs). A TEP is a group of stakeholders and experts who provide technical input in areas that an organization may be in need of for a broader perspective on a topic. Specific tools and meetings may be employed to select and engage the panel, assign tasks, and elicit sharing and further development of knowledge. Many federal and national organizations use TEPs such as CMS, ONC, Agency for Healthcare Research and Quality (AHRQ), and the National Quality Forum (NQF).

An example of a TEP involved in healthcare informatics is CMS's Quality Measures TEP. This TEP provides technical input to the measure contractor on the development, selection, and maintenance of measures for which CMS contractors are responsible. TEP members are chosen to provide input to the measure contractor based on their personal experience and training. TEP members are selected to represent a diversity of perspectives and backgrounds. Information on the nomination process, including self-nominations are available on the CMS public Web site (CMS, 2013b).

NI Policy Advocates. In addition to the organizations listed above, knowledgeable policy nursing informaticists work in a variety of settings where policy issues are addressed, such as academia, vendor, consulting and advisory firms, and within government agencies that drive public policy.

Related to federal agencies that are driving the formation of specific policies are the nursing informaticists that work inside agencies such as CMS, ONC, AHRQ, NIH, and others. Another aspect to a key strategy of influencing public policy is strengthening relationships and informing this nursing stakeholder group about the issues, challenges, needs, and gaps. And once again, employing bi-directional communication to provide opportunity to hear their perspectives and how they can be better supported in their efforts that may influence public policy as well.

Increasing nursing informaticists awareness of various avenues for engagement and understanding of how to get involved in the public policy process will help ensure that the nursing voice is heard. Building the skills, competencies, and confidence to engage is part of the critical path to influence public policy.

HOW DO NURSING INFORMATICISITS INFLUENCE PUBLIC POLICY?

Nursing Informatics Shaping the Future of Healthcare

The IOM has released several landmark reports that serve as a continued gateway for nursing informatics to shape the future of healthcare. Three reports of particular relevance are:

1. Future of Nursing Leading Change, Advancing Health
2. Health IT and Patient Safety
3. Best Care at Lower Cost ... The Path to Continuous Learning Healthcare in America

Future of Nursing Report

The Future of Nursing report is not only about nursing but the future of healthcare in the United States. The report outlines nursing as a key factor to successfully achieving improved outcomes, optimal wellness, and overall population health management (IOM, 2010). Because of the breadth and depth of nursing engagement in all aspects of healthcare, nurses are in a key position to influence healthcare reform and the multi-dimensional needs across all care settings. TIGER (Technology Informatics Guiding Education Reform) provided testimony to the Future of Nursing (FON) committee about the important role of healthcare informatics in creating a vision for nursing, "This is an opportunity to integrate informatics within nursing education, practice, and research so nurses are armed with the necessary tools to address twenty-first-century clinical practice, in an effective, efficient, and safe manner, while also holding the highest standards of evidence-based practice" (TIGER, 2009).

Health IT and Patient Safety

The IOM Health IT and Patient Safety Report summarizes existing knowledge of the effects of health IT on patient safety and made recommendations to maximize and promote safety of health IT–assisted care. Findings included (1) Health IT can improve patient safety even though the gaps in potential risks of health IT are not fully understood, (2) Health IT needs to be viewed as part of the larger sociotechnical system, and (3) All stakeholders need to work together for a coordinated effort to identify and understand patient safety risks associated with health IT.

Who better than nursing informatics should engage and lead in efforts to identify and understand patient safety risks associated with health IT? Nursing informaticists are also in prime position to participate in research and the development of standards and criteria for safe design, implementation, and use of Health IT. The ONC was charged with developing an action plan to address the recommendations and released the action plan in mid-2013 after consideration of public comment to include input from nursing informaticists and NI organizations.

Best Care at Lower Cost ... The Path to Continuous Learning Healthcare in America

Best Care at Lower Cost defines the foundational characteristics of a healthcare system that is efficient, delivers increased value, and is continuously innovating and improving in its ability to deliver high value to patients. The reports outlines several recommendation to include (a) the need for a digital infrastructure that supports the capacity to capture clinical, delivery process, and financial data for better care, system improvement, and creating new knowledge and (b) the need to improve data utility by streamlining and revising research regulations to improve care, promote the capture of clinical data, and generate knowledge. Applying these new strategies can support the transition to a continuously learning health system, one that aligns science and informatics, patient–clinician partnerships, incentives, and a culture of continuous improvement to produce the best care at lower cost (IOM, 2012).

This IOM report's findings and recommendations clearly outline opportunity for Nursing Informatics to engage and lead in policy and research aspects to create the right infrastructures to capture clinical and financial data aligning with the delivery process to provide better care, system improvement, and creating new knowledge. The focus on technical and practice standards, as well as analytics strategy, will ultimately support organizations' drives toward accountable care and achievement of the goals and priorities of the National Quality Strategy.

In summary, these IOM report recommendations and execution of recommendations provide for many opportunities for nursing informatics to influence future policy and shape the healthcare landscape. Collaborative efforts among several nursing-related organizations are underway to unify the voice and efforts. Some of these organizations have been outlined in this chapter.

Position Statement: Transforming Nursing Practice Through Technology and Informatics

The IOM Future of Nursing report has stimulated accelerated efforts among nursing organizations to collaborate and unite on behalf of nursing and future care delivery in the United States. In alignment with the ANA and the Alliance for Nursing Informatics (ANI), this HIMSS Position Statement, "Transforming Nursing Practice Through Technology and Informatics," provides background on key-related issues and identifies specific recommendations for eliminating barriers and addressing nursing's role in transforming healthcare through the use of IT, particularly in regard to the role of nursing informatics. This statement was developed by the HIMSS Nursing Informatics Committee, representing now more than 6500 nurse informaticists, and is supported by HIMSS at large Collaboration and unified messaging among all stakeholders are keys to success. "We (HIMSS) believe that nurses and nursing informatics specialists are vital to accomplishing the goals described in this position paper and advancing healthcare transformation through the use of health IT." (HIMSS, 2011a).

Emerging NI Roles and Call to Action

NI roles continue to evolve, expand, and emerge and are critical to engage in the necessary transformation activities and bridge the new care delivery models into clinical practice with the right technology solutions. However, in order to participate in the public policy process, NI Leaders must be knowledgeable and current in public policy and regulatory initiatives. They must be able to translate the impact of these changes into practice and care delivery while having a voice into planning, implementation, and execution to achieve the requirements of the industry changes.

In summary, Nursing Informaticists increasingly have the opportunity to influence and shape public policy. Meaningful Use and the technology agenda at large while focused on supporting the achievement of the National Quality Strategy will not be accomplished without all nurses. All nurses have a role to unlock the barrier doors that exist today for the necessary changes to achieve the "One voice, One vision" of healthcare transformation.

WORKFORCE IMPLICATIONS

While PPACA takes no action to expressly support or fund nursing informatics, it does include provisions for preparing the workforce for the twenty-first century. Achieving the goals of the Healthcare Reform Bill that relate to health IT would be difficult, or even impossible, if NI is not included as part of the equation. Opportunities for improving awareness of informatics, enhancing Health IT skill levels, and better positioning NI within healthcare policy continue to grow on many different levels.

To assuage any doubt about the expanding influence of NI in the healthcare arena, the provisions of the HITECH Act created a demand for new and highly-skilled employees. Recognizing that healthcare already suffers from a nursing shortage exacerbated by a lack of qualified faculty

(IOM, 2010, p. 8), the Office of the National Coordinator (ONC) was funding for training programs for HIT including funding for informatics programs. While informatics programs continue to increase in size and curriculum development, supplying the demand for qualified nursing informaticist is not fully met as of yet.

Preparing the workforce for the twenty-first century is key and will include an ever-increasing focus on education and usability of technology. Nursing Informatics leaders will need to lead by establishing the strategy and plan for their respective organizations, so technology becomes a natural interwoven aspect of care delivery and workflow. Academia and research settings must be included as well to not only train the future workforce but to support innovations in nursing practice leveraging research-based evidence. NI leader roles are in prime position to bridge research, education, and practice settings to achieve innovations for nursing practice and prepare the workforce for the future.

Skills and Competencies Nursing Informaticists Need to Effectively Communicate with Policy-Makers and Influencers

Advocating for informatics is a complex responsibility that requires in-depth knowledge of both clinical processes and clinical systems. The informatics nurse is advocating not only on behalf of patients, but also on behalf of all nurses and caregivers, as well as known and anticipated technological capabilities. The informatics nurse must recognize and be able to articulate issues of usability, interoperability, standardization, terminology, cost, quality, and safety.

Informatics nurses must be (1) strategists, (2) leaders, and (3) effective communicators; they must (4) engage stakeholders across multiple spectrums to ensure patient, nursing, and technological needs are understood and met. This includes creating buy-in from managers, administrators, and IT within the organization, as well as consultants, developers, and implementation specialists. It further includes those who may be outside the clinical setting, like investors and policy-makers, whose decisions can have a huge impact on clinical systems and processes. According to Suzanne Begeny, Director of Government Affairs at the American Association of the Colleges of Nursing, "In order to effectively shape public policy, nurses need to realize that it takes a significant financial investment to compete on the national level. In addition to money, nurses must act as the impetus for the message, orchestrate support, and prepare our leaders for the political stage." In this way, nursing informatics issues will gain the recognition necessary to be taken seriously as healthcare reform progresses.

Nursing informaticists must be able to convey their concerns about data, and its availability for reporting and dissemination, in terms that are easily understood within the context of the recipient's own constitutional paragon. In other words, nursing informaticists must engage key stakeholders at the intersection of the stakeholder's ability and willingness to influence change. There are many ways to ascertain this understanding: participation in task forces, summits, conferences; creation of white papers; lobbying and support of lobbying efforts; membership in relevant organizations; acting as an expert witness; leading selection committees; and so on. With so many options, it is also necessary that NI leaders are strategic when determining who to engage and with whom to collaborate. They must learn to read others' willingness to assume a shared responsibility for quality informatics, and speak to them in a manner that causes these key players to want to take up the cause. Finally, NI leaders must learn to recognize appropriate engagements, and terms of engagement—even when it comes to their own involvement in promoting a particular cause. Gaining alignment and voice with professional organizations such as HIMSS, AMIA, ANI, ANA, and others creates the power to influence and shape policy that often cannot be achieved as a single individual and/or smaller representation. Not to minimize grassroots efforts, but important to know when to expand grassroots to the next level where organizations typically have more formal venues and channels of influence.

Considerations for Public Health, LTPAC, Home Health, Rural, School, and Community Health Settings and Patient Engagement

Both the ARRA of 2009 and the PPACA of 2010 are transformative pieces of health legislation that aim to stimulate EHR adoption throughout the acute care and physician practice sectors for greater efficiency, patient safety, and improved quality with better coordination of care across providers, venues, and geographies. However, new clinical care delivery strategies and programs are called for that will create accountable care and managing the health of populations. The new models of care must address and mitigate the fragmentation and waste in our siloed healthcare systems while increasing accountability by care delivery team members and patients. These new models and initiatives must also allow for an expanded resource capacity to accommodate the healthcare needs that will be coming from the rapid growth in our elderly population and the increasing populations with chronic diseases. Care settings such as long-term care, post-acute, community-based, and school-based settings have all too often been left behind and excluded in the patient's longitudinal plan of care. Better health, healthier communities, access, and decreased costs will not be achieved without inclusion of these settings. With the rise of ACOs and Population

Health management, improved coordination of care and communication that spans the care continuum is necessary. These new models also require an expanding technology infrastructure supported by health analytics that combines clinical, financial, and operational data. Nursing informatics is needed to engage and lead in defining the necessary technologies and analytics to support future care delivery and the management of individuals and populations health.

HEALTHCARE REFORM

New healthcare delivery and payment models, such as Medical Homes and ACOs, driven by healthcare reform will require an innovative look at how patient and consumer information is captured, exchanged, analyzed, and acted upon.

The medical home is a model for achieving primary care excellence so that care is received in the right place, at the right time, and in the manner that best suits a patient's needs (PCPCC, 2013). Accountable Care Organizations (ACOs) are groups of doctors, hospitals, and other healthcare providers, who come together to provide coordinated high-quality care to a defined group of patients. The goal of coordinated care is to ensure that patients, especially the chronically ill, get the right care at the right time, while avoiding unnecessary duplication of services and preventing medical errors.

NI leaders are needed to engage in ACO strategy development, implementation, and execution. It will be critical for NI leaders to "lead" change management to shape behavior and thinking from current models today which are often physician and/or acute care centric to a cross-continuum coordinated care approach that involves all appropriate care team members. NI leaders are essential stakeholders to orchestrate what information must be provided, captured, and documented to support patient care, and the associated financial and business indicators to monitor and report on outcomes management as well. Technology will continue to be a fundamental enabler to the future care delivery models and NI leaders will be essential to lead the way and to innovate nursing practice through technology.

SUMMARY

Nurse Informaticists must recognize the importance of engaging in the public policy process and advocating for advancements in technology and processes that will promote improved patient care, better health, and lower healthcare costs in the United States. We must take leadership seats at the decision-making table. We must strategically collaborate and plan to have a voice; we must not give away our advocacy voice!

The formation of good public health policy relies on quality, unbiased, substantial data, as well as the expertise of those who provide care within the healthcare environment. We need to lead the charge and engage leadership on every necessary level to ensure that public policy supports NI initiatives. No one is better positioned to collaborate with technology vendors, regulatory bodies, politicians, and others to ensure that healthcare technologies and public policies promote patient care at the extraordinary level we have always ascribed to in nursing.

GLOSSARY

AACN	American Association of Colleges of Nursing
AAN	American Academy of Nursing
ACO	Accountable Care Organization
AHRQ	Agency for Healthcare Research and Quality
AMIA	American Medical Informatics Association
ANA	American Nurses Association
ANIA	American Nursing Informatics Association
ANI	Alliance for Nursing Informatics
ANP-BC	Adult Nurse Practitioner-Board Certified
AONE	American Organization of Nurse Executives
ARRA	American Recovery and Reinvestment Act
ATA	American Telemedicine Association
CAH	Critical Access Hospital
CBO	Congressional Budget Office
CMS	Centers for Medicare & Medicaid Services
CPOE	Computerized Practitioner Order Entry
CQM	Clinical Quality Measures
EH	Eligible Hospital
EHR	Electronic Health Record
EP	Eligible Providers
FAAN	Fellows of the American Academy of Nursing
FAANP	Fellows of the American Association of Nurse Practitioners
FACA	Federal Advisory Committee Act
FNP-BC	Family Nurse Practitioner-Board Certified
FY	Fiscal Year
GAO	U.S. Government Accounting Office
GPO	Government Printing Office
HHS	Department of Health and Human Services
HIE	Health Information Exchange
HIMSS	Healthcare Information and Management Systems Society
HIT	Health Information Technology
HITECH	Health Information Technology for Economic and Clinical Health
HITPC	Health Information Technology Policy Committee
HITSC	Health Information Technology Standards Committee
HPSA	Health Professional Shortage Areas
HRSA	Health Resources and Services Administration
JHU	Johns Hopkins University
MU	Meaningful Use
PA	Physician Assistant

PPACA   Patient Protection and Affordable Care Act
NCVHS   National Committee on Vital and Health Statistics
n.d.   No Date
NI   Nursing Informatics
NIWG   Nursing Informatics Working Group
NP   Nurse Practitioner
NQF   National Quality Forum
ONC   Office of the National Coordinator for Health
          Information Technology
PCPCC   Patient-Centered Primary Care Collaborative
REC   Regional Extension Center
RWJF   Robert Wood Johnson Foundation
TEP   Technical Expert Panel
U.S.   United States of America
WHO   World Health Organization

REFERENCES

Acuff, K. (September 2010). *Definition of health care policy*. Retrieved from http://www.livestrong.com/article/259661-definition-of-health-care-policy/

Agency for Healthcare Research & Quality. (2011, March). *National Strategy for Quality Improvement in Healthcare Report to Congress*.

American Association of Colleges of Nurses. (2013, March 14). *2013 Federal policy agenda*. Retrieved from http://www.aacn.nche.edu/government-affairs/AACN_FedPolicy13.pdf

American Medical Informatics Association (AMIA). (n.d.). *AMIA public policy*. Retrieved from http://www.amia.org/public_policy

American Nurses Association. (2010). *Health care reform: Key provisions related to nursing*. Retrieved from http://www.rnaction.org/site/DocServer/KeyProvisions_Nursing-PublicLaw.pdf

American Nursing Informatics Association. (n.d.). About ANIA. Retrieved from https://www.ania.org/

American Telemedicine Association (ATA). (2014, January). *ATA core guidelines for telemedicine operations*. Retrieved from http://www.americantelemed.org/docs/default-source/standards/core-standards-for-public-comment---draft-for-comment.pdf?sfvrsn=4Comments

Association of American Medical Colleges (AAMC). (2013). *Physician shortages to worsen without increases in residency training*. Retrieved from https://www.aamc.org/download/286592/data/

Centers for Medicare & Medicaid Services (CMS). (2013a, October). *EHR incentive programs*. Retrieved from https://www.cms.gov/ehrincentiveprograms

Centers for Medicare & Medicaid Services. (2013b, October). *Technical expert panels*. Retrieved from http://www.cms.gov/Medicare/Quality-Initiatives-Patient-Assessment-Instruments/MMS/TechnicalExpertPanels.html

Charles, D., King, J., Furukawa, J. F., Patel, V. (2013). Hospital Adoption of Electronic Health Record Technology to

Meet Meaningful Use Objectives: 2008-2012. ONC Data Brief No. 10. Retrieved from http://www.healthit.gov/sites/default/files/oncdatabrief10final.pdf

Congressional Budget Office (CBO). (2012, March). *Updated estimates for the insurance coverage provisions of the Affordable Care Act*. Washington, D.C. Retrieved from http://www.cbo.gov/sites/default/files/cbofiles/attachments/03-13-Coverage%20Estimates.pdf

Federal Advisory Committee ACT (FACA). (1972). Pub. L. 92-463. Retrieved from http://www.gsa.gov/graphics/ogp/without_annotations_R2G-b4T_0Z5RDZ-i34K-pR.pdf

GPO. (2009, February). *Health Information Technology for Economic and Clinical Health (HITECH) Act. Title XIII of Division A and Title IV of Division B of the American Recovery and Reinvestment Act of 2009 (ARRA), Pub. L. No 111-5*. Retrieved from http://www.gpo.gov/fdsys/pkg/PLAW-111publ5/pdf/PLAW-111publ5.pdf

GPO. (2010, January). *Patient Protection and Affordable Care Act. Public Law 111–148*. Retrieved from http://www.gpo.gov/fdsys/pkg/BILLS-111hr3590enr/pdf/BILLS-111hr3590enr.pdf

HRSA. (2010, March 17). *HRSA study finds nursing workforce is growing and more diverse*. Retrieved from http://www.hrsa.gov/about/news/pressreleases/2010/100317_hrsa_study_100317_finds_nursing_workforce_is_growing_and_more_diverse.html

HRSA. (2013, November). *Projecting the supply and demand for primary care practitioners through 2020 in brief*. Retrieved from: http://bhpr.hrsa.gov/healthworkforce/supplydemand/usworkforce/primarycare/primarycarebrief.pdf

Institute of Medicine (IOM). (2010). *A summary of the December 2009 forum on the future of nursing: Care in the community workshop summary*. Washington, DC: The National Academies Press.

Institute of Medicine. (2012). Best Care at Lower Cost: The Path to Continuously Learning Health Care in America. Retrieved from http://www.iom.edu/reports/2012/best-care-at-lower-cost-the-path-to-continuously-learning-health-care-in-america.aspx

Institute of Medicine. (2013). *Reports*. Retrieved from http://www.iom.edu/Reports.aspx

Johns Hopkins University (JHU) Institute for Policy Studies. (2013, October). *What is public policy?* Retrieved from http://ips.jhu.edu/pub/public-policy

McCormick, K. A., Sensmeier, J., Delaney, C. W., & Bickford, C. J. (2013). Introduction to informatics and nursing. In J. D. Bronzino (Ed.), *The biomedical engineering handbook* (4th ed.). *Medical Devices and Systems*. Boca Raton, FL: CRC Press.

National Committee on Vital and Health Statistics (NCVHS). (2013, October). *Public advisory body to the secretary of health and human services*. Retrieved from http://www.ncvhs.hhs.gov/index.htm

ONC Data Brief. (2012b, December). *Physician adoption of electronic health record technology to meet meaningful use objectives: 2009-2012*. Retrieved from http://www.

healthit.gov/sites/default/files/onc-data-brief-7-december-2012.pdf

ONC Data Brief. (2013a, March). *Hospital Adoption of Electronic Health Record Technology to*

ONC Data Brief. (2013b, May). *Regional extension center nurse practitioners and physician assistants: Crucial primary care providers on the path to meaningful use.* Retrieved from http://www.healthit.gov/sites/default/files/onc_databrief_no11_may_2013.pdf

Patient-Centered Primary Care Collaborative (PCPCC). (2013, October). *Defining the medical home.* Retrieved from http://www.pcpcc.org/about/medical-home

Robert Wood Johnson Foundation. (2008, October). Strengthening public health nursing part II: how nurse leaders in policymaking positions are transforming public health. *Charting nursing's future.* Retrieved from http://www.rwjf.org/en/research-publications/

find-rwjf-research/2009/01/charting-nursings-future-archives/strengthening-public-health-nursing-part-ii.html

Stone, D. (2006, December 21). 'Think Tanks and Policy Analysis'. In F. Fischer, G. J. Miller., & M. S. Sidney (Eds.) *Handbook of Public Policy Analysis: Theory, Methods, and Politics. New York, NY:* Marcel Dekker Inc., 149–157.

Technology Informatics Guiding Education Reform (TIGER). (2009, October). *Statement to the Robert Wood Johnson Foundation initiative on the future of nursing: Acute care, focusing on the area of technology informatics.*

U.S. Government Accountability Office (GAO). (2008, February). *Primary care professionals: Recent supply trends, projections, and valuation of Services.* GAO-08-472T. Washington, D.C. Retrieved from http://www.gao.gov/new.items/d08472t.pdf

World Health Organization (WHO). (2013, October). *Health policy.* Retrieved from http://www.who.int/topics/health_policy/en/

19

Communication Skills in Health IT, Building Strong Teams for Successful Health IT Outcomes

Elizabeth (Liz) O. Johnson

• OBJECTIVES

1. Discuss the importance of communication in health IT to achieve adoption of EHR technology.
2. Define the elements of effective communication plans.
3. Identify the stakeholders to consider in communications plans.
4. Describe the federal agencies, regulations, and other factors that affect health IT.

• KEY WORDS

Governance
Communication
Electronic health record
Physicians
Informaticists
Patient

INTRODUCTION

In America's twenty-first century healthcare system, landmark federal reform legislation enacted since 2009 is modernizing care-delivery organizations with new health information technologies (health IT) that regularly begin with the adoption of electronic health records (EHRs). Most notable of these laws are the American Recovery and Reinvestment Act (ARRA) and its Health Information Technology and Economic and Clinical Health (HITECH) Act provision, which established the Centers for Medicare and Medicaid's (CMS) Meaningful Use of EHRs Incentive Programs (Blumenthal & Tavenner, 2010). These programs earmarked more than $22 billion in incentive payments for eligible physicians and healthcare providers who successfully meet increasingly stringent requirements for EHR implementation over the next five years.

The journey to successful integration of health IT by providers industry-wide has been accompanied with challenges. Tremendous complexities exist throughout healthcare organizations working on health IT reform initiatives creating a critical need for effective communication campaigns that run throughout the lifecycles of acquiring, implementing, and adopting EHRs in both inpatient and ambulatory settings. Efforts such as these, with effective communication programs in place as a core strategy, support the goal of achieving the Institute of Medicine's (IOM) six aims for improvement in care-delivery quality, making it safe, equitable, effective, patient centered, timely, and efficient (Institute of Medicine, 2001).

As America's healthcare system strives to be a "continuously learning" system, healthcare leaders and providers realize that communication and improved patient engagement are central to improving the value of healthcare (Institute of Medicine, 2013a). Clinicians, clinical informaticists, health organizations, and health IT policymakers serve as agents of change in the effort to involve patients not only in decision-making, but providing key pieces of health data. To enhance these efforts, IOM began the Evidence Communication Innovation Collaborative, which explores obstacles, solutions, and strategies to enhance patient involvement in healthcare (Institute of Medicine, 2013b). Two projects underway are "shared decision-making strategies for best care" and "patients' attitudes on data sharing," which should provide ways to encourage provider–patient communication and transparency in healthcare.

A number of studies have shown that good physician–patient communication leads to improved patient satisfaction as well as increased willingness of patients to share pertinent data, adhere to medical treatment, and follow advice. Under these circumstances, patients also are less likely to lodge formal complaints or initiate malpractice suits (Ha & Longnecker, 2010).

A strong communication campaign for physicians during the EHR implementation is very important. Without such communication strategies, EHR adoption is far less likely. In 2002, for example, a major west-coast academic medical center that heavily invested in the implementation of computerized provider order entry (CPOE) encountered significant physician resistance. In large part, the clinician revolt occurred because physicians had been insufficiently informed about and inadequately trained in the use of the clinical decision support (CDS) tool being implemented (Bass, 2003). According to David Bates, MD, in a 2006 *Baylor University Medical Center Proceedings* paper, failure to achieve leadership support or clinical buy-in from the large number of providers using the system resulted in strong resistance from an overwhelming majority of physician effectively derailing the entire initiative (Bates, 2006).

Other provider organizations have encountered related challenges with health IT implementations over the past decade (Kaplan & Harris-Salamone, 2009). Such costly, high-risk experiences—especially in an increasingly patient-centric healthcare industry—have underscored the importance of effective, cross-enterprise, patient-focused communication plans and strategies that include physicians and clinicians, administrators, clinical informaticists, IT professionals, and the C-Suite—all of whom play critical roles as new technologies are introduced. As a result, effective communication programs have quickly become a high priority for hospitals and physician practices adopting EHR and CPOE systems throughout the industry. The "continuously learning" healthcare system in America depends on the involvement of all stakeholders—from patients to providers to management to vendors—to manage communications effectively and share them openly within the entire healthcare community. The purpose of this chapter is to provide an overview of communication strategies that have proven effective in driving the implementation of EHRs to support needs of patients, physicians, and the caregiver workforce. Sections in the chapter include (a) the importance of communications in health IT initiatives; (b) a focus on patient-centered, transparent care; (c) components of the communication plan; (d) industry considerations (roles of federal agencies, federal regulations, and the burgeoning role of mobile applications, social media, and health information exchange); and (e) chapter review.

IMPORTANCE OF COMMUNICATIONS IN HEALTH IT INITIATIVES

As Georgia Tech Professor William Rouse noted in a 2008 article entitled "Healthcare as a Complex Adaptive System: Implications for Design and Management," healthcare organizations exist as complex adaptive systems with nonlinear relationships, independent and intelligent agents, and system fragmentation (Rouse, 2008). While variation among them is gradually diminishing through increasing standardization of practices and systems, many provider cultures still struggle with decentralization and reliance on disparate legacy systems (Kaplan & Harris-Salamone, 2009). The majority of healthcare organizations across the nation have implemented EHRs, and providers are working toward meaningful use in their health IT applications, creating the need for effective and tactical communication plans. As the IOM's Evidence Communication Innovation Collaboration notes, "Communication is central to transforming how evidence is generated and used to improve the effectiveness and value of health care" (Halvorson & Novelli, n.d.). The rapid changes in diagnostic and treatment options and the increased number of patients, with varying degrees of health literacy, turning to the Internet for health information only serve to underscore the importance of clear and consistent communication. The following section provides insight into the importance of communications in health IT implementation programs: in governance, the structure of a governance model, and rules for governance efforts.

THE COMPLEXITY OF HEALTHCARE COMMUNICATIONS

Healthcare systems face unique challenges in communications. Unlike corporations or other organizations, healthcare involves a variety of stakeholders, often with competing goals and definitions of quality, in what is called a complex adaptive system (Rouse, 2008). Complex adaptive systems are described by William B. Rouse as follows:

- "They are nonlinear and dynamic and do not inherently reach fixed-equilibrium points. As a result, system behaviors may appear to be random or chaotic." For example, healthcare in America is not governed by a single entity. The federal government provides incentives to providers to implement EHRs, which have financial impact, but the level and timing of compliance is still at the providers' prerogative. Within a community, care providers have different owners and financial structures, i.e., for-profit, not-for-profit, single-owned entity, multi-provider organization, etc., which affects how the EHR fits into their business plans. Communication approaches should be adaptable to environments which will not remain constant.

- "They are composed of independent agents whose behavior is based on physical, psychological, or social rules rather than the demands of system dynamics." The physician population best fits this characterization. Most U.S. hospitals use community-based physicians to service their patients; these physicians are not employees of the hospital and may serve patients in competing hospitals in the community. The hospital's influence over the compliance of these physicians to use the EHR is limited to the physician-perceived benefits of treating patients at that institution. Clear delineation and dissemination of benefits for all stakeholders is an effective approach for affecting independent agents.

- "Because agents' needs or desires, reflected in their rules, are not homogeneous, their goals and behaviors are likely to conflict. In response to these conflicts or competitions, agents tend to adapt to each other's behaviors." Again, physicians provide a good example of this scenario. Take the case where two competing physician cardiology practice groups are serving a hospital that is implementing an EHR system that has built-in standardized decision support to reflect leading clinical practices and to reduce variation in care. However, the two practice groups cannot agree on the standard of care or do not want to share their practices with the other competing group. Being cognizant of this expected behavior should lead to the inclusion of collaboration opportunities as a part of the communication plan.

- "Agents are intelligent. As they experiment and gain experience, agents learn and change their behaviors accordingly. Thus overall system behavior inherently changes over time." Physicians, other clinicians, clinical informaticists, administrators are highly degreed professionals who are required to comply with continuous education requirements in order to maintain their certification. This provides a mechanism for sharing leading practices among their colleagues and changing their knowledge, skill level, and attitudes. The challenge is that the rate of change varies across these groups where we find a continuum of "innovators, early adopters, early majority, late majority, and laggards" as described by Everett Rogers' Technology Adoption Lifecycle model (Rogers, 1962).

- "Adaptation and learning tend to result in self organization. Behavior patterns emerge; they are not designed into the system. The nature of emergent behaviors may range from valuable innovations to unfortunate accidents." When implementing an EHR, we are not just implementing technology; we are also implementing standardized workflows. Although many system users adopt the new workflow, there are also those who develop inappropriate "workarounds" to avoid changing their old behaviors. This requires the clinical leadership use clear messaging to hold their department members accountable for using the new technology in the appropriate manner.

- "There is no single point of control. System behaviors are often unpredictable and uncontrollable, and no one is 'in charge.' Consequently, the behaviors of complex adaptive systems can usually be more easily influenced than controlled." U.S. providers of care reflect a wide spectrum of structures—from small single proprietorships to limited partnerships to large multi-entity corporations. Some are privately owned; others are government owned and operated, such as the Veterans' Administration healthcare system. Within healthcare systems decision-making is rarely a simple single threaded event. Creating successful campaigns for change require understanding the influence structure and leveraging formal and informal communication approaches.

Healthcare is, indeed, a complex adaptive system that cannot be directly controlled. Providers of care must be influenced to do the right thing and to aspire to a common goal. Communications that are planned, strategic, broad-based, and compelling are our best tool in effecting positive changes in our healthcare environment.

LEADERSHIP AND GOVERNANCE

The introduction of EHRs in healthcare organizations drives transformational change in clinical and administrative workflows; organizational structure, i.e., that which exists among physicians, nurses, and administrators; and relationships between the front-line workers, physicians, administrators, and patients (Bartos, Butler, Penrod, Fridsma, & Crowley 2006; Campbell, Sittig, Ash, Guappone, & Dykstra, 2006). Understanding the risks posed by the disruptive facets of organizational and process change is critical to ensuring the effective implementation of EHRs and mitigating risks of failure (Ash et al., 2000). An essential part of risk mitigation in care-delivery reform through health IT is the planning and implementing of organizational communication initiatives that help achieve the aims of an enterprise-wide governance team. To succeed, responsibilities for such communications initiatives should be shared between health system leaders, champions, informaticists, and those charged with oversight of the implementation of health IT systems, all of whom should have a role to play in governance structures whose processes are grounded in a strong communications strategy. A 2012 *Hospital & Health Network* magazine cover story entitled "iGovernance" summarized the importance of such an approach for transforming healthcare organizations as, "This IT governance function, guided from the top but carried out by sometimes hundreds of clinical and operations representatives, will be evermore crucial to managing the escalation of IT in healthcare delivery…." In fact, without such an informed governance process, the article states, "IT at many hospitals and health care systems is a haphazard endeavor that typically results in late, over-budget projects and, ultimately, many disparate systems that don't function well together" (Morrissey, 2012). Accountability begins at the hospital level and rises through the enterprise level. Messaging through electronic, in-person, or video media options from chief executive officers and board members of governance groups solidifies the importance of enterprise-level health IT projects (College of Healthcare Information Management Executives [CHIME], 2010b). However, both governance structures and the communications that support them require tailoring depending on the nature of every health system. Communication leaders from the organization should be involved in developing the governance and communication plan to align with or to evolve the culture of the organization.

Governance models in healthcare organizations provide a structure that engages stakeholders to work through critical decisions and ensure that risks associated with changes in policy, technology, and workflow are mitigated to maintain or improve the quality of patient care. A strong example of a working model is provided by the author's own health system—Tenet Healthcare Corporation. Figure 19.1 illustrates the governance structure of Tenet Healthcare's IMPACT Program (IMPACT: Improving Patient Care through Technology) and the importance of communications as it has been built into all layers.

As shown here, a key to the success of this governance structure is a three-tiered organizational structure that engages the corporation, regional operations, and the hospitals themselves in a coordinated effort. Another key success factor has been early commitment to key roles, including clinical informaticists, physician champions, training and communications leads, and health IT leads. Binding the program together with unified, shared, and consistent messaging continues to be a foundational strategy that supports all aspects of IMPACT's execution (Johnson, 2012).

Barbara Hoehn, RN, MBA, summed up the importance of communications in governance in her 2010 *Journal of Healthcare Information Management* article entitled "Clinical Information Technology Governance." "Today, clinical IT is finally being universally viewed as a critical component of healthcare reform, and we are only going to get one chance to do this right," she wrote. "This means having everyone in the organization, from the Board Members to the bedside clinicians, all focused on the same plan, the same tactical initiatives, and the same outcomes" (Hoehn, 2010).

RULES FOR GOVERNANCE

Enabling governance committees requires a solid set of rules, since hospitals are matrixed organizations comprised of multi-disciplinary staff and leaders from across a healthcare organization. A set of "rules to live by" in "iGovernance" is identified in Table 19.1 (Morrissey, 2012).

The following describes each role:

1. Hardwire the committees: Ensure that the chair of lower-level committees be participants on the next level of committees. Their role is to bring forward recommendations and issues needing higher-level engagement for resolution.

2. Set clear levels of successive authority: Committee responsibilities should be well defined so members know issues they can address and issues beyond their level of authority (Hoehn, 2010).

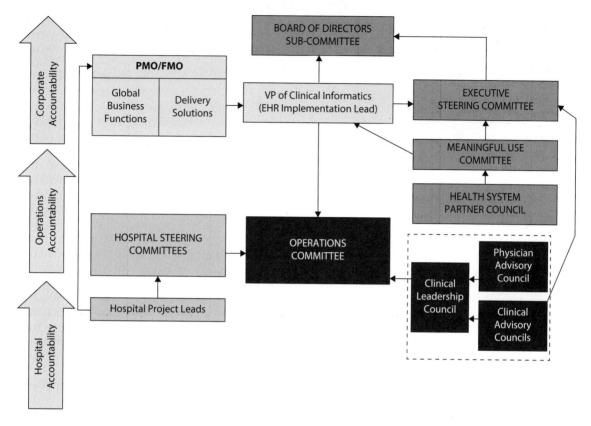

• **FIGURE 19.1.** EHR Implementation and Oversight Governance.

3. Do real work every time: Focus meetings on important issues in need of clinician engagement. If there are no critical items, cancel the meeting and send out status reports electronically.

4. Form no governance before its time: Recognize that different organizations will not be prepared to embrace a governance structure at the same time or to the same degree as others.

5. Put someone in charge that can take a stand: The leader of the top committee must be someone who commands respect and possesses operational authority to enact recommendations.

More specifically for health information technology, the Office of the National Coordinator for Health Information Technology (ONC), knowing that this area requires consensus among many stakeholders, lays out milestones and expected outcomes for governance. In their governance framework, ONC presents milestones and expected outcomes, rather than specific steps, for governance. These goals include organizational transparency and trust for all stakeholders (Office of the National Coordinator for Health Information Technology, 2013).

FOCUS ON CUSTOMERS AND PLAYERS

Those who are engaged in EHR implementation initiatives should also be involved in communications associated with these multi-year programs. Figure 19.2 illustrates the spectrum of customers and players.

TABLE 19.1	Rules to Live by for Governance Participants
1. Hardwire the committees.	
2. Set clear levels of successive authority.	
3. Do real work every time.	
4. Form no governance before its time.	
5. Put someone in charge who can take a stand.	

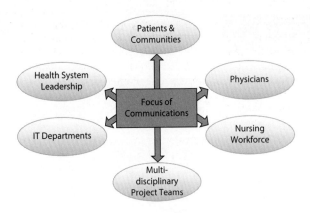

• **FIGURE 19.2.** Focus of Communications.

In the provider setting, each of these groups has a different type of communications engagement. The media and vehicles used may be different, but the strategic focus is the same: improving the quality of patient care through strategic adoption of health IT that is in turn enabled by smart communications.

Patients and Communities

In its 2001 report, *Crossing the Quality Chasm: A New Health System for the 21st Century*, the IOM established the need for patient-centered communications and support as part of the six aims for improving healthcare, as noted in the introduction (Institute of Medicine, 2001). Since then, patient-centric healthcare and the emergence of care-delivery models such as the Patient-Centered Medical Home (PCMH) have become central to health reform. Integral to the PCMH concept are seven joint principles established in 2007, one of which calls for a "whole-person orientation." This means each personal physician is expected to provide for all of a patient's lifetime health service needs. Lifetime engagement related to health drives the requirement for comprehensive physician-to-patient communications and shared decision-making (Patient-Centered Primary Care Collaborative, 2007).

Such communications are also required to support healthcare reform at the community level, as demonstrated in CMS's 2011 establishment of the Three Part Aim for the Medicare Shared Savings Program, e.g., the Medicare ACO, with its focus on "better care for individuals and better health for populations" (Federal Register. I.(C), 2011). In its final rule for the Medicare ACO, CMS mandated the requirement for advancing patient-centered care through accountable care organizations (ACOs), stating, "an ACO shall adopt a focus on patient-centeredness

that is promoted by the governing body and integrated into practice by leadership and management working with the organization's health care teams" (Federal Register II(B)(5), 2011).

Physicians

As discussed in the introduction, adoption of EHRs by health systems or practices cannot be expected to succeed without the endorsement and ownership of the physician community, whose working environment must inevitably adapt to changes to long-established workflows. Furthermore, when included from the outset of any health IT transformation initiative, the deployment of "physician champions" can become powerful and effective communicators, assisting colleagues through health IT adoption.

In fact, a *Government Health IT* story reported that ONC itself, through its regional extension centers, has recruited "physician champions" who are well on their way to becoming meaningful users of EHRs to help others in their area get over the hurdles of digitizing their medical records (Mosquera, 2011). Therefore, the need for communications that supports not only training initiatives and the management of new procedural requirements, but also an understanding of the dynamics of legislated healthcare reform itself, is important from the earliest stages of health IT adoption.

However, such needs are often unmet. An April 2012 *iHealthBeat* article reported, for example, that the results of a recent survey of more than 250 hospitals and healthcare systems demonstrated that significant percentages of respondent physicians had inadequate understanding of Stage 1 meaningful use requirements; others cited a lack of training and change-management issues (Providers Make Progress in EHR Adoption, 2012). As a result of improved programs and communications in organizations such as regional extension centers, 72% of office-based physicians had used an EHR by the end of 2012, and 66% were planning to or had applied for meaningful use (Bendix, 2013). These statistics spotlight the continued need to directly engage physicians in health IT implementations through comprehensive communications initiatives.

Nursing Workforce

For patients in both inpatient and ambulatory settings, nurses constitute the front line of patient care. But for health systems everywhere, they are also on the front line of health IT reform. As Joyce Hahn, Executive Director of the Nursing Alliance for Quality Care, said, "Nurses represent the largest potential users of electronic health records" (Hahn, 2011). As with their physician colleagues, therefore, the role of communications is not limited to training nurses in the use of EHR systems, but rather preparing them to engage fully in the design, testing, and implementation of EHRs to support improved care coordination and continuity of care. Throughout the healthcare industry, health systems CIOs are finding that "the success of large IT implementations will depend not only on the willingness of floor nurses to accept new technology, but also on the strength of the IS-nursing management connection" (Mitchell, 2012). Therefore, engaging nurses through communications both as champions and users of new health IT is a strategic necessity.

The clinical nurse informaticist has become a key role in ensuring the adoption of EHR technology and the sustainment of benefits. This role serves as a key change agent and communicator to all clinical disciplines by facilitating interdisciplinary workflows and using metrics to drive improvements in patient care.

Nursing Advisory Teams (NAT) can function as decision-making bodies—and NAT's decisions will become the standard for the implementation of core clinical EHR applications. The consistent way that these leaders communicate their decisions has proved to be integral to promoting safe, quality patient care and improving outcomes for patients and families while supporting the clinical quality initiatives (Johnson, 2012). Nurses and nursing informaticists can be key persons in the communication approach with physicians. Using their established relationships, nurses are able to remove the barriers and concerns physicians initially express in using EHRs, particularly computerized physician order entry. Provision of key talking points and documented benefits should be formally incorporated into the communication plan.

IT Departments and Multi-disciplinary Project Teams

IT departments and project teams are responsible for meeting the challenges of new-system introductions as well as managing the continuous upgrades to existing ones. To support this work, the teams' roles in communications efforts involve engaging clinicians in staff positions, confirming commitments, managing change, and setting EHR deployment strategies, per *The CIO's Guide to Implementing EHRs in the HITECH Era*, a 2010 paper from the College of Healthcare Information Management Executives (CHIME) (CHIME, 2010a).

Organizational newsletters are effective communication vehicles for sharing best implementation practices, success stories and fostering team cohesiveness across the healthcare organization. For example, *The IMPACT Insider*, Tenet's weekly cross-enterprise e-newsletter for IMPACT program news, features stories from successful hospital CPOE implementations so that upcoming hospitals can take advantage of the lessons learned (Johnson and Browne, 2012). This has resulted in improved training processes and has better prepared the hospitals across the board for changes in the system's EHR system applications. The success stories also fostered healthy competition across the health system to surpass previous CPOE adoption metrics at go-live. Newsletters should be distributed on a consistent basis, have a recognizable template of content that is always included, and provided in a variety of communications mediums such as e-mail, print, and company intranet.

Patients and Consumers

One imperative in the Patient Protection and Affordable Care Act (PPACA) is that providers must encourage patients to engage in their own care and communicate electronically with providers. This is seen as an important step in reducing hospital re-admissions for patients who have certain medical conditions, such as diabetes. However, hospitals face some resistance from patients, who would rather speak directly with their physicians or do not understand the benefits of reviewing and maintaining their own health records.

To combat such challenges, hospitals are creating patient-friendly portals where patients can check their appointments, see their lab results, pay bills, and send secure messages to their physicians. Some hospitals also are interacting directly with private physician offices to ensure follow-up care, which often reduces the need for readmission, and using telehealth services for high-risk patients. In addition, organizations, such as home nursing agencies, are text messaging to check in on pregnant women and new mothers (Versel, 2013). It should be noted that to ensure success, the language and content of patient communication will be different for that used among clinicians. All of the components of health literacy such as reading level, language preference, local naming conventions for health conditions are critical considerations when crafting communications for the patients and consumers.

Another resource that should be considered an effective communication tool and methodology related to patient engagement is the ONC Regional Extension Centers (RECs). These RECs serve as a communication and support resource for providers as they choose, implement, and use EHRs. The centers assist in workflow analysis and help providers connect with their patients using tools like patient portal which is a window to their information in their EHR. As of July 2013, more than 147,000 providers were enrolled with a regional extension center. Of these, more than 124,000 had a live EHR and more than 70,000 had demonstrated meaningful use. Some 85% of REC-enrolled providers were live on an EHR vs. 62% live on an EHR in the general provider population (Office for the National Coordinator of Health Information Technology, n.d.-a).

Healthcare System Leadership

As noted in the section on governance, communications led by an executive-level steering committee, often chaired by a health system's chief executive or operating officer, represent the beginning and the end of successful health IT implementation processes. The top of the organization not only establishes the size of the investment the organization is prepared to make, but also communicates "the broad strategies for IT in advancing business goals and, ultimately, acting on the result of a consistently applied proposal and prioritization regimen" per the 2012 "iGovernance" article cited earlier (Morrissey, 2012).

BUILDING A COMMUNICATIONS PLAN

Kaiser Permanente noted in the 2011 HIMSS Davies Award application for their KP HealthConnect® EHR that they credited their communication initiatives for "creating awareness, building knowledge, managing expectations, motivating end users, and building proficiency" (Health Information Management Systems Society [HIMSS], 2011). As part of their communications plans, they included vehicles such as a central Intranet site, leadership messaging, weekly e-newsletters, regional communication tactics, and videos. Other health systems also employ e-mail updates, end-user training, super-users

who function as subject matter experts, and champions to secure buy-in for system adoption.

A 2009 article by Chad Eckes, CIO, and Edgar Staren, MD, entitled "Communication Management's Role In EHR Success" offers other ideas, such as (Eckes & Staren, 2009):

- Fact Sheets, newsletters, and posters: collateral tailored to clinician audiences
- Road shows: pre-implementation educational demos of forthcoming system capabilities
- Town hall meetings: opportunities for senior leaders to hold question and answer sessions
- Standard meeting reports: detailed status notes of schedules, budget, risks, and progress

An e-newsletter can be used to communicate success stories from hospitals that are further down the road and have successfully implemented EHR systems. Such a vehicle is especially effective for integrated health systems whose hospitals are spread geographically across the country.

Another perspective is provided by a 2005 *JHIM* article by Detlev Smaltz, PhD, FHIMSS, and colleagues, in which they discuss the importance of project communication plans focused on stakeholder groups and meeting their needs. Table 19.2 provides a sample of this plan for three stakeholder groups (Smaltz et al., 2005).

Communicating an EHR implementation plan to physicians, nurses, and providers is essential for EHR success. Unlike many other hospital initiatives, changes that directly affect the responsibilities of providers may be met with ambivalence, passivity, or as in the west-coast medical center mentioned in the introduction, active resistance. Therefore, communication about such changes should

TABLE 19.2	Sample of Health IT Project Communication Plan		
Stakeholder	**Objective**	**Media**	**Content**
Executive Management	Update on cost, benefits, service quality, and milestones	• In-person meeting and briefing	Status update and impact on outcomes
Nursing	Maintain awareness of progress; engage in design effort	• Nurse educators • Nursing leadership • Collateral • Unit meetings • Intranet Web site	• Project methodology • Design participation • Educational info • Outcomes impact
Medical Staff	Maintain awareness of progress; engage in design sessions	• Medical executive committee • Clinical chairs • Targeted newsletter	• Project methodology • Design participation • Educational info • Outcomes impact

include the following four steps, according to Michael Crossnick, *HITECH Answers* (Crossnick, 2012):

1. Create process teams: Create process teams within the staff to define the new workflow processes. These teams get the rest of the staff involved and help educate them as the practice prepares to adopt an EHR. These teams should meet at well-defined intervals on a regular and consistent basis.

2. Communicate the logic for EHR adoption: Explain all the benefits of EHR adoption, how each member of the staff will benefit, and how the patients will ultimately benefit by improved quality of care. Be careful to avoid "because we said so," or "it's a government mandate" statements. While this may be true in some instances, it does not capture the true spirit of EHR adoption.

3. Define measurable success factors: Clearly state what the critical success factors are surrounding the new EHR workflows and processes and follow this with a reporting system to evaluate success and improve the processes once the EHR has been fully deployed.

4. Clearly communicate results: Establish a communication plan to communicate the definition of success. These communications should happen frequently at pre-defined intervals on a regular basis. Be certain to include all successes, as well as areas for opportunity, in these communications. Nothing aligns people faster than gaining success, even if they are initially small accomplishments.

PROJECT PHASES AND THE COMMUNICATION FUNCTIONS

Health IT projects often unfold over multi-year periods with pre-adoption (selection), pre-implementation, implementation (go-live), and post-implementation (outcomes) comprising the four major phases (Rodriguez & Pozzebon, 2011). It is important that communication plans be built and integrated within these phases, because the information needs of stakeholders will vary as projects evolve and mature. Furthermore, a variety of formal and informal communication media will be needed to reach different health-system groups, a point made in a 2009 *Journal of AHIMA* article entitled "Planning Organizational Transition to ICD-10-CM/PCS" (D'Amato, et al., 2009). The article further states that because points of urgency and risks to be mitigated are also critical to key stakeholders, they should also be considered among the key elements of an effective communication strategy.

Patients also should be included in EHR communications. Blackstone Valley Community Healthcare, working with a regional extension center in Rhode Island, created a patient portal named HealthKey, with which patients could schedule appointments and e-mail questions (HealthIT.gov, 2011). Patients coming in for appointments provided their e-mail addresses, which generated invitations to HealthKey. While initial use of the patient portal was modest, those who did use it viewed it favorably. A key issue has been getting patients to complete the second step, which is completing enrollment on the portal. As a result, Blackstone is purchasing kiosk terminals for waiting rooms so patients can complete the enrollment onsite and are planning a patient survey to evaluate HealthKey. Communications strategies may also need some creativity; in late 2013, patients who enrolled in the patient portal were eligible to win a mini iPad (Blackstone Valley Community Healthcare, 2013).

Communication Metrics

The best metrics to measure communication program effectiveness are arguably the same used to present the stories of successful health IT implementations themselves. In Tenet's case, strong governance programs supported by a pervasive and adaptable communications strategy have helped drive EHR/CPOE Meaningful Use go-lives in 49 hospitals across the country by the end of the first quarter of 2014. These results were supported by weekly e-newsletters, hospital site–specific communications campaign, future state workflow localization, change readiness assessments, at-the-elbow support for providers from super-users and subject matter experts throughout the go-live processes, physician partnering, post–go-live support, and 24×7 command centers for 10 days post–go-live.

KEY INDUSTRY CONSIDERATIONS

While much of the communications focus supporting the implementation of new EHR systems and related health IT is directed inside a health system, those responsible for building communication strategies must do so in the context of industry change beyond any hospital's walls. With the arrival and rapid entrenchment of the digital age over the last decade, innovations in mobile devices and social media platforms have broadened, enriching communications options to support successful health IT integration. Furthermore, the actions of the Federal Government to ensure increasing volumes of trusted, secure health information exchange are constantly redefining how and what the healthcare industry can expect to communicate across the continuum of care in the coming days, months, and years. Therefore, communications planning in support of health IT initiatives must reflect the forces driving such change: an expanding world of media, the roles of Federal healthcare agencies, and the adoption of regulatory standards as they are driving the evolution of health information exchange itself.

SOCIAL MEDIA AND eHEALTH INITIATIVES—MEETING THE HEALTH COMMUNICATION NEEDS OF COMMUNITIES

Physicians and clinicians across the industry are increasingly communicating among themselves and with their patients due to an explosion of mobile health device technology. A recent article entitled "Doctors' Tablet Use Almost Doubles in 2012" confirmed through a survey of 3015 physicians that nearly 62% are using some type of tablet platform—with the dominant choice being Apple's iPad. Such technologies are rapidly evolving, and clinicians are increasingly depending upon them to document patient visits, manage clinical workflows, conduct research on technical and clinical issues, and receive alerts regarding patient conditions (Vecchione, 2012).

While the upside to this rapid increase in communication technologies is tremendous, the deployment of such devices in the marketplace may be surpassing the pace for which security precautions can keep up, as noted in a February 2012 *Forbes* article, aptly entitled "How Healthcare's Embrace of Technology has Turned Dangerous" (Lai, 2012). The article acknowledged the "huge potential in helping medical providers diagnose patients more quickly and accurately, improving the patient-provider relationship, and reducing extra paperwork – and the medical errors that are sometimes caused by them." But it also called on hospitals to help "draft up an industry-wide set of best practices governing the use of mobile devices in hospital settings."

To address security issues, the FDA released final guidelines for mobile technology use in September 2013 (Food and Drug Administration, 2013). While these are non-binding guidelines that address mobile medical apps, they provide a roadmap for current use and the development of future medical mobile apps. They may also play a role in other eHealth initiatives as more and more consumers turn to their mobile devices to interface with patient portals to communicate with their providers and maintain their personal health records.

Beyond devices, new digital media vehicles encompass a multitude of healthcare specific social media Web sites such as PatientsLikeMe, Sermo, and Diabetesmine

that have emerged in the Health 2.0/Medicine 2.0 era as defined by Van De Belt and colleagues in their 2010 *Journal of Medical Internet Research* article (Van De Belt, Engelen, Berben, & Schoonhoven, 2010). Keys to enabling productive communications with today's new interactive tools recognizes that "(a) health has become more participatory, (b) data has become the new 'Intel Inside' for systems supporting the 'vital decisions' in health, and (c) a sense of 'collective intelligence' from the network would supplement traditional sources of knowledge in health decision-making" as summarized by Hesse and colleagues in their 2011 article entitled "Realizing the Promise of Web 2.0: Engaging Community Intelligence" (Hesse et al., 2011),

Social media sites bring new opportunities to improve provider-to-provider communications within physician-centric channels. These include sites like Sermo and QuantiaMD, which cater only to the physician community. Other social networking sites support patient communities that bring new opportunities for marketing of services and disseminating best practices, as noted by David Nash, MD, MBA, in a May 2010 article, entitled "Social networking impact on patients, doctors, and non-profits" (Nash, 2010). As with mobile devices, the many positive effects to be gained from participation in social media must be considered alongside concerns for the privacy and security of protected health information. Supported by the HIPAA Privacy and Security Rules passed in 1996, healthcare organizations have become more vigilant in establishing rules and policies governing participation in social media. Such heightened awareness was recently noted in the April 2012 Federation of State Medical Boards, "Model Policy Guidelines for Appropriate Use of Media and Social Networking in Medical Practice." Even so, as these communication platforms evolve in the future, addressing issues of privacy and security will be a key concern for the industry, physicians, health systems, patients, and the healthcare reform movement as a whole (Lewis, 2011).

ROLE OF FEDERAL HEALTHCARE AGENCIES

Healthcare reform during the past decade has been defined, spearheaded, and guided by Federal Government agencies armed with ARRA and HITECH legislation to providing funding, oversight, and industry-level guidance on the implementation and adoption of health IT throughout the United States (Robert Wood Johnson Foundation [RWJF], 2009). Leading the government's healthcare initiatives is the U.S. Department of Health and Human Service (HHS) (Department of Health and Human Services, n.d.).

Two key divisions of HHS are CMS and ONC. In addition to Medicare (the federal health insurance program for seniors) and Medicaid (the federal needs-based program), CMS oversees the Children's Health Insurance Program (CHIP), the Health Insurance Portability and Accountability Act (HIPAA), and the Clinical Laboratory Improvement Amendments (CLIA), among other services. Also, under HITECH, CMS is charged with advancing health IT through implementing the EHR incentive programs, helping define meaningful use EHR technology, drafting standards for the certification of EHR technology, and updating health information privacy and security regulations under HIPAA (Centers for Medicare and Medicaid Services [CMS], n.d.).

Much of this work is done in close conjunction with ONC and the two critically important federal advisory committees that operate under its auspices. The first of these committees is the Health IT Policy Committee, which makes recommendations to ONC on development and adoption of a nationwide health information infrastructure, including guidance on what standards for exchange of patient medical information will be required (Office of the National Coordinator for Health Information Technology [ONC], n.d.-b). The Policy Committee has a number of workgroups that address specific issues, such as governance for a nationwide health information exchange, consumer involvement, and privacy and security measures for EHRs.

The second is the Health IT Standards Committee, which focuses on recommendations from CMS, ONC, and the Health IT Policy Committee on standards, implementation specifications, and certification criteria for the electronic exchange and use of patient health information (PHI) (Office of the National Coordinator for Health Information Technology [ONC], n.d.-c). Many of its workgroups aim to set specific criteria and standards to ease the implementation of new programs and to measure their effectiveness.

Understanding the roles of these agencies and committees—and keeping abreast of their actions—is an important responsibility for those engaged in planning and delivering communications that support health IT adoption. Individually and collectively, they help drive the definition of incentive payment requirements across the three stages of EHR Meaningful Use. Each stage not only creates new health IT performance requirements inside a given health system, but also defines the kinds of information exchange—in themselves forms of communication—that will be required between healthcare entities across the entire continuum of care, including those directly focused on the patient and the community.

Stage 1: Beginning in 2011 as the incentives program starting point for all providers, "Stage 1 meaningful use" consists of transferring data to EHRs and being able to share information, including electronic copies and visit summaries for patients. As of October 2013, 85% of eligible hospitals and 60% of eligible providers have received incentive payments, which means that they have adopted, implemented, and met the criteria for EHR use (Reider & Taglicod, 2013).

Stage 2: To be implemented in 2014 under the current proposed rule and extend to 2016, "Stage 2 meaningful use" includes new standards such as online access for patients to their health information and electronic health information exchange between providers.

Stage 3: Expected to begin in 2017, "Stage 3 meaningful use" is projected to include criteria that demonstrate improvement in the quality of healthcare (Reider & Taglicod, 2013).

ROLE OF REGULATORY STANDARDS AND THE EVOLUTION OF HEALTH INFORMATION EXCHANGE

In today's era of healthcare reform, an increasing number of standards in the area of health, health information, and communications technologies are helping guide the healthcare industry toward interoperability between independent entities and systems. The goal is to support the safe, secure, and private exchange of PHI in ever-increasing volumes to improve the quality of care.

As advised by ONC, CMS, and the Health IT Policy Committee, the Health IT Standards Committee is the primary federal advisory committee working to fulfill this mandate. It is also a committee upon which this author is proudly serving at the appointment of HHS Secretary Kathleen Sebelius. Table 19.3 provides a summary of the duties of this committee as provided by a 2009 Robert Wood Johnson Foundation Report, "Health Information Technology in the US: On the Cusp of Change and the American Recovery and Reinvestment Act" (Robert Wood Johnson Foundation [RWJF], 2009).

The Health IT Standards Committee has established over the course of its deliberations a number of important workgroups as sub-committees to the parent committee. These workgroups meet periodically to discuss their topics, present their findings at Health IT Standards Committee meetings, and make recommendations to this Committee. The agency's sub-committees are formed around subjects such as Clinical Operations, Clinical Quality, Privacy & Security, Implementation, Vocabulary Task Force, Consumer Technology, and the Consumer/Patient Engagement Power Team (Office of the National Coordinator for Health Information Technology [ONC], n.d.-c).

TABLE 19.3	Duties of the HIT Standards Committee
Duties	
Harmonize or update standards for uniform and consistent implementation of standards and specifications.	
Conduct pilot testing of standards and specifications by the National Institute of Standards and Technology.	
Ensure consistency with existing standards.	
Provide a forum for stakeholders to engage in development of standards and implementation specifications.	
Establish an annual schedule to assess recommendations of HIT Policy Committee.	
Conduct public hearings for public input.	
Consider recommendations and comments from the National Committee on Vital and Health Statistics (NCVHS) in development of standards.	

The Implementation Workgroup is dedicated to ensuring that what is being asked of the greater health-system and physician-practice communities is actually feasible in terms of adoption and meaningful use. A strong public communications strategy is core to the work of this workgroup, which holds hearings with broad healthcare industry representation—including health systems, physicians, EHR and other health IT vendors and developers, among others—and maintains active liaison relationships with the sister Health IT Policy Committee.

As a result, the Implementation Workgroup will continue to bring forward "real-world" implementation experience into the Standards Committee recommendations with special emphasis on strategies to accelerate the adoption of proposed standards, or mitigate barriers, if any (Office of the National Coordinator for Health Information Technology, n.d.-d). Currently, the Implementation Workgroup is updating the goals and objectives for Meaningful Use Stage 3.

As are the meetings of the Health IT Policy and Standards Committees, all workgroup meetings are held in public, and notices for each meeting appear on the ONC Web site and in the Federal Register (Office of the National Coordinator for Health Information Technology, n.d-d). Public comment is always welcome.

CHAPTER REVIEW: FUTURE OF COMMUNICATIONS IN HEALTH IT

ARRA, HITECH, and incentives programs supporting the meaningful use of EHRs are helping the healthcare industry make a paradigm shift in care delivery through the accelerated use of health IT. CMS, ONC, and its HIT Policy and Standards Committees are driving communications at the industry level to provide all stakeholders with a common set of rules to follow for selection, design, implementation, and adoption of EHRs. Challenges still persist, however, when effective communication plans are not developed and followed in complex health IT projects that can affect physicians, nurses, administrators, and patients alike.

This chapter has addressed issues regarding the importance of communications and the development of effective communication strategies in strengthening initiatives ranging from governance efforts to physician-to-patient partnerships—all as part of successful EHR implementations. Key takeaways to consider in the conclusion of this chapter include the following:

- Coordinated, cross-enterprise communications strategies are critically important parts of health IT implementations, including the development of governance structures supporting the introduction and adoption of EHR systems.

- The customers and players engaged in communications include patients and communities, physicians, nurses, clinical informaticists, project teams and IT departments, and health system leadership. Remember that patient-centricity, the Meaningful Use program, and physician and nurse engagement are all critical points in the communication initiatives for these participants.

- Vehicles in a communications plan can include an Intranet, print media, road shows, Town Hall meetings, and standard meetings to be used through all phases of a project and the success of such projects can be the best measure of the communication plan's effectiveness.

- Some of the most powerful forces driving change include social media, mobile devices, and continued healthcare reforms and should be considered when developing communications plans.

- The ONC's committees, the HIT Policy and Standards Committees, and sub-committees, such as the Implementation Workgroup, are key drivers of national communications important to all stakeholders involved in working toward the meaningful use of EHRs.

America's healthcare system is a complex, expensive system that needs to learn and adopt continuously to improve the quality of care and outcomes, protect patient safety, and reduce inefficiencies (Institute of Medicine, 2013a). One of the major ways these goals can be accomplished is through the increased use and development of health IT. Health IT can increase providers' abilities to share and retain patient information and can support initiatives in patient engagement, care coordination, Meaningful Use, and eHealth. As the healthcare industry grows increasingly interconnected through health IT and other technologies, effective communication plans will remain essential parts of the process. With a commitment to the development and execution of communications strategies around the implementation of emerging health IT, higher levels of ownership and commitment by professionals will help ensure the success of the U.S. healthcare reform movement in years to come.

REFERENCES

Ash, J. S., Anderson, J. G., Gorman, P. N., Zielstorff, R. D., Norcross, N., Pettit, J., & Yao, P. (2000). Managing change: Analysis of a hypothetical case. *Journal of the American Medical Informatics Association: JAMIA, 7*(2), 125–134.

Bartos, C. E., Butler, B. S., Penrod, L. E., Fridsma, D. B., & Crowley, R. S. (2006). Negative CPOE attitudes correlate with diminished power in the workplace. *AMIA ... Annual Symposium Proceedings/AMIA Symposium, 6*, 36–40.

Bass, A. (2003). Health-care IT: A big rollout bust. *CIO Magazine*. Retrieved from http://www.cio.com/article/29736/Health_Care_IT_A_Big_Rollout_Bust. Accessed on June 1, 2003.

Bates, D. W. (2006). Invited commentary: The road to implementation of the electronic health record. *Proceedings (Baylor University. Medical Center), 19*(4), 311–312.

Bendix, J. (2013). Meaningful use stage 2: Ready or not here it comes. *Medical economics*. Retrieved from http://medicaleconomics.modernmedicine.com/medical-economics/news/meaningful-use-stage-2-ready-or-not-here-it-comes. Accessed on October 25.

Blackstone Valley Community Healthcare. (2013). Pawtucket, RI. Retrieved from http://www.blackstonechc.org/calendar/detail/112/Win-a-iPod-mini.

Blumenthal, D., & Tavenner, M. (2010). The "meaningful use" regulation for electronic health records. *The New England Journal of Medicine, 363*(6), 501–504.

Campbell, E. M., Sittig, D. F., Ash, J. S., Guappone, K. P., & Dykstra, R. H. (2006). Types of unintended consequences related to computerized provider order entry. *Journal of the American Medical Informatics Association: JAMIA, 13*(5), 547–556.

Centers for Medicare and Medicaid Services (CMS). (n.d.). *SearchHealthIT*. Baltimore, MD. Retrieved from http://searchhealthit.techtarget.com/definition/Centers-for-Medicare-Medicaid-Services-CMS

CHIME. (2010a). Chapter 3: Assessing the organization's current state in IT, charting a new course; Chapter 7: considering new role players for your EHR implementation. *The CIO's guide to implementing EHRs in the HITECH era.* CHIME Report. CHIME, Ann Arbor, MI. pp. 13, 31.

College of Healthcare Information Management Executives (CHIME). (2010b). Chapter 9: Communication dispels fear surrounding the EHR conversion. *The CIO's guide to implementing EHRs in the HITECH era.* CHIME Report. Retrieved from http://www.cio-chime.org/advocacy/CIOsGuideBook/CIO_Guide_Final.pdf

Crossnick, M. (2012). EHR implementation process requires communication. *HITECH Answers*. Retrieved from http://www.hitechanswers.net/ehr-implementation-process-requires-communication/. Accessed on March 27, 2012.

D'Amato, C., D'Andrea, R., Bronnert, J., Cook, J., Foley, M., Garret, G., … Yoder, M. J. (2009). Planning organizational transition to ICD-10-CM/PCS. *Journal of AHIMA/American Health Information Management Association, 80*(10), 72–77.

Department of Health and Human Services. (n.d.). Healthy people 2020. *Health communications and health information technology.* Washington, DC. Retrieved from http://www.healthypeople.gov/2020/topicsobjectives2020/overview.aspx?topicid=18

Eckes, C. A., & Staren, E. D. (2009). Communication management's role in EHR success. *HealthIT News.* Retrieved from http://www.healthcareitnews.com/blog/communication-management%E2%80%99s-role-ehr-success?page=0,1. Accessed on June 10, 2009.

Federal Register. I.(C). (2011). Overview and intent of Medicare Shared Savings Program. *76*(212), 67804.

Federal Register II(B)(5). (2011). Processes to promote evidence-based medicine, patient engagement, reporting, coordination of care, and demonstrating patient-centeredness. *76*(212), 67827.

Food and Drug Administration. (2013). Mobile medical applications. Silver Spring, MD. Retrieved from http://www.fda.gov/downloads/MedicalDevices/…/UCM263366.pdf. Accessed on September 25, 2013.

Ha, J. F., & Longnecker, N. (2010). Doctor-patient communication: A review. *The Ochsner Journal, 10*(1), 38–43.

Hahn, J. (2011). Nursing and meaningful use: What's the connection? *Center to Champion Nursing in America Blog.* Retrieved from http://championnursing.org/blog/nursing-and-meaningful-use. Accessed on March 21, 2011.

Halvorson, G. C., & Novelli, W. D., chairs. (n.d.). *Evidence communication innovation collaborative: Effective communication about effective care.* Washington, DC: Institute of Medicine, The National Academies. Retrieved from http://iom.edu/~/media/Files/Activity%20Files/Quality/VSRT/Core%20Documents/Evidence%20Communication%20Innovation%20Collaborative.pdf

Health Information Management Systems Society (HIMSS). (2011). Davies Enterprise Award for Kaiser Permanente. Management section. p. 5.

HealthIT.gov. (2011). *Meaningful use case studies.* Retrieved from http://www.healthit.gov/providers-professionals/blackstone-valley-community-health-care-case-study

Hesse, B. W., O'Connell, M., Augustson, E. M., Chou, W. Y., Shaikh, A. R., & Rutten, L. J. (2011). Realizing the promise of Web 2.0: engaging community intelligence. *Journal of Health Communication, 16*(Suppl. 1), 10–31.

Hoehn, B. J. (2010). Clinical information technology governance. *Journal of Healthcare Information Management: JHIM, 24*(2), 13–14.

Institute of Medicine. (2001). Committee on quality of healthcare in America. Executive summary. *Crossing the quality chasm: A new health system for the 21st century* (pp. 5–6). Washington, DC: National Academies Press.

Institute of Medicine. (2013a). *Best care at lower cost: The path to continuously learning healthcare in America.* Washington, DC: The National Academies Press.

Institute of Medicine. (2013b). *Evidence communication innovation collaborative.* Washington, DC. Retrieved from http://www.iom.edu/Activities/Quality/VSRT/2013-DEC-06.aspx

Johnson, E. O. (2012). IMPACT Journey Program Briefing 04/10/12. Tenet Healthcare Corporation internal corporate briefing.

Johnson, L., & Browne, P. (2012). *Tenet IMPACT program overview.* Dallas, TX. Retrieved from http://investor.tenethealth.com/event/webinar/tenet-hosts-health-information-technology-webinar

Kaplan, B., & Harris-Salamone, K. D. (2009). Health IT success and failure: Recommendations from literature and an AMIA workshop. *Journal of the American Medical Informatics Association: JAMIA, 16*(3), 291–299.

Lai E. (2012). How healthcare's embrace of mobility has turned dangerous. *Forbes.* Retrieved from http://www.forbes.com/sites/sap/2012/01/05/how-healthcares-embrace-of-mobility-has-turned-dangerous/. Accessed on January 5, 2012.

Lewis, N. (2011). Healthcare social media sites neglect privacy protections. *Information Week.* Retrieved from http://www.informationweek.com/news/healthcare/patient/229218547. Accessed on February 14, 2011.

Mitchell, M. B. (2012). The role of the CNIO in nursing optimization of the electronic medical record. Health Information Management Systems Society (HIMSS) 2012 Annual Conference Presentation. February 21, 2012.

Morrissey, J. (2012). iGovernance. *Hospitals & Health Networks Magazine.* Retrieved from http://www.hhnmag.com/display/HHN-news-article.dhtml?dcrPath=/templatedata/HF_Common/NewsArticle/data/HHN/Magazine/2012/Feb/0212HHN_Coverstory#.UuwOobSCeJk

Mosquera, M. (2011). Physician champions' help other docs with EHR adoption. *Government HealthIT.* Retrieved from http://www.govhealthit.com/news/physician-champions-help-other-docs-ehr-adoption

Nash, D. (2010). Social networking impact on patients, doctors, and non-profits. *KevinMD.* Retrieved from http://www.kevinmd.com/blog/2010/05/social-networking-impact-patients-doctors-nonprofits.html. Accessed on May 4, 2010.

Office of the National Coordinator for Health Information Technology. (2013). *The Governance framework for trusted electronic health information exchange.* Washington, DC. Retrieved from http://www.healthit.gov/sites/default/files/GovernanceFrameworkTrustedEHIE_Final.pdf

Office for the National Coordinator of Health Information Technology. (n.d.-a). *Regional extension centers.* Washington, DC. Retrieved from http://www.healthit.gov/providers-professionals/regional-extension-centers-recs

Office of the National Coordinator for Health Information Technology (ONC). (n.d.-b). *Health IT Policy Committee.* Washington, DC. Retrieved from http://www.healthit.gov/policy-researchers-implementers/health-it-policy-committee

Office of the National Coordinator for Health Information Technology (ONC). (n.d.-c). *Health IT Standards Committee.* Washington, DC. http://www.healthit.gov/policy-researchers-implementers/health-it-standards-committee

Office of the National Coordinator for Health Information Technology. (n.d.-d). *Implementation workgroup.* Retrieved from http://www.healthit.gov/policy-researchers-implementers/implementation-workgroup

Patient-Centered Primary Care Collaborative. (2007). *Joint principles of the patient-centered medical home.* Washington, DC. Retrieved from http://www.pcpcc.net/content/joint-principles-patient-centered-medical-home

Providers Make Progress in EHR Adoption. (2012). Challenges remain. *iHealthBeat.* Retrieved from http://www.ihealthbeat.org/articles/2012/4/24/providers-make-progress-in-ehr-adoption-challenges-remain.aspx. Accessed on March 24, 2012.

Reider, J., & Taglicod, R. (2013). Progress on adoption of electronic health records. *Health IT. gov.* Retrieved from http://www.healthit.gov/buzz-blog/electronic-health-and-medical-records/progress-adoption-electronic-health-records/. Accessed on December 6, 2013.

Robert Wood Johnson Foundation (RWJF). (2009). Chapter 4. Recent federal initiatives in health information technology. *Health information technology in the United States: On the cusp of change.* Retrieved from www.rwjf.org/pr/product.jsp?id=50308States.

Rodriguez, C., & Pozzebon, M. (2011). Understanding managerial behaviour during initial steps of a clinical information system adoption. *BMC Medical Informatics and Decision Making, 11*, 42.

Rogers, E. (1962). *Diffusion of innovations.* New York, NY: Free Press of Glencoe, Macmillan Company.

Rouse, W. B. (2008). Healthcare as a complex adaptive system: Implications for design and management. *The bridge.* Retrieved from http://www.learningace.com/doc/1970137/8976864da1ed77c7b52f24baf451face/rouse-naebridge2008-healthcarecomplexity

Smaltz, D. H., Callander, R., Turner, M., Kennamer, G., Wurtz, H., Bowen, A., & Waldrum, M. R. (2005). Making sausage—effective management of enterprise-wide clinical IT projects. *Journal of Healthcare Information Management : JHIM, 19*(2):48–55.

Van De Belt, T. H., Engelen, L. J., Berben, S. A., & Schoonhoven, L. (2010). Definition of health 2.0 and medicine 2.0: A systematic review. *Journal of Medical Internet Research, 12*(2), e18.

Vecchione, A. (2012). Doctors' tablet use almost doubles in 2012. *Information Week*. Retrieved from http://www.informationweek.com/news/healthcare/mobile-wireless/240000469. Accessed on May 16, 2012.

Versel, N. (2013). Hospitals grapple with patient engagement. *US News and World Report*. Retrieved from http://health.usnews.com/health-news/hospital-of-tomorrow/articles/2013/11/05/hospitals-grapple-with-patient-engagement. Accessed on November 25, 2013.

20

Assessing the Vendors

Mark D. Sugrue

• OBJECTIVES

1. Describe an approach to evaluate the vendor marketplace for health information technology solutions.
2. Discuss the evolution of the healthcare technology market place.
3. Distinguish the custom development or "build" approach from the purchasing of commercially available solutions or "buy" approach.
4. Identify two or more criteria that may be used to differentiate one vendor from another.
5. List the key Guiding Principles of a Vendor Analysis Methodology.

• KEY WORDS

Best of breed
Change management
Return-on-Investment (ROI)
Request for Information (RFI)
Request for Proposal (RFP)
Single vendor

INTRODUCTION

Assessing the Healthcare Information Technology market can be a daunting task. It is estimated that the global health IT market will reach $56.7 billion by 2017, an increase from the 2012 market value of $40.4 billion (Pedulli, 2013). In the United States alone, more than 1000 vendors exhibit at the Health Information Management Systems Society (HIMSS) annual conference. Navigating the field of potential vendors and assessing solution require a skilled and experienced leader and a team committed to a fair, unbiased, and thoughtful analysis.

Build vs. Buy

In the early days of Healthcare Information technology, many pioneering organizations elected to develop and support their own electronic health record software. The idea of developing in-house applications, often referred to as the "build" approach, was necessary at a time when commercial options were limited. The benefits of the build approach included the ability to program specifications to the organization's unique requirements and the flexibility to apply future updates or enhancements whenever they were needed.

The cost of the build approach, however, was great and many organizations could not compete within their market for the technical resources required to develop and support home grown solutions. There was also great institutional risk associated with this approach. Mission critical applications, for example, programmed by an employee could result in a single point of failure should that individual no longer be available to the organization.

The commercial healthcare information technology vendor market began to flourish in the middle of the twentieth century with many of the early solution offerings focused on financial and back office functions. As technology continued to evolve so too did the market. Demand for solutions increased steadily and over time vendors began to diversify their portfolios to include more and more applications across different settings.

Today, there are many categories of vendors in the market offering a wide variety of solutions. The competition has helped make purchasing or buying a solution the more popular choice by far. This "buy" option as it is commonly referred to has created a robust and thriving health IT marketplace.

Vendor Assessment Methodology

Effectively assessing the vendor marketplace requires a data-driven methodology and approach that will guide the organization through a vendor analysis process. The graphic in Fig. 20.1 represents a Vendor Assessment Methodology. Throughout the methodology Key Guiding Principles are embedded to ensure that proven best practices are adhered to.

Understanding the steps of the methodology along with the Key Guiding Principles and incorporating these into a well-developed and well-managed project plan will help ensure that the organization is applying a fair and unbiased approach to assessing potential vendor solutions.

Key Guiding Principles

The Key Guiding principles include:

1. Manage the Change; Communicate
2. Maintain and Document Objectivity
3. Think Process; Not Department

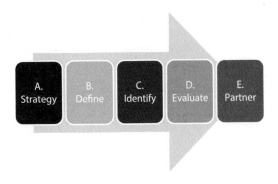

• **FIGURE 20.1.** Vendor Assessment Methodology.

4. Use the Data; Trust your Gut
5. Make a Commitment

VENDOR ASSESSMENT METHODOLOGY

Whether large or small the introduction of new technology into an environment will have an impact on users and potentially patients. Effectively managing this change at both the individual and institutional levels will be a critical success factor (Sugrue, 2010).

In many ways the selection project itself is an opportunity to engage users and begin the process of introducing change. As the team begins to assemble its plan to assess vendors it should remember that communication with all stakeholders is important. While it is not possible to have every stakeholder or employee of the organization actively participating in each step of the process, it is possible and highly recommended for teams to effectively communicate status and inform all of progress.

> **GUIDING PRINCIPLE #1**—Manage the Change; Communicate

Guiding Principle #1 is "Manage the Change; Communicate" and this cannot be stressed enough.

Large-scale transformation efforts such as new technology implementations may begin with an Organizational Change Readiness Assessment prior to a Vendor Assessment. In today's rapidly changing healthcare environment the pace and degree of change can be overwhelming for the organization and for individuals. An Organizational Change Readiness Assessment provides a mechanism to understand the organization's appetite and capacity for change and can help inform the Vendor Assessment effort. For an example of a Readiness Assessment for a physician practice environment see http://www.HealthIT.gov (HealthIT.gov: EHR Implementation Steps March, 2014).

It has been said that successful implementation of technology begins with early end-user engagement. A Change Management Strategy grounded in solid communication that is incorporated throughout the project is the best defense against resistance to change that may occur in any organization. Examples of communication strategies used during a vendor assessment include:

1. Newsletter publication on project goals and status
2. E-mail or intranet communication about the project

3. Town hall meetings led by organization leaders to provide status and answer questions
4. Posters communicating the anticipated timeline and reasons for change
5. Contests to name or internally brand the project

A. Strategy

The first major step in the Vendor Assessment Methodology is "Strategy." This phase of the methodology is typically led by leadership and is intended to provide the structure and strategic alignment and direction necessary to support the entire effort. The Strategy phase typically focuses on four key strategic considerations. These are:

- Business Drivers
- Future State Operational and IT Vision
- Independence and Compliance
- Financial and Return-on-investment

1. Business Drivers ("Why are we doing this?"). An important first step in assessing the vendor market place is to ask "why?" or what are the business or clinical drivers behind the organization's need to evaluate vendor solutions in the first place? Establishing the need for change and having it clearly articulated by leadership is also an important element of an effective people and organizational change management strategy.

There may be a number of reasons why an organization needs to assess the health IT vendor market. Some of these reasons may include:

a. New or pending regulatory requirements unmet by current vendor, such as meaningful use or ICD10
b. Current solution outdated, no longer supported (e.g., Application retired)
c. Changing business needs not met by current solution
d. Merger with another institution on a different platform
e. New enabling technology required to support improved care delivery/practice
f. Leadership decisions to change or introduce new technology
g. Current solution no longer meets business/clinical requirements, such as personalized healthcare
h. Poor service or instability of current vendor

Understanding the organization's unique business drivers for assessing the market and documenting these as part of a Vendor Assessment project charter is essential.

2. Future State ("What are we going to look like in the future?"). It is important for organizations making investments in technology solutions to consider the long-term outlook and impact. Most organizations will have a strategic plan which can provide some insight into the future direction of the enterprise. Leadership must fully consider the technology implications of various business strategies. Consider, for example, the potential technology impacts for the following healthcare-related strategic initiatives:

a. Becoming an Accountable Care Organization: *Increased need to manage data on populations and predictive analytics to support transitions of care*
b. Merger and acquisitions activity: *Data migration and integration of technology platforms across an enterprise*
c. Changing payment models focused on quality: *Data and quality reporting needs*
d. Clinician talent acquisition strategies: *Technology and tools to enable and support leading clinical practice*
e. Patient Engagement Initiatives: *Technology tools such as patient portals and data and information to effectively engage patients and families*

The operational vision helps describe what the future operational environment of the organization may look like. In addition to the operational vision it is important to also understand the overall Information Technology strategy and vision during the initial phase of the Vendor Assessment Methodology. Among other things, the IT strategy will often describe the organization's overall approach to vendor solutions and products in the context of an existing or future IT portfolio.

In recent times, there has been an effort to minimize the number of vendors included in an IT environment. In the past, organizations that embraced the **best-of-breed** model found that managing communication and integration between multiple vendors was challenging. On the other hand, it is well understood that there is not a **single vendor** who meets all of the functional and technical needs of a healthcare enterprise. Today, most organizations are attempting to minimize the number of vendors in their portfolio in the hope of achieving better interoperability between key systems. Where an organization is and most importantly where they want to be in the future along this continuum between best of breed and single vendor is an important strategic element to understand.

Both the Operational and IT strategies are important inputs for the Vendor Assessment Methodology. Anticipated solution benefits should be clearly defined and aligned with the organization's overall strategic direction.

Leadership involvement is essential in order to ensure this alignment of the institutional goals and objectives with expected solution benefits.

3. Independence and Compliance ("Is the process fair and defensible?"). One of the key strategic principles of a well-structured vendor analysis is independence. Merriam-Webster dictionary defines independence as "freedom from outside control or support" (Merriam Webster Online Dictionary: Independence, 2014). An independent vendor analysis process would be free of bias and would result in an objective decision for the organization. It is important for all members of the team to abide by guidelines established to ensure strict independence. These guidelines might include:

a. Acknowledging any real or apparent personal conflicts of interest. Team members who have relationships with representatives from one of the vendors under consideration or members holding a financial interest in one of the companies would be examples of a personal conflict.

b. Having a well-defined and adhered to vendors' "no gift" policy.

c. Agreeing to no outside contact policy during the procurement such that vendors cannot circumvent established communication channels.

d. Strictly managing internal and external communication and ensuring that information is shared with vendors in a timely, consistent, and professional manner.

Oftentimes organizations pursuing large-scale vendor assessments will look to external consulting firms to assist in guiding the organization through the process. The consulting firm selected as well as the resources assigned to the team should be held to the same standards relative to independence and bias.

With healthcare organizations' spending and investing tens and even hundreds of millions of dollars on technology solutions there is an increase in oversight and scrutiny from multiple stakeholders. Public and private boards, for example, may require detailed information regarding the selection of a particular vendor. It is necessary for those who lead these efforts to maintain and document objectivity throughout the process. This documentation would include a project charter, a work plan, timelines, status reports, correspondence, and meeting minutes to name a few. Project documents should be maintained in a secure place, they should provide a detailed chronology of all activity and they should be written with sufficient detail to stand alone upon review. The team should anticipate that all project documents will come under some degree of scrutiny by those outside of the project in the future.

> **GUIDING PRINCIPLE #2**—Maintain and Document Objectivity

Some of the indicators of a fair and objective system selection process are:

- All vendors respond to the same RFI/RFP format.
- There is a single point of contact for vendor questions.
- Vendors are asked not to interact with others in the organization.
- RFI/RFP released to vendors at the same time with same deadlines.
- Any questions asked by and responded to are shared with all vendors.
- Demonstration scripts are provided at pre-determined intervals in advance so that each vendor is provided the same amount of preparation time.
- Demonstration environment and timing is as consistent as possible for all vendors.
- Demonstrations are managed and facilitated fairly and consistently.

In some instances there may be local or regional requirements that must be considered from a compliance perspective. A Certificate of Need (CON) process, for example, is required in some states under certain conditions. According to the National Council of State Legislatures CONs "…are aimed at restraining healthcare facility costs and allowing coordinated planning of new services and construction" (Certificate of need state health laws and programs, 2013). These laws authorizing such programs are one mechanism by which state governments seek to reduce overall health and medical costs (Fig. 20.2).

4. Financial and Return-on-investment ("What are the costs and benefits?"). Lastly, and equally as important, the leadership team must provide some parameters around anticipated solution costs and benefits. Oftentimes with large-scale investments the organization's Board of Directors including the Finance and Investment committees may be involved to help provide some strategic guidance for the leadership and the Vendor Assessment project team as it relates to financial matters. This may also include the need to seek funding from external sources including capital and bond markets.

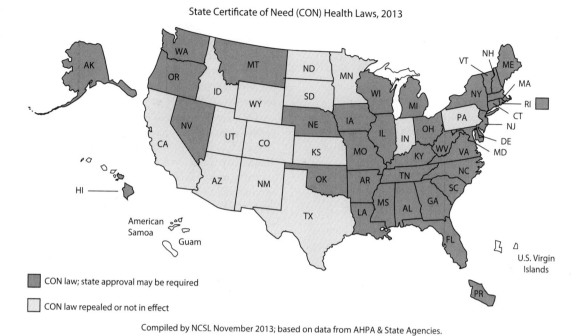

State Certificate of Need (CON) Health Laws, 2013

■ CON law; state approval may be required

☐ CON law repealed or not in effect

Compiled by NCSL November 2013; based on data from AHPA & State Agencies.

• **FIGURE 20.2.** State Requiring CON and those that Do Not. (Reproduced, with Permission. Copyright © National Conference of State Legislatures.)

The leadership team and the Board of Directors are often focused on the anticipated Return-on-investment (ROI) model of the proposed solution. To the extent that they exist the Vendor Assessment project team should fully understand any preliminary assumptions made relative to solution costs and benefits. It will be vitally important for the team to secure data early in the effort that help support and compare the projected financial impact analysis to an actual estimate based on data directly from the vendors. Cost estimates will be discussed further in the Define phase.

B. Define

The Define phase of the Vendor Assessment Methodology is intended to create the list of prospective vendors, to document the functional and technical solution requirements, and to formally request information or a formal proposal from targeted solution providers.

The major tasks in this phase are:

- Conduct market research and understand key market differentiators.

- Develop functional and technical requirements.

- Develop and Submit RFI/RFP.

1. Conduct Market Research and Understand Key Market Differentiators. Conducting a market scan of potential vendors is an important first step of the Define phase. An effective high-level market scan is as much an art as it is a science. While there are many resources available within the industry, the best and most reliable way to attain an appreciation of any vendor and solution is through networking and relationships.

Reaching out to colleagues or networking with peers who have "been there; done that" is a recommended first step in a successful market scan. Participating in trade shows or industry conferences at a local or national level can also provide an opportunity to connect with colleagues and to speak candidly with vendors who attend or exhibit. Lastly, there is a lot of information available on the Internet with varying degrees of reliability. Searching targeted vendor Web sites and/or user groups is often helpful in obtaining baseline information but should be reviewed with an eye toward bias, reliability, and credibility.

It is also recommended to conduct a formal literature review. As health information technology continues to evolve there is an ever-increasing body of knowledge in the formal, peer reviewed literature. While the literature may not have vendor-specific information, it may provide some insight into solutions and anticipated benefits.

A team considering a new acute care Electronic Health Record (EHR), for example, may search the formal literature on Computerized Prescriber Order Entry (CPOE). This research will provide a sound basis not only for the selection but for the identification of key benefits of the new technology.

This review may also alert the selection team to potential unintended consequences of new technology. Together these documented benefits and unintended consequences help inform the understanding of the market and the solution being considered.

For a fee, industry and market research firms offer another way to gain information about vendors and their solutions. Several examples of industry resources are provided in Table 20.1.

As the team begins to understand the market they will find that the vendors in the health information technology market differentiate themselves across several dimensions. Among others, there are business, technical, and solution differentiators that should be considered as part of the Define phase of a vendor assessment.

Business Differentiators

Privately held vs. Public companies: Some health IT vendors are privately held businesses and in some cases wholly owned by the founders. These types of organizations typically make decisions about their business and their solutions based on the company's internal management and leadership. Other vendors in the health IT market are publically traded organizations who ultimately report to external shareholders. Decisions in these organizations are often highly focused around quarterly earnings targets.

Software vs. Services vs. Hardware: There are vendors who function purely as software developers. That is, they develop software solutions but are not as interested in generating revenue from other solution components such as hardware or services. Services vendors, on the other hand, are focused on providing management consulting, staff augmentation, or other high demand skills and expertise and do not usually develop software product. Hardware vendors generate revenue primarily from the sale and support of the hardware component of a solution offering and often partner with other firms for software or services.

It should be noted that these business differentiators are dynamic and can change as a vendor's business evolves. It is also true that a single vendor may differentiate across multiple dimensions. There are software vendors, for example, who also offer services and hardware. Just as there are hardware vendors who market, sell, and support software applications. During a vendor analysis, it is important to understand the potential vendors' primary business differentiators and motivators so that an informed decision can be made.

Industry focus: Another important business differentiator to consider is industry alignment. There are vendors who focus 100% on the healthcare marketplace and others who include industries outside of healthcare in their portfolio. There are pros and cons for each. A healthcare focus offers assurance that a vendor appreciates the unique challenges the healthcare industry faces. On the other hand, the diversity of a company that serves multiple industries could offer innovative solutions to bring forward into healthcare.

Understanding which industries the vendors focus on by asking probing questions and looking at their market penetration and research and development investments can provide insightful information about the organization's past as well as its long-term commitment to providing innovative solutions to the healthcare industry.

Technical Differentiators. There are multiple categories of technical differentiators to consider. Some of these include

TABLE 20.1	Health IT Market Resources	
Resource	**Description**	**URL**
KLAS	Vendor performance data based on customer feedback	http://www.klasresearch.com/
Gartner	Industry research firm	http://www.gartner.com
Forrester	Industry research firm	http://www.forrester.com
HIMSS Analytics	Industry research firm	http://www.himssanalytics.org
U.S. Department of Health and Human Services	Certified Health IT product list	http://www.healthit.gov

those related to the development of software products, product-line growth strategies, or the solution delivery mechanisms the vendor supports.

Development Model: When evaluating vendors it is necessary to understand the underlying solution development model that is used. The development model for software vendors, for example, may involve open source software (OSS) or a proprietary, vendor-controlled approach. For more information on OSS, please refer to Chap. 5. While there is no right or wrong answer for one development model over another it is important to understand the vendors' approach to development and to recognize how that approach is or is not aligned with the organization's current and future IT strategy.

Product Line Growth: A vendor's overall strategy to building its product line is another technical differentiator to consider. Some vendors develop all of their solutions internally while other rapidly acquire technologies from others sources and essentially act as a system integrator. Understanding the technical architecture on which the solution is built as well as the history of all solution components can provide valuable information to the team considering a vendor's solution.

Solution Delivery: Today there are many options for the delivery of technical solutions to organizations. Software solutions and electronic health records, for example, may reside on computers or servers on the physical premises or they may be hosted remotely. In addition, many solutions are now being offered by application service providers (ASP) via the Internet through such mechanisms as Software-as-a-service (SaaS). The team evaluating vendors will need to consider the delivery mode that makes the most sense for the organizations. It is not unusual for vendors to offer multiple delivery options and all should be considered by the team as appropriate.

Solution Differentiators. Solution differentiators are those characteristics of the vendors' products that distinguish them from competitors. These differentiators include the market segments served, product evolution, integration, functionality, and future product development plans.

Market segments served: While many vendors claim to offer a "comprehensive" portfolio of solutions most serve relatively small market segments and have a narrow product line. In healthcare, some

vendors, for example, may provide solutions for the ambulatory market while others focus exclusively on the needs of the acute, inpatient setting. Further narrowing can be seen with what is typically referred to as "niche" vendors who service a very specific need. Peri-operative, Maternal Child Health, Behavioral Health, Radiation oncology, Emergency services are all examples of environments where niche vendors offer solutions.

With the continued consolidation within the industry and the movement toward new models of care delivery, it is important to consider current and future business and clinical needs when analyzing vendors. An organization that operates as an acute care facility today may find that its future includes becoming part of an Accountable Care Organization (ACO) model, for example, where environments such as post-acute, long term, rehabilitation, and others will need to be considered.

Product evolution: Understanding the historical perspective of a vendor's product is an essential element of a comprehensive vendor analysis. One Electronic Health Record vendor, for example, may have established roots by developing inpatient clinical solutions while another may have started out as a vendor focused on radiology systems. Understanding this historical perspective is important in developing an appreciation of the vendor's core competencies and a better understanding of how the solution has evolved over time.

Integration: While some vendors claim to offer an "integrated" solution what they really provide is a franchise model where they purchase or acquire various legacy applications and attempt to integrate them and sell them as a single solution offering. (See "Technical Differentiators" above.) It is vitally important to track each product or application back to its genesis to understand more fully whether a solution was developed as part of a single, integrated platform or is a patchwork of interfaced legacy systems.

Functionality: All solutions that enter a commercial market go through a maturity cycle. In the beginning, there are wide differences in the features and functions and a limited number of vendors offering the solution. Over time, however, as the product matures and more vendors enter the market, competition creates a leveling of functional differentiators.

An assessment of the now mature electronic health record market in the United States would show that the vendors who have led the market all have products that are similar in their features and functions but differentiate on other elements. This Darwin-like survival of the fittest phenomenon is one of the key benefits of having a competitive, commercial market for solutions.

Nonetheless, functionality is a key element of any Vendor Assessment. Functional requirements will be explored in more detail in the "Develop Functional and Technical Requirements" section that follows.

Future Product Development plans: One of the most important differentiators to understand about a vendor is where they are headed with their product line. In many cases, the partnership with vendors can last years or decades. As such, it is important to develop a sense of where the vendor plans to focus development efforts in the next 5 to 10 years. As mentioned previously in the Strategy phase, alignment of the vendors' strategy with an organization's strategic plan is an important step in assessing a vendor's compatibility to partner with an organization over the long term. This is especially true with understanding the vendors' short- and long-term product development plans.

2. Develop Functional and Technical Requirements.

Requirements definition is a very important step in the Vendor Assessment methodology. Requirements can serve multiple purposes. First of all, they help define current state workflows requirements. They also help organize the desired future state features and functions. Often referred to as the "wish list," future state requirements provide an opportunity for the Vendor Assessment team to see if a vendor's solution can support the desired future state environment.

Requirements may also serve a purpose during the contract negotiations phase. Gaps in functionality, for example, may inform any custom modifications that may be contractually obligated. In addition, some institutions may contractually bind the vendor's response to requirements.

As discussed, solution requirements can be divided into functional and technical capabilities. Functional requirements refer to those features and functions that support workflow of end users. Examples of functional requirements in a healthcare software application might include: "Ability to log onto the system," "Ability to register a patient," "Ability to enter an order," "Ability to generate a claim," etc. The U.S. federal government offers a host of templates, best practices, and examples of functional and technical requirements and many other great resources in

the "How to implement EHR's" section of the HealthIT. gov Web site. See Step 3: Select or upgrade to a certified EHR (HealthIT.gov: Step 3 Select or Upgrade Certified EHR, March, 2014; AHRQ, n.d.).

Technical requirements focus less on workflow and more on technical capabilities within the solution. These might include "Ability to interface to Laboratory system," "Supports Window Active Directory," "Ability to send and/or receive HL7 messages," "Complies with HIPAA Technical Security standards," etc.

Requirements can be very specific and detailed or they can be high level. When the team develops requirements consideration is generally given to the current state as well as the potential or desired future state workflow.

A Key Guiding Principle that applies to requirements development is to "Think Process; Not Department." While this principle, like all others, can be applied throughout the Vendor Assessment Methodology, it is particularly important for requirements development.

> **GUIDING PRINCIPLE #3**—Think Process; Not Department

As such, functional requirements should be developed from a process perspective and not a departmental or silo perspective. It is important, for example, when developing requirements for medication administration to consider the implications from the patients' perspective as well as the physicians' (ordering), pharmacists' (verification and dispense), and nurses' (administration and evaluation) perspectives. Approaching requirements from a single discipline, a single department or one step of the workflow would only partially define what is needed.

Nursing represents the largest segment of the healthcare workforce. In the United States, it is estimated that there are 3.1 million Registered Nurses (Nursing by the numbers fact sheet, 2013). Table 20.2 highlights some sample requirements organized around the Nursing Process. Again, it is important to consider the process and not the department or in this case the nursing perspective alone. Assessment requirements, for example, may lead to an impact for nutrition, respiratory, or rehabilitation services. Keeping this broader, process-focused perspective will ensure that functional requirements are comprehensive (see Table 20.2).

Technical requirements can be complex. Requirements in this section generally pertain to the technical aspects that your system must fulfill, such as performance-related issues, system reliability, and availability issues. This

TABLE 20.2	Sample Functional Requirements
Nursing Process	**Sample Functional Requirement**
Assessment	Ability to capture admission assessment data
	Supports Braden Skin Scale Assessment
Diagnosis	User can enter and modify Nursing Diagnoses
	System supports multiple Nursing terminologies
Plan	Supports Nursing and inter-professional plans of care
	Capture user-defined outcomes
Implement	Nursing work lists generated by system
	System displays status of all tasks
Evaluate	Supports analytics related to nursing sensitive quality
	Ad hoc reporting capabilities

TABLE 20.3	Sample Technical Requirements
Hardware	Describe the hardware support model
Implementation	Will the system be available 99.99% of the time for any 24-hour period?
Regulatory Compliance	Is the system Meaningful Use certified?
Report Writing	Is the report writer native to the core application?
Interfaces	Do you support HL7?
Technical Security	System supports alphanumeric passwords?
Backups and Downtime	Can a single record be recovered?
Support	Do you offer 24 × 7 × 365 technical support?

section may include multiple categories of questions that may or may not be able to fit into the structured response (see above) requirement. It is important to develop these requirements in collaboration with subject matter experts from the organization who understand the requirements (Agile Modeling, n.d.).

Sample Technical Requirements (Table 20.3)

Structured Responses. It is important to structure the response to functional and technical requirements where possible to alleviate ambiguity and facilitate requirements analysis. Best practice is to phrase requirements such that they can be answered in a Yes/No response format. This can be difficult for some requirements but will provide for a more effective response analysis.

Soliciting a Yes/No response is not as simple as it may seem. Recognizing that they are being scored and competition exists, vendors will want to respond to requirements with a "Yes" response. This may introduce some ambiguity, however, and responses should be structured to add clarity.

To help alleviate concerns about this ambiguity, vendors should be instructed to respond more accurately through a structured response approach. This may look like those described in Table 20.4.

The scope of the Vendor Assessment project will determine the work effort involved in developing requirements. A focused assessment of a Laboratory solution, for example, would involve a narrower set of requirement than a full Electronic Health Record and Revenue Cycle evaluation.

It may be helpful to start with a pre-defined list of requirements and validate those against your existing workflows. Colleagues who have been through similar efforts may be able to provide sample requirements. An organization may also gather requirements from an external source. The Health Resources and Services Administration (HRSA), for example, offers a number of resources to consider including Electronic Health Record system requirements (HRSA, n.d.). In large-scale efforts it is not unusual to seek out the services of a consulting partner to help manage some of the key steps of a Vendor Assessment. Consultants often have libraries of requirements that they can leverage as part of their work. Regardless of the source of the requirements, it is always recommended to validate these with the operational areas. This not only ensures the

TABLE 20.4	Sample Structured Response Definitions
Response	**Description**
YC	Yes, Current release fulfills
YF	Yes, Future release fulfills (note version # and release mm/yy)
NM	Not standard, custom Modification available if agreed upon by vendor
ND	Not standard, requires further Discussion
NN	Not standard, custom modification Not available
OI	Other third-party software, supports via Interface
ON	Other third-party software, No interface

requirements are correct but it can be an important step in the user engagement process as well.

3. Develop and Submit RFI/RFP. A Request for Information (RFI) is generally used to gather initial information about a vendor and solution offerings and may be used to qualify certain vendors to participate in further analysis. The RFI is often used as a precursor or in conjunction with more formal requests such as a Request for Proposal (RFP), Request for Tender (RFT), or Request for Quotation (RFQ). RFQ is used oftentimes by the government when the product is approved for purchase, but the local authority must spend the money to purchase and install the software. An RFT, on the other hand, is usually an open invitation for suppliers to respond to a *defined* need as opposed to a request being sent to selected potential suppliers.

An RFP is a generally considered a more formal document of solicitation made, often through a formal and structured bidding process. An RFP may be issued by an agency or company interested in procurement of a product, service, or other valuable asset. In the case of a federal or state agency the RFP may be posted to a procurement Web site.

The use of an RFI or an RFP offers several benefits. An RFI/RFP:

a. Informs vendors that an organization is looking to purchase products and/or services and encourages them to participate

b. Requires the organization to specify what it proposes to purchase. If the Requirements Analysis has been prepared properly, it can be incorporated quite easily into the Request document (see below).

c. Alerts vendors that the selection process is competitive

d. Allows for wide distribution and response

e. Ensures that suppliers respond factually to the identified requirements

f. Follows a structured evaluation and selection procedure, so that an organization can demonstrate impartiality—a crucial factor in public and private sector procurements

g. May be used as part of future contract negotiations

Table 20.5 shows a sample RFI/RFP outline.

C. Identify

During the Identify stage each vendor's eligibility for further participation is determined and the vendor finalists are identified. While the RFI/RFP may have been sent to a large number of vendors the goal is to limit the field to three to five qualified vendors for the upcoming and more resource intense Evaluation phase. A review of the RFI/RFP responses is conducted and inclusion criteria are established.

TABLE 20.5	Sample RFI/RFP Outline	
	Section	**Description**
1	Executive Overview	A high level summary of the request
2	Organizational Background	Vital statistics and rationale for selection
3	Response	Instructions for the vendors to follow
4	Evaluation Criteria	Describes what the vendors will be evaluated on
5	Vendor Response	This section explains to the vendor how to respond
	Executive Summary	Response to executive-level questions
	General Information	Response to background information on the vendor
	Application Functions/ Features	Response to functional requirements (one for each functional area in scope with structured responses)
	Technical Requirements	Response to technical requirements (may be several pages and may not be in Yes/No or free text format)
	System Implementation	Provide timelines and resources for deployment
	System Documentation	Provide supporting documentation
	Other	Additional information the vendor would like to provide
	Costs	Response to detailed system cost information (usually provided in a structured format)
6.	Attachments	Templates for the vendor to use or additional information

Quantitative and qualitative analyses are conducted on the RFI/RFP responses, including the functional and technical requirements.

Eliminating vendors from the process can be difficult but should be conducted with transparency and open communication. Once the decision to eliminate a vendor has been made, the vendor should be notified verbally and through a formal written response. Vendors may be holding resources in preparation for demonstrations and should have the opportunity to re-deploy those resources should they not be invited to demonstrate their solution.

D. Evaluate

During the Evaluation phase, the remaining field of vendors and solutions are looked at more closely. During this phase vendor demonstrations, site visits, and reference calls may occur to further inform the team and identify the vendor of choice.

1. Demonstrations. Conducting demonstrations is a significant investment in time and resources for the organizations and vendors. When conducting demonstrations, it is important to strike a balance between the organizations' need to objectively evaluate each vendor and the vendors' desire to show the best features of their product. All of this needs to be considered in the context of time and resource availability as well as competing priorities for both the organization and the vendor.

It is recommended to establish demonstration dates very early in the process; even before final vendors are known. Depending on the size of the effort and resources demonstration dates should be set, rooms reserved, and communication to hold the dates delivered to vendors in the RFI/RFP.

It is important that the demonstrations are fair for all participants. Where possible the same or similar facility should be used at the same time of day for the same duration and with a consistent list of participants. This level of rigor is required to provide an "apples to apples" comparison of demonstration results.

Scripts or scenarios developed by the organization are often used to help guide the demonstration and to capture quantitative and qualitative data for evaluation. Having process-oriented scripts that highlight key system requirements provides an opportunity to see how the system is used to achieve organizational goals. Scripts for clinical systems should be oriented around the patient experience and care delivery. It is a common mistake to overengineer the script which makes it challenging for the vendor to demonstrate to an overly prescriptive process and hard for participants to evaluate.

Rather high-level scripts can be developed that guide the vendor, allow for some flexibility, and provide a mechanism to capture quantitative and qualitative data. The U.S. government's HealthIT.gov Web site offers sample demonstration scripts (Health IT.gov: EHR Demonstration Scenario, Evaluation and Vendor Questions, January, 2013).

2. Site Visits. Site visits are generally conducted with a limited number of organizations due to the commitment of time and expense for both the host facility and the organization considering the solution. It is important for site visits to be planned in advance with specific goals and objectives identified. Site visits are time limited and vary in duration based on the extent of the solution being considered. Vendor participation in site visits varies as does the number of participants. In general, it is better to keep the group small but also important to be inclusive with good representation from key stakeholders. The primary objective is to see the solution deployed in an operational environment and to hear direct and candid feedback from the host facility.

Typically, a site visit agenda will include the following:

a. Introduction and Overview

b. Solution Discussion

c. Facility Tour

d. Questions and Answers

The introduction and overview is intended to introduce the host site and visitors to each other and to reiterate the goals and objectives of the visit. A solution discussion typically follows which describes the host organization's experience with the solution from the beginning. This discussion should include the issues the organization was looking to resolve, the decision process used to identify the selected vendor, the implementation of the solution, the relationship with the vendor, and whether or not expected benefits have been achieved. The mix and number of participants is governed in a large part by the scope of the solution being considered. Key stakeholders should be well represented. It is recommended for the participants to debrief immediately following the site visit and not wait for the return home. Debriefing together and documenting observations immediately ensure that the team accurately captures their thoughts. Observations related to the workflow integration as well as general observations about the host facility are important to document. When multiple site visits occur and time passes it can be difficult to remember details from facility to facility.

3. Reference Calls. Reference calls should be conducted in order to appreciate the perspective of customers who have successfully implemented the vendor solution. When requesting references, it is important to find organizations that are as similar as possible so that a comparison can be completed. It is recommended that at least three (3) reference calls are conducted. References are completed with those organizations that the vendor has provided as a qualified reference. A reference call questionnaire should be developed so that the same questions are captured for each reference.

4. Due Diligence. Due diligence refers to a process of further and deeper investigation of a company prior to contract signing. Much of the information required to support due diligence should have been requested in the RFI/RFP. In some instances, it may be necessary to engage a third party to conduct due diligence and to more thoroughly investigate the financial status of a potential vendor partner.

The quantitative and qualitative data collected throughout the process are used to support and inform the vendor of choice decision. As with most major decisions, however, there is a need to do a "gut check." If despite the data collected the vendor does not "feel" like the right partner during the selection and pass the teams gut check it is unlikely that they will meet the organizations' needs once a contract is signed. While the data are helpful in the end, the instincts of the team and leaders involved in the process are the most valid indicator of future success.

> **GUIDING PRINCIPLE #4**—Use the Data; Trust your Gut

A major deliverable of the Evaluation phase is the Summary Analysis. The Summary Analysis brings together data from all parts of the methodology in a clear and concise format that is ready for executive review. A sample Summary Analysis appears in Fig. 20.3.

E. Partner

In a well-structured vendor selection process, the winner or "Vendor of Choice" often emerges as the clear answer.

In the past, some organizations elected to enter into contract negotiations with multiple potential solution providers in order to increase leverage and provide for a more competitive bidding environment. In practice, however, this strategy seldom achieves the intended results and more often creates unnecessary tension between the organization and its potential future business partner.

> **GUIDING PRINCIPLE #5**—Make a Commitment

As in any relationship, once a partner is identified it is important for both parties to make a commitment to each other's success. Contract negotiations may begin as soon as the preferred vendor is identified. At this stage, it is common for organizations to include legal representatives who are familiar with health information technology contracts as part of the team.

In some cases, early planning activities will occur in parallel with contract negotiations. Data gathered throughout the analysis may be used to inform planning and contract discussions. Some organizations, for example, may include the vendor's response in the requirements as part of the contract in order to hold the vendor accountable for their answers.

Stakeholder communication is vital throughout the life cycle of a vendor selection. Oftentimes the team will be expected to provide a summary of the analysis and current status. The audience for these presentations can range all the way from front-line staff to the organization's board of directors or creditors. Effective communication and presentation skills are essential. The team should anticipate questions and be prepared to respond with short notice to any and all stakeholders. A well-thought-out communication plan during the selection effort will set the stage for ongoing communication during the planning and implementation phases.

SUMMARY AND BEST PRACTICES

In conclusion, it is immense responsibility to lead or participate in the selection of a new vendor partner for an organization. Following a data-driven and evidence-based Vendor Assessment Methodology provides the opportunity for a thoughtful and objective analysis of the vendor marketplace.

The Key Steps of the Vendor Assessment Methodology are:

A. Strategy

B. Define

C. Identify

D. Evaluate

E. Partner

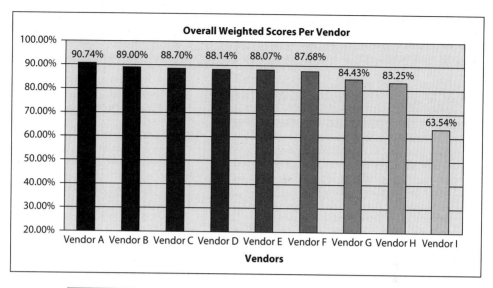

Overall Weighted Scores Per Vendor

90.74% 89.00% 88.70% 88.14% 88.07% 87.68% 84.43% 83.25% 63.54%

(Vendor A, Vendor B, Vendor C, Vendor D, Vendor E, Vendor F, Vendor G, Vendor H, Vendor I)

Vendors

		Vendor A	Vendor B	Vendor C	Vendor D	Vendor E	Vendor F	Vendor G	Vendor H	Vendor I
1)	Live POE solution	✓	✓	β	✓	β	✓	β	✓	β
2)	Live Pharmacy solution	✓	✓	✓	β	✓	✓	✓	✓	NP
3) a.	POE Software License Cost	$15,172,299	$23,866,807	$19,780,000	$16,025,000	$4,424,000	$9,229,000	$5,850,000	$9,503,000	$10,658,000
b.	Pharmacy Software License Cost	I	I	N/A	$1,433,900	$980,000	$3,902,250	$1,604,000	I	NP
c.	Total Proposed Start-up Cost	$18,449,745	$25,054,748	$34,439,268	$25,771,424	$10,600,000	$44,973,980	$24,117,936	$110,568,870	$72,000,000
4)	POE Key Functional Requirements									
iv.a.1.f	Ability to enter orders via PDA	F	F	N	F	✓	N	F	N	N
v.a.2.f	Dose Calculator based on documented patient weight	✓	✓	F	✓	✓	N	✓	✓	✓
v.a.2.r	Supports Adult TPN ordering with templates	✓	✓	F	F	✓	N	✓	N	✓
v1.1.n	Flag orders entered remotely	✓	✓	N	✓	N	N	✓	✓	N
vii.1.d	Require countersignature based on intervention	✓	✓	✓	N	✓	N	✓	✓	✓
vii.5.l	Escalation Rule	✓	✓	F	N	N	N	✓	N	✓
ix.a.l	Ability to modify drug database	✓	✓	N	✓	✓	N	✓	✓	✓
5)	Largest Relative Bedsize >500	✓	✓	✓				✓	✓	
6)	Pharmacy system is stand-alone			✓	β	✓	✓	✓		

Legend

✓	Operational
β	Beta
NP	No Product/System
I	Included in POE cost
F	Future: Available prior to Q4 2003
N	Not Available or Future without date

• **FIGURE 20.3.** Sample Summary Analysis.

Remember to consider and apply the Key Guiding Principles throughout the lifecycle of the Vendor Assessment:

1. Manage the Change; Communicate
2. Maintain and Document Objectivity
3. Think Process; Not Department
4. Use the Data; Trust your Gut
5. Make a Commitment

REFERENCES

Agile Modeling (n.d.). Technical (non-functional) requirements: An agile introduction. Retrieved from http://www.agilemodeling.com/artifacts/technicalRequirement.htm

AHRQ (n.d.). Application and system development requirements. Retrieved from http://www.ahrq.gov/research/publications/pubcomguide/pcguide2apa.html

Certificate of need: State health laws and programs. (2013). Retrieved from http://www.ncsl.org/research/health/con-certificate-of-need-state-laws.aspx

HealthIT.gov (January, 2013). *EHR demonstration scenario, evaluation and vendor questions.* Retrieved from http://www.healthit.gov/providers-professionals/implementation-resources/ehr-demonstration-scenario-evaluation-and-vendor

HealthIT.gov (March, 2014). *Step 3: Select or upgrade certified EHR.* Retrieved from http://www.healthit.gov/providers-professionals/ehr-implementation-steps/step-3-select-or-upgrade-certified-ehr

HealthIT.gov (March 20, 2014). *EHR implementation steps.* Retrieved from http://www.healthit.gov/providers-professionals/ehr-implementation-steps/step-1-assess-your-practice-readiness. Accessed November 22, 2014.

HRSA (n.d.). What are the specific functionalities that are needed in an EHR? Retrieved from http://www.hrsa.gov/healthit/toolbox/ruralhealthittoolbox/getting started/ehr.html. Accessed November 22, 2014.

Health Resources and Services Administration. (September 2010). The Registered Nurse Population: Findings From the 2008 National Sample Survey of Registered Nurses. Washington, DC: U.S. Department of Health and Human Services.

Merriam Webster Online Dictionary. (2014) *Independence.* Retrieved from http://www.merriam-webster.com/dictionary/independence

Pedulli, L. (2013). *Report global health IT market to hit $56.7 billion by 2017.* Retrieved from http://www.clinical-innovation.com/topics/clinical-practice/report-global-health-it-market-hit-567-billion-2017

Sugrue, M. (2010). Clinical leaders and the adoption of health IT. *Nursing Management,* 2010 Sep, 18–21.

21

Nurse Scheduling and Credentialing Systems*

Karlene M. Kerfoot / Kathleen Smith

• OBJECTIVES

1. Describe the history of staffing and current scheduling gaps.
2. Identify the requirements for an intelligent integrated workload management system (WMS).
3. Discuss the new era of healthcare reform and the challenge to staffing and credentialing.
4. Identify challenges for nursing informatics in the future.

• KEY WORDS

Accountable care act
Credentialing
Electronic Health Records (EHR)
Patient acuity systems
Predictive analytics
Safe staffing mandates
User centered staffing
Workload Management Systems (WMS)

ABSTRACT

Historically nurse scheduling was a function of assigning personnel on an equitable basis. These tasks were paper and pencil schedules with little accommodation for variation. The number of personnel assigned to a unit was based on historical patient occupancy rates. In the early 1970s, several commercial systems containing a patient acuity system were available for use. As Electronic Health Records developed, new applications for scheduling nurses became available. In addition to the scheduling functions, software began to provide workforce management functions. There has been a demand to provide minimum staffing levels, and some state laws mandate these levels. In today's environment, there is an increasing need to prove value for nursing care and to use nursing skill to provide improved patient outcomes, manage costs of patient care, and ensure that the appropriate nursing skill is provided through credentialing techniques. This chapter will address some of the issues, and provide a call to action to provide integrated evidence-based systems for nursing's use.

*Disclaimer: The views expressed in this chapter are those of the author(s) and do not necessarily reflect the official policy or position of API.

INTRODUCTION

Historically, nursing work commitment was a function of employment (nurses agreed to work required pattern of weekends, and rotating shifts). The function of nurse scheduling was to try and provide an equitable number of nurses for an assigned shift and honor special requests if at all possible. Special requests were pieces of paper (or later sticky notes) handed to the nurse manager or schedule coordinator, and the nursing schedules were completed using paper and pencil. Usually, allowing the staff nurses to self-schedule was too complicated to manage. The nursing supervisor accomplished shift changes in staffing for callouts, overs-taffing, and under-staffing. Oftentimes, temporary agency nurses were utilized to provide required patient care. In many instances, the use of agency personnel doubled the cost of nursing care. In the early 1960s, Connor and others from The Johns Hopkins University begin to describe a nursing workload measurement system. This three-category classification was based on observable physical and emotional care requirements of patients. Based on the classification, an estimate of nursing care time requirements for the patients was assigned within each category. Other significant findings of the Connor study included:

- Nursing workload was based on the number of patients in each category of care
- A wide variety in care requirements varied from day to day on the same ward or unit
- The number of class 3 or intensive patients was the main determinant of nursing workload (Edwardson & Giovanneti, 1994, p. 97)

Nursing Workload, nursing classification, patient acuity, and nursing intensity are among the terms used to differentiate the number of nurses required to provide optimal care to a group of patients. By the 1980s, a number of computerized systems were developed to assist in the measurement of nursing workload. Patient profiles, nursing task documents, and critical indicators of care were used to develop these measurements. Early systems used time and motion measurement studies based on activities of daily living, e.g., how long to bathe, feed, ambulate a patient, etc. Some of the early computerized scheduling and nursing workload systems included GRASP, Medicus, PRN, ANSOS, Van Slyke, and the Navy Workload Management System (BUMED Instruction 5220.4, 1995; Edwardson, & Giovanneti, 1994, p. 99).

THE GAP BETWEEN PRESENT REALITY AND THE NEEDS OF THE NEW HEALTHCARE SYSTEM IN STAFFING

Today, the predominant mode of scheduling and staffing continues to be on paper via spreadsheets and other similar methods. Using this outdated method of staffing means critical employee information is likely kept in many disparate locations and databases. Without database integration, a Workload Management System (WMS) is not possible. An automated WMS should provide at a minimum:

- Licensure information
- Certification skills information such as PALS, ACLS
- Current contact information
- Employee work preferences
- Competency to "float" or work on a variety of units
- Ability to assess and match the competencies of the nurse with the needs of the patient
- Prospective and predictive analytics for effective staffing
- Integrate quality metrics with staff outcomes

Paper-Based Systems

Outdated staffing and scheduling methods also come with a significant financial cost. Without access to information about number of hours worked, scheduling managers risk assigning overtime hours to a nurse who has worked more than 80 hours in a two-week pay period. This can create poor financial outcomes for the organization. Additionally, there is a growing body of evidence that nurse fatigue poses a serious threat to patient safety (Kane, Shamliyan, Mueller, Duval, & Wilt, 2007; Rogers, Hwang, Scott, Aiken, Dinges, 2004). Many states including California, Massachusetts, and New York have implemented safe staffing requirements limiting the number of consecutive hours a nurse can be on duty. Just as it is possible to aggregate and integrate patient data into an Electronic Health Record (EHR) from a variety of data sources, it is possible to aggregate and integrate information into a WMS that can be integrated with scheduling and staffing, human resource, financial, quality, and other systems. Workforce management technology makes it possible to embed alerts and reminders based on data and evidence integrated from many sources that enable organizations to move from making staffing decisions based on pure opinion to decisions based on data and evidence.

Assessing the Needs of the Patient

In this metrics heavy, care quality focused market; the ultimate goal of staffing and scheduling should be to match the needs of the patient with the abilities of the nurse in order to create excellence in clinical outcomes and operational excellence. Staffing by ratios or matrixes does not capture the unique needs of the individual patient. For example, the needs of an 80-year old with pancreatitis differ greatly from that of a 40-year old with the same diagnoses. The 80-year old needs help with ambulation, has a complicated medication regime, and has a risk of falls and pressure ulcers. Without clearly knowing the needs of the patient, staffing systems fail to keep the needs of the patient as the focus is on staffing and scheduling. Now acuity systems can pull information directly from the medical record to calculate hours of care, eliminating the variation between nurses in the manual system. This integrated technology also saves significant time on the scheduling process as a whole.

Assessing and Matching the Competencies of the Nurse

Nurses have varying skills, experience, competency, abilities, and preferences to care for different types of patients. In traditional staffing systems, there often is not much information available about the nurse to effectively match those competencies with the needs of the patient. Expiration dates for licensure, required certifications, and other expiration dates can sometimes be found but are often stored in another system, such as the human resources system, and are not communicated to staffing managers or those responsible for matching patients to caregivers. Likewise, certifications such as chemotherapy, PALS, and ACLS might be found in information stored on the unit or in a learning management system that is also kept separate from, and not communicated to, the staffing system. Without a fully integrated and dynamic system that makes this information available at the point of assignment of the nurse to the patient, the scheduling process happens without the necessary information to make a good assignment. Bad assignments can be detrimental to an organization's bottom line, not just from a safety standpoint, but also from a quality care measurement standpoint. Manually identifying critical employee information stored on separate systems

takes time and can be difficult, making it impossible to accomplish in a timely manner. If efficiency is the goal, scheduling managers, who are often nursing department leaders, should be spending less time on staffing and scheduling and more time on patient care.

Evidence is mounting about the effect nurse fatigue has on patient care. For example, the likelihood of a nurse making an error is three times higher after working a shift lasting more than 12 hours (Rogers et al., 2004). More hours of RN time spent on direct patient care results in shorter length of patient stays and fewer failures to rescue (Kane et al., 2007). For each full-time equivalent (FTE) nurse per patient day, the absolute risk of mortality decreases by 0.25% (Shilling, Campbell, Englesbe, & Davis, 2010).

Intelligent staffing systems track the amount of hours a nurse has worked, and send alerts and stop to prevent scheduling a nurse approaching excessive hours, which will create patient safety problems. Financially, costs can be reduced by systems that alert scheduling managers to prevent unnecessary overtime by scheduling a nurse who if scheduled, will be in overtime to the exclusion of one who is not given similar competencies. These systems can also ensure that equitable assignments are made by balancing the workload of all the people in a unit by using the information from the patient classification system and nurse competencies. It is not uncommon to see new nurses given difficult and heavy assignments while experienced nurses are under-utilized and not assigned to the patients they can care for best. Nurse satisfaction is tightly tied to assignments. Without data about the competencies of the nurse to effectively make equitable and safe assignments, nurses will more than likely become less than satisfied over time. Without question nurses who are unhappy affect patient satisfaction and engagement. Nurse turnover is an expensive item in the budget, with replacement costs amounting to as much as 250% of their salary. It also accounts for major quality issues. Patient assignments are extremely important when the goal is to generate the best quality and financial outcomes and best nurse satisfaction and retention rates.

Prospective/Predictive Analytics

Effective staffing and scheduling depends on information from a variety of sources such as projected admissions, acuity of patients, and expected length of stay. By integrating and analyzing information from the sources of data that affect staffing and scheduling, it is possible to predict staffing needs and create better and more effective processes. The amount of associated staffing information that is collected and stored is very large. With the modern technology that is designed to analyze large data sets, we now have the opportunity to turn that data into predictable and actionable information.

Integrating Quality Metrics With Staffing Outcomes

With the ability to integrate quality data from several sources, and pull it into a staffing system, it is now possible to integrate quality data with the staffing process. Technology allows us to see in advance what kind of nursing care a particular patient needs, based on an assessment pulled from the documentation in the medical record. By integrating all of these data safer, more effective care is provided. In today's market, where quality standards are given equal measure against financial goals, the clinical and financial sides of the business must work together, or long-term sustainability will suffer.

THE NEW ERA OF HEALTHCARE AND THE CHALLENGE OF STAFFING

The multiple influences of quality performance initiatives, performance targets for patient quality, nurse satisfaction, budget/financial controls, and unanticipated events reflect the ever-increasing complexity of the healthcare system now and in the future. The principles and realities of complexity and complex adaptive systems provide an excellent framework upon which to determine strategies and processes in a rapidly advancing digital world. The recognition of the unpredictable nature of scheduling and staffing as normative, and the importance of the multiple relationships among nurses, staffers, and informaticists supporting computerized systems can only enhance the effectiveness of future systems.

Among the top concerns for nursing executives today are patient satisfaction/patient experience, quality of care, patient safety, and controlling costs (HealthLeaders Media, 2011). Advancements in technology have fostered the creation of more robust EHR solutions, which is giving providers more comprehensive, real-time access to information about a patient's healthcare status. This information has vastly improved patient safety, and ultimately yielded more long-term positive patient outcomes.

The pervasive use of EHRs has been accelerated by the passage of the American Reinvestment and Recovery Act (ARRA), in 2009. Commonly known as the "economic stimulus," the ARRA contained provisions under the Health Information Technology for Economic and Clinical Health (HITECH) Act establishing a foundation for every American to benefit from an EHR as part of a modernized, interconnected, and vastly improved system of care delivery (HealthLeaders Media, 2011). Specifically, Title IV, Division B of the HITECH Act establishes incentive payments under the Medicare and Medicaid programs for EPs and EHs that meaningfully use Certified EHR Technology (CEHRT) (HealthLeaders Media, 2011). This incentive provision is directly responsible for the fundamental industry shift to emphasize and measure quality care standards. The HITECH Act of 2009 has created a fundamental shift in priority toward prevention and community, which is supported through the emphasis on quality care goals tied to more positive patient outcomes.

Achieving long-term financial sustainability in this new marketplace will be impossible for organizations tied to outdated and inefficient workforce scheduling, staffing, and assignment systems. There is an acute need to recognize that a transformational workforce is necessary to meet the needs of the next generation of healthcare.

Moving From Volume to Value

For the better part of the last 50 years, the healthcare industry adhered to a simple, easy-to-measure, fee-for-service model. Today, the focus is moving toward a value-based model that relies heavily on metrics tied to high-quality outcomes. Technology such as the EHR can play a significant role in ensuring patients are not only receiving the highest quality care, but the right care and that information can be linked to a WMS. The average portion of a health system's operating budget devoted to human resources or labor is 54.2% (Becker's Hospital Review, n.d.).

From Site Based to the Continuum of Care Focus

Historically, our healthcare system has been organized around a single site of care. Without a way to track a patient's progress before or after that single site visit, certain quality measures, such as care consistency, were very difficult to achieve. Before EHRs, the ability to follow and integrate the care needs of a patient throughout their healthcare journey was difficult at best. Similarly, without a comprehensive workforce management strategy, ensuring consistency of care across the continuum becomes equally as challenging. With both of these components tied directly to patient satisfaction and care quality metrics, it makes perfect business sense to invest in the technology that will enable complete integration of care needs and staffing across a patient's entire journey.

A coordinated workforce plan allows for scheduling across all units, departments and facilities, regardless of location. Without this coordination the risk for patients and organization costs increase.

Implementing solid staffing practices across entire organizations is critical. At the root of every staffing best practice is the need for accurate, timely information about both patients and caregivers. When staffing decisions are backed by solid data and based on actual patient care needs and staffing skill sets, patient outcomes improve and labor costs are controlled. While staffing is a complex, dynamic, and continuous process, using data driving staffing standards and best practices can lead to staffing plans that consistently match the right caregivers with the right patients, no matter where they are on their healthcare journey.

Implementing Coordinated Care Through Intra-Professional Teams Across the Continuum

The traditional model of staffing has been to assign nurses in isolation without consideration of the complete care team made up of hospitalists, intensivists, social workers, care coordinators, Advanced Practice Nurses, physicians, etc. However, there is now evidence to support that staffing and caring for patients in silos is not as effective as an integrated workforce management strategy across the continuum of care. The WMS entails storing, managing, and maintaining all employee information in a single, fully integrated suite of solutions, replacing disparate systems and incomplete information with a more complete organizational workforce management picture.

UTILIZING DATA AND BEST PRACTICES BASED ON EVIDENCE TO CREATE BETTER OUTCOMES

Evidence-driven protocols are now widely accepted as a means of directing the work of the physician and other clinicians. In today's market, it is expected that staffing needs be based on data and evidence. Staffing and patient care needs are deeply entwined with a hospital's bottom line, and accurate, effective nurse staffing and acuity strategies can help health systems reach their patient care and financial goals. By pairing nurse talents, skills, and experience with specific patient needs through acuity-based staffing, hospitals are able to maintain low readmission rates, deliver exceptional patient care, and remain financially successful.

Nurse staffing and scheduling is a complicated process; from analysis of nurse experience and skill sets to availability and budgeting needs, a great deal of work goes into coordinating staffing plans. Acuity-based staffing

models make it possible to evaluate actual patient care needs in order to make data-driven decisions.

Nurse workload, shift turnover, and inefficient patient matching can directly impact patient care in hospitals. Researchers examined data from 197,961 admissions and 176,696 nursing shifts at an academic medical center and found patient mortality increased as unit shift hours rose and nurse staffing levels dropped (Buerhaus et al., 2011). It has been found that patient deaths cost hospitals approximately $20 billion every year (AHRQ, 2009).

According to a 2013 study in Health Affairs, staffing is the single most significant factor in reducing readmissions. Health systems with higher nurse employment had a 25% lower chance of receiving penalizations for readmissions through HRRP than those that had lower nurse staffing levels (McHugh, Berez, & Small, 2013). Essentially, the higher nurse workloads are and the less nurse managers and staffing coordinators utilize acuity when assigning shifts, the more at-risk patients are for being readmitted.

Moving to User-Centered Staffing

Nurse burnout, retention, and satisfaction directly affect the hospital's bottom line. Nurses put great stake in being able to treat all of their patients safely, effectively, and compassionately, and they feel the impact physically, emotionally, and mentally when the workload is not balanced. So when nurses are not matched correctly with their patients—either they do not have the necessary qualifications to provide adequate care or have too much work for the number of patients they have to treat—they can quickly become dissatisfied with their jobs.

According to the Agency for Health Research and Quality (AHRQ), the risk of nurse burnout increases by 23% and dissatisfaction by 15% for each additional patient a nurse receives (Furillo & McEwan, 2014). However, when hospitals have accurate staffing, nurse burnout and dissatisfaction can drop significantly. Staff turnover is also costly. Replacing a healthcare employee can cost up to 250% of their salary (Goedert, 2013). Taking into account the rate of nurse turnover, hospitals can lose between $3.74 million and $4.98 million every year (NSI Nursing Solutions, 2013).

Technology that empowers nurses to control their own work/life balance is a critical but important investment for organizations seeking to keep turnover rates low, employee satisfaction rates high, and patient outcomes positive. By placing the decision-making process directly on the employee, through user-centered staffing strategies, organizations create a sense of balance for their most critical group of employees.

Achieving these objectives can be done, but it requires the use of technology to provide data and evidence for decisions. Without an electronic employee record that integrates all the information needed to do effective staffing in an intelligent record, the challenges of this new healthcare market cannot be met. The gap to get there is significant and must be closed immediately.

INTEGRATED WORKFORCE MANAGEMENT SYSTEM REQUIREMENT FOR NURSING

In this new healthcare marketplace, it is a real possibility that caregivers will have the opportunity to work across several venues, especially as more organizations merge and consolidate, creating integrated, complete health systems. For the most part, local and regional staffing pools do a good job of addressing the fluctuating census, however there is still a need for contingent labor, especially as budgets become tighter and internal resources decline. As the patient moves throughout the continuum, it is imperative that their medical records travel with them. It is also equally as imperative that an electronic employee record for caregivers be available so that consistent care can be achieved. Providing exceptional patient care in today's accelerated environment is dependent in large part on the management of staff resources and tremendous amounts of employee-related information. The process includes accessing, tracking, managing, and analyzing labor data on-demand to enhance the decision-making process.

Just as the EHR collects information about the patient from a variety of sources, the WMS does the same for the caregiver. When data from the EHR integrate with information from the WMS, the goal of excellence in staffing and scheduling can be achieved. The electronic employee record streamlines workflows that are used each and every day throughout the health system. That streamlining equates to a more satisfied, cost-effective workforce that is empowered to provide high-quality patient care. Implementing a successful, integrated, and intelligent WMS is contingent on several minimal requirements.

Integration Across the Continuum

Just as an EHR follows the patient through their journey across the healthcare system, the WMS should follow caregivers throughout their tenure with their health system employer. Employee-related information from throughout the enterprise including supplemental and contingent staffing sources can be used to review, identify, manage, and maintain processes more effectively for the entire workforce. This strategy makes it possible to eliminate duplicate data maintenance, manual processes, and

costly interfaces while increasing information accuracy and efficiency. Integrating employee information into a seamless data flow makes it possible to track trends and create forecasts that improve human resource utilization. With this enterprise-wide employee data management strategy, the end result will be heightened efficiency and an improved bottom line. Communication between dispirit systems is critical to evolve the WMS. Techniques used to communicate data between systems include:

- Health Level 7 (HL7) Messaging
- Service-Oriented Architecture (SOA)
- Publish-Subscribe Architecture (Pub-Sub)

Increasing use of data will only increase the need for sharing it among software systems. There are varieties of options to consider when building data sets sourced in different software systems. Nursing Informatics needs to understand both the purpose of the data and the options for making the data available, when and where they are needed to allow for the right, and best, choice to be made when the care for the patient requires it.

Centered on the Needs of Patients

Staffing and scheduling activities should be focused solely on creating a safe and healing healthcare experience for the patient. In order to accomplish this efficiently and effectively, it is critical that we leverage acuity data and match them with competency data from the WMS.

Provides Actionable Information About the Caregiver to Create Safe and Fulfilling Work

Access to employee-related data is important for several reasons. Real-time information regarding active licensure, certifications, and demonstrated competencies are important to ensuring safe, quality patient care. In addition, knowing a nurse's preferences for what type of patient they are best suited to care for can make the difference between a great nurse–patient relationship and a poor one. When this type of information is available for consideration, a better patient match can happen. The history and type of hours worked is also important to monitor potential nurse fatigue, excessive overtime, and fairness of assignments such as requests to float when necessary and equitable assignments. The process of staffing and scheduling must be based on national scope and standards such as the American Nurses Association's *Principles of Nurse Staffing*, 2nd Edition (American Nurses Association, 2012). When considered as a whole, all of these elements equate to a better working experience overall, which leads to improved morale and a more satisfied workforce. When this information is stored in separate systems, without a way to integrate and communicate between them, scheduling managers are at a distinct disadvantage. A dynamic system that brings all of this vital information together, in real time, is the key to workforce optimization.

Integrated With Quality and Financial Measures and Outcomes

With increasing evidence correlating effective staffing with patient outcomes, it is critical that we leverage systems that utilize information to support the idea that staffing assignments should provide better outcomes for patients. When more information is accessible regarding patient care needs and the optimal way to deliver that care, the financial realities of healthcare can be balanced with high-quality patient care.

Financial outcomes can be improved with proactive information about the most efficient way to staff and schedule. Over- and under-staffing can create unwanted financial outcomes, as well as unwanted quality outcomes. Integrated staffing systems that can provide information about the financial cost of a staffing decision in real time are imperative to achieving long-term financial sustainability in a highly competitive marketplace.

With a strong clinical-financial connection, productivity measures are more accurate and include cost-of-shift data. With all of that information available and evaluated before the start of the shift, projected overtime and excessive use of contingent labor can be avoided while patient care needs are met. And, with real-time productivity information, discrepancies between budget and actual staffing numbers and labor costs are explained with clinically based justification and actual patient need data. With this complete, multi-dimensional picture of actual patient care needs and the clinical workforce that will meet those needs, organizations can make solid staffing decisions that optimize patient care and minimize labor costs. Clinical leaders are able to align their goals, delivering patient care that achieves both positive clinical outcomes and a healthier bottom line. Systems that can guide the staffing process based on the evidence will provide the beginning level of intelligence needed for a revised business model that depends heavily on excellence in patient outcomes for reimbursement.

Robust Analytical Capabilities

With multiple sources of data available to supply an integrated WMS, there are many opportunities to integrate that data with proactive suggestive analytics and automatic

retrospective reports that will lead to better quality and financial outcomes. Rather than simply pointing out inefficiencies, technology should provide the information necessary to improve efficiencies. Not only is it expensive to deploy more resources than necessary, it becomes a quality issue if the right resources are not in place, which is why it makes good business sense to leverage technology that aligns financial and clinical goals.

THE CHALLENGES FOR NURSING INFORMATICS IN THE FUTURE

Much of the work of nursing informatics has been associated with the patient Electronic Health Record for very good reason. However, with the advent of additional research on the relationship of staffing to patient outcomes, we must now turn our attention to the nurse/caregiver. Certain elements, such as competencies and preparedness to manage a particular type of patient, can dramatically impact patient outcomes. Technology allows us the ability to develop staffing systems that can gather information from many different data sources and match the needs of the patient with the competencies of the nurse. In the past, staffing has been the under-represented frontier of technology development. In this new quality-driven, highly competitive marketplace, we need to focus our attention on skill development of nurses in informatics in order to achieve operational excellence.

Create Awareness That the Healthcare Worker Is the Keystone for Excellence in Outcomes

Staffing and scheduling is a very complicated process that must synthesize many unrelated variables into a coherent understanding that creates excellence in patient outcomes. Without effective staffing, the elegant work of the EHR becomes wasted. Without the right staff to apply the care requirements dictated by the EHR, the patient will not benefit. Given the breadth of most health systems, and likely its sizeable number of employees on staff, it is impossible to adequately synthesize all the necessary employee qualification information without the aid of holistic, integrated technology. An effective, integrated electronic staffing and scheduling system is achieved when information from the WMS integrates with information contained in the patient's medical record.

Staffing and scheduling is a body of knowledge not readily available to the clinical nurse and to nursing informatics practitioners who do not have the background in management. Learning staffing operations is usually an "on-the-job" training experience, and does not include access to the operational literature and available evidence that supports excellence in outcomes. Without that knowledge, it is difficult for the nursing informaticist to understand and advocate for integrated electronic staffing systems that include an electronic employee record.

Elevate the Needs of the Caregiver to Ensure Support for the Individual as a Professional Whole

Collectively all of the information in the WMS is necessary to provide the best staffing. However, in addition to supporting the pursuit of quality patient outcomes, there must also be support for the caregiver. There is increasing evidence available about the impact of nurse fatigue, post-traumatic syndrome, compassion fatigue, and burnout. For example, it is normal for a nurse to feel grief when a patient dies. However, if the nurse is not supported emotionally, the ability to work through the grief will be hampered. In addition, nurses who make mistakes due to nurse fatigue from over-scheduling often face guilt over their error. In reality, the root cause for the error was failure to schedule based on the evidence. Had an electronic employee record been utilized, it would have predicted this kind of untoward outcome. To support efforts for making the WMS ubiquitous, it helps point out that an integrated and holistic staffing and scheduling solution that includes a WMS can send out alerts, reminders, and hard stops to ensure that nurses work in a healthy environment rather than a toxic one that brings harm to patients, and ultimately the organization.

Expand the Focus of Nursing Informatics to Include the Electronic Health Record and Develop Workforce Systems That Are Robust and Real Time

WMS continue to grow and evolve. The challenge today is that we are finding that while we have the critical employee data, are stored across many disparate databases that are not integrated with each other. Thanks to what we know about the technology that runs the EHR, we can develop an intelligent staffing and scheduling system that leverages multiple databases of critical employee information to ensure the most effective staffing assignments. The implication is that schools of nursing and Informatics departments in healthcare organizations must accept the challenge to do for our workforce what we have done for the patient: use technology to ensure optimal outcomes.

As we consider the role technology plays in how we learn to care for patients from a clinical standpoint, it is equally important that we consider the role technology plays in learning about the characteristics of nurses. In today's business climate, these two elements are inextricably linked. An understanding of the nurse–patient relationship needs to be part of the knowledge base of nursing informatics if we are also going to understand the clinical knowledge associated with patient care.

SUMMARY

We are poised on the edge of incorporating the evidence, data, and information about the nurse/caregiver into healthcare in the same manner that we have done with the EHR. With the advent of the WMS for caregivers, the opportunity to match the needs of the patients with the competencies of the nurse is possible within a data/evidence-driven system. Within an intelligent electronic staffing and scheduling system that integrates information about the patient from the EHR with information about the nurse/caregiver in the WMS, it is now possible to balance the workload of the nurse and match the needs of the patients with the nurse/caregiver. In addition, the opportunity to retrospectively evaluate staffing through analysis of the large data sets that the process of staffing generates to improve quality and financial outcomes is vast. The goal of developing predictive models to more accurately predict patient census, acuity and matching that data with the availability and competency of the nursing/caregiver staff is enormous. We are now on the edge of effectively developing and utilizing technology that can provide information to optimize the integration of the nurse with the patient effectively.

Additional Contributors:
Richard Robinson, BA, BS, BSN, Kathy Malloch, PhD, MBA, RN, FAAN

Lisa LaBau

REFERENCES

AHRQ. (2009). *Patient deaths in hospitals cost nearly $20 billion*. Retrieved from http:// archive.ahrq.gov/ news/newsroom/news-and-numbers/110409.html. Accessed on December 31, 2013.

American Nurses Association. (2012). *ANA's principles for nurse staffing* (2nd ed.). Silver Springs, MD: Nursesbooks.org.

Becker's Hospital Review (n.d.). Retrieved from www. beckershospitalreview.com/racs-/-icd-9-/10/10-statistics-on-hospital-labor-costs-as-a-percentage-of-operating-revenue.html

Buerhaus, P., Harris, M., Leibson, C., Needleman, J., Pankratz, S., & Stevens, M. S. (2011). Nurse staffing and inpatient hospital mortality. *The New England Journal of*

Medicine: March 17, 2011. Retrieved from http://www.nejm.org/doi/full/10.1056/NEJMsa1001025. Accessed on January 2, 2014.

BUMED Instruction 5220.4. (1995). Retrieved from http://www.med.navy.mil/directives/externaldirectives/5220.4.pdf

Edwardson, S. R., & Giovanneti, P. B. (1994). Nursing workload measurement systems. *Annual Review of Nursing Research. 12.* Springer Publishing Co. Retrieved from http://books.google.com/books?id=9YLKNIXuhg4C&pg=PA122&dq=grasp+nursing+workload+management+system&hl=en&sa=X&ei=KOsqU_eIBa_I2wX2oIGwDw&ved=0CG4Q6AEwCQ#v=onepage&q=grasp%20nursing%20workload%20management%20system&f=false

Furillo, J., & McEwan, D. (2014). State-mandated nurse staffing levels alleviate workloads, leading to lower patient mortality and higher nurse satisfaction *AHRQ.* Retrieved from http://www.innovations.ahrq.gov/content.aspx?id=3708

Goedert, J. (2013). Keeping your best employees when others want them. *Health Data Management.* Retrieved from http://www.healthdatamanagement.com/news/HIMSS13-retaining-top-HIT-talent-45651-1.html?zkPrintable=truHealthLeaders. Media 2011 industry

survey, nurse leaders. Retrieved from http://www.healthleadersmedia.com/industry_survey/

Kane, R. L., Shamliyan, T., Mueller, C., Duval, S., & Wilt, T. J. (2007, March). Nurse staffing and the quality of patient care. *AHRQ.* www.ahrq.gov. Publication No. 07-E005.

McHugh, M. D., Berez, J., & Small, D. S. (2013, October). Hospitals with higher nurse staffing had lower odds of readmissions penalties than hospitals with lower staffing. *Health Aff (Millwood).* 32(10), 1740–1747. doi:10.1377/hlthaff.2013.0613. Retrieved from http://www.ncbi.nlm.nih.gov/pubmed/24101063

NSI Nursing Solutions. (2013). *2013 National Healthcare & RN Retention Report.* Retrieved from http://www.nsinursingsolutions.com/Files/assets/library/retention-institute/NationalHealthcareRNRetentionReport2013.pdf

Rogers, A. E., Hwang, W. T., Scott, L. D., Aiken, L. H., & Dinges, D. F. (2004, July/August). The working hours of hospital staff nurses and patient safety. *Health Affairs.* 202–212.

Shilling, P. L., Campbell, D. A., Englesbe, M. J., & Davis, M. M. (2010). A comparison of in-hospital mortality risk conferred by high hospital occupancy, differences in nurse staffing levels, weekend admission, and seasonal influenza. *Medical Care, 48*(3), 224–232.

22

Informatics and the Healthcare Industry

Amy J. Barton

This chapter highlights the transformations in healthcare and education within the context of advances in computing and communications technologies. The goals of this chapter are twofold: to explore how eHealth innovations will transform healthcare, education, and research and to present the challenges and issues as a result of these potential transformations. The chapter covers the progression of eHealth applications; eHealth and other associated concepts; future innovations in advanced practice, education, and research; and the challenges and issues arising as a consequence of these transformations.

HISTORICAL CONTEXT OF eHEALTH

The rudimentary roots of telemedicine extend back to ancient times where simple forms of distance communication, such as the use of light reflections and smoke signals, were used to relay messages about external threats, famines, and disease. Long-distance communication evolved from these modest beginnings to systems such as the telegraph, radio, and onward to advanced digital communication and communication systems (Bashshur & Shannon, 2009).

Telehealth applications have evolved from simple communications to sophisticated, pervasive, and widespread systems in the home that make use of wireless, wearable, robotic, and multi-sensorial technologies. In the past, trends in telehealth applications were grouped according to the various media: voice, data, and video. But with the convergence of these technologies, newer technologies merge across these media. Despite these newer technologies, voice applications remain a mainstay of telehealth applications. The tools of telemedicine offer effective and efficient solutions for remote monitoring of the chronically ill, as well as an avenue to allow for diagnosis and treatment of individuals who have no access to healthcare because of geographic limitations (Bashshur & Shannon, 2009).

THE CONCEPT OF eHEALTH

eHealth is an emerging field of medical informatics, referring to the organization and delivery of health services and information using the Web and related technologies. In a broader sense, the term characterizes not only technical development, but also a new way of working, an attitude, and a commitment for networked, global thinking to improve healthcare locally, regionally, and worldwide by using information and communication technology. eHealth represents optimism, allowing patients and professionals to do what was previously impossible (Eysenbach, 2001; Oh, Rizo, Enkin, & Jadad, 2005; Pagliari et al., 2005).

eHealth technologies provide opportunities for customized and meaningful communication, enabling patients to receive individually tailored information that can be viewed and responded to at their convenience. Patients can also post their comments and advice to virtual communities (Neuhauser & Kreps, 2010). The World Health Organization (2012) identified that "technological advances, economic investment, and social and cultural changes are also contributing to the realization that the health sector must now integrate technology into its way of doing business" (p. 1).

eHealth can empower consumers and patients, and it opens doors for new types of relationships, such as shared decision-making between a patient and his/her healthcare provider. "e-Health is the single-most important revolution in healthcare since the advent of modern medicine, vaccines, or even public health measures like sanitation and clean water" (Silber, 2003, p. 7).

The Concept of Telehealth

The American Telemedicine Association (ATA) uses the terms *telemedicine* and *telehealth* interchangeably. "Telemedicine is the use of information exchanged from one site to another via electronic communications to improve patients' health status. Closely associated with telemedicine is the term *telehealth*, which is often used to encompass a broader definition of remote healthcare that does not always involve clinical services" (ATA, 2010).

Telehealth can be considered another component of the eHealth concept, with the difference being around the delivery mechanisms, which can include live video conferencing; store-and-forward systems, such as those used to store digital images; telephone conferencing; and remote patient monitoring and e-visits via a secure Web Portal. Teleconferencing and digital networking systems are now merging, giving rise to "group consultation" opportunities (Doty, 2008; Waegemann, 2010).

While variations in the definitions of telemedicine and telehealth exist, there is agreement on the broad conception of this field as, "the delivery of personal and non-personal health services and of consumer and provider education as well as a means for safeguarding the living environment via information and communication technology" (Bashshur & Shannon, 2009, p. 601). Using the broadest definition of telehealth as a foundation, this chapter will explore the past, present, and future innovations as they apply to healthcare delivery, education, and research.

The Concept of mHealth

Another component of eHealth is mobile-health (mHealth), which can be considered a delivery mechanism for eHealth. mHealth typically refers to the use of a wireless communication device that supports public health and clinical practices (Eytan, 2010; TBHome, 2010). mHealth is seen as a valuable tool as the digitization of health and wellness data increases. It is postulated that many tools will be required, as no single tool will serve all needs for all people. As a result, there is a need to stop focusing on the technological components separately and work toward aggregating these communication technologies in an integrated system. Once this is accomplished, an ecosystem for integrated broad-scale deployment of eHealth tools can be achieved (Eytan, 2010; TBHome, 2010).

Waegemann (2010) views mHealth as the new generation of telemedicine that is laying the foundation for a new generation of healthcare. He describes eHealth as having a focus on using electronic medical records and other technologies, while mHealth focuses on behavioral and structural changes. The current idea that telemedicine requires dedicated connections does not fit the new world view of mHealth. The mHealth revolution is introducing patient-centered, communication-based care in a system that includes wellness and healthcare providers (Bloch, 2010). The healthcare model itself is moving from a provider-driven one to a largely participatory model including all stakeholders such as long-term caregivers, dentists, insurance companies, hospitals, public health officials, primary care providers, consumers, and health systems involved in wellness (Bloch, 2010).

It is crucial to note that these changes will be global in distribution. mHealth is going to allow basic care to be provided that might not otherwise be available in regions of African, Asia, and South America. In developing countries, mobile phones far outnumber personal computers, and they offer support services on both health and technology fronts. The power of these technologies to improve health and the human condition cannot be underestimated: "Modern telecommunications, and the creative use of it, has the power to change lives and help.... solve some of the world's biggest challenges" (United Nations Foundation, Vodafone Group Foundation, & Telemedicine Society of India, 2008). For most of the world, this will be the only computer they will own; it is on the Web and they can carry it everywhere. The impact on healthcare could be great (The doctor in your pocket, 2005).

As mHealth continues to progress, nursing care will need to evolve. Traditionally, nurses have been hands-on caregivers; now, nurses are challenged with developing new models for nursing care that address "care at a distance" using innovations such as mobile phones and text messaging. Communication is at the core of nursing care, and the methods of communication are rapidly changing and growing. Nurses will be able to utilize text messaging over a secure network to send automated appointment reminders, health tips, and messages about available resources in the area. Nurses will need to consider their standards of care and the impact these new modalities will have on care delivery.

eHEALTH APPLICATIONS

Telehealth has both clinical and non-clinical uses. Non-clinical applications include professional education; healthcare administrative duties; research; and the aggregation of health data, excluding patient-specific medical treatments and decisions. Clinical uses include medical decisions involving patient care, diagnostics, and treatments. However, these two categories are somewhat blurred, as patients and providers exchange e-mail communications that are being stored in the patient's computerized record (Bauer, 2009).

Clinical applications for telemedicine can be provided at the point of service or at another location (e.g., in the home for patients who may be home-bound, who reside in rural communities, or who are living in correctional facilities). Telehealth applications can be specialized, such as with telepathology, telepsychology, or remote patient monitoring services for ICUs in acute care facilities. Telehealth is forging new relationships between patients and all types of practitioners; it is moving care out the physician-centric perspective into the twenty-first century model of healthcare that will see more consumer empowerment.

Impact of the Web

Today, 85% of American adults (ages 18 and older) are using the Web; 70% of them access via broadband connections at home, and 61% connect wirelessly to the Web via their laptops or 56% with smart phones (Zickuhr & Smith, 2013). A 2010 Pew Internet and American Life Project study indicates 89% of adults with no chronic diseases go online, while only 72% of adults living with chronic disease are likely to access to the Web (Fox & Duggan, 2013). These findings are in line with trends in public health and technology adoption. Chronic disease is typically associated with being older, African American, less educated, and living in a lower-income household. While Internet use is associated with being younger, white, college educated, and living in a higher-income household (Fox & Duggan).

People living with chronic disease have complicated health issues and are disproportionately offline. Those who are online, however, have additional support; they have each other. Two online activities that are common among people living with chronic diseases are blogging and online health discussions. Having a chronic disease significantly increases the likelihood that the user will use the Web to read and share information. "Nuggets" of information are discovered via these online discussion groups; individuals in the groups connect and they "just keep going" (Fox & Duggan, 2013).

Consumer Engagement

The National eHealth Collaborative (2012) developed the Patient Engagement Framework to assist healthcare organizations in developing a strategic plan to incorporate eHealth tools and resources as part of an overall engagement strategy. The framework includes five phases as described in Table 22.1.

Personal Health Records

Personal health records (PHR) are maintained by the patient, in contrast to the medical record that is maintained by providers at the various clinical agencies caring for the patient. The PHR facilitates patient access to information about his/her health and healthcare experiences. Use of a PHR encourages patients to track care encounters and collect relevant health information to share in care management. Google Health is a Web-based personal health record. Users can build health profiles, import records from hospitals and pharmacies, share their records, and explore online health services (Google Health, 2010).

Managing Health Conditions and Accessing Resources

Electronic resources are being used increasingly to learn about and manage health conditions. Health seeking

TABLE 22.1	The Patient Engagement Framework (National eHealth Collaborative, 2012)
Phase	**Description**
Inform me	The focus is on providing information to assist patients in obtaining relevant materials. Examples include use of mobile devices for directory services, access to basic health information for wellness and prevention, electronic access to standard forms (HIPAA, insurance forms, etc.), and specific information about tests, medications, and procedures.
Engage me	The focus is on providing patients with specific information concerning their care needs. Examples include electronic tools to facilitate tracking of health and fitness behaviors, online tools to schedule appointments, and access to the electronic health record.
Empower me	The focus is on enhancing patient involvement in the care process. Examples include secure messaging and virtual coaching. In addition, patients could have the capability of generating their own data for the health record.
Partner with me	The focus is on tools for shared decision-making and coordination of care across sites. Examples include home monitoring devices and specific directives for patient preferences and intolerances.
Support my e-community	The focus is on enhanced information exchange. Examples include online e-community support forums and e-visits with providers.

behaviors of adults with chronic conditions are notably different from those of adults in general. Specifically, "when controlling for age, income, education, ethnicity, and overall health status, internet users living with one or more conditions are *more likely* than other online adults to:

- Gather information online about medical problems, treatments, and drugs.
- Consult online reviews about drugs and other treatments.
- Read or watch something online about someone else's personal health experience" (Fox & Duggan, 2013).

Those with chronic conditions are more likely to fact check information found on the Internet with their clinicians as well as track personal data related to health and wellness.

Transforming the Practice of Healthcare

Wearable and Portable Monitoring Systems. Remote patient monitoring, considered experimental a few years ago, is now maturing, with a number of applications available. The VitalJacket is one example that utilizes microelectronics in a wearable T-shirt that continuously monitors electrocardiogram waves and heart rate. The shirt can be used for patients or for healthy subjects involved in fitness activities or sports (Biodevices, 2009; Blanchett, 2008).

A system available today from BodyMedia is a wearable monitoring system that focuses on weight loss, health, and fitness. The armband has sensors that collect heat flux, galvanic skin response, skin temperature, as well as an accelerometer. Utilizing a USB cable, one can sync the data with Activity Management software where it is stored and can be tracked by the user (Terry, 2010).

The Health Buddy System is a remote monitoring platform that provides a daily interface between care coordinators and patients with chronic illnesses; this system has a proven track record over the past decade. The appliance can also connect glucose meters, weight scales, blood pressure cuffs, and other medical devices so additional patient data are sent to the healthcare professionals. Health Buddy has been used with a variety of patients including coronary artery bypass graft (Zimmerman, Barason, Nieveen, & Schmaderer, 2004), chronic heart failure (LaFramboise, Todero, Zimmerman, & Agrawat, 2003), diabetes (Cherry, Moffat, Rodriguez, & Dryden, 2002), and asthma (Guendelman, Meade, Benson, Chen, & Samuels, 2002). Care providers access data that can provide an early alert of warning signs that the patient is deteriorating; it addresses gaps in care before the patient becomes critical.

Telenursing and Decision Support Tools. Telenursing is broadening the role of nurses and advancing their value in the chain of healthcare delivery to consumers in remote regions or to homebound patients. Home health nursing via visual communication is a technique that provides accessible care and reduces both travel time and expense. Using videophones, the nurse and patient can establish a more personal relationship. Images can be transmitted interactively from the patient's home directly to attending physicians, improving follow-up and treatment for things such as leg wounds. This technology can be used to plan care interventions and to train patients and their caregivers. Utilizing field notes, photos, and video-recorded dialogs, all care providers can easily follow any changes in leg wounds (Jönsson & Willman, 2008).

Teletriage is a component of telenursing. Decision support tools have been developed as a guide for the teletriage nurse assessing a patient. These tools provide the nurse with structure around the teletriage processes. Utilizing these decision support tools, along with nursing judgment and critical thinking skills, helps minimize risk when providing telephone assistance. For example, the Medicare Quality Improvement Community (MedQIC) Web site has a free online teletriage resource toolkit to support consistent and appropriate teletriage assessments for many conditions including adverse drug reaction; breathing difficulty; depression; feeding tube problems; nausea, vomiting, and fluid loss; wound drainage; and pain management (QualityNet, 2006/2007).

Possibility of Virtual Worlds. Web-based 3D virtual worlds are currently being investigated as a potential tool to engage a variety of audiences in healthy behavior and lifestyle choices regardless of location. These tools are also being used as a new educational method for the healthcare professions that will help facilitate learning through interactive, collaborative learning environments (Skiba, 2007).

The 3D worlds are created online using a virtual persona, or avatar, which interacts with other avatars in the online world. The Centers for Disease Control and Prevention (CDC) has established a Second Life island where users can see streaming videos and access links to information on CDC.gov. The island has a virtual lab and conference center (CDC Home, 2009).

Health Portals and Web 2.0. Web 2.0 social networking sites such as Facebook, Twitter, YouTube, and MySpace are proliferating. Health consumers feel empowered and now want to participate in decisions about their healthcare. Support groups are using the Web as a new platform to organize, share experiences, seek online counseling, and simply connect with others. Web sites are now being utilized by healthcare providers as a place to engage with colleagues on clinical and non-clinical issues.

Hospital portals are being developed where patients can make appointments, renew prescriptions, and review test results and their medical records online. An example is My Health*e*vet, which offers veterans, active duty service members, their dependents, and caregivers access anytime to VA healthcare information and services that include tracking tools and journals to help the user track their health activities (My Health*e*vet, 2010).

WebMD is a consumer portal that is a leader in providing online health information. It provides the ability to browse condition-specific and wellness-related topics. Individuals have the ability to participate in moderated exchanges where they can get expert feedback on a variety of topics such as osteoporosis, skin problems, and gynecology problems. There are also member-created exchanges where users discuss parenting issues or participate in a diet club (WebMD, 2010).

PatientsLikeMe is a popular social networking site. This site contains communities that have been developed to allow patients to become proactive. The community forums include patients, doctors, and organizations. Users learn about treatments and symptoms, and can participate in the forum or have one-on-one discussions. The site was developed for individuals with life-changing diseases such as Amyotrophic Lateral Sclerosis (ALS), Parkinson disease, and epilepsy (PatientsLikeMe, 2010).

mHealth Applications. The rapid and pervasive worldwide adoption of mobile cell phones is going to drive tremendous growth in handheld healthcare over the next decade. Wireless communication technologies are forcing a transformation in how and where healthcare is delivered. The abilities to collaborate, share high-resolution images, and even have live broadcasting of surgeries are all enabled by new technologies.

Applications areas for mHealth include consumer education, emergency response systems, professional and patient communications (e.g., text messaging, e-mail, social networking), health promotion and community mobilization, and public and population health (Waegemann, 2010).

mHealth growth has been around the world with significant demand from "bottom-of-the-pyramid" consumers located in rural areas. Pilot projects are ongoing in countries such as Indonesia, Brazil, Sudan, and Uganda. In Africa, health personnel use mobile phones to provide emergency medical care; their phones use solar charges. A toll-free mobile service is being launched in remote areas of Tanzania, Kenya, and Uganda. In developing economies, mHealth will be a major part of eHealth. mHealth will need to be integrated into the training of healthcare workers, so professionals have the knowledge and skills required to use the technology safely and effectively (Ganapathy & Ravindra, 2008).

IMPACT OF eHEALTH APPLICATIONS

Transforming the Way We Learn

Web-based educational programs are changing the way consumers and healthcare providers learn. These programs continue to proliferate, providing the opportunity for interactive learning and simulations with the ability to have multi-user discussions and presentations in a collaborative learning environment. Faced with limited funds, nursing schools now have the ability to form partnerships and share their resources via the virtual classroom. The Web allows nurses and students the ability to access the most up-to-date research and knowledge facilitating evidence-based practice. Technological innovations, such as video streaming and virtual reality 3D displays, are providing more sophisticated formats in which to deliver educational materials. Web-based educational programs can reach remote students who otherwise would be unable to attend class (Brantley, Laney-Cummings, & Spivack, 2004; Sakraida & Draus, 2003; Simpson, 2003; Smith-Stoner & Willer, 2003).

The role of the nurse as a patient and consumer educator in the digital age is evolving as well. Online educational materials can be tailored to an individual's literacy level and presented in a bilingual format (Lewis, 2003). The advent of Massively Open Online Courses (popularly known as MOOCs) provides accessible and free learning across the globe. Major universities are considering offering credit for these courses (Skiba, 2013). Remote interactive telehealth networks have been shown to be effective in providing pre-operative patient education to rural locations and are increasingly being used for disease management (Roupe, 2004; Thomas, Burton, Withrow, & Adkisson, 2004).

Transforming Healthcare Delivery

Electronic Data Exchange. Advances in eHealth and the growing use of electronic health records have contributed to the realities of health data exchange. During the 1990s, hospitals attempted to create community health information networks to share information at the community level. However, concerns for patient privacy, the high costs of system implementation, and access to information by competing organizations prevented widespread use and acceptance of this innovation .(Thornewill, Dowling, Cox, & Esterhay, 2011).

In the United States, the federal government took a leadership role in health information exchange when the National Committee for Vital and Health Statistics published a report titled "A Strategy For Building a National Health Information Infrastructure" in 2001. This report indicated that "such a capability would improve response in individual and public health emergencies, reduce unnecessary care, decrease the likelihood of adverse events, improve patients' self-management capabilities, and generally enable improve management of chronic disease" (Kuperman, 2011, p. 678). Further federal

leadership occurred in 2004, when President George Bush created the Office of the National Coordinator for Health Information Technology to connect clinicians and improve population health (Shapiro, Mostashari, Hripcsak, Soulakis, & Kuperman, 2011). Funding for the effort became available through the Health Information Technology for Economic and Clinical Health (HITECH) Act, part of the American Recovery and Reinvestment Act of 2009, which provided over $19 billion with incentives for electronic health record implementation further supporting the possibility of electronic health information exchange (Barton, 2012a).

Payment Reform Through Meaningful Use. The HITECH Act also introduced the concept of "meaningful use." The idea was that not only should providers use electronic records within their practices, they should make use of the information available to enhance patient care outcomes. "Per statute, a provider must demonstrate meaningful use by (1) use of certified EHR technology in a meaningful manner such as e-prescribing; (2) that the certified EHR technology is connected in a manner that provides for the electronic exchange of health information to improve the quality of care; and (3) in using this technology, the provider submits to the secretary information on clinical quality measures and such other measures selected by the secretary" (Barton, 2011, p. 8). The funding makes $27 billion available in incentives for eligible providers (maximum $44,000 per provider) who participate in Medicaid and Medicare programs during the five-year, phased implementation period beginning in 2011 (Blumenthal & Tavenner, 2010). Providers who fail to attest to meaningful use will be assessed penalties beginning in 2015. Attestation requires providers to meet 15 core measure requirements such as recording vital signs, using electronic prescribing, and maintaining an electronic problem list. An initial evaluation of the program indicates that providers are successfully meeting requirements and even exceeding thresholds established by the Centers for Medicare and Medicaid Services (Wright, Feblowitz, Samal, McCoy, & Sittig, 2014).

Research Opportunities

Much is written on how eHealth applications may help provide care for an aging population, improve care in rural areas, and decrease healthcare disparities in the United States and increasingly around the world. There is an increasingly important need to look at the impact of eHealth applications on the care provider–patient relationship and how these applications affect outcomes (McGowan, 2008; Merrell & Doarn, 2010).

There is a need to study symptom management and effectiveness of "distant" clinical assessments to identify standardized best practices. The effectiveness of electronic communication methods as avenues to provide healthcare will need to be researched. Nursing research will need to adapt to this ever-evolving landscape of technologies (McGowan, 2008).

Nguyen (2010) identifies unique methodologic research issues and challenges for nursing around the use of information and communication technologies (ICT). The focus of research efforts needs to be on "understanding what intervention component, through what mechanism, for whom, and under what conditions will produce the most optimal health outcome" (p. 31).

Specification of the research focus will facilitate more refinement of individual ICT components that appear to be effective (Nguyen, 2010). Gibbons and colleagues (2009) found three factors in consumer health applications that had a significant effect on health outcomes: (1) individual tailoring, (2) personalization, and (3) behavioral feedback. While randomized controlled trials provide evidence for effectiveness of an intervention relative to a control, there is difficulty in finding consistency of control groups when studying ICT applications. With the increasing pervasiveness of eHealth, nurse researchers will have to evolve their scientific approaches in order to produce the practice-based evidence that is going to be needed (Nguyen, 2010).

Another gap in current research is on the use of telehealth applications for emergency and disaster preparedness and response. There are opportunities for interdisciplinary research on public health surveillance networks to determine pattern recognition algorithms that address threats to public health including flu outbreaks, environmental disasters, and man-made threats such as terrorist attacks (Alverson et al., 2010).

Transforming Emergency Preparedness and Response

During a disaster situation, the use of telehealth technology would allow clinicians to provide healthcare services remotely. A locally based network of clinicians linked via modern communication would help reduce major disruptions in healthcare. Protocols need to be developed for mobile communication devices before disasters so they can be rapidly deployed to provide routine care, triage, and shelter-in-place medical care (Ackerman, 2010; Bloch, 2010).

Advanced wireless electronic technologies are the quickest vehicles to communicate needs during emergency situations. State, federal, and international emergency efforts have not evolved as rapidly as these new technologies.

However, some communities are turning to subscription services to notify residents of threats related to severe weather (Media Weather Innovations, LLC, 2010).

eHEALTH CHALLENGES AND ISSUES

Innovations in eHealth do not come without challenges and issues that healthcare professions must address. As the transformation of healthcare moves toward patient-centric models, the healthcare professionals must resolve some key challenges and issues. These issues concern on legal, ethical, and public policy arenas.

Licensure

The lack of infrastructure for interstate licensure was a key impediment to the growth of telehealth. The U.S. Congress contracted with the Center for Telemedicine Law for a background paper concerning telehealth licensure issues in early 1997 (Telemedicine Report to Congress). Alternative approaches to licensure outlined in that report include consulting exceptions, endorsement, mutual recognition, reciprocity, registration, limited licensure, national licensure, and federal licensure. Additionally, in 2010, the Centers for Medicare and Medicaid Services (CMS) proposed a rule that would allow a streamlined credentialing and privileging process for physicians and practitioners providing telemedicine services (Telehealth Law Center, 2010).

Ethical Issues

The predominant ethical issues concerning telehealth are privacy, confidentiality, and security. The following definitions have been set forth by the American Society for Testing and Materials Committee E31 on Healthcare Informatics, Subcommittee E31.17 on Privacy, Confidentiality, and Access (1997):

Privacy. "The right of individuals to be left alone and to be protected against physical or psychological invasion or the misuse of their property. It includes freedom from intrusion or observation into one's private affairs, the right to maintain control over certain personal information, and the freedom to act without outside interference."

Confidentiality. The "status accorded to data or information indicating that it is sensitive for some reason, and therefore it needs to be protected against theft, disclosure, or improper use, or both, and must be disseminated only to authorized individuals or organizations with a need to know."

Data Security. "The result of effective data protection measures; the sum of measures that safeguard data and computer programs from undesired occurrences and exposure to accidental or intentional access or disclosure to unauthorized persons, or a combination thereof; accidental or malicious alteration; unauthorized copying; or loss by theft or destruction by hardware failures, software deficiencies; operating mistakes; physical damage by fire, water, smoke, excessive temperature, electrical failure or sabotage; or a combination thereof."

System Security. "Security enables the entity or system to protect the confidential information it stores from unauthorized access, disclosure, or misuse, thereby protecting the privacy of the individuals who are the subjects of the stored information."

It is imperative that providers and healthcare systems establish policies concerning privacy, confidentiality, and security as they create systems to facilitate patient-centered care through the provision of eHealth.

EMERGING ISSUES AND CHALLENGES

For all the possibilities it presents, eHealth does come with challenges including privacy concerns, equity across populations, and the need to define a new type of relationship between the patient and the healthcare provider (Eysenbach, 2001). Other issues include integration and networking interoperability, and usability. Finally, there is the challenge to determine what impact these new technologies will ultimately have on patient outcomes.

Disparities in healthcare and access to care still persist and a true solution eludes us. Underserved communities can benefit from improved access to clinical expertise in specialties such as oncology, radiology, infectious disease, and psychiatry. Further, reimbursement for telehealth interventions and a positive cost–benefit ratio are necessary before providers can consider adopting technological innovation into their practice environments. Health systems may want to fund programs if telemedicine visits prevent trips to congested emergency departments. As the healthcare industry is forced to deliver more with less, flexible telemedicine will need to come to the mainstream (Enrado, 2009).

Regulation of mHealth Applications

A recent development regarding mHealth is ruled by the U.S. Food and Drug Administration (FDA, 2013) to regulate a small segment of these applications. The FDA is interested in regulating mobile medical applications that meet the definition of a medical device, are intended to be used as an accessory to a regulated medical device, or transform a mobile platform into a regulated medical device. Specifically:

- Mobile applications that are an extension of one or more medical device(s) or displaying, storing, analyzing, or transmitting patient-specific medical device data

- Mobile applications that transform the mobile platform into a medical device by using attachments, display screens, or sensors or by including functionalities similar to those of currently regulated medical devices

- Mobile applications that allow the user to input patient-specific information and through the use of formulas or processing algorithms, output a patient-specific result, diagnosis, or treatment recommendation to be used in clinical practice or to assist in making clinical decisions (Barton, 2012b, p. 2).

Public Policy

The American Telemedicine Association (2014) outlined guidelines to "advance the science, to assure uniform quality of service to patients, and to promote reasonable and informed patient and provider expectations." These guidelines include administrative, clinical, and technical recommendations designed to provide a safe, quality, telehealth experience.

CONCLUSION

Without a doubt, eHealth applications will proliferate in the future. Healthcare professionals need to seize the opportunities made possible by advanced technologies and create powerful and human-centered applications to facilitate consumers' full participation in health and wellness. To evolve this process, healthcare professional need to be actively involved in resolving challenges, shaping public policy, and evaluating health outcomes.

REFERENCES

Ackerman, K. (2010, April 22). New toolkit for disaster response: Social media, mobile tools & telehealth. *iHealthBeat*. Retrieved from http://www.ihealthbeat.org/features/2010/new-toolkit-for-disaster-response-social-media-mobile-tools--telehealth.aspx

Alverson, D. C., Edison, K., Flournoy, B. A., Korte, B., Magruder, C., & Miller, C. (2010, January/February). Telehealth tools for public health, emergency, or disaster preparedness, and response: A summary report. *Telemedicine and e-Health, 16*(1), 112–114. Retrieved from http://www.liebertonline.com/doi/pdf/10.1089/tmj.2009.0149

American Society for Testing and Materials Committee E-31 on Healthcare Informatics, Subcommittee E-31.17 on Privacy, Confidentiality, and Access. (1997). *Standard guide for confidentiality, privacy, access, and data security principles for health information including computer-based patient records.* Philadelphia, PA: ASTM (Designation E-1869-97).

American Telemedicine Association (ATA). (2010). *What is Telemedicine?* Retrieved from http://www.americantelemed.org/about-telemedicine/what-is-telemedicine#.VG0s-taug2I

American Telemedicine Association (ATA). (2014). *Core guidelines for telemedicine operations.* Retrieved from http://www.americantelemed.org/docs/default-source/standards/core-standards-for-public-comment---draft-for-comment.pdf?sfvrsn=4Comments

Barton, A. J. (2011). The Electronic health record and "meaningful use": Implications for the clinical nurse specialist. *Clinical Nurse Specialist, 25*, 8–10. doi:10.1097/NUR.0b013e3182011f14.

Barton, A. J. (2012a). Health information exchange: Implications for the clinical nurse specialist. *Clinical Nurse Specialist, 26*(1), 10–11. doi:10.1097/NUR.0b013e31823c7ea7.

Barton, A. J. (2012b). The regulation of mobile health applications. *BMC Medicine, 10*, 46.

Bashshur, R., & Shannon, G. W. (2009). *History of telemedicine: Evolution, context, and transformation.* New Rochelle, NY: Mary Ann Liebert, Inc.

Bauer, K. (2009) Healthcare ethics in the information age. In R. Juppicini & R. Adell (Eds.), *Handbook of research on technoethics.* (Vol. 1, pp. 171–172). Hershey, PA: IGI Global.

Biodevices. (2009). *Vital Jacket® knowing your heart.* Retrieved from http://www.vitaljacket.com

Blanchett, K. (2008, March). Remote patient monitoring. *Telemedicine and e-Health, 14*(2), 127–130. Retrieved from http://www.acnpweb.org/i4a/pages/index.cfm?pageid=3470

Bloch, C. (2010b, April 21). UTMB responds to disasters. *Federal Telemedicine News.* Retrieved from http://telemedicnenews.blogspot.com/2010/04/utmb-respons-to-disasters.html

Blumenthal D., & Tavenner, M. (2010). The "meaningful use" regulation for electronic health records. *New England Journal of Medicine, 363*(6), 501–504.

Brantley, D., Laney-Cummings, K., & Spivack, R. (2004). *Innovation, demand and investment in telehealth.* U.S. Dept. of Commerce: Office of Technology Policy. Retrieved from http://www.technology.gov/reports/TechPolicy/Telehealth/2004Report.pdf

CDC Home. (2009, August 10). *Social media at CDC—Virtual worlds.* Retrieved from http://www.cdc.gov/SocialMedia/Tools/VirtualWorlds.html

Cherry, J. C., Moffat, T. P., Rodriguez, C., & Dryden, K. (2002). Diabetes disease management program for an indigent population empowered by telemedicine technology. *Diabetes Technology & Therapeutics, 4*(6), 783–791.

Doty, C. A. (2008, November). Delivering care anytime, anywhere: Telehealth alters the medical ecosystem. *California Healthcare Foundation.* Retrieved from http://www.chcf.org/publications/2008/11/delivering-care-anytime-anywhere-telehealth-alters-the-medical-ecosystem

Enrado, P. (2009, August 19). California telemedicine shortage aims to alleviate nurse shortage. *Healthcare IT News.* Retrieved from http://www.healthcareitnews.com/news/california-telemedicine-program-aims-alleviate-nurse-shortage

Eysenbach, G. (2001). What is e-Health? *Journal of Medical Internet Research, 3*(2), e20.

Eytan, T. (2010, February 18). *Six reasons why mhealth is different than eHealth* [Web log post]. Retrieved from http://www.tedeytan.com/2010/02/18/4731

Fox, S., & Duggan, M. (2013, September). The diagnosis difference. *Pew Internet & American Life Project.* Retrieved from http://pewinternet.org/Reports/2013/The-Diagnosis-Difference.aspx

Ganapathy, K., & Ravindra, A. (2008, July 13–August 8). mHealth: A potential tool for healthcare delivery in India. *Making the eHealth Connection.* Retrieved from http://www.ehealth-connection.org/files/conf-materials/mHealth_A%20potential%20tool%20in%20India_0.pdf

Gibbons, M. C., Wilson, R. F., Samal, L., Lehmann, C. U., Dickersin, K., Lehmann, H. P., & Bass, E. B. (2009, October). *Impact of Consumer Health Informatics Applications.* Evidence Report/Technology Assessment No. 188. (Prepared by Johns Hopkins University Evidence-based Practice Center under contract No. HHSA 290-2007-10061-I) AHRQ Publication No. 09(10)-E019. Retrieved from http://www.ahrq.gov/downloads/pub/evidence/pdf/chiapp/impactchia.pdf

Google Health. (2010). *About Google Health.* Retrieved from http://www.google.com/intl/en-US/health/about

Guendelman, S., Meade, K., Benson, M., Chen, Y. Q., & Samuels, S. (2002). Improving asthma outcomes and self-management behaviors of inner-city children: A randomized trial of the Health Buddy interactive device and an asthma diary. *Archives of Pediatric and Adolescent Medicine, 156*(2), 114–120.

Jönsson, A., & Willman, A. (2008, December). Implementation of telenursing within home healthcare. *Telemedicine and e-Health, 14*(10), 1057–1062.

Kuperman, G. J. (2011). Health-information exchange: why are we doing it and what are we doing? *Journal of the American Medical Association, 18*, 678–682.

LaFramboise, L. M., Todero, C. M., Zimmerman, L., & Agrawat, S. (2003). Comparison of Health Buddy with traditional approached to heart failure management. *Family and Community, 26*(4), 275–288.

Lewis, D. (2003). Computers in patient education. *Computers, Informatics, Nursing, 21*(2), 88–96.

McGowan, J. (2008). The pervasiveness of telemedicine: Adoption with or without a research base. *Journal of General Internal Medicine, 23*(4), 505–507.

Media Weather Innovations, LLC. (2010). *WeatherCall*. Retrieved from http://www.weathercall.net/wc_home.html

Merrell, R. C., & Doarn, C. R. (2010, March). Where is the proof? *Telemedicine and e-Health, 16*(2), 125–126. Retrieved from http://www.liebertonline.com/doi/abs/10.1089/tmj.2010.9995

My HealtheVet. (2010). My HealtheVet home page. *United States Department of Veterans Affairs*. Retrieved from http://www.myhealth.va.gov

National eHealth Collaborative. (2012). *Patient engagement framework*. Retrieved from http://www.nationalehealth.org/patient-engagement-framework

Neuhauser, L., & Kreps, G. L. (2010, February). eHealth communication and behavior change: Promise and performance. *Social Semiotics, 20*(1), 9–27.

Nguyen, H. (2010, April). *Digital Health Consumers: Transforming the Clinical Research Landscape.* Paper presented at the Western Institute of Nursing Annual Communicating Nursing Research Conference, Phoenix, AZ.

Oh, H., Rizo, C., Enkin, M., & Jadad, A. (2005, February 24). What is eHealth?: A systematic review of published definitions. *Journal of Medical Internet Research, 7*(1), e1. Retrieved from http://www.jmir.org/2005/1/e1

Pagliari, C., Sloan, D., Gregor, P., Sullivan, F., Detmer, D., Kahan, J. P., & MacGillivray, S. (2005) What is eHealth? A scoping exercise to map the field. *Journal of Medical Internet Research, 7*(1), e9.

PatientsLikeMe. (2010). *PatientsLikeMe home page*. Retrieved from http://www.patientslikeme.com

QualityNet. (2006/2007). *Tools: Home telehealth reference 2006/2007*. Retrieved from http://www.qualitynet.org/dcs/ContentServer?c=MQTools&pagename=Medqic%2FMQTools%2FToolTemplate&cid=1157485199575

Roupe, M. (2004). Interactive home telehealth: A vital component of disease management programs. *Case Management, 9*(1), 47–49.

Sakraida, T., & Draus, P. (2003). Transition to a Web-supported curriculum. *Computers, Informatics, Nursing, 21*(6), 309–315.

Shapiro JS, Mostashari F, Hripcsak G, Soulakis N, Kuperman G. (2011). Using health information exchange to improve public health. *American Journal of Public Health, 101*(4), 616–623.

Silber D. (2003, May). *The Case for eHealth*. Paper presented at the European Commission's First High-Level Conference on eHealth—European Institute of Public Administration. Retrieved from http://www.epractice.eu/files/download/awards/D10_Award1_ResearchReport.pdf

Simpson, R. (2003). Welcome to the virtual classroom: How technology is transforming nursing education in the 21st century. *Nursing Administration Quarterly, 27*(1), 83–86.

Skiba, D. J. (2007). Emerging technology center: Nursing Education 2.0: Second life. *Nursing Education Perspectives, 28*(3), 156–157.

Skiba, D. J. (2013) On the horizon: The year of the MOOCs. *Nursing Education Perspectives, 34*(2), 36–137.

Smith-Stoner, M., & Willer, A. (2003). Video streaming in nursing education: Bringing life to online education. *Nurse Educator, 28*(2), 66–70.

TBHome. (2010, February 21). *Re: 6 reasons why mHealth is different than eHealth* [Web log comment]. Retrieved from http://tedeytan.com/2010/02/18/4731

Telehealth Law Center. (2010). *Major changes in HIPAA and privacy regulations: What telehealth providers need to know*. Retrieved from http://www.telehealthlawcenter.org/?c=125&a=2187

Telemedicine Report to Congress. (1997). *Legal issues—Licensure and telemedicine*. Retrieved from http://www.ntia.doc.gov/reports/telemed/legal.htm

Terry, M. (2010, March). Wearable health monitors: Real-time, patient-friendly data collection. *Telemedicine and e-Health, 16*(2), 1–5. Retrieved from http://www.liebertonline.com/doi/pdfplus/10.1089/tmj.2010.9994

The doctor in your pocket. (2005, September 15). *Economist*. Retrieved from http://www.economist.com/displaystory.cfm?story_id=E1_QPGRTQD

Thomas, K., Burton, D., Withrow, L., & Adkisson, B. (2004). Impact of a preoperative education program via interactive telehealth network for rural patients having total joint replacement. *Orthopaedic Nursing, 23*(1), 39–44.

Thornewill, J., Dowling, A. F., Cox, B. A., & Esterhay, R. J. (2011). Information infrastructure for consumer health: A health information exchange stakeholder study. *American Journal of Preventive Medicine, 40*(5S2), S123–S133.

United Nations Foundation, Vodafone Group Foundation, & Telemedicine Society of India. (2008, July/August). mHealth and mobile telemedicine—An overview. *Making the eHealth Connection*. Retrieved from http://www.ehealth-connection.org/content/mhealth-and-mobile-telemedicine-an-overview

United States Food & Drug Administration. (September 23, 2013). *FDA issues final guidance on mobile medical apps.* Retrieved from http://www.fda.gov/newsevents/newsroom/pressannouncements/ucm369431.htm

Waegemann, C. P. (2010, January/February). mHealth: Next generation of telemedicine. *Telemedicine and e-Health, 16*, 23–25. Retrieved from http://www.liebertonline.com/doi/pdfplus/10.1089/tmj.2010.9990

WebMD. (2010). *WebMD better Information. Better Health*. Retrieved from http://www.webmd.com

World Health Organization. (2012). *National e-health strategy strategic toolkit.* Retrieved from http://www.who.int/ehealth/publications/overview.pdf?ua=1

Wright, A., Feblowitz, J., Samal, L., McCoy, A., & Sittig, D. (2014). The Medicare Electronic Health Record Incentive Program: Provider performance on core and menu measures. *Health Services Research, 49,* 325–346. doi:10.1111/1475-6773.12134.

Zickuhr, K. & Smith, A. (2013). Home broadband 2013. Pew Internet and American Life Project. Retrieved from http://www.pewinternet.org/2013/08/26/home-broadband-2013/

Zimmerman, L., Barason, S. Nieveen, J., & Schmaderer, M. (2004). Symptom management intervention in elderly coronary artery bypass graft patients. *Outcomes Management, 8*(1), 5–12.

PART 5

Advanced Nursing Informatics in Practice

Gail E. Latimer

23

Structuring Advanced Practice Knowledge: An Internet Resource for Education and Practice

Mary Ann Lavin / Eileen Healy / Mary Lee Barron

• OBJECTIVES

1. Articulate support for the advanced nursing, healthcare technologic, and organizational science domains of advanced practice.
2. Create structures that reflect the integration of doctor of nursing practice knowledge/competencies between and within domains.
3. Select reliable and appropriate Web-based content within advanced practice knowledge/competency domain categories.

• KEY WORDS

Advanced practice
Nursing
Reflection
Structures
Domain(s)
Categories
Healthcare
Technology
Informatics
Organization
Knowledge
Competencies
Curriculum
Education
Database
Pain
Management

IMPROVING HEALTH AND HEALTHCARE THROUGH NURSING

Advanced practice nurses manage information. Information comes in many shapes and forms. One form revolves about initiatives aimed at improving health and healthcare through nursing. This movement received its greatest impetus in *The Future of Nursing* (Institute of Medicine, 2010), with its brief on the *Focus on Scope of Practice* (Institute of Medicine, 2011a). It calls for the States to remove inconsistent barriers to practice and the federal government to advance the reforms needed through the work of Congress and regulatory agencies. The chair was Donna Shalala, President of the University of Miami and former Secretary of the Department of Health and Human Services; the Vice-Chair was Linda Burnes Bolton, DPH, RN, FAAN. This report led to a "Campaign for Action," a joint endeavor by AARP and the Robert Wood Johnson Foundation (2014). Actions were directed toward building a stakeholder base, initiating action at local, state, and national levels, communicating the call to action, and monitoring of results (Illinois Campaign for Action, 2011). Campaign progress is available on a dashboard (Robert Wood Johnson Foundation and AARP, 2010–2011).

Coalitions are active within the majority of states (Robert Wood Johnson Foundation and AARP, 2012). In December 2013, AARP in Virginia announced its part in a 4.5 million dollar program, funded by the Robert Wood Johnson Foundation. This program helps states move forward in advancing the goals of the *Future of Nursing* to improve health and healthcare, most notably access, quality, and cost. Nine other states received funding at the same time. These were Alabama, Alaska, Arkansas, Illinois, Minnesota, Nevada, Ohio, South Carolina, and Vermont (AARP and Robert Wood Johnson Foundation, 2013).

A powerful voice in support of advanced practice is found in the 2014 Miller Center Report, Cracking the Code on Health Care Costs. Its recommendations include the elimination of individual state scope of advance practice barriers and the establishment of a place at the cost table for all stakeholders, including providers, (Miller Center of Public Affairs, 2014).

The authors of the Miller Center report were the members of State Health Cost Containment Commission. There were no nurses on the Commission. On the one hand, this may seem to be a contradiction on the part of a Commission recommending a place at the table for all stakeholders. On the other hand, the Commission consisted of healthcare system CEOs and was chaired by two former governors, one of whom is also a former Secretary of the Department of Health and Human Services under President George W. Bush, the Honorable Michael O. Leavitt. In brief, the report is a strong endorsement for eliminating scope of practice barriers by a highly competent, politically influential, non-nurse healthcare commission. It is a document well worth quoting in every State, where nurses are acting to eliminate scope of practice barriers, attain voice at the table, and provide quality care while working to contain healthcare costs.

STRUCTURING KNOWLEDGE AND ITS RELATIONSHIP TO ADVANCED PRACTICE

Much of informatics involves reflection. Reflection upon a single question led to the First National Conference on the Classification of Nursing Diagnoses in 1973 and the birth of NANDA. The question was: How are nursing data going to be entered into the computer? (Lavin, 2002). Reflection helps people create advances in health information technology. The number, kind, and design of self-management apps require hours of individual and group reflection. Reflection helps people adapt to technology as it influences the acceptance of scientific information (van Prooijen & Sparks, 2014). Reflection on professional practice deepens when routine practice benchmarks are available for review (McKay, Coombs, & Duerden, 2014). Reflection is central whenever change is anticipated, created, required to improve practice or adjust to technological change (Boulus & Bjorn, 2010).

While informatics may begin with reflection, it does not end with reflection. One product of reflection is the structuring of information. Reflection on the structure of advanced practice nursing education and practice at the doctoral level led ultimately to a three-dimensional model presented in this chapter. It is a model that combines knowledge and competencies within three domains. It also serves as a framework for creating a Web-based information databases to assist either the academician or practitioner. Let us begin, however, with a word on the meaning of knowledge structures.

Because some readers may operate more concretely than conceptually, it is important to provide some examples of the structuring of knowledge and its several ramifications. Structuring is what we do when we categorize, recognize categories or classes, place categories within domains, or identify domains and classes within a taxonomy and display results graphically.

Structuring also occurs when we recognize or name clusters within an actual or mathematically imposed space. We examine the relationship of one cluster to other clusters. Statistically, we think of cluster analysis. Astronomically, we think of the Milky Way. Epidemiologically, we think of cluster maps showing the spread of infectious disease.

Finally, we structure knowledge when we look at its various dimensions. Knowledge is not one dimensional. It may be pictured within two dimensions as in a matrix. Knowledge may be distributed within dimensions. It may be poly-dimensional/polygonal, like the facets of a diamond, changing slightly as light or perspective changes. Knowledge may be Web-like as that built by a spider, which glides, climbs, leaps from one knowledge strand to another, all the while remaining connected to its center.

This imaginative exercise has meaning. The ability to structure knowledge facilitates learning. For example, the American Nurses Credentialing Center (ANCC) structures or outlines the categories of knowledge covered by the Nurse Practitioner Certification Exams (American Nurses Credentialing Center, 2013). Each of the many specialties has its own structure, its own content outline. The ANA structures nursing practice with its standards (American Nurses Association, 2010). The nursing terminologies structure nursing concepts within classifications. The purpose of this chapter is to structure the knowledge base of the doctorally prepared advanced practice nurse.

COMPARISONS OF ADVANCED PRACTICE LEARNING AND PRACTICE STRUCTURES

Knowledge structures evolve as our ability to articulate knowledge evolves. This kind of evolution can be seen in Figs. 23.1 through 23.4. Figure 23.1 describes progression through a DNP curriculum. Figure 23.2 describes the integration of content within a DNP capstone project. Figure 23.3 presents a newer model for assessing performance of any program, intervention bundle or intervention. It is only Fig. 23.4 that presents a structure that represents

knowledge undergirding both a DNP curriculum and DNP practice.

We will explore Fig. 23.1 first. Some graduate curricula describe course progression linearly, first lower level foundational courses followed by higher level courses, requiring increasing integration of content (Fig. 23.1). One issue with this method of visualizing academic progression is that it assumes that integration of content occurs linearly, step by step. The model implies that having climbed all steps, a graduate emerges and proceeds to practice all that has been learned. Pictorially, education has ended; practice has begun.

Some advanced practice courses describe integration of content within a matrix. This kind of two-dimensional structure is presented in Figure 23.2. The matrix structure allows for the tracking of knowledge integration within each DNP capstone project. It is recognized that the nature of the integration will differ with each project. This type of structure goes beyond the linear progression we see in Fig. 23.1. Table 23.1 allows the user to see not only what courses have been completed but how the course knowledge shapes an end product, the DNP capstone. Its matrix display depicts, in computer language, input (DNP courses) to output (capstone outline sections).

The number of capstone projects produced is an output measure. However, ideally, each capstone project has output, outcome and impact measures. In this case, "output" as described in Figure 23.3 refers to what we may call "process outcomes." To explain this more simply, let's refer to the work of Florence Nightingale. We know from her work during the Crimean War that she was interested in process outcomes or output. That is, she evaluated how well nurses maintained a hygienic or clean patient environment (Nightingale, 1859). Additionally, Nightingale evaluated patient *outcomes* (i.e., did the patient develop an infection); and she measured impact (i.e., decreases in overall infection and mortality rates)

Capstone project

700 level courses, e.g., interprofessional collaboration, clinical informatics, health policy, health systems, evidence based practice, healthcare systems

500 level courses covering specialty-specific content areas e.g., chronic illness and disease management, geriatric syndromes, preconception/pregnancy management, acute care patient management, and family psychiatric disorder prevention and treatment, advanced practice role, and other cognates.

Core or foundational 500 level courses, e.g., nursing and healthcare ethics, health promotion, advanced pathophysiology, advanced pharmacology, advanced health assessment and clinical decision making, health promotion, principles of practice management, general research methods and epidemiology.

· **FIGURE 23.1.** Linear or Step-Wise Progression of Advanced Practice BSN to DNP Courses.

Saint Louis University School of Nursing DNP Risk Reduction Capstone Project								
DNP Courses that Impact Development and Implementation of Capstone Project	Outline of Capstsone Process							
	Select topic/ question	Intro-duction	Specific Aims	Back-ground	Literature Review	Methods	Analysis	Discussion and Conclu-sions
Introduction to the risk reduction capstone project (0 credits – first semester)								
Courses that contribute to development of topic area								
Ethics in Nursing and Health Care								
Pathophysiology								
Pharmacology								
Health Promotion and Disease Prevention								
Practice Management								
Fluids and Electrolytes								
Family and Child Development								
Leadership in Health Care								
Health Care Delivery System								
Interprofessional Collaboration								
Health Care Policy and Advanced Practice Nursing								
Courses that Contribute to Methods								
General Research Methods								
Principles of Epidemiology								
Evidence-Based Practice								
Clinical Informatics								
Cost and Quality Outcomes								

• **FIGURE 23.2.** Saint Louis University School of Nursing DNP Risk Reduction Capstone Project: Original Matrix Illustrating the Opportunities for Knowledge Synthesis and Integration Within the DNP Risk Reduction Capstone Project. (Reproduced, with permission, from Saint Louis University School of Nursing).

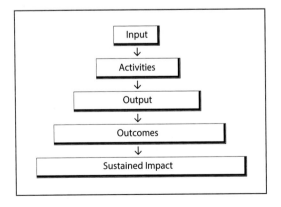

• **FIGURE 23.3.** Assessing Performance, Using United Nations Development Program Terminology, Associated With Results-Based Management (RBM).

(Lavin, Avant, Craft-Rosenberg, Herdman, & Gebbie, 2004). It is likely that Nightingale would have agreed with the terms, a *culture of results* or *results based management (RBM)*, now being advocated by the United Nations Development Programme (UNDP, 2007). Figure 23.2 presents an illustration of the UNDP performance signposts.

If these terms are to be used clinically, it helps provide a context. **Input** refers to structural, financial, human, or technical resources. Examples include staffing, NP educational background/experience. **Activities** are tasks or processes employed to produce an output, e.g., emergency department processes and treatment of patients seeking care for an infection. The **outputs** are the end products of the activities, whether on or off target. For example, an output is the answer to a question like: What is the proportion of multiple urgent sepsis therapies (MUST)–compliant records among ED patients, who

TABLE 23.1	Selected Web sites Illustrating Healthcare Technology Content Within Its Two Classes: Informatics and Healthcare Technology Research, Development, and Entrepreneurship

HEALTHCARE TECHNOLOGY DOMAIN

Informatics

Nursing informatics roles
http://healthit.ahrq.gov/search/nursing%20informatics%20roles

Electronic health record
http://healthit.ahrq.gov/search/electronic%20health%20record

Meaningful use
http://www.cms.gov/Regulations-and-Guidance/Legislation/EHRIncentivePrograms/Meaningful_Use.html

Clinical quality measures
CMS (http://www.cms.gov/Regulations-and-Guidance/Legislation/EHRIncentivePrograms/2014_ClinicalQualityMeasures.html)
HEDIS 2015 HEDIS measures: Summary table of measures, product lines, and changes. http://www.ncqa.org/Portals/0/HEDISQM/Hedis2015/List_of_HEDIS_2015_Measures.pdf)

National Database of Nursing Quality Indicators
http://www.nursingworld.org/MainMenuCategories/ThePracticeofProfessionalNursing/PatientSafetyQuality/Research-Measurement/The-National-Database/Nursing-Sensitive-Indicators_1

Healthcare data
http://www.healthdata.gov/
http://www.forbes.com/sites/oracle/2014/03/03/heathcares-next-innovation-the-answer-is-in-the-data/

Filter development, use and evaluation
http://www.ncbi.nlm.nih.gov/pmc/articles/PMC545129/?report=reader

Foundations of practice analysis: epidemiology and biostatistics
Epidemiology and analysis, including EpiInfo software and health disparities reports:
http://wwwn.cdc.gov/epiinfo/index.htm
http://www.cdc.gov/mmwr/pdf/other/su6001.pdf

Convergence of electronic health record technologic and nursing and documentation standards
http://mnnurses.org/nurses-guide-electronic-health-records-ehr-0

Information management, including taxonomy
http://ana.nursingworld.org/npii/terminologies.htm

knowledge and information structuring and standardizing knowledge
http://www.bsigroup.com/en-GB/our-services/developing-new-standards/Structuring-Knowledge-Standards-Development-Briefing/

Privacy, security, and ethics
http://am.asco.org/ethical-principles-and-use-electronic-health-records

Use of health information technology to reduce patient risk and improve patient care, e.g., http://www.ncbi.nlm.nih.gov/pmc/articles/PMC3444311/

Internet tools and resources
http://healthit.ahrq.gov/health-it-tools-and-resources

University of Toronto, Center for Global eHealth Innovation
http://www.jmir.org/

Health technology research, development, and entrepreneurship

Current health information technology and industry trends and innovations
http://www.innovations.ahrq.gov/

University of Wisconsin Living Environments Laboratory
http://wid.wisc.edu/research/lel/

University of Pennsylvania Health Technology Innovation Incubator
http://www.nursing.upenn.edu/innovation/health-technology-lab/Pages/default.aspx

University of California-Los Angeles, Wireless Pain Intervention Program for At Risk Youth With Sickle Cell Disease, E. Jacob, PhD
http://medicinex.stanford.edu/jacob-abstract/

University of Toronto, Center for Global eHealth Innovation
http://www.jmir.org/

(1) are admitted to the ED for infection, (2) exhibit at least two signs of systemic inflammatory response syndrome, and (3) exhibit at least one sign of hypoperfusion (Horeczko & Green, 2013; Picard, O'Donoghue, Young-Kershaw, & Russell, 2006). The **outcomes** are the intermediate effects of the activities, e.g., length of stay/patient, complications/patient, cost/patient, or sepsis-related mortality rates. **Impact** refers to macro numbers, e.g., institutional, healthcare system, state or national effects in terms of decline in sepsis-related mortality rates and costs.

To the extent that the UNDG outcome terminology adds clarity to the way in which we, as advanced practice nurses, articulate and measure outcomes, then we should consider its use clinically, as described above, and educationally. For example, the current Saint Louis University DNP capstone project, as described in Fig. 23.2, is aimed not just at improving process outcomes, but at reducing patient risk or improving what it refers to as *patient outcomes*. However, clarity is increased if it were to state that the DNP project aim is to reduce patient risk (or improve patient outcomes) and to impact the healthcare system positively, where the system may be a clinic, a nursing unit, an institution, a healthcare system, state or national healthcare statistics.

Matrices are powerful structures for presenting information about two discrete but related sets of data, even though they do not capture depth the way a cube or other multidimensional structures do. For our purposes here, in this chapter, a three-dimensional rectangle will suffice in making this point (Fig. 23.4). Its three dimensions (height, length, and width) display the healthcare technology knowledge, organizational science, and nursing science and practice domains within a BSN to DNP curriculum. These may be considered advanced practice knowledge domains.

As in any taxonomy, domains have classes. The classes within each of these domains are course competencies. Each may be cross-indexed with its AACN Essentials of Doctoral Education for Advanced Practice Nursing (American Association of Colleges of Nursing, 2006, 2011). Just as the AACN aligns DNP education with practice, so does Fig. 23.4. It is not as if the DNP student simply progresses through a curriculum to achieve DNP status as in Fig. 23.1. Nor is it as if knowledge is tracked as in the matrix in Fig. 23.2. Rather, as displayed in Figure 23.4, the DNP student is introduced to, is immersed in, and progresses through an advanced practice program of learning. Although at a certain point, a DNP degree will be conferred, the conferral just further commits the graduate to lifelong growth within the same knowledge and competency domains: advanced nursing science and practice, organizational science and healthcare technology.

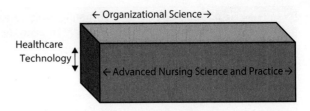

• **FIGURE 23.4.** Saint Louis University Doctor of Nursing Practice Curriculum Displayed as a Three-Dimensional Structure. Technologic science courses are clinical informatics courses, epidemiology, biostatistics, and patient care technology. Organizational/population science courses are healthcare policy, leadership, healthcare ethics, healthcare delivery systems, organizational climate, and inter-professional teamwork. Nursing science courses are advanced physiology, pharmacology, and physical assessment, evidence-based practice. I. principles and II. Applications; health and wellness promotion; clinical (illness and disease) management courses; inter-professional collaboration, including quality improvement methods; and the capstone project. Note: The care of diverse populations and cultural sensitivity is threaded throughout all three dimensions.

This academic structure reflects knowledge and competencies specified in four main documents:

- The Essentials of Doctoral Education for Advanced Practice nursing (American Association of Colleges of Nursing, 2006).

- Core Nurse Practitioner Competencies, identified by the National Organization of Nurse Practitioner Faculties (National Organization of Nurse Practitioner Faculties, 2012).

- Sample test content outlines, such as the Family Nurse Practitioner Board Certification Examination (American Nurses Credentialing Center, 2013). Consensus Model for APRN Regulation: Licensure, Accreditation, Certification, and Education (National Council of State Boards of Nursing, 2014).

These documents do not refer to three domains of advanced practice nursing knowledge at the doctoral level. Rather, with remarkable consistency, they refer to similar, if not identical, knowledge areas and related competencies. We merely group these knowledge areas and competencies into three main categories and create the domains (Fig. 23.4). It is not inconceivable that these three knowledge domains become basic departments within Schools of Nursing.

KNOWLEDGE STRUCTURES FACILITATE THE CREATION OF ADVANCED PRACTICE INTERNET DATABASES

Referring again to Figure 23.4, note that each domain refers to a knowledge base or content area. Each of these can be developed into its own database of hyperlinks to reliable and accurate sources of information. Let us take the **healthcare technology domain** first. It has two classes, at present: *Informatics* and *health technology research, development, and entrepreneurship*.

Informatics for the advanced practice nurse does not go into the same depth nor breadth of content as do informatics courses for the informatics specialist. Table 23.1 shows the kinds of content to be included in advanced practice informatics courses. At the doctoral level, the primary intent of informatics is to support evidence-based practice and quality improvement initiatives to improve patient outcomes and reduce risk. Table 23.1, like the other tables in this chapter, is intended to be a springboard for practice learning. For example, there is only one electronic health record Web site listed. It is the federal HealthIT Web site. There is no mention of Web sites dealing with vendor and IT issues, documentation, efficiency, safety, standards, or security issues—nor even of free, cloud-driven electronic health software now available. In brief, the Web site outlines content areas. Each content area is capable of being further developed into its own information/knowledge Web. The authors place epidemiology and biostatics within the informatics section of the healthcare technology domain. Each represents analytical knowledge basic to the measurement of improvement in healthcare processes and patient outcomes or reduction in patient risk, let alone the measurement of the larger impact such improvements have on society.

Table 23.1 also presents information on the *health technology research, development, and entrepreneurship*. Perhaps most notable is the work being conducted at the University of Wisconsin in the creation of the Living Environments Laboratory and at the University of Pennsylvania in the creation of a Health Technology Incubator, where nurses are developing innovative, point-of-patient contact devices/sensors, mHealth apps, simulations, social media/Web-based uses, and newer software/systems. Finally, Table 23.1 identifies AHRQ Web sites, which support technical innovations to enhance health in every aspect of life today.

The **organizational science domain** has several classes: epidemiology and biostatistics, healthcare policy, leadership, ethics and care delivery systems, and organizational climate. By definition, classes within a domain should be discrete with no overlap. In the biological and chemical world, this is possible. Within the healthcare and nursing education and practice worlds, the classes are not discrete. For example, *epidemiology* and *biostatistics* are integral content within the healthcare technology domain, but they also represent tools used within the organizational science domain. Areas of overlap are substantial among the classes or content areas within each domain as well.

Just as health technology research, development, and entrepreneurship are exploding within the health technology domain, *policy* is exploding within the organizational science domain. Within advanced practice there are two converging policy thrusts. The first is the IOM (2010) report on the Future of Nursing, with its message that nurses practice to the full extent of their education and training. The second is the APRN consensus model promoted by the National Council of State Boards of Nursing (2014), with its intent to license as independent practitioners those who have been properly educated and board certified within at least one of six population foci. The overriding purpose of each endeavor is to increase access of the population to qualified healthcare providers and to improve the health status of the nation. This is also the purpose of the Affordable Care Act (ACA), the foundation of current healthcare policy and reform.

For nursing, at this moment in history, the meaning and intent of leadership is transformation. The transformative power of nursing leadership is acknowledged in the IOM commentary by Fineberg and Lavizzo-Mourey (2013). Transformative leadership is advanced by the ANA and the Robert Wood Johnson Foundation in their respective support for nursing leadership development. The study of transformative leadership is one of the pillars of advanced practice nursing and education.

Healthcare ethics and healthcare delivery systems are inextricably intertwined to the extent that the ethics of healthcare professionals is manifest in the performance of the healthcare system. Performance may be measured by degree of patient safety, but also by compliance with regulations, e.g., the Health Insurance Portability and Accountability Act (HIPAA); Occupational Safety and Health Administration (OSHA); Clinical Laboratory Improvement Amendments (CLIA); and the CDC regarding, for example, mandatory notifiable diseases. How well a healthcare delivery system performs is also a function of the model it follows. For example, accountable care organizations (ACOs) are incentivized by the Centers for Medicaid and Medicare for keeping patients well.

While nursing and medical processes (outputs) and patient outcomes have been measured and while various healthcare policies have been implemented and different delivery systems tried, until now little systematic focus has been on the organizational climate of the practice or delivery system. Led by Dr. Poghosyan at Columbia, a team of investigators developed, tested and is using an organization climate questionnaire to evaluate practice settings, including advanced practice nursing settings in primary care.

This section concludes with a word on inter-professional practice. Healthcare practice today is a collaborative effort among overlapping teams of professionals, dedicated to the well-being of the patient and quality of care being delivered. That said, it behooves all to take advantage of available tools as we commit ourselves to APRN education and practice and to the improvement of health and healthcare in the nation (Tables 23.1 and 23.2).

There are many unobtrusive measures of the transformative changes occurring in nursing today. One is that this very chapter on advanced practice was previously focused on content presented in the Appendix,

Advanced Nursing Science and Practice Domain (available at MHProfessional.com/Nursing). The content in this domain is central to advanced practice and to DNP programs, nationwide. Evidence guides its practice. Its structured approach is standards based. The transformative change in advanced practice, however, is this: While doctorally prepared professionals may be informaticists, policy experts, leaders, healthcare technologists, qualitative improvement specialists, risk managers, organizational consultants, and researchers, the doctor of nursing practice is, at core, a clinician whose clinical science is integrated with high-level healthcare technology and organizational science skills. There is no attempt here to diminish the core of DNP practice by relegating its database to an appendix, but rather to capture the breadth

TABLE 23.2	Selected Web sites Illustrating Content Within the Classes of the Organizational Science Domain of Advanced Practice

ORGANIZATIONAL SCIENCE DOMAIN

APRN-Related Healthcare Policy

American Association of Nursing Practitioners. (2012-2015). NP Policy Essentials
    NP Policy Essentials
    https://www.aanp.org/legislation-regulation/policy-toolbox/np-policy-essentials
    Position Statements and Papers
    https://www.aanp.org/publications/position-statements-papers

National Organization of Nurse Practitioner Faculties: Statements and Papers
http://www.nonpf.org/?page=83

National Council of State Boards of Nursing: APRN Consensus Model Map
https://www.ncsbn.org/2567.htm

American Nurses Association, Overview of APRN Consensus Model
http://www.nursingworld.org/consensusmodel

ANCC APRN Consensus Model and Licensure, Accreditation, Certification, and Education (LACE)
http://www.nursecredentialing.org/Certification/APRNCorner

Institute of Medicine (2010). *The future of nursing: Leading change, advancing health*. Washington, DC: National Academies Press.
http://www.iom.edu/Reports/2010/The-future-of-nursing-leading-change-advancing-health.aspx

AARP Future of Nursing Campaign for Action
http://campaignforaction.org/

American College of Physicians (2009).
Nurse Practitioners in Primary Care: A Policy Monograph by the American College of Physicians
http://www.acponline.org/acp_policy/policies/nursepractitioners_pc_2009.pdf

Miller Center Report: Cracking the code on healthcare costa: http://web1.millercenter.org/commissions/healthcare/
    HealthcareCommission-Report.pdf

Affordable Care Act: Healthcare.gov Web site
https://www.healthcare.gov/marketplace/individual/?gclid=CK-o7Lm38bwCFRAV7AodLCUAZA

Affordable Care Act, Federal Register, (2014). Patient Protection and Affordable Care Act; Exchange and Insurance Market Standards
    for 2015 and Beyond.
https://www.federalregister.gov/articles/2014/05/27/2014-11657/patient-protection-and-affordable-care-act-exchange-and-
    insurance-market-standards-for-2015-and

(continued)

TABLE 23.2	Selected Web sites Illustrating Content Within the Classes of the Organizational Science Domain of Advanced Practice *(continued)*

Leadership

IOM (2011). *The future of nursing: Leading change, advancing health*
http://www.iom.edu/Reports/2010/The-future-of-nursing-leading-change-advancing-health.aspx
The future of nursing: A look back at the landmark IOM report
http://www.iom.edu/~/media/Files/Perspectives-Files/2013/Commentaries/EO-Nursing.pdf
University of Washington Global Nursing Leadership Toolkit
http://collaborate.uw.edu/educators-toolkit/global-nursing-leadership-toolkit.html-0
ANA Leadership Institute (2014)
http://www.ana-leadershipinstitute.org/
Robert Wood Johnson Foundation Nurse Faculty Scholars Program
http://www.nursefacultyscholars.org/

Healthcare ethics

VA online learning modules in healthcare ethics
http://www.ethics.va.gov/integratedethics/onlinemodules.asp
ANA Center for Ethics and Human Rights
http://www.nursingworld.org/ethics/
Key ethical principles
http://www.ascensionhealth.org/index.php?option=com_content&view=article&id=47&Itemid=171

Healthcare delivery systems and their management

Care Delivery Models 2010
    http://www.nursingworld.org/Content/HealthcareandPolicyIssues/Agenda/ANAsHealthSystemReformAgenda.pdf
    http://innovation.cms.gov/initiatives/aco/
    http://www.kaiserhealthnews.org/stories/2011/january/13/aco-accountable-care-organization-faq.aspx
IOM Report: Healthcare system reform and nursing workforce 2011
http://www.nursingworld.org/Content/HealthcareandPolicyIssues/Agenda/ANAsHealthSystemReformAgenda.pdf
Statutes, regulations and healthcare practice compliance
    HIPAA http://www.hhs.gov/ocr/privacy/
    CLIA http://www.cms.gov/Regulations-and-Guidance/Legislation/CLIA/index.html?redirect=/clia/
    Blood borne pathogen compliance https://www.osha.gov/SLTC/bloodbornepathogens/
    Notifiable disease compliance http://wwwnc.cdc.gov/eid/article/11/3/04-0361_article.htm (page created, updated, and last
      reviewed by CDC, April 2012)

Organizational climate [Google the digital object identifier (doi)_ for abstract; complete article information is in the reference list]

Nurse practitioner organizational climate in primary care settings: Implications for professional practice.
    doi: 10.1016/j.profnurs.2013.07.005
Organizational climate in primary care settings: Implications for nurse practitioner practice. DOI: 10.1111/j.1745-599.2012.00765.x
Development and psychometric testing of the Nurse Practitioner Primary Care Organizational Climate Questionnaire.
    doi: 10.1097/NNR.0b013e3182a131d2

Inter-professional teamwork

American Association of Colleges of Nursing
    Education http://www.aacn.nche.edu/education-resources/ipecreport.pdf
    Practice

and depth of this expanded twenty-first century practice, reasonably, within one chapter.

In the previous paragraph, the term "clinician" was used. This term was not meant to apply to nurse practitioners, alone. The clinical leader is a clinician, but one with a focus of practice different than that of the nurse practitioner. Each must be allowed to practice to the fullest extent of their education and its practice parameters or scope.

STRUCTURING AND EVALUATING A DATABASE FOCUSED ON ONE CLINICAL TOPIC: PAIN

According to the Institute of Medicine report, *Relieving Pain in America* (Institute of Medicine, 2011b), approximately 100 million people in the United States suffer from chronic pain, more than diabetes, coronary heart disease, stroke and cancer patients combined. It is estimated that pain costs in the United States are over $600 billion dollars annually in medical bills, lost productivity, and missed work.

Pain is one of the only symptoms common to all specialties. Pain is one of the most frequently given reasons an individual gives when seeking out a healthcare professional. Pain is often under-treated. The reasons for under-treatment of pain include lack of formal professional education in pain, lack of knowledge regarding treatment and management, not believing a patient is in pain, not understanding the physiological and pathophysiological origins of pain, and attitudinal/cultural issues, e.g., not appreciating the variety of responses to pain. One way of addressing at least some of these deficiencies in education is by creating an accessible and easily retrievable pain information database, organized in keeping with the ANA Standards of Professional Nursing Practice.

Six reviewers, experienced in one or more aspects of pain management, evaluated 64 Web sites, categorized within the ANA Standards of Professional Nursing Practice, according to a five-point Likert-based scale. The criteria for the scale were based on the work of Alexander and Tate (1996–2005), who applied five commonly used criteria to evaluate the written word and applied them to information found on a Web page. The criteria were accuracy, authority, objectivity, currency, and coverage. According to Alexander and Tate (1996–2005), the higher the "yes" score, the higher the quality of information on the Web site. Their work may be accessed at http://www.widener. edu/about/campus_resources/wolfgram_library/evaluate/ default.aspx. It is important to note that these criteria are used by the United Nations Framework Convention on Climate change (2014) to evaluate Web resources (https:// unfccc.int/essential_background/library/items/1420.php).

Currently, the most widely used system to evaluate the trustworthiness of a healthcare-related Web site is the HONcode (Health on the Net Foundation, 2013; 2014). HON is a certifying body for healthcare-related Web sites. It uses eight criteria: authoritative, complementary, privacy, attribution, justifiability, transparency, financial disclosure, and advertising policy. If the Web site is accepted, the seal for HON, along with the date it was evaluated, will be displayed on the home Web site page. HON works in congruence with the University Hospitals of Geneva and the Swiss Institute of Bioinformatics (http://www. healthonnet.org/HONcode/Conduct.html).

The main differences between Alexander and Tate's (1996–2005) work and the most commonly used certification method used by HON is that the former is a reviewer evaluation of the quality of the information on the website. The primary quality indicator is information accuracy. The latter, HON, is a certifying body, used only for healthcare sites, to evaluate the site's trustworthiness.

When we evaluated our Web sites we used the five criteria according to Alexander and Tate's definitions but we went one step further. We asked our expert reviewers to quantify the five criteria based on a five-point Likert scale with one being "strongly disagree" and five being "strongly agree." Each expert rated each Web site for each criterion within each of the ANA standards. We kept "accuracy" as the gatekeeper. If a Web site did not average a 4.0 or greater from all the expert reviewers it was eliminated and not included in the database. In inter-rater reliability terms, this meant that 100% of the raters had to score the site at 4.0 or greater. Furthermore, Table 23.3 represents an even higher inter-rater reliability measure. It includes only those with scores ≥4.80 on the 5.0 scale. Finally, the Web sites are coded by the ANA Standard of Practice to which they refer. More complete results are available on the Pain Database page of the nlinks.org Web site. NLINKS stands for Network for Language in Nursing Knowledge (Lavin, Krieger, Meyer, et al., 2005).

Structuring knowledge-based data, even when framed according to ANA practice standards, does not guarantee that the structure or information will be used as designed or, even more importantly, change practice or patient outcomes (Hyppönen et al., 2014; Müller-Staub, Lavin, Needham, & van Achterberg, 2006).

If structured information is to be used, it needs to be available, its usage tracked, within-system patient outcomes and ultimately population-based impact evaluated. The availability and use of such structured pain information for clinical decision support purposes may be tracked using electronic healthcare record data from within a large healthcare system, however. Only when we track these within-system changes in patient outcomes as

TABLE 23.3	Most Highly Scored Pain Information Web sites[a] (Accuracy Averages ≥4.80) Within the ANA Nursing Standards[b]			
Web site Name	**ANA Standard**	**Category**	**Accuracy Average**	**Web site URL**
IASP: Curriculum Outline on Pain for Nursing	Standard 1. Assessment	Education	4.83	http://www.iasp-pain.org/Education/CurriculumDetail.aspx?ItemNumber=2052
IASP: Classification of Chronic Pain	Standard 2. Diagnosis	Practice	4.83	http://www.iasp-pain.org/files/Content/ContentFolders/Publications2/FreeBooks/Classification-of-Chronic-Pain.pdf
FDA Drug Safety Communication: Prescription Acetaminophen Products to be Limited to 325 mg Per Dosage Unit; Boxed Warning Will Highlight Potential for Severe Liver Failure	Standard 5B. Health Teaching and Health Promotion Practice	Education	4.83	http://www.fda.gov/Drugs/DrugSafety/ucm239821.htm
Centers for Disease Control and Prevention (CDC): Prescription Painkiller Overdoses in U.S.	Standard 5D. Prescriptive Authority and Treatment (APRN)	Education	4.83	http://www.cdc.gov/vitalsigns/PainkillerOverdoses/
ASPMN: Pain Management in Patients with Substance Abuse Disorders	Standard 5D. Prescriptive Authority and Treatment (APRN)	Education	4.80	http://www.aspmn.org/documents/PainManagementinthePatientwithSubstanceUseDisorders_JPN.pdf
City of Hope Pain & Palliative Care Resource Center: IV. Pain and Symptom Management. C. Complementary, Alternative, and Integrative Approaches	Standard 5A. Coordination of Care	Practice	4.67	http://prc.coh.org/complementary.asp

[a]For a listing of the scores of all Web sites evaluated, go to www.nlinks.org and click on the Pain Database button.
[b]Within some ANA standard categories, there were no pain education/practice Web sites with accuracy scores ≥4.0, which was used as the initial cutoff in this original work.

a function of information use do we advance healthcare. Only when we track changes across systems of healthcare can we measure the impact on pain reduction in the population as a whole, increases in return-to-productivity, and decreases in healthcare costs. Structuring and evaluating the accuracy and overall value of clinical information on pain is one among many steps forward.

The **advanced nursing science and practice domain** (Appendix) is unchanged insofar as it remains divided into categories according to the ANA Standards of Practice. It is changed insofar as two new emphases are added. The first is that the definition of "diagnosis" is expanded to include the documentation of illness diagnoses, nursing diagnoses, additions/deletions to problem list, preventive care needs (including evidence-based screenings and vaccinations), medication reconciliation and adverse event review conclusions, and functional assessment conclusions. The second is to emphasize the need to document use of evidence-based, often templated, health education materials. Experienced clinical say, "We do this." They report that such needs are addressed verbally or that such needs are met by computer work-a-rounds as they prefer their own methods to computer-generated evidence-based alerts or download. However, the goal of electronic health records is to standardize care so that evidence-based practice is delivered and documented, and hence healthcare outcomes are improved and costs reduced. If evidence-based care is not standardized across healthcare system, healthcare will not be advanced. Furthermore, if documentation is deficient, then when electronic health records are reviewed in the aggregate, the value of advanced practice is underestimated. Nursing, is not visible unless it is documented.

Another section that is added in this edition's database of Internet tools for advanced practice is a section on opioid-related adverse events and deaths. That there is a problem is certain. That some of the remedies will increase the severity of pain in the population is a risk. Advanced practice nurses must help lead the healthcare and nursing communities to evidence-based solutions. It is hoped that the section on opioid therapy in the Appendix will assist in this endeavor.

REFERENCES

AARP and Robert Wood Johnson Foundation. (2013). *Virginia Action Coalition receives grant from Robert Wood Johnson Foundation.* Retrieved from http://states.aarp.org/vnfgrant/. Accessed on January 20, 2015.

AARP and Robert Wood Johnson Foundation. (2014). *Future of Nursing: Campaign for Action.* Retrieved from http://campaignforaction.org/. Accessed on January 20, 2015.

Alexander, J., & Tate, M. (1996–2005). *Original Web evaluation materials (1999–2005).* Widener University. Retrieved from http://www.widener.edu/about/campus_resources/wolfgram_library/evaluate/default.aspx. Accessed on January 20, 2015.

American Association of Colleges of Nursing. (2006). *The essentials of doctoral education for advanced nursing practice.* Retrieved from http://www.aacn.nche.edu/dnp/Essentials.pdf. Accessed on January 20, 2015.

American Association of Colleges of Nursing. (2011). *Core competencies for interprofessional collaborative practice.* Retrieved from http://www.aacn.nche.edu/education-resources/ipecreport.pdf. Accessed on January 20, 2015.

American Nurses Association. (2010). *Nursing: Scope and standards of nursing practice.* Silver Spring, Maryland: American Nursing Association.

American Nurses Credentialing Center. (2013). *Family Nurse Practitioner Board Certification Examination: Test content outline August 6, 2013.* Retrieved from http://www.nursecredentialing.org/FamilyNP-TCO. Accessed on January 20, 2015.

Boulus, N., & Bjorn, P. (2010). A cross-case analysis of technology-in-use practices: EPR-adaptation in Canada and Norway. *International Journal of Medical Informatics, 79*(6), E97–E108.

Fineberg, H. V., & Lavizzo-Mourey, R. (2013). *The future of nursing: A look back at the landmark IOM report.* Institute of Medicine. Retrieved from http://www.iom.edu/Global/Perspectives/2013/The-Future-of-Nursing.aspx. Accessed on January 20, 2015.

Health on the Net Foundation. (2013). HON code of conduct for medical and health websites. Retrieved from http://www.healthonnet.org/HONcode/Conduct.html. Accessed on January 20, 2015.

Health on the Net Foundation. (2014). HON services for the medical professionals. Retrieved from http://www.hon.ch/pat.html. Accessed on January 20, 2015.

Horeczko, T., & Green, J. P. (2013). Emergency department presentation of the pediatric systemic inflammatory response syndrome. *Pediatric Emergency Care, 29*(11), 1153–1158.

Hyppönen, H., Saranto, K., Vuokko, R., Mäkelä-Bengs, P., Doupi, P., Lindqvist, M., & Mäkelä, M. (2014). Impacts of structuring the electronic health record: A systematic review protocol and results of previous reviews. *International Journal of Medical Informatics, 83*(3), 159–169.

Illinois Campaign for Action. (2011, March 1). *Future of Nursing: Campaign for Action.* Retrieved from http://nursing.illinois.gov/PDF/2011-03-07_RAC_Campaign_Overview_2pgs.pdf. Accessed on January 20, 2015.

Institute of Medicine. (2010). *The future of nursing: Leading change, advancing health.* Washington, DC: National Academies Press. Retrieved from http://www.iom.edu/Reports/2010/The-Future-of-Nursing-Leading-Change-Advancing-Health.aspx. Accessed on January 20, 2015.

Institute of Medicine. (2011a). *Relieving pain in America: A blueprint for transforming prevention, care, education, and research.* Washington, DC: National Academies.

Institute of Medicine. (2011b). *Report at a glance. The future of nursing: Focus on scope of practice.* Washington, DC: National Academies Press. Retrieved from http://www.iom.edu/reports/2010/the-future-of-nursing-leading-change-advancing-health/report-brief-scope-of-practice.aspx. Accessed on January 20, 2015.

Lavin, M. A. (2002). President's address. *Nursing Diagnosis, 13*(2), 62–65. Retrieved from http://onlinelibrary.wiley.com/doi/10.1111/j.1744-618X.2002.tb00167.x/abstract. Accessed on January 17, 2015.

Lavin, M. A., Avant, K., Craft-Rosenberg, M., Herdman, T. H., & Gebbie, K. (2004). Contexts for the study of the economic influence of nursing diagnoses on patient outcomes. *International Journal of Nursing Terminologies and Classifications, 15*(2), 39–47.

Lavin, M. A., Krieger, M. M., Meyer, G. A., Spasser, M. A., Cvitan, T., Reese, C. G., … McNary, P. (2005). Development and evaluation of evidence-based nursing (EBN) filters and related databases. *Journal of Medical Library Association, 93*(1), 104–115.

McKay, R., Coombs, T., & Duerden, D. (2014). The art and science of using routine outcome measurement in mental health benchmarking. *Australas Psychiatry, 22*(1), 13–18.

Miller Center of Public Affairs. (2014, January). *Cracking the code on health care costs.* Charlottesville, Virginia:

University of Virginia. Retrieved from http://web1.millercenter.org/commissions/healthcare/HealthcareCommission-Report.pdf. Accessed on January 20, 2015.

Müller-Staub, M., Lavin, M. A., Needham, I., & van Achterberg, T. (2006). Nursing diagnoses, interventions and outcomes - application and impact on nursing practice: Systematic review. *Journal of Advanced Nursing, 56*(5), 514–531.

National Council of State Boards of Nursing. (2014). About NCSBN. *APRN Consensus Model Map*. Retrieved from https://www.ncsbn.org/736.htm. Accessed on January 20, 2015.

National Organization of Nurse Practitioner Faculties. (2012). *Statements & papers*. Retrieved from http://www.nonpf.org/?page=83. Accessed on January 20, 2015.

Nightingale, F. (1859). *A contribution to the sanitary history of the British army during the late war with Russia*. London: Harrison and Sons.

Picard, K. M., O'Donoghue, S. C., Young-Kershaw, D. A., & Russell, K. J. (2006). Development and implementation of a multidisciplinary sepsis protocol. *Critical Care Nurse, 26*(3), 43–54.

Robert Wood Johnson Foundation and AARP. (2010–2011). *Future of Nursing: Campaign for Action Dashboard*. Retrieved from http://campaignforaction.org/sites/default/files/CFA-dashboard-20130103.pdf. Accessed on January 20, 2015.

Robert Wood Johnson Foundation and AARP. (2012). *Future of Nursing: Campaign for Action, action coalition leaders*. Retrieved from http://www.thefuture-ofnursing.org/sites/default/files/Action%20Coalition%20%20Leaders%2006-25-2012.pdf. Accessed on January 20, 2015.

United Nations Development Programme (UNDP). (2007). *Evaluation of results-based management at UNDP*. New York: Suazion, Inc. Retrieved from http://web.undp.org/evaluation/documents/thematic/RBM/RBM_Evaluation.pdf. Accessed on January 20, 2015.

United Nations Framework Convention on Climate Change. (2014). *Criteria used in evaluating Web resources*. Retrieved from https://unfccc.int/essential_background/library/items/1420.php. Accessed on January 20, 2015.

van Prooijen, A. M., & Sparks, P. (2014). Attenuating initial beliefs: Increasing the acceptance of anthropogenic climate change information by reflecting on values. *Risk Analysis, 34*(5), 929–936. doi:10.1111/risa.12152.

BIBLIOGRAPHY

Agency for Healthcare Research and Quality. (n.d.). *Search: Nursing informatics roles at health information technology: Best practices transforming quality, safety and efficiency*. Retrieved from http://healthit.ahrq.gov/search/nursing%2520informatics%2520roles. Accessed on January 19, 2015.

Agency for Healthcare Research and Quality. (n.d.). *AHRQ Healthcare Innovations Exchange*. Retrieved from http://www.innovations.ahrq.gov/. Accessed on January 19, 2015.

Agency for Healthcare Research and Quality. (n.d.). *Search: Electronic health record at health information technology: Best practices transforming quality, safety and efficiency*. Retrieved from http://healthit.ahrq.gov/search/electronic%2520health%2520record. Accessed on January 19, 2015.

Agency for Healthcare Research and Quality. (n.d.). *Health IT tools and resources*. Retrieved from http://healthit.ahrq.gov/health-it-tools-and-resources. Accessed on January 19, 2015.

American Association of Nurse Practitioners. (n.d.). *NP Policy essentials*. Retrieved from https://www.aanp.org/legislation-regulation/policy-toolbox/np-policy-essentials. Accessed on January 19, 2015.

American Association of Nurse Practitioners. (n.d.). *Position statements & papers*. Retrieved from https://www.aanp.org/publications/position-statements-papers. Accessed on January 19, 2015.

American Nurses Association. (2006). *ANA recognized terminologies and data element sets*. Retrieved from http://ana.nursingworld.org/npii/terminologies.htm. Accessed on January 19, 2015.

American Nurses Association. (2008). *Health System Reform Agenda*. Retrieved from http://www.nursingworld.org/Content/HealthcareandPolicyIssues/Agenda/ANAsHealthSystemReformAgenda.pdf. Accessed on January 19, 2015.

American Nurses Association. (2014a). *Center for Ethics and Human Rights*. Retrieved from http://www.nursingworld.org/ethics/. Accessed on January 19, 2015.

American Nurses Association. (2014b). *Nursing-sensitive indicators*. Retrieved from http://www.nursingworld.org/MainMenuCategories/ThePracticeofProfessionalNursing/PatientSafetyQuality/Research-Measurement/The-National-Database/Nursing-Sensitive-Indicators_1. Accessed on January 19, 2015.

American Nurses Association. (2010, 2015). *Scope and standards of nursing, practice*. Retrieved from http://www.nursingworld.org/scopeandstandardsofpractice. Accessed on January 20, 2015.

American Nurses Credentialing Center. (2006). *The essentials of doctoral education for advanced nursing practice*. Retrieved from http://www.aacn.nche.edu/publications/position/DNPEssentials.pdf. Accessed on January 19, 2015.

American Nurses Credentialing Center. (2013). *Family Nurse Practitioner Board Certification Examination: Test content outline August 6, 2013*. Retrieved from http://www.nursecredentialing.org/FamilyNP-TCO. Accessed on January 19, 2015.

American Nurses Credentialing Center. (2014). *APRN Consensus Model and licensure, accreditation, certification, and education (LACE)*. Retrieved from http://www.

nursecredentialing.org/Certification/APRNCorner. Accessed on January 19, 2015.

American Society of Clinical Oncology (ASCO). (n.d.). *Ethical principles and the use of electronic health records.* Retrieved from http://am.asco.org/ethical-principles-and-use-electronic-health-records. Accessed on January 19, 2015.

American Society for Pain Management Nursing. (n.d.). *ASPMN: Pain management in patients with substance abuse disorders.* Retrieved from http://www.aspmn.org/organization/position_papers.htm. Accessed on January 19, 2015.

APRN Consensus Work Group & the National Council of State Boards of Nursing APRN Advisory Committee. (2008). *Consensus Model for APRN Regulation: Licensure, accreditation, certification & education.* Retrieved from https://www.ncsbn.org/Consensus_Model_for_APRN_Regulation_July_2008.pdf. Accessed on January 19, 2015.

Ascension Health. (n.d.). *Key ethical principles.* Retrieved from http://www.ascensionhealth.org/index. php?option=com_content&view=article&id=47& Itemid=171. Accessed on January 19, 2015.

British Standards Institution (BSI). (2014). *Structuring knowledge: Standards development briefing.* Retrieved from http://www.bsigroup.com/Global/our-services/developing-standards/Standards-development-briefing.pdf. Accessed on January 19, 2015.

Centers for Disease Control and Prevention (CDC). (2010, October 27). *Epidemiology and Analysis Program Office.* Retrieved from http://www.cdc.gov/osels/eapo/analytic_methods.html.

Centers for Disease Control and Prevention. (2011, November 1). *Prescription painkiller overdoses in U.S.* Retrieved from http://www.cdc.gov/vitalsigns/PainkillerOverdoses/. Accessed on January 19, 2015.

Centers for Disease Control and Prevention. (2013). Summary of notifiable diseases—United States, 2011. *Morbidity and Mortality Weekly Report (MMWR), 60*(53), 1–118. Retrieved from http://www.cdc.gov/mmwr/PDF/wk/mm6053.pdf. Accessed on January 19, 2015.

Centers for Medicare and Medicaid Services. (2014a). *Clinical quality measures.* Retrieved from http://www.cms.gov/Regulations-and-Guidance/Legislation/EHRIncentivePrograms/2014_ClinicalQualityMeasures.html. Accessed on January 19, 2015.

Centers for Medicare and Medicaid Services. (2014b). *Accountable care organizations (ACOs): General information.* Retrieved from http://innovation.cms.gov/initiatives/aco/. Accessed on January 19, 2015.

Centers for Medicare and Medicaid Services. (2014c). *Clinical laboratory improvement amendments (CLIA).* Retrieved from http://www.cms.gov/Regulations-and-Guidance/Legislation/CLIA/index.html?redirect=/clia/. Accessed on January 19, 2015.

Centers for Medicare and Medicaid Services. (2014d). *Meaningful USE.* Retrieved from http://www. cms.gov/Regulations-and-Guidance/Legislation/EHRIncentivePrograms/Meaningful_Use.html. Accessed on January 19, 2015.

Foley, J. (2014, March 3). Healthcare's next innovation? The answer is in the data. Forbes. *Forbes Magazine.* Retrieved from http://www.forbes.com/sites/oracle/2014/03/03/heathcares-next-innovation-the-answer-is-in-the-data/. Accessed on January 19, 2015.

Jacob, E. (n.d.). *Stanford intersection of medicine and emerging technologies: Wireless Pain Intervention Program for at risk youth with sickle cell disease.* Retrieved from http://medicinex.stanford.edu/jacob-abstract/. Accessed on January 19, 2015.

Kaiser Health News. (n.d.). *FAQ on ACOs: Accountable care organizations, explained.* Retrieved from http://www.kaiserhealthnews.org/stories/2011/january/13/aco-accountable-care-organization-faq.aspx. Accessed on January 19, 2015.

Minnesota Nurses' Association. (2006). *Nurses' guide to electronic health records.* Retrieved from http://mnnurses.org/nurses-guide-electronic-health-records-ehr-0. Accessed on January 19, 2015.

National Organization of Nurse Practitioner Faculties (NONPF). (2013). *Nurse practitioner core competencies.* Retrieved from http://c.ymcdn.com/sites/www.nonpf.org/resource/resmgr/competencies/npcorecompetenciesfinal2012.pdf. Accessed on January 19, 2015.

NCQA. (n.d.-a). *2015 HEDIS measures: Summary table of measures, product lines, and changes.* Retrieved from http://www.ncqa.org/Portals/0/HEDISQM/Hedis2015/List_of_HEDIS_2015_Measures.pdf. Accessed on January 19, 2015.

Poate, D. (n.d.). *Evaluation of results-based management at UNDP.* Evaluation Office, United Nations Development Programme. Retrieved from http://web.undp.org/evaluation/documents/thematic/RBM/RBM_Evaluation.pdf. Accessed on January 19, 2015.

Poghosyan, L., Nannini, A., & Clarke, S. (2013). Organizational climate in primary care settings: Implications for nurse practitioner practice. *Journal of the American Association of Nurse Practitioners, 25*(3), 134–140.

Poghosyan, L., Nannini, A., Stone, P. W., & Smaldone, A. (2013). Nurse practitioner organizational climate in primary care settings: Implications for professional practice. *Journal of Professional Nursing, 28*(6), 338–349.

Poghosyan, L., Nanninik, A., Finkelstein, S. R., Mason, E., & Shaffer, J. A. (2013). Development and psychometric testing of the nurse practitioner primary care organizational climate questionnaire. *Nursing Research, 62*(5), 325–334.

Sochalski, J., & Weiner, J. (2011). Appendix F. Health *care* system reform and the nursing workforce: Matching nursing practice and skills to future needs, not past demands. *The future of nursing: Leading change, advancing health* (pp. 375–400). Washington, DC: National Academies.

University of Pennsylvania School of Nursing. (2014). *Health technology innovation incubator.* Retrieved from http://www.nursing.upenn.edu/innovation/health-technology-lab/Pages/default.aspx. Accessed on January 19, 2015.

University of Toronto, Centre for Global eHealth Innovation. (2014). *Journal of Internet Medical Research.* Retrieved from http://ehealthinnovation.org/. Accessed on January 19, 2015.

University of Washington. (2014). *Global Nursing Leadership Toolkit.* CHSIERP. Retrieved from http://collaborate.uw.edu/educators-toolkit/global-nursing-leadership-toolkit.html-0. Accessed on January 19, 2015.

University of Wisconsin - Madison. (2014). *Wisconsin Institute for Discovery: Living environments laboratory.* Retrieved from http://wid.wisc.edu/research/lel/. Accessed on January 19, 2015.

U.S. Department of Health and Human Services. (2014a). HealthData.gov. Retrieved from http://www.healthdata.gov/. Accessed on January 19, 2015.

U.S. Department of Health and Human Services. (2014b). *The Health Insurance Portability and Accountability Act of 1996 (HIPAA) privacy, security and breach notification rules.* Retrieved from http://www.hhs.gov/ocr/privacy/. Accessed on January 19, 2015.

U.S. Department of Labor, Occupational Safety and Health Administration (OSHA). (2014). *Bloodborne pathogens and needlestick prevention.* Retrieved from https://www.osha.gov/SLTC/bloodbornepathogens/. Accessed on January 19, 2015.

U.S. Department of Veteran Affairs. (2014). *Online learning modules on general ethics topics.* Retrieved from http://www.ethics.va.gov/integratedethics/onlinemodules.asp. Accessed on January 19, 2015.

U.S. Food and Drug Administration. (2014). *FDA drug safety communication: Prescription acetaminophen products to be limited to 325 mg per dosage unit; boxed warning will highlight potential for severe liver failure.* Retrieved from http://www.fda.gov/Drugs/DrugSafety/ucm239821.htm. Accessed on January 19, 2015.

24

Nursing Informatics in Retail Clinics

Frances (Fran) M. Spivak / Sandra Festa Ryan

• OBJECTIVES

1. Understand the evolution of the retail industry and the need for innovation.
2. Understand the mission and the foundational characteristics of affordable, high-quality, easily accessible healthcare.
3. Understand the key services offered and how clinics operate and adjust services to meet consumer needs.
4. Understand the use of technology and innovation to validate the quality of care delivered in retail clinics.

• KEY WORDS

Retail clinics
Convenient care clinics
Quality/HEDIS
EHR
Patient engagement

Desktop computers replacing mainframes, smartphones displacing desktop computers and laptops, e-mail ousting "snail" mail as the communication method of choice around the world: These are more than just examples of how technology has advanced to bring us smarter, faster, more usable ways to live and work. These are also examples of disruptive innovations. Disruptive innovation can occur to fulfill a need in a market that traditional services have been unable to satisfy. These innovations often take a market by surprise, just like the retail clinic movement did to the traditional healthcare landscape. Retail clinics meet the definition of disruptive innovation in that they are a new way of delivering an existing service or product that enables a larger population of skilled but less expensive people to do in a more convenient, less expensive setting things that historically could be performed only by expensive specialists in centralized inconvenient locations (Christensen, Bohmer, & Kenagy, 2000).

Disruptive innovation has influenced healthcare like it has other industries. The current healthcare model is a business-centric not patient-centric delivery approach that is not transparent or easy for the patient to navigate. Patients must go to the medical office at a time convenient to the physician, not necessarily the patient. There are few consumers who would blindly purchase a product without first asking the cost yet this is the norm for how we access healthcare instead of the exception. To achieve our goals of affordable accessible quality care changes to our healthcare delivery model are occurring. These changes are focused on innovations that will enable (Townsend, 2013):

1. The utilization of skilled but less expensive healthcare personnel to provide appropriate levels of care

2. A shift away from traditional healthcare venues like hospitals and physician offices into other lower cost and/or more accessible settings like community-based retail clinics

3. Information technology to support individualized patient care, coordination of care across multiple care venues, and accessibility to care via new technologies like telehealth and ehealth

A growing as well as aging population with multiple chronic disease care needs and the expanded insurance coverage, as a result of the Affordable Care Act, are frequently cited as the causes of the expanded need for primary healthcare services. While demand for healthcare is growing the traditional workforce, primary care providers to meet this demand are not keeping pace. HRSA projects a 16% increase in the demand for primary care physicians by 2020 which will not be offset by the projected 8% increase in supply (United States Department of Health and Human Services, 2013).

The projected shortage of primary care physicians may be mitigated by the anticipated growth in the supply of Nurse Practitioners and Physician Assistants. By 2020 the number of NPs delivering primary care is projected to increase by 30% while the number of Physician Assistants delivering primary care is anticipated to increase by 58% (United States Department of Health and Human Services, 2013). Whether these growing provider groups can meet our nation's demands for primary care is dependent on whether their roles can be successfully integrated into the primary care delivery system and whether they will be allowed to practice at the highest level of their education and licensure.

The literature suggests that simply improving the supply of primary care providers will not meet the market demand for primary healthcare (Bodenheimer & Smith, 2013). Obsolete delivery models that do not address patient needs for accessible, convenient cost-effective care as well as the availability of the workforce delivering that care create additional barriers to delivering primary care services. To meet the demand for primary care services calls for a change to existing care delivery models. This change will be facilitated by clinical innovation that challenges or disrupts the status quo and information technology that improves provider productivity and enhances the quality of care.

RETAIL CLINICS: DISRUPTIVE INNOVATION FOR PRIMARY HEALTHCARE DELIVERY

Convenient, coordinated, high-quality, and affordable healthcare services remain unmet needs for many Americans. Retail clinics, also known as convenient care clinics, are a disruptive innovation designed to address these unmet needs.

Despite healthcare reform the rising cost of healthcare is a frequently identified issue for patients. While healthcare reform may alleviate this concern to some extent for the uninsured, insured workers' out of pocket expenses for healthcare have also continued to increase. As a result many patients with healthcare coverage are finding healthcare increasingly unaffordable (Berry & Mirabito, 2010).

Inconvenient and limited access to healthcare is another source of frustration for many patients. Planning activities in our lives means juggling time for work, family, education, and other related activities. Technology has facilitated our daily activities bringing to the average user the ability to access information, schedule and plan activities, work, and shop and even learn online. Consumers and businesses have embraced technology as a means to better use of time and resources and accessibility to services. This improved accessibility to products and services is available to virtually every facet of our lives except healthcare. When we need to access healthcare is not necessarily something easily planned for. Being able to see a physician where and when we want to is often difficult. As a result patients either wait longer than desirable to see their primary care physician or access care through already overburdened and not necessarily appropriate venues such as emergency departments. Fragmented care is also a possibility if a patient's primary care provider does not have the ability to access the record of healthcare provided outside his/her office.

The inception of retail clinics came from consumer demand for convenient, easily accessible, affordable quality healthcare. The first retail clinics opened their doors in 2000 and since that time have grown to more than 1400 clinics (Cunningham, 2013). Clinics are usually located in community-based retail locations such as drugstores, food stores, and other retail settings and offer a range of services. Given their retail and community-based locations, most clinics are open 7 days/week, 12 hours/day, 360 plus days/year. No appointments are necessary, even though some operators have appointments for some services, and walk-ins are welcome. Nearly half of retail clinic visits take place on weekends and during weekday hours when primary care offices are typically closed, reflecting their convenience and consumer focus (Hansen-Turton & Ridgeway, 2013). Most clinics see patients 18 months or older and visits take an average of 15 to 25 minutes. Visits range from preventative services such as sports physicals, wellness screenings, and vaccination to the majority of visits being acute episodic in nature such as otitis media, sinusitis, and urinary tract infections. Retail clinic costs are very transparent to the patient. Lower overhead costs are associated with retail clinics due to reduced administrative staffing needs, the utilization of NPs and PAs, and the smaller physical footprint needed for clinic operations. Lower overhead costs are also reflected in lower fees for similar care services in comparison with traditional primary care practices. Services and their associated fees are transparent at the clinic and are posted on LCD screens and on check-in Kiosks; they are also posted on company Web sites, so that patients have the information they need to make informed choices. Also readily available either on the clinic Web sites or in the retail establishments are locations and hours of operations for all clinics in a geographic area and nationally. While most clinic visits are handled on a walk-in basis, some operators additionally allow for scheduled appointments for clinic visits via the clinic Web sites or a centralized call in location.

Between 2007 and 2009, there was a sixfold increase in the number of visits to retail clinics (Ashwood et al., 2011). Several studies have been conducted to identify factors that would cause patients to favor using retail clinics over a traditional primary care provider. Convenience, decreased wait time, and lower cost of care were the primary reasons patients were "voting with their feet" by seeking care at retail clinics (Ashwood et al., 2011; Susman et al., 2013). Analysis of patient surveys regarding their experience with their retail clinic visit found 51% of patients would have used an emergency room or urgent care center had the retail clinic not been an option for a visit (Hunter, Weber, & Wall, 2009). Survey Respondents in a study examining provider preferences respondents preferred to see physicians vs. alternate providers (NPs, PAs) if the wait time was equal. However, if wait times were different most preferred to see the NP or PA instead of waiting for an appointment with the physician (Dill, Pankow, Erikson, & Shipman, 2013).

The retail clinic model is primarily staffed by Nurse Practitioners and to a lesser extent by Physician Assistants. Physicians collaborate with clinic providers in accordance with state law and regulation. Unlike physician offices, however, retail clinics are a single provider model where one provider handles all aspects of a patient's visit including registration, diagnosis, treatment, fee collection, discharge, and follow-ups, etc. Some clinics may also have ancillary

help, such as a medical assistant, to assist with some of this process depending on the typical volume of patients seen in the clinic.

From their inception, retail clinic operators planned for the use of technology as part of their clinic operations to address the lack of administrative and ancillary support typically found in primary care provider office visits. A typical physician office has many staff managing the patient's end-to-end visit. An office visit usually begins with administrative staff registering the patient, accessing the patient charts to update demographics and insurance information, determining insurance eligibility before the patient is handed off to medical staff for initial screening (height/weight/vital signs, documentation of chief complaint, etc.). The patient is then ready to see the doctor/provider and waits for his/her examination, diagnosis, and subsequent treatment if indicated. The provider's administrative or medical staff may then perform additional follow-ups such as referrals, scheduling for other visits, and collect the fee for service. This same visit workflow exists in retail clinics but is facilitated by a variety of integrated practice management, EMR, decision support, and patient facing technologies in order to meet the goals of convenient cost-effective quality care.

Retail clinics have always been committed to quality of care. In 2006, retail clinic operators met to form an association, the Convenient Care Association (CCA). The association and industry stakeholders placed a high priority on developing the 10 CCA Quality and Safety Standards for the industry. The first standard requires all clinic personal to be credentialed and licensed providers. Second, clinic operators demonstrate their commitment to high-quality care through peer review collaborating physician review and use of evidence-based practice guidelines. Third, all clinic operators must use EHRs which contribute to efficiency, accuracy, and continuity of care. In addition, clinic providers must establish relationships with local physicians, including primary care providers (PCPs), specialists, and emergency service providers, to ensure appropriate patient care in the event a patient presents with a condition outside the scope of the clinic's capability to address. Fourth, in the event a patient does not have a PCP, the patient will be encouraged to establish a relationship with a PCP. Fifth, the clinics will adhere to industry standards and regulations for healthcare providers such as OSHA, CLIA, HIPAA, etc. Sixth clinics are committed to assisting the patient to manage their health and wellness by providing patient education and counseling and a copy of their records for the encounter. The seventh standard addresses the importance of EHRs in supporting the continuity of care for a patient. EHR used in the clinics allows for the sharing of patient information with the patient's designated healthcare providers electronically via a direct interface using industry standards (HL7) and/or health information exchanges. The eighth and ninth standards address a safe clinic environment and emergency procedures are in place to ensure the safety of the patient. The tenth standard requires transparency of the cost of care so that the patients can make informed choices about their care (Hansen-Turton, Ridgway, Ryan, & Nash, 2009). These standards demonstrate the commitment to delivering quality care on the part of retail clinic operators as well as the value they place on technology to achieve their quality goals.

TECHNOLOGY USE IN RETAIL CLINICS TO DELIVER QUALITY CARE

Providing healthcare is a labor-intensive, knowledge-intensive, skill-intensive, and time-intensive activity (Berry & Mirabito, 2010). In a retail clinic one-provider-one-clinic-model information technology is used to streamline workflows and sharing of data across a variety of applications in order to reduce unnecessary work and streamline the time to deliver care. EHRs present to providers a longitudinal view of the patient's record and appropriate evidence-based clinical guidelines as well as decision support algorithms to support the diagnosis and treatment of the patient.

In retail clinics technology supports patient self-management, practice management, and clinical care delivery workflows.

Patient Self-Management

Engaging the patient in managing their care begins with empowering the patient to access their care where and when they need it. The community-based locations of retail clinics bring healthcare to where patients work, shop, and live. Clinic operators utilize similar models of delivery across their facilities which ensure a somewhat uniform patient experience regardless of where the patient seeks care. For retail clinics, with a national footprint not only can patients who travel have that experience in other parts of the country but their patient record can also be accessed as well.

Online or mobile accessed scheduling systems are being used in many industries to assist consumers in effectively utilizing their services. Consumers access scheduling systems to select convenient dates and times for services such as car repairs, haircuts, and restaurant reservations. Many patients feel comfortable using appointment technology

for their day-to-day activities and embrace the idea of using similar applications to access their healthcare services. For retail clinics, this means balancing the walk-in model of care with allocated time slots for appointments to maintain the flow of patients in a given clinic and efficient use of clinic resources. Part of any scheduling system is appointment reminders. Using secure text or e-mail messaging and/or other messaging options such as telephony, patients can receive reminders of upcoming clinic appointments. Reminders can increase the likelihood of the patient showing up for the visit or allow the patient to cancel the visit, thus freeing up the timeslot for another patient. Patient-managed scheduling also provides the clinic with the first opportunity to capture patient demographic data such as patient name, age, reason for visit, etc. This information can then be utilized in downstream workflows and/or applications to validate the identity of the patient and inform the provider of the reason for visit prior to meeting the patient so he/she can be prepared to deliver the services based on visit reason type.

When the patient arrives at a clinic he/she utilizes a variety of technology-based applications to begin the visit prior to interfacing with the provider. The patient is greeted not by an administrative staff but by kiosks and additional display hardware and applications which provide the information and instructions needed to begin the registration process.

Kiosks are used at clinics to begin the registration process and to inform the patient of wait times and approximate costs of service. A kiosk is a computer terminal with a specialized software application used to capture data that supports a specific business need or process. The kiosk serves two purposes: they replace the administrative staff role in traditional practices, thus supporting the one-clinic-one-provider model, and capture visit-specific data that can be shared with downstream applications such as the EHR to facilitate the provider workflows. Clinics may have more than one kiosk, thereby facilitating the check-in process for multiple patients waiting to see the provider. If the patient has scheduled the visit in advance on check-in patient and visit-specific data can pre-populate the kiosk to facilitate the registration process. During registration the kiosk captures key demographic data about the patient, i.e., name, address, date of birth, gender, as well as the reason for the patient's visit. From the kiosk the patient can find the fee schedule associated with the service they are seeking. If the kiosk captures insurance information the data can be used in conjunction with other financial applications to check for insurance eligibility for the service requested. Usability of the kiosk is an important consideration in the registration process. User experience design of the kiosk screens and flow take into account readability and comprehension as the patients move through the data capture screens. Some retail clinic operators support both English and Spanish versions of the kiosk. User experience design also facilitates easy edit of data entered either on the current or prior displays. Consent capture and financial responsibility information (how the patient will pay for the visit) finish the registration process for the patient and places the user in the queue of patients waiting to be seen by the provider.

The patient is asked to return to the kiosk at the end of the visit to participate in a survey measuring patient engagement and satisfaction with the visit. This information is used as part of a continuous quality improvement effort both personally for the provider and operationally for the clinic in general.

Queue monitors are another device frequently found in retail clinics. Typically these large screen wall mounted monitors reflect the number of patients waiting to be seen by the provider and any individual patient's place in that queue. Some queue systems can calculate approximate wait times for patients based on the reasons for visits of other patients in the queue. Queue monitors are a high patient satisfier for walk-in clinic traffic. As a patient registering for a visit you know exactly how many patients the provider must see before it is your turn and an approximate wait time.

Also found in some retail clinics is additional health information, often displayed on monitors for easy viewing in the waiting areas of the clinic. Information displayed on these monitors includes services provided by the clinic, fees related to the services, as well as general health information such as information about vaccinations.

The final step in the registration and queue management process is alerting the provider that a patient is waiting to be seen. The system will maintain a patient queue list that the provider can access and review prior to meeting the patient. Patient data in the queue list will reflect the data entered by the patient in the kiosk. The queue information helps the provider plan for the next visit and beyond, seeing the full patient load at any given point in time

Once a provider selects a patient from the queue there are two workflows the provider must follow to successfully complete a patient visit, both of which are heavily dependent on information technology. The provider must satisfy the business side of the visit, administrative, billing, reporting, etc., functionality typically defined and supported by practice management software. The provider must also be able to capture relevant clinical information, diagnosis and treatment plans for a patient, functionality typically defined and supported by electronic health records. In a one-clinic-one-provider model these workflows are intertwined and

the information technology that supports the flows must be integrated as well.

Practice Management

Retail clinics utilize technology to support several practice management tasks. Integration of patient demographic data captured in the kiosks feeds the next step in the visit process which is capture of patient insurance and financial information. Several input devices can be used to capture these data. Manual entry of insurance information and scanning of patient insurance documents are the two most common data entry techniques. This implies a scanning device must be available to the provider that is capable of capturing the data from insurance documents clearly and shared with downstream financial applications to support the visit billing process. As more insurers utilize "virtual insurance card" new input devices will be needed by the clinics to capture insurance information from patient smartphones or other mobile devices. The ability to read barcodes or sync with these devices from clinic hardware is an upcoming challenge for retail clinics as these virtual insurance cards become more common.

Once captured the insurance data are shared with an eligibility and verification system. If the service is not covered by the insurer the patient is responsible for payment and is informed accordingly. The ability to capture and verify eligibility for insurance must occur for all insurance carriers for the patient. If there is a payment due by the patient the system also manages pre-payment processing to capture payment due for the services provided. The insurance capture and pre-payment processing occurs prior to the patient being examined. Well-integrated concurrent processing of the various steps helps move the patient through the insurance data capture phase of the process quickly.

Administrative management tasks occur at various milestones throughout the clinical evaluation and documentation of the patient's visit. Once the patient exam has been conducted and a diagnosis and treatment plan identified the system facilitates billing functions including determination and selection of visit charges and codes, collection of payment due.

Evaluation and Management Coding, also known as E&M Coding, is the standardized medical billing process for patient encounters. Retail clinics also follow the E&M coding process for their patient encounters. The E/M codes are based on the American Medical Association's CPT or Current Procedural Terminology codes. To correctly code a visit per the standard the information system utilizes an algorithm that takes into account the documented data for the patient's health history (history of present illness, review of systems, past, family, and social history), physical exam findings, and the level of medical decision-making on the part of the provider needed to address the patient's healthcare issues. The more complex the patient's health history, the more detailed the physical exam may cause a more involved decision-making process on the part of the provider. If this is the case the provider can code the visit to reflect that complexity and be compensated for the level of work needed to address the patient's issues. Rules can be applied to clinical documentation that facilitates this coding process by suggesting billing codes to the provider based on documentation in the EHR. While it is always up to the provider to select the correct billing code, the system is using documented data to determine, based on standard E&M coding logic, the most likely billing code. If the provider believes the code is too high or low for the patient's encounter it is an opportunity to revisit the documentation to determine if clinical information accurately reflects the patient's status. Automating the calculation process facilitates assigning the correct billing code for the encounter.

One of the final steps in any practice is collecting payment from the patient. How the patient prefers to pay for the visit is first captured in registration with the kiosk. If the patient is insured that information along with the additional insurer data (i.e., copay) is carried forward to a final billing process step. The system determines fees for the services provided and calculates the bill for the patient. A bill is generated and payment calculated based on preferred payment method of the patient taking into account copays or other payment options.

Integration of this information with downstream financial billing systems allows for the correct billing of insurers, if applicable, for that visit as well as follow-up billing to patients for costs not covered by insurers.

To manage the administrative practice components of retail clinics requires capturing and processing patient demographic, financial, and clinical data. Clinical data capture occurs in the EHR utilized by the retail clinics. These EHRs facilitate data integration with internal (i.e., billing) and external (i.e., HIEs, Lab, etc.) to achieve continuity of care for the patient.

Clinical Documentation Management

EHRs are fundamental to the success of the retail clinics model of care. Like all practice EHRs, those developed for retail clinics support the assessment, diagnosis, and treatment workflows of the provider. The goal of the retail EMR is to help providers practice autonomously, streamlining administrative functions, while suggesting clinically appropriate actions generated from evidence-based practice guidelines and clinical documentation (Ryan, 2009).

All retail clinic visits begin with documentation of a core set of clinical data related to a patient's health history (past medical, family, social, and procedure), allergies, and medication and immunization history. This core information is captured for each patient on initial visit to the clinic and retrieved and updated as needed in subsequent encounters. These data are used as input to rules that drive suggested actions to a provider and focused documentation templates.

Historically retail clinics have provided a defined scope of services relative to acute episodic illness (i.e., sinusitis, urinary tract infections) and wellness activities (i.e., vaccinations). This emphasis is reflected in the retail EMR with a structured assessment process around commonly seen clinical problems. Focused assessment templates, i.e., vaccination specific, upper respiratory focused, etc., are created that drive data collection for a patient's problem. Rules are run on the data and associated values collected via these focused assessments to suggest treatment plans and patient education documentation as well as generate billing codes and provider follow-up tasks.

To complete the billing process providers must be able to assign the correct ICD code(s) for a clinical encounter. In traditional office practices diagnosis coding is usually done by coding experts. These experts review physician charts and assign the correct diagnosis code based on clinical documentation. In retail clinics coding assistance is built into the EHR system. Robust search functionality allows a provider to quickly find and select a code for the encounter. Quick pick lists of commonly used codes or the ability to save favorite codes facilitate the code selection process. As the country moves to utilizing ICD-10 the enhancements to EHR search as well as clinical documentation functionality will reflect the increased specificity of the diagnosis codes.

As part of the diagnosis and treatment plan a provider may need to order additional tests and/or medications to treat the patient's problem. The retail EHR will utilize industry standards to transmit orders from the system to external applications such as lab and radiology systems. In turn these systems will result back to the EHR the findings for the patient. The system integrates these externally sourced results into the patient record for review by the provider. System-generated tasks alert the provider that follow-ups are required for a patient ensuring timely action occurs.

E-prescribing or electronic prescribing is a technology by which a provider can electronically write and send prescriptions to a pharmacy from their EHR. E-prescribing has had a dramatic impact in improving the quality of patient care. A recent study of physicians in community-based office practices found 50% lower error rates for the practice one year after adopting an e-prescribing system (Abramson, et al. 2012). For retail clinics e-prescribing is integrated into the EHR and provides many benefits to the patient. E-prescribing allows the provider to access a patient's benefit information and choose medications that are covered by the patients' insurance provider. When a provider orders a medication drug interaction checking occurs, and if a contraindication is found it alerts the provider of the problem. E-prescribing also allows a provider to access a patient's medication history. This information facilitates the medication reconciliation process for the patient as well as informs the provider of potential patient health issues. E-prescribing systems also allow the provider to route the prescription to the patient's pharmacy of choice. An electronically transmitted prescription removes safety issues that occur with handwritten prescriptions and saves time in the prescribing process.

One of the quality standards all retail clinics are committed to is sharing a discharge summary of the encounter with the patient's primary care provider to ensure continuity of care. If the provider's system is capable the discharge summary can be transmitted electronically to their EHR in an HL7. The retail EMR is also capable of an integrated faxing solution, e-faxing the discharge summary to providers incapable of receiving it electronically. Reporting of immunizations to state registrations is mandated in many states. The retail EHR is able to support that regulatory mandate via standardized interface transactions.

RETAIL CLINIC ROLE IN PATIENT-CENTRIC CARE

The healthcare reform movement hopes to achieve its goals of quality care at reduced costs through coordinated primary care delivery systems and promotion of medical homes. Accountable Care Organizations (ACOs) are networks of providers with unified governance that assume risk for the quality and total cost of the care they deliver (Burns & Pauy, 2013). Common strategies ACOs employ to achieve these goals are improved care coordination, use of non-physician providers such as nurse practitioners and other health professions, formation of patient-centered medical homes, and use of information technology.

Patient-Centered Medical Home (PCMH) is being promoted as the future of primary care practice. Retail clinics are well positioned to become a key component of ACOs and PCMH. Clinics, through their network of community-based sites, can identify primary care needs of the newly insured population. Closing the gaps in care for these patients occurs when the clinic providers help the patients

find a medical home. Affiliations between retail clinics and community-based providers facilitate referrals to PCMH and extend the reach of PCMH as they utilize retail clinics as treatment options. These affiliations also have the potential to expand the retail clinic's scope of services, for example, chronic disease management, as retail clinics partner in the management of the patient's health with PCMH.

Retail clinics and PCMH will utilize information technology to manage care across their separate but linked venues. Technology will allow retail clinics and PCMH to share patient information, coordinate care across different providers, and better involve patients in the healthcare process (Colpas, 2013). There are several IT capabilities retail clinics have in common with PCMH to deliver coordinated patient care. Utilization of Electronic Health Records enables documentation and tracking of patient conditions as well as coordination of care through shared information. Clinical decision support systems improve the decision-making of providers, reduce medication errors through e-prescribing, and facilitate the use of evidence-based guidelines when incorporated into retail and practice EHR systems. Communication tools facilitate care transitions when data can be shared seamlessly between organizations via health or other data exchanges. Shared information will further strengthen a team-based approach to care, where PCPs see clinic providers as extensions of their practices, not competitors (Morrissey, 2013).

As retail clinics become partners in PCMH networks additional technology needs will arise. Patient engagement tools that incorporate patient self-reported data will help clinicians manage patient conditions. Both retail clinics and PCMH will look to online or mobile applications to involve patients in their care process. Patients will continue to look for healthcare options that are convenient and new technologies such as telehealth will allow clinic and PCMH providers to manage greater caseloads of patients and/or interact at times and places most convenient for the patient.

FUTURE OF RETAIL CLINICS

The rapidly changing healthcare market is providing a unique opportunity for advanced practice nurses to provide high-quality, cost-effective accessible care via retail clinic practices. Retail clinics are a disruptive innovation because they operate outside conventional physician offices, disrupting existing models of primary care (Glabman, 2009). Technology, EHRs, e-prescribing, data exchange are drivers in consumer acceptance of retail clinic services.

From their inception retail clinics have viewed themselves as one member of the care team that a patient can access to meet their healthcare needs. Healthcare access, productivity, and effectiveness can be improved through a team approach to care (Berry & Mirabito, 2010). When the patient utilizes the right care venue with the appropriate level provider and technology facilitates the communication necessary for coordinated care all involved parties—patient, retail clinic, and PCMH—benefit.

Information technology is the foundation upon which the retail clinic business has been built. This foundation enables retail clinics to rapidly respond to market demands of its consumers and care delivery partners.

REFERENCES

Abramson, E. L., Bates, D. W., Jenter, C., Volk, L. A., Barron, Y., Quaresimo, J., ... Kaushal, R. (2012). Ambulatory prescribing errors among community-based providers in two states. *Journal American Medical Informatics Association, 19*(4), 644–648.

Ashwood, J. S., Reid, R. O., Steodji, C. M., Weber, E., Gaynor, M., & Mehrotra, A. (2011). Trends in Retail Clinic Use Among the Commercially Insured. *The American Journal of Managed Care, 17*(11), e443–e448.

Berry, L. L., & Mirabito, A. M. (2010). Innovative healthcare delivery. *Business Horizons, 53,* 157–169.

Bodenheimer, T. S., & Smith, M. D. (2013). Primary care: Proposed solutions to the physician shortage without training more physicians. *Health Affairs, 32*(11), 1881–1886.

Burns, L., & Pauy, M. (2013). Accountable care organizations may have difficulty avoiding the failures of integrated delivery networks of the 1990s. *Health Affairs, 31*(11), 2407–2416.

Christensen, C. M., Bohmer, R., & Kenagy, J. (2000, September–October). Will disruptive innovations cure health care? *Harvard Business Review, 78*(5), 102–112,199.

Colpas, P. (2013, July). Accountable care organizations help to coordinate care. *Health Management Technology, 34*(7), 6–9.

Cunningham, R. (2013, October 22). Health workforce needs: Projections complicated by practice and technology changes. *Issue Brief (George Washington University. National Health Policy Forum). 851,* 1–15.

Dill, M., Pankow, S., Erikson, C., & Shipman, S. (2013). Survey shows consumers open to a greater role for physicians assistants and nurse practitioners. *Health Affairs, 32*(6), 1135–1142.

Glabman, M. (2009, January). Disruptive innovations that will change your life in healthcare. *Managed Care.* Retrieved from http://www.managedcaremag.com/archives/0901/0901.disruptive.html

Hansen-Turton, T., & Ridgeway, C. G. (2013). The future of accessible, affordable, quality health care. In J. Riff, S. F. Ryan, & T. Hansen-Turton (Eds.), *Convenient care clinics the essential guide to retail clinics for clinicians, managers, and educators* (pp. 1–9). New York, NY: Springer.

Hansen-Turton, T., Ridgway, C., Ryan, S. F., & Nash, D. (2009). Convenient care clinics: The future of accessible health care—The formation years 2006-2008. *Population Health Management, 12*(5), 231–240.

Hunter, L., Weber, C., & Wall, J. (2009). Patient satisfaction with retail health clinic care. *Journal of the American Academy of Nurse Practitioner, 21,* 565–570.

Morrissey, J. (2013, May). Medical home: Health IT's next evolution. *Hospitals & Health Networks, 87*(5), 22–23.

Ryan, S. F. (2009). Providing high tech patient care. *The Nurse Practitioner, 34*(10), 6–7.

Susman, A., Dunha, L., Snower, K., Hu, M., Martilin, O., Shrank, W., ... Brennan, T. (2013). Retail clinic utilization associated with lower total cost of care. *The American Journal of Managed Care, 19*(4), e148–e157.

Townsend, J. C. (2013, April 23). Disruptive innovation: A prescription for better healthcare. *Forbes.* Retrieved from http://www.forbes.com/sites/ashoka/2013/04/23/disruptive-innovation-a-prescription-for-better-health-care/

United States Department of Health and Human Services. (2013). *Projecting the supply and demand for primary care practitioners through 2020.* Retrieved from http://bhpr.hrsa.gov/healthworkforce/supplydemand/usworkforce/primarycare/projectingprimarycare.pdf

25

Care Delivery Across the Care Continuum: Hospital–Community–Home

Charlotte A. Weaver / Laura Heermann Langford

• OBJECTIVES

1. Define the post-acute care delivery continuum and their contribution to the *Triple Aims* of increased quality at reduced costs, improved patient experience, and improved population health.
2. Identify the current state of standards needed for care coordination across post-acute care delivery.
3. Describe how healthcare policy and regulations require participation of all care delivery sites including post-acute care to accomplish full care coordination.
4. Explain the current functionality and adoption of electronic health record tools available to and used by post-acute care providers.

• KEY WORDS

Care Delivery
Post-acute care
Care planning
Care plan
Care coordination
Care transition
Quality improvement
National quality strategy
Community
Inpatient-Rehabilitation Facilities (IRF)
Skilled Nursing Facilities (SNF)
Long-Term Care Providers (LTCH)
Home Health Agencies (HHA)
Hospice
Standards Development Organizations (SDOs)

INTRODUCTION

This chapter focuses on a little known, often overlooked, and poorly understood segment of our healthcare system—post-acute care. As decision-makers in care planning and care coordination, nurses' and physicians' formal education often does not include training in these clinical settings nor is the subject covered adequately in curriculum. Consequently, many health professionals carry an insufficient understanding of the post-acute care providers and how they can augment their care plan for a given patient. As we move into the new health reform initiatives mandated under the Patient Protection and Affordable Care Act (ACA) (United States Congress, 2010), a major challenge in achieving the *Triple Aims* of increased quality at reduced costs, improved patient experience, and improved population health is our ability as a healthcare system "to integrate its work over time and across sites of care"(Berwick, Nolan, & Whittington, 2008).

In this chapter, we provide a detailed overview of the post-acute providers recognized and reimbursed for their care by CMS, and placed in the context of the current health reform environment. We highlight the primary entities driving reform and describe the role each plays and their area of contributions. We link the reform initiatives to reimbursement changes and describe how these payment mechanisms are driving new care delivery models that require tight integration with post-acute care providers for optimal outcomes. Informatics is front and center to health reform because care delivery system integration and care coordination require a sophisticated information infrastructure beyond where we are today (Rudin & Bates, 2014). In our current state electronic health record (EHR) systems' review of the post-acute industry, we emphasize the gaps in functionality needed to support standards, care transitions, and coordination. Most importantly, we look at the near-future policy directions for new care delivery methods that require shared care plans, with the ability to send and receive patient information, and to generate outcome reporting. In support of these new technology requirements, we give an update on the progress being made by standards development organizations, and specifically the work being done by the Office of the National Coordinator's (ONC) Standards and Integration Framework (S&I Framework) (Office of the National Coordinator, 2014b).

HEALTHCARE REFORM

The fragmentation of the United States (U.S.) healthcare delivery system is well documented (Bodenheimer, 2008; Mehrotra, Forrest, & Lin, 2011; Shih et al., 2008).

And despite the United States having the highest spending per person of all the industrialized countries, it falls below the majority of the Organization for Economic Co-operation and Development (OECD) nations on major health indices, including having the highest rates for obesity (Organization for Economic Co-operation and Development, 2013; World Health Organization, 2013). In 2011, the United States spent $8500 per person, nearly double that of all other OECD nations and $2800 higher than the next highest, Norway (Hess & Sauter, 2013; World Health Organization, 2013). Similarly, the United States has the highest spending per GDP (Gross Domestic Product) of the OECD nations, 17.7% compared to the next highest country, the Netherlands, at 11.9% (Hess & Sauter, 2013; World Health Organization, 2013). The imperative to reform our healthcare system is driven by these economics.

Development of the National Strategy for Quality Improvement

The current reform framework and changes in reimbursement policies have been pushed forward by a number researchers, private institutes, and government agencies building upon each other's work. Most notable are the contributions from Berwick and colleagues from the Institute of Healthcare Improvement (Berwick et al., 2008) and the work of the Commonwealth Fund's Commission on High Performance Healthcare System (Shih et al., 2008). Taken together, these two bodies of work redefined what should be the focus of care delivery—the Triple Aims (Berwick et al., 2008), and detailed how a "high performance healthcare system" needs to operate and deliver care to achieve value (Shih et al., 2008). The policy recommendations from both Berwick's and Shih's groups informed the guiding aims and priorities adopted by the Department of Health and Human Services (HHS) in its National Strategy for Quality Improvement's framework for change (Agency for Health & Research Quality, 2013a). This reform framework, first published by the Agency for Health and Quality Research (AHRQ) in March 2011 as the National Quality Strategy (NQS), is based on a translated version of IHI's triple aims of "better care, healthy people/healthy community, and affordable care" and six priorities that target making care safe, coordinated, based on evidence of clinical effectiveness, development of new care delivery and reimbursement models, and community level focus for healthier living (Agency for Health & Research Quality, 2013a).

Significantly, for post-acute care providers, one of the six national priorities targets care coordination with expectations for managed care transitions and communication across care settings (Agency for Health & Research Quality, 2013b). Patients with chronic illness and disability are to have a current and shared care plan used by all providers, coordinated through primary care with extensions into community-based providers. NQS includes that there is to be shared accountability of every member of the care team and organizational entity. Access to patient information is to be readily available to every team member, including the patient, and measurements and reporting requirements are required from each integrated partner. The implications of these care delivery mandates for the level of functionality, standards and interoperability needed in our EHR systems across all sectors represent both opportunity and challenge for all of us (Agency for Health & Research Quality, 2012).

Affordable Care Act's Operational Arms

The two most influential health policy bodies created by mandate of the 2010 Affordable Care Act (ACA) are the CMS Innovation Center (Centers for Medicare and Medicaid Services Innovation Center, 2014) and the Patient-Centered Outcomes Research Institute (PCORI) (Patient-Centered Outcomes Research Institute, 2014). The CMS Innovation Center is focused on patient populations using Medicare, Medicaid, or Children's Health Insurance Program (CHIP). Its charge is to test *"innovative payment and service delivery models to reduce program expenditures …while preserving or enhancing the quality of care"* (Centers for Medicare and Medicaid Services Innovation Center, 2014). The CMS Innovation Center is driving structural, care delivery initiatives, such as "Accountable Care Organizations" with the concepts of payment linked to "bundling" of services across a care continuum to manage a given population's health outcomes (Centers for Medicare and Medicaid Services, 2013c; Centers for Medicare and Medicaid Services Innovation Center, 2014; Linehan, 2012; Medicare Payment Advisory Commission, 2010). And complementing this payment system reform focus is PCORI's mandate to *"increase the quantity, quality, and timeliness of usable, trustworthy comparative research information; to accelerate the implementation and use of research evidence; and to exert influence on research funded by others to make it more patient-centered and useful"* (Selby & Lipstein, 2014, p. 592). PCORI funds comparative clinical effectiveness research on treatment methods, drugs, devices, and systems, and mechanisms for the rapid dissemination of these research findings for them to be put into practice rapidly (Selby & Lipstein, 2014). Funding levels for the first three years of PCORI from 2010 to 2013 was $316 million for 192 studies, with the next three years funded at $1.5 billion (Selby & Lipstein, 2014). These two important HHS health policy entities are driving rapid change within our healthcare practice structures linked as they are to new reimbursement incentives and penalties.

INTRODUCING THE POST-ACUTE PROVIDERS

It can be confusing and difficult to those outside of the post-acute care sector to differentiate between the unique services each provides from those that overlap. While not the sole providers of post-hospital care, traditionally CMS includes home health agencies, skilled nursing facilities, inpatient rehabilitation facilities, and long-term care hospitals in this "post-acute care" category (Medicare Payment Advisory Commission, 2012b). To assist in this overview, Table 25.1 (Centers for Medicare and Medicaid Services, 2012; Centers for Medicare and Medicaid Services, 2013a; Medicare Payment Advisory Commission, 2012a, 2012b; Medicare Payment Advisory Commission, 2013a, 2013b) lists each CMS recognized entity, the type of patient services provided, differences, patient eligibility requirement, payment structure, and episode period. Medicare and Medicaid pay the significant portion of care expense for care delivered in the post-acute sector. The Medicare benefit pays for skilled care, therapy, and other services delivered by inpatient rehabilitation facilities (IRF), skilled nursing facilities (SNF), long-term care providers (LTCH), home health agencies (HHA), and hospice. Patients accessing the post-acute providers instead of ambulatory centers or clinics are those who are home bound, or have need of inpatient level of care, have restricted mobility, or are at six months or less at end of life.

Just the sheer numbers of post-acute care providers and the volume of patients that each serves per year show that we cannot reach the goal of an integrated healthcare system at community levels without their inclusion in healthcare reform. As listed at the bottom of Table 25.1, if nursing homes are included in post-acute care providers, there are over 44,500 organizations in this sector (Centers for Medicare and Medicaid Services, 2012; Medicare Payment Advisory Commission, 2013a). In 2012, approximately 3.5 million Medicare beneficiaries, or 10.6% of the 37.2 million Medicare beneficiaries, used home health services representing an average annual increase of 3.1% since 2002 (Centers for Medicare and Medicaid Services, 2013a; Medicare Payment Advisory Commission, 2013a). Similarly, hospice use between 2000 and 2012 has increased annually an average of 8.7%, with just under 1.3 million Medicare beneficiaries served in 2012 as compared to 513,000 in 2000 (Centers for Medicare and Medicaid Services, 2013a). Skilled Nurses Facilities paid

TABLE 25.1 Post-Acute Care Providers, Defining Characteristics, Criteria for Admission, and CMS Reimbursement

Category	Long-Term Acute Care Hospital (LTAC)	Inpatient Acute Rehabilitation (IRF)	Skilled Nursing Facility (SNF)	Home Health (HHA)	Palliative	Hospice	Nursing Home (NH)
FOCUS	Patients with multiple comorbidities, exacerbation of chronic illness, or catastrophically injured. High medical acuity	Restoration of functional independence	Step-down medical/rehab care (skilled care)	Health services are provided in their places of residence for the purpose of promoting, maintaining, or restoring health, or maximizing the level of independence, while minimizing the effects of disability and illness, including terminal illness. Home bound: Normally unable to leave home unassisted To be homebound means that leaving home takes considerable and taxing effort	Patient living with serious and complex chronic illness(es) with significant burden that may last for years Homebound to qualify for Home Health Palliative Services Can continue to seek aggressive treatment	Disease directed therapies are no longer working Projected terminal within six months Four Levels of Care: *Routine Care: in the home scheduled intermittent visits—hospice staff available on-call *Continuous Care—home setting—crisis intervention staff may stay in home for many hours *Respite Care: allows break for caregiver. Transfer to a facility for up to five days. *General Inpatient Care: more complex needs—cannot be managed in the home.	Long-Term Supportive Care (Custodial) Considered patient's home
Anticipated Length of Stay	25 days or greater	10 to 15 days	15–20 days or greater	Per episode (Acute or Chronic). And had a skilled need	Not dependent on life expectancy	six months or less	Indefinite—Patient's Home
Program for Medically Complex Patients	YES	NO	SOME	YES	YES	YES	NO
Program for Patients Requiring Ventilator Weaning	YES	NO	NO	SOME	High Flow Oxygen Needs	NO	NO

24-Hour Respiratory Therapy	YES	NO	NO	NO	NO	Depending on Level of Care Needs	NO
Telemetry Monitoring	YES	NO	NO	Telehealth Monitoring of Vital signs and weight	Telehealth Monitoring of Vital signs and weight	SOME—Vital Signs	NO
Nursing Activity	At least 6.5 hours per patient day	Three to five hours per patient day Requires daily skilled care	Based on Skilled Nursing need	Based on Skilled Nursing number of days per week	Based on Skilled Nursing number of days per week	Based on Skilled Nursing need	Variable. Custodial care
Daily Physician visits	YES May also have consultants Assessment or Intervention Daily	YES but minimally Three times per week (Physiatrist) may also have a consultant	NO As needed and Minimally every 30 days	NO Requires a Face-to-Face 90 days prior to admission to home health or within 30 days of admission to home health	NO Requires a Face-to-Face 90 days prior to admission to home health or within 30 days of admission to home health	Depending on Level of Care Needs	NO. As needed and Minimally every 30 days
Program for Rehabilitative Services	YES	YES Must be able to tolerate three hours per day	YES as needed, no minimum	YES Based on Therapy Assessment Functional Needs	YES Depending on Functional Level Assessment	NO	YES as needed, no minimum
License	Acute Hospital	Acute Rehab Unit/Hospital	Skilled Nursing	Home Health Agency	Level of Care offered through Home Health Agency	Hospice	Skilled Nursing
Therapy Program	Optional	Three hours or more per day at least five days per week	Optional—usually one to two hours per day five days a week	Core	Depending on Functional Level Assessment	NO	Optional
Patient Profile	Medically Complex	Functionally impaired/Medically Stable	Chronic Medical/Functional Conditions	Acute Medical and Chronic Medical/Skilled Nursing and Functional Conditions	Patient requires relief from the symptoms, pain, and stresses of a serious illness—whatever the diagnosis	Patient has a terminal illness and prognosis is six months or less that is certified by the physician	Chronic Medical/Functional Conditions

(continued)

TABLE 25.1 Post-Acute Care Providers, Defining Characteristics, Criteria for Admission, and CMS Reimbursement *(continued)*

Category	Long-Term Acute Care Hospital (LTAC)	Inpatient Acute Rehabilitation (IRF)	Skilled Nursing Facility (SNF)	Home Health (HHA)	Palliative	Hospice	Nursing Home (NH)
General Admission Criteria	Intensive medical/surgical treatment Medical complexity and 24-hour intermediate critical care/acute medical surgical No minimum short-term acute stay required	Medically stable 24-hour rehab nursing Must be able to tolerate three hours of therapy per day No acute hospital stay required	Medically stable 24-hour rehab nursing or restorative care, therapy as needed Three-day acute care stay prior to admission is required Medically complex with comorbidities Can discharge to Home Health or Hospice	Willing and able caregiver Skilled home care services for assessment, treatment, monitoring, or education and/or Skilled therapy need Medically stable Homebound	Willing and able caregiver Skilled home care services for assessment, treatment, monitoring, or education and/or Skilled therapy need Medically stable Homebound	Patient has a terminal illness and prognosis is six months or less Willing and able caregiver	Medically stable 24-hour rehab nursing or restorative care, therapy as needed Three-day acute care stay prior to admission is required from STACH
Patient Assessment Data Set	CARES	IRF-PAI	MDS	OASIS—C1	Uses either Hospice or HHA	HIS	MDS
Case Mix System		CMG (Case Mix Group)	RUG (Resource Utilization Groups)	HHRG (Home Health Resource Groups)	Uses either Hospice or HHA	Level of Care	RUG (Resource Utilization Groups)
Unit of Payment	Discharge	Discharge	Day	60-Day Episode	Uses either Hospice or HHA	Day	Day
Average LOS	26.6 days	13.1 days	27 days	Two episodes	No data	86 days (Median = 18 days)	≥1 year
Average Payment per Unit	$38,582	$17,085	$10,808	$2,691	No data	$11,321	Medicaid
Number of Organizations in 2012	437	1,166	15,139	12,225		3612	15,671

Sources:

MedPAC. (2013, March). *Report to Congress: Medicare Payment Policy*, Chapter 12: Hospice, p. 270. Retrieved from http://www.medpac.gov/chapters/mar13_ch12.pdf. Accessed on February 24, 2014.

MedPAC. (2012). A data book: Health Care Spending and the Medicare program. June 2012.

MedPAC. (2013). A data book: Health Care Spending and the Medicare Program, June 2013. Retrieved from http://www.medpac.gov/documents/Jun13DataBookEntireReport.pdf. Accessed on February 24, 2014.

MedPAC. (2012). *Payment basics series for skilled nursing facility, home health agency, inpatient rehabilitative facility, and long-term care hospital services*, 2012. Retrieved from www.medpac.gov

CMS (2012). *Nursing Home Data Compendium, 2012.* Retrieved from https://www.cms.gov/Medicare/Provider-Enrollment-and-Certification/CertificationandComplianc/downloads/nursinghomedatacompendium_508.pdf. Accessed on March 1, 2014.

for under the Medicare benefit was almost $27.6 billion in fiscal year 2012 and served 1.7 million Medicare beneficiaries (Centers for Medicare and Medicaid Services, 2013a). The 2012 Medicare spend for post-acute care was about 12% of total program expenditures: SNF at 6%; home health at 3.6%; hospice at 2.1%; and IRFs and LTHCs at just about 1.5% (Centers for Medicare and Medicaid Services, 2013a; Medicare Payment Advisory Commission, 2013a). The marked growth in the use of post-acute care over the last decade is due in part to the unprecedented growth in the number of Americans aged 65 or older. In addition to Americans just living longer, the impact of the post-World War II baby boom is expanding the proportionate percentage of elderly in our U.S. demographics. Starting January 1, 2011, each and every day about 10,000 Americans have turned 65 years old, and this trend is projected to continue through to 2030 when about 72 million people will be over 65, or about 20% of Americans (Centers for Disease Control and Prevention, 2013).

As detailed in Table 25.1, every post-acute care setting carries eligibility requirements that must be met to be paid by CMS under Medicare. Long-term care hospitals (LTCH) and inpatient rehabilitation facilities (IRFs) must meet the same conditions of participation that acute care hospitals are held to for admissions and facilities criteria (Linehan, 2012). Unique to IRFs is the requirement that 60% of their patients must have one of 13 diagnoses specified by Medicare and this is referred to as the "60 percent rule". In addition to patients needing inpatient care, they must need and be expected to improve with intensive rehabilitation therapy three hours or more per day/five days per week. LTCH's only program requirement for patients is that their average length of stay must be greater than 25 days (Linehan, 2012). Patients in need of skilled nursing facilities services commonly are those recovering from orthopedic surgeries, or other medical conditions requiring short-term skilled nursing care and rehabilitation services, such as stroke, neurological conditions, or acute pneumonia. Rehabilitative therapies include physical therapy, occupational therapy, and importantly for stroke and neurological patients' access to speech-language services that address safe eating, swallowing, and communication. Most SNFs are part of a nursing home that treats patients who have exceeded the SNF 100-day limit, and generally, are given less intensive, long-term care services than the skilled services required for Medicare coverage.

Home healthcare is the largest of all the post-acute care providers and continues to grow annually. Eligibility is tied to home-bound status, defined as requiring "considerable and taxing effort" to leave the home, and to the need for skilled nursing care or therapy to maintain or improve their health status and/or functional capacities.

Over the past decade, home health agencies are becoming less of a post-hospital admission provider, and are taking an increasing percentage of their referrals from physician's offices, clinics, and community-based Assisted Living Facilities. Between 2001 and 2009, home health episodes not preceded by an inpatient stay increased from 52% to 65% (Medicare Payment Advisory Commission, 2012b, p. 213). Hospice eligibility is linked to certification by an attending physician and a hospice medical director that the person is terminal and at the end-stage of their disease trajectory with six or less months to live. Hospice is also covered under the Medicare benefit, but until recently, was seldom used as a discharge destination from a hospital stay.

The Role for Post-Acute Care Providers

Increasingly, as Care Transitions demonstration projects mandated under the 2010 Affordable Care Act (ACA) have generated lessons learned in care coordination, other post-acute care providers, such as Hospices and Kidney Dialysis Centers, have started to be included in planning (Linehan, 2012; Medicare Payment Advisory Commission, 2012b). For example, in Care Transition partnerships between home health agencies (HHA) and hospitals, these teams quickly learned how imperative it was to have a clinical profile tool with risk criteria that could differentiate and identify individuals at the "end-of-life" stage of a chronic disease from those with longer term trajectories. Without this specificity, these terminal patients were referred to providers with a rehabilitative or curative mandate post-discharge, such as home health or a Skilled Nursing Facility (SNF). Because these patients are those projected as having a six months' life expectancy, they are inherently not medically stable and the result is frequent Emergency Room visits and rehospitalizations (Advisory Board, 2010).

This advancement in care transitions initiatives required care planning changes that depended on informatics and data analysis. In these early initiatives, the partners had to have the ability to tract patients who had to be readmitted within 30 days from hospital discharge and report back to their partners. This meant that the SNF's or HHA's clinical information system had to have the ability to capture patients' clinical profiles, protocol treatment outcomes, and clinical data with the ability to share with the hospital partner. This level of functionality is largely missing in today's systems (Agency for Health & Research Quality, 2012; Bates & Bitton, 2010; Resnick & Alwan, 2010; Weaver & Moore, 2011). What most organizations report is that the functionality limitations needed to support care transitions and coordination are being compensated for by staff doing some portion of tracking and reporting manually. The second major change that was informed by the data was for hospitals to actively include hospice as a post-hospital destination and to take on the hard conversations with physicians, patient, and family to have that option available to the patient. Once organizations made the leap to start looking for end-of-life criteria and defined hospice as an appropriate discharge placement (if patient and family agreed), progress was made. Doing appropriate discharge planning for hospice eligible individuals rather than referring to home health has helped mitigate rehospitalizations in this vulnerable population as well as improving the individuals' experience from their care. It is in understanding the services that each post-acute care provider offers, that will allow us to align patients' post-discharge care plan with their needs and wishes. It is essential to know which setting offers what services on the curative, rehabilitative to preventative and palliative care continuum to match patients wishes to correct setting and achieve a healthcare system that embodies the means to deliver on the Triple Aim goals.

CLINICAL INFORMATION SYSTEMS IN POST-ACUTE CARE

Just as Meaningful Use (MU) incentives are impacting acute and ambulatory care providers, they are also affecting the post-acute care providers even though they are not included as eligible providers for payment incentives (Blumenthal & Tavenner, 2010; Office of the National Coordinator for Health Information Technology, 2014). Under MU, hospital organizations and physician offices are financially rewarded to adopt and use EHR functionality. In just over a decade, EHR adoption has profoundly impacted how clinicians work, document, and use data in support of clinical decisions and care planning in these settings. Accordingly, expectations for data exchange and empowering data analytics are expanding beyond the medical center and are being placed upon the post-acute care community (Centers for Medicare and Medicaid Services, 2013d).

Through the ACA legislation, quality measure definition work of the National Quality Forum, and in conjunction with CMS' power of reimbursement sanctions, the last five years have seen a rapidly changing health policy landscape. Quality measures in support of Triple Aim goals are required and linked to reimbursement. The most disruptive measure to the status quo being readmission rates for conditions that call for post-discharge, care coordination to avoid risk of rehospitalization within 30 to 60 days (Centers for Medicare and Medicaid Services, 2013d;

Jencks, Williams, & Coleman, 2009; Remington, 2014). As hospitals strive to address this risk to their revenues, they are beginning to reach out to Skilled Nursing Facilities, Home Health and Rehabilitation Facilities with the ask for data exchange, care planning and reporting that is catching the post-acute EHR industry unprepared for this level of functionality or sophistication (Pearson & Bercovitz, 2006).

While the majority of post-acute organizations have information systems that include clinical documentation, these are designed largely to function as data captures for billing and CMS' mandatory minimum data base sets. Each post-acute provider has a mandatory minimum data set that must be submitted to CMS at regular intervals for each patient admission and discharge (see Table 25.1) as a condition for reimbursement by CMS. This regulatory requirement has driven the way systems have been built for the post-acute market over the past 30 years and is fundamental to understanding the current state. Home health illustrates this evolution and why there is a lack of functional parity between the EHR systems serving the post-acute market as compared to those for acute and ambulatory care.

Case Example: Evolution of Clinical Information Systems in Home Health

In 2000, CMS moved home health to prospective payment reimbursement that was linked to a new documentation tool—the Outcome and Assessment Information Set (OASIS) to be used at admission. Few legacy systems offered a clinical solution to capture even the routine visit notes in the home at this time. Patient records and clinical documentation were collected on paper and agencies' medical records were paper-based. In anticipation of the 2000 OASIS introduction, agencies started looking to their legacy billing and ADT (admission/discharge/transfer) system vendors to provide OASIS documentation capture. Vendors quickly responded by developing documentation systems that would allow for clinicians to capture the OASIS data and pass it directly into the back-end billing system, eliminating the need for office staff to reenter the OASIS documentation. Billing and ADT system vendors adopted a "bolt-on" approach to capture OASIS documentation. Consequently, the structure of the clinical documentation was based on a task concept that organized the patient record by visit note type in chronologic order, with each discipline having their separate documentation tasks. More than a decade later, the remnants of this developmental approach are evident in the system offerings in the marketplace today. Current state still has limited workflow support functionality, integrated patient record views, multi-discipline team workflow and patient care data views, clinical decision support, structured terminologies, and/or flexible quality reporting capabilities.

Unfortunately, the health information technology (HIT) software suppliers for the home health industry reflect the cottage industry nature of home health itself. There are a myriad of small vendors who supply their local markets with systems developed to cover the basic front office and billing functions with added OASIS capture functionality. These basic systems require minimal capital outlay and are affordable for the thousands of small-sized agencies (over 10,000) that make up the bulk of the home health industry (Medicare Payment Advisory Commission, 2012a). However, that segment of the market with bigger buying power—the larger home health agencies and organizations, the Veterans Administration system, and the hospital-based agencies—has driven demand for and development of more comprehensive clinical systems with advanced functionality to integrate with their referral sources and the demands of Meaningful Use functionality (Weaver & Teenier, 2014).

While the HIS vendors have matured their products to deliver point of care, clinical documentation, these systems still have a strong focus on driving the reimbursement process rather than supporting clinical workflow and decision support. Lack of structured clinical data still characterizes the industry today and has long challenged home health provider organizations' ability to provide quality and clinical outcome measures. The most mature products offer the ability to maximize reimbursement by managing the number of patient visits and identifying patients at risk of re-hospitalization, and clinician views are still task and note based, siloed by discipline. Most of the major vendor systems in the market today remain on their original 1980s technical platform architectures and programming languages. However, a very hopeful new development is the entry of new start-up vendors who have built their solutions as a Web-based platform, using cloud technology and i-Pad devices with the added advantage of leveraging off of Apple built applications. These twenty-first century tools and architectures allow for rapid development, nimbleness, and options to plug into the side application market for Apple devices, with a very low cost of ownership (Weaver & Teenier, 2014). These new market developments offer a way forward for home health and the other post-acute providers and gives hope for significant progress and catch up to MU functionality levels over the next five years.

EHR Adoption Levels in Home Health

From 2000 to 2013, there have been three national surveys conducted on the levels of EHR adoption in the home health industry. These are the 2000 National Home and Hospice Care Survey (NHHCS) (Pearson & Bercovitz, 2006); the 2006-2007 American Association of Homes and Services for the Aging (Resnick & Alwan, 2010); and Fazzi Associates' 2013 survey of over 1000 HHA agencies (Fazzi Associates, 2013). Tracking across these surveys shows a shift from only 32% of HHAs having clinical systems with the basic EHR functions in 2000 to 58% as reported in the 2013 survey. This means that a bit more than 40% of the agencies sampled in 2013 are still in paper mode for clinical documentation, and of those, only 42% reported that they would be looking to buy a system in the next 12 months (Fazzi Associates, 2013).

Missing from these benchmarks, however, is the degree to which the specific functionality that is basic to EHR standards today is in the systems being used. This functionality includes clinical decision support; flexibility of views of patient care information; point-of-care support for clinical documentation; telemedicine and standardized, structured terminologies; and ability to send and receive patient information with other external providers. Resnick and Alwan (Resnick & Alwan, 2010), the authors of the 2007 survey study, tried to answer this question by looking at the functionality used in the EMR systems. They reported the following: patient demographics—95%; point-of-care clinical documentation—29%; clinical notes—34%; clinical decision support—34%; and physician's ability to electronically sign orders on the plan of treatment order form—50%. Resnick and Alwan also found that sharing of health information data with other providers was almost negligible in 2007 stemming from the lack of enabling functionality, such as the Consolidated Clinical Document Architecture (C-CDA) tool in the home health EHR systems at that time (Office of the National Coordinator, 2014a). While Fazzi's 2013 survey did not address the question of functionality (Fazzi Associates, 2013), the major vendors in the industry have moved to embrace the C-CDA tool since the 2007 survey.

STANDARDS NEEDED FOR CARE COORDINATION

Standards for clinical information systems apply to the ways data are named, stored, and shared as well as to promote accuracy and to work more efficiently. Ultimately, standardized systems can improve patient safety and lower healthcare costs (Thompson, Classen, & Haug, 2007). When aspects of care coordination are standardized, it is easier to collect data and share data pertinent to care across multiple sites by various care providers. Care Coordination has been a topic of interest for standard development and implementation organizations for many years, such as government agencies like CMS and HHS agencies such as the ONC Standards & Interoperability Framework, and by non-profit agencies such as Health Level 7 (HL7), and Integrating the Healthcare Enterprise (IHE).

The Continuity Assessment Record and Evaluation (CARE) Tool was created by CMS as part of the Post-Acute Care Payment Reform Demonstration (PAC-PRD) authorized by the Deficit Reduction Act of 2005 (Centers for Medicare and Medicaid Services, 2013b; Office of the National Coordinator, 2014a). The purpose of the CARE tool was to standardize patient assessment information from PAC settings to better understand differences of care provided to similar patients at different settings and guide payment polices. The CARE tool uses Web-based technology to develop an interoperable data reporting systems for the Medicare program. The Web-based technology allows for future changes in the data sets to incorporate advances in evidence-based care. The CARE tool is designed to minimize the provider burden and only includes items related to severity, payment, or monitoring the quality of care. The CARE tool was developed based on previous tools in use such as OASIS, MDS, and IRF-PAI in 2006 (Centers for Medicare and Medicaid Services, 2013d). The tool was tested in a two-phased demonstration project during 2008–2010 (Centers for Medicare and Medicaid Services, 2013d). Its initial use was required by CMS for Long-Term Care Hospitals in the fall of 2012. Additional pieces have been and will be continued to be required as the CMS continues to roll out additional quality measures (Centers for Medicare and Medicaid Services, 2014).

Another major focus of Standards Development Organizations (SDO) has been defining the shared care plan. The care plan has great potential for facilitating coordination of care across settings and between multiple disciplines. It is one centralized location where all care team members can see a patient's individualized health goals. There is potential for the care plan to be exchanged between settings allowing for continuity of care provided. Standardization of care plan elements is key to facilitating this exchange. Many SDOs are addressing the needs of care plan definition and organization. Care Plan elements have been the topic of standardization efforts for several years at HL7. The HL7 Patient Care, Structured Documents, and the Services Oriented Architecture Working Groups have all sponsored projects related to the care plan. Projects have ranged from describing a conceptual model for the care plan and determining standard messages to communicate key care plan elements to defining a service-oriented architecture. In addition, the IHE's Patient Care Coordination (PCC) workgroup and the Office of the National Coordinator (ONC) Standards & Interoperability Framework (S&I Framework) have also

done considerable work to define a standard care plan that can serve multiple care transition use cases, and population management of individuals with chronic diseases.

The Consolidated Clinical Document Architecture (C-CDA) is the result of a harmonization project addressing overlapping efforts of HL7, IHE, Health Information Technology Standards Panel (HITSP), and the Health Story Project. CMS adopted the C-CDA as a tool that gave provider organizations a means to accomplish patient information exchange, and for EHR vendors to embed in their products to meet ONC's certification requirements. CMS' Medicare and Medicaid EHR Incentive Program (commonly referred to as MU) rewards eligible providers for EHR adoption through incentive payments. Acute and ambulatory care providers can only qualify for CMS incentive payments by using EHR systems that have met ONC's EHR Certification Criteria. In this instance, the functionality for the exchange of patient care summaries and other patient information needed for care coordination. Initially available for the exchange of clinical summaries, the C-CDA has also been reviewed and revised to support its use for the exchange of care plans (Office of the National Coordinator for Health Information Technology, 2014).

The 2014 Edition Certification Program for Health Information Technology (Office of the National Coordinator for Health Information Technology, 2014) specifically calls for the use of the HL7 C-CDA to be used for capturing and exchanging patient summary information. Implementation guides (IGs) are tools created by the HL7 community to provide guidance on how the standards developed by the organization are to be implemented. In some cases, however, the IGs are insufficient for implementers and questions to the use of the standard remain (S&I Framework, 2014). In some cases, if these questions are answered by each site implementing their unique interpretation of the standard, these independent solutions result in the inability to exchange information even when the standard was followed. The S&I Framework's Transition of Care Initiative took this challenge on and produced a companion guide to supplement the Consolidated Clinical Document Architecture (C-CDA) Implementation Guide (C-CDA IG). This deliverable is useful for those implementing C-CDA by providing samples of clinically relevant documents and suggested testing procedures.

Some of these SDOs have completed their standards development process and others are still being publically reviewed and revised. Completed and published HL7 Standards are found at http://www.hl7.org/implement/standards/index.cfm?ref=nav. HL7 standards still under development and reviewed are best found by contacting the working groups through their respective co-chairs (http://www.hl7.org/about/hl7cochairs.cfm). IHE has the unique role of providing more specific information related to integrating and implementing standards created by the SDOs. There are multiple domains, clinical and other non-clinical healthcare domains, represented in IHE. The Patient Care Coordination (PCC) domain is specifically concerned with identifying, clarifying, and testing standards related to coordinating care across settings and disciplines. The framework maintained by IHE-PCC provides technical specifications with clinical use cases and examples specifically describing the implementation of standards to facilitate care coordination. IHE tests each of the technical specifications proposed for inclusion into the framework by inviting vendors to participate in an annual "Connectathon" event. At this event, vendors implement the proposed specification as either a "creator" or a "receiver" of the content included in the specification and demonstrate a successful exchange of the content with other participating vendors. The IHE -PCC committee has created several specifications related to care coordination including Care Management (CM), Cross-enterprise Basic eReferral Workflow Definition (XBeR-WD), Patient Care Plan (PtCP), and Patient Plan of Care (PPOC). These and other IHE PCC supplements for trial implementation are found at http://www.ihe.net/ Technical_Frameworks/#pcc.

The ONC launched the S&I Framework in January 2011 to engage community involvement on interoperability challenges critical to meeting Meaningful Use objectives (http://wiki.siframework.org/). The Transitions of Care (ToC) Initiative was one of the first teams to be organized. This workgroup focused primarily on building consensus toward the exchange of clinical summaries. The ToC also quickly expanded its focus to address the usefulness and need for the exchange of the care plan for the overall success of care coordination. This care plan focus led to the formation of the Longitudinal Care Coordination (LCC) Initiative which has been dedicated to identifying and validating a standards-based framework for care management of chronic disease populations across multiple settings and disciplines (http://wiki.siframework.org/ Longitudinal+CC+WG+Charter). The LCC Initiative has consisted of several related sub-workgroups. These workgroups have addressed or are in the midst of addressing and refining several aspects of patient information exchange in the longitudinal care space. These areas of focus include functional and health status assessments, patient and care team goals and desired outcomes, and the interoperable care plan. The deliverables of these community-led initiatives include identifying use cases and the key data elements and functional requirements supported by key assessment areas and a longitudinal care plan, and addressing key longitudinal care planning gaps in existing and evolving standards. Additionally, the LCC provides

guidance to community outreach pilot programs to implement evolving care coordination tools in real-world situations to identify policies required for operational systems.

For all this standards development work and despite efforts on the parts of many committed individuals and organizations to collaborate and harmonize across the different standards organizations, there is not yet one data set or set of definitions identified for the requirements of patient information exchange for care coordination or for the care plan. Effort has been made in many instances toward consensus on items like LOINC (Logical Observation Identifiers Names and Codes®) but different templates, timing of development, review processes, engaged team members, and international involvement often affect the end result. Future work in the area is needed, however, to harmonize data sets and definitions identified for care coordination to minimize confusion and maximize information exchange for optimal care coordination. The road to complete interoperability is not yet complete. Progress has been made through standardized tools such as the CARE tool and the C-CDA, but it is just a beginning. IHE has demonstrated interoperable success through events such as the Connectathon, but day-to-day use of interoperable Care Plans between acute and post-acute care areas is not yet happening. Complete implementation and use of standardized interoperable care plans is challenged by the long history of different definitions and use of care plans over many decades. There are as many definitions and clinical processes for care planning as there are unique sites of care and individual care providers. Physicians, bedside nurses, care managers, physical therapists, nutritionists, etc., all use care plans consisting of data elements and workflow specific to their own care domains. Care plans have served more as a tool for the specific discipline to meet their purposes or regulations than ever applied as a patient-centered tool crossing care setting or discipline boundaries. Many standards development and implementation organizations have focused their efforts on specifying the data elements and the definitions to be in a care plan. And implementation organizations have worked to demonstrate the ability to exchange care plan content across disparate clinical information systems. In some cases (HL7 and IHE), the SDOs clearly state that their work is not to determine governance or clinical process for care planning but to define the content and the tools allowing them to be used for care coordination regardless of governance or clinical process.

The impact to vendors of the standards development related to care coordination varies based on their current tools in place. Meeting requirements for CMS Certification for use in meeting MU incentive payments is the greatest focus for most. For Stage 2 MU this means that the exchange of certain data elements related to care coordination, such as problems, goals, and instructions. The standards communities and vendors try to anticipate upcoming regulations and clinical needs for healthcare information exchange. Regardless, there is often some scrambling within and between the organizations and vendor communities between the times a regulation is announced and the initial implementation date.

Nursing has been represented in all phases and environments of standards development for care coordination. Each of the SDOs reviewed here embraces wide engagement from all disciplines. The SDOs encourage clinicians and clinical informaticists to contribute in leadership roles, and also as contributors, reviewers, testers, and/or implementers. Nurses engaged in these development projects represent the full spectrum of nursing including acute care, pediatric care, chronic care, care management, and post-acute care.

DISCUSSION

U.S. healthcare spending puts an unsustainable burden on taxpayers who fund Medicare and Medicaid, employers who fund healthcare insurance as an employment benefit, and individuals doing self-pay. If the Healthcare Exchanges mandated under the 2010 Patient Protection and Affordable Care Act (United States Congress, 2010) become an operational reality, then the United States will lose the dubious distinction of being the only industrialized nation that does not provide universal health insurance to its population. Regardless of how the United States pays for its healthcare, reforming how care is delivered and reimbursed to achieve value for dollar spent is now well underway. System reform holds opportunity for post-acute care to be tightly integrated partners at community levels for the first time. Care coordination is multidimensional and essential to preventing adverse events, ensuring efficiency, and making care patient centered (Bodenheimer, 2008). Patients in greatest need of care coordination include those with multiple chronic medical conditions, concurrent care from several health professionals, many medications, extensive diagnostic workups, or transitions from one care setting to another. Effective care coordination requires well-defined multi-disciplinary teamwork based on the principle that all who interact with a patient must work together to ensure the delivery of safe, high-quality care. This integration calls for fairly sophisticated levels of electronic health record system capabilities, and this may present challenges for most organization given the current state of information systems in the post-acute market.

The U.S. healthcare system is in the process of dramatic and rapid change. Health policy and reimbursement reform is being driven on multiple legislative and regulatory fronts. The areas most impactful to the post-acute care sector are those under the National Quality Strategy's priority for care coordination and the management of care transitions. These aims and priorities are currently defined through readmission outcome metrics that are linked to significant CMS reimbursement penalties. To date these reimbursement penalties have applied to hospitals for just three conditions (acute myocardial infarction, heart failure, and pneumonia). But CMS will be adding additional readmission measures to include Hospital-Wide All Cause Unplanned Readmission Measure (HWR measure) to apply to LTHCs, IRFs, and all acute and critical access hospitals; hip/knee arthroplasty, and chronic obstructive pulmonary disease for FY2015; strokes for FY 2016; and MedPAC proposed readmission penalties for Home Health and SNF (Remington, 2014).

Just as these forces for change are making operational expertise within one sector insufficient, clinicians and informaticists alike must be informed of the full care continuum. This knowledge is fundamental to our ability to do effective and appropriate care planning with coordination that includes the patient and family in decision-making today and going forward. For those that design, build, test, implement, and support clinical systems use in organizations, these broader understandings of integrated and coordinated care are essential (Rudin & Bates, 2014). Also, to deliver care and information systems that support care that is coordinated, inclusive of patient, cost-effective and achieves highest outcomes, we have to be able to work as a team that goes where the patient and family go—out into community and mostly home. It could be easily argued that the majority of healthcare that makes a difference in health levels happens where the patient lives (Bates & Bitton, 2010; Jenkins, Kouri, & Weaver, 2010). Yet in the United States, we have tended to think of care delivery as a place a patient goes to, a hospital, Emergency Room, Doctor's office or Clinic. Current economic imperatives, changing demographics of our aging population, and healthcare policy are all driving rapid innovation in our healthcare delivery methods that call for an expansion out into community and home. And home may be in Assisted Living Facilities, Senior Living residences, Group Homes, Memory Care Facilities, or Nursing Homes.

Informatics has a major role to play in reaching the NQS goals of a healthcare system that delivers value for money spent and a healthier population. Detailed information technology requirements are needed for functionality that must be in place in a cross-continuum to support care coordination, communication and access data collection, measurements, and reporting—all infrastructure capabilities that are missing in some degree in our electronic health records (EHR) systems today across care settings (Agency for Health & Research Quality, 2012; Rudin & Bates, 2014). Nursing and nursing informatics are optimally positioned to be leaders in the teams that design, build, and implement these new health and IT systems that enable care coordination.

REFERENCES

Advisory Board. (2010). *Preventing unnecessary readmissions: Transcending eh hospital's four walls to achieve collaborative care coordination.* The Advisory Board, 2010, # 21139. Retrieved from www.advisory.com

Agency for Health & Research Quality. (2012). Chapter 8: Health system infrastructure. *National Healthcare Quality Report, 2011,* pp. 200–220. Rockville, MD: AHRQ Publication 12-0005. Retrieved from http://www.ahrq.gov/research/findings/nhqrdr/nhqr12/nhqr12_prov.pdf

Agency for Health & Research Quality. (2013a). *Annual progress report to Congress: National strategy for quality improvement in health care.* Retrieved from http://www.ahrq.gov/workingforquality/nqs/nqs2013annlrpt.htm. Accessed on March 2, 2014.

Agency for Health & Research Quality. (2013b). Chapter 6: Care coordination. *National Healthcare Quality Report, 2012,* pp. 159–168. Rockville, MD: AHRQ Publication 13-0002.

Bates, D. W., & Bitton, A. (2010). The future of health information technology in the patient-centered medical home. *Health Affairs, 29*(4), 614–621.

Berwick, D. M., Nolan, T. W., & Whittington, J. (2008). The triple aim: Care, health, and cost. *Health Affairs, 27*(3), 759–769.

Blumenthal, D., & Tavenner, M. (2010). The "meaningful use" regulation for electronic health records. *The New England Journal of Medicine, 363,* 501–504. Retrieved from http://healthcarereform.nejm.org/?p=3732&query=home

Bodenheimer, T. (2008). Coordinating care—A perilous journey through the health care system. *The New England Journal of Medicine, 358*(10), 1064–1071.

Centers for Disease Control and Prevention. (2013). *The state of aging and health in America 2013.* Atlanta, GA: CDC, US Dept. of Health and Human Services. Retrieved from www.cdc.gov/aging

Centers for Medicare and Medicaid Services. (2012). *Nursing home data compendium.* Retrieved from https://www.cms.gov/Medicare/Provider-Enrollment-and-Certification/CertificationandComplianc/downloads/nursinghomedatacompendium_508.pdf. Accessed on March 1, 2014.

Centers for Medicare and Medicaid Services. (2013a). *Medicare and medicaid statistical supplement.* Retrieved from http://www.cms.gov/ Research-Statistics-Data-and-Systems/Statistics-Trends-and-Reports/MedicareMedicaidStatSupp/2013.html. Accessed on March 8, 2014.

Centers for Medicare and Medicaid Services. (2013b). *CMS CARE item set and B-CARE.* Retrieved from http://www.cms.gov/Medicare/Quality-Initiatives-Patient-Assessment-Instruments/Post-Acute-Care-Quality-Initiatives/CARE-Item-Set-and-B-CARE.html. Accessed on February 20, 2014.

Centers for Medicare and Medicaid Services. (2013c). *Overview of the medicare post-acute care payment reform initiative.* Retrieved from http://www.cms.gov/Medicare/Demonstration-Projects/DemoProjectsEvalRpts/Downloads/PACPR_RTI_CMS_PAC_PRD_Overview.pdf. Accessed on February 20, 2014.

Centers for Medicare and Medicaid Services. (2013d). *Overview of the medicare post-acute care payment reform initiative.* Retrieved from http://www.cms.gov/Medicare/DemonstrationProjects/DemoProjectsEvalRpts/Downloads/PACPR_RTI_CMS_PAC_PRD_Overview.pdf. Accessed on February 20, 2014.

Centers for Medicare and Medicaid Services. (2014). *LTCH data submission specifications overview, Version 1.01.1.* Retrieved from http://www.cms.gov/Medicare/Quality-Initiatives-Patient-Assessment-Instruments/LTCH-Quality-Reporting/LTCHTechnicalInformation.html. Accessed on March 8, 2014.

Centers for Medicare and Medicaid Services Innovation Center. (2014). Retrieved from http://innovation.cms.gov/about/index.html. Accessed on February 24, 2014.

Fazzi Associates. (2013). *State of the home care industry study.* Retrieved from http://www.fazzi.com/id-2013-state-of-the-home-care-industry-study.html

Hess, A. E. M., & Sauter, M. B. (2013). 10 countries spending the most on healthcare. *WSJ.* Retrieved from http://www.marketwatch.com/story/10-countries-that-spend-the-most-on-health-care-2013-07-30. Accessed on July 30, 2013.

Jencks, S. F., Williams, M. V., & Coleman, E. R. (2009). Rehospitalizations among patients in the Medicare Fee-for-Service program. *The New England Journal of Medicine, 360*(14), 1418–1428.

Jenkins, M., Kouri, P., & Weaver, C. A. (2010). Informatics for personal health management. In C. A. Weaver, C. W. Delaney, P. Weber, & R. L. Carr (Eds.), *Nursing and informatics for the 21st century: An international look at practice, education and EHR trends* (pp. 25–44). Chicago, IL: HIMSS Publishing.

Linehan, K. (2012). Medicare's post-acute care payment: a review of the issues and policy proposals. *Issue brief/National Health Policy Forum,* Issue Brief # 847, Washington, DC: George Washington University. Retrieved from www.nhpf.org. Accessed on February 22, 2014.

Medicare Payment Advisory Commission. (2010, March). *Report to the Congress: Medicare Payment Policy,* p. 213. Retrieved from www.medpac.gov/documents/Mar12_EntireReport.pdf

Medicare Payment Advisory Commission. (2012a). *Payment basics series for skilled nursing facility, home health agency, inpatient rehabilitative facility, and long-term care hospital services.* Retrieved from www.medpac.gov

Medicare Payment Advisory Commission. (2012b, June). *A data book. Health care spending and the medicare program.* Retrieved from www.medpac.gov/documents/Jun12DataBookEntireReport.pdf

Medicare Payment Advisory Commission. (2013a, June). *A data Book: Health care spending and the medicare program.* Retrieved from http://www.medpac.gov/documents/Jun13DataBookEntireReport.pdf. Accessed on February 24, 2014.

Medicare Payment Advisory Commission. (2013b, March). *Report to Congress: Medicare Payment Policy.* Chapter 12: Hospice, p. 270. Retrieved from http://www.medpac.gov/chapters/mar13_ch12.pdf. Accessed on February 24, 2014.

Mehrotra, A., Forrest, C. B., & Lin, C. Y. (2011). Dropping the baton: Specialty referrals in the United States. *The Milbank Quarterly, 89*, 39–68.

Office of the National Coordinator. (2014a). Health IT. *Introduction to C-CDA and corresponding 2014 edition certification criteria.* Retrieved from http://www.healthit.gov/policy-researchers-implementers/consolidated-cda-overview

Office of the National Coordinator. (2014b). Standards and interoperability framework. *List of current standards initiatives in process.* Retrieved from http://wiki.siframework.org/Introduction+and+Overview. Accessed on February 24, 2014.

Office of the National Coordinator for Health Information Technology. (2014). *ONC fact sheet: 2014 Edition standards & certification criteria (S&CC) final rule.* Retrieved from http://www.healthit.gov/sites/default/files/pdf/ONC_FS_EHR_Stage_2_Final_08212.pdf. Accessed on February 20, 2014.

Organization for Economic Co-operation and Development. (2013). *OECD health statistics.* Retrieved from www.oecd.org/health/healthdata. Accessed on March 1, 2014.

Patient-Centered Outcomes Research Institute. (2014, Feb 13). Perspective from The New England Journal of Medicine—PCORI at 3 Years—Progress, Lessons, and Plans. Retrieved from http://www.pcori.org/blog/pcori-at-3-years-progress-lessons-and-plans/. Accessed on February 24, 2014.

Pearson, W. S., & Bercovitz, A. R. (2006). Use of computerized medical records in home health and hospice agencies: United States, 2000. *Vital and Health Statistics, 13*, 1–14.

Remington, L. (2014). Readmission prevention and quality: What's ahead? *The Remington Report, 22*(2), 4–6.

Resnick, H. E., & Alwan, M. (2010). Use of health information technology in home health and hospice agencies: United States, 2007. *Journal of the American Medical Informatics Association, 17*(4), 389–395.

Rudin, R. S., & Bates, D. W. (2014). Let the left hand know what the right is doing: a vision for care coordination and electronic health records. *Journal of the American Medical Informatics Association, 21*, 13–16.

S&I Framework. (2014). Standards and interoperability framework, office of the national coordinator. *Companion guide to consolidated CDA for MU2.* Retrieved from http://wiki.siframework.org/Companion+Guide+to+Consolidated+CDA+for+MU2. Accessed on February 22, 2014.

Selby, J., & Lipstein, S. H. (2014). Perspective: PCORI at 3 years—Progress, lessons, and plans. *The New England Journal of Medicine, 370*, 592–595. Retrieved from http://www.nejm.org/doi/full/10.1056/NEJMp1313061

Shih, A., Davis, K., Schoenbaum, S., Gauthier, A., Nuzum, R., & McCarthy, D. (2008). *Organizing the U.S. health care delivery system for high performance.* Commission on a High Performance Health System, New York, NY: The Commonwealth Fund. Retrieved from http://www.commonwealthfund.org/usr_doc/Shih_organizingushltcaredeliverysys_1155.pdf. Accessed on March 1, 2014.

Thompson, D. I., Classen, D. C., & Haug, P. J. (2007). EMRs in the fourth stage: The future of electronic medical records based on the experience at intermountain healthcare. *Journal of Healthcare Information Management, 21*(3), 49–60.

United States Congress. (2010). *Patient Protection and Affordable Care Act.* Retrieved from http://www.gpo.gov/fdsys/pkg/BILLS-111hr3590enr/pdf/BILLS-111hr3590enr.pdf

Weaver, C. A., & Moore, J. V. (2011). Home health: The missing ingredient in healthcare reform. In V. K. Saba & K. A. McCormick (Eds.), *Essentials of nursing informatics* (5th ed., pp. 289–300). New York, NY: McGraw Hill.

Weaver, C. A., & Teenier, P. (2014). Rapid EHR development and implementation using Web and cloud-based architecture in a large home health and hospice organization. *Proceedings of the 10th International Nursing Informatics Conference, June 2014* (pp. 251–262). Amsterdam: ISO Press, in press.

World Health Organization. (2013). *World health statistics.* Retrieved from http://www.who.int/gho/publications/world_health_statistics/2013/en/

26

Foundation of a Nursing Plan of Care Standard

Luann Whittenburg / Virginia K. Saba

• OBJECTIVES

1. Describe structure for Plans of Care (PoC) in health information system.
2. Describe the complexity of nursing care and knowledge.
3. Discuss the Nursing PoC standard for use in coded nursing care plans.
4. Describe educational framework for health information standards' initiatives.
5. Discuss standard for information retrieval of nursing PoC information.
6. Clarify nursing process standard to which nurses are held accountable.

• KEY WORDS

Nursing Plan of Care (PoC)
Clinical Care Classification (CCC) System
Meaningful use
Nursing process
Information standard
Integrating the Healthcare Enterprise (IHE)
American National Standards Institute (ANSI)
Healthcare Informatics Standards Panel (HITSP)

BACKGROUND

A Nursing Special Interest Group (SIG) was initiated in 2006 within the Integrating the Healthcare Enterprise (IHE), an International Standard Development Organization, to reflect the importance of communication integrity and continuum of care during patient/client transfers. The Institute of Medicine has identified the highest risk of errors affecting patients occur at the point-of-care transfer. The group represented acute, home health, psychiatric, and long-term care entities. Use cases were written. Agreements included the need for evidence-based documentation and started with initial assessment details based on regulatory body requirements. In October 2007, a proposal came to the Planning and Technical Committee of the Patient Care Coordination Domain, requesting the approval of an IHE nursing subcommittee and the IHE Nursing Sub-committee came into existence mid-2008. The Nursing Sub-committee began moving forward with a profile to demonstrate use of nursing process to illustrate documentation of plan of care elements illustrating patient progress along the health-illness continuum (Dickerson & Veenstra, 2010). This focus was demonstrated in 2010 when a nursing plan of care (PoC) profile standard was successfully balloted as a patient plan of care (PPOC). However, because the PPOC did not specify nursing it has been interpreted by IHE members as referring to all health professionals providing care to a patient even though the PPOC used a nursing terminology, Clinical Care Classification System, and followed the nursing process as illustrated in Fig. 26.1.

Medical diagnoses cannot be expected to explain the nursing care of patients nor function as the primary framework for documenting patient care and professional nursing data for communities, families, and individuals. The goal of nursing care is to improve health and the Nursing Plan of Care standard describes the complexity of nursing care. The Nursing PoC is a reference standard for the implementation of structured nursing data in electronic healthcare information systems. The Nursing PoC standard was developed by informatics nurse specialists to encourage Standard Development Organization

interest in the information exchanges of the largest group of healthcare professionals—nurses!

Nursing standards reflect the information insights of Florence Nightingale who through her groundbreaking work in informatics founded nursing as a theory-based, scientific profession with an independent body of knowledge and wisdom (Nightingale, 1860). Nightingale focused on quality indicators of patient care and the measures of care which lead to the development of nursing standards as the framework for care accountability in nursing. These standards, based on empirical evidence and experience, were used by Nightingale to develop powerful analytical displays of data to support performance-based nursing—early evidence-based practice

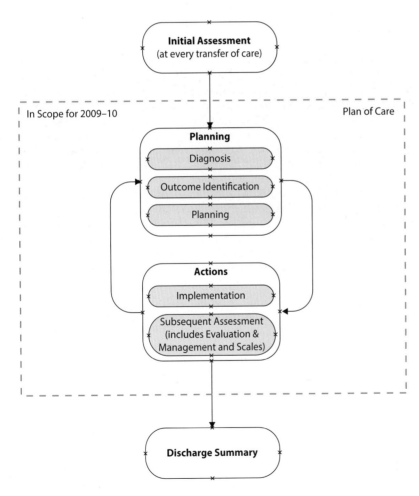

· **FIGURE 26.1.** Patient Plan of Care (PPOC) Model.

and the current foundation of nursing care and practice (Rehmeyer, 2008).

In the early 1900s, nursing standards were based primarily on the educational levels of the nurses and the standards of performance were embodied in the early state nursing licensing statutes. However, the American Nurses Association (ANA) recognized the need for evidence to measure the relationship of clinical documentation on patient care and provided the authority and support for standardizing nursing practice. In 1970, the ANA recommended the "nursing process" become the professional standard of nursing practice. And, as computer technology advanced so did nursing's awareness of the need for structured documentation of nursing practice. In 1992, ANA Database Steering Committee "recognized" the first four nursing terminologies: (1) Clinical Care Classification (CCC) System; NANDA International Inc. (NANDA-I); (3) Nursing Intervention Classifications (NIC); and (4) OMAHA System as well as approving a new nursing specialty, "Nursing Informatics." (American Nurses Association, 1992, p16; Baker, 2012; Saba & McCormick, 1996). The ANA subsequently developed the *Scope and Standards of Nursing Informatics Practice* which endorsed the nursing process' six standards (phases) for Nursing Informatics Practice (ANA, 2008, 2010). The ANA also recognized the need for quantitative evidence to measure the relationship of clinical documentation to the impact on patient care, and a scientific foundation for evidence-based practice.

In 2008, O'Kane et al. noted that the fundamental building block of any high-performance health system is reliable information about the effectiveness of care. Yet, electronic health record (EHR) systems are not designed for documenting a dynamic plan of care following the nursing process at the point of care. For example, in many health information record systems the information flow for nursing is disjointed, largely focusing on tasks rather than the individual care needs of the patient. The effect on the patient care in the acute setting is that the documentation of the admission nursing assessment does not inform nor connect to patient treatment orders. Currently, electronic nursing plans of care are generally "textbook" protocols not uniquely designed for a specific patient and display the nurses' workflow or conversely nursing plans of care are written as free-text, paper-based, nursing notes without any framework or structure. The purpose of this chapter is to provide nursing initiatives focusing on the Nursing Plan of Care (PoC) standard to strengthen the use of nursing standards in inpatient hospitals' Electronic Health Record (EHR) Systems. The Chapter will:

1. Examine the nursing plan of care within the current federal "Meaningful Use" regulations

2. Identify organizations involved in the selection of information management standards for the healthcare industry including nursing

3. Provide an example of a standard-based nursing plan of care following the nursing process that is easily implemented in any EHR system The chapter will also describe the use of the Clinical Care Classification (CCC) System as an example of a nursing terminology—a data integrator and standard for the exchange of nursing documentation among and across health information technology systems

INTRODUCTION

Federal Initiatives

The federal government began to focus on computer-based healthcare technology with the Institute of Medicine (IOM) report on *The Computer-based Patient Record* (Institute of Medicine, 1997). The IOM asserted that the computerization of the patient records could improve the quality and safety of patient care. This landmark document as well as the *To Err in Human* (IOM, 1999) and *Preventing Medication Errors* (IOM, 2006) reports affirmed that electronic healthcare record systems could reduce the number of medication errors and death in hospitals and prevent medication errors. These reports and numerous other initiatives addressing this issue led to Executive Order No. 13335, *"Incentive for the Use of Health Information Technology and Establishing the Position of the National Health Information Technology Coordinator"* that established the Office of the National Coordinator (ONC) (Exec. Order No 13335, 2004). The Office of the National Coordinator (ONC) was legislatively mandated under the Health Information Technology for Economic and Clinical Health (HITECH) Act of 2009, part of the American Recovery and Reinvestment Act (ARRA) of 2009, a $789 billion dollar economic stimulus package (Hitt & Weisman, 2009) implemented during the global economic decline. The HITECH Act allocated $19 billion to hospitals and physicians who demonstrate the "meaningful use" of electronic medical records (U.S. 111th Congress, 2009).

In 2005, the ONC mandated the American National Standards Institute (ANSI) establish a strategy for reviewing and recommending healthcare technology standards which resulted in the dissolution of the ANSI Healthcare Informatics Standards Board (HISB) (ANSI, 2003; ANSI, 2005a) and the formation of the Healthcare Information Technology Standards Panel (HITSP) (ANSI, 2005b). The HITSP mission was to identify the healthcare standards that would be required for the electronic documentation of patient care and interoperable with other systems (HITSP, 2005). The strategy used by HITSP, a public consensus panel composed of industry stakeholders, was to review and analyze specific "Use Cases" and identify standard terminologies based on an objective and well-defined business process approach and criteria. The selected HITSP standards were produced through agreement by a group of experts, publicly vetted to ensure 'fit' for intended purpose, availability of accessible format, and an ongoing review and revision process.

In analyzing the "Use Cases" for Biosurveillance, nurses noted most terminology standards in hospitals were used for the reimbursement of medical services and terminology used for the documentation of the patient care processes performed by the nurses was overlooked and a missing "gap" from the national dialog. As a result, the HITSP Biosurveillance Committee analyzed, vetted, and selected the Clinical Care Classification (CCC) System as the first national nursing terminology that was interoperable for the documentation of patient care. And upon recommendation from the Office of the National Coordinator for Health Information Technology (ONC) and by HITSP, the CCC System was adopted as an interoperable national nursing standard by the Secretary of Health and Human Services, Michael O. Leavitt (2005–2009). (Alliance for Nursing Informatics [ANI], 2007; Health Information Management and Systems Society [HIMSS], 2007); Leavitt, 2007; U.S. Department of Health and Human Services, 73 FR 3973, 2008).

In total, 58 terminology and interoperability standards were selected by HITSP for the computer processing of patient care for the Secretary of the United States of the DHHS. Subsequently, the number was reduced to 28 standards for the implementation of the HITECH ACT of 2009 "Meaningful Use" (MU) legislative regulations (U.S. Department of Health and Human Services, 74 FR 3599 E9-1068, 2009). The standards selected were primarily selected for the reimbursable services of inpatient departments such as laboratory, pharmacy, radiology, etc. Nursing documentation and services were again excluded because nursing is not yet a reimbursable patient care service. Nursing labor continues to be invisible in the billable rate of the inpatient room rate or obscured in the administrative (G&A) costs of outpatient and other facility settings.

Development of a Nursing Plan of Care

Once HITSP selected a nursing standard for the documentation of patient care, the informatics nurses engaged in HITSP, solicited the Integrating the Healthcare Enterprise (IHE, 2008) to use the HITSP selected nursing terminology, and developed a methodology for the documentation of patient care. As a result, the Nursing Plan of Care (PoC), under the name of the *Coded Nursing Documentation Plan of Care,* was proposed and accepted by IHE as a New Work Item Proposal (NWIP). The NWIP underwent additional development by nursing and technical experts and using the consensus process was publicly vetted under the name of the Patient Plan of Care (PPOC) that recognized the patient-centric focus of healthcare (Fig. 26.1). The PPOC is an IHE profile describing the data concepts needed by nurses for documentation in the electronic health record. The Patient Plan of Care (PPOC) explicitly formalized the data requirements of nurses for the efficient and timely capture of care events at or near the bedside acknowledging the patient-centric healthcare environment. The intent was to interpret for non-clinicians usual and customary nursing workflows, data and documentation concepts, and the nursing process structure used in documenting nursing events at the point of care. The PPoC provided the context for nursing data using common scenarios following the American Nurses Association (ANA) Nursing Process standard (six phases) represented by the information model and terminology (vocabulary) of the CCC System.

The CCC System was used repeatedly as an exemplar of structured, coded, nursing terminology. The use of the CCC System for the IHE profile standard was an extension of the interoperability conformance recognition of the CCC by Health Level Seven (HL7) interoperability for electronic transmission and the integration of the CCC System in the Unified Medical Language System (UMLS) for all clinical settings. The CCC, specifically designed for computer-based systems, conforms to the Cimino criteria for standardized terminology (Cimino, 1998).

The Nursing PoC identified a missing and essential professional component for the electronic documentation of nursing practice. The Nursing PoC standard used the CCC System to name, describe, and code the nursing *"essence of care"* which refers to "documentation of the primary reason including the essential nursing care needs" (Saba, 2007) for providing patient care for a specific condition. Thus, the PoC was evaluated and accepted as a Standard Development Organization (SDO) work program initiative. Several of the Nursing Informatics

(NI) Committees and Nursing Special Interest Groups supported and promoted the Nursing PoC integration into the Centers for Medicare and Medicaid Services (CMS) MU Regulations.

Meaningful Use

Currently in the Meaningful Use (MU) requirements (Office of the National Coordinator for Health Information Technology, n.d.) is the term Eligible Professionals (EPs) and defined by CMS as "responsible for the diagnosis and treatment of patients prescribing medications, laboratory tests, radiology procedures, other care modalities, activities and services" (U.S. Department of Health and Human Services, 77 FR 53967, 2012). The definition in the regulation encompasses traditional nursing practice responsibilities: (1) provide individualized patient care, (2) coordinate care with other providers, (3) provide caring practices, (4) use the nursing process (integration of singular actions of assessment, diagnosis, and identification of outcomes, planning, implementation, and evaluation) to provide and document patient care, and (5) provide quality healthcare and achieve optimal outcomes. Professional nurses are also responsible for the implementation of medical provider orders and the collaboration with allied health professionals: Physical, Occupational, Respiratory, Speech Therapists, etc.

Meaningful Use Stages 1 and 2

Initially, one of the four proposed denominators in the Stage 1 MU objectives omitted and excluded the eligible providers of patient care and/or the caring process (Whittenburg & Saba, 2012). As stated above, the MU focus was on provider orders for reimbursable special services in Computerized Provider Order Entry (CPOE) systems. For example: "Number of orders for medications, laboratory tests and radiology" were entered in the EHR system and if the application was implemented successfully, the hospital/facility received federal funds from the ONC technology program. The process continued in MU Stage 2 and which focused on quality indicators.

How a Nursing Plan of Care Could Impact Meaningful Use

In the public comment periods for MU Stages 1 and 2, written recommendations were made to CMS for endorsement of the IHE Nursing PoC standard to achieve interoperable healthcare data for quality indicators. These recommendations cited the implementation of PoC standard to advance the MU impact on quality, safety, and the outcomes of patient care needed to evaluate

the episode of illness. By adding a Nursing PoC to the MU "Number of Orders" denomination, the denominator could standardize the various terms used to describe the care process: care plan, plans of care, treatment plan, etc. Second, the Nursing PoC using the Nursing Process framework provides a complete minimum requirements for a care plan field: "problem" (focus of the care plan) with (1) Assessment, (2) Diagnosis, (3) Goal (target outcome)/Expected Outcome, (4/5) Planning and Implementation ("instructions" for Interventions and Actions), and (6) Expected Outcome (target or measure/outcomes achieved). Third, with the Nursing PoC included in the MU patient care reporting, the Nursing PoC could generate a status report of the status of the patient at any point in time, updated and revised based on specific clinical requirements, and addressed in the clinical decision support systems. For CMU and MU, the Nursing PoC offered a readily available standard to summarize the quality care as part of each Clinical Quality Measure's Description (based on six phases) for the transition of care (ToC) along the continuum of care. The recommendation was deferred to MU Stage 3.

Meaningful Use Stage 3

Meaningful Use Stage 3 is poised to identify the requirements for care coordination and sharing of information across multiple provider groups—from long-term care and post-acute care to behavioral health and other allied services (Whittenburg & Saba, 2012). There is growing recognition of the need for and the benefits of fully interoperable health information technology system's capabilities across provider groups (Reynolds & Sutherland, 2013) and of the importance of the information or data needs of the medically complex and/or functionally impaired individuals within provider groups service. Effective, collaborative partnerships among service providers and individuals are necessary to ensure that individuals have the ability to participate in planning their care and that their wants, needs, and preferences are respected in healthcare decision-making. The identification and harmonization of standards for the longitudinal coordination of care will improve efficiencies and promote collaboration by:

- Improving provider's workflow by enabling secure, single-point data entry for the Transfer of Care (ToC) and Care Plan exchange including a Nursing PoC

- Eliminating the large amount of time wasted in phone communication and the frustrations and dissatisfaction of the receiving provider in not always obtaining care transition and care planning information in a timely manner

- Reducing paper and fax transmissions, and corresponding labor intensive, manual processes during a ToC or Care Plan exchange including a Nursing PoC

- Supporting the timely transition of relevant clinical information at the start of home healthcare and as the patient's condition changes

- Enabling sending and receiving provider groups to initiate and/or recommend changes to patient interventions more promptly

In 1991, Carpenito cited the benefits of care planning: (1) ability to provide written directions rather than verbal communication to reinforce patient safety in hand-offs of care, (2) ensures continuity of care, (3) prioritizes problems, (4) provides a means to review and evaluate care, and (5) demonstrates the complex role of professional nurses in the health settings. Almost 25 years later, legislation is bringing nurses closer to standard-based care planning.

NURSING PLAN OF CARE FRAMEWORK AND NURSING PROCESS

The theoretical framework for a fully operational Nursing PoC is the Nursing Process. "The common thread uniting different types of nurses who work in various areas of nursing practice is the nursing process—the essential core of practice for the registered nurse to deliver holistic, patient-focused care" (ANA, 2010). The Nursing Process encompasses all significant nursing actions—the process forms the foundation of the nurse's professional practice and decision-making.

The nurse is required to apply nursing knowledge systematically and logically to interpret, analyze, and use data to determine the appropriate plan of care based on knowledge of the physical, biological, and behavioral sciences. As part of academic preparation, nurses have biochemistry, biophysics, microbiology, anatomy, physiology, psychology, and sociology courses. This basic knowledge of the sciences enables nurses to recognize patient problems and determine how the patient's health is disrupted by a health problem.

The Nursing "PoC" using the nursing process provides a clinical decision support tool to enhance patient care outcomes. Nurses have the ability to improve the quality of patient outcomes by maximizing data interoperability using the CCC System as the example, so knowledge is accessible for nursing practice and documentation on the Nursing PoC. As patients transition through the healthcare system, the nursing plan of care data is modified and communicated. Not only do Nursing PoC data support a continuum of care for the patient, they also provide a source of knowledge for care providers which may increase efficiency in the care process, improve care quality, and decrease the cost of care across care settings. The Nursing PoC provides nurses with a nursing process framework to care for patients that complements the patient's treatment plan and creates a healthcare environment of safety and patient-focused practice.

The Nursing Process is the standard of practice and includes the following six phases: **assessment** which includes the collection of comprehensive data pertinent to the patient's health or condition. The data are then analyzed to determine the nursing **diagnosis** or problem. The nurse then identifies the **expected outcomes** (goals) for each diagnosis for development of a care **plan** to attain the expected outcomes. The registered nurse **implements** the identified plan with ongoing **evaluation** of progress toward the attainment of the identified **outcomes** (Fig. 26.2).

The nursing process focuses on patient care processes provided by nurses and allied health personnel in clinical practice settings (Saba 2007, 2011).

The nursing process operationalizes and demonstrates the art and science of nursing. The six phases of the nursing process describe the standard levels of nursing care and encompass all significant actions taken by nurses to

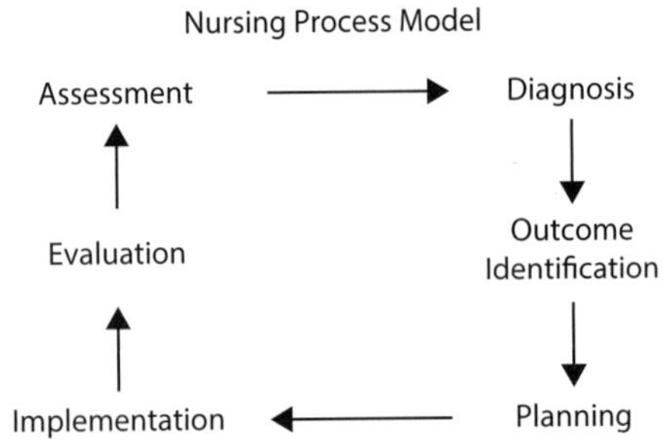

Nursing Process Model

• **FIGURE 26.2.** Nursing Process Model. (ANA, 1998). (Reproduced, with permission, from American Nurses Association. (2010). *Nursing's Social Policy Statement: The Essence of the Profession*, 3rd ed. (p. 23). Silver Springs, MD: nursesbooks.org. © 2010 American Nurses Association.)

provide care to patients/clients, and form the basis for clinical decision making.

The Nursing Process provides the framework for the Nursing PoC and requires continual assessment and reassessment and the evaluation of patient responses or nursing interventions to achieve the identified nursing outcomes. Essentially there is no end to the Nursing Process or Nursing PoC processes until a patient's healthcare needs are met. The Nursing Process remains focused on Nursing PoC of the patient and adapted to meet patient needs and concerns.

Other characteristics of the Nursing PoC and Nursing Process framework include:

Universally Applicable: Nursing Process framework is appropriate for any patient, of any age, with any clinical diagnosis, at any point on the health continuum, and in any setting (e.g., school, clinic, hospital, or home) across all nurse specialties (e.g., hospice, maternity, pediatric, etc.).

Goal-oriented: Nursing Process interventions are determined by the nursing diagnoses and chosen for the purpose of achieving the nursing outcome.

Cognitive Process: Nursing Process involves nursing judgment and decision-making.

The current twenty-first century use of an electronic Nursing PoC supports the role of nursing as a caring profession and dispels the depiction of technical and menu-driven profession and the computable structure of the CCC System promotes standard upgrades and versioning in existing clinical documentation systems. The implementation of a structured, standard, coded nursing terminology offers organizations a return on investment through transparency and insight into the value of nursing care (workload), resources (staffing), and care outcomes. The Nursing PoC provides crucial information about patient care in healthcare regardless of the clinical setting. The Nursing PoC informs healthcare professionals about care delivery plans among nursing, allied health providers for the integration of care, and a data-driving understanding of care decision effects on quality outcomes.

DESCRIPTIONS OF "OTHER PLANS OF CARE"

A Nursing PoC is an information standard "blueprint" for nursing and serves nurses and allied health professionals.

A Nursing PoC is a dynamic plan directly related to a patient's medical condition under clinical treatment and encouraged nurses to address "whole person" patient diagnosis(es) and problems that contributes a level of completeness in understanding nursing's contributions to patient care outcomes by providing a structured, coded, systematic view of patient-centered processes (Klebanoff & Hess, 2013).

Currently, there are numerous commercial organizations and publishing corporations that are offering commercial electronic nursing plans of care for uses in the EHR systems; however, that are similar to textbook chapters of nursing plans of care being used in schools of nursing for educational purposes. The electronic plans of care being offered generally are not using a coded nursing terminology compatible with the EHR system and thus retrieval of meaningful data for measuring outcomes is questionable. In fact meaningful data for analysis, reuse, and/or aggregation to conduct research on and to generate evidence-based information may not be achievable. As a result the current focus is still on the standards organizations that are attempting to address the needs of MU Stage 3 for a "patient care plan" as described below by the HL7 Nursing Sub-committee and the IHE Patient Care Coordination (PCC) Committee. This new initiative has as a resource the PPOC approved by the IHE in 2010 as a possible model.

CARE PLANNING PROPONENTS

Health Level Seven International (HL7)

Health Level Seven International (HL7) is a Standard Development Organization that states: **"Care planning is a conceptual framework with many interrelated dependencies and antecedents"** (Outstanding Issues, n.d., para 1). The HL7 Nursing Sub-committee is collaborating with the IHE Patient Care Coordination (PCC) Committee on the details of a Care Plan that can be used by all healthcare professionals. The committees are discussing the "significant confusion and extensive debates over the different types of Care Plans: Care Plan, Plan of Care, and Treatment Plan" (Introduction, n.d., para 1).

Such care plans are likely to be understood and used in different ways depending on the preference, context of use, funding model, etc., under which they operate. "For example: medicine generally refers to 'management plans' or 'treatment plans', midwifery has 'birthing plans', social care has 'support plans' and nursing and many other health and social professions refer to 'Care Plans', or 'Intervention

Plans'. Increasingly guidance is proposing just one 'Care Plan' that can be used by all groups and by using a discipline identification code. Application functionality and descriptions may need to reflect these varying needs whilst combining the record together as an integrated care record." (Introduction, n.d., para 3).

"The benefit of care planning is enabling a multi-professional care plan used by teams across organization boundaries (primary, secondary, tertiary care). A universal approach to care plan content will give a broad base to inform care plans and this approach should reduce the variation in care planning to support consistent, high quality, evidence based delivery of care" (Outstanding Issues, n.d., para 2). Once finalized the multi-professional care plan is proposed to be integral component of MU Stage 3 which will be introduced in late 2014 and/or 2015.

Standards and Interoperability Framework

The Standards & Interoperability (S&I) Framework approach from the Office of the National Coordinator for Health Information Technology (ONC), Office of Standards & Interoperability, is another initiative to create better care, better health, and cost reduction by care delivery improvements (Berwick, Nolan & Whittington, 2008).

The S&I Framework states:

> A Care Plan is a consensus-driven dynamic plan that represents all of a patient's and Care Team Members' prioritized concerns, goals, and planned interventions. It serves as a blue print shared for all Care Team members, including the patient, to guide the Care Team Members (including Patients, their caregivers, providers and patient's care. A Care Plan integrates multiple interventions proposed by multiple provider and disciplines for multiple conditions. (Care Plan Framework, n.d., para. 1)

HEALTHCARE INFORMATICS STANDARD GROUPS

In 2008, Raths notes: "If health information exchange is to get to the next level, formulating standards will be an absolute key" (Raths, 2008, p.34). The interest and involvement of the Standard Development Organizations (SDOs) in demonstrating the implementation of data terminology standards for nursing care across all settings of care

is crucial to providing the evidence of nursing care outcomes. The catalyst for the Nursing PoC is the six standards or Phases of the nursing process for documenting professional nursing practice using a standardized nursing terminology such as the CCC System. Descriptions of key informatics groups focusing on Meaningful Use standards are summarized below.

Office of the National Coordinator for Health Information Technology

The Office of the National Coordinator for Health Information Technology (ONC; www.healthit.gov) is a division of the Office of the Secretary, U.S. DHHS with a focus on coordinating the adoption, implementation, and use of health information technology, including the electronic exchange of health information, to achieve the **"Triple Aims Framework"** of reform: 1) **"Better Care**: (improve the overall quality, by making health care more patient-centered, accessible, and safe); 2) **Healthy People/Health Communities**: (Improve the health of the U.S. population by supporting proven interventions to address behavioral, social, and environmental determinants of health in addition to delivering higher-quality care); and 3) **Affordable Care**: (Reduce the cost of quality health care for individuals, families, employers, and government reducing per capita costs of health care) (Health Information Technology [HIT] Policy Committee, 2011).

In order to provide funding to hospitals and Eligible Professionals for the demonstration of the "Meaningful Use" of electronic medical records, ONC developed the Nationwide Health Information Network (NHIN to advance the nation's health information infrastructure (Nationwide Health Information Network, n.d., para 1). The NHIN set standards and policies to enable a diverse set of federal agencies and non-federal organizations to securely exchange electronic health information over the Internet. The NHIN is now the eHealth Exchange managed by non-federal, non-profit industry coalition (Sullivan, 2012).

Standards & Interoperability Framework (S&I Framework)

The Standards & Interoperability (S&I) Framework (http://www.siframework.org) was formed to enable healthcare stakeholders to improve the quality of healthcare through greater health information exchange. The S&I

Framework, established by the DHHS, ONC, is a public, private community forum focused on solving healthcare interoperability challenges through the establishment of "harmonized interoperability specifications that support national health outcomes and healthcare priorities, including MU, and the ongoing efforts to create better care, better population health and cost reduction through delivery improvement" (Standards & Interoperability Framework Explored, n.d., para 1).

The S&I Framework has two key initiatives involving care plans: the S&I Longitudinal Coordination of Care (LCC) initiative that is focused on improving the transitions of patients across acute and post-acute care settings and the S&I Transition of Care (ToC) initiative created to identify and develop healthcare standards that would enable the electronic exchange of core clinical information among providers, patients, and other authorized entities to meet Stage 1 and Stage 2 MU ToC requirements.

Longitudinal Coordination of Care Initiative

The S&I Framework Longitudinal Coordination of Care (LCC) Initiative provides an infrastructure to standardize transitions of care and care plan exchange across the continuum of care (Background, n.d., para 1). The value of this initiative will be measured through the attainment of the following immediate and long-term outcomes (Target Outcomes & Expected Deliverables, n.d., para 1) listed below:

1. Identification of functional requirements from a Use Case describing key conditions and business rules to enable transitions of care and care plan exchange, while protecting privacy and confidentiality

2. Development of concise architectural guidance using easy-to-understand documentation, user-friendly tooling, and formal models to assist providers, software vendors, and others in applying technical requirements for transitions of care and the interoperable exchange of care plans

3. Execution of one or more pilots to evaluate the specific use case for transitions of care and care plan exchange

4. Development or identification of new national standards building upon existing and validated S&I ToC standards, and specific for patient

assessment summaries; priority transitions of care across the continuum of care; and care plan exchange

Transitions of Care Initiative

"The mission of the Transitions of Care (ToC) Initiative is to improve the exchange of core clinical information among providers, patients and other authorized entities electronically in support of meaningful use and IOM-identified needs for improvement in the quality of care" (Purpose and Goals, n.d., para 1). The initiative supports national health initiatives, key healthcare stakeholders, and healthcare priorities and is driven by one compelling question: "What if every care transition was enabled by an unambiguously defined core set of high-quality clinical data?" The ToC Initiative seeks to support MU 1 that specifies the exchange of key clinical information among providers of care and with patients and other authorized entities electronically based on level of system capability, i.e., human readable, unstructured text, or full interoperable structured data (Purpose and Goals, n.d., para 1). "The ToC Initiative standards target specific provider groups or disciplines—eligible providers (EPs) and eligible hospitals (EHs)—and the software developers and vendors who would design or upgrade EHR systems to enable the exchange" (Initiative Overview, n.d., para 2).

The S&I LCC Initiative "builds on the ToC Initiative standards and aims to address identified gaps in transitions of care and care planning" (Background, n.d., para 3).

SUMMARY

The voluntary participation by nurses in healthcare standards activities, groups, and committees achieved an increased level of data visibility of nursing in the healthcare standard activities. As the nation moves toward fully operational health information record systems, nurses must know and understand how nursing care actions relate to other electronic data elements in the synthesis of information to improve patient care. The Federal Office of Management & Budget current models of care are not aligned with the objective to provide the right care to the right patient at the right time (Trends in Health Care Cost Growth and the Role of the Affordable Care Act, 2013; Brief Description of the Problem, 2008, para 3).

Patient care data represent one of the largest gaps of data required by the CMS for inpatient hospital care which includes clinical documentation and the complexity of care performed by professional nurses. Gordon (2005) noted that clinical documentation may be the most critical factor in a patient's treatment and recovery and understanding the impact of care on outcomes may be the key to improving quality in today's healthcare system. The ability to understand the relationship of nursing contributions to improving healthcare quality and the outcomes of patient care is uniquely nursing. A description of the effects of nursing practice on patients through the analysis of standardized, coded nursing concepts benefits nurses by emphasizing the importance of collected, analyzed, and retrieved nurse data to support nursing practice recommendations for patient care.

The future for healthcare information systems involves expanding the capture of coded nursing data using a nursing terminology that follows the nursing process for each patient. Nurses can use the Nursing PoC to begin to tell a cohesive and accurate electronic patient story

in an EHR that can be used for the Continuity of Care: Ambulatory Care, Long-Term Care, and Rehabilitation Care (all care settings), for the Physician/Provider's office, and for the Patient at home. Using coded nursing data allows for the analysis of nursing and patient outcomes data. Clinicians will be able to use informatics tools and analytics to analyze the patient story (screened and filtered) and nurses can tell a patient's story and capture nursing data in coded manner at the point of care at the same time. Nurses then have the quantitative evidence needed to measure the relationship of nursing interventions and actions documented to the nurse's impact on patient care using analytical displays of data to support performance-based nursing—and a scientific foundation for evidence-based practice.

The Use Case of a PoC using the CCC System mapped to SNOMED CT for interoperability is presented with description in Box 26.1 and Sample Care Plan in Box 26.2.

BOX 26.1:   USE CASE—NURSING PLAN OF CARE: CCC SYSTEM AND SNOMED CT

The CCC System/SNOMED CT Nursing Plan of Care is written as an inpatient scenario for Acute Care Hospitals (inpatient care). The Nursing PoC follows the six phases of the Nursing Process for the electronic nursing documentation of the Nursing Plan of Care (PoC) based on discrete concepts (data/elements). Generally a typical hospital inpatient plan of care will have multiple nursing diagnoses requiring multiple nursing interventions and actions required during an episode of care delivery. Within a hospital, when a patient is transferred, the Nursing PoC remains active with revisions and/or updates continuing to carry out the care processes and provide continuity of care across care settings.

SNOMED / CCC System Plan of Care Scenario
A 70-year-old male is admitted to a hospital unit after presenting to the Emergency Department (ED) with productive cough, acute rib pain with coughing, increased work of breathing, pulse oximetry saturation of 88%, temperature of 102.2 degrees, heart rate of 108, blood pressure of 156/88. Chest x-ray done in ED showed bilateral lower lobe and right middle lobe infiltrates. Medical diagnosis is Pneumonia

The step-by-step process of creating a Nursing PoC for a patient with Pneumonia using the CCC system Nursing Terminology mapped to SNOMED CT is below. A patient is admitted to a hospital for the emergency room with a medical condition (Pneumonia) requiring hospital and nursing care. A Nurse reviews the Provider's Orders and develops an individualized Nursing PoC for the patient based on the Nursing Process. The Nurse developed a Nursing PoC using the CCC System, a coded, nursing standardized, point-of-care, user interface terminology mapped to SNOMED CT reference terminology. During the inpatient stay, the Nurse reviews the patient's Nursing PoC shift by shift and/or at a minimum reviews the Nursing PoC daily to ensure that patient progress and quality care are maintained and nursing intervention actions are evaluated. When there is a change in the patient's medical condition, or when a patient is transferred within the facility, the Nursing PoC is updated and revised as needed. The electronic Nursing PoC is active as long as the patient remains an inpatient and until the patient is discharged when it becomes a Summary Record for Continuity of Care.

BOX 26.2:   USE CASE SAMPLE—NURSING PLAN OF CARE USING THE CCC SYSTEM VERSION 2.5 AND MAPPED TO SNOMED CT. (SABA, 2011)

Nursing Plan of Care	Care Component / Signs and Symptoms (Assessment)	Nursing Diagnoses	Expected Outcomes	Nursing Interventions (Planning)	Nursing Action Types (Implementation)	Actual Outcomes (Evaluation)	Evidence
1	**Respiratory: L**	**Respiratory Alteration: L26.0**	L26.0.2	**Pneumonia Care: L36.0**	L36.0.2	L26.0.2	(1a) Ribs splinted for coughing: Day 1 and Day 2; (1b) Bed elevated 30 degrees: Day 1, Day 2, and Day 3 *(Not coughing, able to get out of bed)*
	Productive Cough and Pneumonia	Change in or modification of breathing function	Stabilize	Actions performed to support pulmonary hygiene	PERFORM *(Splint ribs for coughing)*	**Stabilized** (Status of Nursing Diagnosis Outcome)	
				Positioning Therapy: A61.1	**A61.1.2**		
				Process to support changes in body positioning	PERFORM *(Elevate bed 30 degrees per day)*		
SNOMED CODES		Respiratory Alteration **Code:12/989/3005**		Respiratory Care Adjustment (procedure): **Code 12/48/4000** Positioning patient (procedure): **Code 22/982/408**		**409052007** Stabilization of status	

(continued)

BOX 26.2: USE CASE SAMPLE—NURSING PLAN OF CARE USING THE CCC SYSTEM VERSION 2.5 AND MAPPED TO SNOMED CT. (SABA, 2011) (CONTINUED)

Nursing Plan of Care	Care Component / Signs and Symptoms (Assessment)	Nursing Diagnoses	Expected Outcomes	Nursing Interventions (Planning)	Nursing Action Types (Implementation)	Actual Outcomes (Evaluation)	Evidence
2 (cont.)	Respiratory: L	Breathing Pattern Impairment: L26.2	L26.2.1	Breathing Exercises: L36.1	L36.1.3	L26.0.1	Taught use of breathing inhaler four times per Day 1; Day 2 and Day 3 two times per day *(Able to breathe normally)*
	Difficulty breathing	Inadequate inhalation and exhalation	Improve	Actions performed to provided therapy on respiratory or lung exertion	TEACH *(Use of breathing inhalator four times per day)*	Improved	
SNOMED CODES		Ineffective Breathing Pattern *Code:20/55/3003*		Breathing Exercise Education (Regime Therapy): *Code 38/584/9007*		390771008 Improvement of status	
3 (cont.)	Respiratory: L	Gas Exchange: L26.3	L26.3.1	Oxygen Therapy Care: L35.0	L35.0.2	L26.3.1	Regulated humidified oxygen (O$_2$) per nasal cannula and titrated to be kept at oxygen greater than 92% on room air for Day 1 and Day 2 and stopped on Day 3 *(Oxygen no longer needed)*
	Pulse Oximetry Saturation of 88%	Imbalance of oxygen and carbon dioxide transfer between lung and vascular system	Improve	Actions performed to support the administration of oxygen treatment	PERFORM *(Regulate humidified oxygen per nasal cannula and titrate to keep pulse ox greater than 92% on room air on Day 1 and Day 2 and stopped on Day 3 (Oxygen no longer needed)*	Improved	

SNOMED CODES					
	Impaired Gas Exchange (Finding) Code:70/94/4005	Q45.1.1	Oxygen Therapy (Procedure): **Code 57/48/5005**	**390771008** Improvement of status	
4	**Sensory: Q**	Q45.1.1	**Q47.0.2**	**Q45.1.1**	(1a) Pain scale score was less than 3 and medicated with Demerol; (1b) Demerol 50 mg three times a day on Day 1 & 2; twice on Day 3 (rib pain ended and Demerol stopped) *(Pain relieved)*
	Acute Pain: Q45.1		**Acute Pain Control: Q47.0**		
Acute rib pain when coughing/pneumonia	Physical suffering or distress to hurt	Improve	PERFORM *(Apply pain scale)*	PERFORM *(Apply pain scale)*	
			Medication Treatment: H23.4	**H23.4.2**	
			Actions performed to administer drugs or remedies regardless of route	PERFORM (Give pain medication, Demerol 50 mg, with patient input when pain scale score greater than 3)	
SNOMED CODES	Acute Pain (Finding) **Code: 27/466/3001**		Pain Control (Procedure): **Code 22/578/2006** Administration Medication (Procedure): **Code 18/62/9005**	**Improved** **390771008** Improvement of status	

(continued)

BOX 26.2: USE CASE SAMPLE—NURSING PLAN OF CARE USING THE CCC SYSTEM VERSION 2.5 AND MAPPED TO SNOMED CT. (SABA, 2011) (CONTINUED)

Nursing Plan of Care	Care Component / Signs and Symptoms (Assessment)	Nursing Diagnoses	Expected Outcomes	Nursing Interventions (Planning)	Nursing Action Types (Implementation)	Actual Outcomes (Evaluation)	Evidence
5	Physical Regulation: K	Physical Regulation Alteration: K25.0	K25.0.1	Vital Signs: K33.0.2	K33.0.2	K25.0.1	Vital signs taken every four hours on Day 1 and Day 2; every 12 hours on Day 3 (Vital signs normal) Gave antibiotics (PCN 1GM IM) on Day 1 and Day 2 and stopped on Day 3 (Temperature normal; PCN discontinued)
	Vital Signs	Change in or modification of somatic control	Improve	Actions performed to measure temperature, pulse, respirations, and blood pressure	PERFORM (Take vital signs every four hours until normal)	Improved	
				Medication Treatment: H23.4	H23.4.2		
				Actions performed to administer drugs or remedies regardless of route	PERFORM (Administer antibiotic (Penicillin [PCN] 1GM IM) until temperature normal		
SNOMED CODES		Physical Regulation Alteration (Finding) **Code: 12/985/6004**		Vital Signs (Procedure): **Code 61/74/6007** Administration Medication (Procedure): **Code 18/62/9005**		390771008 Improvement of status	

REFERENCES

Alliance for Nursing Informatics (ANI). (2007). *Nationwide health information technology standard for nursing: A nationally endorses nursing standard selected by the Healthcare Information Technology Standards Panel (HITSP) and American Health Information Community (AHIC).* Retrieved from http:// www.allianceni.org/docs/ news012007.pdf

American National Standards Institute. (2003). *ANSI Healthcare Informatics Standards Board survey highlights industry challenges and successful standards.* Retrieved from http://www.ansi.org/news_publications/news_story. aspx?menuid=7&articleid=529

American National Standards Institute. (2005a). *ANSI Healthcare Informatics Standards Board supports the national health information infrastructure.* Retrieved from http://www.ansi.org/news_publications/news_story. aspx?menuid=7&articleid=f6608739-9569-4092-a2d0-7e2ea1756b50

American National Standards Institute. (2005b). *Healthcare Information Technology Standards Panel.* Retrieved from http://www.ansi.org/standards_activities/standards_boards_panels/hisb/hitsp.aspx?menuid=3

American Nurses Association. (1992). Council on Computer Applications in Nursing. Report on: *The designation of nursing informatics as a nursing specialty.* Congress of Nursing Practice. Unpublished report. Washington, DC, ANA.

American Nurses Association. (1998). *Standards of clinical nursing practice* (2nd ed.). Silver Springs, MD: American Nurses Association.

American Nurses Association. (1994, 1998, 2008). *Scope and standards of nursing practice: Nursing informatics.* Silver Springs, MD: American Nurses Association.

American Nurses Association. (2010). *The Nursing Process: A common thread amongst all nurses.* Retrieved August 16, 2010, from https://nursingworld.org/EspeciallyForYou/StudentNurses/Thenursingprocess.aspx?css=print

Background. (n.d.). Longitudinal coordination of care. *WG charter.* Retrieved from http://wiki.siframework.org/Longitudinal+CC+WG+Charter

Baker, J. D. (2012). Nursing informatics. *Perioperative Nursing Clinics, 7*(2), 151–160.

Berwick, D. M., Nolan, T. W., & Whittington, J. (2008). The triple aim: Care, health, and cost. *Health Affairs, 27*(3), 759–769. doi:10.1377/hlthaff.27.3.759

Brief Description of the Problem. (2008, September 10). *IHE PCC profile proposal, Clinical documentation of patient assessments using a coded nursing terminology.* Retrieved from Wiki.ihe.net/images/7/75/IHE_Clinical_Documentation_Proposal_10Sep08_vks_law_(2)_(3).doc

Care Plan Framework. (n.d.). Standards & interoperability framework [S&I]. *Care Plan (new).* Retrieved from Wiki.siframework.org/file/view/20130808_C-CDA.docx/444014444/20130808_C-CDA.docx

Carpenito, L. J. (1991). *Nursing care plans and documentation: Nursing diagnoses and collaborative problems.* Philadelphia, PA: J.B. Lippincott Company.

Cimino, J. J. (1998). Desiderata for controlled medical vocabularies in the twenty-first century. *Methods of Information in medicine, 37*(4-5), 394–403.

Dickerson, A., & Veenstra, M. (2010). *History of the IHE nursing subcommittee.* Chicago, IL: Health Information Management and Systems Society.

Exec. Order No 13335, 69 C. F. R. 24059 (2004, April 27). Retrieved from http://www.gpo.gov/fdsys/pkg/FR-2004-04-30/pdf/04-10024.pdf

Gordon, S. (2005). *Nursing against the odds: How healthcare cost cutting, media stereotypes, and medical hubris undermine nurses and patient care.* Ithaca, NY: Cornell University Press.

Health Information Management and Systems Society (HIMSS). (2007). *HHS Secretary Leavitt's acceptance of HITSP interoperability standards paves the way for progress and opportunities for the industry.* Retrieved from http://www.himss.org/News/NewsDetail.aspx?ItemNumber=16370&navItemNumber=17442

Health Information Technology (HIT) Policy Committee. (2011, April 13). *National strategy for quality improvement in health care.* Retrieved from www.healthit.gov/sites/default/files/archive/HIT Policy Committee/2011/2011-04-13/NQSStakeholderEngagementBriefing_04-13-2011.ppt

Healthcare Information Technology Standards Panel (HITSP). (2005). *About HITSP.* Retrieved from http://www.hitsp.org/about_hitsp.aspx

Hitt, G., & Weisman, J. (2009). Congress strikes $789 billion stimulus deal. *Online Wall Street Journal.* Retrieved from http://online.wsj.com/news/articles/SB123436825805373367

Initiative Overview. (n.d.). *Interoperable Care Plan Exchange, Use Case v2.0, longitudinal coordination of care.* Retrieved from Wiki.siframework.org/file/view/SIFramework_LCC_UC2 2013-06-06.docx/436956246/SIFramework_LCC_UC2 2013-06-06.docx

Institute of Medicine. (1997). *The Computer-based patient record: An essential technology for health care.* Washington, DC: The National Academies Press.

Institute of Medicine. (1999). *To err is human: Building a safer health system.* Washington, DC: The National Academies Press.

Institute of Medicine. (2006). *Preventing medication errors: Quality chasm series.* Washington, DC: The National Academies Press.

Integrating the Healthcare Enterprise. (2008). *Coded nursing documentation (CND; CDOC-NT).* Retrieved from http://webcache.googleusercontent.com/search?q=cache:JayqoP-FwDcJ:wiki.ihe.net/images/8/8c/Detailed_Proposal_Coded_Nursing_Documentation_Profile_Oct22_2008.doc+&cd=2&hl=en&ct=clnk&gl=us

Introduction. (n.d.). *Health Level Seven international, Types of plan—differentiation and definitions.* Retrieved from http://wiki.hl7.org/index.php?title=Differentiations_and_Definitions

Klebanoff, N. A., & Hess, D. (2013). Holistic nursing: Focusing on the whole person. *American Nurse Today.*

Retrieved from http://www.americannursetoday.com/article.aspx?id=10830&fid=10780

Leavitt, M. O. (2007, January 22) [*Letter to Community Members*]. Health and Human Services [HHS]. Washington, DC.

NANDA International Inc. (n.d.). Retrieved from http://www.nanda.org/nanda-international-about-our-name.html

Nationwide Health Information Network. (n.d.). *HealthIT.gov interoperability portfolio*. Retrieved from http://www.healthit.gov/policy-researchers-implementers/nationwide-health-information-network-nwhin

Nightingale, F. (1860). *Notes on nursing: What it is, and what it is not.* New York, NY: D. Appleton & Company.

O'Kane, M., Corrigan, J., Foote, S. M., Tunis, S. R., Isham, G. J., Nichols, L. M., … Tooker, J. (2008). Crossroads in quality. *Health Affairs, 27*(3), 749–758. doi: 10.1377. Retrieved from http://content.healthaffairs.org/content/27/3/749.full

Office of the National Coordinator of Health Information Technology. (n.d.). *Meaningful Use. What do you think?*. Retrieved from http://www.healthit.gov/policy-researchers-implementers/meaningful-use-regulations

Outstanding Issues. (n.d.). *Health Level Seven international. Types of plan—Differentiation and definitions*. Retrieved from http://wiki.hl7.org/index.php?title=Types_of_Plan_-_Differentiation_and_Definitions

Purpose and Goals. (n.d.). *Interoperable care plan exchange, Use Case v2.0, Longitudinal coordination of care*. Retrieved from Wiki.siframework.org/file/view/SIFramework_LCC_UC2 2013-06-06.docx/436956246/SIFramework_LCC_UC2 2013-06-06.docx

Raths, D. (2008). Setting the standards stage. *Healthcare Informatics, 25*(3), 34–35. Retrieved from http://www.healthcare-informatics.com/article/setting-standards-stage?page=show

Rehmeyer, J. (2008). Florence nightingale: The passionate statistician. *Science News*. Retrieved from http://www.sciencenews.org/view/generic/id/38937/title/Math_Trek_Florence_Nightingale_Thepassionate_statistician

Reynolds, H. W., & Sutherland, E. G. (2013). A systematic approach to the planning, implementation, monitoring, and evaluation of integrated health services. *BMC Health Services Research, 13*(20130531), 168, doi:10.1186/1472-6963-13-168.

Saba, V. K. (2007). *Clinical Care Classification (CCC) System manual: A guide to nursing documentation.* New York, NY: Springer Publishing.

Saba, V. K. (2011). *Clinical Care Classification (CCC) System: Version 2.5* (2nd ed.). New York, NY: Springer Publishing. Retrieved from http://www.sabacare.com/Tables/?PHPSESSID=be25d6c15991cbfda29a5eaa0ceb0e7c

Saba, V. K., & McCormick, K. A. (1996). *Essentials of computers for nurses* (2nd ed.). New York, NY: McGraw-Hill Publishing Company Ltd.

Standards & Interoperability Framework Explored. (n.d.). *What is the S&I framework.* Retrieved from http://www.siframework.org/framework.html

Sullivan, T. (2012). eHealth exchange is now a non-federal entity. *Government Health IT*. Retrieved from http://www.govhealthit.com/news/ehealth-exchange-now-non-federal-entity

Target Outcomes & Expected Deliverables. (n.d.). Longitudinal coordination of care. *WG Charter*. Retrieved from http://wiki.siframework.org/Longitudinal+CC+WG+Charter

Trends in Health Care Cost Growth and Role of the Affordable Care Act. (2013). Retrieved from www.whitehouse.gov/sites/default/files/docs/healthcostreport_final_noembargo_v2.pdf

U.S. 111th Congress. (2009). *American Recovery and Reinvestment Act of 2009*. Publication No. H.R.1: Government Printing Office: Washington, DC. Retrieved from http://www.gpo.gov/fdsys/pkg/BILLS-111hr1enr/pdf/BILLS-111hr1enr.pdf

U.S. Department of Health and Human Services, 73 FR 3973. (2008, January 23). Office of the National Coordinator for Health Information Technology (ONC), DHHS. *Notice of availability: Secretarial recognition of certain Healthcare Information Technology Standards Panel (HITSP) interoperability specifications and the standards they contain as interoperability standards for health information technology.* Retrieved from http://www.gpo.gov/fdsys/pkg/FR-2008-01-23/pdf/08-234.pdf and https://www.federalregister.gov/articles/2008/01/23/08-234/notice-of-availability-secretarial-recognition-of-certain-healthcare-information-technology#h-9

U.S. Department of Health and Human Services, 74 FR 3599 E9-1068. (2009, January 21). Office of the National Coordinator for Health Information Technology (ONC), HHS. *Notice of availability: Secretarial recognition of certain Healthcare Information Technology Standards Panel (HITSP) interoperability specifications and the standards they contain as interoperability standards for health information technology.* Retrieved from http://federal.eregulations.us/fr/notice/1/21/2009/E9-1068

U.S. Department of Health and Human Services, 77 FR 53967. (2012). Centers for Medicare and Medicaid Services (CMS). *Medicare and Medicaid Programs; Electronic Health Record Incentive Program—Stage 2: Health information technology: standards, implementation specifications, and certification criteria for electronic health record technology,* (2014 Edition). Revisions to: *The Permanent Certification Program for Health Information Technology; Final Rules (45 C.F.F. Part 170; 42 C. F. R.412; 42 C.F.F. 413; 42 C.F.R 495)*. Retrieved from http://www.gpo.gov/fdsys/pkg/FR-2012-09-04/pdf/FR-2012-09-04.pdf

Whittenburg, L., & Saba, V. K. (2012, March 20). [*Letter to the Department of Health and Human Services, Centers for Medicare & Medicaid Services 77 FR 53967 (09/04/2012)*] Copy in possession of Dr. Luann Whittenburg.

27

Computerized Provider Order Entry

Emily B. Barey

- OBJECTIVES

  1. State two reasons why CPOE is different from other healthcare information technology implementations.
  2. State at least three common barriers to a successful CPOE implementation.
  3. State at least three strategies to ensure a successful CPOE implementation.
  4. State at least two future possible directions of CPOE.
  5. State three core competencies required of the nurse informaticist working with CPOE.

- KEY WORDS

  CPOE
  ARRA
  HITECH
  Meaningful Use
  Change management

INTRODUCTION

Much of the attention paid to Computerized Provider Order Entry (CPOE) has historically been associated with early adopters at academic medical centers such as Brigham and Women's Hospital and leading community sites such as El Camino Hospital reporting on their experience with clinical information systems in the 1980s and 1990s. Then, in 2000–2001, through the publications of the Institute of Medicine's *To Err is Human* (Institute of Medicine [IOM], 2000) and *Crossing the Quality Chasm* (IOM, 2001) and the subsequent focus of The Agency for Healthcare Research and Quality on preventing medical errors this past decade, CPOE received renewed attention as a patient safety tool. The private sector, simultaneously through employer organizations such as the Leapfrog Group for Patient Safety, has also pursued a similar agenda (The Leapfrog Group, 2010). Each consistently recommends the use of CPOE to improve healthcare quality. Benefits often highlighted range from the simple help of physician order legibility to the more complex decision support related to allergy and interaction checking, medication dosing guidance, and in some cases culminating in an overall decrease in patient mortality and significant financial return on investment (Kaushal et al., 2006; Longhurst et al., 2010; Poissant, Pereira, Tamblyn, & Kawasumi, 2005).

A new dimension of CPOE has emerged with the passage of The Health Information Technology for Economic and Clinical Health Act of 2009 (HITECH). As part of the American Recovery and Reinvestment Act of 2009 (ARRA), the aim of HITECH is to promote the adoption and meaningful use of health information technology (HIT). Included in HITECH are financial incentives to physicians and healthcare organizations that utilize electronic health records (EHR), including CPOE. These incentives initially have come in the form of increased reimbursement rates from the Centers for Medicaid and Medicare Services (CMS), but will ultimately result in a penalty if adoption and meaningful use of the EHR are not met. The Department of Health and Human Services (DHHS) has now published two sets of criteria and objectives for the meaningful use of EHR technology. The first set was published in July 2010, the second in September 2012. A third set is expected to be published sometime in 2016. The three stages are intended to promote data capture and sharing across healthcare entities, advance clinical processes, and improve clinical outcomes (DHHS, 2013).

This chapter discusses a brief history of CPOE and its recently renewed significance on a national level with the passage of HITECH. Benefits of CPOE have been long established; however, the HITECH offers new incentives to promote widespread adoption more rapidly. A successful CPOE implementation methodology is critical to fully realizing the vision of the HITECH. This chapter will address common barriers to a successful implementation of CPOE and strategies to overcome those barriers. A patient safety framework will also be reviewed in order to avoid any unintended consequences that arise as the result of a new technology implementation. Finally, the chapter sets the stage for the future of CPOE, including the required core competencies of the nurse informaticist to leading this type of implementation today and tomorrow.

The significance of CPOE cannot be underestimated. Although CPOE implies a physician or a provider-centric tool, the workflow and subsequent management of those patient care orders involves the entire inter-disciplinary team, with the nurse at the center as patient care coordinator. CPOE is also often the foundation for standardizing care delivery and best clinical practices, along with being an important component of advanced decision support. As such, in addition to the broader backdrop of patient safety, quality, and now financial incentives, it is essential to recognize the impact of CPOE on the work of the nurse and the significance of the nursing informaticist in obtaining a core competency in CPOE.

DEFINITION OF CPOE

CPOE is often used as an abbreviation to represent how an EHR system requires an end user to electronically enter patient care orders and requests. There have been electronic order communication tools available in the past that allowed for the transmission of lab, radiology, medication, and other types of orders to downstream ancillary systems; however, they relied largely on the transcription of a handwritten physician note by a department secretary, nurse, or pharmacist and offered limited rules checking or clinical decision support (CDS) capacity.

The "P" in CPOE has most commonly stood for Provider, but will also appear as Physician or Prescriber. This is what makes CPOE different from basic electronic order submission. The transcription step is removed, and the provider places the order directly into the system. By using Provider it is also implied that the user placing the order is authorized to give or sign that order and leaves room for other disciplines in addition to physicians who have a scope of practice that supports CPOE, such as advanced practice nurses and physician assistants.

CPOE is also different in that it is inherently tied to a CDS system that enables the checking and presentation of patient safety rules during ordering, such as drug–drug interaction checking, duplicate checking, corollary orders, and dose calculations (Tyler, 2009). The "E" is also sometimes replaced by an "M" and stands for computerized physician order management or computerized provider order management, further implying that these orders are no longer once and done, but will require ongoing review and updating in the context of rules, alerts, and other feedback mechanisms an EHR may provide that paper and pen cannot. Management of an order also implies that it is more than simply entered, but also communicated to other care team members, reviewed, and acted upon.

In 2005, Dr. Michael McCoy proposed three types of CPOE: basic, intermediate, and advanced (McCoy, 2005). Basic incorporates order entry with simple decision support features such as allergy or drug–drug interaction checking. Intermediate level CPOE includes additional relevant results display at the time of ordering and the ability for providers to save their order preferences. Dr. McCoy considered advanced CPOE to represent advanced clinical order management, and it is here that more sophisticated decision support in the form of "guided ordering" or "mentored ordering" would be available (McCoy, 2005, p. 11).

The definition chosen for CPOE is important to clarify, as it will impact the scope of the CPOE implementation and the related design, build, testing, and training requirements. Will it be basic or advanced? Will it include physicians only or all clinicians more broadly? The definition and standards are also significant as healthcare organizations are now required to benchmark themselves to national HITECH Meaningful Use metrics.

IMPLEMENTATION

Implementing CPOE, in many ways, is not unlike other health information technology projects. It requires a project plan, with appropriate time to complete workflow analysis, build, testing, and training. Like other HIT projects, the most successful implementations have a change management plan that facilitates end-user adoption of the new technology. CPOE, however, is unlike other HIT projects in that it often impacts the healthcare organization on a much broader and deeper scale than, for example, activating a clinical data repository, Picture Archiving and Communication System (PACS), or a clinical notes dictation system. CPOE is at the heart of patient care and cannot be done in isolation to one department or discipline as it ultimately demands not only a new medium in which providers will work—the EHR—but also a new way in which to work. Babbott et al. discuss that physicians working with a fully functioning EHR including CPOE could be presented with multiple tasks ranging from preventative health reminders to required documentation, and that although this may lead to a more accurate assessment than on paper it calls into question if current practice patterns can sustain this "contemporary" approach (2014, p. 4). CPOE has only recently become an accepted tool as routine as using a stethoscope for new healthcare professionals.

COMMON BARRIERS TO SUCCESSFUL ADOPTION

Despite the recent, rapid expansion of CPOE in the wake of Meaningful Use, a review of the literature suggests that there are still segments of providers where the "digital divide" persists and adoption remains low. Those at greatest risk include small, primary care practices, frequently owned by physicians and with some evidence suggesting a greater proportion of patients that are Medicaid, minority, or uninsured (Ryan, Bishop, Shih, & Casalino, 2013). These sites frequently do not have the practical knowledge to implement a CPOE system, apply quality improvement methods to achieve benefits from it, or sustain maintenance. Critical access and smaller hospitals are also at risk due to a low patient volume that limits the organization's ability to apply operational resources to a CPOE implementation, recruit and retain skilled IT personnel, and difficulty finding a suitable vendor that can successfully accommodate these limitations (Desroches, Worzala, & Bates, 2013).

The literature also suggests that "four main drivers influence a providers' decision on electronic health records: affordability; product availability; practice integration; and provider attitudes. HITECH addresses the first three, but providers' attitudes [that are] critical to the success of the act, are beyond the legislation's control" (Gold, McLaughlin, Devers, Berenson, & Bovbjerg, 2012). And that despite established benefits of an EHR; the implementation can still be disruptive and require a steep learning curve for providers to use the features effectively (Ryan, Bishop, Shih, & Casalino, 2013).

STRATEGIES FOR A SUCCESSFUL ADOPTION

A number of studies and reports have been written about successful implementation strategies for CPOE. Written in 2000, *A Primer on Physician Order Entry* cited executive leadership, physician involvement, a multi-disciplinary approach to implementation, good EHR system response time, and flexible training strategies as the keys to a successful CPOE implementation (Drazen, Kilbridge, Metzger, & Turisco, 2000). A more recent study that focused on supporting those provider practices most at risk for successful CPOE adoption reinforced those strategies with eight specific implementation tactics including building relationships to gain the trust of providers that will support the change, hiring staff that understand the domain of the physician practice, setting realistic expectations and obtainable goals, ensuring there is enough physical space for hardware so that providers may work effectively, aligning the organization's vision with the goals of the implementation, developing a business case to identify the expected benefits of CPOE, planning for provider practice redesign, and creating a sustainable support model for ongoing improvement efforts (Torda, Han, & Scholle, 2010).

Given the barriers to and strategies for successful adoption of CPOE outlined here, the work of a nurse informaticist in a CPOE implementation will draw on all aspects of nursing informatics practice as defined by the American Nurses Association, however, as a consultant the nurse informaticist may add the greatest value to solving the complex issues of CPOE through expert domain knowledge, change management theory and planning, process improvement methods, and patient safety review (ANA, 2008).

DOMAIN KNOWLEDGE

Nurses understand many of the physicians' work processes and along with nurse informaticists are in a unique position to assess the impact of new CPOE workflows through communication, coordination, and knowledge sharing (Ghosh, Norton, & Skiba, 2006). Two observations from nurse leaders highlight the importance of this role for ensuring no interruption to patient care, effective care team processes and generally aiding the provider using CPOE for the first time.

The first leader said: "the planning team spent a great deal of time learning all that nurses did to actualize a physician order prior to CPOE. We also recognized the importance of focusing on the output of CPOE to ensure that it supports effective nursing practice" (Ghosh et al., 2006, p. 928). The second leader explained: "our nursing staff was part of the initial phase roll out of CPOE. This built in support system has been a critical factor in driving physician adoption" (Ghosh et al., 2006, p. 928).

CHANGE MANAGEMENT

In addition to ensuring a reliable order management workflow, nurses' domain knowledge also enables the nurse informaticist to plan and support an effective series of change management activities. Change management and communication activities should be a part of each implementation phase starting as early as planning and continuing past the activation of the new system; as project milestones, each activity should build on each other toward unifying providers and the entire care team, solidifying their readiness for a new way of working with CPOE. The requirement of a comprehensive change management plan is well stated by Studer who completed an extensive literature review of effectiveness of EHR implementations and concluded that organizational factors must be considered before, during, and after the implementation in order to promote successful adoption (2005).

One of those organizational factors is readiness for change. "In practical terms, readiness for change requires both a willingness and capacity to change" (Holt, Helfrich, Hall & Weiner, 2010, p. 50). Holt et al. suggest three broad dimensions of organizational readiness to be considered when planning an implementation project and in selecting a method for assessing it. These include psychological factors, structural factors, and the level of analysis (Holt et al., 2010). Several instruments are available to assess readiness to change and the nurse informaticist may help identify the best tool by assessing those being asked to change, the factors under which the change is being made, and the level of impact the change will be felt by either the individual or the organization (Holt et al., 2010).

The need for a sustained change management plan after the implementation was supported in a survey of providers using an EHR. The "high EMR cluster" of providers had a significant correlation to higher stress levels and lower job satisfaction (Babbott et al., 2014, p. 4). Achieving the expected benefits of CPOE is dependent on a provider's ability not only to survive but also thrive in the "high EMR cluster." The nurse informaticist may apply basic usability theory and process improvement methods to identify areas of work redesign that may ease the transition and promote realizing benefits sooner.

USABILITY, PATIENT SAFETY, AND PROCESS IMPROVEMENT METHODS

Despite the many positive outcomes related to EHR implementations, the literature does note negative, unintended consequences of system implementations that cannot be ignored (Ash et al., 2007; Han et al., 2005). Along with reports of usability also being a barrier to adoption of EHR and the expected increase in EHR development and use as a result of HITECH, the Agency for Healthcare Research and Quality (AHRQ) funded research in 2009 and 2010 to establish a common set of recommendations, use cases, policy, and research agenda items related to the usability of EHR systems (AHRQ, 2010). AHRQ categorized the functions of an EHR into four roles: memory aid, computational aid, decision support aid, and collaboration aid (Armijo, McDonnell, & Werner, 2009). How well the EHR can support these functions and a clinician using them in a complex care environment is a direct result of the system's design and usability (Armijo et al., 2009).

Usability is a quality attribute that assesses how easy user interfaces are to use (Nielsen, 2003). There are many quality attributes that represent usability, and for the purposes of CPOE usability, those to focus on include learnability, efficiency, errors, satisfaction, and utility (Nielsen, 2003). Usability expert Jakob Nielsen stresses that it is better to run several small tests in an iterative approach, where five end users are typically enough to identify the most important usability problems (2003). With this in mind, there are three types of testing activities that will promote system usability: a gap analysis between current and future state content and workflows, shadowing a provider real-time working in current state with the new CPOE system testing future state and care team simulation. AHRQ further recommends that these types of tests are organized around a specific framework of use cases including acute episodes, chronic conditions, preventative and health promotion, and undifferentiated symptoms. The combination of measuring these usability attributes through different types of testing activities that are organized around common use cases should capture the high-risk and high-volume workflows related to CPOE and EHR use broadly.

Any usability problems that arise from testing should be seen as an opportunity to drive possible work redesign, CPOE system enhancements, and training and change management efforts. If problems cannot be solved, then goals and expectations of the CPOE implementation must be recalibrated to reflect something more realistic including the potential of not implementing a specific feature or workflow if the risk to safe and reliable patient care may be compromised.

Sustained process improvement methods post-live implementation will further support new usability case studies and successful adoption. The Plan-Do-Study-Act or PDSA model as developed by Associates in Process Improvement can be a helpful framework for guiding this type of work (Langley, Nolan, Nolan, Norman, & Provost, 2009). The PDSA approach would facilitate assembling a team to define the problem, set an improvement goal, brainstorm possible solutions, choose and test a subset of solutions in order to identify which solutions are most effective, and then spread those changes to address the problem broadly. The process may be iterative and starting small and then expanding scope ensures both judicious use of resources and acceptance of the change.

Although the primary goal of these activities is to ensure a safe, reliable CPOE system technical build and to anticipate and plan for the work redesign required of providers, a secondary goal is equally important. These activities also engage the providers and those end users impacted by the changes made by CPOE in a way that enables building relationships of trust with the informatics and information technology team. This is accomplished by identifying and meeting the provider and care team needs that surface during the testing and improvement work, and if unable to meet the needs clearly communicating a risk mitigation plan. The work also simultaneously develops the core competencies required to not only configure and maintain a CPOE system technically, but also to lead and manage professionally through this enormous change for the entire healthcare organization. The cumulative benefits, and subsequent risk mitigation, of usability testing and post-live PDSA efforts make the investment well worth the expense for guiding the CPOE implementation toward healthcare transformation and away from simple automation of current state practice.

FUTURE DIRECTIONS

There is no doubt that CPOE will be an important feature and function of EHRs for the foreseeable future. As noted previously, recent, renewed attention to the adoption of CPOE at a national level with the passage of ARRA has solidified CPOE's position as significant to the delivery of healthcare of the future. The increased number of providers using CPOE alone will change the course of future development in this area, not to mention advances in software, hardware, and interoperability standards.

As coordinated care becomes the gold standard for healthcare delivery, pharmacists and nurses are working to their full scope of practice and partnering with physicians to facilitate key CPOE processes such as medication reconciliation and orders management. Pharmacists and pharmacy techs are collecting medication history, dispensing discharge prescriptions to ensure continuity of care and educating patients on medication management. Nurses and other inter-disciplinary team members such as respiratory therapists and nutritionists are now not only clarifying orders and implementing prescribed interventions, but are also making recommendations through order entry as pended, protocoled, or suggested sets that a physician may accept or decline. This collaboration will only continue to grow and will support both improved provider productivity with CPOE and greater accuracy in the plan of care for a patient.

Increasing patient engagement is another core component to healthcare reform and may include a new role for patients in the future of CPOE. Although medication reconciliation has historically been the domain of providers, a recent pilot study conducted by the VA Boston Healthcare System enabled patients to electronically verify their medication list post-discharge. This virtual medication reconciliation avoided potential adverse drug events and reinforced the patient's desire to partner directly with their physician in all aspects of their care (Heyworth et al., 2014).

The focus of CPOE software development has been oriented to improving basic usability and addressing specific workflow concerns, such as medication reconciliation. In the future, the focus will be on making CPOE systems smarter and able to better anticipate the providers' next action based on past patterns of use. In addition, clinical decision support will continue to become more robust and patient specific, but with it will be a more elegant management of alerting to avoid alert fatigue.

Hardware platforms for personal computing are an exciting area to watch for the future of CPOE. Providers will be able to choose from a wide range of devices in size and portability that will be increasingly enabled for touch screen and tailored to the unique information needs of a specialty, such as intensive care, surgery, or oncology. There will be continued improvement of integration between telecommunication systems and EHR software that will facilitate increased remote alerting, monitoring, and access capabilities.

As interoperability standards between EHR systems improve, it is quite possible that resurgence in a "best of breed" vendor approach to EHR software modules could occur. It would require a significant expansion of data exchange standards beyond medication, allergy, and problem lists, but it is not unfathomable, considering the leaps in HIT standardization in the past five years alone. In the meantime, it is certain that interoperability will expand the provider's accountability for considering and reconciling patient historical data as EHR systems are already passing discreet medication, allergy, and problem list data to be consumed downstream by other EHRs and the providers using them.

Research related to the impact of CPOE adoption on this new scale, along with the use of electronic health records broadly by setting and type of provider will be critical to guiding the future of CPOE, and the nurse informaticist has much to contribute to shaping that future as leaders of health information technology implementations (Hogan & Kissam, 2010).

CORE COMPETENCIES OF THE NURSE INFORMATACIST IN CPOE

Sensmeier summarized the demand for nursing informatics professionals in 2006 and quoted the American Medical Informatics Association (AMIA) Chair, Charles Safran, M.D., as stating that "every hospital and care setting needs one [nurse informaticist] in order to meet the government's vision for EHRs" (2006, p. 169). This is further reinforced in the 20th Annual HIMSS Leadership Survey where "half of healthcare IT professionals indicated that a focus on clinical systems will be their organizations' top IT priority in the next year, with a specific focus on EMR and CPOE technology" (Health Information Management Systems Society [HIMSS], 2009, p. 7). A significant barrier identified by the survey was a lack of IT staffing, particularly in application level support and process/workflow design (HIMSS, 2009).

Application level knowledge represents the ability to assemble the building blocks of a clinical information system in the most effective way to meet the needs of the end user. This skill will primarily rely on the nurse informataticist's ability to assess, plan, and implement. In the case of CPOE, this will require not only technical competency for the purposes of designing and building the workflows to deliver patient care orders into the application, but also content management knowledge to standardize those orders and reinforce them with evidence-based practice. More broadly, application level knowledge also includes the ability to assess the integration points and impact of a particular application like CPOE with other applications like a results interface or pharmacy information system.

As discussed, the nurse informataticist as consultant will also possess the domain knowledge of CPOE workflows and clinical process that is essential for successfully translating and aligning the needs of the end user, the patient,

and the healthcare organization into the application, and leveraging its features and functions to meet those needs. As no single nurse informaticist can know everything about all of an organization's processes or physician practice, workflow analysis skills draw on the nurse's underlying ability to interview clients for their history, complete an assessment, and collaborate across disciplines to meet a common goal. These are skills that would have been learned in nursing school for the purposes of patient care, and here scale for the purposes of ensuring the best outcomes for the organization utilizing the CPOE being implemented. For example, a nurse would never implement a plan of care for a patient simply based on diagnosis alone. So too a nurse informaticist would never implement CPOE simply based on one provider or one department.

The nurse informaticist as consultant can also assess the need for and establish a change management plan for CPOE. These skills are also learned by nurses early in their clinical careers, as they relate to providing patients with education about their plan of care. This may include anticipatory guidance for changes large and small to a patient's lifestyle, daily routine, relationships, and perception of themselves. The nurse's ability to establish a healthy, trusting relationship with the client is at the core of successful patient education. Preparing an organization for the changes related to CPOE is at its core fundamentally not that different; however, the scale is significantly bigger and broader as the learning styles, motivators, and metrics of success for the CPOE implementation will vary widely across providers, patients, the inter-disciplinary team, and the organization itself. Subsequent "coping mechanisms" for the CPOE changes will also vary by organization based on culture, infrastructure, available resources, and the ability to apply those resources. The nurse informatacist working with CPOE is competent in assessing an individual's and an organization's readiness to change, can employ basic usability and process improvement methods to anticipate the impact of the change and lead through the change in a positive, constructive way.

Ensuring a usable system that promotes patient safety and provider adoption is another primary requirement for the nurse informaticist implementing CPOE. Familiarity with the heuristics of usability along with the ability to assess common high-risk and high-volume use cases for unintended consequences will ensure that benefits of the implementation are realized reliably and without causing undue harm.

National healthcare policy review has often been reserved to the scope of practice of nurse leaders in management or academia. The expert nurse in CPOE, however, can no longer isolate him- or herself from the of work government on healthcare information technology.

As stated previously, the implications of healthcare reform and HITECH are now more than ever tightly intertwined with the daily care of patients and the clinical information systems that support that care delivery. While an advanced degree in healthcare policy is not necessary, the competent nurse informaticist should understand the regulatory and compliance landscape, and its impact on clinical processes and applications as this will always be an influence on his or her future work.

CONCLUSION

CPOE remains one of the most challenging areas within healthcare IT today, and yet it has the promise of significant benefits to both the patient and the provider, making it an area of potential great professional reward. CPOE systems have improved over the years and will only continue to become more user-friendly and sophisticated in their clinical decision support capabilities as the demand increases from broader adoption. Cultural barriers to CPOE implementation will also shift as adoption becomes required to demonstrate meaningful use of an EHR. With core competencies of systems knowledge, workflow analysis, change management, usability theory, process improvement methods, human factors, and healthcare policy, the nurse informaticist will be well positioned to support CPOE implementations today and shape the systems of tomorrow.

REFERENCES

Agency of Healthcare Research and Quality. (2010). *Use of dense display of data and information design principles in primary health care information technology systems.* Washington, DC: Author. Retrieved from http://healthit.ahrq.gov/ahrq-funded-projects/use-dense-display-data-and-information-design-principles-primary-care-health

American Nurses Association. (2008). *Nursing informatics: Scope and standards of practice.* Washington, DC: American Nurses Publications.

Armijo, D., McDonnell, C., & Werner, K. (2009). *Electronic health record usability: Evaluation and use case framework.* AHRQ Publication No. 09(10)-0091-1-EF. Rockville, MD: Agency for Healthcare Research and Quality.

Ash, J. S., Sittig, D. F., Poon, E. G., Guappone, K., Campbell, E., & Dykstra, R. H. (2007). The extent and importance of unintended consequences related to computerized provider order entry. *Journal of the American Medical Informatics Association, 14*(5), 415–423.

Babbott, S., Manwell, L. B., Brown, R., Montague, E., Williams, E., Schwartz, M., … Linzer, M. (2014). Electronic medical records and physician stress in primary care: Results from the MEMO study. *Journal of the Medical Informatics Association, 21*(e1), e100–e106.

Department of Health & Human Services. (2013). *EHR incentives and certification: How to attain meaningful use.* Washington, DC: Author. Retrieved from http://www.healthit.gov/providers-professionals/how-attain-meaningful-use

Desroches, C. M., Worzala, C., & Bates, S. (2013). Some hospitals are falling behind in meeting meaningful use criteria and could be vulnerable to penalities in 2015. *Health Affairs, 32*(8), 1355–1360.

Drazen, E., Kilbridge, P., Metzger, J., & Turisco, F. (2000). *A primer on physician order entry.* Oakland, CA: California HealthCare Foundation.

Ghosh, T., Norton, M., & Skiba, D. (2006). Communication, coordination and knowledge sharing in the implementation of CPOE: Impact on nursing practice. *American Medical Informatics Association Annual Symposium Proceedings, 928.*

Gold, M. R., McLaughlin, C. G., Devers, K. J., Berenson, R. A., & Bovbjerg, R. R. (2012). Obtaining providers buy-in and establishing effective means of information exchange will be critical to HITECH's success. *Health Affairs, 31*(3), 514–526.

Han, Y. Y., Carcillo, J. A., Venkataraman, S. T., Clark, R. S. B., Watson, R. S., Nguyen, T. C., … Orr, R. A. (2005). Unexpected increased mortality after implementation of a commercially sold computerized physician order entry system. *Pediatrics, 116*(6), 1506–1512.

Health Information Management Systems Society. (2009). *20th annual HIMSS leadership survey.* Chicago, IL: Author. Retrieved from http://www.himss.org/files/HIMSSorg/2010SURVEY/DOCS/20thAnnualLeadershipSurveyFINAL.pdf

Heyworth, L., Paquin, A. M., Clark, J., Kamenker, V., Stewart, M., Martin, T., & Simon, S. R. (2014). Engaging patients in medication reconciliation via a patient portal following hospital discharge. *Journal of the American Medical Informatics Association, 21*(e1), e157–e162.

Hogan, S. O., & Kissam, S. M. (2010). Measuring meaningful use. *Health Affairs, 29*(4), 601–606.

Holt, D. T., Helfrich, C. D., Hall, C. G., & Weiner, B. J. (2010). Are you ready? How health professionals can comprehensively conceptualize readiness for change. *Journal of General Internal Medicine, 25*(Suppl. 1):50–55.

Institute of Medicine. (2000). *To err is human: Building a safer health system.* Washington, DC: National Academies Press.

Institute of Medicine. (2001). *Crossing the quality chasm: A new health system for the 21st century.* Washington, DC: National Academies Press.

Kaushal, R., Jha, A. K., Franz, C., Glaser, J., Shetty, K. D., Jaggi, T., … Bates, D. W. (2006). Return on investment for a computerized physician order entry system. *Journal of the American Medical Informatics Association, 13*(3), 261–266.

Langley, G. L., Nolan, K. M., Nolan, T. W., Norman, C. L., Provost, L. P. (2009). *The improvement guide: A practical approach to enhancing organizational performance* (2nd ed.). San Francisco, CA: Jossey-Bass Publishers.

Longhurst, C. A., Parast, L., Sandborg, C. I., Widen, E., Sullivan, J., Hahn, J. S., & Sharek, P. J. (2010). Decrease in hospital-wide mortality rate after implementation of a commercially sold computerized physician order entry system. *Pediatrics, 126*(1), e1–e8. Retrieved from http://www.pediatrics.org

McCoy, M. J. (2005). Advanced clinician order management—A superset of CPOE. *Journal of Healthcare Information Management, 19*(4), 11–13.

Nielsen, J. (2003). *Usability 101: Introduction to usability.* Fremont, CA: Author. Retrieved from http://www.useit.com/alertbox/20030825.html

Poissant, L., Pereira, J., Tamblyn, R., & Kawasumi, Y. (2005). The impact of electronic health records on time efficiency of physicians and nurses: A systemic review. *Journal of the American Medical Informatics Association, 12*(5), 505–516.

Ryan, A. M., Bishop, T. F., Shih, S., & Casalino, L. P. (2013). Small physician practices in New York needed sustained help to realize gains in quality from use of electronic health records. *Health Affairs, 32*(1), 53–62.

Sensmeier, J. (2006). Every organization needs them: Nurse informaticians. In C. A. Weaver, C. W. Delaney, P. Weber, & R. L. Carr (Eds.), *Nursing and informatics for the 21st century* (pp. 169–178). Chicago, IL: Healthcare Information and Management Systems Society.

Studer, M. (2005). The effect of organizational factors on the effectiveness of EHR system implementation—what have we learned? *Electronic Healthcare, 4*(2), 92–98.

The Leapfrog Group. (2010). *Factsheet: Computerized physician order entry.* Washington, DC: Author. Retrieved from http://www.leapfroggroup.org/media/file/FactSheet_CPOE.pdf

Torda, P., Han, E. S., & Scholle, S. H. (2010). Easing the adoption and use of electronic health records in small practices. *Health Affairs, 29*(4), 668–675.

Tyler, D. (2009). Administrative and clinical health information systems. In D. McGonigle & K. G. Mastrian (Eds.), *Nursing informatics and the foundation of knowledge* (pp. 205–218). Sudbury, MA: Jones and Bartlett Publishers.

28

Physiological Monitoring and Device Interface

R. Renee Johnson-Smith

• OBJECTIVES

1. Describe importance of medical device connectivity.
2. Define components of medical device interfaces devices.
3. Understand issues and challenges of infusion management and Smart Pumps.
4. Introduce Smart Room technology.
5. Describe importance of alarm fatigue in medical device connectivity.
6. Explore the challenges with medical device connectivity.

• KEY WORDS

Medical device connectivity
Interoperability
HL7
Middleware
MDDS
Device association
Data validation

In today's healthcare climate of increasing patient acuity, decreasing resources, and increased financial restraints, the use of medical devices interfaced with each other as well as the electronic health record are imperative for the safety and quality of care of today's patients.

SCENARIO

A patient is newly admitted to an intensive care unit from the emergency department at a suburban hospital. The patient is placed on a physiologic monitor and a ventilator in the ICU. The nurse associated the patient to the monitor so that she could automatically chart vital signs in the EHR. The patient has labs drawn and resulted every two hours via a POC (Point-of-Care)

device. The patient had radiology exams in the ED prior to arriving in the ICU. An interactive infusion pump (Smart Pump) administers medications intravenously and interacts with the EHR to record titration of the medications automatically in real time. Twenty-six miles away, at a remote monitoring center (tele-ICU) stationed in a large metropolis hospital is also monitoring the patient. An alarm sounds from the physiologic monitor at the bedside while a secondary alert sounds within the tele-ICU unit alerting staff at the patient's bedside as well as in the tele-ICU that the patient has gone into VT (Ventricular Tachycardia), a lethal heart arrhythmia that requires immediate intervention. While the care givers at the bedside start advanced cardiac life-saving measures, the remote clinician can begin searching the electronic health record for the patient's most recent lab results, pertinent medical history, medication history, as well as radiology results. The remote clinician has special software that enables the remote clinician to review real-time vital signs, track and review trends, and recognize changes. The remote clinician can view the activities occurring in the patient room via a two-way camera with audio as well as call a code for the bedside, thus allowing the bedside clinician to remain at the bedside providing direct patient care. The bedside and remote clinicians methodically work together to resolve the issue, convert the patient, and stabilize the patient....

The aforementioned scenario is real and possible today due to advancements in medicine, technology, and legislation. According to Medical Strategic Planning, Inc., over the last decade the number of devices that need to be interfaced has grown from a handful to over 400 major devices (MSP Industry Alert, 2009). The medical device connectivity market was worth $3.5 billion in 2013 and is projected to reach $33 billion by 2019, which is a growth rate of 37.8% (Miliard, 2013). Medical device connectivity is expected to increase efficiency and productivity, improve clinical workflow, lower costs while improving patient quality and safety.

MEANINGFUL USE

The Health Information Technology for Economic and Clinical Health (HITECH) Act signed into law on February 17, 2009, as part of the American Recovery and Reinvestment Act (ARRA) of 2009 stimulated adoption of the electronic health record (EHR) (US Department of Health and Human Services, 2013; Williams, 2012). The HITECH Act allows eligible providers and eligible hospitals to qualify for the Center for Medicare Medicaid Services (CMS) incentive payments if they achieve "meaningful use" of certified EHR technology to provide patient care (Center for Medicaid and Medicare Services, 2013). EHR vendors are incented to obtain ARRA certification for their EHR products. It is not enough for healthcare providers to have purchased and implemented a certified EHR, providers must also demonstrate meaningful use. The Centers for Medicare & Medicare Services (CMS) and the Office of the National Coordinator for Health Information Technology (ONC) are providing meaningful use criteria for both acute care (hospital/ER) and provider practices (clinic) settings. Eligible providers and eligible healthcare facilities that comply will receive incentive payments. In time, those failing to comply will be penalized.

Meaningful Use is a three-phased approach building upon each other. HITECH does not provide incentives specifically for medical device connectivity in itself but connectivity drives the adoption of EHR use and thereby meaningful use adoption.

INTEROPERABILITY

Medical device connectivity generally refers to the integration of medical devices with hospital information systems (HIS) to facilitate functions (ECRI Institute, 2012). Advancements in technology have expanded medical device connectivity from connecting a device to an EHR, to connecting disparate medical devices so that they all may communicate with each other also known as **interoperability**. According to HIMSS, "interoperability describes the extent to which systems and devices can exchange data, and interpret that shared data. For two systems to be interoperable, they must be able to exchange data and subsequently present that data such that it can be understood by a user" (HIMSS, 2013).

STANDARDIZED COMMUNICATION

The ability of medical devices to talk to each other requires a standard language or communication structure, the most common in healthcare being **HL7** or Health Level Seven. According to Interface, HL7 is by definition "an ANSI (American National Standards Institute) standard for healthcare specific data exchange between computer applications. The name comes from 'Health Level 7,' which refers to the top layer (Level 7) of the Open Systems Interconnection (OSI) layer protocol for the health environment. The HL7 standard is the most widely used messaging standard in the healthcare industry around the world" (Interfaceware, 2013).

MIDDLEWARE

Device connectivity and operability require middleware. **Middleware** is a term with broad implications. For purposes of this chapter, **middleware** enables integration of data between two or more programs, devices, or information systems. **Middleware** facilitates communication and data sharing. While the following is not all-inclusive, several types of middleware will be discussed *such as integration engines, gateways, medical device data systems, and Class II medical devices for active monitoring.*

INTEGRATION ENGINE

Often *integration engine* or *interface engine* are terms used interchangeably. In the healthcare industry, integration engines use HL7 to characterize their ability to manage all interfaces. The engines aggregate and share data regardless of the transmission protocol. They are responsible for message routing and translation.

GATEWAY

Data can also be transferred through a device *gateway*. These are usually transferred through a central server that consolidates and collates data and then forwards the information to the aggregator or EHR (Day, 2011).

MEDICAL DEVICE DATA SYSTEMS

Unfortunately not all medical devices use or know how to speak native HL7 so a medical device connectivity solution (MDCS) or a **medical device data system** (MDDS) is required (Table 28.1 provides the FDA description of MDDS). Medical device connectivity solutions are

TABLE 28.1	Medical Device Data Systems (MDDS)

Medical Device Data Systems (MDDS) are hardware or software products that transfer, store, convert formats, and display medical device data. An MDDS does not modify the data or modify the display of the data, and it does not by itself control the functions or parameters of any other medical device. MDDS are not intended to be used for active patient monitoring.

Examples of MDDS include:

- Software that stores patient data such as blood pressure readings for review at a later time
- Software that converts digital data generated by a pulse oximeter into a format that can be printed
- Software that displays a previously stored electrocardiogram for a particular patient

The quality and continued reliable performance of MDDS are essential for the safety and effectiveness of healthcare delivery. Inadequate quality and design, unreliable performance, or incorrect functioning of MDDS can have a critical impact on public health.

http://www.fda.gov/MedicalDevices/ProductsandMedical Procedures/GeneralHospitalDevicesandSupplies/Medical DeviceDataSystems/default.htm

available via the EHR vendor, medical device vendors, and third-party vendors. Typically the EHR solution and medical device vendor solutions only work with its own solution whereas third-party solutions are designed to be agnostic to the medical devices and can interface with a multitude of devices, sometimes referred to as *enterprise-wide connectivity*. The advantage of third-party vendors for a medical device connectivity solution is it allows a single vendor to manage the interface between the enterprise-wide medical device data and the EHR rather than the facility managing a multitude of interfaces for each type of device (ECRI Institute, 2012). It also enables hospitals to choose any vendor for patient care–related devices regardless of the of integration issues.

CLASS II MEDICAL DEVICES

According to FDA regulatory requirements in the healthcare information space, MDDS classified devices are limited to data transfers to an EHR only. MDDSs are precluded from use in active patient monitoring and alarming (Johnson, 2012). While an MDDS can have alarms related to its own operational status (ECRI Institute, 2012) it cannot analyze. Solutions that collect, process, and distribute medical device data for surveillance, alarms, analytics, and decision support are not considered an MDDS but are regulated by the FDA as a Class II medical device (Johnson, 2012). A Class II medical device used for active monitoring is utilized in the aforementioned ICU scenario as the software that allows the remote clinicians to review real-time vital signs, track and review trends, and recognize changes.

POINT OF CARE

The bedside medical device and how data are transmitted from the medical device characterizes point-of-care (POC) connectivity solutions. The POC solution serves as middleware where the POC device or component associates the patient to the medical device and compiles the information from the medical device to send to a server (DiDonato, 2013) to be translated into an appropriate inbound language, generally HL7, for the EHR to accept and store. POC devices generally link to the medical device via a wired serial connection or wirelessly. The association of the medical device data to a specific patient is generally referred to as *patient context* or *patient association* (ECRI Institute, 2012). POCs contain *device drivers* that allow them to understand the proprietary data of the medical device POC (ECRI Institute, 2012).

PERIODIC/EPISODIC DEVICES

Periodic or *episodic devices* are those that obtain a single set of measurements from a patient at single points in time or spot checks (DiDonato, 2014; ECRI Institute, 2012). Episodic devices are generally mobile and used with multiple patients. Examples of common episodic devices are portable vital sign monitors, glucose meters, pulse oximetry, and ECG machines.

CONTINUOUS NETWORKED DEVICES

Continuous devices are divided into stand-alone or networked devices. Continuous networked devices are commonly stationed in a patient room to treat a single patient over a continuous time span. They are generally hardwired and connected to a vendor specific central server negating the need for a POC component/Solution. An example is a bedside physiologic monitor such as the one in the aforementioned scenario.

CONTINUOUS STAND-ALONE DEVICES

Continuous stand-alone medical device solutions are used to continuously monitor a single patient over a period of time but the device is portable and not hardwired or networked to a vendor-specific server, thereby requiring a POC component within the patient room or attached to the medical device itself. In the scenario, the ventilator and infusion pump were continuous stand-alone devices. Table 28.2 provides a diagram illustrating the medical device connectivity architecture.

PATIENT-TO-DEVICE ASSOCIATION (P2DA)

Consider the aforementioned scenario, the patient has multiple devices in the ICU but how do the medical device and related POC solution know which patient the data are coming from in order to correctly translate them and direct them to the correct patient record in the EHR? The

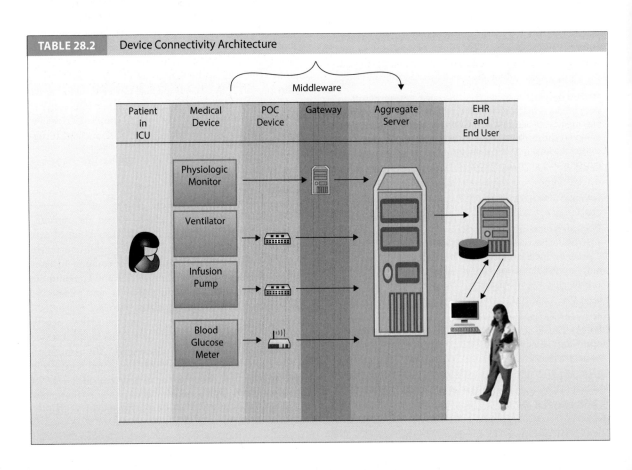

TABLE 28.2   Device Connectivity Architecture

TABLE 28.3	P2D2
PPID	Positive Patient Identification
PPA	Positive Patient Association

linking of the medical device data with the right patient is referred to as *patient association*. There are historically two approaches to patient association: patient centric and location centric (ECRI Institute, 2012). Table 28.3 identifies common association terms.

PATIENT-CENTRIC IDENTIFICATION

Patient-centric identification involves associating a medical device with a patient based on a unique patient ID number, often the patient's unique medical record number. In our scenario the patient in the ICU is associated to the physiologic monitor. The bedside nurse in our scenario manually entered the patient's unique ID number into the monitor when the patient was admitted which "associated" the right patient to the right device so the right data will be available for documentation. Often the medical device may also have an ADT list to choose the correct patient. The nurse in the scenario also associated the Smart Pump to the patient using bar code technology by scanning the patient's wrist band and scanning the infusion pump so the patient is now associated to the pump. Lastly, the nurse associated the ventilator.

LOCATION CENTRIC

In *location-centric* association the patient is typically identified by a location such as a room or bed. This type of association can be unreliable and thereby unsafe especially when a patient is moved often such as in an emergency department or surgical area. In 2009, the Joint Commission added criteria to the NPSG.01.01.01 "Identifying Patients Correctly" goal that states, "The patient's room number or physical location is not used as an identifier" (www.jointcommission.com). With clear direction from the Joint Commission, coupled with the increasing meaningful use objectives, most vendors and healthcare institutions are moving away from location-centric association and identifying better means to support unique patient identifiers to provide safer patient to device communication.

AUTO-ID

While our scenario focuses on a patient in an ICU where many devices are fixed or unique to critical care patients and continuous, imagine a typical medical/surgical acute

care unit where vital sign monitors or blood glucose meters are used in multiple rooms on multiple patients for spot checks. Manually entering a unique patient ID or selecting a patient from a list can be time intensive and allows room for error. Auto-ID technologies such as bar code scanning and passive RFID is becoming increasingly useful and available as a means to assist with mobility and periodic device use (McAlpine, 2011). Table 28.4 provides a more comprehensive overview of RFID from the FDA.

TABLE 28.4	Radio Frequency Identification (RFID) (Food and Drug Administration, 2014)

Description

Radio Frequency Identification (RFID) refers to a wireless system comprised of two components: tags and readers. The reader is a device that has one or more antennas that emit radio waves and receive signals back from the RFID tag. Tags, which use radio waves to communicate their identity and other information to nearby readers, can be passive or active. Passive RFID tags are powered by the reader and do not have a battery. Active RFID tags are powered by batteries.

RFID tags can store a range of information from one serial number to several pages of data. Readers can be mobile so that they can be carried by hand, or they can be mounted on a post or overhead. Reader systems can also be built into the architecture of a cabinet, room, or building.

Uses

RFID systems use radio waves at several different frequencies to transfer data. In healthcare and hospital settings, RFID technologies include the following applications:

- Inventory control
- Equipment tracking
- Out-of-bed detection and fall detection
- Personnel tracking
- Ensuring that patients receive the correct medications and medical devices
- Preventing the distribution of counterfeit drugs and medical devices
- Monitoring patients
- Providing data for electronic medical records systems

The FDA is not aware of any adverse events associated with RFID. However, there is concern about the potential hazard of electromagnetic interference (EMI) to electronic medical devices from radio frequency transmitters like RFID. EMI is a degradation of the performance of equipment or systems (such as medical devices) caused by an electromagnetic disturbance.

http://www.fda.gov/Radiation-EmittingProducts/RadiationSafety/ElectromagneticCompatibilityEMC/ucm116647.htm

DATA VALIDATION

In the above scenario, the patient is associated to a monitor and per the association discussion we learned that the nurse manually associated the monitor to the patient with the patient's unique identifier. There is still a question as to how does the EHR know which vital signs to record or which vital signs are accurate? How does the EHR know not to record the blood pressure that was false because the cuff failed, or not to record the pulse oximetry reading of 75% that occurred when the pulse oximetry came off while the patient was turned? Since data are continuously being sent to the EHR, the nurse must validate which data are accurate and should be recorded within the permanent patient medical record. This process of manual verification of data and recording them into the medical record is known as **data validation**. The accuracy of the data is extremely important. Data verification can occur at the POC component, within a separate application or within the EHR.

CONNECTIVITY DIRECTION

Historically device connectivity solutions were unidirectional, or the flow of information was from the medical device to the EHR only; this is also often referred to as *classic* or *one-way connectivity*. The emergence of bi-directional connectivity is mounting quickly as a viable solution in healthcare. Bi-directional connectivity not only exports data from bedside medical devices to the EHR, but also allows the EHR to export data back to the bedside medical devices.

SMART PUMPS

An emerging trend in acute healthcare settings is the use of *Smart Infusion Pumps* and *Interactive Smart Pumps*. Smart pumps use drug libraries which allow infusion pumps to perform functions that assist with programming and calculating dose and rate delivery as adapted by a healthcare institution and to patient care areas (Cummings & McGowan, 2011). Hard and soft limits or *guardrails* are programmed within Smart Pumps for medications. Soft limits can generally be overridden after a clinician acknowledges a safety alert whereas hard limits are generally set for high-risk medications (Cummings & McGowan, 2011). Smart Pumps may have software that allows automatic transmission to the EHR. Taking technology to the next level, a Smart Pump that has bi-directional communication is often referred to as an *Interactive Smart Pump* and allows pre-populating the infusion orders from the EHR to the infusion pump,

TABLE 28.5	Smart Pump Complications
User Error	**Device Error**
• Improper programming of the medication including incorrect dose rate • Selecting incorrect drug • Not reviewing alerts • Programming the wrong pump channel	• Software defects— pre-programmed alarms do not activate or alarms active in absence of an issue • Over- or under-infusion • Out-of-date drug library

thus saving the nurses' time in programming the pump and reducing keying errors while programming ultimately increasing patient safety and efficiency.

Smart Pumps are not without complications and not intended to replace the human touch of a healthcare provider. Smart pumps errors can be classified into user error or device error. Table 28.5 lists common complications related to both classifications of errors.

SMART ROOMS

Gaining traction is the growth of *Smart Rooms*. The University of Pittsburgh Medical Center (UPMC) was the first to pilot such technology in a medical surgical unit (Orlovsky, 2013) in June 2011. The Smart Rooms at UPMC use real-time location solutions (RTLS) tracking to bring patient information from the EHR to a computer in the patient room. The clinicians were identified when entering the room by ultrasound-enabled badges identifying them to the patient and families, eliminating the need for white boards. Each patient room has a patient- and family-centered screen that can be used to identify caregivers, provide a schedule of the day activities for the patient, as well as access to view educational programs. Lastly the rooms include a direct care touch screen which aids in documentation and provides important clinical attributes such as allergies, labs, and meds (Cerrato, 2011; Hagland, 2011).

As Smart Room technology has matured (grown) the desire for interaction and development has also grown. From a clinical perspective, caregivers request more interfacing of devices including smart beds, single sign-on, RTLS that identifies where a patient is when off the unit or where a commonly used medical device is located such as an ECG machine. Families have more concierge-type requests such as entertainment (movies and games), electronic notepads, Web cams, or video conferencing with patients from remote locations. While Smart Rooms are in their infancy stages, as healthcare demands more interoperability and patients demand better safety and quality service the use of Smart Room technology will continue to mature.

ALARMS

Alarms are intended to alert a caregiver when an immediate or potentially adverse event occurs or could occur. A caregiver is then expected to acknowledge the alarm and respond appropriately. As the number of medical devices increases so has the number of alarms generated from medical devices. Caregivers are challenged with responding to multiple alarms produced from multiple devices. Considering our scenario of the patient in the ICU, alarms could be emitted not only from the physiologic monitor, infusion pump, and ventilators but the nurse must also respond to call lights, bed-exit devices, feeding pumps, sequential compression devices, telephone calls, texts/pages, etc. (Cvach, 2012).

According to the Joint Commission, there may be several hundreds of alarms per day per patient depending on the patient's location (Sentinel Event Alert, 2013). Many alarms are false alerts or nuisance alarms. A nuisance alarm does not usually indicate immediate intervention is needed. An example could be that a patient's physiologic monitor alerts because the patient turned in the bed and there was a jump in the patient's heart rate while the patient turned. It is estimated that 85% to 99% of alarms do not require intervention (Sentinel Event Alert, 2013).

ALARM FATIGUE

Due to the aforementioned issues, many caregivers become immune or desensitized to the alarms and are not as timely to respond to alarms (Sentinel Event Alert, 2013). In some scenarios, alarms may be intentionally and unintentionally silenced or turned off. Either desensitization or silencing alarms leads to patient harm.

USE ALARMS SAFELY

The Joint Commission has taken a position in deterring patient harm due to alarm errors and has added alarms back into the 2014 National Patient Safety Goals, NPSG.06.01.01, Use Alarms Safety, requiring improvements to ensure that alarms from medical devices are heard and responded to timely (The Joint Commission, 2013). While much of the ownership of alarm fatigue and adverse events related to alarms is placed on the caregivers and healthcare institutions, medical device companies are exploring technology to develop safer and more effective alarm management. Medical device vendors are

seeking to improve parameter acquisition techniques as well as improve alarm and alert designs to reduce non-clinically significant alarms (ACCE Healthcare Technology Foundation, 2013). Medical device vendors are researching and implementing *smart alarms* which are alarms that are built upon algorithms that consider multiple physiologic parameters. Lastly, efforts are being created around middleware that could route alarms from various devices to central call systems either location based or through a mobile nurse call system.

CHALLENGES

While there have been huge advancements in medical device integration there are just as many challenges that still need addressed as the industry matures.

Cost

From a vendor standpoint, it is timely and costly to research and develop devices, device drivers, and software. Once the software or devices are available on the market, it is expensive for healthcare facilities to replace or purchase new equipment. It can also be very time consuming to test and install updated software. From a structural standpoint, it can be very costly to add network components after a structure is constructed so as healthcare facilities expand or rebuild, infrastructure of existing network as well as the future of the networks need to be considered.

Risk Management/Security

Healthcare institutions' information systems transmit and store a great deal of sensitive and protected information; therefore, mitigating risks and safely securing the information are as important as safely caring for the patient. However, medical IT and device interoperability industry lacks mature communication standards and governance. While the FDA regulates the classification of medical devices, there is room for growth in how the devices interface and communicate. Table 28.6 lists some of the Healthcare IT advocacy associations and standards.

Clinician Adoption

Device vendors and healthcare providers must work together to continue development of automation that will enhance patient care, safety, and workflows. When new types of technology or devices are introduced in the healthcare setting, it must increase efficiency or adoption will not occur. Typically there is not a one-size-fits-all approach

TABLE 28.6	Healthcare IT Advocacy Associations and Standards
AAMI	Advancing Safety in Medical Technology
CIMIT	Center for Integration of Medicine and Innovative Technology
IEC 80001	Application of Risk Management for IT-Networks Incorporating Medical Devices
IHE	Integrating the Healthcare Environment
ISO/IEEE 10073	Medical Informatics—Medical Device Information
MD PnP	Medical Device Plug N Play

because workflows vary immensely between settings and units. Workflows and challenges with workflows must be thoroughly considered and tested prior to implementation.

SUMMARY/CONCLUSION

Over the last decade, the medical device industry has experienced an explosion in the types and numbers of devices needed to care for patients. Traditionally medical devices were concentrated to high acuity areas such as intensive cares, emergency departments, or surgical suites, however much of the medical device surge is related to caring for patient outside the walls of high acuity areas and even outside the walls of the hospital. Device integration and connectivity is moving into the ambulatory and home care space where patients can be monitored with mobile technology. Advancements in wireless technology and mobile technology have implications not even considered yet.

SCENARIO REVISITED

The patient recovered from her life-threatening arrhythmic event and is ready for discharge from the hospital. Due to having a life-threatening cardiac event, she will be discharged with a wireless home holter monitor and pulse oximetry. A visiting nurse will visit and download the information from the holter monitor and oximetry weekly. In the meantime, the patient will record all her activity, rest, and recovery.

REFERENCES

ACCE Healthcare Technology Foundation. (2013). *Impact of clinical alarms on patient safety*. White Paper. Retrieved from http://thehtf.org/white%20paper.pdf

Center for Medicaid and Medicare Services. (2013). *Meaningful use.* Retrieved from http://www.cms.gov/Regulations-and-Guidance/Legislation/EHRIncentivePrograms/Meaningful_Use.html.

Cerrato, P. (2011). *Hospital rooms get smart.* Commentary. Retrieved from http://www.informationweek.com/hospital-rooms-get-smart/231901129. Accessed on July 26, 2013.

Cummings, K., & McGowan, R. (2011). Smart infusion pumps are selectively intelligent. *Nursing*, 59.

Cvach, M. (2012). Monitor alarm fatigue an integrative review. *Biomedical Instrumentation and Technology.* 46(4), 268–277.

Day, B. (2011). Standards for medical device interoperability and integration. *Patient Safety and Quality Healthcare.* Retrieved from http://www.psqh.com/januaryfebruary-2011/739-standards-for-medical-device-interoperability-and-integration.html. Accessed on July 2013.

DiDonato, S. (2013). Open communication. Integrating medical equipment with electronic health records. *Health Facilities Management.* Retrieved from http://www.hfmmagazine.com/hfmmagazine/jsp/articledisplay.jsp?domain=HFMMAGAZINE&dcrpath=HFMMAGAZINE/Article/data/03MAR2013/0313HFM_FEA_technology

DiDonato, S. (2014). *Understand the complexities of integrating your technologies.* Retrieved from http://1technation.com/ecri-update-medical-devices-talking/. Accessed on January 10, 2014.

ECRI Institute. (2012). Guidance article. Making connections. *Health Devices.* 102–115.

Food and Drug Administration. (2014). *RFID.* Retrieved from http://www.fda.gov/Radiation-EmittingProducts/RadiationSafety/ElectromagneticCompatibilityEMC/ucm116647.htm. Accessed on January 4, 2014.

Hagland, M. (2011). Smart rooms, smart care delivery. *Healthcare Informatics.* Retrieved from http://www.healthcare-informatics.com/article/smart-rooms-smart-care-delivery. Accessed on July 26, 2012.

HIMSS. (2013). *What is interoperability.* Retrieved from http://www.himss.org/library/interoperability-standards/what-is?navItemNumber=17333

Interfaceware. (2013). *HL7 Standard.* Retrieved from http://www.interfaceware.com/hl7-standard/#sthash.78dH9VhJ.dpuf

Johnson, R. (2012). Medical device connectivity beyond MDDS, case study.

McAlpine, B. (2011). Improving medical device connectivity. *Health Management Technology.* 32(5), 18–9.

Miliard, M. (2013). Big Growth seen for device integration. *Healthcare IT News.* Retrieved from http://www.healthcareitnews.com/news/big-growth-seen-device-integration

MSP Industry Alert. (2009). MDDS—Key to clinical data integration at the point-of-care. www.medsp.com. *Medical Strategic Planning. 11*(1), 5–11.

Orlovsky, C. (2013). Smart rooms raise health care IQ. Nursesone.com. Retrieved from http://www.nursezone.com/Nursing-News-Events/devices-and-technology.aspx?ID=17500. Accessed on July 26, 2013.

Sentinel Event Alert. (2013). Medical device alarm safety in hospitals. *The Joint Commission, Issue 50.*

The Joint Commission. (2013). *National patient safety goals.* Retrieved from http://www.jointcommission.org

U.S. Department of Health and Human Services. (2013). *Health information privacy.* Retrieved from http://www.hhs.gov/ocr/privacy/hipaa/administrative/enforcementrule/hitechenforcementifr.html

Williams, J. (2012). Achieving interoperability: What's happening out there? *Biomedical Instrumentation & Technology.* 46(1), 14–23.

29

Health Information Technology: Striving to Improve Patient Safety*

Patricia P. Sengstack

• OBJECTIVES

1. Describe the current state of the evidence in relation to health IT and patient safety.
2. Discuss the federal government's involvement in assisting to improve patient safety using health IT.
3. Describe at least three resources that organizations can use to evaluate the safety of their IT systems.

• KEY WORDS

Health IT
Patient safety
Errors
Electronic Health Record (EHR)
Computerized Provider Order Entry (CPOE)
Unintended consequences
HITECH Act
Office of the National Coordinator for Health IT (ONC)
Patient safety organizations
Common formats

INTRODUCTION

The first Electronic Health Record (EHR) with Computerized Provider Order Entry (CPOE) was introduced in 1971, over 40 years ago (Goolsby, 2002). Since then, adoption of these systems in both acute and ambulatory settings has been relatively slow, until the signing of the American Reinvestment and Recovery Act (ARRA)

*Dr. Sengstack is the Chief Nursing Informatics Officer in the Center for Clinical Excellence and Innovation for the Bon Secours Health System in Marriottsville, MD. She is also the current President of the American Nursing Informatics Association and is on the faculty and teaches informatics at Vanderbilt University School of Nursing.

in 2009. The ARRA included the authorization of the Health Information Technology for Economic and Clinical Health (HITECH) Act which allocated over $17 billion to stimulate the adoption of quality health IT systems or EHRs that demonstrate meaningful use (U.S. Department of Health & Human Services, 2014).

While these financial incentives to increase adoption appear to be working, issues from rapid implementation have surfaced over the last decade including several related to patient safety. As these systems have evolved and increased in sophistication, evidence supporting the view that EHRs reduce medication errors has been documented (Kaushal, Shojania, & Bates, 2003). On the

419

other hand, conflicting studies have provided evidence that these systems can actually increase errors, attributing them to poor design or implementation (Koppel et al., 2005). The recent focus has been on the adoption of EHRs to achieve incentive payments from the HITECH Act, with less of a focus on patient safety. The HIT industry, the federal government, and other watchdog agencies have begun to take notice. This chapter will provide background information in the area of health IT and patient safety as it has evolved over the last decade. It will review the government's response in addressing the health IT safety issue. Involvement by other professional organizations will be briefly reviewed followed by an offering of tools and resources that organizations can utilize in their practice settings to assist in ensuring that health IT is as safe as possible.

BACKGROUND—HEALTH IT SAFETY

Since its publication in 1999, The Institute of Medicine's *To Err Is Human* has been a driving force for improvements in patient safety across the nation. The evidence cited clearly indicates the seriousness of the situation in terms of lives lost and money wasted as a result of errors that occur in our healthcare organizations. There have been multiple solutions offered, but a common and resounding theme continues to be the use of technology and the application of EHRs with CPOE systems (Kohn, Corrigan, & Donaldson, 2000). Literature supporting the use of electronic records to reduce errors has been evolving and includes several systematic reviews as well as stand-alone studies (Ammenwerth, Schnell-Inderst, Machan, & Sievert, 2008; Franklin, O'Grady, Donyai, Jacklin, & Barber, 2007; Kohn et al., 2000; Reckmann, Westbrook, Koh, Lo, & Day, 2009; Shulman, Singer, Goldstone, & Bellingan, 2005). Evidence demonstrates that they really can reduce errors. This positive outlook has driven healthcare's key stakeholders to proceed with development, adoption, and oversight, including EHR vendors, hospitals, ambulatory practices, home health agencies, long-term care facilities, and the federal government. With the signing of the ARRA in 2009, organizations became increasingly eager to adopt EHRs and receive sizeable incentive payments. In fact, hospital adoption of at least a basic EHR system has more than tripled since 2009, with a concomitant increase in the total percentage of hospitals with certified EHRs from 72% to 85%. Additionally in 2012, nearly three-quarters (72%) of office-based physicians adopted an EHR, up from 42% in 2008 (The Office of the National Coordinator for Health Information Technology [ONC] Update, 2013).

While the studies mentioned above support the benefits and enhanced safety features that can be realized with an EHR along with a CPOE system, there have been articles published that indicate a potential negative side, one that points to the EHR as the actual cause of errors. A popular study that was published in the *Journal of the American Medical Association* by Koppel et al. in 2005 reported that CPOE systems actually facilitate medication errors. This article ran contrary to what most believed, but identified, using quantitative and qualitative methods, 22 types of medication error risks associated with the use of CPOE (Koppel et al., 2005). In a retrospective study by Walsh et al. researchers attempted to determine the frequency and types of pediatric medication errors attributable to design features in a CPOE system. The rate of identified computer-related errors was 10 errors per 1000 patient days, and the rate of "serious" computer-related errors was 3.6 errors per 1000 patient days (Walsh et al., 2006). Another study highlights how an EHR perpetuated a deadly IV order of potassium that was left unchecked. In this case study, a patient received a total of 316 mEq of KCL over 42 hours despite the fact that all KCL orders during that time period were entered via a CPOE system (Horsky, Kuperman, & Patel, 2005). And in a study by Han et al. (2005) researchers observed an unexpected increase in mortality in a pediatric ICU that coincided with the implementation of their CPOE system (Han et al., 2005).

In a qualitative study by Campbell, Sittig, Ash, Guappone, and Dykstra, researchers attempted to identify the types of unintended consequences seen with the implementation of EHR systems with CPOE. This study involved an expert panel using an iterative process that took a list of adverse consequences of CPOE, and sorted them into categories. One category labeled "Generation of New Kinds of Errors" indicated that new kinds of errors appear when CPOE is implemented. Examples of items in this category include juxtaposition errors when users select an item next to the intended choice; a wrong patient being selected; desensitization to alerts (alert overload); confusing order option presentations; and system design issues with poor data organization and display. Users get frustrated trying to find the right spot to enter a particular data element and end up entering orders on generic screens, bypassing any rules and alerts configured, all potentially leading to medication errors (Campbell, Sittig, Ash, Guappone, & Dykstra, 2006). While all of these studies, both positive and negative, provide valuable insight into how EHRs are configured, each one of them reports limitations with the studies and admits that it would be difficult to generalize the findings.

NATIONAL HEALTH IT SAFETY INITIATIVES

Institute of Medicine—Health IT and Patient Safety Report

Recognizing the need to increase focus on implementing EHRs safely, the Office of the National Coordinator for Health Information Technology (ONC) requested that the Institute of Medicine (IOM) form a team of experts to assess the current state of EHRs and their ability to improve patient safety. In November 2011, the IOM published "Health IT and Patient Safety: Building Safer Systems for Better Care". This 235-page document provides a comprehensive description of the state of electronic health records and their ability to improve safety with a goal of making health IT–assisted care safer, putting our nation in the best position to realize the potential benefits of health IT (Institute of Medicine [IOM], 2012). It provided the 10 recommendations found in Table 29.1.

After their review and analysis, the IOM panel of experts found little published evidence to quantify the magnitude of the risk, but believe that if designed and implemented inappropriately, EHRs could lead to unintended adverse consequences. They reported that literature on the topic was limited and lacked what was needed to truly define and assess the current situation of health IT safety. They recognized the current dissatisfaction with poor user interface design, poor workflow support, and complex data interfaces as being threats to patient safety. Also identified as a contributing factor to unsafe conditions was the lack of system interoperability and the need for clinicians to review data from multiple systems (Institute of Medicine [IOM], 2012).

It is clear in this report that the need is to develop strategies that will standardize the reporting of health IT–related errors. The depth and breadth of the problem cannot be measured or analyzed when error reporting structures are heterogeneous, not mandated, and often swept under the carpet. There is also an emphasis on increasing the transparency in that reporting from both vendors and system users as the industry learns and improves. It points out the need for a multi-faceted approach and calls for vendor participation, IT user involvement, and governmental support and oversight. Safer implementation and use of health IT is a complex, dynamic process that requires a shared responsibility between vendors and healthcare organizations. The importance of this work was evident in one of the IOM recommendations which requested the development of an action plan by the ONC within 12 months to ensure that improvements proceed in a strategic way.

TABLE 29.1	IOM—Health IT and Patient Safety Recommendations

1. The Secretary of Health and Human Services (HHS) should publish an action and surveillance plan within 12 months that includes a schedule for working with the private sector to assess the impact of health IT on patient safety and minimizing the risk of its implementation and use.

2. The Secretary of HHS should ensure insofar as possible that health IT vendors support the free exchange of information about health IT experiences and issues and not prohibit sharing of such information, including details (e.g., screenshots) relating to patient safety.

3. The ONC should work with the private and public sectors to make comparative user experiences across vendors publicly available.

4. The Secretary of HHS should fund a new Health IT Safety Council to evaluate criteria for assessing and monitoring the safe use of health IT and the use of health IT to enhance safety. This council should operate within an existing voluntary consensus standards organization.

5. All health IT vendors should be required to publicly register and list their products with the ONC, initially beginning with EHRs certified for the meaningful use program.

6. The Secretary of HHS should specify the quality and risk management process requirements that health IT vendors must adopt, with a particular focus on human factors, safety culture, and usability.

7. The Secretary of HHS should establish a mechanism for both vendors and users to report health IT–related deaths, serious injuries, or unsafe conditions.

8. The Secretary of HHS should recommend that Congress establish an independent federal entity for investigating patient safety deaths, serious injuries, or potentially unsafe conditions associated with health IT. This entity should also monitor and analyze data and publicly report results of these activities.

9a. The Secretary of HHS should monitor and publicly report on the progress of health IT safety annually beginning in 2012. If progress toward safety and reliability is not sufficient as determined by the Secretary, the Secretary should direct FDA to exercise all available authorities to regulate EHRs, health information exchanges, and PHRs.

9b. The Secretary should immediately direct FDA to begin developing the necessary framework for regulation. Such a framework should be in place if and when the Secretary decides the state of health IT safety requires FDA regulation as stipulated in Recommendation 9a above.

10. HHS, in collaboration with other research groups, should support cross-disciplinary research toward the use of health IT as part of a learning healthcare system. Products of this research should be used to inform the design, testing, and use of health IT.

Office of the National Coordinator for Health Information Technology—Safety Plan

In July 2013, ONC published their response to the IOM report in the form of the Health Information Technology Patient Safety and Action & Surveillance Plan (Office of the National Coordinator for Health Information Technology, 2013a). They iterate the challenge of discerning if health IT is the true cause of a medical error given the limitations on the recent research. There are many unknowns and the need to clearly define health IT–related errors of both omission and commission is still needed. For example, if allergy alerting in an EHR has not been configured or turned on, and a patient experiences an adverse allergy event—is that a health IT–related error? What about when a system user opens a patient list for an inpatient unit and the patient at the top of the list is already pre-selected by default. If orders are accidently placed on this patient—is that a health IT–related error? Many errors such as these have been identified, while many others are still lurking, yet to be recognized when a near miss or adverse event occurs. With this in mind, the ONC action and surveillance plan addresses the need to focus on learning and assessing the current status prior to developing the solution. It calls for strong leadership at all levels to continue to take on the task of realizing the potential of these systems that can improve patient safety with a goal of inspiring confidence and trust in health IT.

The ONC's Action and Surveillance plan has two main objectives: (1) Use health IT to make care safer and (2) Continuously improve the safety of health IT (Office of the National Coordinator for Health Information Technology, 2013). They emphasize the importance of a shared responsibility between clinicians, administrators, IT staff, quality improvement staff, patients, government, health IT vendors, usability experts, patient safety organizations, accrediting bodies, academic institutions, health insurers, professional organizations, and publishers. It will truly take all of these key stakeholders working together to ensure health IT is used as safely as possible and is optimized to reduce errors.

The plan revolves around three key areas: Learning, Improving, and Leading. Recognizing the fact that there is much to learn in this area, the ONC is aiming to increase the quantity and quality of data and knowledge about health IT safety. While organizations may internally discover, report, and correct health IT–related errors, there lacks a standard methodology for reporting that will benefit patients at large. The establishment of processes and mechanisms that facilitate reporting among users and vendors of health IT is recommended along with strengthening the use of state and national Patient Safety Organizations (PSOs) to help collect and report on these issues. Additionally, the need is recognized that not only do we need standard terminologies to report health IT–related errors, but we need processes to report them centrally and a method to aggregate and analyze the data. The goal is to make it easy for clinicians to report patient safety events to PSOs using standard terminologies such as the Agency for Healthcare Research and Quality's (AHRQ) Common Formats. AHRQ develops and maintains a set of Common Formats that include a set of common definitions and reporting formats that allow organizations to collect and submit standardized information regarding health IT–related patient safety events and hazards (PSO Privacy Protection Center, 2013). The ONC proposes to support PSOs in their work to collect, aggregate, and analyze the data related to health IT safety. On a broader scale, ONC will continue their work in support of the National Quality Strategy to identify opportunities to learn and ultimately make care safer thought the use of health IT.

In addition to growing the body of knowledge related to health IT and patient safety, the ONC plans to focus on improvement efforts. The goal is to develop resources and evidence-based corrective actions to improve health IT safety and patient safety. To establish priorities in health IT safety work, the ONC intends to align with the National Quality Strategy (NQS), the Meaningful Use program as part of the HITECH Act, and the Centers for Medicare and Medicaid Service's (CMS) Partnership for Patients initiative. Through goals established by the NQS, an emphasis is recommended in areas such as strategies for how technology can assist in the reduction of hospital readmissions and preventable hospital-acquired conditions (Office of the National Coordinator for Health Information Technology, 2013). Supporting these goals are the 10 patient safety domains set forth by CMS's Partnership for Patients. These domains include (1) Adverse drug events, (2) Catheter-associated urinary tract infections, (3) Central-line associated blood stream infections, (4) Readmissions, (5) Ventilator-associated pneumonia, (6) Pressure ulcers, (7) Surgical line infections, (8) Obstetrical adverse events, (9) Venous thromboembolism, (10) Injuries from falls and immobility. Utilizing health IT to improve in these areas will help drive the patient safety effort. The plan additionally intends to continue the work of the Meaningful Use program that supports and encourages safe and meaningful use of health IT. This effort includes configuring EHRs with CPOE to reduce medication errors using allergy alerting, dose range checking, improving reconciliation of medications across care settings, and many other methods to assist in error reduction (Office of the National Coordinator for Health Information Technology, 2013a).

Other improvement efforts considered important and included in the plan address the need to incorporate safety into certification criteria for health IT software as well as into education and training on the safe use of health IT for all healthcare professionals. The need to support health IT research and the development of tools is also emphasized. ONC has begun work in this area by contracting with research teams to develop tools that can be used by organizations that use these systems as well as vendors who produce them. Some of these tools will be described later in this chapter.

Driving safety improvements requires leadership and the ONC spells out a number of strategies to address the direction that needs to be supported. In addition to providing methods to engage all key stakeholders, ONC is planning to develop a strategy and recommend an appropriate, risk-based regulatory framework for health IT. This framework includes working collaboratively with other federal agencies such as the Food and Drug Administration and the Federal Communications Commission (Office of the National Coordinator for Health Information Technology, 2013).

Encouraging state governments to get involved and incorporate health IT into their patient safety oversight program is included in this plan with an emphasis on statewide adverse event reporting. Including the patient and family caregivers as part of the solution is listed as a focus that ONC will address in order to more effectively engage patients in using health IT to make care safer. And lastly as part of leading this effort, the ONC will establish a Safety Program that coordinates these efforts among all stakeholders to ensure cohesive progress is being made as the plan is implemented. Through efforts coordinated by ONC, The Department of Health and Human Services (HHS) will monitor the Health IT Safety Program and strive toward the goal of patients and providers having confidence in the safety of health IT (Office of the National Coordinator for Health Information Technology, 2013).

Agency for Healthcare Research and Quality—Common Formats

In addition to the many areas of healthcare that AHRQ participates, they have taken a significant interest in the area of health IT over the last several years in partnership with the ONC. One area of focus has been the development of what are called Common Formats for reporting patient safety events. Their vision, along with the ONC, is that the reporting of health IT safety issues will occur not just at the organizational level, but at the national level as well. In using the Common Formats for reporting, it is hoped that standardized aggregate data will provide valuable analysis and trending that can lead to more focused efforts and significant improvements in patient safety. To assist in this effort many states have now formed Patient

Safety Organizations (PSOs) that have emerged as part of the Patient Safety and Quality Improvement Act of 2005. At present there are 77 PSOs in 29 states listed by AHRQ. It is these organizations that will help in the collection of data on patient safety and submit non-identified data to AHRQ's Network of Patient Safety Databases (NPSD) (The Office of the National Coordinator for Health Information Technology [ONC] Update, 2013). In addition to the PSOs, providers and other entities can voluntarily contribute non-identified patient safety events to the NPSD.

The Common Formats for standardized reporting of health IT–related errors are actually not found on AHRQ's Web site, but on the PSO Privacy Protection Center's Web site, and are a bit challenging to find. Descriptions and contributing factors for health IT safety issues are listed and can be used when reporting incidents, near misses, and unsafe conditions. For example, a "4.3 Contributing Factor" of an incident may be related to "4.3.2 Equipment/device function" that resulted in "4.3.2.1 Loss or delay of data." As software evolves to more efficiently capture health IT safety events, it is hoped that Common Formats will be utilized as the norm to aid in our learning as we continue to improve our clinical systems.

In 2011, AHRQ announced the completion of another tool called the Health IT Hazard Manager after extensive beta testing, which gives healthcare providers a method of capturing and managing hazard data in software that includes near miss errors and actual errors, according to the AHRQ Web site (AHRQ Hazard Manager, 2012). The AHRQ tool, funded with a $750,000 grant led by Abt Associates with the ECRI Institute and Geisinger Health System's Patient Safety Institute, does not allow healthcare providers to share data collected with the tool among themselves, but to see only their own reports. Vendors, however, will receive the safety reports relevant to their products. According to AHRQ, healthcare organizations, vendors, policy-makers, and researchers will be able to request access to view de-identified, aggregate reports of hazard attributes (AHRQ Hazard Manager, 2012). The terms used in the Hazard Managers are mapped to those in the Common Formats so data can be aggregated and analyzed. While the Hazard Manager tool itself has not yet been released, the research surrounding its development is available for those interested in health IT safety and its reporting.

Food and Drug Administration

While the U.S. Food and Drug Administration (FDA) has been concerned with patient safety since its inception, they have only recently explored the area of EHRs. For decades, the FDA has received several hundred thousand medical device reports (MDRs) of suspected device-associated deaths, injuries or system malfunctioning. These MDRs have been entered into the Manufacturer and User Facility Device Experience or MAUDE database for centralized housing, analysis, and reporting (U.S. Food and Drug Administration, 2013b). A limitation of this database is its age. Because it is so old, its capabilities to conduct real-time reporting and analysis are limited, hindering any attempts to discover unknown adverse events. This, in turn, affects its ability to generate and evaluate evidence. A new database will soon take its place according to a press release statement from September 17, 2013, called the Pharmacovigilance Report Intake and Managed Output (PRIMO) software system (Gaffney, 2013).

In July 2012, Congress enacted the Food and Drug Administration Safety and Innovation Act (FDASIA). Section 618 of FDASIA instructs the Secretary of HHS, acting through the FDA Commissioner and in collaboration with ONC and the Federal Communications Commission (FCC), to issue a report by January 2014 on a proposed strategy that includes recommendations on an appropriate risk-based regulatory framework for health IT. The intent is for the framework to promote innovation, protect patient safety, and avoid regulatory duplication. The report will be informed by input from the public as well as the ONC's Health IT Policy Committee and will incorporate what the agencies learn about risk, safety, and opportunity for innovative technologies to support improved health and safety outcomes. The agencies will consider how to make it easier for innovators to understand the regulatory landscape, ways to minimize regulatory burden, and how to design an oversight approach that supports innovations and patient safety (U.S. Food and Drug Administration, 2013a).

The Institute for Safe Medication Practices

The Institute for Safe Medication Practices (ISMP) is devoted entirely to medication error prevention and safe medication use. They have been in existence for over 30 years, helping healthcare practitioners keep patients safe. Their mission is to lead efforts to improve the medication use process. They have published multiple guidelines and tips for the designers of EHRs as they configure medication orders and order sets. The ISMP's Guidelines for Standard Order Sets provides a five-page checklist that allows organizations to evaluate the safety of their CPOE systems (Institute for Safe Medication Practices, 2010). This guide includes recommendations for screen layout, use of symbols and abbreviations, and order set content development. ISMP also has a robust voluntary error-reporting program called the Medication Errors Reporting Program (MERP). This is a system where practitioners can report any errors

related to medication use. The goal for this program is to learn about errors occurring nationwide, understand their origins, and share lessons learned with the healthcare and health IT community. Each year, ISMP receives hundreds of error reports from healthcare professionals. Additionally, ISMP is certified as a Patient Safety Organization (PSO) by AHRQ (Institute for Safe Medication Practices, 2014).

ECRI Institute

For 45 years, ECRI Institute, a non-profit organization, has focused on scientific research to discover the effectiveness of medical procedures, devices, drugs, and processes, all to improve patient care. ECRI Institute is also a PSO; in fact it is one of the first to be federally certified. In December 2012, they conducted an evaluation of health IT–related events and unsafe conditions with the goal of improving the understanding of technology's impact on healthcare delivery. In this publication "ECRI Institute PSO's Deep Dive: Health Information Technology" included more than 170 health IT–related events reported by 36 healthcare organizations over a nine-week period. The events included wrong patient data entries, users ignoring alerts, and gaps in reporting critical test results due to poor system interoperability. Some events involved multiple safety issues and in total identified 211 patient safety issues that were grouped into 22 event categories. The five most frequently identified health IT–related problems identified were (1) System interface issues, (2) Wrong input, (3) Software issue/system configuration, (4) Wrong record retrieved, and (5) Software issue/functionality (ECRI Institute, 2013a). This report was followed by a whitepaper titled "Anticipating Unintended Consequences of Health Information Technology and Health Information Exchange: How to Identify and Address Unsafe Conditions Associated with Health IT." In this report several examples of commonly encountered health IT–related incidents are shared. Examples include The user ignored or overrode an alert; test results were sent to the wrong provider causing a delay in action; text entries were not shared due to poorly designed interfaces between systems; and an item from an outside source was scanned into the wrong patient record. It further explores these phenomena of health IT and patient safety, but strongly advocates for using standardized reporting methods that funnel up to PSOs. Issues to be addressed by healthcare managers are listed that provide a foundation for a solid health IT safety program. These issues include a checklist of questions a manager should ask as health IT safety is evaluated. Questions include topics of how adverse events are reported; if a standard terminology is used in the reporting; what processes are in place for follow-up after an incident; policies/procedures in place for system corrective action, and the existence of a budget to support health IT safety activities (ECRI Institute, 2013a, 2013b).

Leapfrog Group

Another CPOE opinion leader, The Leapfrog Group, represents a coalition of healthcare purchasers that has been a driving force in the improvement of healthcare quality. They are strong advocates for the use of CPOE systems. They have developed a CPOE "standard" including a requirement that organizations operating CPOE systems should demonstrate (via testing scenarios) to ensure that their inpatient CPOE system can alert physicians to at least 50% of common serious prescribing errors. In an article by Kilbridge, Welebob, and Classen, the development of these standards are described including the description of a framework with 12 different categories of CPOE-based decision support that have the potential to prevent a prescribing error (Kilbridge, Welebob, & Classen, 2006). Organizations are asked to conduct this test in a development or practice database that is similar to their production CPOE system. Configuration elements of the system that are tested include duplicate ordering, single- and cumulative-dose levels, allergy checking, drug–drug interaction, contraindications based on patient diagnosis, contraindications based on relevant laboratory values, and dose levels based on radiology studies. This test is Web based and self-administered, but can only be taken if the organization also participates in Leapfrog's general hospital survey.

HEALTH IT SAFETY TOOLS AND RESOURCES

Resources for organizations to turn to for help in not only developing health IT safety strategic plans but for assessing their current situation have been emerging over the last several years. These tools provide excellent information for those in charge of health IT safety with varying levels of expertise. Tools include the Web-based Guide to Reducing Unintended Consequences in Health Information Technology, the Safety Assurance Factors for EHR Resilience (SAFER) Guides, ECRI Institute's "How to Identify and Address Unsafe Conditions Associated with Health IT, The CPOE Design Recommendations Checklist, and the Pick-list Checklist.

AHRQ's Guide to Reducing Unintended Consequences of Electronic Health Records

AHRQ's Guide to Reducing Unintended Consequences of Electronic Health Records is an online resource designed to help organizations anticipate, avoid, and address problems that can occur when implementing and using an electronic health record (EHR). The purpose in developing the Guide was to provide practical knowledge, troubleshooting tools and resources. The guide provides multiple resources and addresses both future and current EHR users. It provides information on how to survive a system downtime and includes a copy and paste toolkit as organizations struggle to address the complexities of allowing this functionality in EHRs. Case examples are provided on safety-related topics along with potential remediation solutions to several challenges in health IT (Jones et al., 2011).

SAFER Guides

The SAFER guides consist of nine guides organized into three categories. These guides enable healthcare organizations to conduct self-assessments of their EHR safety in a variety of areas. The guides identify recommended practices to optimize the safety and safe use of EHRs. Each guideline contains a listing of recommended practices. See Table 29.2 for the categories and high-level descriptions of the nine recommendation guides. These recommended practices are then broken down further into associated rationale, suggested sources of input for reviewing the practice, and examples of potentially useful practices or scenarios. An emphasis is placed on the need to review and analyze these recommendations with all key stakeholders at the table. A multi-disciplinary approach with IT staff, clinicians, risk managers, administrators, and other appropriate team members, all at the table is believed to be ideal for the success of working through these guides (Office of the National Coordinator for Health Information Technology, 2013b).

CPOE Design Checklist/Pick-List Checklist

Two additional checklists that address health IT safety and provide tools for evaluating a current EHR include the CPOE Design Checklist and the Pick-list Checklist. These tools include checklists for configuring a CPOE system and creating Pick lists, or drop-down lists that are based on published health IT safety evidence. The CPOE Design Checklist is a 46-item list and provides a tool that can be used during software selection, design, or evaluation. The items in the list fall into four categories: Clinical Decision Support, Order Form Configuration, Human Factors Configuration, and Workflow Process Configuration (Sengstack, 2010). Examples of some of the checklist items included in the CPOE Design Checklist are found in Table 29.3.

TABLE 29.2	SAFER Guides
Foundational Guides	**Description**
High Priority Practices	Identifies "high risk" and "high priority" recommended safety practices intended to optimize the safety and safe use of EHRs
Organizational Responsibilities	Identifies individual and organizational responsibilities (activities, processes, and tasks) intended to optimize the safety and safe use of EHRs
Infrastructure Guides	**Description**
Contingency Planning	Identifies recommended safety practices associated with planned or unplanned EHR unavailability—instances in which clinicians or other end users cannot access all or part of the EHR
System Configuration	Identifies recommended safety practices associated with the way EHR hardware and software are set up ("configured")
System Interfaces	Identifies recommended safety practices intended to optimize the safety and safe use of system-to-system interfaces between EHR-related software applications
Clinical Process Guides	**Description**
Patient Identification	Identifies recommended safety practices associated with the reliable identification of patients in the HER
Computerized Provider Order Entry with Decision Support	Identifies recommended safety practices associated with Computerized Provider Order Entry (CPOE) and Clinical Decision Support (CDS)
Test Results Reporting and Follow-up	Identifies recommended safety practices intended to optimize the safety and safe use of processes and EHR technology for the electronic communication and management of diagnostic test results
Clinician Communication	Identifies recommended safety practices associated with communication between clinicians and is intended to optimize the safety and safe use of EHRs

TABLE 29.3	CPOE Design Recommendations (Examples)

Display alert when an allergy has been documented or an allergy to another drug in the same category is documented.

Provide alert of potential allergy at time of order entry, not order submission.

Display alert when the same medication is ordered and when separate doses of the same medication are to be given within a "closely spaced time."

Display alert when order specifying a route of administration that is not appropriate for the ordered medication (e.g., Antifungal topical cream ordered with route of IV).

Create an alert informing users ordering potassium when there has not been a serum potassium value recorded in the past 12 hours or if the most recent potassium value is greater than 4.0.

All ordering screens should be designed in a similar fashion. Fields for drug, dose, route, frequency, etc., should be in the same place on all screens.

Do not use field labels that require a negative answer for a positive response (e.g., Is IV contrast contraindicated?).

Use alternate line colors between patients to help visual separation of names.

Provide way to alert caregivers to new orders.

The Pick-List Checklist

In the 2011 IOM report, Health IT and Patient Safety: Building Safer Systems for Better Care, one of the 10 recommendations mentioned earlier emphasizes the need to conduct more research in the area of health information technology and patient safety. They specifically state that there should be more research in the area of "the pick-list problem." A review of the literature finds relatively little information on how to properly configure a pick list in an EHR, and no research studies have been conducted to date on the pick list itself. The limited information gleaned in the literature is offered in an 11-item Pick-list Checklist that can be used by all levels of informatics specialists to assess current configuration based on the best evidence available. An easy-to-use checklist such as this has multiple benefits and represents a starting point for informatics specialists to evaluate and improve the systems that care providers rely on to deliver safe patient care. Examples of items contained within this checklist include not truncating items on the pick list, do not put similar terms on top of one another, do not by default pre-select an item on the list, and use alternating line colors between patient names to help in the visual separation of names (Sengstack, 2013). We need to configure our systems so that our users choose the right thing the first time. Each of the items listed in The Pick-list Checklist do not seem to be rocket science, but taken collectively, they have the potential to strengthen the quality and safety that clinical systems were meant to deliver.

CONCLUSION

Think nationally, act locally. This is a mantra we should adopt when it comes to health IT. Our federal government and professional organizations can only do so much. It will take each organization working in partnership with the government, health IT vendors, and PSOs to drive improvements in patient safety using health IT. Tools, knowledge, and resources offered in this chapter can help lay the foundation for a strong health IT strategic plan that can assist organizations as they strive to capture the full potential of their systems. In summary, healthcare organizations need to ensure the safety of their health IT systems. All stakeholders must become involved and increasingly transparent as they learn and share their safety lessons from the implementation and use of health IT. In light of the fact that the EHR is fast becoming the standard in healthcare today, it is imperative that organizations commit time, energy, and funding to ensure that these clinical systems are integral to reaching their error reduction goals.

REFERENCES

AHRQ. (2012, March). Health IT Hazard Manager: Design & Demo. Retrieved from http://www.ahrq.gov/news/events/conference/2011/walker-hassol/index.html

Ammenwerth, E., Schnell-Inderst, P., Machan, C., & Sievert, U. (2008). The effect of electronic prescribing on medication errors and adverse drug events: A systematic review. *Journal of the American Medical Informatics Association, 15*(5), 585–600.

Campbell, E. M., Sittig, D. F., Ash, J. S., Guappone, K. P., & Dykstra, R. H. (2006). Types of unintended consequences related to computerized provider order entry. *Journal of the American Medical Informatics Association, 13*, 547–556.

ECRI Institute. (2013a). *Anticipating unintended consequences of health information technology and health information exchange how to identify and address unsafe conditions associated with health IT.* Retrieved from http://www.healthit.gov/sites/default/files/How_to_Identify_and_Address_Unsafe_Conditions_Associated_with_Health_IT.pdf

ECRI Institute. (2013b). *ECRI institute PSO uncovers health information technology-related events in deep dive analysis.* Retrieved from https://www.ecri.org/Press/Pages/Health-Information-Technology-HIT-Deep-Dive.aspx

Franklin, B. D., O'Grady, K., Donyai, P., Jacklin, G., & Barber, N. (2007). The impact of a closed-loop electronic prescribing and administration system on prescribing errors, administration errrors and staff time: a before and after study. *Quality and Safety of Health Care, 16*, 279–284.

Gaffney, A. (2013). *So long, MAUDE: CDRH selects PRIMO as Adverse Event Reporting Replacement System.* Retrieved from http://www.raps.org/regulatoryDetail.aspx?id=9436

Goolsby, K. (2002). *CPOE odyssey: The story of evolving the world's first computerized physician order entry system and implications for today's CPOE decision makers.* Retrieved from http://www.outsourcing-center.com/2002-08-cpoe-odyssey-article-38166.html

Han, Y. Y., Carcillo, J. A., Venkataraman, S. T., Clark, R. S., Watson, R. S., Nguyen, T. C., … Orr, R. A. (2005). Unexpected increased mortality after implementation of commercially sold computerized physician order entry system. *Pediatrics, 116*, 1506–1512.

Horsky, J., Kuperman, G. J., & Patel, V. L. (2005). Comprehensive analysis of a medication dosing error related to CPOE. *Journal of the American Medical Informatics Association, 12*, 377–382.

Institute for Safe Medication Practices. (2010). *Guidelines for standard order sets.* Retrieved from http://www.ismp.org/newsletters/acutecare/articles/20100311.asp

Institute for Safe Medication Practices. (2014). *The National Medication Errors Reporting Program (ISMP MERP).* Retrieved from https://www.ismp.org/orderforms/reporterrortoismp.asp

Institute of Medicine (IOM). (2012). *Health IT and patient safety: Building safer systems for better care.* Washington, DC: The National Academies Press. Retrieved from http://www.iom.edu/Reports/2011/Health-IT-and-Patient-Safety-Building-Safer-Systems-for-Better-Care.aspx

Jones, S. S., Koppel, R., Ridgely, M. S., Palen, T. E., Wu, S., & Harrison, M. I. (2011, August). Guide to reducing unintended consequences of electronic health records prepared by RAND corporation under contract No. HHSA290200600017I, task order #5. Agency for Healthcare Research and Quality (AHRQ). Rockville, MD.

Kaushal, R., Shojania, K. G., & Bates, D. W. (2003). Effects of computerized physician order entry and clinical decision support systems on medication safety. *Archives of Internal Medicine, 163*, 1409–1416.

Kilbridge, P. M., Welebob, E. M., & Classen, D. W. (2006). Development of the Leapfrog methodology for evaluating hospital implemented inpatient computerized physician order entry systems. *Quality and Safety in Health Care, 15*, 81–84.

Kohn, L. T., Corrigan, J. M., & Donaldson, M. S. (Eds.). (2000). *To err is human: Building a safer health system.* Washington, DC: National Academy Press.

Koppel, R., Metley, J. P., Cohen, A., Abaluck, B., Localia, A. R., Dimmel, S. E., & Strom, B. L. (2005). Role of computerized physician order entry systems in facilitating medication errors. *Journal of the American Medical Association, 5*(293), 1197–1203.

Office of the National Coordinator for Health Information Technology. (2013a). *Health Information Technology Patient Safety Action & Surveillance Plan.* Retrieved from http://www.healthit.gov/sites/default/files/safety_plan_master.pdf

Office of the National Coordinator for Health Information Technology. (2013b). *Safety assurance factors for EHR resilience: SAFER guides.* Retrieved from http://www.healthit.gov/policy-researchers-implementers/safer

PSO Privacy Protection Center. (2013, Spring). *AHRQ common formats.* version 1.2. Retrieved from https://www.psoppc.org/web/patientsafety/commonformats

Reckmann, M. H., Westbrook, J. I., Koh, Y., Lo, C., & Day, R. O. (2009). Does computerized provider order entry reduce prescribing errors for hospital inpatients? A systematic review. *Journal of the American Medical Informatics Association, 16*(5), 613–622.

Sengstack, P. (2010, Fall). CPOE configuration to reduce medication errors: A literature review on the safety of CPOE systems and design recommendations. *Journal of Health Information Management, 24*, 26–34.

Sengstack, P. (2013). The pick-list checklist: Reducing adjacency errors in health information technology. *Journal of Health Information Management, 27*(2), 68–71.

Shulman, R., Singer, M., Goldstone, J., & Bellingan, G. (2005). Medication errors: A prospective cohort study of hand written and computerised physician order entry in the intensive care unit. *Critical Care, 9*, R516–R521.

The Office of the National Coordinator for Health Information Technology (ONC) Update. (2013, June). *On the adoption of health information technology and related efforts to facilitate the electronic use and exchange of health information a report to Congress.* Retrieved from http://www.healthit.gov/sites/default/files/rtc_adoption_of_healthit_and_relatedefforts.pdf

U.S. Department of Health & Human Services. (2014). Office of the National Coordinator for Health Information Technology. Certification and EHR Incentives, HITECH Act 2009. Retrieved from http://www.healthit.gov/policy-researchers-implementers/hitech-act

U.S. Food and Drug Administration. (2013a). *Food and Drug Administration Safety and Innovation Act (FDASIA).* Retrieved from http://www.fda.gov/regulatoryinformation/legislation/federalfooddrugandcosmeticactfdcact/significantamendmentstothefdcact/fdasia/ucm20027187.htm

U.S. Food and Drug Administration. (2013b). *MAUDE—Manufacturer and user facility device experience.* Retrieved from http://www.accessdata.fda.gov/scripts/cdrh/cfdocs/cfmaude/search.cfm

Walsh, K. E., Adams, W. G., Bauchner, H., Vinci, R. J., Chessare, J. B., Cooper, M. R., ... Landrigan, C. P. (2006). Medication errors related to computerized order entry for children. *Pediatrics, 118*, 1872–1879.

30

The Role of Technology in the Medication-Use Process

Matthew C. Grissinger / Michelle M. Mandrack

• OBJECTIVES

1. Describe factors that will influence the adoption of technology in healthcare.
2. Describe the challenges and rewards related to implementing a computerized prescriber order entry system (CPOE).
3. Recognize the benefits and limitations of barcode-assisted medication administration (BCMA) technology as it relates to overall efforts to reduce medication errors, including errors using these systems.
4. Define the benefits and limitations of automated dispensing cabinets (ADCs) in healthcare and their application to the medication-use process.
5. Describe the benefits and limitations of smart infusion pump technology.
6. Recognize the value of and a methodology for assessing an organization's readiness for implementing technology.

• KEY WORDS

Automated dispensing cabinet
Barcode-assisted medication administration technology
Computer prescriber order entry
Failure mode and effects analysis
High-alert medications
Medication error
Smart infusion pump delivery systems

INTRODUCTION

Due to the numerous steps required in the care of patients, the healthcare industry is inherently error prone and fraught with opportunities for mistakes to occur. This concept was confirmed in the oft-quoted 1999 Institute of Medicine (IOM) report, *To Err Is Human: Building a Safer Health System,* where the authors extrapolated that between 44,000 and 98,000 patients die each year in the United States from preventable medical error. These deaths were the results of practitioner interactions with "bad systems" (Kohn, Corrigan, & Donaldson, 1999). The authors emphatically state that the healthcare industry must place safety as the number 1 national priority and work diligently toward this goal. One explicit recommendation emanating from the first of a series of IOM reports on healthcare is to improve the safe design of systems as is presently being employed in the aerospace and nuclear industries, which are also highly error-prone fields. These industries not only acknowledge and accept the notion that individuals will make errors from normal mental slips and lapses in memory, but recognize that enhancing safety system design through the use of technology is an invaluable tool in the prevention of potentially life-threatening mistakes. Estimates on the financial impact of adverse drug events (ADEs) attribute $2 billion of increased hospitalization costs to preventable ADEs (Adachi & Lodolce, 2005). The 2006 IOM report, *Preventing Medication Errors,* noted that to deliver safe drug care, healthcare organizations should make effective use of well-designed technologies, which will vary by setting. Although the evidence for this assertion is strongest in the inpatient setting, the use of technology will undoubtedly lead to major improvements in all settings (Aspden, Wolcott, Bootman, & Cronenwett, 2006). In 2009, the American Recovery and Reinvestment Act (ARRA) invested $25.8 billion into healthcare to incentivize the adoption, standardization, and meaningful use of health information technology (S1, 2009).

TECHNOLOGY AND HEALTHCARE

In the past, the majority of technology acquisitions have consisted of basic stand-alone computer systems, which were primarily used for data input to increase each department's efficiency with financial accountability measures. These computers were generally installed in the pharmacy, radiology, and laboratory departments, and could also be found in the administration and business offices. Each department was allowed to evaluate and purchase their own unique computer system, preventing any integration of data or dissemination of critical patient information, which is indispensable in providing safe care (Leape et al., 1995). But even as improving technologies have emerged allowing for seamless integration of information to occur, organizations are challenged with the huge costs associated with replacing their non-integrated computer systems. According to an American Society of Health-System Pharmacists (ASHP) survey in 2011, 66.7% of the responding hospitals stated that they had the components of an electronic medical record (EMR), but completely digital hospitals with fully implemented EMRs is far in the future, considering only 8% of hospitals were fully digital (without paper records). An estimated 34.2% of hospitals were using computerized prescriber order entry systems (CPOE) with decision support, 50.2% use barcode medication administration, and 67.9% were using intelligent infusion devices (smart pumps) (Pedersen, Schneider, & Scheckelhoff, 2011).

INFLUENCES ON THE ADOPTION OF TECHNOLOGY

Consumers have become increasingly concerned that hospitals are less than safe following the numerous mass media reporting of medical mistakes, which have resulted in patient harm and deaths. In 1995, there were television and newspaper accounts that reported the tragic death of a patient from a preventable ADE due to an inadvertent administration of a massive overdose of a chemotherapy agent over four days. This particular error became a watershed event for patients, practitioners, and healthcare organizations alike, not only because it occurred at the world renowned Dana Farber Cancer Institute, but also because it happened to the prestigious *Boston Globe* healthcare reporter, Betsy Lehman. How could a mistake of this proportion occur in a leading healthcare facility where each practitioner is specifically educated in the care and treatment of cancer patients? A root cause analysis of the error revealed that there was no malpractice or egregious behavior, but that excellent, conscientious, and caring pharmacists and nurses simply interpreted an ambiguous handwritten chemotherapy order incorrectly. In retrospect, if technology had been available, the physician could have entered the medication order into a CPOE system and this heartbreaking error may not have happened.

Unfortunately, this example is by far not an isolated case. According to a 1994 American Medical Association report, medication errors related to the misinterpretation of physicians' prescriptions were the second most prevalent and expensive claim listed on malpractice cases filed over a seven-year period on 90,000 malpractice claims between 1985 and 1992 (Cabral, 1997). Also, it has been estimated in the outpatient setting that indecipherable or unclear orders resulted in more than 150 million telephone calls from pharmacists and nurses to prescribers requiring clarification, which not only is time consuming for practitioners, but estimated to cost healthcare systems billions of dollars each year. Thus, the availability of critical clinical information needed at the point of care (during prescribing, dispensing, and administering) can not only improve time management and contribute to cost savings through improved utilization of medications, staff and patient satisfaction, but most importantly, reduce the incidence of error.

The first organized attempt to move acute care organizations toward improving patient safety through technology began from an initiative by The Leapfrog Group. Composed of more than 150 private and public organizations providing healthcare benefits, this group felt that they had a significant financial investment in preventing errors for their employees, thus increasing productivity by contracting only with those organizations that had hospital-wide adoption of CPOE technology. Yet, a survey by Leapfrog completed in 2003 showed that not only did this financial incentive result in no increase from the 2002 survey in the number of hospitals that had implemented CPOE, but there was also a drop of 17% in hospitals now fully committed to CPOE implementation before 2005

(Stefanacci, 2004). According to Leapfrog, 26% of the 1244 hospitals that completed their survey in 2009 report having a CPOE system in at least one inpatient department (Leapfrog, 2010). Even if an organization implements CPOE, this does not mean that the system will catch incorrect medication orders entered into the system. Another report from Leapfrog, based on a study between June 2008 and January 2010 of 214 hospitals from across the United States who completed Leapfrog's CPOE evaluation tool, revealed that these systems potentially missed half of the routine medication orders and one-third of potentially fatal medication orders (Leapfrog). Because little research is available on the effectiveness of CPOE on medication error prevention, other organizations such as the Joint Commission, a non-profit organization that is the nation's leading standards-setting and accrediting body in healthcare, and the National Quality Forum (NQF) are presently refraining from uniformly requiring its adoption.

Probably the most important development to promote the implementation of technology is the announcement by the Centers for Medicare & Medicaid Services (CMS) of a proposed rule to implement provisions of the American Recovery and Reinvestment Act of 2009 (Recovery Act) that provide incentive payments for the meaningful use of certified electronic health records (EHR) technology. The Medicare EHR incentive program will provide incentive payments to eligible professionals, eligible hospitals, and critical access hospitals that are meaningful users of certified EHR technology. The Medicaid EHR incentive program will provide incentive payments to eligible professionals and hospitals for efforts to adopt, implement, or upgrade certified EHR technology or for meaningful use in the first year of their participation in the program and for demonstrating meaningful use during each of five subsequent years (CMS, 2010).

Interest in the use of barcoding technology increased due to the Food and Drug Administration's (FDA's) February 25, 2004 ruling, which required medications to have machine-readable barcodes. In an optimally acute care, barcoded environment, a nurse would scan his or her barcode identification badge at the beginning of each medication administration time, the patient's barcode identification band, and the intended drug's barcoded label with a barcode scanner. A mismatch between the patient, the drug packaging applied during manufacturing/repackaging, an incorrect time, dose or route, and the patient's medication record would trigger a warning, prompting the nurse to investigate the discrepancy before administering the medication. One of the first healthcare facilities to adopt barcode technology was due to the inspiration of a nurse at the Department of Veterans Affairs (VA) in Topeka, Kansas. Her insight resulted in a 74% improvement in errors caused by the wrong medications being administered, a 57% improvement in errors caused by incorrect doses being administered, a 91% improvement in wrong patient errors, and almost a 92% improvement in wrong time errors between 1993 and 1999. Additional examples of evolving technology used to prevent medication errors include automated dispensing cabinets (ADCs) and smart infusion pumps. As more technology systems are introduced into healthcare, it is important that nurses understand their benefits and problems, and how technology will affect their practice. As noted by the IOM report, *Keeping Patients Safe: Transforming the Work Environment of Nurses*, despite its potential, patient safety experts caution that technology by itself is not a panacea. While able to remedy some problems, technology may also generate new forms of error and failure (Institute of Medicine, 2004).

Computerized Prescriber Order Entry (CPOE)

To a large degree, healthcare practitioners still communicate information in the "old-fashioned way." According to the aforementioned ASHP technology survey, 34.2% of U.S. hospitals had a CPOE system in 2011, which was a 45% increase from the preceding year. The survey showed that more larger hospitals had a CPOE system compared to smaller hospitals (Pedersen et al., 2011).

Many factors demonstrate the need for a shift from a traditional paper-based system that relies on the practitioners' vigilance to automated order entry, record keeping, and clinical care. These factors include accessing patient information spread across multiple organizations that may be unavailable, especially in large organizations and, therefore, medical care would be provided without pertinent patient information. The structure of the patient's record often makes it difficult to locate valuable information as well as illegible handwritten entries by healthcare practitioners, and for those patients with chronic or complex conditions, the records can increase to multiple volumes over many years. These problems result in a variety of communication breakdowns when providing healthcare to patients from the duplication of services, delays in treatment, increased length of stay, and increased risk of medical errors. Additionally, human memory–based medicine can be inaccurate or not recalled.

There are also many barriers that lead to ineffective communication of medication orders that include issues with illegible handwriting, use of dangerous abbreviations and dose designations, and verbal and faxed orders. Studies have shown that as a result of poor handwriting, 50% of all written physician orders require extra time to interpret. Sixteen percent of physicians have illegible handwriting (Cohen, 2007). Illegible handwriting on medication orders has been shown to be a common cause of prescribing errors and patient injury and death have actually resulted from such errors (ASHP, 1993; Brodell, 1997; Cabral, 1997). In a study at a large teaching hospital, published in 2005, one in three house physicians and medical students who believed their orders were always legible had been asked to clarify them because of poor legibility (Garbutt, Highstein, Jeffe, Dunagan, & Fraser, 2005). Illegible orders may also lead to delays in the administration of medications. To clarify these illegible orders, the healthcare practitioner's workflow is typically interrupted (Cohen, 1999).

The use of a CPOE system has the potential to alleviate many of these problems. CPOE systems allow physicians to electronically order medications, tests, and consultations. They also provide advice on best practices and alerts to the possible adverse consequences of a therapy, such as an allergy or a harmful combination of drugs (American Hospital Association [AHA], 2007). But there are many other potential enhancements that even a basic CPOE system could offer to further enhance safe medication ordering practices, including features unique to the acute care setting, ambulatory care setting, or both; prescribers access to records and ability to enter orders from their office or home; prescriber selectable, standardized single orders or order sets; implementation of organization-specific standing orders based on specific situations such as before or after procedures; menu-driven, organization-specific lists of medications on formulary; and passive feedback systems that present patient-specific data in an organized fashion, such as test results, charges, reference materials, and progress notes, or active feedback systems to provide clinical decision-making tools by providing specific assessments or recommendations through alerts and reminders or even therapeutic suggestions at the time the order is entered.

CPOE systems offer many other advantages over the traditional paper-based system. They can improve quality, patient outcomes, and safety by a variety of factors such as increasing preventive health guideline compliance by exposing prescribers to reminder messages to provide preventive care by encouraging compliance with recommended guidelines, identifying patients needing updated immunizations or vaccinations, and suggesting cancer screening and diagnosis reminders and prompts. Other advantages include reductions in the variation in care to improve disease management by improving follow-up of newly diagnosed conditions, reminder systems to improve patient management, automating evidence-based protocols, adhering to clinical guidelines, or providing screening instruments to help diagnose disorders. Order entry systems can improve drug prescribing and administration by driving formulary usage, improving antibiotic usage,

suggesting whether certain antibiotics or their dosages are appropriate for use. Medication refill compliance can be increased using reminder systems to increase adherence to therapies. Drug dosing could be improved, especially for those medications whose dosing is based on laboratory results, such as heparin or warfarin, to maintain adequate anticoagulation control.

Many studies have demonstrated a reduction in ADEs with the use of CPOE. For example:

- Bates and colleagues showed that serious medication errors were reduced by 55% and preventable ADEs were reduced by 17% (Bates, Leape & Cullen 1998).

- Another study has shown that non-missed-dose medication errors fell from 142/1000 patient-days to 26.6/1000 patient-days (Bates et al., 1999). The same study showed a reduction of non-intercepted serious medication errors from 7.6/1000 patient-days to 1.1/1000 patient-days.

- A study of a pediatric critical care unit found a 41% reduction in potentially dangerous errors after implementation of CPOE (Potts, Barr, Gregory, Wright, & Patel, 2004).

- An evaluation of the potential benefit of CPOE over pharmacist review for ordering errors demonstrated that CPOE could reduce potentially dangerous prescribing errors but would have no effect on administration errors, which have a high risk of patient injury (Wang et al., 2007).

- In a meta-analysis of 12 original investigations that compared rates of prescribing medication errors with handwritten and computerized physician orders, 80% of those studies reported a significant reduction in total prescribing errors, 43% in dosing errors, and 37.5% in ADEs (Shamliyan, Duval, Du, & Kane, 2008).

- A study of a neonatal intensive care unit in a tertiary care center showed that the number of orders with no opportunity for errors improved from 42% to 98% after the implementation of CPOE (Jozefczyk et al., 2013).

In addition, errors of omissions would be reduced, such as failure to act on results or carry out indicated tests. Handwriting and interpretation issues would be eliminated. There would be fewer handoffs if the CPOE system was linked to information systems in ancillary departments which would eliminate the need for staff members to manually transport orders to the pharmacy, radiology department, and laboratory, resulting in fewer lost or misplaced orders and faster delivery time. The system has also eliminated the need for staff members in those departments to manually enter the orders into their information systems, reducing the potential for transcription errors (Healthcare Information and Management Systems Society, 2002). Medical data capture and display would be improved, enabling a more comprehensive and accurate documentation by prescribers and nurses. Access to pertinent literature and clinical information from knowledge bases and literature sources would enable ready access to updated drug information. These obvious improvements to patient care would not only improve patient safety but also increase efficiency, productivity, and cost-effectiveness.

CPOE systems can offer a variety of solutions to help reduce the cost in providing healthcare and making more appropriate utilization of services. In the outpatient setting, reductions in hospitalizations and decreased lengths of stay can be obtained from automated scheduling of follow-up appointments to reducing unnecessary diagnostic tests. Better use of formulary and generic drugs can be achieved by providing feedback of prescribing charges and patterns to encourage prescribers to substitute generic medications for more expensive branded medications. Properly designed systems can show an improvement in workflow and time-saving measures for prescribers, if the program makes sense to the prescriber and follows a rational process while performing order entry, by improving the availability and responses to information regarding diagnosis and treatment. Savings related to the storage of paper medical records could be substantial, compared with the cost of storing computerized backup storage devices. Entering medication and diagnostic orders into a computer system would allow for instantaneous capturing of charges, therefore enhancing revenue. Costs associated with the use of transcription notes would be eliminated as well by using an electronic patient record system. Lastly, there is patient and user satisfaction. For example, the admission process for patients from the outpatient setting into an acute care organization can be a cumbersome and time-consuming process. Electronic systems would improve communication, if connected to an outpatient clinical referral system, by decreasing the amount of time needed to complete the referral process in addition to providing important patient information such as patient allergies and diagnosis. The time spent searching for or organizing paper-based information would be substantially reduced, thus improving prescriber and nurse satisfaction as well.

Despite the many documented benefits of using a computerized system, many roadblocks and safety issues exist. One primary area of concern revolves around the costs of implementing CPOE, which are estimated to be about $8 million, with $1.35 million in annual maintenance for a 500-bed hospital. For a 720-bed tertiary hospital, the cost was estimated to be $11.8 million for the development, implementation, and operation of CPOE over a 10-year period (Wietholter, Sitterson, & Allison, 2009). Investing in a CPOE system is not analogous to purchasing software off the store shelf, and it involves far more resources than spending money on a software package. Hospitals will need a minimum infrastructure to support its use, such as a fiber optic backbone network; time, space, and manpower to provide adequate staff education and development; and workstations and high-speed Internet access. The process of selecting the vendor is a costly and difficult process, especially if a vendor cannot address the organization's specific needs. In addition, staff resources will be needed to develop and program organization-specific rules, guidelines, or protocols and to implement the system, plus provide ongoing support for any needed enhancements or changes to the system. It is also difficult to prove or demonstrate any quantifiable benefits or returns on investment because it is hard to accurately measure the actual costs of using paper-based records. Benefits such as provider convenience, patient satisfaction, and service efficiency are not easily captured on the bottom line in terms of increase in revenue, decrease in expense, or avoidance of expense. Add on top of these competing priorities, including other forms of automation to enhance medication safety, such point-of-care barcoding systems and smart infusion pumps that are currently on the market. Another challenge involves the integration of "legacy" systems, those that have been in institutions for many years, which already exist in healthcare organizations. Many organizations are risk averse, waiting to let others be the clinical pioneers before they invest in these systems. Finally, despite the prospects of enhanced workflow and reduction in medication errors, there are real and potential problems with even the best CPOE systems.

As previously mentioned, CPOE systems have demonstrated a reduction in ADEs. Unfortunately, unsafe prescribing practices and medication errors are still possible with these systems. Some organizations, in fear of alienating prescribers, have an active CPOE system but the clinical order screening capability of warnings and alerts have been turned off. The capability to build rule-based safety enhancements, or clinical decision support (CDS), is often available in the software but the actual rules, such as prompts for prescribers to order potassium replacement for patients with laboratory results below normal potassium levels, are not provided by the vendor nor are they typically programmed for use by organizations. CDS is a method for delivering clinical knowledge and intelligently filtered patient information to clinicians and/or patients for the purpose of improving healthcare processes and outcomes. CDS includes knowledge-delivery interventions, such as targeted documentation forms and templates, relevant data presentation, order and prescription creation facilitators, protocol and pathway support, reference information and guidance, and alerts and reminders (Osheroff, 2009).

The Leapfrog CPOE evaluation tool has been promoted as a means of monitoring the efficacy of hospitals systems and their CDS. Results from a study designed to determine the relationship between Leapfrog scores and the rates of preventable ADEs and potential ADEs indicated that scores from the Leapfrog CPOE evaluation tool closely relate to actual rates of preventable ADEs and that Leapfrog testing may alert providers to potential vulnerabilities and highlight areas for further improvement (Leung et al., 2013).

A study by Nebeker and colleagues showed that high rates of ADEs may continue after CPOE implementation if the system lacks CDS for drug selection, dosing, and monitoring (Nebeker, Hoffman, Weir, Bennett, & Hurdleet, 2005). Studies have shown those prescribers, using only the basic CPOE system alone, order appropriate medication doses for patients 54% of the time. By comparison, prescribers using the CPOE system with decision support tools prescribed appropriate doses 67% of the time. The addition of the decision support tools also increased the percentage of prescriptions considered ordered at appropriate intervals to 59%, from 35% with the basic CPOE system (Kaushal et al., 2001). A national sample of 62 hospitals voluntarily used a simulation tool designed to assess how well safety decision support worked when applied to medication orders in computerized order entry. This simulation detected only 53% of the medication orders that would have resulted in fatalities and 10% to 82% of the test orders that would have caused serious adverse drug events (Metzger, Welebob, Bates, Lipsitz, & Classen, 2010).

Complex and time-consuming order entry processes can often lead to practitioner frustration as evidenced by potential increases in the use of verbal orders, another error-prone process in communicating medication orders. Computer issues such as error messages, frozen screens, slow access to information, and other issues lead to problems of accessing critical patient or drug information as well as adding to prescriber frustration. It is important to have the ability to access past patient histories, particularly previous ADEs and comorbid conditions, yet some systems are unable to access prior patient care encounters. Problems may arise if drug information updates are not performed on a timely basis or if this information is difficult to access. One key error reduction strategy is the ability to install user-defined warnings (e.g., "look-alike/ sound-alike" drug name alert), yet some systems do not allow for this type of customization.

New types of medication errors can occur with the use of CPOE such as wrong patient errors, when the wrong patient is selected from a menu list of similar patient names; wrong drug errors, when the wrong medication is selected from a list due to look-alike similarity in either the brand or generic name; or orders intended for laboratory levels that are filled as medications. In a study that compared the manifestations, mechanisms, and rates of system-related errors associated with two electronic prescribing systems showed that 27.4% of system-related errors manifested as timing errors, 22.5% wrong drug strength errors, and selection errors accounted for 43.4% (34.2/100 admissions) (Westbrook et al., 2013). Another study that attempted to quantify the frequency and analyze risk factors for patient mis-selection errors when entering orders revealed many contributing factors, including similarly spelled last names when picking patient names from a list, having multiple charts opened at the same time, and distractions (Levin, Levin, & Docimo, 2012).

Even though CPOE systems are intended for use by prescribers, their presence in organizations will affect nursing and other personnel as well. CPOE systems will affect or even change the work of nurses in many ways, both negative and positive (AHA, 2000). First, like prescribers, these systems will require nurses to possess basic computer skills. Depending on the design of the system, nurses may find it difficult to know when new orders have been entered into the system, a special concern with respect to "STAT" or other new orders. Nurses sometimes see off-site entry of orders by prescribers as detrimental, because it reduces the opportunity to communicate information or ask questions face-to-face with prescribers with regard to the care of patients. In some situations, prescribers are reluctant to enter orders and use verbal orders as a way of "getting around" entering orders into the CPOE system and, in fact, nurses may end up entering verbal orders from prescribers.

But there are many beneficial aspects of these systems for nurses. Providing the capability for computerized physician order entry and making patient education material available electronically to nurses also have been identified as strategies to facilitate communication. With computerized physician order entry, nurses do not have to engage in transcription or verification of orders. Electronic patient education materials, unlike printed materials, are easily modifiable to meet clinician and patient needs; it is also possible to track which materials were given and by whom, assess follow-up and comprehension, and link education activities and documentation (Case, Mowry, & Welebob, 2002).

Nurses may have more time with patients due to enhanced productivity due to a reduced frequency in contacting prescribers to clarify orders. Additionally, there would be reductions in time wasted in transcribing duplicate orders for the same medication or test; greater standardization of orders, lessening the need to understand and adhere to diverse regimens and schedules; improved efficiency when ordering tests or procedures, thus reducing time devoted to carrying out redundant orders; and less need to enter voice orders into the system as prescribers gain access to the system from other units and remote locations. Finally, orders would be usually executed faster, medications would be available more quickly, and patients receive care more promptly. It is important for healthcare administration and nurses to understand that for a CPOE system to work as intended, it must be fully utilized by prescribers.

Barcode-Assisted Medication Administration (BCMA)

Nurses play a vital role in the medication-use process, ranging from their involvement in the communication of medication orders to the administration of medications. As nurses know well, the administration of medications can be a labor-intensive and error-prone process. One study showed that 38% of medication errors occur during the drug administration process (Leape et al., 1995). While about half of the ordering, transcribing, and dispensing errors were intercepted by the nurse before the medication error reached the patient, almost none of the errors at the medication administration stage were caught. In another study of medication administration errors in 36 healthcare facilities, Barker et al. found that some type of medication administration error occurred in almost 20% of medication doses administered (Barker, Flynn, Pepper, Bates, & Mikeal, 2002). In addition, nurses are burdened with larger patient loads and are caring for patients with higher degrees of acuity than ever before. To make matters worse, the number of medications that have reached the market has grown 500% over the past 10 years to more than 17,000 trademarked and generic drugs in North America (Institute for Safe Medication Practices [ISMP], 2000). Rapid advances in technology have helped make this process more efficient and safe. One form of technology that will have a great impact on medication safety during the administration process is barcode-assisted medication administration (BCMA) technology.

For more than 20 years, barcode technology has clearly demonstrated its power to greatly improve productivity and accuracy in the identification of products in a variety of business settings, such as supermarkets and department stores. Proven to be an effective technology, it quickly spread to virtually all other industries. Yet, many organizations in the healthcare industry have not fully embraced this valuable technology as a method to enhance patient safety.

The 2011 ASHP National Survey reported that approximately 50% of hospitals stated using barcode technology (Pedersen et al., 2011). This number has increased significantly over the past year, with implementation rates improving by 45%. This survey showed that all Veterans Affairs hospitals used BCMA, and general and children's medical-surgical hospitals with 100 to 399 beds were more likely to have BCMA to verify the accuracy of medication administration at the point of care. The reasons for these few numbers are varied and may include the cost of implementation, challenges integrating with current informatics systems, and prioritization among other information technology projects. The survey also revealed that larger hospitals (400 or more staff beds) had adopted CPOE before starting to adopt BCMA.

For the healthcare industry, the potential effect of implementing barcode technology to improve the safe administration of medications is enormous. As previously stated, the VA Healthcare System, a pioneer in the use of barcode technology, looked at their medication error rate based on the number of incident reports related to medication errors before and after implementation of the BCMA system. The study showed that following the introduction of the BCMA, reported medication error rates declined from 0.02% per dose administered to 0.0025%. This is almost a 10-fold reduction in errors over eight years (Johnson, Carlson, Tucker, & Willette, 2002). In a study that used the direct-observation methodology to monitor medication administration before and after the deployment of electronic medication administration records (eMARs) and BCMA systems showed a 54% reduction of medication administration errors (Paoletti et al., 2007). In another study that assessed rates of errors in order transcription and medication administration on units before and after implementation of the BCMA, observers noted an 11.5% error rate in medication administration on units that did not use the BCMA versus a 6.8% error rate on units that did use it—a 41.4% relative reduction in errors. The rate of potential ADEs (other than those associated with timing errors) fell from 3.1% without the use of the BCMA to 1.6% with its use, representing a 50.8% relative reduction (Poon et al., 2010). Procedural areas and emergency departments (EDs) are oftentimes excluded from the implementation of BCMA systems due to distinct differences from typical patient care areas. One recent study showed that, in addition to being feasible, the implementation of a BCMA system was associated with a relative reduction of medication administration errors by 80.7% (Bonkowski et al., 2013).

BCMA can improve medication safety through several levels of functionality. At the most basic level, the system helps verify that the right drug is being administered to the right patient at the right dose by the right route and at the right time. On admission, patients are issued an individualized barcode wristband that uniquely identifies their identity. When a patient is to receive a medication, the nurse scans their barcoded employee identifier and the patient's barcode wristband to confirm their identity. The Joint Commission has stated that a barcode with two unique, patient-specific identifiers will provide health-care organizations a system that complies with the 2014 National Patient Safety Goal requirement of obtaining two or more patient identifiers before medication administration (Joint Commission, 2014). Prior to medication administration, each barcoded package of medication to be administered at the bedside is scanned. The system can then verify the dispensing authority of the nurse, confirm the patient's identity, match the drug identity with their medication profile in the pharmacy information system, and electronically record the administration of the medication in an eMAR system.

The use of an eMAR is likely to be more accurate than traditional handwritten MARs. One study showed that by using BCMA, the medication-verification component greatly facilitates the documentation process for nurses and may be an important factor for its acceptance (Poon et al., 2008). In a survey of nurses who worked in a variety of clinical settings, the nurses believed that using barcoding and eMARs at the bedside was more time consuming, but they acknowledged that the extra time was worth it to ensure verification. Saving time on transcribing orders or trying to read handwritten, paper-based medication sheets was seen by many to be a significant positive change (Hurley et al., 2007). Furthermore, the barcode scanner can enable nurses to have greater accuracy in recording the timing of medication administration, as the computer generates an actual "real-time" log of medication administration. Additional levels of functionality can include some of the following features:

- Up-to-date drug reference information from online medication references. This could include pictures of tablets or capsules, usual dosages, contraindications, adverse reactions, and other safety warnings, pregnancy risk factors, and administration details.
- Customizable comments or alerts (e.g., look-alike/sound-alike drug names, special dosing instructions [e.g., 2 tablets = 10 mg]) and reminders of

important clinical actions that need to be taken when administering certain medications (e.g., do not crush; respiratory intubation is required for neuromuscular blockers).

- Monitoring the pharmacy and the nurse's response to predetermined rules such as alerts or reminders. This includes allergies, duplicate dosing, over-/underdosing, checking for cumulative dosing for medications with established maximum doses such as acetaminophen.
- Reconciliation for pending or STAT orders (i.e., a prescriber order not yet verified by a pharmacist). The ability of the nurse to enter a STAT order into the system on administration that is linked directly to the pharmacy profile and prevents the duplicate administration of the same medication.
- Capturing data for the purpose of retrospective analysis of aggregate data to monitor trends (e.g., percentage of doses administered late; alerts that were overridden). However, this analysis should *not* be used to assess employee performance, especially if it could lead to punitive action.
- Verifying blood transfusion and laboratory specimen collection identification.
- Increased accountability and capture of charges for items such as unit stock medications.

It is important to understand that the successful implementation of an effective BCMA system "forces" nurses to accept and change some of their long-held practices when administering medications to achieve a higher level of medication safety. When BCMA technology is used correctly, it drives compliance with the proper identification of patients, it documents real-time administration, and acts as a double-check. It is also vitally important to its success that affected staff members, and specifically frontline nurses, are involved in all the decisions related to the purchase, education, and implementation of barcode technology. Before embarking on a BCMA implementation, it is critical to anticipate potential failures and develop contingency plans for unexpected results. In a study that evaluated the workflow variables related to a bedside barcode technology-based medication administration process, the authors concluded that nurses were found to be primarily engaged in tasks performed at the bedside. However, tasks such as retrieving missed medications and routinely updating patients' vital assessment records added workflow blocks to the medication administration process (Dasgupta et al., 2011). And second study revealed that the introduction of BCMA in an intensive care unit (ICU) resulted in nursing spending less time on the documentation process and more time conversing with patients during the medication administration process (Dwibedi et al., 2012).

Of course, a stringent testing phase should also be built into the system rollout phase using a technique such as failure mode and effects analysis (FMEA) to proactively address potential sources of breakdowns, work-arounds, or new sources of medication errors. One study noted significant changes to workflow that occurred during the implementation of a BCMA system at VA hospitals that might lead to the use of work-arounds (Patterson, Cook, & Render, 2002). Negative effects and corresponding work-arounds include the following:

- Nurses were sometimes caught "off guard" by the programmed automated actions taken by the BCMA software. For example, the BCMA would remove medications from a patient's drug profile list four hours after the scheduled administration time, even if the medications were never administered.

- Inhibited coordination of patient information between nurses and physicians. Before the BCMA was implemented, the prescriber could quickly review the handwritten MAR at the patient's bedside or in the unit's medication room.

- Nurses found it more difficult to deviate from the routine medication administration sequence with the BCMA system. For example, if a patient refused a medication, the nurses had to manually document the change since the medication had already been documented as given when it was originally scanned.

- Nurses felt that their main priority was the timeliness of medication administration because BCMA required nurses to type in an explanation when medications were given even a few minutes late. Particularly in long-term care settings, some nurses were observed to scan and pre-pour medications for unavailable patients so that they would appear "on time" in the computer record, thereby relying on memory to administer unlabeled medications when the patient returned to the unit.

- Nurses used strategies to increase efficiency that circumvented the intended use of BCMA. For example, some nurses routinely entered a patient's social security number by typing the numbers rather than scanning the patient's barcode wristband, because typing seemed to be quicker. This was especially true if the nurse experienced difficulty in scanning the patient's barcode arm band (i.e., curvature of the barcode on the patient's wrist band on patients with small wrists, or damaged barcodes) (Patterson et al., 2002).

The interaction between nurses and technology at the bedside is important and must be continually evaluated for safety. As previously mentioned, nurses tend to develop work-arounds for ineffective or inefficiently designed systems. Koppel, Wetterneck, Telles, and Karsh (2008) sought to identify reasons for work-arounds and found three categories that capture this phenomenon: (a) omission of process steps, (b) steps performed out of sequence, and (c) unauthorized process steps. The authors identified 15 types of work-arounds, including, for example, affixing patient identification barcodes to computer carts, scanners, doorjambs, or nurses' belt rings; carrying several patients' pre-scanned medications on carts. The authors identified 31 types of causes of work-arounds, such as unreadable medication barcodes (crinkled, smudged, torn, missing, covered by another label); malfunctioning scanners; unreadable or missing patient identification wristbands (chewed, soaked, missing); non-barcoded medications; failing batteries; uncertain wireless connectivity; emergencies. The authors found nurses overrode BCMA alerts for 4.2% of patients charted and for 10.3% of medications charted. The possible consequences of the work-around include wrong administration of medications, wrong doses, wrong times, and wrong formulations. Shortcomings in BCMA design, implementation, and workflow integration encouraged work-arounds.

One medication error reported to ISMP caused by a work-around (overriding an alert), involved a mix-up with an order for digoxin elixir (used for congestive heart failure), which was stocked on the unit as a 0.05 mg/mL, 60 mL multi-dose bottle (usual dose is 0.125–0.25 mg [2.5–5 mL]). The nurse not only misinterpreted the dose of digoxin elixir as 60 mL, but accidentally retrieved a bottle of doxepin (used for depression), which was available as 10 mg/mL (usual dose is 75–150 mg per day [7.5–15 mL]) from unit stock and attempted to administer what she thought was digoxin elixir. This error occurred because she scanned the barcode on the bottle, which generated an error window on the laptop computer screen stating "drug not on profile" and did not investigate the error. The system allowed the nurse to manually enter the wrong medication's national drug code (NDC) number (a medical code set that identifies prescription drugs and some over-the-counter products), ignoring the correct drug NDC number that had been entered by the pharmacy which appeared on the laptop screen and administered

60 mL of doxepin elixir. This allowed the nurse a method to bypass the check system and simply type in numbers and administer a drug, whether it was the right or wrong ordered medication.

Alerts that are generated by BCMA systems often may not be noticeable. For example, a system may generate a visual display of the alert but not provide a distinct auditory alert. If a nurse does not look at the screen for any alerts after scanning a patient's wristband and/or barcoded medications, errors will ensue. Additionally, the alerts are not hard-stops, meaning that the system does not physically stop a practitioner from proceeding with scanning or administering a medication (Pennsylvania Patient Safety Authority [PSA], 2008). Problems have also occurred when other processes surrounding medication administration have broken down. Although the steps directly involved with the scanning of the medication and patient may be completed, errors can be introduced if distractions occur or medications are laid down after the scanning process.

One major issue that initially hindered the widespread implementation of BCMA systems was with the pharmaceutical industry's unwillingness to adopt a universal barcode standard and apply a barcode consistently to the container of all medications, including unit-dose packages. But in February 2004, the FDA established a new rule that requires a barcode on most products in a linear format that meets the Uniform Code Council (UCC) or Health Industry Business Communications Council (HIBCC) standards. This barcode must contain the product's NDC number, but the expiration date and lot numbers are optional (ISMP, 2004).

Further complicating the issue is the unavailability of unit-dose packaging for some medications. At this point, if hospital pharmacies that employ barcode technology cannot purchase medications that are packaged in a unit-dose system, they must re-package these medications and re-label each with a barcode. This can only be done at considerable cost in manpower and/or automated repackaging equipment. In addition, the chance of a medication error occurring is increased because doses must be taken from their original container and then re-packaged or re-labeled, and there could be an error in the application of the correct barcode label or in choosing the right medication. One medication error reported to ISMP includes a scenario where a facility utilized a BCMA system for their inpatients where not all injectables had manufacturers' barcodes on the vials or ampules, and pharmacy technicians had to generate computer-printed barcodes for those products. Prior to the intubation of a patient, a vial of succinylcholine chloride with an incorrect dose label was discovered. The printed label read 20 mg/10 mL,

whereas the manufacturer's label read 20 mg/mL. Had the patient received the incorrect dose, it would have been 10 times the dose needed.

The use of BCMA systems can possibly introduce new types of medication errors. Although few medication errors have been reported with these systems, it can be hypothesized that some of the following types of errors could occur, especially if the system includes only the most basic of functionality:

- **Wrong dosage form**: Certain drug shortages may force a pharmacy to dispense a different strength or concentration (mg/mL) other than what is entered in the BCMA software.

- **Omissions**: After the patient's barcode armband and medication have been scanned, the dose is inadvertently dropped onto the floor. This results in a time lapse between the documentation that the medication was supposedly administered and the actual administration after obtaining the new dose.

- **Extra dose**: An extra dose may be given when there are orders for the same drug to be administered by a different route. For example, if one nurse gives an oral dose and is called away and the covering nurse administers the dose intravenously (IV). The problem arises when there is no alert between profiled routes of administration indicating that the medication was previously administered by one route that is different than the second route.

- **Wrong drug**: In situations when the nurse received an alert indicating that the wrong medication was selected, but the alert is overridden and the medication is administered.

- **Wrong dose**: These systems are limited in their capability to verify the correct volume (e.g., 1 mL) of oral or parenteral solutions to administer. Most systems prompt a nurse to manually enter the volume that was administered.

- **Unauthorized drug**: An order to hold a medication unless a lab value is at a certain level such as an aminoglycoside (i.e., elevated gentamicin drug level).

- **Charting errors**: Distinguish the indication for the administration of the medication (Tylenol 650 mg every four hours as needed for pain or fever).

Automated Dispensing Cabinets (ADCs)

Traditionally, hospital pharmacies provided medications for patients by filling patient-specific bins of unit-dose medications, which were then delivered to the nursing unit and stored in medication carts. The ADC is a computerized point-of-use medication-management system that is designed to replace or support the traditional unit-dose drug delivery system. The devices require staff to enter a unique logon and password to access the system using a touch screen monitor or by using finger print identification. Various levels of system access can be assigned to staff members, depending on their role in the medication-use process. Once logged into the system, the nurse can obtain medications from drawers or bins that open after a drug is chosen from a pick list.

Many healthcare facilities have replaced medication carts or open unit-stock systems with ADCs. The results of an ISMP survey showed that 94% of hospital respondents were utilizing ADCs in their facilities; of those, more than half (56%) were using the technology as the primary means of drug distribution (ISMP, 2008a). The 2011 ASHP national survey of pharmacy practice provided further evidence of a trend toward decentralized automated systems using ADCs to distribute patient medications. While the ASHP survey results showed that only 22% of hospitals in 2002 employed ADCs as the primary method of drug distribution, by 2011 this figure had increased significantly to include 63% of hospital respondents (Pedersen et al., 2011).

The rationale behind the wide acceptance of this technology may include:

- **Improved pharmacy productivity**: The use of ADCs may promote streamlining of the pharmacy dispensing process due to the reduced number of steps from filling each patient's individual medication bin to filling a centralized station. It also has the potential to reduce time needed to obtain missing medications.

- **Potential to enhance nursing productivity**: In a study that was designed to assess how nurses spend their time, nurse location and movement, and nurse physiologic response, approximately two-thirds of all time spent on medication administration was related to drug delivery to the patient (46.7 minutes). The other third (24.9 minutes) was spent preparing drugs for administration. The authors concluded that process improvements could reduce the time required for this step (Hendrich, Chow, Skierczynski, & Zhenqiang, 2008). Therefore, the time spent gathering or obtaining missing medications could be reduced with an automated decentralized drug distribution model using ADCs. Also, the turnaround time in obtaining newly ordered medications may be decreased.

- **Improved charge capture**: ADCs that are interfaced with the accounting department allow for the capture of all patient charges associated with administered medications.

- **Automated inventory control**: ADCs that utilize barcode technology can interface with the wholesaler for improved inventory control. In addition, the use of barcode technology increases the accuracy and efficiency of the ADC stocking process.

- **Improved security of controlled substances**: ADCs can be used to comply with regulatory requirements by tracking the storage, dispensing, and use of controlled substances.

- **Timelier drug availability**: ADCs can speed up delivery time for first and stat doses. In fact, a study found that storing key antibiotics in the ED ADC can significantly reduce order-to-antibiotic time and increase the percentage of severely septic patients receiving antibiotics within the recommended three hours from arrival to the ED (Hitti et al., 2012).

- **Enhanced patient quality and safety**: ADC systems often allow for organization-specific, user-generated alerts to prevent medication errors such as warnings related to potential errors associated with high-alert medications and with look-alike/sound-alike medication names.

However, such systems cannot improve patient safety unless cabinet *design* and *use* are carefully planned and implemented to eliminate opportunities for wrong drug selection and dosing errors. According to the PSA, nearly 15% of all medication error reports cited ADCs as the source of the medication, and 23% of those reports involve high-alert medications. Many of the reports described cases in which the design and/or use of ADCs had contributed to the errors. The types of errors reported included wrong drug errors, stocking/storage errors, and medications being administered to patients with a documented allergy (PSA, 2005).

Some documented unsafe practices with the use of these devices include **the lack of pharmacy screening of medication orders prior to administration**, which negates an independent double-check of the original order. In the aforementioned ASHP survey conducted in 2011, 96.2% of hospitals had ADCs that used patient-specific medication profiles, which limits user access to those medications with active orders for the specified patient after the order has been reviewed by the pharmacist. However, of those hospitals that used patient-specific profiles with their ADCs, it is estimated that 12.2% of medications are dispensed as overrides (the manual action taken to counteract or bypass the normal operation) (Pedersen et al., 2011). Unless a situation is emergent (in which waiting for a pharmacist to review the order before accessing the medication could adversely impact the patient's condition) medication orders should be screened by the pharmacy for the appropriateness of the drug, dose, frequency, route of administration, therapeutic duplication, real or potential allergies or sensitivities, real or potential interactions between the prescription and other medications, food, and laboratory values, and other contraindications prior to removal from the ADC. This is particularly problematic when medications, which are considered "high-alert," are removed on override in these devices* (Table 30.1). For example, in a medication error submitted to ISMP that occurred in a small hospital after the pharmacy was closed, an order was written for "calcium gluconate 1 g IV." The nurse, however, misread the label and believed that *each 10 mL* vial contained only 98 mg. Thus, she thought she needed 10 vials when actually each mL actually contained 98 mg, or 1 g/10 mL vial. A 10-fold overdose was avoided because the drug cabinet contained only six vials of calcium gluconate. Fortunately, this error was detected when the nurse contacted a pharmacist at home to obtain additional vials.

Choosing of the wrong medication from an alphabetic pick list is a common contributing factor in medication errors, which arises from medication names that look alike. For example, in a report submitted to ISMP, one organization described three errors regarding mix-ups between diazepam and diltiazem removals from ADCs in their intensive care units. In one case, diazepam was given at the ordered diltiazem dose and, in another case, a physician noted the amber color of the diazepam vial as the nurse was drawing up the dose (meaning to obtain diltiazem). The organization concluded that once the wrong drug was chosen, the cabinet seemed to "confirm" that the correct drug was selected since the nurse assumed the correct drug was chosen from the menu and thought the correct drug was in the drawer that opened. The nurse "relied" on her ability to choose the right drug from the pick list.

Medications, especially high-alert drugs, placed, stored, and returned to ADCs are problematic. The process of placing and re-stocking medications into an ADC is primarily a pharmacy function. Unfortunately, studies have indicated that an independent double-check (one individual supplies the cabinet with the medication and a second individual independently checks that the correct medication was placed into the appropriate location) does not always occur. In the 2011 ASHP survey, 86.5% of the hospitals with ADCs had pharmacists check the accuracy and integrity of the medications in the ADC either before or after they are stocked (Pedersen et al., 2011). A significant advance in the safe use of ADCs is the incorporation of barcode technology, which can effectively increase the accuracy of the ADC medication replenishment process. This survey also showed that 43% of hospitals use barcode technology when loading ADCs. Scanning medications when stocking ADCs can minimize the possibility of pharmacy staff placing medications in the incorrect pocket (Pedersen et al.). For example, in a case reported to ISMP, a patient had orders for both MS Contin (morphine sulfate *controlled* release) 15 mg tablets and for morphine sulfate *immediate* release 15 mg tablets. A pharmacy technician loaded both medications in the ADC in the patient care unit. The person loading the medications inadvertently loaded the MS Contin in the pocket for the morphine sulfate immediate release and the morphine sulfate immediate release in the pocket for the MS Contin. Some doses of each medication were actually administered to a patient. Fortunately, the patient suffered no apparent adverse effects from this incident. A second nurse discovered the error when removing the medication for the next dose.

Another report involved the need to refill unit stock in an ADC with furosemide 40 mg/4 mL. A pharmacy technician selected what was thought to be vials of furosemide 40 mg/4 mL from the stock in a satellite pharmacy and then, without a pharmacist double-check, left the pharmacy and filled the ADC. A nurse on the unit went to the cabinet to fill an order for furosemide 240 mg. She obtained six vials out of the ADC and drew them into a syringe. After drawing up the sixth vial, the nurse noticed a precipitation. At that point, the nurse checked the vials to find that she had five vials of furosemide 40 mg/4 mL and one 5 mL vial of phenylephrine 1%. Both these medications were available in the same size amber vials with very little color or marking differentiation. These types of errors may have been avoided if barcode scanning technology had been utilized in the ADC refilling process.

Storage of medications with look-alike names and/ or packaging next to each other in the same drawer or bin is a contributing factor of errors involving ADCs. A common cause of these mix-ups is what human factors experts call "confirmation bias," where a practitioner reads a drug name on an order or package and is most likely to see that which is most familiar to him, overlooking any disconfirming evidence. Also, when confirmation bias occurs, it is unlikely that the practitioner would question what is being read. This can occur both in the re-stocking

---

*High-alert medications can be defined as medications that, when involved in medication errors, have a high risk of injury or death. There is no documentation that the occurrence of medication errors is more common with high-alert medications than with the use of other drugs but the consequence of the error may be far more devastating (Cohen, 2007). Examples of high-alert medications can be found in Table 30.1.

TABLE 30.1

Classes/Categories of Medications	Specific Medications
Adrenergic agonists, IV (e.g., **EPINEPH**rine, phenylephrine, norepinephrine)	Epoprostenol (Flolan), IV
Adrenergic antagonists, IV (e.g., propranolol, metoprolol, labetalol)	Magnesium sulfate injection
Anesthetic agents, general, inhaled, and IV (e.g., propofol, ketamine)	Methotrexate, oral, non-oncologic use
Antiarrhythmics, IV (e.g., lidocaine, amiodarone)	Opium tincture
Antithrombotic agents, including:	Oxytocin, IV
• Anticoagulants (e.g., warfarin, low-molecular-weight heparin, IV unfractionated heparin)	Nitroprusside sodium for injection
• Factor Xa inhibitors (e.g., fondaparinux)	Potassium chloride for injection concentrate
• Direct thrombin inhibitors (e.g., argatroban, bivalirudin, dabigatran etexilate, lepirudin)	Potassium phosphates injection
• Thrombolytics (e.g., alteplase, reteplase, tenecteplase)	Promethazine, IV
• Glycoprotein IIb/IIIa inhibitors (e.g., eptifibatide)	Vasopressin, IV or intraosseous
Cardioplegic solutions	
Chemotherapeutic agents, parenteral and oral	
Dextrose, hypertonic, 20% or greater	
Dialysis solutions, peritoneal and hemodialysis	
Epidural or intrathecal medications	
Hypoglycemics, oral	
Inotropic medications, IV (e.g., digoxin, milrinone)	
Insulin, subcutaneous and IV	
Liposomal forms of drugs (e.g., liposomal amphotericin B) and conventional counterparts (e.g., amphotericin B desoxycholate)	
Moderate sedation agents, IV (e.g., dexmedetomidine, midazolam)	
Moderate sedation agents, oral, for children (e.g., chloral hydrate)	
Narcotics/opioids	
• IV	
• Transdermal	
• Oral (including liquid concentrates, immediate and sustained-release formulations)	
Neuromuscular blocking agents (e.g., succinylcholine, rocuronium, vecuronium)	
Parenteral nutrition preparations	
Radiocontrast agents, IV	
Sterile water for injection, inhalation, and irrigation (excluding pour bottles) in containers of 100 mL or more	
Sodium chloride for injection, hypertonic, greater than 0.9% concentration	

Reproduced, with permission, from the Institute for Safe Medication Practices. © ISMP 2012. Report medication errors or near misses to the ISMP Medication Errors Reporting Program (MERP) at 1-800-FAIL-SAF(E) or online at www.ismp.org.

process of the ADC and in the removal of medications. One example includes a situation where a physician asked for ePHEDrine, but a hurried nurse picked EPINEPHrine from the ADC, drew up the medication into a syringe, and handed it to the primary nurse who administered the EPINEPHrine. The patient suffered a period of hypertension and chest pain but eventually recovered. In another example, a prescriber wrote an order for morphine via a patient-controlled analgesia (PCA) pump. The nurse used the override function to remove a PCA syringe containing meperidine from the ADC. When pharmacy reviewed the override medication removal report the next morning, the error was discovered. The PCA pump still had the meperidine cartridge in place, but the pump settings were for morphine, resulting in an inappropriate dose. An example that made national news involved three premature infants who died in a Midwestern hospital after receiving an overdose of heparin. Vials of heparin 10,000 unit/mL 1 mL were placed incorrectly into a unit-based ADC where 1 mL, 10 units/mL vials were normally kept. Several nurses requested 10 unit/mL vials to prepare an umbilical line flush and were directed to that drawer, but did not notice that the vials contained the wrong concentration (ISMP, 2006).

Another important improvement in the safety of ADCs is the use of lidded pockets, which can minimize the risk of these types of stocking and selection errors. Lidded pockets restrict access to only the medication selected, thereby minimizing the possibility of picking a medication from the wrong pocket, taking other doses than the one needed for a specific patient, or having the pharmacy staff load or return medications to the wrong pocket. The 2011 ASHP national survey found that 62% of hospitals utilized ADCs with lidded pockets (Pedersen et al., 2011).

The development of "work-arounds" for ineffective or inefficient systems can be devastating to patient safety. The interaction between a nurse and technology is very important and often is not considered when various forms of automation, including ADCs, are purchased, installed, and employed on the nursing unit. When the device does not respond as expected, nurses often find various ways of working around the system to obtain medications. In the PCA medication selection error discussed above, overrides were established by the organization that allowed nursing to obtain certain medications without review by a pharmacist. Overrides usually are needed with medications used in emergency situations. Unfortunately, when overused, overrides also serve as an "extended" pharmacy in order to obtain and administer medications prior to verification by the pharmacy. One study involving the use of an expert panel that developed criteria for override access and revised the override medication list showed a reduction in the number of medications and dosage forms on the override list by 42% (from 119 different medications in 244 different dosage forms to 92 different medications in 163 different dosage forms), resulting in a significant decrease in opioid override rates (Kowiatek, Weber, Skledar, Frank, & DeVita, 2006).

Additional error reports involving work-arounds include the removal of medications using the inventory function (used to determine the number of doses on hand of a particular medication) to obtain medications for patients without pharmacy screening, removal of a larger quantity of medications than ordered for one patient, and removal of medications for multiple patients while the cabinet is open.

In spring 2007, ISMP convened a national forum of stakeholders to create inter-disciplinary guidelines for ADCs. These associated core processes are intended to be universally incorporated into practice in an effort to promote safe ADC use and subsequently improve patient safety:

1. **Provide Ideal Environmental Conditions for the Use of ADCs.** The physical environment in which the ADC is placed can have a dramatic effect on medication errors. Specifically, the work environment and a busy, chaotic work area were cited as the top two contributing factors in medication errors.

2. **Ensure ADC System Security.** Security processes must be established to ensure adequate control of medications outside of the pharmacy and to reduce the potential for medication diversion from ADCs.

3. **Use Pharmacy-profiled ADCs.** The use of a "profiled" ADC allows the pharmacist to clinically review new drug orders for appropriateness prior to the medication being accessed by the nurse or other healthcare professional.

4. **Identify Information That Should Appear on the ADC Screen.** Having sufficient patient information and drug information when dispensing and administering medications is key to the safety of the medication use process. Because there is limited space available on the ADC screens, it is important to focus on presenting the information that is of the greatest value to practitioners, allowing for the clear identification of specific patients, their active medication profiles, and supporting information for safe drug use.

5. **Select and Maintain Proper ADC Inventory.** The ADC inventory should be determined based on the needs of the patient population served and replenished on a regular schedule. Medications should be routinely reviewed and adjusted considering medication prescribing patterns, drug utilization, and specific unit needs (taking into account typical patient ages and diagnoses). Standard stock medications should be identified, and approved, for each patient care area, with the goal to limit the variety of drug concentrations, avoid bulk supplies, and provide medications in ready-to-use unit doses.

6. **Select Appropriate ADC Configuration.** Restricting access to medications limits the potential for inadvertently selecting the wrong medication.

Medications stocked in ADCs may be high alert or high cost, and it is important to ensure that only the right drug is selected. For these reasons, it is important to maximize the use of high-security drawer configurations such that each drug has its own unique and segregated location within the ADC, and so access is limited to only the specific drug needed.

7. **Define Safe ADC Re-stocking Processes.** The re-stocking process encompasses a number of sub-processes that can involve both pharmacy and nursing staff. It is important that the process contain redundancies to ensure that the correct medication is placed in the correct location within the ADC. It is also important that the process be defined and organized so staff involved can only follow the correct pathway and the potential for process variation is limited. Consider systems that utilize barcode scanning technology during stocking, which can minimize the risk of misplacement errors.

8. **Develop Procedures to Ensure the Accurate Withdrawal of Medications From the ADC.** Processes must be developed that reduce the risk or mitigate the harm associated with the administration of the wrong medication, dose, route, or frequency due to ADC medication retrieval errors. Of particular importance is the ability and expectation for the nurse to access the medication administration record when selecting medications from the ADC. In addition, the contents (variety, concentrations, and volume) and configuration of the ADC play a large role in the practitioner's ability to safely select and remove medications from the ADC.

9. **Establish Criteria for ADC System Overrides.** Use of ADC overrides should be situationally dependent, and not based merely on a medication or a list of medications. Criteria for system overrides should be established that allow emergency access in circumstances in which waiting for a pharmacist to review the order before accessing the medication could adversely impact the patient's condition. Routinely run and analyze override reports to help track and identify problems.

10. **Standardize Processes for Transporting Medications from the ADC to the Patient's Bedside.** A process should be developed that reduces the risk of medications being administered to the wrong patient at the wrong time during the transportation of medications from the ADC to the patient. Supporting safety may require the availability of additional ADCs or the placement of ADCs in strategic locations to prevent work-arounds. Not having sufficient ADCs, or having them located far from patient rooms, fosters the at-risk behavior of taking medications for more than one patient at a time or taking medications for more than one scheduled administration time. The safety of this practice also is impacted by the organization's ability to secure medications during transport between the ADC and the patient's bedside.

11. **Eliminate the Process for Returning Medications Directly to Their Original ADC Location.** Instead, return all medications to a common, secure one-way return bin that is maintained by pharmacy, not to an individual pocket or bin within the ADC. Occasionally practitioners inadvertently return medications to the wrong pocket, either because of user distraction, look-alike and sound-alike medications in a matrix bin, or a slip in procedure.

12. **Provide Staff Education and Competency Validation.** All ADC users must be educated and have regular competency validation in the proper operation of the device in order to meet expectations for safe use. Most often this education occurs during the practitioner's orientation period, or upon ADC installation, but an annual update may be required in order to ensure ongoing appropriate use. Users who are not properly oriented to the device may develop practice habits and device work-arounds that are considered unsafe (ISMP, 2008b).

Smart Infusion Pump Delivery Systems

Infusion pumps are primarily used to deliver parenteral medications through IV or epidural lines and can be found in a variety of clinical settings ranging from acute-care and long-term care facilities, patient's homes, and physician's offices. Among ADEs, the significant potential for patient injury and death related to IV medication errors is well known (ASHP, 2008; Aspden et al., 2006; Cohen, 2007).

A study conducted in an academic medicosurgical intensive care unit found that up to 21 separate errors might have occurred in association with a single dose of an IV medication, and one of the most common occurring errors related to a discrepancy between the medication order as recorded in the patient's chart and the IV medication that was being infused (Summa-Sorgini et al., 2012). An Australian study designed to identify the prevalence of medication administration errors and their related causes found that errors in the administration of continuous IV infusions occurred in almost one out of five infusions, and the most common error (79.3%) was wrong administration rate (Han, Coombes, & Green, 2005).

Adachi & Lodolce showed that the most common reason for the administration of wrong doses of intravenous medications was an error in programming IV infusion pumps (41%), and this step in the medication-use process was associated with the highest impact (2005). Husch and colleagues (2005) examined IV administration errors specifically associated with IV pumps and of the 426 medications observed infusing via an IV pump, 66.9% had one or more errors related to their administration. Causes of these IV administration errors were diverse in nature.

In addition, Pettus and Vanderveen (2013) warn that a single wrong keystroke when programming an infusion pump can result in a 10- or 100-fold overdose with tragic results, further calling it "death by decimal." Highlighting these concerns, ECRI (a non-profit organization that evaluates medical device safety) announced that medication administration errors using infusion pumps placed second on its annual list of Top 10 Health Technology Hazards for 2013 (ECRI, 2012). Conversely, infusion pumps with dose error reduction software (DERS), often referred to as smart pumps, can reduce medication errors, improve workflow, and provide a new source of data for continuous quality improvement by identifying and correcting these pump-programming errors.

The administration of parenteral medications has traditionally been based on a calculation of a volume to be infused per hour of delivery. Infusion pumps are capable of delivering a wide range of delivery rates, ranging from 0.01 mL/hour to as much as 1 L/hour, which could result in the device being programmed all too easily in error to deliver a 10- or 100-fold overdose. For example, one such error reported to ISMP occurred when a nurse attempted to program an infusion pump for a baby receiving parenteral nutrition (PN) by inputting 13.0 mL/hour. The decimal point key on the pump was somewhat worn and difficult to engage. Without realizing it, the nurse programmed a rate of 130 mL/hour. Fortunately, the error was discovered within one hour. The baby's glucose rose to 363, so the rate of the PN infusion was decreased for a period of time and the infant then stabilized.

Confusion with dosing nomenclature has been another source of error. A medication may be inadvertently programmed to be administered as micrograms per kilogram per minute (mcg/kg/min) instead of micrograms per minute (mcg/min), a 24-hour dose may be delivered over one hour, or a missing decimal point or an additional zero may result in a 10-fold overdose. Infusion pumps are specifically designed to have maximum flexibility, so they can be used in multiple areas of the facility. Consequently, a pump used today for a 200-kg patient in the adult ICU may also be used on a 3 kg infant in the ED.

In other cases, mis-programming of a medication's concentration has resulted in significant error. One such example involved HYDROmorphone 20 mg/100 mL (0.2 mg/mL) intended to be infused at 2.5 mg/hour. For the institution, this was a custom concentration and required programming of the infusion as volume over time instead of selecting the concentration from the smart pump drug library. When programming the pump, the nurse mistakenly entered 2.5 mg/100 mL as the concentration instead of 20 mg/100 mL. Based on the incorrect programming, the pump delivered the medication at a rate of 100 mL/hour instead of 12.5 mL/hour. The entire 20 mg bag of HYDROmorphone was delivered to the patient in one hour. The outcome of this patient is unknown (ISMP, 2012). Other programming errors have resulted in additional monitoring and medical intervention. For example, a heparin infusion 25,000 units/250 mL was dispensed from the pharmacy in a concentration that was available in the smart pump library. However, the nurse selected the custom concentration option erroneously entering 800 units/250 mL. The ordered dose of 800 units/hour should have infused at 8 mL/hour, but instead infused at 250 mL/hour. The patient received the entire bag in one hour and required treatment with IV protamine (ISMP, 2012).

The common denominator in many of these and other cases was a single wrong entry or button pressed. The use of a smart infusion pump, programmed with patient and drug parameters, provides the ability to recognize an error before the infusion even begins. In a study to assess the impact of infusion pump technologies, comparing traditional infusion pumps with smart pumps, the number of nurses who remedied "wrong dose hard limit" errors was higher when using the smart pump (75%) than when using the traditional pump (38%) (Trbovich, Pinkney, Cafazzo, & Easty, 2010).

The introduction of smart infusion technology has changed the paradigm of infusion therapy by removing the reliance on memory and human input of calculated values to a software-enabled filter to prevent keystroke errors in programming infusion devices for delivery of parenteral medications. Smart pumps can include comprehensive libraries of drugs, usual concentrations, dosing units (e.g., mcg/kg/min, units/hour) and dose limits as well as software that incorporate institution-established dosage limits, warnings to the practitioner when dosage limits are exceeded, and configurable settings by patient type or location in the organization (i.e., ICU, pediatric ICU [PICU]). Such systems make it possible to provide an additional verification at the point of care to help prevent medication errors.

Current smart pump software enables the infusion system to provide an additional verification of the programming of medication delivery. The user receives an alert when the dose is below or above the organization's pre-established limits. The limits can be set as either "soft" (can be overridden) or "hard" (one that will not let the nurse go any further without reprogramming the pump). The drug library in the system generally requires the practitioner to confirm the patient care area, drug name, drug amount, diluent volume, patient weight (as appropriate), dose, and rate of infusion. The system can allow organizations to configure unit-specific profiles, which include customized sets of operating variables, programming options, and drug libraries.

Although not widely available at the present time, smart infusion systems could also incorporate barcode technology to advance the safe programming of IV medications. Specifically, IV interoperability is a process which integrates the eMAR, BCMA, and smart pump into a barcode-driven workflow. This technology automatically populates the smart pump with the pharmacy verified, provider order. In addition, it allows infusion-specific data from the smart pump to be electronically recorded in the eMAR at time of administration. One study found that the integration of IV interoperability reduced medications errors, involved pharmacists in checking infusion rates, and simplified nursing workflow (Prusch, Suess, Paoletti, Olin, & Watts, 2011).

Another significant benefit associated with smart pump technology is the ability to access transaction data from the infusion device for quality improvement efforts. Continuous quality improvement logs in the software record the close calls (programming errors) averted by the system. Practitioners can use these data to assess current practices and identify ways of improving safe use of medications. For each safety alert, a record can be generated with the time, date, drug, concentration, programmed rate, volume infused, and limit exceeded, as well as the clinician's response to the warning (i.e., continue at the current settings or change the programming). Similar data for infusions delivered with traditional settings for rate and volume can also be captured, along with other transactional data generated as a result of pump use (e.g., alarms, air in line). Thus, the system can be used to show whether potential infusion errors were detected and to assess current practice to determine if improvements can be made to optimize care and reduce costs.

Documented examples of errors prevented using smart pump technology have been published. For example, in an event reported to ISMP, a physician in the ED wrote an order for Integrilin (eptifibatide) but inadvertently prescribed a dose appropriate for ReoPro (abciximab). The Integrilin infusion was initiated and continued for approximately 36 hours after the patient was transferred to a medical/surgical unit. During this time, the patient's mental status was deteriorating. Coincidentally, at that time, the hospital was switching to a smart pump infusion system. As the nurse was transferring the infusion parameters from the old infusion system to this new system, safety software incorporated in the device alerted the nurse that there was a "dose out of range." The pump would not allow the nurse to continue until a pharmacist was called and the mistake was corrected. In another case, a hospital's heparin protocol called for a loading dose of 4000 units followed by a constant infusion of 900 units/hour. The loading dose was administered correctly, but the nurse inadvertently programmed the continuous dose as 4000 units/hour. Since the pump limit for heparin as a continuous infusion was set at 2000 units/hour, the infusion device would not start until the dose was corrected. In both cases, these mistakes may have gone undetected without preprogrammed limits and patient harm might have resulted.

Smart pump technology is also not without limitations. If the smart pump drug library is bypassed, and the infusion rate and volume is manually entered, the dose error reduction software will not be in place to prevent a potential error. Engaging in this at-risk behavior reduces the likelihood that an error will be identified since no alerts will be triggered (ISMP, 2009). In a prospective, randomized time-series trial, Rothschild and colleagues (2005) noted that intravenous medication errors were frequent and could be detected using smart pumps. The authors found no measurable impact on the serious medication error rate with smart infusion pumps, likely in part due to poor compliance. Violations of infusion practice during the intervention periods included bypasses of the drug library (25%). Numerous events have been reported to the PSA that include examples of errors associated with the use of smart infusion pumps. Some examples include similar types of errors that may occur with the use of general infusion pumps:

- Organizations that did not standardize the concentrations of high-alert medications
- Practitioners inadvertently switching IV lines between separate infusion pumps or dual-chambered infusion pumps
- Wrong-dose errors when inaccurate patient weights were used to calculate and program weight-based doses
- Inadvertent selection of a wrong drug or the wrong unit of measure in the smart pump's library (PSA, 2007)

Thus, prior to implementation, it is important to use proactive approaches such as FMEA and clinical simulations to identify potential clinical practice issues and risk of error with IV drug administration utilizing smart infusion pumps. Implementation should be coordinated by a multi-disciplinary team (including frontline nurses) that can determine best practices. This team should institute changes in policies and procedures that reflect the installation of smart infusion technology. Asking a nurse to choose from among many concentrations, dosing units, or remembering several possible drug names will increase the risk of error with smart pump use. Therefore, standardization of IV-related policies and procedures, standardization of concentrations, dosing units (e.g., mcg/min vs. mcg/kg/min), and drug nomenclature is essential. These items should be consistent with those used on the MAR, CPOE system, pharmacy computer system, electronic medical record, and pharmacy labels, if applicable.

Many drug references provide information on the maximum dose over a 24-hour period but do not provide the minimum and maximum doses that can be administered over one hour, so the team should develop dosage limits for infusions and boluses based on current policy and practice, the literature, and common references used in medical practice. In addition, there needs to be a determination of which dose limits require a "soft" or a "hard" stop. Existing best practices and policies and unit-based dosage limits should then be used to develop data sets based on patient care areas, for example, adult ICU, adult general care, neonatal intensive care unit (NICU), PICU, pediatric general care, labor and delivery, and anesthesia. Different configurations can be created for each area. It will also be important to include a procedure for the nursing staff to follow in the event a drug must be given which is not in the library or if a non-standardized concentration must be used. Lastly, there must be a clear expectation for staff to maximize the use of the DERS to fully realize the safety benefits of this technology.

Utilizing a well-planned, multi-disciplinary approach to smart pump implementation which maximizes the use of the DERS has the potential to significantly reduce IV medication administration errors and patient harm.

IMPLEMENTATION OF TECHNOLOGY

Implementing any form of technology in a healthcare organization can be an imposing task. Many organizations have purchased various forms of automation, with little or inadequate planning and/or preparation, which can lead to errors as well as the development of serious problems. Therefore, it is vitally important to thoroughly plan for necessary workflow changes and to remember your goal is to improve clinical processes, which can be facilitated by technology. Foremost, the process will require total commitment from the organization's executive and medical leadership as well as all staff members who will be affected by the implementation. It is essential that leadership sends a clear message that the new technology is important to patient safety and that they provide their unwavering support and financial backing as the project evolves. Providing this level of commitment will greatly increase the success of the project.

Identifying physician champions at a very high level in the organization is crucial and involving them in the decision-making and planning process will help persuade practitioners to "buy into" technology. In addition, an inter-disciplinary team of key individuals who can collaborate on an effective and realistic plan for implementation should be organized to provide ongoing project direction and oversight. Important key players include the chief information officer, information technology, risk managers, medical staff, frontline practitioners, and other support staff who may interact directly with the technology. The multi-disciplinary implementation team will need to address the following issues:

- Outline goals for the type of automation to be implemented (e.g., to improve safety, decrease costs, eliminate handwritten orders). Consider identifying primary and secondary goals.

- Develop a wish list of desired features and determine which, given budgetary constraints, are practical.

- Investigate systems that are presently available. Find out about successes and failures by talking with or visiting individuals from other organizations who have implemented similar systems. Determine whether the new system will interface with your current information systems and to what extent customization will be required.

- Analyze the current workflow and determine what changes are needed. This may include any changes that will occur in the current processes as well as the organizational culture. A lack of fit with clinical process and practice can be a downfall because healthcare practitioners tend to resist process changes that produce inefficiencies, complicate their work, or do not provide clear benefits.

- Policies and procedures for both the implementation and ongoing use must be defined prior to rollout. There will be numerous workflow changes that must be carefully planned to address the multiple operational transitions during the rollout such as when:

- ○ Each care area transitions from a paper-based system to an automated system

- ○ Patients are transferred from the automated units to areas with no automation

- ○ Healthcare providers move from areas with automation to areas without automation (California HealthCare Foundation, 2000)

• Identify the required capabilities and configuration of the new system. If the system allows for the creation of rules, protocols, guidelines, or drug dictionaries, individuals that will be affected by these changes need to develop these items before the system is implemented.

• "Sell" the benefits and objectives of automation to staff. Do not try to justify the new system by promising that it will allow the institution to decrease the number of staff members, because it most likely will not. A good system, though, should enhance safety and improve efficiency by decreasing the number of repetitive and mundane tasks. You may see the number of steps in the medication-use process decrease, but the remaining steps will require highly educated, competent personnel who understand and can deal with the complexity and importance of those steps.

• Develop an implementation plan. Set realistic timeframe expectations. Extensively test the system for accuracy and safety before implementation. Focus on efficiency and safety. Healthcare practitioners will not use a system, which is perceived as less efficient than the existing system.

Once the system has been implemented within the organization, there are still many issues that need to be considered. Plan on many years of system development and enhancement after the product is initially piloted. As soon as the system is installed, it is important to commit in a meaningful way to its continual monitoring and improvement. The healthcare environment is a dynamic one in which opportunities for new and different errors with technology will likely arise. Identify key measures that will help you determine whether your systems are really improving safety and quality and reducing costs. Beware of cumbersome features that may provoke users to override features or develop work-arounds with the system. Finally, do not be discouraged by initial dissatisfaction among staff members, and do not interpret initial negative reactions as failures.

CONCLUSION

Nurses have the responsibility to become familiar with the availability of "safety" technology, its advantages and disadvantages, and to work in collaboration with other healthcare stakeholders in the search for new and innovative technologic solutions to improve patient safety.

REFERENCES

Adachi, W., & Lodolce, A. E. (2005). Use of failure mode and effects analysis in improving the safety of i.v. drug administration. *American Journal of Health-System Pharmacy, 62*, 917–920.

American Hospital Association. (2000). *AHA guide to computerized physician order-entry systems.* (2000). Retrieved on 9 March, 2014 from http://www.aha.org/content/00-10/CompEntryA1109.pdf

American Hospital Association. (2007). *Continued progress hospital use of information technology.* Retrieved from http://www.aha.org/aha/content/2007/pdf/070227-continuedprogress.pdf. Accessed on February 21, 2014.

American Society of Health-System Pharmacists. (1993). ASHP guidelines on preventing medication errors in hospitals. *American Journal Hospital Pharmacists, 50*, 305–314.

American Society of Health-System Pharmacists. (2008). Proceedings of a summit on preventing patient harm and death from i.v. medication errors. *American Journal of Health-System Pharmacy, 65*, 2367–2379.

Aspden, P., Wolcott, J. A., Bootman, L., & Cronenwett, L. R. (Eds.). (2006). *Preventing medication errors: quality chasm series.* Washington, DC: The National Academies Press.

Barker, K. N., Flynn, E. A., Pepper, G. A., Bates, D., & Mikeal, R. (2002). Medication errors observed in 36 healthcare facilities. *Archives of Internal Medicine, 162*, 1897–1903.

Bates, D. W., Leape, L. L., & Cullen, D. J. (1998). Effect of computerized physician order entry and a team intervention on prevention of serious medication errors. *Journal of American Medical Association, 280*, 1311–1316.

Bates, D. W., Teich, J. M., Lee, J., Seger, D., Kuperman, M. D., MaLuf, N., … Leape, L. (1999). The impact of computerized physician order entry on medication error prevention. *Journal of the American Medical Informatics Association, 6*(4), 313–321.

Bonkowski, J., Carnes, C., Melucci, J., Mirtallo, J., Prier, B., Reichert, E., … Weber, R. (2013). Effect of barcode-assisted medication administration on emergency department medication errors. *Academic Emergency Medicine, 20*, 801–806.

Brodell, R. T. (1997). Prescription errors. Legibility and drug name confusion. *Archives of Family Medicine, 6*, 296–298.

Cabral, J. D. (1997). Poor physician penmanship. *Journal of American Medical Association, 278*, 1116–1117.

California HealthCare Foundation. (2000). *A primer on physician order entry.* Retrieved from http://www.chcf.org/publications/2000/09/a-primer-on-physician-order-entry. Accessed on February 20, 2014.

Case, J., Mowry, M., & Welebob, E. (2002). *The nursing shortage: Can technology help?* Oakland, CA: California HeathCare Foundation.

Centers for Medicare & Medicaid Services. (2010). *Fact sheets: Medicare and medicaid health information technology: Title IV of the American Recovery and Reinvestment Act.* Retrieved from http://www.cms.gov/Newsroom/MediaReleaseDatabase/Fact-Sheets/2009-Fact-Sheets-Items/2009-06-16.html. Accessed November 24, 2014.

Cohen, M. R. (1999). Preventing medication errors related to prescribing. In M. R. Cohen (Ed.), *Medication errors* (p. 8.2). Washington, DC: American Pharmaceutical Association.

Cohen, M. R. (2007). Preventing prescribing errors. In M. R. Cohen (Ed.), *Medication errors* (2nd ed., p. 189). Washington, DC: American Pharmaceutical Association.

Dasgupta, A., Sansgiry, S. S., Jacob, S. M., Frost, C. P., Dwibedi, N., & Tipton, J. (2011). Descriptive analysis of workflow variables associated with barcode-based approach to medication administration. *Journal of Nursing Care Quality, 26*(4), 377–384.

Dwibedi, N., Sansgiry, S., Frost, C., Johnson, M., Dasgupta, A., Jacob, S. M., … Shippy, A. A. (2012). Bedside barcode technology: impact on medication administration tasks in an intensive care unit. *Journal of Hospital Pharmacy, 47*(5), 360–366.

ECRI Institute. (2012). Top 10 health technology hazards for 2013. *Health Devices, 41*(11), 1–23.

Garbutt, J. M., Highstein, G., Jeffe, D. B., Dunagan, W. C., & Fraser, V. J. (2005). Safe medication prescribing: training and experience of medical students and housestaff at a large teaching hospital. *Academic Medicine, 80,* 594–599.

Han, P. Y., Coombes, I. D., & Green, B. (2005). Factors predictive of fluid administration errors in Australian surgical care wards. *Quality and Safety in Healthcare, 14,* 179–184.

Healthcare Information and Management Systems Society. (2002). Gaining MD buy-in: Physician order entry. *Journal of Healthcare Information Management, 16,* 67.

Hendrich, A., Chow, M., Skierczynski, B., & Zhenqiang, L. (2008). A 36-hospital time and motion study: How do medical-surgical nurses spend their time? *Permanente Journal, 12,* 25–34.

Hitti, E. A., Lewin, J. J., Lopez, J., Hansen, J., Pipkin, M., Itani, T., & Gurny, P. (2012). Improving door-to-drug antibiotic time in severely septic emergency department patients. *Journal of Emergency Medicine, 42*(4), 462–469.

Hurley, A. C., Bane, A., Fotakis, S., Duffy, M. E., Sevigny, A., Poon, E. G., & Gandhi, T. K. (2007). Nurses' satisfaction with medication administration point-of-care technology. *Journal of Nursing Administration, 37,* 343–349.

Husch, M., Sullivan, C., Rooney, D., Barnard, C., Fotis, M., Clarke, J., & Noskin, G. (2005). Insights from the sharp end of intravenous medication errors: Implications for infusion pump technology. *Quality and Safety in Healthcare, 14,* 80–86.

Institute of Medicine. (2004). *Keeping patients safe: transforming the work environment of nurses.* Washington, DC: National Academies Press. Retrieved from http://www.nap.edu/catalog.php?record_id=10851

Institute for Safe Medication Practices. (2000). *A call to action: eliminate handwritten prescriptions within 3 years.* Retrieved from http://www.ismp.org/Newsletters/acutecare/articles/WhitepaperBarCodding.asp. Accessed on August 9, 2010.

Institute for Safe Medication Practices. (2004). ISMP applauds final FDA bar code rule. *ISMP Medication Safety Alert!, 9*(4), 1.

Institute for Safe Medication Practices. (2006). Infant heparin flush overdose. *ISMP Medication Safety Alert!, 11*(19), 1–2.

Institute for Safe Medication Practices. (2008a). ADC survey shows some improvements, but unnecessary risks still exist. *ISMP Medication Safety Alert!, 13*(1), 1–2.

Institute for Safe Medication Practices. (2008b). *Guidance on the interdisciplinary safe use of automated dispensing cabinets.* Retrieved from http://www.ismp.org/Tools/guidelines/ADC_Guidelines_Final.pdf. Accessed on February 20, 2014.

Institute for Safe Medication Practices. (2009). *Proceedings from the ISMP Summit on the Use of Smart Infusion Pumps: Guidelines for Safe Implementation and Use.* Retrieved from http://www.ismp.org/Tools/guidelines/smartpumps/comments/printerVersion.pdf. Accessed on February 20, 2014.

Institute for Safe Medication Practices. (2012). Smart pump custom concentrations without hard "low concentration" alerts - a perfect storm for patient harm. *ISMP Medication Safety Alert!, 17*(4), 1–3.

Johnson, C. L., Carlson, R. A., Tucker, C. L., & Willette, C. (2002). Using BCMA software to improve patient safety in Veterans Administration Medical Centers. *Journal of Healthcare Information Management, 16*(1), 46–51.

Jozefczyk, K. G., Kennedy, W. K., Lin, M. J., Achatz, J., Glass, M. D., Eidam, W. S., & Melroy, M. J. (2013, August). Computerized prescriber order entry and opportunities for medication errors: comparison to tradition paper-based order entry. *Journal of Pharmacy Practice, 26*(4), 434–437.

Kaushal, R., Bates, D. W., Landrigan, C., Mckenna, M. S., Clapp, M. D., Federico, F., & Goldmann, D. A. (2001). Medication errors and adverse drug events in pediatric inpatients. *Journal of American Medical Association, 285,* 2114–2120.

Kohn, L., Corrigan, J., & Donaldson, M. (Eds.). (1999). *To err is human: Building a safer health system.* Washington, DC: National Academy Press.

Koppel, R., Wetterneck, T., Telles, J. L., & Karsh, B. T. (2008).Workarounds to barcode medication administration systems: Their occurrences, causes, and threats to patient safety. *Journal of the American Medical Informatics Association, 15,* 408–423.

Kowiatek, J. G., Weber, R. J., Skledar, S. J., Frank, S., & DeVita, M. (2006). Assessing and monitoring override medications in automated dispensing devices. *Journal on Quality and Patient Safety, 32,* 309–317.

Leape, L. L., Bates, D. W., Cullen, D. J., Cooper, J., Demonaco, H. J., Gallivan, T., et al. (1995). Systems analysis of adverse drug events. *Journal of the American Medical Association, 274,* 35–43.

Leapfrog. (2010). *Leapfrog Group report on CPOE evaluation tool results June 2008 to January 2010.* Retrieved from http://www.leapfroggroup.org/news/leapfrog_news/4778021. Accessed on 16 August, 2010.

Leung, A. A., Keohane, C., Lipsitz, S., Zimlichman, E., Amato, M., Simon, S. R., … Bates, D. W. (2013, June). Relationship between medication event rates and the Leapfrog computerized physician order entry evaluation tool. *Journal of the American Medical Informatics Association, 20*(e1), e85–e90.

Levin, H. I., Levin, J. E., & Docimo, S. G. (2012). "I meant that med for Baylee not Bailey!": a mixed method study to identify incidence and risk factors for CPOE patient misidentification. *AMIA Annu Symp Proc.* 2012;2012:1294–1301. Epub 2012 Nov 3.

Metzger, J., Welebob, E., Bates, D. W., Lipsitz, S., & Classen, D. C. (2010). Mixed results in the safety performance of computerzied physician order entry. *Health Affairs, 29,* 655.

Nebeker, J. R., Hoffman, J. M., Weir, C. R., Bennett, C. L., & Hurdleet, J. F. (2005). High rates of adverse drug events in a highly computerized hospital. *Archives of Internal Medicine, 165,* 1111–1116.

Osheroff, J. (Ed.) (2009). *Improving medication use and outcomes with clinical decision support: a step-by-step guide.* Chicago, IL: Healthcare Information and Management Systems Society.

Paoletti, R. D., Suess, T. M., Lesko, M. G., Feroli, A. A., Kennel, J. A., Mahler, J. M., … Sauders, T. (2007). Using bar-code technology and medication observation methodology for safer medication administration. *American Journal of Health-System Pharmacy, 64,* 536–543.

Patterson, E. S., Cook, R. I., & Render, M. L. (2002). Improving patient safety by identifying side effects from introducing bar coding in medication administration. *Journal of the American Medical Informatics Association, 9,* 540–553.

Pedersen, C. A., Schneider, P. J., & Scheckelhoff, D. J. (2011). ASHP national survey of pharmacy practice in hospital settings: Dispensing and administration-2011. *American Journal of Health-System Pharmacy, 69,* 768–785.

Pennsylvania Patient Safety Authority. (2005). Problems associated with automated dispensing cabinets. *Pennsylvania Patient Safety Advisory, 2,* 122–126.

Pennsylvania Patient Safety Authority. (2007). Smart infusion pump technology: don't bypass the safety catches. *Pennsylvania Patient Safety Advisory, 4,* 139–143.

Pennsylvania Patient Safety Authority. (2008). Medication errors occurring with the use of bar-code administration technology. *Pennsylvania Patient Safety Advisory, 5,* 21–23.

Pettus, D. C., & Vanderveen, T. (2013, November/December). Worth the effort? Closed-loop infusion pump integration with the EMR. *Biomedical Instrumentation & Technology, 47*(6), 467–477.

Poon, E. G., Keohane, C. A., Bane, A., Featherstone, E., Hays, B. S., Dervan, A., … Gandhi, T. K. (2008). Impact of barcode medication administration technology on how nurses spend their time providing patient care. *Journal of Nursing Administration, 38,* 541–549.

Poon, E. G., Keohane, C. A., Yoon, C. S., Ditmore, M. B., Bane, A., Levtzion-Korach, O., … Gandhi, T. K. (2010). Effect of bar-code technology on the safety of medication administration. *New England Journal of Medicine, 362,* 1698–1707.

Potts, A. L., Barr, F. E., Gregory, D. F., Wright, L., & Patel, N. R. (2004). Computerized physician order entry and medication errors in a pediatric critical care unit. *Pediatrics, 113,* 59–63.

Prusch, A. E., Suess, T. M., Paoletti, R. D., Olin, S. T., & Watts, S. D. (2011). Integrating technology to improve medication administration. *American Journal of Health-System Pharmacists, 68,* 835–842.

Rothschild, J. M., Keohane, C. A., Cook, E. F., Orav, E. J., Burdick, E., Thompson, S., … Bates, D. W. (2005). A controlled trial of smart infusion pumps to improve medication safety in critically ill patients. *Critical Care Medicine, 33,* 533–540.

S1—111th congress: A*merican Recovery and Reinvestment Act of* 2009. Retrieved from http://www.recovery.gov/arra/About/Pages/The_Act.aspx. Accessed on February 20, 2014.

Shamliyan, T. A., Duval, S., Du, J., & Kane, R. L. (2008). Just what the doctor ordered. Review of the evidence of the impact of computerized physician order entry system on medication errors. *Health Services Research, 43,* 32–53.

Stefanacci, R. (2004). Public reporting of hospital quality measures. *Health Policy Newsletter, 17,* 4.

Summa-Sorgini, C., Fernandes, V., Lubchansky, S., Mehta, S., Hallett, D., Bailie, T., … Burry, L. (2012). Errors associated with IV infusions in critical care. *Canadian Journal of Hospital Pharmacy, 65*(1), 19–26.

The Joint Commission. (2014). *2014 National patient safety goals.* Retrieved from http://www.jointcommission.org/assets/1/6/HAP_NPSG_Chapter_2014.pdf. Accessed on 20 February, 2014.

Trbovich, P. L., Pinkney, S., Cafazzo, J. A., & Easty, A. C. (2010). The impact of traditional and smart pump infusion technology on nurse medication administration performance in a simulated inpatient unit. *Quality & Safety on Healthcare, 19,* 430–434.

Wang, J. K., Herzog, N. S., Kaushal, R., Park, C., Mochizuki, C., & Weingarten, S. R. (2007). Prevention of pediatric medication errors by hospital pharmacists and the potential benefit of computerized physician order entry. *Pediatrics, 119,* e77–e85.

Westbrook, J. I., Baysari, M. T., Li, L., Burke, R., Richardson, K. L., & Day, R. O. (2013, November-December). The safety of electronic prescribing: manifestations, mechanisms, and rates of system-related errors associated with two commercial systems in hospitals. *Journal of the American Medical Informatics Association, 20*(6), 1159–1167.

Wietholter, J., Sitterson, S., & Allison, S. (2009). Effects of computerized prescriber order entry on pharmacy order-processing time. *American Journal of Health-System Pharmacists, 66,* 1394–1398.

31

The Magnet Model

Andrea Mazzoccoli / Susan H. Lundquist

• OBJECTIVES

1. Identify the five components of the ANCC Magnet Model.
2. Describe how technology has influenced the professional practice environment.
3. Describe some ways nursing informatics as a specialty can support the achievement of magnet standards and emerging demands of professional practice.

• KEY WORDS

Transformational leadership
Structural empowerment
Exemplary professional practice

The nursing practice environment is being challenged to rapidly respond to internal and external demands. Value-driven, patient-centered healthcare outcomes across the continuum amid the landscape of increasing complexity of care are the requirement for today's delivery systems. New models of care are emerging that require empirical, evidence-based accountable care. These new models will not be accomplished, without the use and integration of informatics to track and quantify cost of care, improve the process and workflows of care, and more transparently communicate outcomes of care. Incorporating healthcare information technology and the expertise of nursing informatics into future models will ensure patient care is safer, more efficient and effective, and promote excellence in nursing practice. Nursing excellence is promoted and recognized through the American Nurses Credentialing Center (ANCC) Magnet Recognition Program. The Magnet Commission has defined a vision for Magnet organizations to serve as the fount of knowledge and expertise for the delivery of nursing care globally by striving for discovery and innovation to lead the reformation of healthcare and the discipline of nursing (American Nurses Credentialing Center, 2008, 2014). Sources of evidence

used to define and evaluate the organization's achievement of the magnet standards identify informatics and technology as necessary components of the structures and processes to achieve the anticipated benefits.

Essential elements for excellence in professional nursing practice are defined within the ANCC Magnet Recognition Program. The Magnet model defines five components that when fully disseminated and enculturated throughout organization create professional practice environments that yield positive patient, nurse, and organizational outcomes. The five components are ***transformational leadership, structured empowerment, exemplary professional practice, new knowledge and innovation, and empirical outcomes*** (http://www.nursecredentialing.org/magnet/programoverview/new-magnet-model). The essential elements are described along with the structures and processes known to develop professional nursing practice as a core competency and contribute to patient and provider outcomes for organizational effectiveness. The Magnet Model informs nursing informatics practice to serve as a driver to practice excellence. Nursing informatics fully enculturated in the practice environment supports development of high-performing nursing organizations, clinical practice in addition to most importantly, supporting the ability to define, measure, and report outcomes at an individual, department, population, or organizational level. The following paragraphs will define the specific domains defined within the ANCC Magnet Recognition Program Magnet model and describe the influence and relationship between practice and informatics.

TRANSFORMATIONAL LEADERSHIP

Transformational leadership can be defined many ways. The ANCC Magnet Model defines the transformational leader as one who develops a strong vision for the practice and creates an environment where nurses at every level has a voice to advocate for resources, fiscal, and technology, to support their practice. The transformational nurse leader articulates a future vision where patient care is supported and accelerated through access to information and interoperability of the technology. The patient care vision supports the alignment of people, process, and technology. The leader is accountable to assure the provision of the highest quality of care, which positions the chief nurse executive to serve as the organization's executive project sponsor for the implementation of technology solutions and electronic health record. Most importantly, the nurse leader is responsible for the strategic nursing platform, which requires reformation of our care delivery systems and relationships between and among providers, patients, and community.

A strategic vision for practice that is supported by informatics promotes the development of innovative approaches to care by improving the work of the nurse through improved access to information and opportunities and new ways for the nurse to communicate and interact with other providers and the patient. The use of informatics science to drive the design of new models and roles for nursing practice requires a different set of skills and competencies for nursing leaders.

All health systems today are being influenced by the growth in technology. One of the sources of evidence organizations must be able to demonstrate is the work of the nursing leader and department in strategic planning. Specifically, how the nursing mission, vision, strategic and quality plans aligns with the overall organization's strategic goals. This plan must demonstrate the structure and processes used by nursing to improve efficiency and effectiveness. Without the strong influence of informatics, organizations would struggle to meet this standard. Many organizations use their strategic information technology initiatives as evidence of their effort in this aspect of the magnet standards.

For organizations to achieve successful implementations of health information technology there must be leadership buy-in and sponsorship and engaged nurse executives. It is now widely acknowledged that the implementation of a clinical IT solution is a clinical project requiring the vision and commitment of clinical leadership. The nurse executive is a key stakeholder in the IT implementation to ensure the alignment with the strategic vision and plan for the professional nursing practice. In this role, the nurse executive is also a champion to positively influencing acquisition, implementation, and adoption of IT within the organizations.

The American Organization of Nurse Executives (AONE) has included informatics in its recent update of competencies for nursing executives. The competencies will support the application of informatics to create a new way of thinking and defining practice excellence. The competencies AONE has developed include guiding principles for nurse executives which serve as a tool for nurse executives as they engage in IT initiatives within their organization. AONE first addressed technology with the development of the AONE Guiding Principles for Defining the Role of the Nurse Executive in Technology Acquisition and Implementation (AONE Guiding Principles for Defining the Role of the Nurse Executive in Technology Acquisition and Implementation, American Organization of Nurse Executives, 2007, 2009). Advancing that work they also developed AONE Guiding Principles for the Nurse Executive to Enhance Clinical Outcomes by Leveraging Technology (American Organization of Nurse Executives, 2009).

The role of the Chief Nursing Informatics Officer (CNIO) has emerged to support and help translate the science of informatics for all nursing roles. Associated with a specific set of standards for practice in the ANA Scope and Standards for Nurse Informatics, the CNIO role provides a partner to the role of the chief nurse executive. The partnership described by Swindle and Bradley describes an engagement between the roles where the CNIO provides direction and oversight for clinical informatics programs aligned with the vision for practice and operations led by the CNO (Swindle & Bradley, 2010). The area of informatics provides a dimension within our profession for ongoing professional development. The field of informatics is recognized as a dimension for professional growth in nursing. The incorporation of informatics expertise into organizational structures will support the alignment of our people, processes, and technology. Leveraging technology to support the alignment of practice and operations will lead to more creative and successful solutions to improve workflow, and process changes that improve communication and care coordination to improve outcomes.

STRUCTURAL EMPOWERMENT AND EXEMPLARY PROFESSIONAL PRACTICE

The voice, autonomy, and decision-making authority of direct care nurses are at the core of the structural empowerment and exemplary professional practice components of the ANCC Magnet model. Structural empowerment is evidenced through flat, flexible organization where the flow of information is fluid between the bedside and leadership. Improvements in practice settings and nurses' involvement in decision-making groups are critical.

In defining shared governance structure organizations may choose to include informatics across various councils to ensure the efforts and activities evaluated by the council consider how technology can play a supporting role. In others, the organization may additionally create an Informatics Council, including representation from multiple disciplines, where aspects of the IT implementation and adoption are reviewed and agreed upon. The involvement of nurses at all levels in these councils and the integration of information technology within the activities of the councils supports the key aspects of structural empowerment within the Magnet program.

Magnet organizations are required to demonstrate improvements in practice settings across the continuum that have occurred as a result of the use of data and information. Examples of this may include the use of technology to identify patients are risk for pressure ulcers, clinical summaries designed as hand-off tools, and alerts to ensure core measures are addressed in a timely manner. Selection and use of technology that supports practice promote structure and process components defined in the magnet framework. The changes to workflow process that improve care support the evidence of how those structures and processes result in improved outcomes that can be measured and reported.

Exemplary professional nursing practice within the magnet framework is supported through a professional practice model and care delivery system that delineate the role of the nurse as a fully accountable provider responsible for care that is patient centered, safe, effective, efficient, and equitable. Inter-disciplinary collaboration within magnet facilities demonstrates the need for collegial and respectful alignment of all disciplines focused on the needs of the patient. This requires new methods to support inter-disciplinary planning, communication, and coordination. In addition, this will require the effective use of information systems and technology to support clinical care planning, execution, and documentation. The effective use of informatics to improve inter-disciplinary care communication and coordination positions the care team to respond to the growing need to increase patient involvement in their own care.

At the core of achieving exemplary professional nursing practice is the ability to monitor care for effectiveness by having access to data to analyze and evaluate against national benchmarks and respond to improve. There are standards designed to evaluate how nurses investigate, develop, implement, and systematically evaluate standards of nursing practice. This requires evidence that nurses are using a data-driven approach focused on outcomes to evaluate their practice on a regular basis. Technology influences improvements in workflow and care processes associated nursing informatics transcends the areas defined within exemplary professional nursing practice: inter-disciplinary care, privacy, security and confidentiality, culture of safety, and quality-of-care monitoring and improvement. There are many specific patient care initiatives (restraint use, falls, pain) that Magnet organization's use to demonstrate their efforts and each organization is required to provide evidence that demonstrates how information systems and technology used to support clinical care is integrated and evaluated. Magnet organizations are expected to outperform mean or median benchmark performances and to lead the creation of a new delivery system through continuous improvement and research efforts. The use of technology to provide access to information through dashboards and business intelligence will assist in the development of new knowledge that will support new care delivery models based on exemplary practice.

With the new models of care evolving to support the shift toward accountable care technology will be a tool that can help providers coordinate care across settings with the increasing utilization of health information exchanges. Organizations will leverage their technology investments to engage patients and families within the community and to connect them with providers in an effort to address care delivery as well as health and wellness. Exemplary practice will increasingly be about care of the patient where they are connecting them to care across the continuum.

NEW KNOWLEDGE, INNOVATION, AND EMPIRICAL QUALITY OUTCOMES

The demand for exceptional performance and continuous improvement requires Magnet organizations to integrate the current evidence into practice. Nurses at the bedside drive and champion the adoption of new practices in an effort to provide the best care for their patients. The impact of technology to support the use of evidence and decision support at the point-of-care is powerful. The use of data and evidence to drive improvements in care can be found throughout magnet organizations. It is, in part, due to the nurse's involvement in decisions related to technology and information systems that lead to these improvements in care. There are many areas where technology can be used to support improvement in care coordination and outcomes such as medication reconciliation, provider order entry, and transition of care management. The magnet framework supports an environment of creating and applying new knowledge to create the future.

Organizations must demonstrate activities to support research and innovation and that nurses are involved with the design and implementation of technology to enhance the patient experience and nursing practice. Nurses play a critical role in system design, selection, implementation, and optimization of information technology and through this work will impact patient safety and quality. Their involvement will influence the acceptance and adoption of technology to fully allow for the support of informatics, a driver of quality of care, and enhanced patient outcomes. Informatics will be critical as hospitals and health systems attempt to leverage their electronic medical records to respond to and achieve the "meaningful use" criteria to receive incentives. Nurses across care settings and roles must be better equipped to understand information technology process to fully optimize to meet the needs of clinicians and patients. Magnet standards unified with the informatics objective to improve nursing practice through the use of technology provide a compelling transformative nursing agenda. Magnet organizations are poised to lead this effort as demonstrated by their ongoing commitment to practice excellence.

Pathway to Excellence

The ANCC Pathway to Excellence program is a program which recognizes a positive nurse practice environment. Pathway to Excellence evolved from the former Texas Nurses Association's Texas Nurse Friendly Hospital initiative. Under the ANCC Pathway to Excellence program

12 practice standards considered essential to a positive nurse practice environment provide the foundation. Like the Magnet program, as part of the process, organizations must demonstrate their ability to address these practice standards. The Pathway program focuses on improving the quality-of-care delivery and the professional satisfaction of nursing.

Exemplars in Practice

The ANCC's Magnet and Pathway to Excellence programs both highlight nursing excellence in the delivery of quality patient care. The ability to design, deliver, and innovate care organizations and the nursing department must have information technology as an integral component.

Exemplars where IT initiatives support the Magnet model:

- In addressing the Magnet model components around new knowledge, innovations, and improvements an organization established the goal of having their nurses provide evidence-based practice more consistently. Collaboration between the Nursing Practice Council, Information Technology, and Nursing Leadership fostered the strategy for greater adoption of evidence. After selecting an evidence-based content provider they completed analysis to begin populating their electronic health record with the evidence. Initially this began with the placement of links in the electronic health record where evidence would be most beneficial to the nurse and quickly advanced to specific notes and references to evidence-based practice for specific performance measures. Today, all patient plans of care have been developed using evidence-based content. Changes in practice, process, and IT have led to the successful adoption of evidence-based practice across the organization

- In addressing Exemplary professional practice an organization developed intra-professional councils to drive IT and changes to IT. Utilizing their council structure including nursing and other disciplines they review aspects of care delivery and how to leverage IT to support those efforts. Nursing Practice Council reviews all documentation practices, including content and defines areas requiring updates and where technology can be used to support practice. The IT Nursing Steering Committee reviews all applications used by nursing across the health system. Nursing practice support by information technology is able to monitor clinical performance so clinicians can see how they are doing and what is happening supporting changes and adjustments in clinical process as needed.

REFERENCES

American Nurses Credentialing Center. (2008, 2014). *Magnet recognition program application manual.* Silver Spring, MD: American Nurses Credentialing Center.

American Organization of Nurse Executives. (2007, 2009). *AONE guiding principles defining the role of the nurse executive in technology acquisition and implementation.* Washington, DC: American Organization of Nurse Executives.

American Organization of Nurse Executives. (2009). *AONE guiding principles for the nurse executive to enhance clinical outcomes by leveraging technology.* Washington, DC: American Organization of Nurse Executives.

Swindle, C. G., Bradley, V. M. (2010). The newest O in the C-suite: CNIO. *Nurse Leader, 8*(3), 28–30.

32

Public Health Practice Applications

Judy D. Gibson / Janise Richards / Arunkumar Srinivasan / Derryl E. Block

• OBJECTIVES

1. Define public health informatics and the public health nurse informatician.
2. Describe the National Electronic Disease Surveillance System.
3. Describe two public health electronic information systems with implications for the public health nurse.
4. Discuss the public health informatician role and the emerging role of the public health nurse informatician in case studies.

• KEY WORDS

Public health informatics
Electronic public health surveillance
Electronic public health information systems
Interoperability standards
Office of National Coordinator for Health Information Technology
National Electronic Disease Surveillance System

OVERVIEW

For many years, public health practitioners stated the belief that if nobody thought about public health, then public health must be doing its job. The battles that health practitioners waged against infectious diseases (such as malaria, tuberculosis [TB], and leprosy), chronic diseases, and environmental health hazards were often not highlighted in the media. In recent years, after recent outbreaks of SARS and Influenza A virus (H1N1), dramatic large-scale foodborne disease outbreaks, and the explosion of chronic illnesses that are linked to multiple vectors such as obesity, public health is frequently in the media limelight. The continuing need to be alert to emerging public health problems, responsive in emergencies, and accountable to the public has intensified health departments' efforts to collect data and information from multiple sources.

Health departments are collecting and analyzing data on a scale that was inconceivable even 10 years ago (Fig. 32.1) (Centers for Disease Control and Prevention [CDC], 2013a). To be able to manage this overwhelming deluge of data and information, public health practitioners have tapped into information technology. During 2000–2010, information systems have become widely adapted to fit the special needs within public health. Recognizing the importance of linkages among clinical care (also known as direct care), clinical care information systems, laboratory information systems, and other data sources to better understand and improve the state of the nation's health, public health has helped establish data and information exchange standards to support system interoperability.

This chapter provides an overview of the application of informatics to public health, describes legislation that

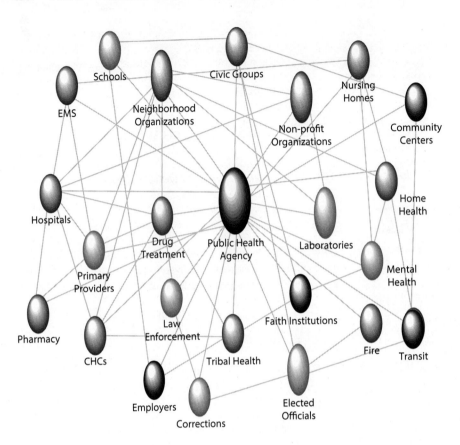

• **FIGURE 32.1.** Local Public Health Information and Data Exchange Entities. (Reproduced from OSTLTS (2009). National Public Health Standards Program. Centers for Disease Control and Prevention. http://www.cdc.gov/ostlts/.)

has affected public health information systems, and provides examples of electronic data exchange between clinical care and public health. The chapter also introduces the emerging role of the Public Health Nurse Informatician (PHNI) and gives examples of differentiating the public health nurse (PHN) and the PHNI.

PUBLIC HEALTH, PUBLIC HEALTH INFORMATICS, PUBLIC HEALTH NURSING, AND THE PUBLIC HEALTH NURSE INFORMATICIAN

In 1920, C.-E. A. Winslow defined public health as "the science and art of preventing disease, prolonging life and promoting health through the organized efforts and informed choices of society, organizations, public and private, communities and individuals" (Winslow, 1920).

The roots of public health were established in the United States when the Public Health Service (PHS) was established in 1798 by the Marine Hospital Service Act. In 1944, with the passage of the Public Health Service Act [Title 42 U.S. Code], the PHS mission was broadened to protect and advance the nation's physical and mental health. To accomplish this mission, public health had to define the activities clearly that would lead to this desired outcome.

In a seminal study by the Institute of Medicine, *The Future of Public Health*, the functions of public health were described as assessment, policy development, and assurance (Institute of Medicine, 1988). Assessment includes activities of surveillance, case finding, and monitoring trends, and is the basis for the decision-making and policy development by public agencies. Policy development is the broad community involvement in formulating plans, setting priorities, mobilizing resources, convening constituents, and developing comprehensive public health policies. Assurance covers activities that verify the implementation of mandates or policies, and guarantees that the provision of necessary resources is provided to reach the public health goals. To enhance further the core public health functions, a committee of public health agencies and organizations convened by the U.S. Public Health Service described the 10 essential services of public health (Public Health Functions Steering Committee, 1994). Figure 32.2 (Centers for Disease Control and Prevention [CDC], 2013a) describes the relationship between the core functions and essential services of public health.

The essential governmental role in public health is guided and implemented by a variety of federal, state/territorial, and local regulations and laws as well as federal, state/territorial, and local governmental public health agencies. At the local level, tens of thousands of governmental units at the county, municipality, township, school district, and other special jurisdiction levels must interact to provide public health services. This complex array of public health functions, services, responsibilities, and interactions is not a static environment, but one that is constantly changing.

Information forms the basis of public health. To make informed decisions and policies, public health practitioners require timely, quality information. The 1996 World Health Report cites the continuing need to "disseminate

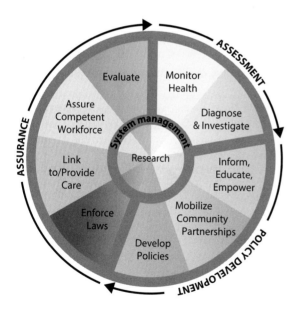

• **FIGURE 32.2.** Three Core Functions and 10 Essential Services of Public Health. (See ASTDN, 2000. Reproduced from Public Health Functions Steering Committee (1994). Public Health in America. DHHS. http://www.health.gov/phfunctions/public.htm.)

health information widely, in the sharing of epidemiological and statistical data, reports, guidelines, training modules and periodicals" (World Health Organization, 1997). Although there are numerous sources of public health data and information, the sources lack standardization in data organization, nomenclature, and electronic transmission. Innovative methods for storing, organizing, exchanging, and disseminating the millions of pieces of data gathered during public health activities have provided the foundation for the field of public health informatics.

Public health informatics has been defined as "the systematic application of information and computer science and technology to public health practice, research, and learning" (Friede, Blum, & McDonald, 1995). Public health informatics, like public health, focuses on populations. In public health informatics, population-level data and information are collected, analyzed, and disseminated with the ultimate goal of supporting preventive, as opposed to curative, interventions.

The demarcation between public health and clinical healthcare systems is frequently blurred, especially given legislation that has provided the funding and legal platforms to build the information systems needed to protect and advance the nation's physical and mental health. The provision in the 2004 Health Insurance Portability and Accountability Act (HIPAA) that generally prohibits disclosure of an individual's medical record and payment history without expressed authorization of the individual is known as the Privacy Rule. For public health purposes, the law provides for the disclosure of patient information to public health without authorization from the patient, for the purpose of preventing or controlling disease, injury, or disability, and for conducting public health surveillance, public health investigations, and public health interventions (Health Insurance Portability and Accountability Act [HIPAA], 2002). The 2010 Patient Protection and Affordable Care Act (PPACA) established policies and technically interoperable and secure standards for federal and state health and human services programs (DHHS, 2010). As public health, clinical care, information science, computer science, and information technology continue to come together, the field of public health informatics will continue to expand to support the public health functions of assessment, policy development, and assurance to promote a healthy nation.

Public Health Nursing

Public health nursing practice "focuses on population health through continuous surveillance and assessment of the multiple determinants of health with the intent to promote health and wellness; prevent disease, disability, and premature death; and improve neighborhood quality of life. These population health priorities are addressed through identification, implementation, and evaluation of universal and targeted evidence-based programs and services that provide primary, secondary, and tertiary preventive interventions. Public health nursing practice emphasizes primary prevention with the goal of achieving health equity" (American Nurses Association, 2013).

The *Public Health Informatician (PHI)* is a "public health professional who works either in practice, research, or academia and whose primary work function is to use informatics to improve population health. The role requires more expertise than the multi-highly functional public health professional that assists with informatics-related challenges or supports personal productivity with information technology" (U.S. Department of Health and Human Services, CDC, 2013).

Nursing informatics (NI) "is a specialty that integrates nursing science, computer science, and information science to manage and communicate data, information, knowledge, and wisdom in nursing practice. NI supports consumers, patients, nurses, and other providers in their decision-making in all roles and settings. This support is accomplished through the use of information structures, information processes, and information technology" (American Nurses Association, 2008).

The proposed role of the *Public Health Nurse Informatician (PHNI)* combines the competencies of PHI and nursing informatics. A PHNI is a PHN who has specialized in nursing informatics and has skills in supporting the establishment of systems to improve public health surveillance through access to clinical care information. Further, the PHNI has advanced skills in using nursing taxonomies and nomenclatures as a tool for nursing informatics in public health practice. PHNIs ensure that data needs are adequate to measure performance for multiple determinants of health. These are examples of the differences between the PHN and the PHNI that will be described in this chapter.

The Public Health Surveillance Landscape

The public health mission is to promote the health of the population rather than to treat individuals. In support of this mission, public health workers collect data on the determinants of health and health risks from factors in the pre-exposure environment, the presence of hazardous agents, behaviors, and exposures (Centers for Disease Control and Prevention [CDC], 2013b; World Health Organization, 2010). Public health workers monitor the occurrence of health events, conditions, deaths, and the activities of the healthcare systems and their effects on

health. Public health professionals use these data to inform decisions about the most effective mechanisms for interventions. Information from multiple, sometimes incompatible, systems or sources must be combined for an accurate depiction of problems (Fig. 32.1) (Centers for Disease Control and Prevention [CDC], 2013a). There is a need for rapid and comprehensive access to data across system boundaries, that is, the system at all levels as well as the healthcare industry systems (Koo, Morgan, & Broome, 2003).

Data collection and sharing in public health occur at three levels: local, state/territorial, and federal (e.g., Centers for Disease Control and Prevention [CDC]). Programs at each level have similar organization and management structures. Since most funding is based on programmatic need, many information systems have been built to support specific programs, thereby creating "silo"-like systems. To be productive, the program-oriented funding streams and information systems need to flow together.

Efforts are underway to assist healthcare providers in overcoming barriers to data collection and sharing through the implementation of regional, state/territorial, and local health information exchanges (HIEs) (Wild, Hastings, Gubernick, Ross, & Fehrenbach, 2004) and the National Electronic Disease Surveillance System (NEDSS) (CDC, 2013c) initiative. This comprehensive rather than disease-specific approach to data collection and sharing is the foundation of public health informatics and warrants further inspection.

Infectious Disease Electronic Surveillance

The three levels of the organizational structure of public health have distinct data collection and sharing roles in support of the electronic surveillance system (Fig. 32.3) (Birkhead & Maylahn, 2000). Each year, the Council of State and Territorial Epidemiologists (CSTE) and the CDC jointly update a list of reportable diseases and conditions. The CSTE recommends that all states and territories enact laws (statue or rule/regulation as appropriate) to make nationally reportable conditions reportable in their jurisdiction (Council of State and Territorial Epidemiologists [CSTE], 2010). The local (city or county) health department—the frontline of public health—interacts most closely with clinicians and agencies in the community, gathers reports of communicable diseases, tracks and monitors cases, conducts investigations, and often provides direct services (STD testing, vaccines, contact tracing, directly observed therapy, case management). The state health department uses legislation as well as regulations to require reporting by healthcare entities: to report certain illnesses, to require vaccinations for school entry,

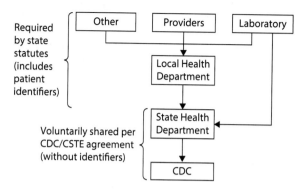

Required by state statutes (includes patient identifiers)

Other | Providers | Laboratory

Local Health Department

State Health Department

Voluntarily shared per CDC/CSTE agreement (without identifiers)

CDC

• **FIGURE 32.3.** Notifiable Disease Surveillance Data Flow to Public Health. (Data from Birkhead & Maylahn, 2000.)

to coordinate statewide disease surveillance, and to monitor incoming reports from counties, and then submit those reports, voluntarily and minus names, to the CDC. The state prioritizes problems and develops programs, runs the state public health laboratory, and serves as liaison between the CDC and local level. The CDC publishes national surveillance summaries and conducts research and program evaluations to produce public health recommendations. The CDC provides grants to states for specific programs, technical assistance, and, by invitation, outbreak response for state and local partners (Birkhead & Maylahn, 2000).

National Electronic Telecommunications System for Surveillance (NETSS)

In 1984, the CDC, in cooperation with the CSTE and epidemiologists in six states, began testing the Epidemiologic Surveillance Project. The project's goal was to demonstrate the effectiveness of computer transmission of public health surveillance case-based data between state health departments and the CDC. By 1989, all 50 states were participating in the reporting system. The Epidemiologic Surveillance Project was renamed the National Electronic Telecommunications System for Surveillance (NETSS) to reflect its national scope (CDC, 2013d). The NETSS system includes 22 core data elements for reportable disease conditions. The CDC analyzes these data and disseminates them in the *Morbidity and Mortality Weekly Report (MMWR)*. This overwhelming volume of data to be managed by health departments led to the National Electronic Disease Surveillance System (NEDSS) initiative, which provides guidance for the technical architecture and standards for nationally reportable condition reporting. When the CDC decided to transition from NETSS to NEDSS, it

was determined that no further modification to NETSS would be made. NETSS differs from NEDSS in several ways. NETSS was case based; NEDSS is person based. In addition, NETSS used proprietary codes, but NEDSS is based on standards so it can capture data already in electronic healthcare data streams. These differences precipitated the need to transition to NEDSS.

National Electronic Disease Surveillance System (NEDSS)

In 1999, the CDC, the CSTE, and state and local public health department staff began work on information system standards for the NEDSS initiative (National Electronic Disease Surveillance System Working Group, 2001). The NEDSS initiative uses standards to advance the development of efficient, integrated, and interoperable surveillance systems at the state and local levels. This initiative facilitates the electronic transfer of information from clinical information systems in healthcare, reduces the provider's burden of providing data, and enhances the timeliness and quality of information provided.

Implementation of the NEDSS initiative was supported by the CDC. States were funded to assess their current systems and develop plans to implement criteria compatible with the NEDSS initiative. The criteria included browser-based system data entry, an Electronic Laboratory Results (ELR) system for laboratory staff to report results to health departments as authorized, and a single repository for integrated databases from multiple health information systems. Also supported were system-wide electronic messaging upgrades for sharing the data. Finally, the CDC developed a platform called the NEDSS-Base System (NBS) for public health surveillance functions, processes, and data integration in a secure environment. States then had the option to choose this platform or another NEDSS-compatible system.

Some states developed systems using specified NEDSS standards, while other states used a CDC-developed system. To understand better how the NEDSS initiative meets its mission, we will examine the NBS role in supporting public health surveillance.

Healthcare Providers Role and the NBS

Healthcare providers are responsible for providing clinical care and reporting state-designated reportable conditions to public health departments. As a registered user of the NBS, a healthcare provider can directly enter data from case and laboratory reports into the state's electronic surveillance system at the point of care. In addition to the direct entry of data, healthcare providers can securely query the database, verify completeness of reporting using analysis tools, and ensure compliance with state public health laws. Healthcare providers can send electronic case reports using the Health Level Seven Clinical Document Architecture (HL7 CDA) format when their electronic health record (EHR) is equipped to report in the standard format.

Clinical Laboratories and the NBS

Staff members in public and private laboratories are required by law to notify public health departments of state reportable conditions. Timely reports are critical to public health surveillance because they prompt investigations of cases of reportable diseases or outbreaks. Registered laboratory users of the NBS system enter reports directly using the Web-based laboratory reporting function of the NBS. This report is then readily available to the public health NBS users to conduct the investigation (Levi, Vinter, & Segal, 2009).

Public Health Practitioner Role and the NBS

The local or state public health practitioner responds to incoming data on reportable conditions and implements appropriate public health case finding, tracking, and monitoring. Public health practitioners, who are registered users of the NBS, may review reports from laboratories and healthcare providers for patients residing within their jurisdictional boundaries. The public health practitioner may create an "alert" function for new data received in the NBS (such as for reports of meningococcal disease). Upon receipt of a new report, the public health practitioner may order a public health field investigation. Clinical, laboratory, epidemiologic, and follow-up data are entered at point of care and stored in the NBS. Stored data can be read, analyzed, and shared. The public health practitioner classifies the case, based on stored data and standard case definitions, and forwards the notification to CDC using the NEDSS messaging format, HL7, or NETSS (if no messaging guide exists). A data transfer function in the NBS allows users to notify another jurisdiction when a patient moves and to transfer records for follow-up.

Federal (CDC) Role and the NBS

A key part of the public health surveillance process is assessment of population health in the United States. The capabilities of the NBS support public health investigations and interventions at the state level and allow reporting of nationally notifiable diseases in a more complete

and standardized manner and in near real time for analysis by CDC program areas. This supports effective policy formation at the national level when events of public health significance happen. The data are disseminated through the *Morbidity and Mortality Weekly Reports (MMWR)*.

Privacy Protection and the NBS

In order to protect personally identifiable information, the NBS requires user authentication, authorization, and auditing protocols. To verify the identity of the user, the NBS supports custom authentication. Once authenticated, the NBS application authorizes access to data based on user role, geographical area(s), disease(s), public health event(s), and action(s). For example, a local public health practitioner may be assigned access to Foodborne and Diarrheal (FDD) investigations and laboratory reports for a public health jurisdiction. The supervisor can be assigned access to multiple public health jurisdictions across multiple families of diseases (e.g., FDD and hepatitis). The NBS creates an audit file containing a fingerprint trail with a timestamp of the user's activities.

Value of Information Solutions to Surveillance Practice

NEDSS-compatible infectious disease electronic surveillance systems change how public health departments at all levels communicate to perform their mission. Access to data repositories is no longer limited to a central location. Rather, epidemiologists, registered as the NBS users, may have data access at all public health levels. These systems enhance the capacity of local and state public health agencies to react quickly to disease occurrences.

Future Directions for Infectious Disease Surveillance

State public health programs face major funding and infrastructure challenges in adopting the standards-driven information systems for electronic disease surveillance. The CDC encourages adequate and sustained funding by public health programs for the NEDSS initiative and encourages partners and clinical providers at the point of care to adopt standards and create a uniform, interoperable, and bi-directional process for electronic disease surveillance. Initiatives such as the CDC's Public Health Informatics Fellowship Program train professionals to apply information science and technology to the practice of public health (CDC, 2013e).

Because public health informatics requires the integration of computer science, information science, and information technology into the public health system and with clinical care, one method to better understand how public health information systems work is to examine their application in collecting, organizing, exchanging, and disseminating data and information. The following two cases illustrate public health information systems applied in the context of an immunization information system and a TB electronic surveillance system.

Using Informatics in an Immunization Information System

Public health has been an advocate for immunization to prevent disease for decades. Currently, vaccine-preventable diseases are at, or near, record lows (Roush, Murphy, & Vaccine-Preventable Disease Table Working Group, 2007). The Every Child By Two organization provides some basic facts regarding the need for immunization registries. In the United States, there are around 4 million births each year (11,000/day); by age 2, a child will need to have up to 20 vaccinations; 2.1 million children are under-immunized; and 22% of American children see two immunization providers in their first 2 years (Every Child By Two, 2010).

Immunization records and registries began as paper forms that were completed by hand at the point of service. The immunization record was kept with the patient's file, and an official copy was given to the patient or patient's guardian. On a periodic basis, usually once a month, all the immunizations records were aggregated by hand (or calculator) with patient demographics and vaccine information written into a registry that was shared with the local health agency. This time-consuming process contained many vulnerable points where the data could be wrongly entered, incorrectly calculated, or not included in the overall tally.

Newer immunization registries are based on electronic Immunization Information Systems (IIS). These IIS are confidential, computerized information systems that allow for the collection of vaccination histories and provide immediate access by authorized users to a child's current immunization status. One impetus for IIS arose from the *Healthy People 2010* objective (14.26), which stated that 95% of children younger than 6 years of age would be registered in a fully operational IIS (U.S. Department of Health and Human Services, 2010). "Nationally, 19.2 million U.S. children aged <6 years (84%) participated in an IIS in 2011. Child participation in IIS has increased steadily, from 63% in 2006 to 84% in 2011. Of the 54 grantees with available data in 2011, 24 (44%) reported that >95% of children aged <6 years in their geographic area participated in their IIS. An additional 13 (24%) grantees reported child participation rates ranging from 80% to 94%" (CDC, 2013f).

Benefits of the implementation of an IIS for the public include having a private and secure place to safeguard important immunization information from multiple providers that will be used throughout a person's life; receiving timely immunization reminders; and eliminating duplicate immunizations. Benefits for healthcare providers include consolidating immunization records from different sources; automatically calculating the immunizations needed; easily providing official copies of immunization records; reducing chart pulls for coverage assessments and Healthcare Effectiveness Data and Information Set (HEDIS) reviews (National Committee for Quality Assurance [NCQA], 2013); automating vaccine inventory and ordering procedures; allowing for vaccine tracking during vaccine shortages or manufacturer recalls; flagging high-risk patients for timely vaccination recalls; and assisting with vaccine safety and adverse event reporting. To accomplish these activities, the IIS must be able to exchange data and information.

Data, vocabulary, and transmission standards are critical to IIS success. A core IIS dataset has been defined, current procedural terminology (CPT) codes have been mapped to CVX (vaccine codes), and MVX (manufacturers of vaccines) codes have been developed to facilitate immunization data exchange between IIS, billing and administrative systems, inventory management systems, and other support systems. In addition, HL7 standards are used for codes as well as patient demographics, appointment scheduling, file synchronization, and other data management transactions produced and received by the systems.

The IIS has been successfully implemented in many states. Examples include the Michigan Care Improvement Registry (Michigan Care Improvement Registry [MCIR], 2013), the Oregon Immunization ALERT system (Oregon DHHS, 2013), the Wisconsin Immunization Registry (WIR) (Wisconsin Immunization Program, 2013), the Iowa Immunization Registry Information System (Iowa Department of Public Health, 2013), and the Louisiana Immunization Network for Kids Statewide (LINKS) (Louisiana Immunization Network for Kids Statewide [LINKS], 2013).

Challenges to moving IIS forward include funding and human capacity to build and manage the system. The HITECH Act (American Recovery and Reinvestment Act [ARRA], 2009) that provides funding and educational programs focusing on informatics will help nurses and others develop skills refine and effectively use this important public health information system.

Using Informatics in a Tuberculosis Electronic Information System

Tuberculosis is a chronic bacterial infection caused by *Mycobacterium tuberculosis*. The most common site of infection is the lung, but other organs may be involved. Healthcare providers are required by laws in all 50 states to report patients with TB and other conditions on the state's list of notifiable conditions. Confirmed TB cases are reported by clinicians and laboratory staff to local health departments and then to statewide disease surveillance programs connected to state health departments. A confirmed case of TB is one that meets the clinical case definition or is laboratory confirmed. Reporting is also recommended for patients who have suspected respiratory TB prior to laboratory confirmation, to expedite contact tracing and TB transmission control.

Multiple systems are involved in electronic TB reporting. Data reporting systems include the National TB Surveillance System (Division of TB Elimination, 2013a), the TB Genotyping Information Management System (Division of TB Elimination, 2013b), and the Electronic Disease Notification System (CDC: Division of Global Migration and Quarantine, 2013).

The National TB Surveillance System is an electronic incidence surveillance system that collects 49 data items on newly diagnosed verified cases of TB in the United States. The appropriate authority transmits the data from the state or designated health jurisdiction to CDC at three intervals: initially at the time of case verification, at receipt of initial test results for drug susceptibility, and at treatment closure. Formats for reporting TB cases have evolved over decades from paper-based reporting beginning in 1952, to electronic reporting introduced in the mid-1980s, to an NEDSS-compatible, electronic surveillance system, using HL7 messaging, operational in 2010 for verified TB cases reported in 2009.

The TB Genotyping Information Management System (TB GIMS) builds upon the established infrastructure of the CDC's National TB Surveillance System and incorporates genotype data to create a centralized database and reporting system. State public health laboratories submit isolates from culture-confirmed cases to one of two designated genotyping laboratories for molecular characterization, which helps with identifying recent transmission and potential outbreaks.

The Electronic Disease Notification System alerts state and local health department programs of refugees and immigrant arrivals to their jurisdictions and provides overseas medical screening results and treatment follow-up information. Each refugee or immigrant with a TB classification is referred to the TB program for medical screening and treatment follow-up.

CDC uses data from these reporting systems to disseminate performance measurement reports for national TB-related performance indicators (NTIP). CDC shares these reports electronically with health department programs receiving federal funding for TB prevention and control. The national reports are used by state programs to set performance targets, measure performance, and evaluate the program's capacity to control and prevent TB (Division of TB Elimination, 2012).

Work continues on managing data quality to improve accuracy, completeness, consistency in collecting data, and timeliness of reporting in the National TB Surveillance System. Additionally, future applications are needed to automate data exchange between the TB reporting systems and to standardize laboratory data for direct reporting to the National TB Surveillance System.

The Public Health Informatician and the Emerging Roles for Public Health Nurse Informatician

The emerging role of the PHNI is illustrated in case studies to demonstrate the core public health functions of assessment and assurance performed by the PHNI and the PHI. In the first case study, the PHI ensured the retrieval of destroyed health records (immunization data) for displaced Hurricane Katrina communities by linking people with their records through informatics. By retrieving health records, the PHI enforced the rules regarding immunization record requirements while ensuring provision of needed immunizations. In the second case study, the PHI, while participating in assessment activities to monitor health status and health problems in displaced Hurricane Katrina communities, identified a norovirus outbreak. The PHI developed and used a simple data checklist of symptoms, and compiled daily information reports and environmental risk information to evaluate the ongoing effectiveness and quality of emergency public health services. In the third case study, the PHNI designed an assessment activity for barriers to adherence behaviors with TB treatment. The PHNI described a clinical nursing information system (CNIS) for a behavioral adherence model adapted to TB program literature. The resulting dataset can be used to manage data, monitor the performance plan, and evaluate the effectiveness and quality of personal health services.

CASE STUDY 32.1. IMMUNIZATION REGISTRIES AND EMERGENCY RESPONSE AFTER HURRICANE KATRINA

Hurricane Katrina made landfall in Louisiana on August 29, 2005. To escape the storm, more than 200,000 residents of New Orleans and the surrounding area evacuated to shelters in Houston, Texas. In their hurry, they left behind most personal belongings, including immunization records or medical records. Since the hurricane landed as the fall school session was about to begin, state and local school boards in Texas agreed to accept the displaced children into schools without proof of immunization, but stated that proof of immunizations would be necessary to remain in school.

To assist families in finding their children's records, the Houston-Harris County (Texas) Immunization Registry (HHCIR) staff contacted their vendor, who was also the vendor for the Louisiana Immunization Network for Kids Statewide (LINKS), to investigate the possibility of linking the two IIS. In less than 24 hours, the HHCIR, vendor, and LINKS personnel had developed a technological bridge built on HL7 standards connecting the two systems. Ten days later, they had created a mechanism that allowed health authorities to acquire child and adolescent immunization histories from LINKS. This merged Web-based immunization registry was made available to public health officials and selected healthcare providers in temporary clinics in the Astrodome and George R. Brown Convention Center. Originally, the new IIS was a "search and view" only system; the HL7 data exchanges capability was added to allow the LINKS-HHCIR connection to exchange patient data and information from one system to the other.

Over the next month, more than 20,000 records were searched and approximately 10,000 were successfully matched for displaced children in the greater Houston area. By September 2006, one year later, nearly 19,000 records had been successfully matched. The estimated cost savings of this on-the-fly, hybrid IIS, just in vaccines for these children, is slightly over $1.6 million. These costs do not factor in the savings in time, pain, and lost work time or missed school that would have occurred if the children had needed to be re-immunized. Nor do the costs reflect the societal costs that may have occurred if the children had not been allowed to attend school (Boom, Dragsbaek, & Nelson, 2007). The use of the IIS immunization registry post-Katrina empowered patients, parents, and healthcare providers to know immunization history.

CASE STUDY 32.2. NOROVIRUS OUTBREAK IN PERSONS DISPLACED BY HURRICANE KATRINA

Collecting and sharing data and information is essential for public health practice. In September 2005, nearly 1000 evacuees from Hurricane Katrina and relief workers in numerous facilities had symptoms of acute gastroenteritis. A checklist of symptoms was used to collect data

on an intake form in medical facilities setup to provide care on an outpatient basis. This information was gathered and entered into a database, and results were distributed each morning.

On September 2, staff observed an increase in adults and children with symptoms of acute gastroenteritis. On some days, nearly 21% of adults and 40% of children visiting one clinic had acute gastroenteritis. They conducted enhanced surveillance to improve identification of acute gastroenteritis, investigated the apparent outbreak, identified the infectious agent, and implemented control measures.

The reported epidemiologic and laboratory findings suggested that an outbreak of norovirus gastroenteritis had affected individuals in numerous facilities. These outbreaks are not associated with contaminated food or water, but spread through person-to-person contact or from fomites in crowded settings. This information was used to provide a health alert for epidemiologic features and clinical presentation, and to promote rehydration treatment and measures to prevent secondary transmission (CDC, 2005).

CASE STUDY 32.3. USING INFORMATICS FOR PUBLIC HEALTH PROGRAM EVALUATION

A diagnosis of TB disease or latent TB infection in a child represents recent transmission of *M. tuberculosis*; therefore, trends in TB disease and latent TB infection in young children are important indicators to assess the effectiveness of TB prevention and control efforts. Investigations of persons having infectious pulmonary TB can avert TB in children who have been infected with *M. tuberculosis* by finding and treating these children before they progress to TB disease (Lobato et al., 2008).

Monitoring standardized nursing activities (investigation and adherence) can help identify missed opportunities for preventing TB in young children. For example, when a child develops TB disease or latent TB infection, how timely was the exposed child identified or screened for TB (case interview/investigation adequacy)? Was the child recommended for TB treatment but did not start or did not complete treatment (caregiver adherence issues)? Was the person having infectious pulmonary TB and exposing the child recommended for treatment, but did not start or did not complete treatment (adherence issues)?

PHNs use a clinical nursing information system (CNIS) dataset, constructed with standardized nursing terminology recognized by the American Nurses Association, to account for nursing activities, to manage program outcomes, and to describe a planned approach to nursing care. Although PHNs use the CNIS dataset to generate data on patient assessments and to characterize healthcare provider interactions with patients, authors looked for a CNIS dataset specifically adapted for identifying barriers to investigation and adherence to treatment.

PHNs can select from various CNIS datasets. They selected a vendor application of CNIS for the public health programs in Maine and Minnesota. The CNIS in Maine is a statewide PHN initiative within the public health system. It is used to document clinical care and to inform program evaluation. Common tools are used for nursing care and education plans, flow sheets, and encounter forms for individual client services (TB, MCH, childhood lead poisoning) (Correll & Martin, 2009). In Minnesota, the Omaha system contributes to the outcomes management program in local public health departments by providing quantitative data and graphs for program planning, evaluation, and communication with administrators and local government officials (Monsen, Martin, Christensen, & Westra, 2009).

PHNs in the TB program described components of a planned approach to overcome adherence barriers and support completion of long-term TB treatment. PHNIs are in an excellent position to identify, describe, and label the issues associated with health outcomes as well as to

identify, describe, and label interventions that affect those outcomes. The Patient-Centered Care (PCC) Model for Perceived Barriers to Adherence with TB Treatment helps the nurse identify and document multiple determinants of adherence behavior and useful interventions (Table 32.1) (Gibson, Boutotte, Wilce, & Field, 2011).

FUTURE DIRECTIONS IN PUBLIC HEALTH INFORMATION SYSTEMS

Although public health information systems have matured over the past decade, many challenges remain. In general, public health practitioners have not taken an active role in the development of health information systems within their jurisdictions. Since the bulk of public health activities occur within state/territorial level and local health departments, public health practitioners must provide support and leadership to local healthcare systems in the emerging concept of multiagency responsibility for health. Local agencies and institutions such as managed care organizations, hospitals, laboratories, environmental health agencies, nursing homes, police staff, community centers, pharmacies, civic groups, corrections staff, drug

TABLE 32.1	Patient-Centered Care Model (PCC Model) for Barriers to Patient Adherence With Taking Medication and Keeping Appointments for Tuberculosis Treatment (Gibson, Boutotte, Wilce, & Field, 2011)	
Patient Diagnosis (NANDA-I)	**Nursing Interventions (NIC)**	**Patient Outcomes (NOC)**
Ineffective health maintenance	Sustenance support	Social support
Ineffective protection	Infection control	Immune status
Adjustment impaired/Risk-prone health behavior	Decision-making support	Well-being
Decisional conflict: whether to participate in treatment	Mutual goal setting	Participation in healthcare decisions
Defensive coping	Patient contracting	Coping
Fear (stigma)	Emotional support	Fear self-control
Powerlessness: perceived threat	Patient's rights protection	Health beliefs: perceived ability to perform
Ineffective therapeutic regimen management	Medication management	Medication response
Ineffective family therapeutic regimen management	Discharge planning	Family participation in professional care
Noncompliance	Health policy monitoring	Compliance
Knowledge deficit	Teaching	Knowledge of
• Disease process	• disease process	• disease process
• Treatment regimen	• treatment regimen	• treatment regimen
Communication impairment	Culture brokerage	Communication ability

NANDA-I, Nanda International; NIC, Nursing Interventions Classifications; NOC, Nursing Outcomes Classification.
Reproduced, with permission, from Gibson, J.D., Boutotte, J., Wilce, M., & Field, K. (2010). A patient-centered care model for perceived barriers to adherence with tuberculosis treatment. (Unpublished Work.)

treatment centers, EMS staff, and home health agencies are partners in maintaining the public's health. Figure 32.1 (Centers for Disease Control and Prevention [CDC], 2013a) illustrates entities involved in local data/information exchange. Additionally, public health practitioners have the expertise needed to inform developers of the health information system about specific data and information needs for population-based analyses to recognize emergent issues in the community, to assist in diagnostic and treatment decisions, and to understand better methods to improve the health of the community. Federal agencies involved in public health can provide the leadership and expertise in developing consensus on data and health information technology (HIT) standards that will allow for the exchange of public health data and information across public health jurisdictions creating a "network of networks" that function as a national public health information system.

Using data in innovative ways through the use of data visualization and decision support systems will increase public health's ability to understand disease trends, make decisions, and apply the appropriate resources where needed. The use of decision support based on clinical and prevention guidelines can integrate prevention messages into primary care.

As some HIT stabilizes and other technology innovations occur, public health can be the beneficiary of the focus and funding that are driving healthcare reform. As clinical care and public health continue to integrate and support each other's goal of keeping people healthy, HIT will provide the platform to improve the health of the nation.

The Future of the Public Health Nurse Informatician Role

"The PHN practice specialty needs a deeper understanding of informatics theories and methods to practice more effectively" (American Nurses Association, 2013). While the Scope & Standards of Nursing Practice for Nursing Informatics (American Nurses Association, 2008) and the Competencies for Public Health Informaticians (Association of Schools of Public Health, University of Washington Center for Public Health Informatics, 2013) have been published, literature review did not identify scope and standards of public health nursing informatics (PHNI) or competencies for public health nursing informaticians. It is necessary to describe the nursing profession's contributions to addressing national public health priorities and initiatives.

The workforce capacity for public health surveillance is limited but necessary to identify public health needs so that interventions to improve individual, community,

and population health can be planned. Health reform and related funding is driving the HIT platform. In response, fellowship programs and internships in surveillance and public health informatics are addressing those needs (Drehobl, Roush, & Stover, 2012; CDC; *ASPH partner fellowship programs*; *ASPPH Graduate Training Program fellowships and internships*; *MELDI-Public Health Informatics Fellowship Program*; *NIH Nursing Informatics Internship*; *Informatics university programs*; *American College of Medical Informatics [ACMI] fellowship*).

Health reform promises the eliciting of evidence-based practice to improve health (Agency for Healthcare Research and Quality [AHRQ], 2013). Therefore, HIT must capture interventions by multiple providers including nurses. Many promising practice-based interventions are addressed by nursing practice (Spencer, Schooley, & Anderson, 2013).

PHN leaders, working in partnership with other stakeholders, monitor and evaluate program performance. They clarify and describe practice-based interventions linked with achieving partnership goals and objectives. For example, The COPE Healthy Lifestyles Teen intervention for the national priority of Nutrition, Physical Activity, Obesity (CDC, 2013g) links the nursing role and responsibilities with program goals and objectives by tracking nurse-sensitive indicators for BMI and pedometer step (Melnick, Jacobson, & Kelly, 2013). As healthcare reform continues to evolve, PHN leadership will need to take an active role in the development of the scope and standards of public health nursing informatics practice and informatician competencies associated with these accountabilities.

SUMMARY

In summary, public health, public health informatics, public health information systems, and the ever-increasing integration of public health and healthcare present many opportunities to improve the Nation's health. Recent legislation has provided the guidance and funding platforms to create a seamless integration of health information systems to assist with better decision-making in patient care and in policy development. The development of individual data and information system standards is occurring less frequently as nationally recognized HIT and data exchange standards are stabilizing. Efforts supporting the certification of the information technology used in health have an impact on the adoption and integration of these standards by information system vendors. Successful implementations of standards-based information systems have demonstrated enormous cost savings in time and money.

PHNs contribute data to the standards-based data exchange systems; use information to target care for individuals, families, groups, and populations; and then evaluate programs by means of the information systems. The PHNI seeks partners to understand variables of concern to nurses in clinical care, such as barriers to adherence behaviors, in the development of the standards-based data exchange systems. The PHNI provides leadership to the PHNs in the use of health information technology to improve the health of the nation.

REFERENCES

Agency for Healthcare Research and Quality (AHRQ), U.S. Preventive Services Task Force. (2010). *Guide to community preventive services*. Washington, DC: Author. Retrieved from http://www.thecommunityguide.org/library/book/Front-Matter.pdf

American Nurses Association. (2008). *Nursing informatics: Scope and standards of practice*. Silver Spring, MD. Retrieved from Nursebooks.org

American Nurses Association. (2013). *Public health nursing: Scope and standards of practice*. Silver Spring. MD. Retrieved from Nursebooks.org

American Recovery and Reinvestment Act (ARRA). (2009). Department of Health Human Services, Pub. L. No. 111-5 (Feb. 17, 2009). Washington, DC. Retrieved from http://frwebgate.access.gpo.gov/cgi-bin/getdoc.cgi?dbname=111_cong_bills&docid=f:h1enr.pdf

Association of Schools of Public Health, University of Washington Center for Public Health Informatics. (2013). *Competencies for public health informaticians 2009*.

Birkhead, G. S., & Maylahn, C. M. (2000). State and local public health surveillance. In S. M. Teutsch & R. E. Churchill (Eds.), *Principles and practice of public health surveillance* (2nd ed., p. 253). Oxford University Press.

Boom, J. A., Dragsbaek, A. C., & Nelson, C. S. (2007). The success of an immunization information system in the wake of hurricane Katrina. *Pediatrics, 119*(6), 1213.

CDC. (2005). Norovirus outbreak among evacuees from hurricane Katrina—Houston, Texas, September 2005. *MMWR—Morbidity and Mortality Weekly Report, 54*(40), 1016.

Centers for Disease Control and Prevention (CDC). (2013a). *National Public Health Performance Standards Program: 10 essential public health services*. Retrieved from http://www.cdc.gov/nphpsp/essentialservices.html/

Centers for Disease Control and Prevention (CDC). (2013b). *National environmental health data tracking network*. Atlanta, GA. Retrieved from http://ephtracking.cdc.gov/showHome.action

CDC. (2013c). *National Electronic Disease Surveillance System (NEDSS)*. Retrieved from http://wwwn.cdc.gov/nndss/script/nedss.aspx/

CDC. (2013d). *National Electronic Telecommunications System for surveillance (NETSS)*. Atlanta, GA. Retrieved from http://www.cdc.gov/ncphi/disss/nndss/netss.htm

CDC. (2013e). *Public health informatics fellowship program*. Atlanta, GA. Retrieved from http://www.cdc.gov/phifp/

CDC. (2013f). Progress in Immunization Information Systems—United States, 2011. *Morbidity and Mortality Weekly Report. 62*(03), 48. Retrieved from http://www.cdc.gov/mmwr/preview/mmwrhtml/mm6203a2.htm

CDC. (2013g). *Winnable battles*. Retrieved from http://www.cdc.gov/winnablebattles/

CDC: Division of Global Migration and Quarantine. (2013). Disease surveillance among newly arriving refugees and immigrants—Electronic Disease Notification System, United States, 2009. *Morbidity and Mortality Weekly Report, 62*(SS07), 1. Retrieved from http://www.cdc.gov/mmwr/preview/mmwrhtml/ss6207a1.htm

Correll, P. J., & Martin, K. S. (2009). The Omaha System helps a public health nursing organization find its voice. *Computers, Informatics, Nursing, 27*(1), 12.

Council of State and Territorial Epidemiologists (CSTE). (2010). *Modification of the process for recommending conditions for national surveillance*. 10-SI-02. CSTE, 1–4. Atlanta, GA. Retrieved from http://c.ymcdn.com/sites/www.cste.org/resource/resmgr/PS/10-SI-02.pdf

DHHS. (2010, March 23). *The Patient Protection and Affordable Care Act (PPACA)*. Pub. L. No. 111–148. Retrieved from http://www.gpo.gov/fdsys/pkg/PLAW-111publ148/pdf/PLAW-111publ148.pdf

Division of TB Elimination. (2012). *National TB indicators project (NTIP)*. CDC. Atlanta, GA. Retrieved from http://www.cdc.gov/tb/publications/factsheets/statistics/NTIP.htm

Division of TB Elimination. (2013a). *Tuberculosis information management*. CDC. Atlanta, GA. Retrieved from http://www.cdc.gov/tb/programs/tims/default.htm

Division of TB Elimination. (2013b). *TB genotyping information management system (TB GIMS) fact sheet*. CDC. Atlanta, GA. Retrieved from http://www.cdc.gov/tb/programs/genotyping/tbgims/implementation_statelab.htm

Drehobl, P. A., Roush, S. W., Stover, B. H., Koo, D. (2012). Public health surveillance workforce of the future. *Morbidity and Mortality Weekly Report, 61*(3), 25.

Every Child By Two. (2010). *About registries (Immunization Information Systems)*. Retrieved from http://www.ecbt.org/index.php/strategies_and_resources/index.php/

Friede, A., Blum, H. L., & McDonald, M. (1995). Public health informatics: How information-age technology can strengthen public health. *Annual Review of Public Health, 16*, 239.

Gibson, J. D., Boutotte, J., Wilce, M., & Field, K. (2011). A patient-centered care model for barriers to patient adherence with taking medication and keeping appointments for tuberculosis treatment. In V. K. Saba & K. A. McCormick (Eds.), *Essentials of nursing informatics* (5th ed., p. 508). New York, NY: McGraw Hill.

Health Insurance Portability and Accountability Act (HIPAA). (2002). *Privacy Rule.* DHHS. 45, CFR Parts 164. Retrieved from http://www.hhs.gov/ocr/privacy/hipaa/administrative/privacyrule/

Institute of Medicine. (1988). *The future of public health.* Washington, DC: National Academy Press.

Iowa Department of Public Health. (2013). *Immunization Registry Information System (IRIS).* Des Moines, IA. Retrieved from http://www.idph.state.ia.us/immtb/Immunization.aspx?prog=Imm&pg=Iris

Koo, D., Morgan, M., & Broome, C. V. (2003). New means of data collection. In P. W. OCarroll, W. A. Yasnoff, M. E. Ward, L. H. Ripp, & E. L. Martin (Eds.), *Public health informatics and information systems* (p. 379). New York, NY: Springer.

Levi, J., Vinter, S., & Segal, L. M. (2009). *Ready or not? Protecting the public's health from diseases, disasters, and bioterrorism.* Biosurveillance—NEDSS compatibility. Trust for America's Health, 24. Robert Wood Johnson Foundation. Retrieved from http://healthyamericans.org/reports/bioterror09/pdf/TFAHReadyorNot200906.pdf

Lobato, M. N., Sun, S. J., Moonan, P. K., Weis, S. E., Saiman, L., Reichard, A. A., ... Zero Tolerance for Pediatric TB Study Group. (2008). Underuse of effective measures to prevent and manage pediatric tuberculosis in the United States. *Archives of Pediatrics & Adolescent Medicine, 62*(5), 426.

Louisiana Immunization Network for Kids Statewide (LINKS). (2013). Retrieved from https://linksweb.oph.dhh.louisiana.gov/linksweb/main.jsp/

Melnick, B. M., Jacobson, D., Kelly, S., Belyea, M., Shaibi, G., Small, L., ... Marsiglia F. F. (2013). Promoting healthy lifestyles in high school adolescents: A randomized control trial. *American Journal of Preventive Medicine, 45*(4), 407.

Michigan Care Improvement Registry (MCIR). (2013). *Michigan care improvement registry.* Retrieved from http://www.mcir.org/

Monsen, K. A., Martin, K. S., Christensen, J. R., & Westra, B. (2009). Omaha System data: Methods for research and program evaluation. *Studies in Health Technology and Informatics, 146,* 783.

National Committee for Quality Assurance (NCQA). (2013). *HEDIS and quality measurement.* Washington, DC. Retrieved from http://www.ncqa.org/HEDISQualityMeasurement.aspx

National Electronic Disease Surveillance System Working Group. (2001). National Electronic Disease Surveillance System (NEDSS): A standards-based approach to connect public health and clinical medicine. *Journal of Public Health Management & Practice, 7*(6), 43.

Oregon DHHS. (2013). *Oregon immunization alert system.* Retrieved from http://www.immalert.org/new/

Public Health Functions Steering Committee. (1994). *Public health in America.* DHHS. Retrieved from http://www.health.gov/phfunctions/public.htm

Roush, S. W., Murphy, T. V., & Vaccine-Preventable Disease Table Working Group. (2007). Historical comparisons of morbidity and mortality for vaccine-preventable diseases in the United States. *Journal of the American Medical Association, 298*(18), 2155.

Spencer, L. M., Schooley, M. W., Anderson, L. A., Kochtitzky, C. S., DeGroff, A. S., Devlin, H. M., & Mercer, S. L. (2013). *Seeking best practices: a conceptual framework for planning and improving evidence-based practices.* Atlanta, GA. Retrieved from http://www.cdc.gov/pcd/issues/2013/13_0186.htm

U.S. Department of Health and Human Services. (2010). *Healthy people 2010: Understanding and improving health* (2nd ed.).

U.S. Department of Health and Human Services, CDC. (2013). Retrieved from http://www.cdc.gov/informaticscompetencies/

Wild, E. L., Hastings, T. M., Gubernick, R., Ross, D. A., & Fehrenbach, S. N. (2004). Key elements for successful integrated health information systems: lessons from the states. *Journal of Public Health Management & Practice,* (Suppl.), S36–S47.

Winslow, C. E. A. (1920). The untilled fields of public health. *Science New Series, 51*(1306), 23.

Wisconsin Immunization Program. (2013). *Wisconsin immunization registry (WIR). Wisconsin Department of Health Services.* Retrieved from http://dhs.wisconsin.gov/immunization/WIR.htm

World Health Organization. (1997). *The world health report 1996—Fighting disease, fostering development.* Retrieved from http://www.who.int/whr/1996/en/index.html

World Health Organization. (2010). *The determinants of health, World Health Organization.* Retrieved from http://www.who.int/hia/evidence/doh/en/

PUBLIC HEALTH INFORMATICS EDUCATION PROGRAMS

American College of Medical Informatics (ACMI) fellowship. (n.d.). Retrieved from http://www.amia.org/programs/acmi-fellowship

ASPH partner fellowship programs. (n.d.). Retrieved from http://www.asph.org/document.cfm?page=751&JobProg_ID=20

ASPH Graduate Training Program fellowships and internships. (n.d.). Retrieved from http://www.asph.org/document.cfm?page=752

CDC. (n.d.). *Public health informatics fellowship program.* Retrieved from http://www.cdc.gov/phifp/

Informatics university programs. (n.d.). *Includes some fellowships at universities.* Retrieved from http://www.amia.org/education/programs-and-courses

MELDI-Public Health Informatics Fellowship Program. (n.d.). Retrieved from http://meldi.snre.umich.edu/node/1166

NIH Nursing Informatics Internship. (n.d.). Retrieved from http://www.cc.nih.gov/dcri/education.html

33

Informatics Solutions for Emergency Planning and Response

Elizabeth (Betsy) Weiner / Capt. Lynn A. Slepski

• OBJECTIVES

1. Describe the contributions that informatics can provide to emergency planning and response.
2. Illustrate various ways that informatics tools can be designed and used to support decision-making and knowledge base building in emergency planning and response efforts.
3. Utilize the 2009 H1N1 example as a case study in how informatics was used to plan and respond to this pandemic event.
4. Project areas of emergency management and response that would benefit from informatics assistance.

• KEY WORDS

Emergencies
Disasters
Public health informatics
Bioterrorism
Biosurveillance

INTRODUCTION

Unfortunately, both natural and manmade disasters have catapulted us into a world that has resulted in making emergency planning and response a high priority need. There has been a documented rise in terrorism incidents, as well as natural disasters worldwide. Natural events have ranged from earthquakes, tsunamis, floods, hurricanes, typhoons, to pandemic disease events affecting billions. Conflicts and nuclear disasters have added to the complexities. In addition to natural disasters, political and social upheavals massively disrupt the lives and livelihoods of populations and result in the forced displacement of millions of people. The World Health Organization (WHO,

2014) reported that during 2013 they responded to three major crises: Syria, where 9.3 million people were in need of urgent humanitarian assistance; the Philippines, where Typhoon Haiyan/Yolanda killed nearly 6000 people, devastated the lives of millions, and destroyed over a million homes, and the Central African Republic where rising tensions between Muslim and Christian communities and the collapse of the state have left the entire population of the country in fear and affected by the crisis. These emergencies can have extensive political, economic, social, and public health impacts, with potential long-term consequences sometimes persisting for years after the emergency (WHO, 2013). As a result, both planning and response efforts have taken on new importance in relation to emergencies and disasters. The purpose of this chapter is to explore the intersection between informatics and emergency planning and response in order to determine current and future informatics contributions.

The United States is not immune from this increased emphasis on emergency preparedness. The events of September 11, 2001, forced the United States into the realization that the country was not adequately protected from terrorism. Then, within a short window of time, the anthrax outbreaks stressed the public health infrastructure to the point that bioterrorism arose as an additional deadly threat. As a result of these two experiences, the government of the United States responded at an unprecedented pace to better prepare and manage terrorist events. Furthermore, the pandemic H1N1 incident in 2009 created data collection challenges that caused public health officials to creatively provide solutions for meaningful data acquisition in order to be able to effectively manage the event. Events such as the mass shooting in Newtown, Connecticut, Hurricane Sandy on the eastern coast of the United States, and the horrific tornado in Moore, Oklahoma, serve as recent illustrations of how response efforts have had to be altered to meet varied situations. Hemingway and Ferguson (2014) reflected on lessons learned during the Boston Marathon bombing and concluded that emergency preparedness plan updates must reflect the changing types of disasters, changing communication technologies, and the changing workforce.

Early contributions by the informatics community focused on surveillance of threat detection. However, as informaticists became more familiar with emergency planning and response, it became clear that contributions toward efficiency, analysis, remote monitoring, telemedicine, and advanced communications would be valued. The most consistent challenge for emergency and disaster response continues to be communication and information management. Effective response requires high situational awareness analyzing real-time information to assess needs and available resources that can change suddenly and unexpectedly. There is a critical interdependence between data collected in the field about a disaster incident, casualties, healthcare needs, triage, and treatment and the needed community resources such as ambulances, emergency departments, hospitals, and intensive care units. Concurrently, information from the various inpatient facilities and ambulance resources alters the management and disposition of victims at the scene of a disaster. Opportunities abound for new telecommunication technologies. Smart devices, wireless connectivity, and positioning technologies are all advances that have application during disaster events. These technologies are being used and evaluated to improve patient care and tracking, foster greater safety for patients and providers, enhance incident management at the scene, coordinate response efforts,

and enhance informatics support at both the scene of the disaster and at the community resource levels.

The 2004 earthquake and tsunami that devastated parts of Southeast Asia illustrated the uncoordinated invasion of people and organizations that resulted in unnecessary duplication, competition, and failure to assist many of the victims in need (Birnbaum, 2010). Subsequently, the Interagency Standing Committee (IASC) of the United Nations Office for the Coordination of Humanitarian Affairs (UN-OCHA) initiated changes called the "humanitarian reform." This reform effort organized clusters whose principal mission was to assist the impacted government with coordination of all responses and with evaluations of the impact of interventions. The World Health Organization was appointed as the lead agency for health, which includes coordination and production of health information (WHO, 2009, p. 8). Three of the eight strategic areas of their five-year programme required informatics: (3) improve health information and operational intelligence; (4) provide baseline information on health risks, health risk reduction, and emergency preparedness; and (7) build emergency preparedness knowledge and skills through training, guidance, research, and information services. This organization at the global level was aimed at discouraging individual and organizational response efforts that were not part of this coordinated response. The United States has also organized their planning and response efforts for the same reasons, and informatics is increasingly taking on more important roles in these efforts.

THE FEDERAL SYSTEM FOR EMERGENCY PLANNING AND RESPONSE

Most disasters and emergencies are handled by local and state responders. The federal government provides supplemental assistance when the consequences of a disaster exceed local and state capabilities.

Under the Homeland Security Presidential Directive 5 (HSPD5) (White House, 2003), the Secretary of Homeland Security, as the principal Federal official for domestic incident management, coordinates Federal actions within the United States to prepare for, respond to, and recover from terrorist attacks, major disasters, and other emergencies. Coordination occurs if and when any one of the following four conditions applies: (1) a Federal department or agency acting under its own authority has requested the assistance of the Secretary; (2) the resources of State and local authorities are overwhelmed and Federal assistance has been requested by the appropriate State and local authorities; (3) more than one Federal department or agency has become substantially involved in responding to the incident; or (4) the Secretary has been directed to assume responsibility for managing the domestic incident by the President. Further, HSPD5 directs Federal department heads to provide their full and prompt cooperation, support, and resources to the Secretary in protecting national security.

The National Response Framework, enacted in January 2008, established a comprehensive, national, and all-hazards approach to respond to disasters and emergencies (Department of Homeland Security, 2008a). Built on its predecessor, the National Response Plan, it includes guiding principles that detail how federal, state, local, tribal, and private sector partners, including the healthcare sector, prepare for and provide a unified domestic response, improving coordination and integration. The Framework emphasizes preparedness activities that include planning, organizing, training, equipping, exercising, and applying lessons learned and assigns lead federal agencies to each of 15 Emergency Support Functions (ESF) (Department of Homeland Security, 2008b).

The ESF group functions are used to provide Federal support during a response (Table 33.1), and assigns leads for each functional area. The Department of Health

TABLE 33.1	Emergency Support Functions by Lead Department and Scope	
Function	**Lead Department/ Agency**	**Scope**
ESF #1— Transportation	Transportation	Aviation/airspace management and control Transportation safety Restoration/recovery of transportation infrastructure Movement restrictions Damage and impact assessment
ESF #2— Communications	Homeland Security/Federal Emergency Management Agency	Coordination with telecommunications and information technology infrastructures Restoration and repair of telecommunications infrastructure Protection, restoration, and sustainment of national cyber and information technology resources Oversight of communications within the Federal incident management and response structures
ESF #3—Public Works and Engineering	Defense/U.S. Army Corps of Engineers	Infrastructure protection and emergency repair Infrastructure restoration Engineering services and construction management Emergency contracting support for life-saving and life-sustaining services
ESF #4— Firefighting	Agriculture/ Fire Service	Coordination of federal firefighting activities Support to wildland, rural, and urban firefighting activities
ESF Scope ESF #5— Emergency Management	Homeland Security/Federal Emergency Management Agency	Coordination of incident management and response efforts Issuance of mission assignments Resource and human capital Incident action planning Financial management
ESF #6—Mass Care, Emergency Assistance, Housing, and Human Services	Homeland Security/Federal Emergency Management Agency	Mass care Emergency assistance Disaster housing Human services
ESF #7—Logistics Management and Resource Support	Homeland Security/Federal Emergency Management Agency	Comprehensive, national incident logistics planning, management, and sustainment capability Resource support (facility space, office equipment and supplies, contracting services, etc.)

(continued)

TABLE 33.1	Emergency Support Functions by Lead Department and Scope *(continued)*	
Function	**Lead Department/ Agency**	**Scope**
ESF #8—Public Health and Medical Services	Health and Human Services	Public health Medical Mental health services Mass fatality management
ESF #9—Search and Rescue	Defense Homeland Security/Federal Emergency Management Agency	Life-saving assistance Search and rescue operations
ESF #10—Oil and Hazardous Materials Response	Homeland Security/ U.S. Coast Guard	Oil and hazardous materials (chemical, biological, radiological, etc.) response Environmental short- and long-term cleanup
ESF #11— Agriculture and Natural Resources	Agriculture Interior	Nutrition assistance Animal and plant disease and pest response Food safety and security Natural and cultural resources and historic properties protection and restoration Safety and well-being of household pets
ESF #12—Energy	Energy	Energy infrastructure assessment, repair, and restoration Energy industry utilities coordination Energy forecast
ESF #13—Public Safety and Security	Justice	Facility and resource security Security planning and technical resource assistance Public safety and security support Support to access, traffic, and crowd control
ESF #14—Long-Term Community Recovery	Homeland Security/ Federal Emergency Management Agency Urban Development Small Business Administration	Social and economic community impact assessment Long-term community recovery assistance to states, local governments, and the private sector Analysis and review of mitigation program implementation
ESF #15—External Affairs	Homeland Security/Federal Emergency Management Agency	Emergency public information and protective action guidance Media and community relations Congressional and international affairs Tribal and insular affairs

Reproduced from Department of Homeland Security (2008b).

and Human Services leads public health and medical responses, including biosurveillance.

The Federal Emergency Management Agency (FEMA) received critical public feedback following their poor response efforts during the 2005 Hurricane Katrina. Since that time, the agency has creatively added new social media sites, ways to crowdsource disasters, and centralized places to get information. Examples include an interactive emergency kit checklist with information about what to do during specific hazards; a disaster reporter feature where users upload disaster photos with GPS features for posting on a public map; and a new social hub (FEMA, 2013). In addition, they have recently added the FEMA LinkedIn page and the U.S. Fire Administration Facebook page where there are job listings, stories about what a "day in the life" looks like at FEMA, other training resources, and tips for assisting fire departments or firefighters.

CASE STUDY 33.1. INFORMATICS AND 2009 H1N1

Although there have been other viruses that have surfaced with the potential to become pandemic, the 2009 H1N1 influenza pandemic continues to be the most recent pandemic and illustrates how informatics can contribute to an emergency response. Initially concerned that a circulating H5N1 virus (Avian Influenza A) was mutating and could cause a human pandemic, global experts had focused efforts over the last several years on rapidly developing catastrophic plans even though a pandemic virus had not emerged. There were significant concerns, given that during the twentieth century three flu pandemics were responsible for more than 50 million deaths worldwide and almost a million deaths in the United States (Department of Health and Human Services [DHHS], 2005) (Table 33.2). The CDC estimates that 43 million to 89 million people had H1N1 between April 2009 and April 2010, and they estimate between 8870 and 18,300 H1N1 related deaths (DHHS, 2014a). On August 10, 2010 the WHO declared an end to the global H1N1 flu pandemic (WHO, 2010).

Many governments believed that if a pandemic-capable virus emerged, there would be rapid worldwide spread as the 1918 Pandemic had spread across countries and continents in less than one year in a time without commercial air travel to facilitate the spread of disease (DHHS, 2005). It was understood that a worldwide influenza pandemic occurring in this century could have major effects on the global economy, especially travel, trade, tourism, food, consumption, and eventually, investment and financial markets and could lead to widespread economic and social disruptions. As a result, many countries engaged in detailed pandemic planning and prepared to adopt draconian-like measures to delay but not stop the arrival of the virus, such as border closures and travel restrictions.

Here in the United States, modelers predicted catastrophic death estimates (Table 33.3). The 1918–1919 flu pandemic, to date the most severe, had caused the deaths of at least 675,000 Americans and affected about one-fifth of the world's population. Researchers believed that if a pandemic of similar severity occurred today, 90 million Americans could become ill, quickly exceeding available healthcare capacity and result in approximately 2 million Americans deaths (DHHS, 2005).

Preparedness planners assumed that all populations were at risk. They believed that disease would be widespread, affecting multiple areas of the United States and other countries at the same time preventing the redistribution of resources. The world would experience multiple waves of outbreaks potentially occurring for an extended period of time (over 18 months), affecting the entire United States for a period of 12 to 16 weeks with community waves each lasting 6 to 8 weeks (DHHS, 2005). One to three pandemic waves would occur (Occupational Safety and Health Administration [OSHA], 2007). Further, planners believed that a pandemic could affect as many as 40% of the workforce during periods of peak flu illness, predicting that employees could be absent because of their own illness, or would be caring for sick family members or for children if schools or daycare centers are closed. They also recognized that workers would be absent if public

TABLE 33.2	History of Pandemics by Deaths, Causative Strain, and At-Risk Population			
Pandemic	**Estimated U.S. Deaths**	**Estimated Worldwide Deaths**	**Influenza A Strain**	**Populations at Greatest Risk**
1918–1919	500,000	40 million	H1N1	Young, healthy adults
1957–1958	70,000	1–2 million	H2N2	Infants, elderly
1968–1969	34,000	700,000	H3N2	Infants, elderly

Reproduced from Department of Health and Human Services Pandemic Influenza Plan (2005), p. B-7.

TABLE 33.3	Estimates of Numbers of Episodes of Illness, Healthcare Utilization, and Death Associated With Moderate and Severe Pandemic Influenza Scenarios* in the United States	
Characteristic	**Moderate (1958/68-like)**	**Severe (1918-like)**
Illness	90,000,000 (30%)	90,000,000 (30%)
Outpatient Medical Care	45,000,000 (50%)	45,000,000 (50%)
Hospitalization	865,000	9,900,000
ICU Care	128,750	1,485,000
Mechanical Ventilation	64,875	742,500
Deaths	**209,000**	**1,903,000**

Reproduced from Department of Health and Human Services Pandemic Influenza Plan (2005), p. 18.
*Estimates based on extrapolation from past pandemics in the United States. Note that these estimates do not include the potential impact of interventions not available during the twentieth-century pandemics.

transportation was disrupted or if they were afraid to leave home (Department of Homeland Security, 2007).

Adopting a "worst case scenario," government experts rapidly developed a number of strategies to help local governments plan, stating that the Federal government would not likely be able to provide any assistance during the actual pandemic. For example, DHHS (2007) developed a Pandemic Severity Index (PSI) to characterize the severity of a pandemic. It was designed to predict the impact of a pandemic and provide local decision-makers with standardized triggers that were matched to the severity of illness impacting a specific community (Table 33.4). The severity index was based on a case-fatality ratio to measure the proportion of deaths among clinically ill persons. Recommended actions were identified in advance, and communicated to the public in hopes of increasing their understanding and compliance. Using the PSI, a severe pandemic influenza, similar to the 1918 Pandemic, was defined as a category 4 or 5, with 20% to 40% of the population infected. For a severe pandemic, HHS recommended that localities be prepared to dismiss children from schools and close daycares for up to 12 weeks, as well as initiate adult social distancing, which included suspension of large public gatherings and modification of the work place schedules and practices (e.g., telework and staggered shifts).

The Centers for Disease Control and Prevention, part of HHS, monitors influenza activity and trends and virus characteristics through a nationwide surveillance system as well as estimates the burden of flu illness using statistical modelling (CDC, 2010). On April, 29, 2009, the CDC began reporting cases of respiratory infection with swine-origin influenza A (H1N1) viruses transmitted through human-to-human contact (CDC, 2009a, 2009b). It established the case definition for 2009 H1N1 as an acute febrile respiratory illness in a person and laboratory-confirmed swine-origin influenza A (H1N1) virus infection at CDC by either of the following tests: real-time reverse transcription-polymerase chain reaction (rRT-PCR), or viral culture (CDC, 2009a). The CDC began tracking and reporting the number of cases, hospitalizations, and deaths at state, local, and national levels using standard state reporting mechanisms. It was soon apparent that using actual case counts resulted in dramatically underreported disease.

On July 24, 2009, CDC abandoned initial case counts, when it recognized that those numbers represented a significant undercount of the actual number of 2009 H1N1 cases. They found that 2009 H1N1 was less severe and caused fewer deaths than expected when compared to the pandemic planning assumptions. As a result, existing plans, which used case fatality numbers as the trigger for initiating response actions, were not effective.

Scientists turned to other means to begin to understand the effects of disease and predict its future course. For example, because trending indicated that children and young adults were at higher risk, the Department of Education began looking at school closures and school absenteeism, examining both teacher and student absences. Each of the critical infrastructure key resource sectors held weekly calls with private sector partners to elicit whether there were trends beginning to indicate business interruption problems, which might forecast social disruptions. The National Retail Data monitoring system tracked the real-time purchase of over-the-counter (OTC) medications, such as fever reducers and influenza treatments, in over 29,000 retail pharmacies, groceries, and mass merchandise stores. This University of Pittsburgh system (2014a) is used to provide early detection of naturally occurring disease outbreaks as well as bioterrorism.

The CDC moved to using estimates. Using the influenza module from BioSense, CDC tracked flu with data from over 500 local and state health departments, hospital emergency rooms, Laboratory Response Network labs, Health Information Exchanges, as well as the Departments of Defense and Veterans Affairs. The Real-Time Outbreak Disease Surveillance (RODS) was designed in 1999 to

TABLE 33.4	Matrix of Community Mitigation Strategies by Pandemic Severity Index		
Interventions by Setting	**1**	**Pandemic Severity Index 2 and 3**	**4 and 5**
Home			
Voluntary isolation of ill at home (adults and children); combine with use of antiviral treatment as available and indicated	Recommend[b,c]	Recommend[b,c]	Recommend[b,c]
Voluntary quarantine of household members in homes with ill persons[d] (adults and children); consider combining with antiviral prophylaxis if effective, feasible, and quantities sufficient	Generally not recommended	Consider[e]	Recommend[e]
School			
Child social distancing			
• Dismissal of students from schools and school-based activities, and closure of childcare programs	Generally not recommended	Consider: ≤ 4 weeks[f]	Recommend: ≤ 12 weeks[g]
• Reduce out-of-school social contacts and community mixing	Generally not recommended	Consider: ≤ 4 weeks[f]	Recommend: ≤ 12 weeks[g]
Workplace / Community			
Adult social distancing			
• Decrease number of social contacts (e.g., encourage teleconferences, alternatives to face-to-face meetings)	Generally not recommended	Consider	Recommend
• Increase distance between persons (e.g., reduce density in public transit)	Generally not recommended	Consider	Recommend
• Modify or cancel selected public gatherings to promote social distance (e.g., postpone indoor stadium events)	Generally not recommended	Consider	Recommend
• Modify work place schedules and practices (e.g., telework, staggered shifts)	Generally not recommended	Consider	Recommend

Reproduced from Department of Health and Human Services (2007), p. 12.

Generally Not Recommended = Unless there is a compelling rationale for specific populations or jurisdictions, measures are generally not recommended for entire populations as the consequences may outweigh the benefits.

Consider = Important to consider these alternatives as part of a prudent planning strategy, considering characteristics of the pandemic such as age-specific attack rate, geographic distribution, and the magnitude of adverse consequences. These factors may vary globally, nationally, and locally.

Recommended = generally recommended as an important component of planning strategy.

[a]All these interventions should be used in combination with other infection control measures including hand hygiene, cough etiquette, and personal protection equipment such as face masks. Additional information on infection control measures is available at www.pandemicflu.gov (DHHS, 2007).

[b]This intervention may be combined with treatment of sick individuals using antiviral medications and vaccine campaigns, if supplies are available.

[c]Many sick individuals who are not critically ill may be managed safely at home.

[d]The contribution made by contact with asymptomatically infected individuals to disease transmission is unclear. Household members in homes with ill persons may be at higher risk and have asymptomatic illness promoting community disease transmission. Therefore, household members of homes with sick individuals would be advised to stay home.

[e]To facilitate compliance and decrease risk of household transmission, this intervention may be combined with provision of antiviral medications to household contacts depending on drug availability, feasibility, and effectiveness; policy recommendations for antiviral prophylaxis are addressed in a separate guidance document.

[f]Consider short-term suspension of classes, that is, less than four weeks.

[g]Plan for prolonged suspension of classes, that is, one to three months; actual duration may vary depending on transmission in the community as the pandemic wave is expected to last six to eight weeks.

collect and analyze disease surveillance data in real time (University of Pittsburgh, 2014b). Interpreting these estimates, one study hypothesized that for every reported lab-confirmed case of H1N1 between April and July 2009, there were an estimated 79 total cases. The same study found that for every identified hospitalized case there were more likely 2.7 hospitalized people (Reed et al., 2009).

Concerned that the limited capacity of the healthcare system would be overwhelmed and finite resources such as H1N1 test kits would be consumed, CDC published updated self-treatment guidance and told the public that H1N1 testing was no longer necessary. Instead, persons with minor flu-like illnesses were assumed to be infected and encouraged to utilize advice lines staffed by nurses to obtain answers to questions rather than to seek appointments with healthcare providers. For the first time, the U.S. government established a one-stop federal Web site (www.flu.gov) that housed information such as frequently asked questions as well as messaging aimed at individuals and families, businesses, and healthcare professionals from across the federal interagency. The Web site contained tailored planning documents for schools and communities, and included targeted information for special populations. One particularly helpful site was a Flu Vaccine Locator, which contained a database that provided the general public with the locations of clinics that had vaccine supplies utilizing zip codes (DHHS, 2014b).

For the first time, HHS used social media to communicate with young people. Recognizing that large numbers of young adults were affected, they launched a Facebook application "I'm a Flu Fighter!" that allowed and encouraged users to spread information about H1N1, such as where they received the H1N1 vaccine, to their Facebook friends (Mitchell, 2010).

Other recent viruses have arisen but cannot be categorized as pandemic because they have not caused sustained and efficient human-to-human transmission. Informatics has been important in this reporting and analysis. H5N1, commonly known as avian influenza ("bird flu"), is such an example. In July 2013, WHO announced a total of 630 confirmed human cases which resulted in the deaths of 375 people since 2003, but did not meet pandemic criteria (WHO, 2013). Also in 2013, the American Academy of Family Physicians (2013) reported that the case numbers of H7N9 stalled in China, but that the pandemic potential remains. H7N9 is an unusually dangerous virus for humans with cases resulting in severe respiratory illness, with a mortality rate of roughly 30% (Li et al., 2014). H7N9 does not kill poultry, which makes surveillance much more difficult. Other recent threats include a new respiratory virus

Middle East Respiratory Syndrome (MERS-CoV), which arose in 2013 in Saudi Arabia (Todd, 2014). Todd concludes that since all viral mutations are unpredictable, it is impossible to predict whether any of these viruses or yet another emerging virus will be the cause of a new pandemic. We must, therefore, continue our diligence in surveillance activities.

Healthcare Consumers Contribute to Surveillance Activities

In the H1N1 case study described above, healthcare consumer data became an important aspect of the disease surveillance model that augmented data collected by the CDC. Why was that the case? Now more than ever before consumers have the opportunity to contribute to surveillance activities. In some cases, the participation is a conscious decision, but in others consumers may be unknowingly contributing to this informatics process.

Part of the advantage of externally generated CDC surveillance mechanisms is that they shorten the typical lag time to publication for CDC's publicly reported data which is currently estimated to be from 10 to 14 days (Ginsberg et al., 2009). Telephone triage data are now being used to help track influenza in a specified geographic location with the added advantage that the data are real time in nature. In addition, patient demographics and disease symptoms can also be captured in a standard format. Another new mechanism for data capture about influenza is through physician group proprietary systems. In these systems, the healthcare providers enter the data for suspected or confirmed influenza patients. By far, the most talked about trend in influenza surveillance for the 2009 H1N1 outbreak was Google's Flu Trends. The assumption made with this system was that there was a relationship between how many people search the Internet for flu-related topics and how many people have flu-like symptoms. In studies conducted by Google.org comparing Google Flu Trends to CDC published data, they found that the search-based flu estimates had a consistently strong correlation with real CDC surveillance data (Ginsberg et al., 2009).

COMPETENCY-BASED LEARNING AND INFORMATICS NEEDS

In order to provide a successful nursing response effort, nurses must be appropriately and consistently educated to provide the right response. Competency-based education provides an international infrastructure for nurses to learn about emergency preparedness and response. Yet, currently there are no accepted, standardized requirements for disaster nursing training or continuing education (Slepski & Littleton-Kearney, 2010).

There have been, however, a number of competency development efforts geared to different nursing audiences. In collaboration with the CDC, researchers from the Columbia University School of Nursing identified nine objectively measurable skills for public health workers and seven competencies for leaders, followed by an additional three competencies for public health professionals (Columbia University School of Nursing Center for Health Policy, 2001). There were also two competencies identified for public health technical and support staff relating to (1) demonstration of equipment and skills associated with his/her functional role in emergency preparedness during regular drills and (2) description of at least one resource for backup support in key areas of responsibility. In 2003, the International Nursing Coalition for Mass Casualty Education (later renamed the Nursing Emergency Preparedness Coalition, or NEPEC) generated a list of 104 competency statements for all nurses responding to disasters using domains developed by the American Association of Colleges of Nursing (Stanley, 2005). Additional competencies were developed by the University of Hyogo and the International Council of Nurses. All of the competency efforts were considered by a WHO group of nursing experts as they developed competency domains during the first consultation on nursing and midwifery in emergencies (WHO, 2007, p. 10).

Efforts to identify content to match competencies have also proven successful. An additional group of experts met following WHO's first consultation on nursing and midwifery contributions in emergencies to identify possible content that matched the identified competencies at the undergraduate nursing level (WHO, 2008). Online modules produced by NEPEC (http://www.nursing.vanderbilt.edu/incmce/modules.html) and the National Nursing Emergency Preparedness Initiative (NNEPI) (www.nnepi.org) both received international awards from Sigma Theta Tau International for quality computer-based education programs.

The CDC currently sponsors a public health informatics fellowship program that is a two-year paid fellowship in public health informatics (CDC, 2014). The competency-based and hands-on training allows students to apply information and computer science and technology to solving real public health problems.

Informatics and Incident Management

Information technology staff members have long been familiar with emergency planning for disaster recovery related to their systems, but find themselves in a new role as part of a more comprehensive team approach to disasters and emergencies. The incident management system (IMS) was first used by firefighters to control disaster scenes in a multijurisdictional and interdepartmental manner. The IMS calls for a hierarchical chain of command led by the incident manager or commander. Each job assignment is consistently followed by assigned personnel who refer to a specific job action sheet. This system improves communication through a common language, allows staff to move between management locations, and facilitates all responders to understand the established chain of command. The IMS has been adapted for hospital use and is called the Hospital Incident Command System (HICS).

The Emergency Operations Center (EOC) is the physical location where the Incident Management Team convenes to make decisions, communicate, and coordinate the various activities in response to an incident. Accurate, real-time data acquisition regarding patient needs, rescue personnel, and resources available is critical to overall coordination. Table 33.5 presents functions where technology can be used to capture and represent data for purposes of increasing situational awareness in the EOC for the purposes of making the most informed and efficient decisions. In addition, the informatics processing efforts that contribute to the incident management system are also described.

Informatics and Volunteerism

Healthcare volunteers are a necessary component of mass casualty events but also create challenges. How do you count volunteers so that they are only entered once? How do you educate them so that they can perform effectively when needed? How are liability issues dealt with? Are there certain tasks that lend themselves to volunteer efforts? Some states offer their nurses the opportunity to volunteer when they renew their nursing licensure. It is then possible for state-wide volunteer databases to be built, but these are only shared within the state system. Some states require a set number of hours of continuing education in emergency preparedness in order to renew licensure.

The federal government does have a system for organizing teams that are willing to travel to other regions of the country in the event of an emergency. These teams are called disaster medical assistance teams (DMATs). When DMATs are activated, members of the teams are federalized or made temporary workers of the federal government, which then assumes the liability for their services. Their licensure and certifications are then recognized by all states.

TABLE 33.5	Technology and Informatics Contributions to Incident Management	
Functions	**Possible Technologies**	**Informatics Processing**
Data for Incident Command Center	Smart White Board	Organize and detect patterns and trends in data
	Electronic Dashboards	Predict resource needs and safety zones
	Resource Modeling	Access additional data and information
	Internet Access to Information Resources	Record and process decisions for legal and financial purposes
	Staffing and Scheduling Records	Analyze data to determine statistical significance
	Electronic Logs to Capture Data and Decisions	Report and analyze Internet surveillance systems
	Resource Inventories	Promote standardization of data collection and vocabulary
	Resource Distributor Database	
	Online Disaster Manual with Job Action Sheets	
Communications	Landlines	Standardized vocabulary and roles
	Radio Communications	Communication standards set in order to prioritize and determine accuracy of data transmission
	Cell Phones	
	Satellite phones	Data collection from the field is sent back to EOC
	Amateur Radios	Data collection and analysis contributes to situational awareness
	Third and Fourth Generation Wireless Devices	
	Electronic Mail	
	Internet, Twitter, Facebook, YouTube	
	Television and Radio announcements E-commerce	
Patient Tracking	Global Positioning systems (GPS)	Data and Information processed for purposes of triage and transport
	Bar code tracking	Data collected to determine magnitude of disaster
	Radio frequency identification	
Provider Safety	Radiation monitors and badges	Data collection and Monitoring to determine safe radiation levels
	Radio communications	Cellular triangulation to determine location
	GPS devices	
	Cell phones	
Ambulance Tracking	GPS	Monitor for triage and admission purposes
	Cell phones	
	Radio communication	
Patient data acquisition and monitoring	Electronic record	Collect and analyze to determine trends across geographic area
	ED status system	
	Wireless monitoring	
	Pharmacy electronic records	

The Medical Reserve Corps (MRC) and the Emergency System for Advance Registration of Volunteer Health Professionals (ESAR-VHP) both represent initiatives of the Department of Health and Human Services to improve the nation's ability to prepare for and respond to public health emergencies. The MRC is a national network of community-based volunteer units that focus on improving the health, safety, and resiliency of their local communities. MRC volunteers include medical and public health professionals such as physicians, nurses, pharmacists, dentists, veterinarians, and epidemiologists. Many community members—interpreters, chaplains, office workers, legal advisors, and others—can fill key support positions. For example, nurses trained in informatics are often used by MRC units to compile needed databases depending on the response effort at hand. At the time of this writing, there are 991 units composed of 206,770 volunteers, covering 73.69% of the United States (Medical Reserve Corps, 2014).

The national ESAR-VHP program provides guidance and assistance for the development of standardized state-based programs for registering and verifying the credentials of volunteer health professionals in advance of an emergency or disaster (ESAR-VHP, 2014). Each state program collects and verifies information on the identity, licensure status, privileges, and credentials of volunteers. These programs are built to a common set of national standards and give each state the ability to quickly identify and assist in the coordination of volunteer health professionals in an emergency. These registration systems include information about volunteers involved in organized efforts at the local level (such as MRC units) and the state level (DMAT and state medical response teams). In addition, individuals who prefer not to be part of an organized unit structure can also be entered into the registry in order to allow for a ready pool of volunteers. State ESAR-VHP programs provide a single, centralized source of information to facilitate the intrastate, interstate, and state-to-federal deployment or transfer of volunteer health professionals. Several collaboration suggestions have been generated in an effort to integrate both the MRC and ESAR-VHP initiatives, including having state coordinators for both initiatives (MRC, 2014).

Most volunteer opportunities require education prior to responding to the event. MRC units have competency-based education requirements. The American Red Cross has a long history of volunteerism during disasters, and has education requirements for nurses depending on what roles they will play in disaster relief. Regardless of the group, nurses are urged to be a part of an organized group rather than simply showing up on the scene of a disaster and contributing to the confusion. All of these initiatives require informatics solutions in order to function effectively. Organizing the results of these efforts into a standardized registry allows for more informed decisions and increased efficiency of services during times of response and relief efforts.

Disaster Electronic Medical Records and Tracking

Expanding the use of the electronic health record should help both patients and their healthcare providers during times of emergencies and disasters. Accessing clinical data for displaced patients should also improve tremendously with interoperable data and the sharing of clinical information, all recent initiatives from the Office of the National Coordinator for Health Information Technology (ONC). One project that emerged from that office during Hurricane Katrina was called KatrinaHealth and illustrated such potential with the pooling of information resources across federal and private sectors. KatrinaHealth.org was a free and secure online service that provided Katrina evacuees their authorized healthcare providers and pharmacists with a list of the prescription medications evacuees were taking before they were forced to leave their homes, lost their medications, and the medical records (Markle Foundation, American Medical Association, Gold Standard, RxHub, & SureScripts, 2006).

Another situation served to illustrate the importance of the electronic health record when an EF5 tornado struck Joplin, Missouri, on May 22, 2011 (Abir, Mostashari, Atwal, & Lurie, 2012). Significant damage was inflicted on St. John's Regional Medical Center, claiming the lives of five of its 188 patients and one visitor. The EHR system had been implemented only three weeks earlier, and fortunately had a regional backup in Springfield, Missouri. Besides being able to access patient records, the informatics staff were able to modify the names and beds in the units to reflect the temporary facilities that were needed due to damage in the main facility. A number of regional physician practices were also able to resume caring for patients in alternate sites.

DeMers et al. (2013) describe a secure, scalable disaster electronic medical record and tracking system called the Wireless Internet Information System for medical Response in Disasters (WIISARD). This system is a handheld, linked, wireless EMR system utilizing current technology platforms. Smart phones connected to radio frequency identification readers can be used to efficiently track casualties resulting from the incident. Medical information can be transmitted on an encrypted network to fellow team members, medical dispatch, and receiving medical centers. The authors report that the system has been field tested in a number of exercises with excellent results. This pre-hospital EMR merges data with the receiving hospital EMR using HIPAA-compliant methods. Fayaz-Bakhsh and Sharifi-Sedeh (2013) are critical in noting that one of the most typical consequences of disasters is the near or complete collapse of terrestrial telecommunications infrastructures, resulting in disaster managers having difficulty getting Internet connectivity or cell phone coverage. The WIISARD team recognized those concerns and used an ad hoc field network that could circumvent challenges around damaged or overwhelmed traditional communication network systems (Chan, Griswold, & Killeen, 2013).

Tracking of patient victims is another important function needed during disaster and emergency events. The allocation of various resources over multiple geographical locations makes for a complex decision-making process, thus allocation of patients to hospitals and adequate patient tracking and tracing are major issues. Accurate and current information is critical for situational awareness—the ability to make timely and effective decisions during rapidly evolving events. In order to overcome such challenges, these authors developed a Victim Tracking and Tracing System (ViTTS) (Marres, Taal, Bemelman, Bouman, & Leenen, 2013). Their system design allowed for early, unique registration of victims close to the impact site that was able to later connect to the receiving systems.

Mobile health (mHealth) technology can also play a critical role in improving disaster victim tracking, triage, patient care, facility management, and theater-wide decision-making. Callaway et al. (2012) thought that the delivery of care after disasters like the earthquake in Haiti could be better integrated using mHealth. They chose to develop, deploy, and evaluate a novel electronic patient medical record and tracking system in the immediate post-event setting. An iPhone-based mobile technology platform called iChart was selected. During their implementation, there were 617 unique patient entries into the patient tracker, resulting in an adequate ability to triage patients as they arrived as new transfers. Users rated that the iChart improved provider handoffs and continuity of care, and standardized the information into one language. Given the chaotic nature of volunteer physicians' arrivals and departures, the mobile application also accommodated fluctuating provider schedules by keeping a centralized repository of basic patient information. The online database was also used to generate daily census figures.

Case, Morrison, and Vuylsteke (2012) reviewed the literature to determine ways that mobile technology could help disaster medicine. They classified applications into five types: (1) disaster scene management; (2) remote monitoring of casualties; (3) medical image transmission; (4) decision support applications; and (5) field hospital information technology systems.

Future Advances

While the 2009 pandemic fortunately was far less severe than the "Armageddon-like" event that planners forecasted, it served to highlight many opportunities for the use of informatics to assist in emergency preparedness and response. Health information technology investments are a necessary foundation in healthcare reform, linking potentially valuable information such as vaccination records and subsequent use of healthcare services to provide information about adverse events as well as vaccine effectiveness (Lurie, 2009). Already, the CDC works closely with WHO to make certain that many of the databases link to one another, but over time this will improve as well. Continuing to pay attention to social media for crowdsourcing, for trending, and for analysis of text messages will remain an important contribution to disaster care.

Using "grids" to connect multiple computers across the country will allow data sources to share and view large amounts of health information. Grid participants will be able to analyze data in other jurisdictions without moving the actual data, which is an important step forward in overcoming policy barriers to moving data out of a jurisdiction to protect individual privacy.

Having interoperable patient data is a current goal of the Office of the National Coordinator for Health Information Technology, but it will also serve to improve the data available as victims become dispersed from their typical healthcare environments. Pulling that data closer to the point of care with mobile devices will only enhance the quality of data available for healthcare providers to make critical decisions with limited time and resources. Allowing these data to be transmitted across international lines will most certainly assist in our quest to provide healthcare to victims regardless of where they seek shelter. International communication standards will also become an important factor in improving communication across borders.

SUMMARY

In conclusion, the 2009 H1N1 outbreak was a recent example of emergency preparedness and response. It reinforced the fact that estimating the number of actual flu cases is very challenging as current case counting relies on encounter information, which is prone to underreporting. Informatics is an emerging field that has the potential to immediately support the early identification of a communicable disease such as pandemic influenza, reducing loss of life and the consumption of limited resources. Use of automated case-specific disease monitoring applications such as BioSense, ESSENCE, and RODS and tracking retail data such as OTC medication purchases allow researchers to collect, analyze, and present real-time disease information which allows users to have immediate access to information that previously would have taken days to assemble. Technological developments will further enhance the ability to use informatics to detect the first warning signs during an emergency.

Consumers themselves have assumed surveillance roles in their quest to seek data and information resources. The increase use of social media provides a new mechanism for data collection and trending.

Coordinated response efforts require excellent communication based on efficient decision-making. Informatics can contribute to this agenda, particularly in an era when healthcare resources are dwindling. Informatics infrastructure contributes continuous monitoring of data, standards for combining data, technology-enhanced processing and analysis that help detect significant patterns, centralized diagnostic tool and protocols for treatment, and advanced communication technology. As a result, informatics solutions need to remain central to emergency planning and response efforts.

REFERENCES

Abir, M., Mostashari, F., Atwal, P., & Lurie, N. (2012). Electronic health records critical in the aftermath of disasters. *Prehospital and Disaster Medicine, 27*(6), 620–622. doi:10.1017/S1049023X12001409.

American Academy of Family Physicians. (2013). *H7N9 case numbers stalled, but pandemic potential remains.* Retrieved from http://www.aafp.org/news-now/health-of-the-public/20130516h7n9.html

Birnbaum, M. L. (2010). Stop!!!!!. *Prehospital and Disaster Medicine, 25*(2), 97–98.

Callaway, D. W., Peabody, C. R., Hoffman, A., Cote, E., Moulton, S., Baez, A. A., & Nathanson, L. (2012). Disaster mobile health technology: Lessons from Haiti. *Prehospital and Disaster Medicine, 27*(2), 148–152.

Case, T., Morrison, C., & Vuylsteke, A. (2012). The clinical application of mobile technology. *Prehospital and Disaster Medicine, 27*(5), 473–480.

Centers for Disease Control and Prevention. (2009a). *Update: Swine influenza A (H1N1) infections—California and Texas.* Retrieved from http://www.cdc.gov/mmwr/preview/mmwrhtml/mm5816a7.htm. Accessed on April 2009.

Centers for Disease Control and Prevention. (2009b). *Update: Infections with a swine-origin influenza A (H1N1) virus—United States and other countries.* Retrieved from http://www.cdc.gov/mmwr/preview/mmwrhtml/mm5816a5.htm. Accessed on April 28, 2009.

Centers for Disease Control and Prevention. (2010). *CDC estimates of 2009 H1N1 influenza cases, hospitalizations and deaths in the United States.* Retrieved from http://www.cdc.gov/h1n1flu/estimates_2009_h1n1.htm. Accessed on April 2009–April 10, 2010.

Centers for Disease Control and Prevention. (2014). *Public health informatics fellowship program.* Retrieved from http://www.cdc.gov/PHIFP/About.html

Chan, T. C., Griswold, W. G., & Killeen, J. P. (2013). Author reply. *Prehospital and Disaster Medicine, 28*(6), 647. doi:10.1017/S1049023X13009047

Columbia University School of Nursing Center for Health Policy. (2001, April). *Core public health worker competencies for emergency preparedness and response.* Retrieved from http://www.phf.org/resourcestools/Documents/emergencypreparednesscorecompetencies_Columbia_University.pdf

DeMers, G., Kahn, C., Johansson, P., Buono, C., Chipara, O., Griswold, W., & Chan, T. (2013). Secure scalable disaster electronic medical record and tracking system. *Prehospital and Disaster Medicine, 28*(5), 498–501. doi:10.1017/S1049023X13008686

Department of Health and Human Services. (2005). *HHS pandemic influenza plan.* Retrieved from http://www.flu.gov/planning-preparedness/federal/hhspandemicinfluenzaplan.pdf

Department of Health and Human Services. (2007). *Interim pre-pandemic planning guidance: Community strategy for pandemic influenza mitigation in the United States.* Retrieved from http://www.flu.gov/planning-preparedness/community/community_mitigation.pdf

Department of Health and Human Services. (2014a). *Pandemic flu history.* Retrieved from http://www.flu.gov/pandemic/history/index.html

Department of Health and Human Services. (2014b). *Vaccination & vaccine safety.* Retrieved from http://www.flu.gov/prevention-vaccination/vaccination/index.html

Department of Homeland Security. (2007). *Pandemic influenza preparedness, response, and recovery guide for critical infrastructure and key resources.* Retrieved from http://www.flu.gov/planning-preparedness/business/cikrpandemicinfluenzaguide.pdf

Department of Homeland Security. (2008a). *Introducing the national response framework.* Retrieved from http://www.fema.gov/pdf/emergency/nrf/about_nrf.pdf

Department of Homeland Security. (2008b). *National response framework. Emergency support annexes: Introduction.* Retrieved from http://www.fema.gov/pdf/emergency/nrf/nrf-esf-intro.pdf

ESAR-VHP. (2014). *The emergency system for advance registration of volunteer health professionals.* Retrieved from http://www.phe.gov/esarvhp/Pages/about.aspx

Fayaz-Bakhsh, A., & Sharifi-Sedeh, M. (2013). Electronic medical records in a mass-casualty exercise. *Prehospital and Disaster Medicine, 28*(6), 646. doi:10.1017/S1049023X13009047.

Federal Emergency Management Agency. (2013). *Crowdsourcing disasters and social engagement multiplied.* Retrieved from http://www.fema.gov/blog/2013-08-02/crowdsourcing-disasters-and-social-engagement-multiplied#.Uoa7VOvh-aU.mailto

Ginsberg, J., Mohebbi, M., Patel, R., Brammer, L., Smolinski, M., & Brillant, L. (2009). Detecting influenza epidemics using search engine query data. *Nature, 457,* 1012–1015. doi:10.1038/nature07634.

Hemingway, M., & Ferguson, J. (2014). Boston bombings: Response to disaster. *AORN Journal, 99*(2), 277–288.

Li, Q., Zhou, L., Zhou, M., Chen, Z., Li, F., Wu, H., ... Feng, Z. (2014, February 6). Epidemiology of human infections with Avian influenza (H7N9) virus in China. *The New England Journal of Medicine, 370*(6), 520–532. doi:10.1056/NEJMoa1304617

Lurie, N. (2009). H1N1 influenza, public health preparedness, and healthcare reform. *The New England Journal of Medicine, 361*(9), 843–845. Retrieved from http://content.nejm.org/cgi/content/short/361/9/843

Markle Foundation, American Medical Association, Gold Standard, RxHub, & SureScripts. (2006). *Lessons from KatrinaHealth.* Retrieved from http://research.policyarchive.org/15501.pdf

Marres, G. M. H., Taal, L., Bemelmann, M., Bouman, J., & Leenen, L. P. H. (2013). Online victim tracking and tracing system (ViTTS) for major incident casualties. *Prehospital and Disaster Medicine, 28*(5), 445–453. doi:10.1017/S1049023X13003567

Medical Reserve Corps. (2014). *Find a unit.* Retrieved from https://www.medicalreservecorps.gov/HomePage

Mitchell, D. (2010). *Facebook application "I'm a Flu Fighter" announced by Sebelius.* Retrieved from http://www.emaxhealth.com/1275/90/35120/facebook-application-im-flu-fighter-announced-sebelius.html

Occupational Safety and Health Administration. (2007). *Pandemic influenza preparedness and response guidance for healthcare workers and healthcare employers.* Retrieved from http://www.osha.gov/Publications/OSHA_pandemic_health.pdf

Reed, C., Angulo, F. J., Swerdlow, D. L., Lipsitch, M., Meltzer, M. I., Jernigan, D., & Finelli, L. (2009, December). Estimates of the prevalence of pandemic (H1N1) 2009, United States, April-July 2009. *Emerging infectious disease.* Retrieved from http://wwwnc.cdc.gov/eid/article/15/12/09-1413_article. doi: 10.3201/eid1512.091413.

Slepski, L., & Littleton-Kearney, M. T. (2010). Disaster nursing educational competencies. In R. Powers & E. Daily (Eds.), *International disaster nursing* (pp. 549–559). New York, NY: Cambridge University Press.

Stanley, J, (2005). Disaster competency development and integration in nursing education. *Nursing Clinics of North America, 40*(3), 453–467.

Todd, B. (January, 2014). Middle East Respiratory Syndrome (MERS-CoV). *American Journal of Nursing, 114*(1), 56–59.

University of Pittsburgh. (2014a). *About the National Retail Data Monitor.* Retrieved from https://www.rods.pitt.edu/site/content/blogsection/4/42/

University of Pittsburgh. (2014b). *The RODS open source project.* Retrieved from https://www.rods.pitt.edu/site/content/view/15/36/

White House. (2003, February 28). *Homeland Security Presidential Directive 5: Management of domestic incidents.* Retrieved from http://www.fws.gov/Contaminants/FWS_OSCP_05/fwscontingencyappendices/A-NCP-NRP/HSPD-5.pdf

World Health Organization. (2007). *The contribution of nursing and midwifery in emergencies: Report of a WHO consultation.* WHO Headquarters, Geneva, November 22–24. Retrieved from http://www.who.int/hac/events/2006/nursing_consultation_report_sept07.pdf

World Health Organization. (2008). *Integrating emergency preparedness and response into undergraduate nursing curriculum.* Retrieved from http://whqlibdoc.who.int/hq/2008/WHO_HAC_BRO_08.7_eng.pdf

World Health Organization. (2009, December). *Strengthening WHO's institutional capacity for humanitarian health action: A five-year programme progress report.* Retrieved from http://www.who.int/hac/events/5years_progress_report_brochure.pdf

World Health Organization. (2010). *WHO recommendations for the post-pandemic period.* Retrieved from http://www.who.int/csr/disease/swineflu/notes/briefing_20100810/en/index.html

World Health Organization. (2013). *Cumulative number of confirmed human cases for avian influenza A (H5N1) reported to WHO, 2003-2013.* Retrieved from http://www.who.int/influenza/human_animal_interface/EN_GIP_20130604CumulativeNumberH5N1cases.pdf

World Health Organization. (2014). *Overview of global humanitarian response 2014.* Retrieved from https://docs.unocha.org/sites/dms/CAP/Overview_of_Global_Humanitarian_Response_2014.pdf

34

Federal Healthcare Sector Nursing Informatics*

Capt. Margaret S. Beaubien / Murielle S. Beene / Christine Boltz / Lee Ann Harford / LTC Mike Ludwig / Daniel F. Marsh / Joel L. Parker / COL Katherine Taylor Pearson / Capt. Stephanie J. Raps

• OBJECTIVES

1. Describe the history of Nursing Informatics in the federal healthcare sector.
2. Briefly describe the various roles of nursing informaticists in the federal sector.
3. Articulate how technology supports information sharing and collaboration with emphasis on the unique populations within the federal sector.
4. Discuss the high-risk and high-impact informatics challenges facing the federal government.

• KEY WORDS

Federal Healthcare Sector
Nursing informatics roles and responsibilities
Informatics technology and challenges in federal government
Federal nursing informatics
Military nursing informatics
Veteran affairs nursing informatics

THE EMERGENCE OF NURSING INFORMATICS WITHIN THE FEDERAL HEALTHCARE SECTOR

Introduction

The U.S. Federal healthcare system is one of the largest integrated health delivery entities in the world and is a dynamic "systems of systems" architectural model. The system has a long history of innovation, adoption, research, development, implementation, and evaluation in technological advances. Over six decades, federal nursing informaticists have been at the forefront of various professional development initiatives and computer applications (AMIA, 2013b). The federal healthcare system supports the growth and advancement of professional nursing roles, standards, and technologies. The federal nursing sector supports healthcare informatics in diverse practice settings and agencies, but the focus of this chapter is limited to the Department of Defense (DoD) Military Health Services (MHS) of the Air Force, Army, Navy; the Department of Veterans Affairs (DVA); and the U.S. Public Health Services (USPHS).

---

*Disclaimer: The views expressed in this article are those of the author(s) and do not necessarily reflect the official policy or position of the Air Force, Army, Navy, the United States (U.S.) Department of Defense, the U.S. Department of Veterans, or the U.S. Government.

Federal Sector Ecosystem

The federal healthcare sector often is referred to as the "public" or "government" segment. The discipline of nursing informatics within the federal sector is the origin of numerous innovations and milestones cutting across diverse public healthcare agencies. Collaboration and shared communication among all healthcare professionals are vital to providing the delivery of quality, effective care across the spectrum of nursing care while ensuring the use of nursing processes in the area of informatics. A brief description of the three federal healthcare entities is described next.

Department of Defense (DoD) Healthcare Landscape

The DoD Military Health System (MHS) provides global healthcare services to over 9.6 million beneficiaries to include active duty service members, National Guard and Reserve members, retirees, and their families (Military Health System, 2012). The MHS is composed of over 130,000 Air Force, Army, and Navy healthcare professionals (Military Health System, 2012). The MHS manages individual health benefits and costs through the TRICARE program, similar to private insurance companies such as Blue Cross/Blue Shield. TRICARE brings together the uniformed services resources and supplements them with networks of civilian healthcare professionals, institutions, pharmacies, and suppliers providing access to high-quality healthcare services. A high degree of interaction between the public and private healthcare delivery systems is necessary to various support programs, such as the Wounded Warrior Project which provides care for the severely injured active service members and veterans (TRICARE, 2013).

MHS healthcare professions provide care and treatments in a variety of geographic and technical environments. The community of care system is an interwoven network of 52 "brick and mortar" inpatient hospitals and medical centers; 15 facilities are located in foreign countries. The MHS has over 640 ambulatory surgery/outpatient care clinics and dental clinics. Health Information Technology (HIT) legacy systems and emerging technology are utilized in stateside medical treatment facilities, such as hospital and clinics, and overseas in austere battlefields facilities, tents, hospital ships, and aircrafts used for patient evacuations and aeromedical transport. The various locations and facilities add to the complexity and challenges of using information technology for clinical care. Consequently, Tri-Service nursing informaticists may find themselves practicing in the traditional hospital settings,

in non-traditional settings aboard Navy vessels such as the USNS Mercy or USNS Comfort, on a forward-deployed battlefield, in a humanitarian mission, or recovery support mission from a natural disaster. A few of the many humanitarian missions include operations during the 9/11 attacks in New York; relief to those impacted by Hurricane Katrina in New Orleans; and the response and recovery efforts of the earthquake survivors in Haiti.

Department of Veteran Affairs (DVA) Landscape

The primary mission of the Department of Veteran's Affairs (VA) is to maximize the veteran's activities of daily living throughout the continuum of care. The VA is comprised of an integrated healthcare system reaching across all 50 states and several U.S. Territories, with an eligible population of 22 million veterans of which 8.8 million are enrolled at VA facilities (United States Department of Veterans Affairs, 2012). In 2013, the VA had over 151 acute care hospitals and 827 Community Base Outpatient Clinics (CBOC). Daily, the VA sees over 200,000 outpatients, 6000 emergency room visits, and has an average inpatient census of nearly 11,000. A unique entry point into the VA is through "Vet Centers," which are community-based outreach clinics, where both active duty and veterans can access healthcare benefits including individual and family counseling and educational benefits.

Currently, VA has over 59,000 full- and part-time professional nurses; 283 are recognized as informatics nurses (United States Department of Veterans Affairs, 2012). The VA is known for providing world-class healthcare and is also a leader in informatics and successfully developing information technologies. Examples include Computerized Patient Record System (CPRS), Bar Code Medication Administration (BCMA), and Personal Health record (PHR), discussed later in the chapter. Telehealth and Telehome Care is increasingly used to provide care to veterans (United States Department of Veterans Affairs, 2012).

Department of Health and Human Services (DHHS) Landscape

The DHHS is charged with protecting the health of the American public and providing essential human services, such as Medicare and Medicaid. Within DHHS, the U.S. Public Health Service (USPHS) has programs dedicated to disease prevention and control; biomedical research; food and drug protection as well as medical device safety; mental health and substance abuse management; healthcare system and resource enhancements; and medical care for underserved and special needs populations (USPHS, 2013a). The USPHS Commissioned Corps of uniformed public health professionals respond to public health needs and to advancing the science of public health practices. Many of the USPHS scientists and clinicians were involved with early research studies and innovations in information technology.

The Office of the National Coordinator (ONC) has the distinct role, under DHHS, to oversee national e-Health programs including the adoption and implementation of electronic health records. In particular, the Agency for Healthcare Research & Quality (AHRQ), the National Institutes of Health (NIH), and the National Library of Medicine (NLM) provide research funding supporting the development of clinical informatics and emerging healthcare technologies (USPHS, 2013c). An enormous number of innovations and computer programming technologies received federal grant investments from these agencies.

A Snapshot of Nursing Informatics Pioneers in the Federal Sector

The genetic strands of the nursing profession can be traced back to the Crimean War where Florence Nightingale cared for the soldiers in the battlefields and Clara Barton founded the American Red Cross (Osbolt & Saba, 2008). Both Nightingale and Barton proved to be early informaticists, as evidence through their documentation practices and use of data for early statistical documentation that can be thought of as the "big data" of the 1800s.

A number of contemporary informaticists started their professional nursing careers as military officers or federal public health commissioned nurses. In the 1950s, Army nurse Lieutenant Colonel (Ret.) Harriet Werley served as a nurse researcher at Walter Reed Army Institute of Research her studies included data processing initiatives with IBM and was instrumental in the development of the Nursing Minimum Data Set (NMDS) (Osbolt, 2003). Retired Army Colonel Nancy Staggers, another important military nurse informaticists, earned the first PhD in Nursing Informatics from the University of Maryland and conducted research on human–computer interactions and system usability studies (AMIA, 2013b).

Within the USPHS Commissioned Corps, Virginia Saba, Kathleen McCormick, and Carol Romano were nursing officers who leaned forward and spearheaded nursing informatics into the twenty-first Century. Dr. Saba promoted the use of computer technology to solve problems in administration, education, research, and clinical nursing practice. Dr. Kathleen McCormick began her informatics career at the NIH as an informatics scientist and clinical trial researcher. She conducted early nursing informatics initiatives and achieved major advances in nursing informatics including the development of the

Computerized Clinical Decision Support program for the AHRQ (AMIA, 2013b). Dr. Carol Romano is highly recognized for the design and implementation of one of the first computerized medical information systems in 1976.

The twenty-first century federal nurse informaticists have greatly expanded in scope because of the early efforts and innovations in computer technologies.

Historical Landmarks in Federal Technological Advancements

The journey to nursing informatics as we know it today started in the 1970s with key military and federal innovations and initiatives in computer programming and applications. Early studies at the AHRQ led to healthcare system development to include nursing care planning and clinical documentation. Simultaneously, the DoD designed one of the first clinical computer systems known as the Tri-Service Medical Information System (TRIMIS) (Osbolt & Saba, 2008). In the mid-1970s and early 1980s, both the DoD's Composite Healthcare System (CHCS) and the VA's Veterans Health Information Systems and Technology Architecture (VistA) developed similar but distinct "government off the shelf" (GOTS) electronic medical records using the Massachusetts General Hospital Utility Multi-Programming System (MUMPS) programming language. In the 1980s, the VistA information system was legally declared as open source technology and was available for unrestricted use within both the public and private sectors (Osbolt & Saba, 2008). The federal sector was also responsible for the development of national reference databases such as the NLM Medline and most recently the software-licensing program of SNOMED for both public and commercial entities (Osbolt & Saba, 2008).

Federal Legislative Role in Nursing Informatics

The Federal government plays a critical legislative role in the emergence of healthcare informatics in both the public and private sectors. The primary goal is to share healthcare information. Healthcare reform laws and regulations enacted by Congress expanded the opportunities for nurses to work outside of clinical practice, and to engage in emerging roles like information management and technological. The roles of nursing informaticists were incorporated into healthcare policy, research, consultation, academia, and computer applications. The federal laws are mandated for public healthcare organizations, usually results in early adoption of information technology. These mandates often "pushed" to multiple federal agencies to develop and implement new or immature technology. For example, in 2004, Executive Order (EO) 13335 advanced the development, adoption, and implementation of HIT standards nationally through collaboration among public and private interests (Federal Register, 2004). This mandate provided authority for both public and private healthcare sectors to forge partnerships to established interoperable HIT standards and technologies.

Chapter Overview

The remainder of the chapter discusses the evolution of nursing informatics roles, responsibilities, and competencies in multiple federal agencies. The major information management and technological milestones within specific federal agencies are presented. Finally, the major challenges facing nursing informatics and HIT in the federal health sector are discussed.

FEDERAL NURSING INFORMATICS ROLES AND RESPONSIBILITIES

Nurses in the federal sector have been influential leaders in Health Information Technology (HIT) and informatics for decades. Federal leaders in nursing informatics made significant contributions to the profession and led various aspects of design, testing, implementation, training, and support for a diverse range of clinical information systems and technologies (AMIA, 2013a). Federal entities were early adopters of electronic health records (EHR), computerized provider order entry (CPOE), administrative HIT applicative to include workload management and clinical documentation systems. With the rapid proliferation of HIT, federal nursing informatics specialists continue to be indispensable leaders in the advancement of healthcare in our nation as evidenced by their high level of involvement, adaptability, and management skills.

Federal agencies embrace the role of nurses within HIT, but standardization and formalization of nursing informatics roles and responsibilities are at various stages of maturity within each of the federal agencies (American Nurses Association, 2008). Today, federal informatics nurses serve in roles ranging from direct patient care, where informatics is an additional duty, to that of the expert Informatics Nurse Specialist (INS), serving in enterprise level leadership. Significant efforts have been made to formalize and standardize the role of the INS within the federal agencies. Regardless of the maturity level of the organization with regard to INS role development, INSs are actively engaged throughout all levels of the organization.

Many nurses within the federal sector started their informatics career by serving as a functional representative or "super user" during the development, training, and implementation of a HIT system or application. The responsibilities of the federal nurse informaticist include systems development and implementation, privacy and safety measures, quality initiatives, and informatics education. Under various titles, these experts typically lead or participate in key informatics, documentation, or quality meetings at the facility level, and the level of education and formalization of positions varies between federal services.

The VA and DoD MHS support various forms of nursing informatics involvement at the leadership or strategic level of the organization. Federal nursing informaticists can assume roles such as Chief Medical, Health, or Nursing Information Officer; Chief Information Officer; or clinical informatics consultant. The INS serves as an expert advising authority with regard to all HIT-related issues, and many are involved in the strategic development of numerous initiatives to include informatics workforce development; HIT acquisition, governance, and budgeting; management of clinical systems; policy and program development; workflow analysis and development.

The federal sector also presents unique INS opportunities largely due to the large size of the organizations and the unique missions. Regardless of role or title, nurses with informatics education and training utilize their skills in every healthcare setting, to include military deployments within a combat zone. Recently, DoD initiated research on the role of deployed nurse informaticists which resulted in pilot projects for studying overseas combat deployment positions and which may lead to authorizing formal positions for INSs within these environments. The spectrum of career broadening opportunities for federal INSs ranges from data analysis and business intelligence to that of managing the acquisitions and programs for new "cradle to grave" clinical systems.

Federal agencies build on the foundations established decades ago from early federal informatics nursing leaders by continuing to formalize the roles and responsibilities of the informatics nurse. In the microcosm of the federal government, it is possible to realize the significant potential of an integrated healthcare system. The collaborative nature between and among the different federal agencies have allowed our nursing informatics leaders to learn from the various roles and responsibilities, especially as the roles evolve to ensure the successful development, implementation, and sustainment of our future national electronic health records systems. Today, the federal agencies continue to work together to build a professional roadmap that will meet the needs of new HIT systems while providing the most effective, safe delivery of quality healthcare for our military service personnel and veterans.

Federal Nursing Informatics Competencies

The development and implementation of federal nursing informatics competencies has followed an organizational and facility-specific path. The Army chartered a comprehensive and methodological approach to competencies for healthcare workforce, including nurse informaticists. Their strategy documents several role-specific competencies for each identified role such as the CMIO, clinical workflow analysts, and clinical systems trainer. The strategy also included specific role profiles, integrating position description with competencies for the position. Unique in the workforce-level plan are metrics for proficiency growth, satisfaction, and mentorship, providing valuable feedback for strategy update, refinement, and application.

VA nurses practice in a wide array of informatics-related positions such as Clinical Applications Coordinator, Bar Code Medication Administration Coordinator, Data Analyst, Researcher, Software Development and Portfolio Manager, Terminologist, and Informatics Educator. VA healthcare informatics career development strives toward developing a common base of competencies integral for all health informatics roles, which further supports the multidisciplinary professional arena in which they practice.

The Air Force is currently exploring organized structure options for the future of INS. The current competencies are related to the clinical informatics consultant roles embedded within the Headquarters of the Air Force. Supporting the Office of the Chief Information Officer, these competencies include collaboration in new technology life cycle development, policy formation, deployment of technologies, and business practice optimization. These competencies ensure the nurses are engaged in the strategic implementation of HIT initiatives with the beginnings of operational considerations in workflow analysis and tools that align with business practice optimization.

Navy's approach to nursing informatics competences takes a more local, facility-specific way to identify and build (Health Information and Management Systems Society [HIMSS], 2011) the required roles and competencies to include common training resources from the American Nurses Association, HIMSS, ONC, etc. Frequently the education of the nursing informaticist was based on individual career objectives and resulted in the nurse obtaining a graduate certificate in informatics from an accredited university, informatics certification via the American Nurse Credentialing Center or HIMSS, or acquiring new knowledge from such courses as American Medical Informatics Association's 10 × 10 offering. Competencies for these positions were not centralized and were often integrated into position descriptions, making translation and comparison a challenge. Navy medicine is actively developing the role and training paths for future implementation.

Professional Career Development

The federal healthcare space consists of an array of career paths and workforce maturity for informatics nurses (American Health Information Management Association [AHIMA] and American Medical Informatics Association [AMIA], 2006). However, the federal sector shares the commonality of informatics being a transforming career creating multiple new and unique opportunities in leadership and management of change (Gardner et al., 2009; The Tiger Team, 2007).

One example of new career paths stems from the VA baseline assessment of the "State of the informatics workforce in 2011." The results assisted in developing a comprehensive workforce roadmap to develop health informatics competencies, career paths, and communities that prepare the VA informatics workforce to engage in this transformation. Findings portrayed a VA informatics workforce that was primarily rooted in informal informatics preparation or training that consisted of self-trained individuals. At the time of the study, the workforce did not have clearly defined position descriptions or career paths and the healthcare professionals struggled to define and describe their role within the organization. As a result, several workforce development efforts have been implemented to address these deficiencies to include an online course, "Introduction to Health Informatics," that is based upon the ONC informatics curriculum (The Office of the National Coordinator for Health Information Technology, 2013) and offered in partnership with Washington State Bellevue College. Additional VA efforts include a health informatics video lecture series, and a health informatics certificate program aimed at training thousands of clinicians in applied health and medical informatics within 10 years called AMIA 10 × 10 (AMIA, 2013a).

Similarly, the Department of Defense has a rich history of informatics experience. Army medicine formalized the role of the CMIO in 2008, establishing processes and a workforce structure to support clinical informatics and HIT operations within the Army. With the establishment of the CMIO, the leadership successfully obtained authorization for a multi-disciplinary informatics skill identifier for the clinical informatics workforce. The skill identifier for nursing requires a Master's degree in informatics, completion of an Army-specific functional proponent course, and two years of healthcare informatics experience.

Navy medicine recently began to identify positions for nurse informaticists. The informatics positions are frequently inherent collateral duties embedded to the nurse's primary responsibilities and role. Informatics roles are often specific to the organization's current HIT needs, whether it is implementation of the electronic health record, intranet or patient portals, or facility-specific systems for patient acuity and nurse staffing. Several headquarters and specialty command positions do provide full-time nursing informatics positions in clinical informatics.

The Air Force similarly identified the need for specialty training and focused career broadening experience in nursing informatics. In 2011, the Air Force began the nurse informatics fellowship program. In 2013, the clinical informatics consultant positions were realigned which ultimately created a path at the enterprise and facility level. The tactical level continues to be developed, as those nurses are involved as "super users" and in working groups that serve as additional duties based on interest. The Air Force continues to look at the precedent set by the other federal partners and national organizations as it builds a path that meets the Air Force INS needs for the future (Staggers, 2007).

EVOLUTION OF TECHNOLOGY

The Department of Defense (DoD) and the Department of Veterans Affairs (VA) have been leaders in the development and implementation of electronic health records. The Federal health sector provides a wide range of services to active duty service members, National Guard, Reserve members, veterans, retirees, and their families. Multiple environments and tools actively support developing interoperable systems, as result clinical documentation linking the continuity of care faces many unique challenges.

Department of Defense

The evolution of the EHR, for the DOD MHS, began in 1987 with the government-owned Composite Computerized Healthcare System (CHCS) (Director, Operation, Test and Evaluation, 2000). Deployed in the 1990s, CHCS was a first-generation EHR and supported physician order entry. A nurse's role in using this system was to check or validate physician orders and result retrieval of laboratory and radiology results (Skinner, 2008).

CHCS continues to provide different patient views depending on user roles; clinicians are able to view a patient's current and past medical history and medications. Other outpatient functions include verifying eligibility for care and scheduling appointments.

In 1988, the first application of a commercially developed inpatient record called CIS (Clinical Information Systems) later to be known as Essentris was implemented at an MHS facility. Initially the inpatient documentation was aimed at labor and delivery units and the ability to capture the wave forms from mothers in labor; meeting the critical need to capture and store wave forms, where traditional wax encoded strips deteriorated. System deployments then moved to the critical care units and eventually into the other inpatient units. By 2011, all 58 MHS inpatient facilities worldwide had Essentris installed and implemented (Defense Health Clinical System [DHIMS], 2011).

The MHS began to explore options for an updated electronic documentation process for recording clinician outpatient encounters. By late 1998 a third version of a concept of operations for CHCS II (Composite Healthcare System II), later to be called AHLTA, (Armed Forces Health Longitudinal Technology Application) was being circulated. In 2004 the deployment of AHLTA, the DoD's global EHR, made it the largest ambulatory EHR in the world with a single clinical data repository (CDR), serving over 9 million beneficiaries (Skinner, 2008). AHLTA provides a secure, standards-based, enterprise-wide medical information system that generates, maintains, and provides 24/7 access to the electronic health records of active duty military, their family members, and others entitled to DoD healthcare. Lastly, in 2012 the MHS deployed a Secure Messaging system, similar to e-mail, to communicate with outpatient community. The Air Force took the Secure Messaging system one step further and added a Personal Health Record feature to this system.

AHLTA offered staff a new capability for decision support and predictive analysis through data mining as a result of healthcare providers using a structured taxonomy for writing clinical notes and the capture of the data in a central repository. This data mining used automated computational and statistical tools and techniques to evaluate and analyze large data sets and assist predicting potential disease/illness patterns. AHLTA provides informatics nurses with the ability to search the repository for previous outpatient encounters within the MHS and the ability to retrieve patient data prior to a scheduled outpatient appointment or conduct a follow-up based on care documentation. Some patient information available includes vital signs, allergies, medications, demographics, past medical history, previous encounter notes, problem lists, and lab results.

AHLTA captures information in the fixed facility outpatient environment. The ability to document care onboard ships and within the operational field was later developed to meet the specific needs of the remote/mobile environment. AHLTA-Mobile was designed to capture information on a handheld device and store first responder clinical documentation. Initial injury and illness clinical documentation is then transferred to AHLTA-Theater (used in remote locations) and onto the Theater Medical Data Store (TMDS). Unique features of the mobile application allow for operations in no to low communications environments, ability to pre-populate demographic data (Fact Sheet, n.d.-a). AHLTA-Theater has the same user interface look as AHLTA and operates in a stand-alone environment utilizing a store and forward capability updating information when connected to a network and eventually updating the AHLTA CDR (Fact Sheet, n.d.-b).

A system of considerable note for the deploying forces is the Theater Medical Information Program-Joint (TMIP-J). It is a multi-Service automated system that integrates sustaining bases medical applications for use by deployed forces including all of the variations of AHLTA, CHCS, Defense Medical Logistics Standard Support (DMLSS). The system provides an EHR, medical command and control, medical logistics, and patient movement and tracking for the theater environment (Department of Defense, n.d.).

Department of Veterans Affairs

The VA dates its computerization efforts back to the early 1980s with the advent and subsequent deployment of Decentralized Hospital Computer Program (DHCP) across the VA enterprise. Locally developed applications helped evolve DHCP as new needs and technologies emerged to greatly enhance patient care. DCHP integrated over time and evolved into the Veterans Health Information Systems and Technology Architecture (VistA). VistA is deployed universally across the VA at more than 1500 sites of care, including each Veterans Affairs Medical Center (VAMC), Community-Based Outpatient Clinic (CBOC), Community Living Center, and at nearly 300 VA Vet Centers. A key to the evolution of VistA was the development and deployment of the Computerized Patient Record System (CPRS)—a graphical user interface (GUI) that interacts with the VistA common functions and integrated applications via reusable interfaces. VistA, CPRS, and a variety of other VistA-based applications support day-to-day clinical and administrative operations at local VA healthcare facilities (VistA Evolution Executive Summary, 2013).

In 1992, a registered nurse from the Topeka Kansas VAMC was returning a rental car, and wondered if rental cars could be barcoded and scanned why not medication? This was the origin of the development of Bar Code Medication Administration (BCMA) (Coyle & Heinen, 2005). As a component of the VistA-based electronic medical record and CPOE, the VA implemented BCMA in 1999. Since its inception, BCMA has moved through several versions to evolve into sophisticated solution-driven clinical software. Nurses have continually assisted in the design of the software. Nurses continue to provide input to the software development to create a safe environment for practicing nursing and for ensuring patient safety and to expand the use of the software to other clinical scenarios

such as lab, blood bank, and clinical inventory. Additionally, the Indian Health Service (IHS) Office of Information Technology (OIT) Electronic Health Record (EHR) Deployment Team, Veterans Health Administration's (VHA) Bar Code Resource Office (BCRO), and VA's OIT continue efforts for BCMA implementation to expand the patient safety benefits of BCMA into IHS and tribal facilities through partnering agreements.

My HealtheVet is another key component of the VA's evolution of technology (United States Department of Veterans Affairs, 2013c). My HealtheVet (MHV) is the official Personal Health Record (PHR) of the Department of Veterans Affairs. MHV offers enhanced online health tools, services, and resources for both the user and the clinician 24/7 and 365 days per year.

The VA continues to address the evolution of technology, recognizes the contribution of the Open Source community in the future of Electronic Health Records, and was instrumental in the establishment of the Open Source Electronic Health Record Agent (OSEHRA) (EHR Intelligence, 2012). The VA has enlisted OSEHRA to develop future enhancements to VistA. This decision was part of a joint effort with the DoD to store all veterans' and service members' health records electronically using a single source as part of the Department's pioneering activities in the OSEHRA community, VA has contributed the VistA code to the OSEHRA effort.

Within the VA, the development of the next-generation Electronic Health Record Evolution has been linked to multiple efforts. In 2009, President Barack Obama charged the Departments of Veterans Affairs (VA) and Defense (DoD) to "work together to define and build a seamless system of integration" of electronic health records (EHR) (Lee, 2009). In 2011, the VA and DoD Secretaries committed to developing a single, joint, common, interagency Electronic Health Record (iEHR) by 2017. This approach was intended to overcome certain challenges to system interoperability. In early 2013, the Departments recognized increased costs and risks associated with the initial implementation path and proposed a new strategy. The Departments' redefined efforts as seamless sharing of interoperable health data between EHR systems. Under this new framework, with continued emphasis on interoperability, each agency is responsible for its own EHR system. VA has committed to use existing VA Health Information Systems and Technology Architecture (VistA) and incrementally deliver new functionality through a VistA Evolution Program. The mission of the program is to advance the VistA technical platform to promote improved outcomes to quality, safety, efficiency, and satisfaction in healthcare for Veterans through supporting patient-centered team-based care, enhancing clinical reasoning, and providing EHR system interoperability with the DoD and other healthcare partners (VistA Evolution Executive Summary, 2013).

Interoperability Between the DoD and VA

An additional concept to discuss regarding breakthroughs in technology is the interoperability data sharing initiatives between the DoD and the VA. Here is an overview of some of the most widely used efforts, which will be expanded on in the section on challenges.

The Federal Health Information Exchange (FHIE) Program was the initial interagency initiative between the DoD and the VA (http://www.va.gov/EXHIBIT300/docs/FHIE.pdf, 2009), enabling a secure, one-way transmission of protected electronic health information from DoD to VA on service members who had separated from the Armed Forces. FHIE uses existing clinical systems and began populating the VA repository in 2002 (United States Department of Veterans Affairs, 2002). As more patients began to seek care from both the DoD and VA simultaneously the need for a bi-directional exchange of data in real time created the Bidirectional Health Information Exchange (BHIE). BHIE utilizes a middleware, hardware, and software framework that provides a secure, bi-directional, real-time interagency exchange of clinical data and patient demographics between the DoD and VA health information systems. Once again driven by the need to improve patient safety for those patients seeking care from both the DoD and VA the Clinical Data Repository/Health Data Repository (CHDR) initiative emerged (http://vaww.va.gov/VADODHEALTHCARE/Clinical_Data_Repository_Health_Data_Repository_CHDR.asp). CHDR consists of an interface between DoD's Clinical Data Repository (CDR) of AHLTA and VA's Health Data Repository (HDR). CHDR enables the bi-directional exchange of computable outpatient pharmacy and medication allergy data and enhances decision support by cross-referencing drug–drug and drug–allergy interactions. CHDR was an important step forward toward "interoperability" and represented a departure from "viewable" data.

One last initiative on interoperability is the Virtual Lifetime Electronic Record (VLER). The VLER not only shares data between the DoD and VA but also shares the exchange of data between private healthcare providers. This is a multi-faceted business and technology initiative that includes a portfolio of health, benefits, personnel, and administrative information sharing capabilities (United States Department of Veterans Affairs, 2013b). This functionality provides Veterans, Service members, their families, care-givers, and service providers with a single source of information for health and benefits needs in a way that is secure and authorized by the Veteran or Service member. When VLER is fully implemented, all information needed to quickly and accurately provide services and benefits to our Veterans and Service members will be exchanged electronically and proactively, putting the right information in front of the right people at the right time for them to take action.

The DoD and VA have been early adopters of technologies and in many cases have pushed the nation in the direction of adopting electronic medical records. This section has focused on some of those technologies driven by the needs of the battlefield and en route care of the service member and the long-term care provided by the Veterans Administration. The next section will focus on some of the challenges the DoD and VA have overcome to continue to improve the delivery of healthcare to those they serve.

CHALLENGES

The remainder of this chapter focuses on some of the unique technical and business challenges that are part of the federal healthcare space.

One of the earliest examples of the contributions of the DoD to the information age was the development of the Advanced Research Projects Agency Network (ARPANET) (Ramsaroop, Ball, Beaulieu, & Douglas, 2001). In 1966 the Defense Advanced Research Project Agency (DARPA) contracted with individuals in Cambridge, Massachusetts, on a project to create a wide area network. Using packet switching technology it became the first nationwide digital network and connected academic computer centers working on DoD projects. By 1972 a total of 29 educational institutions were linked to one computer in the DoD. Hence the start of "internetworking" (Ramsaroop et al., 2001) as it was originally known or the Internet. However, once other computer networks began connecting to the network the military's concern for security caused them to break off their segment forming the MILNET in the early 1980s.

Security concerns in relation to the network became even more important to the DoD and now represent one of the unique challenges setting them apart even from the VA. The DoD has the obligation to secure not only protected health information (PHI) or personally identifiable information (PII), but the sensitive data residing on the same network as information considered sensitive but unclassified and is intended for official use only (FOUO). From the original MILNET the DoD now operates two separate segments, the Non-classified Internet Protocol (IP) Router Network (NIPRNet) carrying FOUO information for DoD customers to provide "protected access to the public internet" (Defense Information Systems Agency [DISA], 2013) and the Secret Internet Protocol

Router Network (SIPRNet) which carries classified data. The classified data may include healthcare data from the battlefield.

Although the VA and all federal agencies have the same need to protect PHI and PII just as any private or commercial entity, the uniqueness of the military mission of the DoD creates additional layers of security and strict requirements are in place for personnel to access the network. Information Assurance (IA) is a risk management function to protect information management and information technology (IM/IT) investments by ensuring the Confidentiality, Integrity, and Availability (CIA) of information. In order to do so, the DoD establishes enclaves or a collection of computing environments or services under the control of a single authority or security policy, including personnel and physical security. This may create conflicts with entities, which follow different security policies than the DoD such as the VA and Office of the National Coordinator for Health and Human Services (ONC/HHS) for National Health Information Exchange (HIE).

Any IM/IT capability logically crossing the boundaries of an enclave such as data transfer or exchange requires an "Authority to Connect" (ATC) across that boundary. Across the DoD, there are constraints regarding what policies apply to what type of boundary such as another military service, another agency such as VA, or the Internet. Access by a user directly to data in that enclave requires the use of approved access request processes and technical controls. This includes requirements/constraints, which may not be owned by IM/IT. Examples include background investigations, need to know, management of Foreign Nationals, etc. The challenge to deploying any new software becomes the time involved in making sure that the application and/or system has been properly assessed and permission has been granted to allow access for that system to be connected to the network and can take six months or more, putting a deployment beyond the scheduled start date if these activities are not considered as part of the entire project management plan.

The connectivity to shore-based applications from onboard ships, remote and geographically austere locations is another challenge. Developing applications with the ability to store and forward data when connectivity is available via secure channels from a deployed environment is a way to overcome this challenge. Satellite availability is devoted to ship operations and combatant commanders in the field taking priority over medical operations. Conducting operations with minimal Internet capability, referred to as low or no communications environments, is similar to what healthcare providers in rural areas may experience in remote areas where even cell reception is problematic due to the lack of penetration of wireless networks.

Funding

The ability to fund medical care including the buildings, people, services, equipment, etc., in the federal government is not the same as in the private sector and may introduce new challenges to the informatics nurse. An appropriations bill, which is a legislative motion passed by Congress, is necessary before any government agency can spend money. Appropriations are used to fund discretionary programs and are generally approved on an annual basis. This also means that any funds appropriated must be spent or obligated by the end of the fiscal year and cannot be carried over from year to year. If Congress has not passed a new appropriation, then an appropriation bill called a continuing resolution may be passed which allows for continued spending for a short period of time at the same rate as the previous year. If there is no appropriation, the government faces an Anti-Deficiency Act violation if they try to spend money on any activity for which there is no appropriation.

For the DoD, the National Defense Authorization Act voted on by Congress gives the DoD the ability to spend money and provides specific instructions for the funding. In the H.R. 4310 (112th): National Defense Authorization Act for Fiscal Year 2013 (House of Representatives, 2012) the act divided funding into divisions in which the Department of Defense Authorizations was one of four divisions. Based on these appropriations the breakdown of funding for health information technology is a part of the Defense Health Programs (DHP) budget and is later divided into one of eight categories to include HIT.

The DHP Appropriations for just the health information technology consists of Operation & Maintenance (O&M), Procurement and Research, Development, Test, & Evaluation (RDT&E) funds. Some primarily deployable healthcare activities and research functions are funded by the Military Departments of the Army, Navy, and Air Force through their O&M, Procurement, RDT&E, and Military Personnel (MilPers) appropriations. The health plan comprises the largest portion of the Defense Health Programs budget and is a significant amount of money in the overarching Defense budget. Information Technology (IT) is a smaller portion of that, making the challenge between how to drive efficiencies in spending on sustainment of the budget for HIT and create room for modernization. Many of the HIT projects are created with initial funding as special projects, but the sustainment is rarely funded at the same time causing funding deficits into the future.

Whereas the DoD requires annual appropriations, the VA has some two-year appropriations. The (VA) Budget is also apportioned into six program areas. Two areas are related to informatics, the first is Medical Care Programs, which funds a broad range of primary care, specialized care, and related medical and social services, including education and training for physician residents and other healthcare trainees and medical research and development. The second area is Information Technology, which funds operations and maintenance, staffing, and development. The Assistant Secretary for Information and Technology controls the IT appropriation for information and technology.

The centralized model for HIT funding is unique among federal agencies as many of the other agencies organize HIT funding by business lines. This impacts the degree to which individual Administrations such as Health, Benefits, and Memorials influence and control funding decisions for HIT projects. Prioritization of HIT funding is based on decisions reached by VA leadership and the HIT governance boards, and is based upon the VA Strategic Plan and Agency Priority Goals (United States Department of Veterans Affairs, 2013a). Prioritization is accomplished across the three principal sub-categories of Pay and administrative funding which funds the HIT staff and covers overhead costs of program management; mandatory sustainment and information security which includes necessary but non-critical sustainment efforts to continue or enhance the Office of Information Technology (OIT) operations; and development, including marginal sustainment, to cover development, modernization, and enhancements of projects.

More than half of the appropriation covers expenses for mandatory sustainment and information security, which fund the VA's HIT infrastructure, including computer, hardware, software maintenance, networks, and phone systems at all the VA hospitals, outpatient clinics, regional benefit offices, and cemeteries. Spending for staffing and administration is the second largest category; together, these compromise almost 75% of the HIT budget (United States Department of Veterans Affairs, 2013a). Development and other minor needs comprise the remainder of the HIT budget. VA is challenged with increased sustainment costs, which increasingly limit the funding available for developmental needs. This is due in part to the recent additions of HIT products without a commensurate removal of older legacy systems. Determining a divestiture strategy is a key driver in HIT program planning for the near future.

VA is also challenged with the extra effort required to program funding for HIT needs where there is a difference between Veterans Health Administration (VHA) funding and HIT funding. VHA receives two-year advance appropriations for some of their medical care appropriation accounts (Medical Services, Medical Support and Compliance and Medical Facilities). This affords more stable planning and programming, but can cause difficulties when HIT is only funded with one-year appropriations (United States Department of Veterans Affairs, 2013a).

Standards and Interoperability

Interoperability is a key part of sharing data and there are a number of activities focused on creating interoperable standards. As noted in the previous section DoD and VA have a number of data sharing initiatives, from viewing data such as through FHIE and BHIE to actionable data that triggers decision support via CHDR. To achieve computable semantic interoperability, both agencies standardize their data for each given clinical domain (pharmacy, allergy, etc.) and exchange the standardized data through the interface. DoD and VA standardized data are "mediated" by way of an agreed upon "vocabulary" that enables DoD and VA to use each other's data in decision support applications. For medications, the mediation terminology used is RxNorm. For non-medication allergies the UMLS CUI is used for mediation. For Signs and Symptoms or reactions related to Allergies, SNOMED-CT is utilized. This data mapping can be time consuming and never-ending.

The issue is not unique for the federal partners but the early adoption of data exchanges between the DoD and VA lead to increased awareness of the need to engage with the organizations that develop healthcare-related data exchange standards. Over the years, the DoD and VA along with many of their civilian partners have been very active in implementing standard terminologies and ontologies. Ryan Bosch, MD, (Pedulli, 2013) from INOVA Health System, pointed out that simply linking the 5000 physicians in his system was very difficult due to the proprietary nature of the different labs each facility uses. This scenario highlights that data mapping challenge. Moving away from data mapping to open standards using standardized terminologies will decrease the reliance on proprietary data schemes within electronic health records. The integration of industry definition, codes/terms, and the regulation of medical devices that now attach to hospital networks is a maturing process for healthcare as a business, public or private.

Introduced in 2007, the International Health Terminology Standards Development Organization (IHTSDO) was established to develop, maintain, promote, and enable the uptake and correct use of its terminology products in health systems. The IHTSDO Workbench provides terminology content modelers with a set of tools to author, map, search, browse, and classify terminology, plus undertake workflow and process automation (IHTSDO, 2013). The VA has since undertaken efforts to enhance and extend the IHTSDO Workbench to bolster performance and functionality, improve the general user experience, and promote cooperative modeling of normalized content.

There are a number of joint partnerships between the DoD Informatics community and the VA along with civilian partners in private industry. They are engaged in data mapping and interoperability and have members on various working groups within many of the standards organizations working to drive the nation toward an interoperable, standardized nomenclature. Some of the efforts with Health and Human Service and the Office of the National Coordinator for Health Information Technology have led to the refinement of the data exchange needed for the virtual lifetime electronic record (VLER) (Fridsma, 2011).

The DoD and VA have also been active participants in many of the more well-known standards development organizations driving nationals standards to improve the exchange of information not only from DoD to VA and back, but with commercial partners. Some of these bodies include the Health Level 7 (HL7) Standards Organization where the formatting and data terminologies and ontologies are being specified (Health Level Seven International Standards, 2013), the Logical Observations Identifiers, Names, Codes (LOINC) work group, and SNOWMED-CT which defines clinical terminology and a universal standard for identifying laboratory results and other clinical observations. The ability to exchange laboratory results data since 1994 is a great step in the right direction but more work is needed in this area on the actual sending and receiving of the tests as these remain within the proprietary language of the system being used at a given facility.

Size and Complexity

The initial section of this chapter provided details on the number of facilities and the different environments within which the federal partners work. One of the unique challenges is the geographically dispersed federal sector facilities. The DoD manages hospitals and clinics around the world with staff working in all 24 time zones, creating a time management challenge. Similarly, the VA has clinics in some locations located near former military installations such as in the Philippines and Puerto Rico and some in current locations such as Guam. The Coast Guard has a much further reach than our continental coast including remote locations from Alaska to Hawaii and supporting maritime safety where U.S. Navy ships are located such as foreign ports like Kuwait Naval Base. As for the United States Public Health Service (USPHS) officers who are charged with the health of the entire United States population they serve alongside the military on board ships, in Military Treatment Facilities (MTFs) or public sector partners during time of national disasters such as flood

and fires (United States Public Health Service [USPHS] Nursing, 2013b). Caring for patients utilizing these scattered and diverse networks are a challenge both logistically and physically.

Each agency has specific medical missions that drive their requirements for healthcare in these diverse locations. In order to sustain a fit and medically protected force the DoD operates preventative medicine facilities in undisclosed locations on seven continents. A secondary mission for the DoD is to provide a full-service hospital asset for use by other government agencies involved in the support of disaster relief and humanitarian operations worldwide. This is handled by the hospital ships which were discussed earlier. The VA's healthcare mission covers the continuum of care by providing inpatient and outpatient services, including pharmacy, prosthetics, and mental health; long-term care in both institutional and non-institutional settings and other healthcare programs such as readjustment counseling.

High-Level Requirements and Approval Process

The federal agencies have a prescribed governance process beginning with high-level requirements from the functional community that can come from either the clinical or business owners. For the DoD these requirements are in response to the strategic goals of a medically ready force and a force that is medically ready to deploy. Once a decision is made that the need cannot be satisfied by a policy change and a material solution is necessary, the needs are vetted with the technical communities for potential approaches to meet the requirement. Then a decision is made to add those requirements to a system that already exists or modernize the system, buy a commercial product, or develop the material solution from the ground up. IT must remember that they support the end user and rely on the functional proponent to set the requirements.

Decisions on HIT spending follow the MHS governance processes, which include the military services (Army, Navy, and Air Force) for all clinical and business systems. The ability of a single Service to individually decide to field a system or application to meet a service specific need has been reduced to sustaining only what is currently in their portfolio of activities. Any new system or changes to an existing system must now be a collective discussion concurred on by all the Services before money is spent on any project in sustainment or a new program or change to an existing program is initiated. Prior to funding any expenditure in any given year the money has to be certified by the Deputy Chief Management Officer (DCMO) that the money will actually be spent in the way it was appropriated for and on the programs and projects based on the amount allocated in a given year and for a specific reason such as sustainment, operations, and maintenance of new research and development.

In the VHA, high-level requirements and architecture artifacts are produced based on a top-down and bottom-up approach. Business needs are identified, defined, and delivered in support of the VA Strategic Plan and Agency Priority Goals, as well as in response to requests from end users located in a variety of settings throughout the administration, including medical centers. VHA's business process life cycle leverages requirements and architecture to support investment planning and solution decisions. The volume and complexity of VHA processes, systems, and business rules drive the need for a disciplined approach to identify, approve, and mature VHA requirements management and development processes.

There are a number of unique challenges faced by the business analysts and architects that support high-level requirements development in VHA as well as in the DoD. One is the agencies' healthcare mission and the need for the business analysts to work with a geographically dispersed stakeholder population who employ a diverse number of HIT systems and demand more innovative solutions to improve effectiveness and efficiency of care delivery.

Requests for changes for enhancements to existing systems are gathered from a variety of sources in both agencies including staff in the field via a Web portal, but senior executives responsible for Medical Programs also direct requests. For the VA requests for new services can originate in response to business process issues, transformational initiatives, patient safety alerts, national directives, legislative mandates, regulatory guidelines, VA-defined material weakness findings, and system-wide Office of the Inspector General findings. As a result, requirements team members must have skills that allow them to achieve a balance between programmatic direction and strategic plans, and the functional needs of the end users in the field. They must also apply process re-engineering skills to recommend policy or training initiatives, instead of HIT enhancements where appropriate. However, these challenges are well balanced against a culture that places a high value on nursing informatics within the practice of healthcare and the development of HIT solutions.

The DoD and the VA have been engaged for many years with clinical information management activities and consensus building through the Interagency Clinical Informatics Board (ICIB). The ICIB ensures that clinicians lead the prioritization of recommendations for electronic health data sharing (VA-DoD Interoperability, June 2, 2009 [On-line]. Available: http://www.tricare.mil/dvpco/downloads/20090625/PlenaryJune2IMITstatus interoperableelectronichealthrecord.pdf).

SUMMARY

In summary this chapter provided information on the federal healthcare sector and the development of health informatics within the Department of Defense and the Veterans Administration. It provided some concrete examples regarding the size and complexity of providing care across the globe from austere battlefield condition and aboard ships to fully integrated technologically robust brick and mortar facilities. In addition, it detailed some of the early advances in computerized medical records and networks that make up the integrated health delivery systems that the federal partners utilize and how the federal partners continue to add to the body of knowledge on interoperability and standards while helping drive the nation to implement the next generation of electronic medical records that meet meaningful use. The chapter discussed some of the challenges and opportunities in working as an informatics professional in the federal healthcare sector. Some of those challenges are unique because of the diversity of information technology platforms used to capture data and the infrastructure on which it must be transmitted. Ultimately, it succeeds because despite the challenges, there is an opportunity to make a difference in the ability to provide quality healthcare to all those we all serve.

Additional Contributors:

Diane Bedecarré MS, RN-BC
LTC Benjamin "Eli" Seeley, MSN, RN, RN-BC, CPHIMS, CEN
Robert C. Campbell, MSN, RN-BC, FHIMSS, CPHIMS
Mary Ann Cardinali, MSN, BSN, RN-NEA-BC
Major Amalia M. DiVittorio, MSN, MBA, RN-BC
Elizabeth J. Fleischer, MSN, B.S., RN-BC, NREMT
Linda B. Hebert, MS, RN
Catherine Hoang RN, MS
Chris E. Nichols MHA, RN, LSSBB
Margaret E. Manion, MSN, RN-C
Toni Phillips, RN, MSN
Angela M. Ross, MSN, MPH, RN-BC, PMP
Jeffrey J. Sartori MS, RN
Lynn A. Shuler, MA, RN, CCRC
Ahnnya Slaughter, MSN, CNS, APRN-BC, RN-BC
Andrew P. Spencer, MSN, RN
LTC Angela Stone Icaza, MBA, MS, RN-BC, CCRN
Natasha T. Sutton, MSN, BC-RN
Tiffany N. Sylver, MSN, RN
Major Tammera G. Mattimoe WHNP, MSN, RNBC
Beverly A. Taylor, MSN, RN, CPHQ

REFERENCES

American Health Information Management Association (AHIMA) & American Medical Informatics Association (AMIA). (2006). *Building the workforce for health information transformation*. Retrieved from http://www.amia.org/sites/amia.org/files/Workforce_2006.pdf. Accessed on December 27, 2013.

American Nurses Association (ANA). (2008). *Nursing informatics: Scope and standards of practice*. Silver Spring, MD: American Nurses Association.

AMIA. (2013a). *AMIA 10×10 training heath care professionals to serve as informatics leaders*. Retrieved from http://www.amia.org/education/10x10-courses. Accessed on December 27, 2013.

AMIA. (2013b). *Nursing informatics history project*. Retrieved from http://www.amia.org/programs/working-groups/nursing-informatics/history-project. Accessed on December 20, 2013.

Coyle, G. A., & Heinen, M. (2005). Evolution of BCMA within the Department of Veterans Affairs. *Nursing Administration Quarterly, 29*(1), 32–38.

Defense Health Clinical System (DHIMS). (2011, June). Essentris™ 100% deployment. *The Beat*. Retrieved from http://dhcs.health.mil/docs/newsletter/the_beat_iv_i3_jun2011.pdf

Defense Information Systems Agency (DISA). (2013). *Sensitive but unclassified IP data*. Retrieved from http://www.disa.mil/Services/Network-Services/Data/SBU-IP. Accessed on October 31, 2013.

Department of Defense (DoD). (n.d.). *Theater Medical Information Program—Joint (TMIP-J)*. Retrieved from http://www.globalsecurity.org/military/library/budget/fy2009/dot-e/dod/2009tmipj.pdf. Accessed on January 6, 2014.

EHR Intelligence. (2012). *EHR and the VA: Part 1—History*. Retrieved from http://ehrintelligence.com/2012/04/19/ehr-and-the-va-part-i-history/. Accessed on December 15, 2013.

Fact Sheet [On-line] (n.d.-a). Retrieved from http://dhcs.health.mil/docs/factsheets/factsheet-AHLTA_Mobile.pdf

Fact Sheet [On-line] (n.d.-b). Retrieved from http://dhcs.health.mil/docs/factsheets/20120905-Fact%20Sheet-AHLTA-Theater.pdf

Federal Register. Executive Order 13335—Incentives for the Use of Health Information Technology and Establishing the Position of the National health Information Technology Coordinator, Friday, April 30, 2004.

Fridsma, D. (2011). *Interoperable health information exchange featured at GHIT conference*. Retrieved from http://www.healthit.gov/buzz-blog/from-the-onc-desk/interoperable-health-information-exchange-featured-conference/. Accessed on January 27, 2014.

Gardner, R. M., Overhage, J. M., Steen, E. B., Munger, B. S., Holmes, J. H., Williamson, J. J., … AMIA Board of Directors. (2009). Core content for the subspecialty of clinical informatics. *Journal of the American Medical Informatics Association, 16*(2), 153-157. doi:10.1197/jamia.M3045

Health Information and Management Systems Society (HIMSS). (2011). *HIMSS nursing informatics: Workforce survey*. Retrieved from http://himss.files.cms-plus.com/HIMSSorg/content/files/2011HIMSSNursingInformaticsWorkforceSurvey.pdf. Accessed on December 27, 2013.

Health Level Seven International Standards. (2013). *Introduction to HL7 standards*. Retrieved from http://www.hl7.org/implement/standards/index.cfm?ref=nav. Accessed on October 31, 2013.

House of Representatives. (2012). H.R. 4310 (112th): National Defense Authorization Act Fiscal Year 2013 112th Congress, 2011-2013. Washington, DC.

International Health Terminology Standards Development Organization (IHTSDO). (2013). *Members of IHTSDO*. Retrieved from http://www.ihtsdo.org/members/. Accessed on December 31, 2013.

Lee, J. (2009). *The care they were promised and the benefits that they have earned*. Retrieved from http://www.whitehouse.gov/blog/09/04/09/The-Care-They-Were-Promised-and-the-Benefits-That-They-Have-Earned. Accessed on January 06, 2014.

Military Health System (MHS). (2012). *2012 MHS stakeholder report*. Retrieved from http://www.health.mil/Reference-Center/Reports/2012/12/31/2012-MHS-Stakeholders-Report. Accessed on December 01, 2014.

Osbolt, J. G. (2003). In memoriam: Harriet Helen Werley. *Journal of the American Medical Informatics Association, 10*(2), 224–225.

Osbolt, J. G., & Saba, V. K. (2008). A brief history of nursing informatics in the United States of America. *Nursing Outlook, 56*(5), 199–205. doi:10.1016/j.outlook.2008.06.008

Pedulli, L. (2013). Desperately seeking better standards. *Clinical innovation + technology, 2*(9), 12–14. Retrieved from http://www.clinical-innovation.com/topics/interoperability/desperately-seeking-better-standards. Accessed on October 13, 2013.

Ramsaroop, P., Ball, M. J., Beaulieu, D. B., & Douglas, J. V. (2001). *Advancing federal sector health care: A model for technology transfer (health informatics)*. New York: Springer.

Skinner, J. (2008). Scholarly Paper; Capture the Gap: A Clinical Informatics Assessment and Recommendation for Implementing an Electronic Clinical Documentation Capability in Aeromedical Evacuation.

Staggers, N. T. (2007). *Validating mobilization competencies, for air force clinical nurses* (PB2007107660). Alexandria VA: National Technical Information Service.

The Office of the National Coordinator for Health Information Technology. (2013). *Workforce development programs*. Retrieved from http://www.healthit.gov/providers-professionals/participating-community-colleges. Accessed on December 27, 2013.

The Tiger Team. (2007). *The Tiger Initiative. Revolutionary leadership driving healthcare innovation: The TIGER leadership development collaborative report.* Retrieved from http://www.thetigerinitiative.org/docs/TigerReport_RevolutionaryLeadership.pdf. Accessed on December 27, 2013.

TRICARE. (2013). *About TRICARE.* Retrieved from http://www.tricare.mil/Welcome.aspx. Accessed on December 01, 2014.

United States Department of Veterans Affairs. (2002). *VA/DoD electronic health records addressing interoperability.* Retrieved from http://www.va.gov/opa/pressrel/pressrelease.cfm?id=505. Accessed on January 3, 2013.

United States Department of Veterans Affairs. (2012). *2012 Performance and accountability report.* Retrieved from http://www.va.gov/budget/report/. Accessed on October 15, 2013.

United States Department of Veterans Affairs. (2013a). *Annual budget submission.* Retrieved from http://www.va.gov/budget/products.asp. Accessed on October 13, 2013.

United States Department of Veterans Affairs. (2013b). *Virtual lifetime electronic record (VLER).* Retrieved from http://www.va.gov/VLER/index.asp. Accessed on January 03, 2014.

United States Department of Veterans Affairs. (2013c). *Welcome to my HealtheVet.* Retrieved from https://www.myhealth.va.gov/index.html. Accessed on December 15, 2013.

United States Public Health Service (USPHS) Nursing. (2013a). *Federal Nursing Service Council.* Retrieved from http://phs-nurse.org/federal-nursing-service-council. Accessed on December 20, 2013.

United States Public Health Service (USPHS) Nursing. (2013b). *Nursing: About USPHS.* Retrieved from http://phs-nurse.org/about-usphs. Accessed on December 20, 2013.

United States Public Health Service (USPHS) Nursing. (2013c). *Nursing: Career opportunities with the USPHS.* Retrieved from http://phs-nurse.org/nurse-resource-manual/chapter-3. Accessed on December 20, 2013.

VistA Evolution Executive Summary—unpublished 2013.

35

Consumer/Patient Engagement and eHealth Resources

Barbara B. Frink

• OBJECTIVES

1. Describe the concept of patient engagement from patient, health system, and provider perspectives.
2. Discuss several influences of health policy, specifically the HITECH Act and the American Recovery and Reinvestment Act of 2011, on the development of patient engagement strategies within an EHR framework.
3. Describe three characteristics of a learning healthcare organization, and the potential role of patient engagement.
4. List the primary components and functions of patient portals, and how they differ from other ehealth resources.

• KEY WORDS

Consumer engagement
Patient engagement
eHealth
Meaningful use
Patient empowerment
Patient activation
ePatients
Patient portal
Learning healthcare organizations
Consumer eHealth tools

CONSUMER ENGAGEMENT AND EHEALTH RESOURCES

Introduction

The mission of healthcare clinicians is the improvement and support of the health and healthcare of consumers: patients, families, communities, and populations. In addition to the scientific and technological foundations of contemporary clinical practice, one of the necessary components of achieving that mission is clinician and consumer use of enabling technologies, which include ehealth resources, meaningful use of electronic health records (EHRs), and other electronic health media. Recent developments in health policy, widespread availability of mobile electronic tools, and a shift to value-based healthcare have created a renewed interest in "patient engagement" methods and strategies that lead to improvements in individual and population health. There are both explicit and implicit suggestions in this topic that the current healthcare system is flawed, and at times demonstrates perverse approaches to achieving improved outcomes of care.

Nursing and other clinical informaticists, long involved with clinicians in the design, implementation, and adoption of EHRs, are now finding that they are also more directly involved with patient and family access and use of data from EHRs. One of the ways this is occurring is through the use of secure electronic communication and Web sites, often sponsored by provider organizations. Commonly known as patient portals, these secure Web sites are changing the way that clinicians and patients/consumers communicate in both anticipated and unanticipated ways. Both the new methods of communication and availability of data to patients are having a profound effect on clinicians and on patients. The language used to describe this phenomenon is variable, but is coalescing around the term patient engagement. For that reason, the focus of this chapter is on the complexities of the concept of consumer/patient engagement and the availability of ehealth resources to support that engagement within the context of improving health outcomes.

U.S. HEALTH POLICY INFLUENCES

Although healthcare policy is not the subject of this chapter, a brief review of recent policy influences in the United States, including meaningful use of EHRs as a primary driver of patient engagement, provides the context within which the current emphasis on patient engagement is occurring.

The American Recovery and Reinvestment Act of 2009 and HITECH Act

The American Recovery and Reinvestment Act of 2009 (H.R. 1–111th Congress, 2009) contained within it a provision for major multi-year investments in the U.S. health information technology infrastructure: The Health Information Technology and Economic and Clinical Health (HITECH) Act. Through a combination of significant federal financial investments and extensive criteria specified for measurement in three stages, the HITECH Act has had a profound influence on the implementation and adoption of electronic health records (EHRs) by both eligible healthcare providers and eligible hospitals. By 2013, 80% (>3800) of eligible hospitals had received incentive payments and 50% of 338,000 registered eligible providers received an EHR incentive payment (HealthIT.gov, 2013, April).

Meaningful Use of EHRs.   Meaningful use criteria for eligible providers and eligible hospitals are specified as either core measures (must be met) or menu measures, that is the provider may choose to meet a specified number of measures from a list of choices. The Meaningful Use program has been specified in three stages: Stage One, data capture and sharing: 2011–2012; Stage Two, advanced clinical processes: 2014; and Stage Three, improved outcomes: 2016. A complete description of the meaningful use program, all criteria, and stages is available from the Centers for Medicare & Medicaid (2013). Meaningful use criteria are framed within five domains and five objectives (HealthIT.gov, 2013) which are noted in Table 35.1.

The domains and objectives are specified here to emphasize the influence and drivers for both patient engagement and empowerment. It is not coincidental that there has been intense focus among both providers and hospital organizations on defining patient engagement strategies that would encourage and even ensure that consumers make use of ehealth resources.

The Affordable Care Act of 2011

The Affordable Care Act of 2011 created accountability for the Secretary of HHS to "establish a national strategy to improve the delivery of healthcare services, patient health outcomes, and population health" (Patient Protection and Affordable Care Act [Public Law 111–148], 2011). By March 2011, the national strategy was communicated in a report to Congress (Department of Health and Human Services, 2011), which established that strategy within the context of three aims, known as the National Quality Strategy:

- Better Care: Improve the overall quality of care, by making healthcare more patient centered, reliable, accessible, and safe.

TABLE 35.1	Meaningful Use Domains and Objectives	
Domains		**Objectives**
Improve Quality, Safety, Efficiency		Better Clinical Outcomes
Engage Patients and Families		Improved Population Health Outcomes
Improve Care Coordination		Increased Transparency and Efficiency
Improve Public and Population Health		Empowered Individuals
Ensure Privacy and Security for Personal Health Information		More Robust Research Data on Health Systems

- Healthy People/Healthy Communities: Improve the health of the U.S. population by supporting proven interventions to address behavioral, social, and environmental determinants of health in addition to delivering higher-quality care.

- Affordable Care: Reduce the cost of quality healthcare for individuals, families, employers, and government (Department of Health and Human Services, 2011, p. 1)

Ten guiding principles were identified to ensure that goals and outcomes were specified for the three aims. The first of these principles provides a context for healthcare consumer engagement: "Person-centeredness and family engagement, including understanding and valuing patient preferences, will guide all strategies, goals, and improvement efforts" (AHRQ, 2011, section 1). This principle is further defined as:

> The most successful health care experiences are often those in which clinicians, patients, and their families work together to make decisions. When patients' needs, experiences, perspectives, and preferences are taken into account—and when they get the clear and understandable information and support they need to actively participate in their own care—outcomes and patient satisfaction can improve. How patients rate their experience is now widely used as a measure of high quality care, but more can be done to empower individuals and make sure their needs and preferences are taken into account. (AHRQ, 2011, section 1)

Office of the National Coordinator Strategic Plan 2011–2015

Also in 2011, the Office of the National Coordinator for Health Information Technology (ONC) published its strategic plan for 2011–2015. The fourth goal of that plan is to "Empower Individuals with Health IT to Improve their Health and the Health Care System" (Office of the National Coordinator of Health Information Technology, 2011, p. 5). The intent of the goal is to design health IT policies and programs to meet individual needs and expectations; provide individuals with access to their information; help facilitate a strong consumer health IT market; and better integrate individuals' and clinicians' communications through health IT. The goal statement also includes the caveat that when the public "… is empowered with access to its health information through useful tools, it can be a powerful driver in moving toward patient-centered health care" (Office of the National Coordinator of Health Information Technology, 2011, p. 5).

Institute of Medicine Report 2012

In 2012, the Institute of Medicine published a report supporting the concept that healthcare is on a continuous learning pathway to improve care and lower cost. The authors highlight four recent developments that enable improved care with lowered costs to become a reality: *vast computational power* that makes analysis of actual patient care possible; *connectivity* making communication between and among patients and professionals a reality, as well as continuously available information; *system and organizational science advances* that support improvement and efficiencies in care within highly complex environments; and *empowerment of patients* that "unleashes the potential" for partnerships with professionals in the prevention and treatment activities, particularly those that require behavioral change (The Institute of Medicine, 2012, p. xii).

In these examples from recent healthcare policy, we see the consistent inclusion of consumers empowered and engaged to improve healthcare and health outcomes through the use of information and information tools.

CONSUMERS AND PATIENTS

Throughout this chapter, you will see a consistent theme emerge around the concept of "engagement": multiple words are used as synonyms for engagement, but with imprecise definitions; terms that represent different concepts are often used interchangeably, and from both research and strategic perspectives, the field is young. The title of this chapter is "Consumer Engagement," however you will note that much of the discussion to follow uses the adjective "patient" as opposed to "consumer". Because much of the literature uses "patient" to modify engagement and empowerment, that language is retained in the discussion. However, it is worthwhile to consider the importance of language in conveying meaning, and to at least briefly discuss the subtle and not so subtle differences between the terms "consumer" and "patient" in the context of engagement. Dr. Paul Keckley, writing in the foreword to the Deloitte 2012 U.S. Healthcare Consumer Survey, includes an excellent description contrasting the two terms. He asserts that the term "patient" denotes a primarily passive and reactive role, versus the term "consumer," which implies a role that is more active, and able to influence the healthcare industry. For example, in regard to "level of engagement in decisions about their treatments, patients depend upon physicians to make decisions on their behalf in contrast with consumers who depend on physician recommendation augmented by their own research to confirm or corroborate.

Similarly, for awareness of treatment options and associated costs, patients have a low level of awareness and depend on physician opinion while consumers have a high level of awareness and depend on information sources from online tools and social media. Both patients and consumers have a high level of trust in providers based on personal experience, but consumers add comparison shopping" (Keckley & Deloitte Center for Health Solutions, 2012, p. 1).

As the field of engagement matures within healthcare, the distinctions between the terms patient and consumer will become more precise and useful for measurement and evaluation.

PATIENT-CENTERED CARE, PATIENT EMPOWERMENT, AND CONSUMER/PATIENT ENGAGEMENT

Patient-Centered Care

Although the concept of patient-centered care is not new, over the past 10 to 15 years, the movement to improve quality, effectiveness, and outcomes of healthcare has included a renewed emphasis on patient-centered care. Primary examples of this are the development of new models of primary care delivery—the patient-centered medical home (PCMH) and accountable care organizations. Despite this new focus, there are multiple inconsistencies in how the concept is used and reported. Examples from Hobbs' (2009) dimensional analysis of patient-centered care in nursing include a variety of definitions including personalized meal selections, pleasant environments, emotional support, and inclusive decision-making. It is the concepts of shared decision-making and patient engagement that are consistent links to patient-centered care (Bechtel & Ness, 2010; Beck, Daughtridge, & Sloane, 2002; Roseman, Osborne-Stafsnes, Amy, Boslaugh, & Slate-Miller, 2013; Stewart et al., 2000; Wennberg, Marr, Lang, O'Malley, & Bennett, 2010). Carman et al. (2013, pp. 223–224) consider patient- and family-centered care as a broad term "conveying a vision for what health care should be," which includes concepts of partnership with providers, patients, and families.

Carman et al. (2013) reinforce the fact that the terms patient- and family-centered care are also used interchangeably with patient engagement and patient activation. For this chapter discussion, patient-centered care is a broad term encompassing several characteristics and concepts, often including patient engagement, empowerment, and activation.

Empowerment and Engagement—Aligned but Distinct Concepts

Empowerment has been defined as "the process of increasing the capacity of individuals or groups to make choices and to transform those choices into desired actions and outcomes" (The World Bank, 2014). In the context of health and health informatics, Brennan and Safran describe empowerment as "granting power to a dependent group or enhancing an individual's ability for self-determination" (Brennan & Safran, 2005, p. 8). Although the terms empowerment and engagement are often used interchangeably, there are distinctive differences as well as potential interactions between the two concepts. Patients may become engaged on their own behalf, and are therefore empowered as consumers. On the other hand, there may be an implicit or explicit "granting" of power to patients by healthcare professionals that indicates "we are partners with you (and or your family/caregivers), in managing your health and illness," which may then engage the patient. Exploring the definitions and the relationships between these concepts through research is key to informing appropriate and effective strategies for improving care. As the term "patient engagement" becomes more frequently used to denote healthcare organizational strategies that encourage portal access and involvement of patients in their care, understanding the tactics that effect both empowerment and engagement and their effect on outcomes becomes increasingly important.

The empowerment of individuals is a major theme in both professional and lay literature on patient engagement. The term "ePatient" has become identified with concepts of empowerment and engagement from a patient perspective. The term ePatient was first used in a white paper (Ferguson & E-Patient Scholars Working Group, 2013) describing how health consumers used the Internet. Originally, they defined the "e" as electronic, then the "e" was expanded to include the terms engaged, equipped, enabled, empowered, and later, educated and expert (deBronkart & Sands, 2013). The terms were used to describe an increasing number of healthcare consumers who were using the Internet to research healthcare or disease topics either on behalf of themselves or for friends and family. The feedback from these consumers was that they experienced "better health information and services, and different (but not always better) relationships with their doctors" (Ferguson & E-Patient Scholars Working Group, 2013, p. II).

Consumer/Patient Engagement

The potential for patient engagement to change the trajectory of outcomes of care and cost has been a subject of great interest and research focus within the healthcare community. Patient engagement, referred to as "a block-buster drug," was a theme for an entire issue of *Health Affairs* (Dentzer, 2013), and the framework for an in-depth report on consumer eHealth, contracted for by the ONC in 2012 (Ozbolt, Sands, Dykes, Pratt, Rosas, & Walker, 2012). Both of these sources of literature provide evidence that although the term "patient engagement" is frequently used, there is not yet a common definition or understanding of the concept. This is also supported by Gruman et al. (2010, p. 350) who purport that despite our understanding that there is benefit from patient's actively participating in their care, there has not been a systematic identification of the behaviors that—either implicitly or explicitly—define patient engagement.

The use of the term "patient engagement" has grown exponentially in recent years. Coulter, Safran, and Wasson (2012) state that in 2000, patient engagement was mentioned about 10 times per year on a Google search, versus a 2010 rate of over 100,000 mentions per year. Such volume indicates not only high interest, but also the necessity of clearly defining the concept in order to understand the complex relationships between engagement, health outcomes, and healthcare costs.

In 2012, the National eHealth Collaborative conducted a survey of consumer engagement with health information technology using its 450-member Learning Network. A response rate of 21% (n = 95) yielded results showing a majority ranking consumer engagement as a high priority, however the majority also indicated that the strategies for achieving patient engagement were still being clarified (National eHealth Collaborative, 2012). The report provides detailed information about the goals, definitions, strategies, and measures of success for achieving patient engagement as perceived by the respondent group.

The voice of the patient has also become more active in regard to healthcare engagement and ehealth resources, as reflected in such publications as *Let Patients Help* (deBronkart & Sands, 2013), *Doctor, Your Patient Will See You Now* (Kussin, 2011), and *e-Patients Live Longer* (Finn, 2011). The books are focused on providing information to consumers and providers, particularly on ehealth and communication, for better management and safer healthcare during patient experiences. In *Let Patients Help* (deBronkart & Sands, 2013), written by a patient and his physician, the authors address both patient and provider aspects of seeking, understanding, and acting on health information within the context of the relationship. Tip sheets are included for "how to be an e-Patient and an empowering provider" (deBronkart & Sands, 2013, Chapter 3). By contrast, Finn (2011) writes as a healthcare consumer, using anecdotes, guidelines, and guidance as a method of encouraging patients

to become better agents on their own behalf, and thereby improve healthcare outcomes. In addition to describing multiple methods of digital communication pertaining to healthcare, she includes substantive information on both electronic health records and personal health records, and describes the benefits to the patient of access to these data sources.

Simultaneous to the consumer/patient led emphasis on patient engagement, individuals and groups from the provider community have been offering their perspectives and advocacy. Dr. Daniel Sands, co-founder of the Society for Participatory Medicine, and an early adopter of patient engagement strategies (Sands, 2005), offers a provider perspective: "We healthcare professionals undervalue ourselves if we believe our value to be omniscience in our fields. In fact, our skill (beyond procedural expertise) is in knowing how to find and interpret information and to apply it to an individual patient, as well as to serve as a comforter and healer in the Hippocratic sense." (Sands, 2013, p. xxi). He describes this developing model of care delivery as "participatory medicine"—a relationship-based model of mutual partnership (Sands, 2013). A contemporary definition of participatory medicine is found on that inter-disciplinary Society's Web page (Society for Participatory Medicine, 2014) "… a model of cooperative healthcare that seeks to achieve active involvement by patients, professionals, care givers, and others across the continuum of care on all issues related to an individual's health. Participatory medicine is an ethical approach to care that also holds promise to improve outcomes, reduce medical errors, increase patient satisfaction and improve the cost of care." In this definition, we see a focus on individual patient and caregiver relationships across the full continuum of care as well as an explicit connection to the policy drivers of improved outcomes and lower costs of care.

A similar approach to patient engagement is expressed in the preface to a recently edited collection on patient engagement from the provider and healthcare system perspective (Oldenburg, Chase, Christensen, & Tritle, 2013). In addition to specifying that "patients need to be equipped, enabled, empowered, and engaged, working in partnership with providers to change the system" Oldenburg (2013, p. xxv) includes the necessity of patient's having access to their healthcare data, including medical records, as well as health IT tools.

Patient Engagement and Patient Activation

In addition to the widespread use but imprecise definition of the term patient engagement, another term—patient activation—is sometimes used in the same context, and is also not clearly defined. In their review of the evidence about the effect of patient activation on health outcomes, care, and costs, Hibbard and Greene (2013) define both terms. They state that the terms engagement and activation are used interchangeably, but without clear definition and with different meaning. Patient activation assumes that a patient understands their role in the care process, and has the "knowledge, skill, and confidence to manage their health and health care" (Hibbard & Greene, 2013, p. 207). In contrast, patient engagement includes activation, that is, patient engagement may include strategies to encourage or support activation. Both of these terms assume that an individual is capable of acting on their own behalf, rather than simply complying with medical directions.

Researchers have developed a Patient Activation Measure (Hibbard, Stockard, Mahoney, & Tusler, 2004) which has been used in multiple studies to demonstrate the relationship between degree of patient activation and degree of participation in preventive behavior, healthy lifestyle, and avoidance of harmful behaviors (Hibbard, Mahoney, Stock, & Tusler, 2007; Remmers, Hibbard, Mosen, Wagenfield, Hoye, Jones, 2009; Skolasky, Mackenzie, Wegener, & Riley, 2011). Table 35.2 displays summary directional significance for the results of several studies using the Patient Activation Measure (PAM) to

determine health outcomes (Fowles, Terry, Xi, Hibbard, Bloom, & Harvey, 2009; Hibbard, 2009; Hibbard & Cunningham, 2008; Hibbard & Greene, 2013).

There is some evidence that lower activation scores are also associated with higher costs, and also predictive of higher future costs, however specific utilization patterns have not yet been demonstrated (Hibbard, Greene, & Overton, 2013). Despite the sometimes interchangeable use of these imprecisely defined terms, clarity is being developed through the systematic use of a tested measure, and the exploration of relationships to better outcomes and lower costs.

As a summary to this section on patient engagement, Table 35.3 provides selected examples of definitions of patient engagement, which emphasizes the current complexities of measuring the effect of patient engagement on health outcomes and costs.

PATIENT ENGAGEMENT IN THE CONTEXT OF EHEALTH RESOURCES

Two of the characteristics that are consistently associated with patient engagement are communication and access to information. We use the term "ehealth" as a bridge term to describe categories of resources available to patients, families, and healthcare providers. Such resources are crucial for a true partnership in care to be successful in improving outcomes of care and potentially decrease healthcare costs. For purposes of discussion, the ehealth is defined as:

> …an emerging field at the intersection of medical informatics, public health and business, referring to health services and information delivered or enhanced through the Internet and related technologies. In a broader sense, the term characterizes not only a technical development, but also a state-of-mind, a way of thinking, an attitude, and a commitment for networked, global thinking, to improve health care locally, regionally, and worldwide by using information and communication technology (Eysenbach, 2001, p. 1).

Over time, this concept has been further refined to include the participants in ehealth: healthcare clinicians; patients, families, and caregivers; and consumers managing their health (Keselman, Logan, Smith, Leroy, & Zeng-Treitler, 2008, p. 475). Although there are innumerable ehealth resources that are available to consumers and providers, in this review, ehealth resources that have direct links to patient engagement—patient portals and online resources—are discussed.

TABLE 35.2	Patient Activation Measure Scores and Health Outcome Behaviors
Activation Score	**Behavior**
Less Activation	Three times as likely to have unmet medical needs
	Twice as likely to delay medical care
More Activation	Two to three times as likely to:
	Prepare questions for provider visit
	Know about treatment guidelines for conditions
	Seek out health information
	Compare quality of healthcare providers
Chronically Ill	
More Activation	More likely to:
	Adhere to treatment
	Perform regular self-monitoring
	Seek regular care for chronic condition

TABLE 35.3	Patient Engagement and Patient Activation Definitions	
Concept	**Definition**	**Reference**
Patient Engagement	• Providers and patients working together to "promote and support active patient and public involvement in health and healthcare and to strengthen their influence on healthcare decisions, at both the individual and collective levels"	Angela Coulter (Coulter, 2011, p. 11)
Patient Engagement	• "Actions individuals must take to obtain the greatest benefit from the health care services available to them. Focuses on behaviors of individuals relative to their health care that are critical and proximal to health outcomes, rather than the actions of professionals, or policies of institutions."	Center for Advancing Health (2010, p. 2)
Patient Engagement	• "A partnership including shared decision-making with providers; a mechanism to strengthen the patient voice in deciding what is best for them; and a better way to understand their conditions."	Bechtel and Ness (2010, p. 917)
Patient and Family Engagement	• "A set of behaviors by patients, family members, and health professionals and a set of organizational policies and procedures that foster both the inclusion of patients and family members as active members of the health care team and collaborative partnerships with providers and provider organizations."	AHRQ (Maurer, Dardess, Carman, Frazier, Smeeding, & American Institutes for Research, 2012, p. 10)
Patient Engagement in the context of Patient Activation	• "A broad concept that includes activation; the interventions designed to increase activation; and patient's resulting behavior, such as seeking preventive care…"	Hibbard and Greene (2013, p. 207)
Patient Activation	• "… the degree to which the individual understands they must play and active role in managing their own health and health care, and the extent to which they feel able to fulfill that role."	Hibbard and Mahoney (2010, p. 377)

Patient Portals

A patient portal is an electronic gateway through which patients may access their personal health data and communicate with healthcare providers. The gateway is a secure online Web site, which is often sponsored by individual providers, groups of providers, health systems, or payers. While all portals allow secure access to at least some personal health data, such as lab test or imaging results and secure patient-provider messaging, portals may vary in functionality. Some portals provide a broader menu of available services, such as appointment scheduling and bill payment. The portal technology may be provided by an EHR vendor or other information technology vendor.

Although patient portals, often stand-alone applications, have been in use for several years, it has not been until recently that there has been substantial progress in this area. The specification of Stage 1 meaningful use criteria specifying electronic access to personal health data has provided a major incentive for healthcare systems and/or provider groups to offer electronic access.

Not surprisingly, vendors of certified EHRs are developing "companion" applications that offer patients a secure access to at least portions of the EHR, as well as communication with providers (Goldzweig, 2012; Goldzweig et al., 2013; Sakar & Bates, 2014). Evidence of the effectiveness of patient portals in improving health is insufficient. In a systematic review of the literature, Goldzweig et al. (p. 677) found that although patient attitudes are positive, there may be cultural or health literacy barriers to effective portal use. In addition, they caution that the patient portal is a new technology requiring ongoing study for effectiveness and patient satisfaction.

Meaningful Use and Patient Portals. Meaningful use Stage 2 guidelines specifically promote patient engagement through the use of portal technology required by eligible providers and eligible hospitals to allow patients access to personal health data. The core requirements that are related to the domain of patient engagement and empowerment objectives are listed for reference.

Patient Engagement Core Measure Requirements for Eligible Providers (EP) Stage 2 (Centers for Medicare & Medicaid, 2012b):

- Provide patients the ability to view online, download, and transmit their health information within four business days of the information being available to the EP.
- Provide clinical summaries to patients for each office visit.
- Use clinically relevant information to identify patients who should receive reminders for preventive/follow-up care and send these patients the reminders, per patient preference.
- Use clinically relevant information from Certified EHR Technology to identify patient-specific education resources and provide those resources to the patient.

Patient Engagement Core Measure Requirements for Eligible Hospitals Stage 2 (Centers for Medicare & Medicaid, 2012a):

- Provide patients the ability to view online, download, and transmit information about a hospital admission.
- Use clinically relevant information from Certified EHR Technology to identify patient-specific education resources and provide those resources to the patient.

Consumer Engagement with EHealth Tools

The alignment of meaningful use criteria with increased consumer access to electronic communication and health information resources has created new pressure for the availability of ehealth tools to be on par with other consumer services. Ahern, Woods, Lightowler, Finley, and Houston (2011) predict that consumer behavior in the use of the Internet and wireless technology for healthcare purposes will create a "sea change" in patient engagement (Ahern et al., 2011, p. S163). They also suggest that three conditions need to exist for the achievement of patient oriented meaningful use: 1). "patients need to have access to personally relevant health information and services; 2). patients will need to believe that there is value in using health information technology (HIT); and 3). specific healthcare improvements should be directly attributable to patients' use of HIT" (Ahern et al., 2011, p. S164). Building on this work, Marchibroda and deBronkart (2013) conceptualize three types of electronic health tools for engaging consumers: those that support patient education and

TABLE 35.4	Consumer EHealth Tools: Types and Examples
Type of Consumer EHealth Tool	**Examples**
Support patient education and self-care	• Online education resources, interactive tools for monitoring health such as diet, exercise, blood sugar • Online communities focused on health conditions or caregiving • Social media—Facebook, twitter posts • PHRs—personal health records
Support patient information and transactions associated with care delivery	Patient portals including: • Secure messaging (e-mail), appointment scheduling • Download of personal health data—test results, visit notes, clinical summaries, medication lists • Reordering prescriptions • Bill payment
Support care delivery process	• Remote monitoring devices with automatic data transmission • Reminders based on guidelines or health conditions • Telehealth monitoring or visits • May include online chat or virtual visit with provider

self-care; those that support patient information and transaction needs associated with care delivery; and those that support care delivery (Marchibroda & deBronkart, 2013, pp. 71–73). Table 35.4 displays examples of each of the three ehealth tools (Keselman et al., 2008; Marchibroda, 2013, p. 11; Marchibroda & deBronkart, 2013, pp. 70–73).

These examples provide a very limited high-level view of resource categories. There are multitudes of online content-rich (and poor) health resources available to consumers and providers alike. Examples include symptom management, disease management, decision support, health literature, research results, condition and disease guidelines, and resources for caregivers, to name a few. For an in-depth review of both available consumer health content and methods for determining the quality of that content, please see Zielstorff and Frink (2011).

CONCLUSION

As this chapter is concluded, we suggest that this discussion is one point on a trend line. The status of ehealth resources is continually evolving, as are the roles of consumers, patients, and clinicians in regard to the use of ehealth resources. As presented here, patient engagement, an inclusive term with several definitions, is considered and named to be a major influence on the ultimate outcomes and cost of care. However, distinctive similarities and differences between patient-centered care, consumer/patient engagement, patient empowerment, and patient activation are only beginning to be studied and understood. New technologies, such as the patient portal, have yet to be fully adopted or deployed, and evaluations have been limited. Stage 2 meaningful use is only a few months old. It is a challenging time to be in clinical care and clinical informatics.

There is much to be done in clarifying the interaction between consumer/patient engagement, the use of ehealth resources, and outcomes of care. There is ample opportunity for contribution to:

- Participate in consumer/provider groups to establish criteria for effective e-communication
- Explore the possibilities of providing more effective interactive education content for patient portals
- Partner with consumers in developing governance structures for managing patient and consumer access to institutional ehealth resources
- Establish methods for measuring and evaluating consumer, patient and family, and provider satisfaction with the developing process

It is clear that this is a time of profound change. Concepts such as patient engagement have been infused with meaning and anticipated results that currently outstrip our ability to measure. However, the goal is of high value: working in partnership—consumers, patients and families, and clinician providers—to improve the outcomes of care while contributing to responsible cost reduction.

REFERENCES

Ahern, D. K., Woods, S. S., Lightowler, M. C., Finley, S. W., & Houston, T. K. (2011). Promise of and potential for patient-facing technologies to enable meaningful use. *American Journal of Preventive Medicine, 40*(582), S162–S172.

AHRQ. (2011, March 21). *Principles for the National Quality Strategy.* Retrieved from http://www.ahrq.gov/workingforquality/nqs/principles.htm. Accessed on January 17, 2014.

Bechtel, C., & Ness, D. L. (2010). If you build it, will they come? Designing truly patient-centered health care. *Health Affairs, 29,* 914–920.

Beck, R. S., Daughtridge, R., & Sloane, P. D. (2002). Physician-patient communication in the primary care office: A systematic review. *Journal of the American Board of Family Practice, 15*(1), 25–38.

Brennan, P. F., & Safran, C. (2005). Empowered consumers. In D. Lewis, W. V. Slack, G. Eysenbach, R. Kukafka, P. Z. Stavri, & H. Jimison (Eds.), *Consumer health informatics: Informing consumers and improving health care* (pp. 8–21). New York, NY: Springer Sceince + Business Media.

Carman, K. L., Dardess, P., Maurer, M., Sofaer, S., Adams, K., Bechtel, C., & Sweeney, J. (2013). Patient and family engagement: A framework for understanding the elements and developing interventions and policies. *Health Affairs, 32,* 223–229.

Center for Advancing Health. (2010). *A new definition of patient engagement: What is engagement and why is it important.* Retrieved from http://www.cfah.org/pdfs/CFAH_Engagement_Behavior_Framework_current.pdf. Accessed on January 25, 2014.

Centers for Medicare & Medicaid. (2012a, October). *Stage 2 eligible hospital and critical access hospital (CAH) meaningful use core and menu objectives table of contents.* Retrieved from http://www.cms.gov/Regulations-and-Guidance/Legislation/EHRIncentivePrograms/Downloads/Stage2_MeaningfulUseSpecSheet_TableContents_EligibleHospitals_CAHs.pdf. Accessed on January 25, 2014.

Centers for Medicare & Medicaid. (2012b, October). *Stage 2 eligible provider (EP) meaningful use core and menu measures table of contents.* Retrieved from http://www.cms.gov/Regulations-and-Guidance/Legislation/EHRIncentivePrograms/Downloads/Stage2_MeaningfulUseSpecSheet_TableContents_EPs.pdf. Accessed on January 25, 2014.

Centers for Medicare & Medicaid. (2013). *Meaningful use.* Retrieved from http://www.cms.gov/Regulations-and-Guidance/Legislation/EHRIncentivePrograms/Meaningful_Use.html. Accessed on January 25, 2014.

Coulter, A. (2011). *Engaging patients in healthcare.* New York, NY: McGraw-Hill Education.

Coulter, A., Safran, D., & Wasson, J. H. (2012). From the guest editors: On the language and content of patient engagement. *Journal of Ambulatory Care Management, 35*(2), 78–79. doi:10.1097/JAC.0b013e31824a5676.

deBronkart, R. D., & Sands, D. Z. (2013). *Let patients help! A "patient engagement" handbook - how doctors, nurses, patients and caregivers can partner for better care.* Richard Davies deBronkart, jr. dba "e-Patient Dave". CreateSpace Independent Publishing Platform. www.CreateSpace.com.

Dentzer, S. (2013). Rx for the 'blockbuster drug' of patient engagement. *Health Affairs, 32*(2), 202–202.

Department of Health and Human Services. (2011, March). *Report to Congress: National strategy for quality improvement in health care.* Retrieved from http://www.ahrq.gov/workingforquality/nqs/nqs2011annlrpt.pdf. Accessed on January 15, 2014.

Eysenbach, G. (2001). What is e-Health? *Journal of Medical Internet Research, 3*(2), 1. Retrieved from http://www.jmir.org/2001/2/e20/. Accessed on January 19, 2014.

Ferguson, T., & E-Patient Scholars Working Group. (2013). *E-Patients: How they can help us heal health care.* Retrieved from http://e-patients.net/e-Patient_White_Paper_with_Afterword.pdf. Accessed on January 25, 2014.

Finn, N. B. (2011). *E-Patients live longer. The complete guide to managing health care using technology.* Bloomington, IN: iUniverse, Inc.

Fowles, J. B., Terry, P., Xi, M., Hibbard, J., Bloom, C. T., & Harvey, L. (2009). Measuring self-management of patients' and employees' health; further validation for the Patient Activation Measure (PAM) based on its relation to employee characteristics. *Patient Education and Counseling, 77*(1), 116–122.

Goldzweig, C. L. (2012). Editorial. Pushing the envelope of electronic patient portals to engage patients in their care. *Annals of Internal Medicine, 157,* 525–526.

Goldzweig, C. L., Orshansky, G., Paige, N. M., Towfigh, A. A., Haggstrom, D. A., Miake-Lye, I., ... Shekelle, P. G. (2013). Electronic patient portals: Evidence on health outcomes, satisfaction, efficiency, and attitudes. *Annals of Internal Medicine, 159,* 677–687.

Gruman, J., Holmes, M. H., French, M. E., Jeffress, D., Sofaer, S., Shaller, D., & Prager, D. J. (2010). From patient education to patient engagement: Implications for the field of patient education. *Patient Education and Counseling, 78,* 350–356.

H.R. 1–111th Congress. (2009). *American Recovery and Reinvestment Act of 2009.* Retrieved from http://www.govtrack.us/congress/bills/111/hr1. Accessed on January 25, 2014.

HealthIT.gov. (2013). *Meaningful use definition and objectives.* Retrieved from http://www.healthit.gov/providers-professionals/meaningful-use-definition objectives. Accessed on January 25, 2014.

HealthIT.gov. (2013, April). *A record of progress on health information technology.* Retrieved from http://www.healthit.gov/sites/default/files/record_of_hit_progress_infographic_april_update.pdf. Accessed on January 17, 2014.

Hibbard, J. (2009). Using systematic measurement to target consumer activation strategies. *Medical Care Research and Review, 66*(1 Suppl.), 9S–27S.

Hibbard, J., & Cunningham, P. J. (2008). How engaged are consumers in their health and health care, and why does it matter? *Research Briefs, 8,* 1–9.

Hibbard, J., Greene, J., & Overton, V. (2013). Patients with lower activation associated with higher costs; delivery systems should know their patients' scores. *Health Affairs, 32*(2), 216–222.

Hibbard, J., & Mahoney, E. (2010). Toward a theory of patient and consumer activation. *Patient Education and Counseling, 78,* 377–381.

Hibbard, J., Stockard, J., Mahoney, E. R., & Tusler, M. (2004). Development of the Patient Activation Measure (PAM); conceptualizing and measuring activation in patients and consumers. *Health Services Research, 39*(4 Pt. 1), 1005–1026.

Hibbard, J. H., & Greene, J. (2013). What the evidence shows about patient activation: Better health outcomes and care experiences; fewer data on costs. *Health Affairs, 32*(2), 207–214.

Hibbard, J. H., Mahoney, E. R., Stock, R., & Tusler, M. (2007). Do increases in patient activation result in improved self-management behaviors? *Health Services Research, 42*(4), 1443–1463.

Hobbs, J. L. (2009). A dimensional analysis of patient-centered care. *Nursing Research, 58*(1), 52–79.

Keckley, P. C., & Deloitte Center for Health Solutions. (2012). *2012 U.S. Survey of Health Care Consumers.* Retrieved from http://www.deloitte.com/view/en_US/us/Insights/centers/center-for-health-solutions/research/517f54995c0e7310VgnVCM2000001b56f00aRCRD.htm. Accessed on January 25, 2014.

Keselman, A., Logan, R., Smith, C. A., Leroy, G., & Zeng-Treitler, Q. (2008). Developing informatics tools and strategies for consumer-centered healt communication. *Journal of American Medical Informatics Association, 15,* 473–483.

Kussin, S. Z. (2011). *Doctor, your patient will see you now.* New York, NY: Rowman & Littlefield Publishers, Inc.

Marchibroda, J. M. (2013, July 24). *Health information technology: Using it to improve care* (Statement of Janet M. Marchibroda, Director, Health Innovation Initiative before the United States Senate Committee on Finance). Washington, DC: Bipartisan Policy Center.

Marchibroda, J. M., & deBronkart, D. (2013). The role of information technology in health care. In K. A. McCormick & B. Gugerty (Eds.), *Healthcare information technology* (pp. 61–81). New York, NY: McGraw Hill.

Maurer, M., Dardess, P., Carman, K. L., Frazier, K., Smeeding, L., & American Institutes for Research. (2012, May). *Guide to patient and family engagement: Environmental scan report.* Agency for Healthcare Research and Quality, Rockville, MD. http://www.ahrq.gov/research/findings/final-reports/ptfamilyscan/ptfamilyref.html

National eHealth Collaborative. (2012). *Consumer engagement with health information technology. Summary of NeHC survey results.* Retrieved from http://www.nationalehealth.org/ckfinder/userfiles/files/Consumer Con.Meeting/CE_HIT_Summary3.pdf. Accessed on January 18, 2014.

Office of the National Coordinator of Health Information Technology. (2011, September). *Federal Health Information Technology Strategic Plan 2011-2015.* Retrieved from http://www.healthit.gov/sites/default/files/utility/final-federal-health-it-strategic-plan-0911.pdf. Accessed on December 5, 2014.

Oldenburg, J. (2013). Preface. In J. Oldenburg, D. Chase, K. T. Christensen, & B. Tritle (Eds.), *Engage! Transforming healthcare through digital patient engagement* (pp. xxv–xxix). Chicago, IL: HIMSS Media.

Oldenburg, J., Chase, D., Christensen, K. T., & Tritle, B. (Eds.). (2013). *Engage! Transforming healthcare through digital patient engagement*. Chicago, IL: HIMSS Media.

Ozbolt, J., Sands, D. Z., Dykes, P., Pratt, W., Rosas, A. G., & Walker, J. M. (2012, September 19). *Summary report of consumer eHealth unintended consequences work group activities* . Prepared for the Office of the National Coordinator for Health Information Technology. Rockville, MD. Contract No.: HHSP23320095655WC.

Patient Protection and Affordable Care Act [Public Law 111-148], Detailed Summary. (2011). p.4. http://www.dpc. senate.gov/healthreformbill/healthbill04.pdf. Accessed December 4, 2014.

Remmers, C., Hibbard, J., Mosen, D. M., Wagenfield, M., Hoye, R. E., & Jones, C. (2009). Is patient activation associated with future health outcomes and healthcare utilization among patients with diabetes? *Journal of Ambulatory Care Management, 32*(4), 320–327.

Roseman, D., Osborne-Stafsnes, J., Amy, C. H., Boslaugh, S., & Slate-Miller, K. (2013). Early lessons from four "aligning forces for quality" communities bolster the case for patient-centered care. *Health Affairs, 32*, 232–241.

Sakar, U., & Bates, D. W. (2014). Care partners and online patient portals. *Journal of the American Medical Association, 311*(4), 357–358. doi:10.1001/jama.2013.285825.

Sands, D. Z. (2005). Electronic patient-centered communication: E-mail and other e-ways to communicate clearly. In D. Lewis, W. V. Slack, G. Eysenbach, R. Kukafka, P. Z. Stavri, & H. Jimison (Eds.), *Consumer health informatics: Informing consumers and improving health care*

(pp. 107–120). New York, NY: Springer Science + Business Media.

Sands, D. Z. (2013). Foreword. In J. Oldenburg, D. Chase, K. T. Christensen, & B. Tritle (Eds.), *Engage! Transforming healthcare through digital patient engagement* (pp. xxi–xxiv). Chicago, IL: HIMSS Media.

Skolasky, R. L., Mackenzie, E. J., Wegener, S. T., & Riley, L. H. (2011). Patient activation and functional recovery in persons undergoing spine surgery [Abstract]. *Orthopedics, 34*(11), 888.

Society for Participatory Medicine. (2014). *About us*. Retrieved from http://participatorymedicine.org. Accessed on January 25, 2014.

Stewart, M., Brown, J. B., Donner, A., McWhinney, I. R., Oates, J., Weston, W. W., & Jordan, J. (2000). The impact of patient-centered care on outcomes. *Journal of Family Practice, 49*, 796–804.

The Institute of Medicine. (2012). *Best care at lower cost: The pathway to continuously learning health care in America*. Washington, DC: The National Academies Press.

The World Bank. (2014). *Empowerment*. Retrieved from http://web.worldbank.org/WBSITE/EXTERNAL/TOPICS/EXTPOVERTY/EXTEMPOWERMENT/0,,menuPK:486417~pagePK:149018~piPK:149093~theSitePK:486411,00.html. Accessed on January 18, 2014.

Wennberg, D. E., Marr, A., Lang, L., O'Malley, S., & Bennett, G. (2010). A randomized trial of a telephone care-management strategy. *The New England Journal of Medicine, 363*, 1245–1254.

Zielstorff, R. D., & Frink, B. B. (2011). Consumer and patient use of computers for health. In V. K. Saba & K. A. McCormick (Eds.), *Essentials of nursing informatics* (5th ed. pp. 577–601). New York, NY: McGraw Hill Medical.

PART 6

Nursing Informatics— Complex Applications

Kathleen A. McCormick

36

Healthcare Analytics

Kathleen C. Kimmel

• OBJECTIVES

1. Define healthcare analytics and related terms:
   i. Data
   ii. Information
   iii. Knowledge
   iv. Wisdom
   v. Decision Support
   vi. Business Intelligence
   vii. Knowledge Management
   viii. Performance Management
   ix. Predictive Analytics
2. Describe the difference between report production and analytical drill down evaluations for decision support.
3. Discuss how decision support, business intelligence, and performance management fit.
4. Illustrate how analytics contributes to and fuels rapid-cycle improvement processes.
5. Discuss data governance for optimal use of analytics.

• KEY WORDS

Value-based purchasing
Triple Aim
Quality Metrics
Population health
Accountable care organizations
Middleware
Enterprise data warehouse
Data validity
Key performance indicators
Transactional processing systems
Management information systems
Data visualization tools
Database administrator

INTRODUCTION

Business intelligence, performance management, information technology (IT), and analytics are currently contributing to transformational healthcare reform. When Don Berwick was chief executive officer (CEO) of the Institute for Healthcare Improvement (IHI), he and his organization coined the term, "The Triple Aim" (Berwick et al., 2008; IHI, n.d.). The three components of Triple Aim are:

1. Improve the experience of care
2. Improve the health of populations
3. Reduce the per capita costs of healthcare

In July 2010, Berwick was appointed by President Barack Obama to serve as the Administrator of the Centers for Medicare and Medicaid (CMS) through a recess appointment. He was tapped to implement the Affordable Care Act (ACA), which was enacted in March 2010. (It was later defended and supported by the Supreme Court in June 2013.) In December 2011, Berwick resigned from CMS. Although Berwick's time was short at CMS his legacy remained. He brought with him the concept of the Triple Aim and it stuck. The Triple Aim concepts continue to be the driver of Governmental healthcare policy and funding.

Although the Affordable Care Act (ACA), which was enacted in 2010, occurred three months before Berwick's appointment, the elements of the Triple Aim are highly aligned with the ACA (Table 36.1).

HEALTHCARE ANALYTICS

This chapter deals with what is healthcare analytics. Quite simply, analytics is the science of analysis (Turban, Sharda, & Denlen, 2011). Analytics is akin to the central nervous system of the body, where information is processed and is interpreted (analyzed) by the brain. Analytics is the systematic use of data and related business insights developed through applied analytical disciplines (e.g. statistical, contextual, quantitative, predictive, cognitive, other [including emerging] models) to drive fact-based decision-making for planning, management, measurement, and learning. Analytics may be descriptive, predictive, or prescriptive (Cortada, Gordon, & Lenihan, 2012).

When applied to healthcare, analytics incorporates business intelligence (BI) information from a variety of

TABLE 36.1	Comparison of Triple Aim and the Affordable Care Act
Triple Aim Criteria	**Initiatives in the Affordable Care Act**

Improve the experience of care	• Offer incentives and penalties to improve the experience of care, such as:
	  ○ Meeting the Value-Based Payment (VBP) patient satisfaction goals and the Consumer Assessment of Healthcare Providers and Services (CAHPS)
	  ○ Supplying patient portals

Improve the health of populations	• Provide payment based on quality, such as:
	  ○ Achieving quality metrics, and
	  ○ Meeting Pay for performance/physician quality incentives
	• Establish awards for clinically integrated care, such as:
	  ○ Working Health Information Exchanges
	  ○ Creating disease registries
	  ○ Providing clinician portals
	  ○ Offering Patient Centered Medical Homes
	  ○ Creating and delivering Accountable Care Organizations and Medicare Shared Savings Programs
	  ○ Providing Population Health initiatives that
	  ○ Support and encourage patient engagement
	  ○ Incorporate mobile applications that contribute toward the patient achieving their desired health goals
	  ○ Integrate electronic home device monitoring systems and telemedicine

Reduce the per capita cost of healthcare	• Make adequate health insurance coverage more affordable and available to the public
	• Offer incentives to expand coverage
	  ○ Regulate healthcare coverage (including first dollar coverage for preventative care)
	  ○ Create health insurance exchanges
	• Reform delivery and payment systems to provide better care in a cost-efficient manner
	• Impose employer penalties
	• Structure payment based on quality

TABLE 36.2	Basic Definitions
Term	**Example**
Data—Data consist of the raw facts. Data are meaningless by themselves and require context to be interpreted.	Example: A single data point of a temperature: If the patient's temperature is 100.2°F/37.9°C, what conclusions can you make? More information is needed to make any conclusion. Is the patient a new born or an adult? Is the patient in a bed or is the patient an athlete who has finished running a race?
Information—Data are in a contextually organized state. A collection of data or facts.	Example: An EHR where a patient's vital signs, lab results, radiology information, demographics, medications, treatments, unit, diagnosis, problem statements, medications, and drip rates reside and can be visualized contextually together.
Knowledge—Knowledge is information that can be used to make decisions. It consists of understanding of the information that is discovered and can be put to use.	Example: A control chart type dashboard that shows Meaningful Use data points and associated information in a format that can be used to conduct a root cause analysis or can contribute to performance management by using it for a rapid-cycle improvement process methodology.
Wisdom—Is the application of data, information, and knowledge to make appropriate decisions.	Example: Applied nursing judgment: A nurse notices an elderly, type 1—insulin dependent—diabetic woman, has multiple emergency room visits for diabetes-related emergencies. After noticing the analytical trends the nurse delves deeper. As the nurse questions the patient the nurse learns that the woman has vision problems and is unable to accurately view the amount of insulin she draws in her syringes, which leads to inaccurate insulin doses. The nurse recommends an ophthalmology consult. The patient acquires a pair of prescription glasses that allows her to give herself the appropriate insulin dose. The patient's return ED visits for diabetic issues for the patient drop by 90%.

systems including electronic health records (EHRs); financial systems (e.g., general ledger and billing systems); stand-alone analytical applications; admission, discharge, and transfer (ADT) systems; enterprise resource planning (ERP); time and attendance; scheduling systems; stand-alone clinical department applications, such as laboratory, radiology, OB/GYN, other electronic systems. Analytic applications are able to apply statistics, formulas, modeling, and are expressed with visual analytical tools such as score cards and dashboards with drill down capabilities.

The first step in understanding analytics is to start with a few basic associated definitions shown in Table 36.2.

ANALYTICS IN HEALTHCARE

The use of analytics, clinical and BI, performance management, predictive modeling and simulation and the use of enterprise data warehouses (EDWs) in healthcare are not new. Health insurance plans (also called "payers") have been using EDWs and data marts for 20 years. While seeming new to healthcare, analytics have been used by hospital chief financial officers (CFOs) for well over 10 years. The finance department of hospitals is routinely

monitoring and tracking a variety of financially oriented scorecards and dashboards.

Years ago the payer community realized that having multiple best-of-breed departmental electronic systems, each of which has its own analytical applications for reporting, caused problems when data from different systems needed to be combined and reported together. Because each proprietary best-of-breed department system has different ways of describing, entering, formatting, storing, handling, and reporting data when multiple diverse systems are compared it is the equivalent of the "Tower of Babel" with many different languages and no way to normalize or standardize data. An EDW takes data from multiple source systems, extracts the data, transforms and loads (ETL) the data into one standardized and normalized format. Once the data are normalized and standardized it comprises "one version of the truth" (i.e., a reliable and trusted source of data). Descriptions of the data, including the data source; formats; descriptions; calculations; etc., are stored in the meta-data. (Meta-data is data about the data.) The middle ware, or presentation layer, enables users to access the data. Common-off-the-shelf (COTS) query tools are listed below. In addition, visual application dashboard tools such as Qlikview, Tableau, Spotfire, Microsoft Visual Stack, etc., can be used for dashboards. Common "middleware" or reporting/analytics tools used in hospitals are:

- **Crystal reports**
- **Business Objects**
- **Excel:** Used for analysis, reporting, and manual integration of data
- **SSRS:** SQL Server Reporting Services is used as way of extracting and manipulating data
- **SPSS:** Used for statistical analysis in social science
- **R:** A free software programing language and software environment for statistical computing and graphics. It is used at many academic medical centers
- **RDL:** Report Definition Language used for data reporting
- **Microsoft—Access Database:** Used for storing and manipulating data obtained from other systems
- **PORG:** Personal Option Report Generator used by some financial and payroll systems for reporting and data extraction
- **SQL:** Standard Query Language used to run reports and extract data from relational databases
- **Promodol:** Tool for data simulation

BASIC HEALTHCARE ANALYTICS DEFINITIONS

Analytics falls under the decision support systems (DSS). Often clinicians find this difficult to understand. They are used to limiting their thinking to DSS as being only alerts and reminders that are built into EHRs (Fig. 36.1).

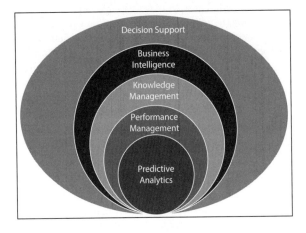

• **FIGURE 36.1.** Decision Support Relationship Diagram.

A broader understanding of DSS is called for. Actually, DSSs are an overarching and all-encompassing term used to describe and computerized system that enables the process of decision-making (Turban et al., 2011). Various types of decision support terms are described in Table 36.3.

THE DIFFERENCE BETWEEN REPORTS AND ANALYTICS

There are often misconceptions associated with analytics and reports. Both reports and analytics are considered to be forms of business intelligence (BI). (Remember, any data or information generated from electronic systems is considered to be BI.) Reports or analytics can be for:

- Quality of care, such as how many pressure ulcers have occurred in the hospital, when they occurred, and what was the patient's age, diagnosis, sex, etc., in order to reduce the number of pressure ulcers

- Service Line analysis, such as for low-birth-weight babies, what was the age of the mother, ethnic group, the presence or absence of prenatal care, economic status, education, zip code, etc., to set the stage for outreach to populations at risk for low-birth-weight babies

- Clinical effectiveness, such as evaluating the time taken in a colonoscopy and correlating the total time of the procedure to incidents of missed diagnoses of colon cancer to lower the rate of patients whose colon cancer was missed during a colonoscopy procedure

- Variation in practice (cost, quality, length of stay, and post-operative complications) when comparing bowel resections performed by general surgeons versus gastroenterology specialists to consult and coach physicians with outcomes that consistently deviate from the outcomes of the top performers

- Operational effectiveness, such as evaluating the time from arrival in the emergency department to admission to a patient floor, to reduce patient wait times

- Improve financial performance, such evaluating the number and reasons for claims denials to lower the number of denials

The greatest shortcoming of reports is that the ability to analyze them is often limited. That is, frequently, when a single report is studied, additional questions arise, such as (1) is this a single incident; (2) is it isolated or is it happening elsewhere; (3) how long has it been occurring; (4) is it occurring all the time or is it occurring on a specific day of the week or time of day; (5) is it universal or

TABLE 36.3	Descriptions of Decision Support Terms
Term	**Description**
Decision Support Systems	A conceptual framework for decision-making. It involves using various computerized applications that apply quantitative models, and simulation models which impact strategy and performance.
Business Intelligence	Business intelligence (BI) systems are a sub-system of DSS. They are any computerized applications that apply analytical tools, applications, and methodologies. The process of BI is based on the process of transforming data to information. In the early 1980s, the term executive information systems (EIS) was used as senior business leaders used multi-dimensional data in either ad hoc or routinely scheduled runs for reporting, forecasting, status against key performance indicators (KPIs). In the 1990s, the term EIS morphed to BI. Included in BI are data warehouses, data marts, online analytical processing (OLAP), dashboards, and scorecards with drill down capabilities.
Knowledge Management Systems (KMS)	Knowledge management systems involve computerized applications to identify, collect, capture, store, manage, and disseminate useful knowledge to workers to support individual or group decision-making. KMSs bring together culture, process and decrease variation in practice. For example, KMSs would be used by an IT support center to inform each of the support line employees of known issues and the proper fix or work-around to provide to the caller. Technologies that support KMSs are artificial intelligence (AI), intelligent agents (AIs), knowledge management in databases (KMDBs), extensible markup language (XML), Web 2.0, electronic document management systems (EDM), enterprise knowledge portals (EKPs), collaborative computing and groupware tools, knowledge serves, knowledge harvesting tools, search engines, and content management systems (CMS).
	Knowledge management is more of a methodology. It is an applied business practice that uses technology. The model includes data, information, knowledge, action, and results (DIKAR). It is important to continuously keep a KMS system up-to-date and relevant. If the data elements are old and out-of-date usage will be poor and users can make errors if out-of-date information is accessed.
Business Performance Management (BPM)	Performance management is a subset of BI. BPM is used to change behaviors related to achieving results. Analytical visual applications such as scorecards and dashboards are used. BPM becomes valuable as it relates to various rapid-cycle improvement processes.
Predictive Analytics	Predictive analytics uses forecasting and simulation models to predict occurrences, trends, or outcomes. Examples of predictive models are the LACE model for predicting patients who are at a high risk for a hospital readmission. LACE is an abbreviation for the four predictive factors:
	• L = length of stay • A = acute admission through the emergency department (ED) • C = co-morbidities • E = ED visits within the past six months (RWJF)
	Another example is the CURB-65 criteria for predicting mortality for Community Acquired Pneumonia in patients 65 or older.
	• C = Confusion of recent onset • U = Urea (BUN > 7) • R = Respiratory rate > 30 breaths per minute • B = Blood Pressure (Systolic < 90 mmHg and Diastolic < 60 mmHg) • 65 = Age 65 or older (MedicalCriteria.com, n.d.)

does it pertain to specific providers; (6) is it occurring at all locations or specific locations; (6) is it seasonal or not; (7) has it happened before? To answer these type of questions additional reports may need to be created. In contrast, analytics often offers the ability to drill down to the lowest level of granularity. Additionally, with analytics, multiple electronic systems can be incorporated to generate a more detailed understanding of the situation and the ability to

uncover a problem that otherwise might not be evident. For example, a static report may show that cardiac ventriculograms have increased, while an analytical analysis may show that 60% of these studies were not reimbursed by the commercial health insurance payers because these tests were considered medically excessive and unnecessary because an echocardiogram was the recommended test for the diagnosis code listed (see Table 36.4.)

TABLE 36.4	Comparison of Reports Versus Analytics
Reports	**Analytics**
A static view of data at a point in time that shows what happened	A malleable view that can drill down to indicate why it is happening, and can assist with determining the root cause
One data source, one view that shows one aspect of the problem or situation	Multi-phasic views that incorporate data and information from other electronic systems, such as clinical information from an EHR and financial systems
Validity and reliability issues as each separate analytical system has its own terminology and description of values	"One version of the truth" where standardized terminology is used and the process for producing the analytics is tracked

Another important element in understanding data and information is the data source and how the reporting applications determine the values used in the reporting functions. Each analytical application has its own vocabulary or meta-data (data about the data). For example, one system may calculate length of stay (LOS) as an occupied hospital bed at midnight. Another system may include observation beds in its LOS calculation or calculate at a different time of day. When a variety of systems have different lexicons, obviously the results are different as the numerators and denominators differ. Physicians, nurses, and other clinical providers often do not understand that variations in how data are captured, organized, stored, and reported depends on how the definitions are structured and that if the same question were asked and reported on by 10 different analytical applications that have different formats the reports would have dissimilar results. The fact that a clinician or executive can ask one question and receive many diverse answers tends to confound clinicians who immediately doubt the veracity and validity of the results. In the world of enterprise data warehouses (EDWs), if clinicians doubt that the results are a true reflection of the data they quickly discount the value of the EDW diminishes. Once doubts of the data's veracity are raised the use of the EDW diminishes. It is important that clinical informatics professionals constantly educate the end users as to how reporting and analytics work and how various conflicting reports can be legitimate based on how the data were entered, compiled, the date they were reported, and the exceptions that were extracted before the report was created and how often the data were refreshed.

It is important to understand the systems where reports originate. That is, is the system a real-time transactional system or is it an analytical application that has a cutoff point for collecting and reporting the data? Most data warehouses and data marts are not real-time transactional systems. Variation in results reported by different systems (and even in the same system) can occur because of the time the report is run. It is important to understand the type of reporting. For example, if an ad hoc report is run at eight o'clock in the morning and the data are refreshed at noon a report run an hour later could differ.

UNDERSTANDING HOW DECISION SUPPORT, BI, AND PERFORMANCE MANAGEMENT FIT

In hospitals and healthcare organizations there are a variety of systems. It is important to understand these systems and how they are used. The major systems are:

- **Transactional processing systems (TPSs):** A TPS is used for operational management. They tend to be real-time systems, such as ADT. For example, a transactional system would have minute-to-minute census information. They are used for operations management.

- **Decision Support Systems:** These systems are not transactional, which means that they are not real time. These systems are used for tactical or strategic management decision. Data marts and data warehouses receive data feeds from transactional systems or operational data stores (ODS) at pre-defined intervals. The frequency of data feeds to a data warehouse or a data mart often depends on the decisions that are being made and how current the data need to be (data latency). For example, a CFO may need to see accounts receivable information daily, while an analytics analysis to calculate financial reserves may only need to be run on a monthly basis. Another example may be a chief quality officer who wants information on the occurrence of hospital acquired conditions (HACs) on a daily dashboard. Business Intelligence systems are a subset of DSS.

- **Management Information Systems (MIS):** A MIS consists of transactional data that process patient data. It includes document management software, health information management systems (HIS), microfiche viewing systems, and telephone systems.

- **Data Visualization Tools:** Dashboards and score-cards are examples of how data and information can be displayed. It is important to determine the type of dashboard, such as financial, clinical outcomes, departmental specific, patient flow, service line, etc. When designing dashboards it is important to select the best format.

  ○ The format of the dashboard can be pie charts, graphs, tables, bubble charts, scatter diagrams, run charts (where information is displayed over time), and control charts (similar to run charts with the addition of upper and lower thresholds). Clinical informatics professionals often need to counsel and discuss with end users which visual application viewing format would work best. Presenting several prototypes and discussing the advantages and disadvantages of each prototype can be valuable. Some BI experts dislike using pie charts because of the limitations associated. Indeed, the pie chart is the least effective visual analytical display (Few, 2007). Vendors of data warehouses, data marts, and analytical applications will have many options for choosing visualization options.

HEALTHCARE ANALYTICS AND THE RAPID-CYCLE IMPROVEMENT PROCESS

Business Performance Management (BPM), also called performance management, focuses more on strategy and objectives. Business Intelligence (BI) is an important element of performance management. Think of BI as the technology and performance management as the additional layer that enables planning, monitoring, and analyzing. Using the core BI applications and tools performance management extends the monitoring and measurement for tracking a variety of metrics such as core measures, accountable care organization (ACO) metrics, value-based purchasing (VBP), hospital-acquired conditions (HACs), and a long list of other quality and outcomes metrics. Each of the metrics would be described as a key performance indicator (KPI). An example of a KPI would be having 100% of vital signs recorded in an EHR.

The goal of performance management is to change behavior. Changing behavior and culture is aided by rapid-cycle improvement processes. Rapid-cycle improvement

processes are a mechanism to promote rapid behavioral changes leading to cultural changes. The most common rapid-cycle improvement processes used in hospitals today are:

- Plan-Do-Check Act (PDCA)
- Six Sigma (Define, Measure, Analyze, Improve, and Control)
- Lean (Voice of the customer, value stream mapping, determination of the value-added and non-value-added steps, create or revise processes)
- Root Cause Analysis (RCA), (Retrospective analysis of a problem or event—asks a series of why questions to determine the root cause)
- Failure Mode Effects Analysis (FMEA), (Process maps current state, identify process failures, estimate effect of identified failures, identify top reasons for failure, and take risk mitigation steps)

Rapid-cycle improvement processes are combined with visual analytical tools, such as dashboards to allow the teams to track progress toward the goals over time. Dashboards are an easy means to determine if the action is working or not and to spark additional questions, which the team can respond to as they work toward achieving the KPIs. A use case scenario follows, which integrates the concepts of business intelligence monitoring of performance management to ensure that the Meaningful Use Smoking Cessation metric is achieved.

USE CASE SCENARIO: PERFORMANCE MANAGEMENT FOR MEANINGFUL USE SMOKING STATUS

There are several steps involved in performance management efforts. This vignette will break down the process into steps. Remember that performance management is essentially a strategic process that is intended to achieve results, produce outcomes, and change behavior. The steps are:

- **Strategic planning situation analysis:** To begin our Meaningful Use smoking status performance management project we start by capturing our baseline. At hospital "A," of a multi-hospital system, smoking status is recorded on 20% of the patients. We find that smoking status resides in the EHR under the "social history" category. In order to comply with Stage 1 of meaningful use (MU) the threshold is to have smoking status recorded on 50% patients who are 13 years of age or older.

The problem with the compliance at hospital "A" is that the nurses are charting smoking status in the wrong cell on their EHR data entry screen. The nurses need to enter it under social history or it will not be captured in the vendor's operational data store (ODS). The EDW is programmed to read and extract this data up from the ODS.

- **Planning horizon:** We have one month to the start of the 90-day reporting period. We have to act quickly to resolve the issue of nurses not entering data in the appropriate field to capture that smoking status was evaluated and charted.

- **Environmental scan:** Our environmental scan indicates huge variability in hospital compliance. Using our dashboards we see that hospital "A" is at 20% and hospital "B" is at 90%. This is a strengths, weaknesses, opportunities, threats (SWOT) analysis. We find huge variability with nurse recording of smoking status and other MU measures. Naturally one asks why the nurses at hospital "A" are at 20% compliance while the nurses at hospital "B" are at 90% for the very same smoking status recording requirement. Are the nurses at hospital "B" much better nurses? Why the variance? This is where research and observation come into play. Upon investigation it is found that the nurses at hospital "A" are focused on smoking cessation rather than smoking status. These are two different variations of smoking. One is reporting *if* the patient smokes and the other is focused on an outcome of ceasing the smoking behavior. Smoking cessation is an old requirement that patients receive smoking cessation education. The nurses at hospital "A" provide every patient with smoking cessation education. Since they give all patients (whether they smoke or not) cessation education they believe that it is redundant to record smoking status if they record they have educated the patient on smoking. That is, the nurses felt it is not necessary for them to complete the smoking status information. The environmental scan indicated that education was required to change behavior.

- **Gap Analysis:** Since hospital A's recording of smoking status is at 20% and they need to be over 50% the gap they need to overcome is 30%.

- **Strategic vision:** The strategic vision is that all hospitals in the system will have 100% compliance with the Meaningful Use thresholds and will in fact exceed them.

- **Business strategy:** The strategies will be education and compliance monitoring to ensure compliance.

- **Identify goals and objectives:** Create an education plan, meet with hospital CNO, hospital clinical informatics professionals, nurse managers, and compliance officers and review each of the MU measures. Inform them of the importance of having nurses enter data appropriately and show where in the EHR product build the data entry cells are located. Explain the monitoring and dashboard systems and explain who will monitor and how often.

- **Communication:** The team agreed that education and communication were the key elements. All nurses were needed to be familiar with meaningful use and how where they entered data in the EHR made the difference. The patient care nurses also needed to see and understand the key performance indicators (threshold attained for each MU measure) and the drill down capabilities.

- **Rewards and incentives:** It is advantageous when pay and performance are linked. At this multi-hospital system the executives and the CNO have a business performance scorecard. Achieving the MU thresholds and receiving the CMS EHR incentive funds is tied to their bonuses.

- **Focus:** The MU threshold compliance dashboard is viewed at all levels—corporate, region, hospital, compliance office, and individual nursing unit.

- **Resources:** Each hospital selects one individual who is ultimately responsible. Most students have experienced situations where a committee is responsible and oftentimes the result is that no one is responsible. At these hospitals the chief operating officer (COO) assumed ultimate responsibility.

- **Key Performance Indicators (KPIs):** The KPIs are the MU 14 Core, 10 Menu, and 15 quality measures. The goal is that the thresholds set by the hospitals, which in most cases exceeds the CMS thresholds, are met. For example, CMS has a 50% threshold for smoking status recording while this hospital system established an internal threshold of 80% that they expect their hospitals to meet.

- **Dashboard:** The hospital system opted for a dashboard to display both the progress bar with red and green to show if they are below (red) or above (green) the CMS threshold. The progress bar allows anyone to view it to see progress toward the goal. The minimum threshold is the line of demarcation between displaying red or green. It also enables users click on one of the measures and see a graphical representation below. The hospital used a control chart as its visual tool. Control charts have upper and lower limits. The upper limit is a line showing the hospital's self-imposed threshold. The lower line of the control chart is the CMS minimum threshold. The control chart also serves as a run chart. You can see that by the end of the reporting period, hospital "A" has achieved 100% compliance with the hospitals' standard of 100% compliance with recording vital signs.

Use Case 1. Performance Management Example for Meaningful Use Smoking Status Metric

Applying Analytics in the Workplace. Meaningful use, accountable care organizations and value-based purchasing (VBP) are areas where healthcare has a need to monitor and measure performance against criteria. When the CMS Meaningful Use final rules were published by CMS in July 2010 it caused pressure on eligible hospitals and critical access hospitals as well as eligible professionals (EPS). It brought with it pressure to have an EHR that would be capable of meeting the 14 Core Measures, five of the 10 Menu Measures, and the 15 quality measures. Eligible hospitals and eligible professionals quickly discovered that they needed computerized support to assist with monitoring and reporting the measures—especially for the 90-day continuous reporting period.

Meaningful Use can be seen as a paradigm shift in clinical decision-making. For many years, decision-making was more of an art than a science. Decisions were based on gut-reactions, intuition, or experience (Turban et al., 2011). This type of decision-making was often the best possible option available to executives because the analytical data upon which to make decisions were often lacking or marginal. Meaningful Use reporting required strict discipline in entering data correctly and reporting and analyzing data.

Healthcare organizations have recognized that technological tools are necessary to support highly complex care delivery and ensure adherence to best practices. Knowledge management systems (KMS) support decision-making by providing access to knowledge assets and sharing them throughout the organization. Intellectual assets are also known as intellectual capital. The use of KMS contributes to high efficiency and fosters a culture of collaboration. KMS include groupware systems, communication tools, collaborative management tools, content management, and document management.

Use Case: Clinical example: Intermountain Health Care's clinical knowledge repository uses validation architecture to ensure documents are valid—Intermountain Health Care's Clinical Knowledge Repository (CKR) provides a central location to store clinical documents. The CKR contains over 8000 unique documents ranging from Clinical Provider Order Entry (CPOE) order sets to clinical protocols. Most of the content in the CKR is represented in eXtensible Markup Language (XML). The authoring tool used to create CKR XML documents is from a third-party XML editor. The authoring tool allows users to create and edit XML documents without requiring them to have knowledge of XML. The XML editor is capable of performing standard XML validations, including verification that the document is well formed and that it is a valid instance of the appropriate XML Schema. In order for the CKR XML documents to operate within their target clinical systems, extensive validation of the content and structure of the XML documents becomes mandatory. A knowledge management validation tool is used. It alerts document authors if they need to fix a document. The result of having the user-friendly error messages is that less than 1% of all documents in Intermountain's knowledge repository are invalid (Hanna, Rocha, & Hulse 2005).

Use Case 2: Use Case Scenario to Ensure Data Are Valid for Knowledge management

Analytics and Governance. The failure rate for enterprise data warehouses (EDWs) is estimated to be as high as 70% to 80% (Kernochan, 2011). Failure is due to a variety of issues. Most importantly the data need to be reliable, well organized, and designed with the end users' needs in mind. Organizations that are embarking on an EDW for the first time usually require expert assistance. Working with an EDW is iterative. It is truly a process in which you learn as you progress. One way to greatly reduce the risk of failure is to use an Agile development approach. Agile is a rigorous, disciplined approach to systems and software development (Douglass, 2012).

Healthcare EDW Readiness Assessment. Before starting a readiness assessment it is important to ensure that the following attributes are in place. The lack of these items can be red flags that can put a project in jeopardy. Success factors for an EDW are having:

- Clearly stated mission and vision as well as objectives, such as KPIs. That is, everyone knows and can articulate the need and value of the EDW.

- Highly stable organization with low volatility (turnover) of key leaders. Because a long-term commitment to an EDW is paramount to success, if the chief executive officer (CEO), CFO, or other senior executive positions are in a state of flux there is greater risk to the EDW project's success. Indeed, when senior leaders change, often the organization's priorities change with them. An EDW is a major commitment and requires stable, solid, and consistent support over the duration of the project.

- Solid, unified, and unwavering support and leadership from the senior executives (i.e., the "C-suite"—CEO, CNO, CFO, CMO, etc.). If there are only occasional pockets of support, the nurse informatics professional is advised to work closely with the C-suite stakeholders to build cohesive support before proceeding. If the organization is prone to "turf wars" where different departments operate in silos and compete with each other for scarce dollars for project funding the risk of failure increases. In this situation the nurse informatics professional may want to create a value-realization chart that identifies how the EDW can benefit each of the various departments. When each department clearly understands and agrees with how the EDW is in their best interest the EDW has a greater chance of a high degree of success.

- Strong and reliable source systems such that data integrity issues are minimized. Most data sources have some integrity issues. The IT term, "garbage in, garbage out" (GIGO) refers to introducing messy data sources. When building an EDW if the data integrity of any one of the core systems is questionable the builders will identify the data problems and provide data to assist the upstream system administrators to improve the data quality. Oftentimes data integrity issues are unknown prior to the start of the EDW building process.

- Appropriate short- and long-term budget allocation. An EDW is an investment. Once the EDW is established the true value is in the ongoing use of the data as they are transformed to information, knowledge, and intelligence to make decisions and change behavior as part of the performance management process. This type of work requires teams and the appropriate funding for staffing teams. If the EDW budget is not protected and allocated over the long term there will be short-term gains that may not be able to be sustained.

- Appropriately skilled and dedicated staff who are able to remain on the project. When corners are cut on staffing and when important resources are pulled off the EDW project and assigned to other work efforts continuity suffers and can delay the project. Too many missed deadlines and delays contribute to a perception of a troubled project. It is sometimes hard to recover from perceptions that the project is not going well.

- Clear communication of the expected functionality at each stage of the project. Setting clear expectations is a critical success factor. Clinicians who have been involved in the role out of an EHR usually understand this principle. It is important to strive for quick wins that impact the strategic or clinical quality priorities. Once success is declared chances are end users see the value and eagerly clamor for additional KPIs that support their specific departments. It is also important to avoid "scope creep." Since EDW projects, by their very nature, are iterative, it is wise to build in a buffer to support a small amount of changes. In the governance structure it is advisable to have a change control board (CCB) that can discuss and approve appropriate changes in scope and to deny or protect the integrity of the project such that major changes to the scope are limited.

- Cooperative vendors that support the project. The lack of vendor cooperation and using data as a weapon for commercial gain are inappropriate. Oftentimes vendors believe their products or platform can compete or approximate the capabilities and functionality of an EDW. Some of these vendors "hold the data hostage" and deny access to data feeds from source systems. This makes it difficult to obtain the data extracts that feed the data warehouse or the data marts. It may be appropriate to ensure that appropriate legal language is included in contracts that stipulates who is the owner of the data—the vendor or the organization. Uncooperative vendors that impose limitations to the organization's access to their data sources and block interoperability should not be tolerated.

- Strong clinical and technical collaboration approach versus a technical development effort. Weekly reporting of tasks, activities, deliverables, and milestones to the appropriate committees and sub-committees is important. An oversight team of stakeholders needs to attend the weekly team meetings. The project manager and clinical sponsor should be hosting these meetings. An Agile development approach versus a traditional "waterfall" approach to the EDW development—where end users are involved throughout the project contributes to meeting expectations—is more effective.

Business Intelligence and Analytics Data Governance.
It is important to have a stakeholder group responsible for
overseeing the EDW. It is advisable to have an analytics
competency center (ACC), which is also often referred to
as a BI competency center (BICC). The role of the ACC is
to champion the BI investments, facilitate data standardization, as well as coordinate and oversee all BI activities,
ensuring that they are aligned and prioritized in accordance
with the overall strategic goals of the organization.
Establishing an ACC is a complex undertaking and before
launching one, one must assess both the challenges,
including an assessment of the current BI state, as well
as the readiness to work as a team in addressing the BI
initiatives of the organization.

There are various approaches to creating an ACC,
such as a centralized, consulting, functional, center of
excellence and a decentralized structure. The various
approaches revolve around how the organizations' data
analysts are arranged as well as their reporting structure.
In a centralized model the analysts are combined into one
department. The consulting model also organizes analysts
in one unit and the various departments who have analytical requests "contract" with the analyst group. Functional
models situate the analysts in specific departments that
routinely use their services, yet in this model consulting services are provided to other departments when
required. Center of excellence models are decentralized
and analysts reside in their specific department of expertise, yet have a dotted-line arrangement to a program
office to respond to requests from various other groups
or teams as needed. The decentralized model places analysts in the departments they are assigned with no connection structure to other analysts (Davenport, Harris, &
Morrison, 2010).

Several committees are recommended for an ACC:

- **Executive Oversight Committee:** The executive
  oversight committee comprises senior executive
  who meet regularly to set strategic analytic
  direction for the organization.

- **ACC Steering Committee:** The ACC steering
  committee monitors the EDW development and
  ensures that the BI and analytics requirements
  are being met. The steering committee members
  represent their respective departments and
  prioritize the KPIs. They evaluate the various
  electronic and legacy systems to determine which
  one is to be "the source of truth." That is, often data
  reside in more than one system. In these situations,
  the committee must decide which system is the one
  that will feed the EDW. This group also decides on
  definitions and data lexicons, such as determining

a consistent definition on how length of stay is
measured and calculated. They also make decisions
and document business rules that govern the data
as well as logic, data consistency, quality, accuracy,
data utilization, and data access. Occasionally
disputes can arise because of conflicting priorities.
This group works to resolve conflicts and establish
a change control process. Another expectation
of the committee is to track issues and monitor
progress toward resolution. Team members consist
of a technical director, an analytics director,
analysts, a database administrator, directors,
and subject matter experts from across the
organization.

In closing, analytics and BI can help organizations
achieve the triple aim and make care safer. The true
beneficiaries of efforts to become an analytics-focused
organization are both individual patients and populations
of patients.

REFERENCES

Berwick, DM, Nolan, TW., & Whittington, J. (May/June,
  2008). The Triple Aim: Care, health, and cost. *Health
  Affairs, 27*(3),759–769.

Cortada, J., Gordon, D., & Lenihan, B. (2012). The value of
  analytics in healthcare. *IBM Executive Report*, (p. 2),
  New York, NY: IBM, Somers.

Davenport, T., Harris, J., & Morrison, R. (2010). *Analytics
  at work* (p. 106). Boston, MA: Harvard Business
  Press.

Douglass, B. (2012). *Top tips to using agile in mission critical
  agile development*. Retrieved from www.ibm.com

Few, S. (2007). Save the pie for dessert. Blog. Retrieved from
  https://courses.washington.edu/info424/2007/readings/
  Save%20the%20Pies%20for%20Dessert.pdf

Hanna, T., Rocha, R., Hulse, N., Del Fiol, G., Bradshaw. R. L.,
  & Roemer L. K. (2005). Customized document validation
  to support a flexible XML-based knowledge management framework. *AMIA Annual Symposium Proceedings*,
  291–295.

Institute for Health Improvement. (n.d.). The Triple Aim.
  Retrieved from http://www.ihi.org/Engage/Initiatives/
  TripleAim/Pages/default.aspx

Kernochan, W. (2011). Why most data warehouses fail.
  Enterprise Apps Today. Retrieved from http://www.
  enterpriseappstoday.com/business-intelligence/why-
  most-business-intelligence-projects-fail-1.html

MedicalCriteria.com. (n.d.). *CURB-65*. Retrieved from
  http://www.medicalcriteria.com/criteria/inf_curb65.htm

Turban, E., Sharda, R., & Denlen, D. (2011). *Decision support
  and business intelligence systems* (pp. 16, 41, 78). Upper
  Saddle River, NJ: Prentice Hall.

37

Planning, Design, and Implementation of Information Technology in Complex Healthcare Systems

Thomas R. Clancy

• OBJECTIVES

1. Define complex systems in the context of General Systems Theory.
2. Describe complex adaptive systems, a special case of complex systems.
3. Illustrate challenges and solutions for planning and designing information technology in complex healthcare systems.
   i. Wicked problems
   ii. High-reliability organizations
   iii. Structured and agile design methods
4. Provide examples of tools and methods used to plan and design information systems in complex healthcare processes.
   i. Computer-Aided Software Engineering
   ii. Discrete Event Simulation
   iii. Network Analysis Tools

• KEYWORDS

Complex adaptive systems
Wicked problems
Agile design
Discrete event simulation
Network science
Nurse informaticist
Electronic Medical Record
Systems analyst

INTRODUCTION

The introduction of information technology into the workflow of clinicians requires thoughtful planning, design, and implementation. Healthcare organizations of today are among some of the most complex systems in the world. They are composed of diverse specialties and multiple providers linked through a complex information network. Understanding and predicting the impact of new technology on healthcare system behavior is an ongoing challenge for nurse informaticists. That is because complex systems are unpredictable and what works in one organization does not guarantee success in another.

Nurse informaticists play a critical role in the successful deployment of healthcare information technology. Their unique blend of clinical knowledge and information systems expertise make them ideal systems analysts. As complex systems research discovers new findings, nurse informaticists must remain informed on how new knowledge can be translated into practice settings. The objective of this chapter is to provide a review of complex systems from the context of a general systems theory and then provide an overview of new strategies to plan, design, and implement information systems in healthcare organizations.

GENERAL SYSTEMS THEORY

A system can be defined as a set of interacting units or elements that form an integrated whole intended to perform some function (Skyttner, 2001). An example of a system in healthcare might be the organized network of providers (nurses, physicians, and support staff), equipment, and materials necessary to accomplish a specific purpose such as the prevention, diagnosis, and treatment of illness. General systems theory (GST) provides a general language which ties together various areas in inter-disciplinary communication. It endeavors toward a universal science that joins together multiple fields with common concepts, principles, and properties. Although healthcare is a discipline in and of itself, it integrates with many other systems from fields as diverse as biology, economics, and the physical sciences.

Systems can be closed, isolated, or open. A closed system can only exchange energy across its borders. For example, a greenhouse can exchange heat (energy) but not physical matter with its environment. Isolated systems cannot exchange any form of heat, energy, or matter across their borders. Examples of closed and isolated systems are generally restricted to physical sciences such as physics and chemistry. An open system is always dependent on its environment for the exchange of matter, energy, and information. Healthcare systems are considered open and are continuously exchanging information and resources throughout their many integrating sub-systems. Some fundamental properties collectively comprise a general systems theory of open systems.

Open Systems

All open systems are goal seeking. Goals may be as fundamental as survival and reproduction (living systems) to optimizing the flow of information across computer networks. To achieve goals, systems must transform inputs into outputs. An input might include the entry of information into a computer where it is transformed into a series of binary digits (outputs). These digits can then be routed across networks to end users more efficiently than other forms of communication. As simple systems interact, they are synthesized into a hierarchy of increasingly complex systems, from sub-atomic particles to entire civilizations (Skyttner, 2001). Levels within the hierarchy have novel characteristics that apply universally upward to more complex levels but not downward to simpler levels. In other words, at lower or less complex levels, systems from different fields share some characteristics in common. For example, both computer and biological systems communicate information by encoding it, either through computer programs or via the genome respectively. It is the inter-relationships and inter-dependencies between and across levels in hierarchies that create the concept of a holistic system separate and distinct from its individual components. As commonly noted, a system is greater than simply the sum of its individual parts.

Complex Systems

System behavior can be related to the concept of complexity. As systems transition from simple to complex it is important for nurse informaticists to understand that system behavior also changes. This is especially important in the management of data and information for clinical and administrative decision-making. Table 37.1 presents some examples of differences between simple and complex systems in healthcare.

As healthcare systems become increasingly complex it becomes progressively more difficult to predict how changes in provider workflow are impacted by new information technology. This is especially important for those individuals responsible for planning, designing, and implementing information systems in the healthcare environment of today.

The evolution of information systems in healthcare is replete with failed implementations, cost overruns, and dissatisfied providers. It is important to understand, however, that healthcare systems of today are some of the most complex in the world. The unpredictable nature of complex healthcare systems results from both structural and temporal factors. The structure of complex systems is composed of numerous elements connected through a rich social network. In hospitals, those interactive elements include both internal entities such as patients, nurses, physicians, technicians, and external entities, such as other hospitals, insurance payers, and regulatory agencies. The way information flows through this complex

TABLE 37.1	Simple Versus Complex Healthcare Systems		
Simple System	**Example**	**Complex System**	**Example**
There are a small number of elements in the system. Elements are parts of the system (people, places, and things).	A one physician, one nurse practice.	There are a large number of elements in the system.	A large academic health center with multiple providers and specialties.
There are few interactions between the elements.	Interactions occur primarily between the nurse and physician, and patient.	Many interactions between elements.	Thousands of interactions occur daily between patients, providers, and machines (computers).
Interaction between elements is highly organized. The number of sub-systems is small and fixed. Information flows primarily in two or three directions.	There is direct communication between the nurse, physician, and patient. These interactions may be enabled through a single, practice-based EHR.	Interactions between elements are loosely organized. There are multiple levels in the hierarchy of sub-systems where information flows in many directions.	Interactions occur between multiple providers. The medical center may have a sophisticated EHR with many applications integrated within it.
System behavior varies little. Day-to-day activities are highly predictable.	Because patient acuity varies little, provider workload remains the same from day to day.	System behavior is probabilistic and it is impossible to predict with certainty.	Because patient acuity can vary considerably, provider workload can change significantly from day to day.
The system does not evolve over time, is largely closed, and is slow to adapt to environmental changes.	The practice is mature and is not accepting new patients.	The system evolves over time. The system is largely open and constantly adapting to the external environment.	The medical center has multiple specialties that accept diverse disease conditions that require ongoing research and new knowledge.
The system is not robust to environmental shocks.	Changes in reimbursement or competitive pressures can quickly eliminate the practice in the marketplace.	Because of its diversity of services, the system can withstand environmental shocks.	Because there are many providers with multiple specialties, the system can withstand significant environmental changes that may impact one area.

Web of channels depends on the technology used, organizational design, and the nature of tasks and relationships (Clancy & Delaney, 2005).

As systems evolve from simple to complex systems a hierarchy of levels emerges within the organization. From a theoretical standpoint, complex systems form a "fuzzy," tiered structure of macro-, intermediary, and micro-systems (Clancy & Delaney, 2005). In hospital environments, for example, nursing units can be understood as micro-systems within the health system. When nursing units are combined into divisions (e.g., critical care, medical-surgical, or maternal-child), the nursing units' internal processes expand beyond their boundaries (for example, the medication usage process) to create intermediary or meso-systems. Major clinical and administrative systems emerge at the macro-level through the aggregation of interactions occurring at lower levels.

At the micro-system level, the relationship between cause and effect is somewhat predictable. However, as the organizational structure expands to include meso- and macro-system levels, causal relationships between stimulus and response become blurred. With increasing levels of complexity, the rich network of interactions between nurses, physicians, pharmacists, and other providers at multiple levels within the organization quickly expands the variability and range of potential states a system might exhibit. This is the driving force behind the unpredictability in complex system behavior.

Complex Adaptive Systems

Complex adaptive systems (CAS) are special cases of complex systems; the key difference being that a CAS can learn and adapt over time (Clancy, Effken, & Persut, 2008).

From biologic to man-made systems, CAS's are ubiquitous. The human body, comprised of its many subsystems (cardiovascular, respiratory, neurologic), is a CAS and continuously adapts to short- and long-term changes in the environment. The same principles can be applied to social organizations such as clinics or hospitals. Organizational learning is a form of adaptation and it has the capacity to change culture. New reporting relationships can alter the structure of a social network and act as the catalyst for adaptation to environmental change. For example, the movement from hierarchical organizational structures to quasi-networked reporting relationships can improve communication both vertically and horizontally.

Complex adaptive systems exhibit specific characteristics that are different than simple systems and the terminology used to define them may be unfamiliar to healthcare providers. Table 37.2 provides a description of terminology used to describe complex system behavior. Each term in the table builds on the previous term to demonstrate how system behavior becomes unpredictable.

As healthcare systems become increasing complex, those individuals challenged with planning, designing,

TABLE 37.2	Complex Adaptive Systems Terminology	
Term	**Description**	**Example**
Combinatorial Complexity	A system with a large number of alternative states.	The medication management process involves many different providers, medications, times, routes, and patients. The many potential combinations of these at any one time can be enormous.
Dynamic Complexity	The degree to which system behavior becomes more complex over time.	Computer provider entry systems can create a network of interactions between the prescription, transcription, dispensing, and administration process that is so complex that errors may become lost in the system. Over time, if not discovered, the effects of the error can amplify and result in serious harm to a patient.
Feedback	The iterative process where system outputs loop back and impact system inputs.	Growth in the complexity of CPOE systems is driven by feedback. Since CPOE systems are composed of combinations of many different applications, new combinations of them create new features adding to overall complexity. Technology actually creates itself out of itself
Exponential Growth	The doubling of an output in a fixed period of time. Exponential growth can be positive or negative.	The computational processing capacity of computers doubles about every 18 months. This phenomenon, known as Moore's Law, has held steady for many years.
Non-linearity	When stimulus and response are unequal. A large stimulus may have little effect on outcomes while a small stimulus may generate a large response.	The introduction of information technology into the traditional workflow of providers can elicit a significant backlash if not carefully managed. The long-term negative effects of provider resistance can far exceed the initial costs of purchasing the system.
Self-organization	The "coming together" of system entities (providers) to achieve a goal without the guidance or influence of a central authority.	Work-arounds are a form of self-organization. For example, if a new bar code medication management system interferes with the workflow of nurses, they may self-organize and apply shortcuts without knowledge by the manager.
Emergence	New patterns of behavior arising from self-organization	A spike in medication errors from work-arounds may emerge as a new pattern on managerial reports.

(continued)

TABLE 37.2	Complex Adaptive Systems Terminology *(continued)*	
Term	**Description**	**Example**
Stochastic	The distribution of events is a mixture of deterministic and random processes.	The sequence of times between medication administrations is a mixture of scheduled (deterministic) and PRN (random) processes. The distribution is neither fully deterministic nor random.
Chaos	Chaos describes a class of systems in which small changes to the initial conditions of the system create deterministic (non-random), but very complex behavior.	The behavior of a system, from simple to complex lies on a continuum from fully deterministic to fully random. Chaos appears random but in fact is deterministic. It is found primarily in natural systems (weather patterns, biologic systems, chemistry) but also in man-made systems. Chaotic behavior often shows itself in the sequence of events in a process, i.e., interarrival rate of admissions to a nursing unit.
Power Law Distributions	A power law distribution is characterized by a few events of enormous magnitude disbursed among many events with much smaller impact.	Pareto's Law where 80% of the output is caused by 20% of the inputs is an example of a power law distribution. For example, 80% of the complaints surrounding a new information system may be verbalized by only 20% of the users.

and implementing information technology must be knowledgeable of complex adaptive system principles as well as the tools and methods to analyze their behavior.

IT IS ALL ABOUT FLOW: FAST AND LONG, SHORT AND SLOW

A key concept to understand is that all systems, whether they are natural (rivers, trees, weather) or man-made (stock markets, the Intranet, health systems), have currents that flow through them. Oxygen and blood flow through animate systems such as trees or humans while water and electricity flow in currents through inanimate systems such as rivers or lightening. Patients flow through hospitals and clinics while information flows through computer networks and electronic health records. Without flow, a *system* cannot exist and to survive, it must evolve in a direction that improves its access to designs that improve the flow of currents through them. In nature, the branching pattern in trees is not accidental. Rather the configuration of branches is the result of natural selection and the search for optimal designs to transport water and oxygen from the ground back to the atmosphere. This treelike branching pattern is so efficient that it is also seen in other structures such as river basins, the human respiratory system, computer networks, and road systems.

Just as water flows *fast* for *long* distances through wide river channels, digitized information flows *fast* for *long*

distances through large cable networks connecting institutions. As rivers fan out to create deltas, smaller channels form and flow *slows* and travels a *shorter* distance. And as computer networks branch out to users within organizations, the flow of digital information also *slows* and travels *shorter* distances as it supplies multiple users. To optimize and maintain flow, fast and long flow must equal short and slow flow. In natural systems such as rivers, the ratio of channels that are slow and short make up about 80% of total channels, while the remaining 20% are fast and long. And this ratio shows up not only in rivers but in tree branches, the human circulatory system, and computer networks! Although flow is faster in large river channels than in smaller tributaries, the total flow is maintained by the creation of numerous tributaries that as a whole are equal to the flow of the larger channels (Bejan & Zane, 2012).

This fundamental concept can also be applied to the flow of electronic data and the design of information systems. When information is delayed, either as a result of poorly designed systems and cumbersome processes and policies, it is usually a mismatch between "short and slow" and "fast and long" information flow. If it is overly time consuming to enter provider orders into an EHR (short and slow) then it delays those orders from being communicated in a timely manner through the health systems computer network to the pharmacy (long and fast). As a result, orders stack up (develop queues) and delay the flow of information. Whenever, delays occur, nurse informaticists should look for imbalances between "short and slow" and "fast and long" information flow.

INFORMATION SYSTEM PLANNING

The inter-relatedness of sub-systems characteristic of complex healthcare processes requires participation by many different stakeholders in the planning cycle. In complex systems, outputs from one process often become inputs to many others. A new admission on a nursing unit (input) can generate orders (output) to pharmacy, radiology, respiratory care, as well as many other departments. As various levels of care (clinic, hospital, long-term care) become increasingly connected, interoperability of computer systems becomes crucial. In addition, as clinical and administrative areas become more specialized, it is essential that domain experts participate in the planning process.

Wicked Problems

Problems encountered in complex systems are commonly described as "wicked." A wicked problem is difficult or impossible to solve because of incomplete, contradictory, and changing requirements that are often difficult to recognize (Rittel, Horst, & Melvil, 1973). Wicked problem are:

- Very difficult to define or formulate
- Not described as true or false, but as better or worse
- Have an enumerable or exhaustive set of alternative solutions
- Inaccessible to trial and error; solutions are a "one shot" deal
- Unique and often a symptom of another problem

Provider order entry (POE) systems often exhibit wicked problem behavior because stakeholders have incomplete, contradictory, and changing requirements. For example, although POE systems have been shown to reduce cycle time for the entire medication management process on a *global* level, individual providers may spend more time *locally*, having to enter orders via a keyboard. Here global and local benefits contradict each other. In addition, commercial vendors cannot allow "test driving" their application before purchase (trial and error). Because of the enormous expense associated in implementation of POE applications, once a system has been installed it is very difficult and costly to remove it (a one shot deal). Finally, because practice patterns vary, each provider wants the system customized to their workflow (each problem is unique). But because there are many providers there are an enumerable number of alternative solutions.

Wicked problems cannot be solved by the common rubric of defining the problem, analyzing solutions, and making a recommendation in sequential steps; the reason being, there is no clear definition of the problem. By engaging all stakeholders in problem solving, those people most affected participate in the planning process and a common, agreed approach can be formulated. Of utmost importance is understanding that different problem solutions require different approaches. For example, bar-coded medication management is one strategy for reducing medication errors. However, to be effective, this strategy must be implemented as part of an overall strategy for reducing medical errors. This strategy might be adopting concepts and principles from high-reliability organizations (HRO). A high-reliability organization assumes that accidents (or errors) will occur if multiple failures interact within tightly coupled, complex systems. Much of the research regarding HRO has been fueled by well-known catastrophes such as the Three Mile Island nuclear incident, the space shuttle Challenger explosion, and the Cuban Missile Crisis (Weick & Sutcliffe, 2001).

High-Reliability Organizations

Key attributes of HROs include a flexible organizational structure, an emphasis on reliability rather than efficiency, aligning rewards with appropriate behavior, a perception that risk is always present, sensemaking (an understanding of what is happening around you), heedfulness (an mutual understanding of roles), redundancy (ensuring there is sufficient flex in the system), mitigating decisions (decision-making that migrates to experts), and formal rules and procedures that are explicit. Employing information technology, such as bar-coded medication administration, must be implemented in the context of an overall strategy to become an HRO. For example, BCMA emphasizes reliability over efficiency and integrates formal rules and procedures into the medication management process. Collectively, these features reduce the probability of multiple failures converging simultaneously.

On the other hand, planning for clinical decision support (CDS) applications may require a different approach than implementation of BCMA. CDS systems link health observations with health knowledge to influence health choices by clinicians for improved healthcare (Garg et al., 2005). These applications cover a broad range of systems from simple allergy alerts to sophisticated algorithms for diagnosing disease conditions. The cognitive sciences inform and shape the design, development, and assessment of information systems and CDS technology. The sub-field of medical cognition focuses on understanding the knowledge structures and mental processes of clinicians during such activities as decision-making and problem solving (Patel, Arocha, & Kaufman, 2001).

Optimizing the capabilities of CDS systems to allow better decision-making requires an understanding of the structural and processing patterns in human information processing. For example, knowledge can be described as conceptual or procedural. Conceptual knowledge refers to a clinicians' understanding of specific concepts within a domain while procedural knowledge is the "how to" of an activity. Conceptual knowledge is learned through mindful engagement while procedural knowledge is developed through deliberate practice. If CDS planners are not careful, they may inadvertently design a system that transforms a routine task such as checking a lab value (procedural knowledge) into a cumbersome series of computer entries. If the clinician is simultaneously processing conceptual knowledge (problem solving and decision-making) and complex procedural tasks, it will place an unnecessary burden on working memory and create frustration.

In summary, the frequent occurrence of wicked problems in complex healthcare systems highlights the challenges faced by information system planners today. Successful planning for the introduction of information technology requires participation by a diverse group of stakeholders and experts. There is no "cookie cutter" solution in system planning. Each application must be aligned with an overall organizational strategy which drives the implementation approach.

INFORMATION SYSTEM DESIGN

The characteristic behavior of complex systems and the emergence of wicked problems have prompted system planners to search for new methods of system design and implementation. The introduction of new information technology in healthcare organizations involves the integration of both new applications and incumbent legacy systems. For example, a new POE application will need to interface with existing pharmacy, radiology, and lab systems. Although, an initial "starter set of orders" usually accompanies the POE application, the task of interfacing it with appropriate departmental systems, creating new order sets, and developing CDS generally falls to an internal implementation team with vendor support. Over time, this development team will design and build a POE system that is much different than the original application.

Structured Design

Historically design and implementation of healthcare information systems relied heavily on structured methods. The most common structured design and implementation

TABLE 37.3	System Design and Life Cycle
Step	**Description**
1	Identify problems, opportunities, and objectives
2	Determine human information requirements
3	Analyze system needs
4	Design the recommended system
5	Develop and document software
6	Test and maintain the system
7	Implement and evaluate the system.

method used is the System Design Life Cycle (SDLC). The SDLC acts as a framework for both software development, and implementation and testing of the system. Table 37.3 presents the broad steps in the SDLC (Kendall & Kendall, 2006)

An SDLC approach prescribes the entire design, testing, and implementation of new software applications as one project with multiple sub-projects (see Table 37.3). Project deadlines can extend over many months and in some cases years. The method encourages the use of standardization (for example, programming tools, software languages, data dictionaries, data flow diagrams, and so forth). Extensive data gathering (interviews, questionnaires, observations, flowcharting) occurs before the start of the project in an effort to predict overall system behavior, after full implementation of the application.

Agile Design

As healthcare systems have become increasingly complex, the SDLC approach has come under fire as being overly rigid. Behavior, characteristic of complex systems (sensitivity to initial conditions, non-linearity, and wicked problems), is often unpredictable, especially after the introduction of information technology in clinical workflow. Equally challenging is the difficulty of trialing the impact of new information systems before having to actually purchase them. Site visits to observe a successful application in one facility are no guarantee of success in another. Many healthcare organizations have spent countless millions in failed system implementations.

To overcome these problems, healthcare organizations are turning to "agile" methods for design and implementation of information systems (Kendall & Kendall, 2006). Agile design is less prescriptive than structured methods and allows for frequent trial and error. Rather than mapping the entire project plan up front, agile methods clearly define future milestones but focus on short-term successes. To do so the implementation team and software developers collaboratively evaluate and prioritize the sequence of task to implement first. Priority is assigned to tasks that can be accomplished within a short time frame, with a minimum of cost while maintaining high quality standards. This "timeboxing" of projects forces the team to search for simple, but elegant solutions. Developers often work in pairs to cross-check each other's work and distribute the workload. Communication is free flowing between developers and the implementation team. Once a solution is developed it is rapidly tested in the field and then continuously modified and improved. There is a philosophy that the interval between testing and feedback be as close as possible to sustain momentum in the project.

Agile design is one example of how to manage information technology projects in complex systems. Rather than trying to progress along a rigid project schedule, simple elegant solutions are rapidly designed, coded, and tested on a continuous basis. Over time, layer upon layer of elegant solutions evolve into a highly integrated, complex information system. Ironically, this is the same process that many natural systems have used to evolve into their current state.

THE SYSTEMS ANALYST TOOLBOX

Whether structured or agile design methods are used during project implementation, systems analysts rely heavily on various forms of modeling software. Modeling applications visually display the interaction and flow of entities (patients, providers, information) before and after implementation of information technology. Models link data dictionaries with clinical and administrative workflow through logical and physical data flow diagrams. Models can be connected through a hierarchy of parent and child diagrams to analyze system behavior locally (at the user level) and globally (management reports). There are many commercial modeling tools available. Table 37.4 presents various types of modeling software and how they are used.

TABLE 37.4	The Systems Analyst Toolbox	
Simulation Method	**Description**	**Healthcare Example**
Flowcharts	Flowcharts represent one of the most basic tools used by system analysts to describe the flow of entities (information, patients, and providers) in a process. Flowcharting software can be found as a stand-alone commercial product or as a feature in word processing, spreadsheet, and project management software.	Prior to the installation of a new clinical documentation system, the current paper documentation process was flow charted and then compared to the new automated process using standard flowchart symbols.
CASE Tools	Computer-Aided Software Engineering is a suite of software applications used for systems design and analysis. CASE tools improve communication, integrate life cycle activities, and are used extensively in the design and implementation of new applications.	CASE tools could be used to develop and implement a package of software application used in the development of an electronic medical record.
Discrete Event Simulation	Discrete event simulation (DES) utilizes mathematical formulas to show how model inputs change as a process evolves over time. Typically the model is built visually using standard flowchart symbols. For example, rectangles may represent processes and diamonds, decision points.	Analyzing cycle time, patient flow, bottlenecks, and non-value-added activities before and after installation of a computerized clinical documentation system in an emergency department. Simulation can be easily incorporated into popular methods of performance improvement such as Six Sigma and Lean.
Network Analysis	The unit of measure in network analysis is the pattern of relationships that exist between entities and the information that flows between them. Network analysis combines theories from sociology and information science (network theory). The field characterizes entities as "nodes" and the relationship or link between them as "ties." The pattern and strength of ties between nodes is then plotted on a graph where the flow of information can be analyzed.	Network analysis tools could be used to quantify access to computer help desks for providers by showing how centralized or decentralized the distribution of Centers are for organizations within a health system.

Discrete Event Simulation

Two software applications that are well suited for the analysis of complex systems are discrete event simulation (DSA) and network analysis (NA). DSA is a software application that allows analysts to flow chart processes on a computer and then simulate entities (people, patients, information) as they move through individual steps. Simulation allows analyst to quickly communicate the flow of entities within a process and compare differences in workflow after the introduction of new technology. DSA applications contain statistical packages that allow analysts to fit empirical data (process times, inter-arrival rates) to theoretical probability distributions to create life-like models of real systems. Pre- and post-implementation models can be compared for differences in cycle time, queuing, resource consumption, cost, and complexity. DSA is ideal for agile design projects because processes can be quickly modeled and analyzed prior to testing. Unanticipated bottlenecks, design problems, and bugs can be solved ahead of time to expedite the agile design process.

Network Analysis

Network analysis applications plot the pattern of relationships that exist between entities and the information that flows between them. Entities are represented as network nodes and can identify people or things (computers on nursing units, handheld devices, servers). The information that flows between nodes is represented as a tie and the resulting network pattern can provide analysts with insights into how data, information, and knowledge move throughout the organization. Network analysis tools measure information centrality, density, speed, and connectedness and can provide an overall method for measuring the accessibility of information to providers. NA graphs can uncover power laws (see Table 37.2) in the distribution of hubs in the organizations network of computers and servers. This can be beneficial in investigating the robustness of the computer network in the event a key hub crashes.

ORGANIZATIONAL FRAGILITY

The potential impact of growing healthcare complexity is enormous. Beyond a certain level, organizational complexity can decrease both the quality and financial performance of a health system. In his book, *Antifragile*, Taleb describes the concept of fragility in complex systems such as healthcare (Taleb, 2012). As certain systems become increasingly complex, unexpected events can create an exponentially negative impact. For example, the death of a patient, as the result of a medication error propagating

across multiple inter-dependent hospital departments, has a much greater impact on a large hospital than on a smaller one. It takes significantly more resources to investigate and make changes in larger hospitals than smaller ones because of the number of people, departments, types of equipment, and so forth that are involved. Thus increasing size (or complexity) promotes "fragile" behavior in health systems: they break easily.

One can get a sense of the impact of size and complexity on the fragility of organizations by scanning The Centers for Medicare and Medicaid's Hospitals Consumer Assessment of Healthcare Providers (HCAHPS) survey scores (HCAHPS Online). The HCAHPS provide a standardized survey instrument and data collection methodology for measuring patients' perspectives on hospital care. The HCAHPS is administered to a random sample of patients continuously throughout the year in hospitals. From "Communication with Nurses" to "Pain Management," of the 10 hospital characteristics publically reported, scores decrease with an increase in hospital bed size in nearly every category. Just as an elephant falling five feet suffers significantly more damage than a mouse, large, complex organizations suffer exponentially greater harm than smaller ones for similar events.

In contrast, certain systems are "anti-fragile" to negative events and actually become stronger as they are stressed. A good example, among many, is the human body's immune system, which creates new antibodies when it is exposed to antigens. The concepts illustrated from these biologic "learning systems" can be translated into man-made systems through continuous learning organizations. By learning from stressors (unanticipated events) and then implementing and revising policies and procedures to prevent them from occurring again the health system actually becomes stronger. To illustrate one example of the concept of fragility the following actual use case is described.

DESIGNING SYSTEMS WITHIN AN INCREASING COMPLEX WORLD—A CASE SCENARIO

In 2005, a large health system located in the Southwest initiated a plan to implement a single vendor, enterprise-wide EHR across its 10 hospitals. The system contained one large academic medical center of 800 beds and 9 hospitals ranging in size from 25 to 475 beds. These hospitals were distributed throughout the state where 50% were in large urban areas and the remainder in rural locations. Although the network of hospitals acted as an integrated delivery system, each implemented their EHR according

TABLE 37.5	EHR Performance Measures

- User satisfaction (survey tool)
- Staffing utilization and overtime (staffing reports)
- Percent utilization of EHR by providers (management reports)
- Provider productivity (patient visits per day)
- Pharmacy to provider callbacks (pharmacy system reports)
- Number and severity of medication errors (risk management reports)
- Evaluation of documentation quality—legibility, completeness, appropriateness
- Compliance with clinical decision support reminders and alerts
- Volume of lab or imaging procedures ordered (lab and radiology system reports)
- Chart pulls (medical record departmental reports)
- Release of information (ROI) response time and backlog
- Billing turnaround times (revenue cycle reports)
- Claim rejections
- CPT E&M code levels
- Documentation of services (CPT codes)
- Patient satisfaction

to their own process and timeline. Thus the success of various EHR implementation strategies used by each hospital could be assessed by measuring specific performance outcomes post-implementation (see Table 37.5)

Complete implementation of the EHR occurred over a three-year period with one hospital at a time going "live" according to a master schedule. One year post-implementation each hospital then compared pre- and post-performance metrics to assess how well strategic objectives were met.

Result of the one-year post-study varied considerably between hospitals and it is beyond the scope of this chapter to review all of the results. However, it is important to note that one hospital significantly outperformed the remaining nine hospitals on nearly all performance metrics. This high-performing, community hospital had a bed size of 475 and utilized an "agile" design strategy as compared to the other hospitals that followed a more traditional systems development lifecycle (SDLC).

As previously described, traditional EHR implementation strategies have followed the SDLC (see Table 37.3) using a structured design process. The SDLC typically maps out the complete planning, design, and implementation of projects in advance. This prescriptive process attempts to anticipate all possible future scenarios and then designs and build the system to accommodate them. Nursing, pharmacy, radiology, and other clinical areas

then work with commercial vendors to create flowcharts that describe their existing workflows and revise them to align with the EHR's new workflow.

There are a number of disadvantages of the SDLC that can lead to an increase in organizational fragility in complex systems such as healthcare. These include:

- It is virtually impossible to anticipate all of the different scenarios that may arise in advance.
- User needs and technology may change during the implementation phase especially if the timeline is delayed.
- Workflows are often designed in silos (nursing, pharmacy, radiology) and do not communicate well when integrated in an overall workflow.

Of the nine hospitals that used the SDLC many of these issues emerged during implementation of the EHR. For example, because of its size and complexity, the 800-bed medical center had a protracted EHR implementation that spanned three years. Because the entire system was fully designed in advance, it was difficult to accommodate changes in technology and new service requirements that occurred during the three-year implementation. The system could not readily adapt to the emergence of wireless mobile devices (tablets, phones, and so forth), consumer informatics (patient portals), and Web-based services. Although clinical documentation was now electronically stored it was not standardized in a way that accommodated reporting requirements for the Accountable Care Act and "meaningful use." And because workflow design had been developed through individual departments (nursing, radiology, pharmacy, and so forth) communication was slow and cumbersome. Provider order entry systems, clinical documentation, and medication administration all took longer than previous paper systems.

The aforementioned use case is an example of a fragile organizational design. When the system was stressed, such as in a sudden increase in admissions, it quickly became overwhelmed and "broke." Medical errors, system downtime, resources, and cost all exponentially increased rather than decreased in response to unanticipated events.

In contrast to other hospitals, the high-performing hospital utilized an agile design process when implementing their EHR. One team of clinicians, vendor consultants, administrators, and hospital programmers developed a project timeline that "loosely" guided the system over a one-year period. This allowed flexibility for unanticipated events that occurred along the way and did not tie the team down to a ridged plan. Rather than implementing the EHR on all units simultaneously, the same team went from unit to unit and designed the system along the way.

The team designed the system in a modular format rather than building the entire system in advance. The modular format allowed system designers to break workflow up into natural use cases. For example, one nursing module might be "New Patient Assessment" while another might be "Patient Discharge." By using the modular format, designers could make changes to one part of the EHR without having to go back and make multiple changes to other areas.

As the design team went from one department to the next it used a rapid design and implementation strategy. The team would meet with key departmental content experts, review the existing workflow, and then quickly design a new workflow. The new workflow would be rapidly piloted on the unit over a one- to two-week period while continuously making changes based on feedback. This process allowed the team to build upon the success of previous units and make recommendations on best practices. In other words, the team was continuously learning from their mistakes and correcting them as they advanced through the organization.

The agile design process used by this hospital is an example of an "anti-fragile" organization. Stressors or unanticipated events actually strengthened the system as the design evolved. That is because an organization that uses feedback to continuously learn, just as in biologic systems, adapts more readily to change and becomes stronger. In high-performing organizations, the design phase never actually ends. It is continuous and always adapting and learning from unanticipated events.

SUMMARY AND CONCLUSIONS

Healthcare complexity is growing at an exponential rate (Clancy, 2010). This, in part, is because new technology itself is composed of combinations of existing technologies. For example, POE systems interface with existing applications (technologies) in pharmacy, lab, and radiology. Each individual departmental application is composed of further sub-components that are themselves technologies. This recursive process continues until it reaches the most basic parts of the system. If each component of this hierarchical tree is considered a technology, then new, novel technologies form from new combinations. For example, voice-activated clinical documentation recently emerged by combining Voice over Intranet (VoIP) technology from other industries with existing EHR systems. Thus as we see new technologies grow at a linearly rate,

the potential combinations of them grow exponentially. The more potential combinations of technologies there are (combinatorial complexity), the higher the probability of discovering new uses for them. Thus, technology actually creates itself out of itself (Arthur, 2009).

The relentless march of technology creates both benefits and challenges for nurse informaticists. As the sheer number of technologies grows, the combinations of them become ever more complex. Simply look at the complexity of EHR systems in hospitals today. These systems are a mixture of new and legacy systems connected through a complex network of customized interfaces. Equally complex is the acceleration in how quickly the underlying processes these technologies execute changes. New knowledge supporting evidence-based practices is growing so fast that new CDS algorithms programmed into today's EHRs can become outdated in a matter of weeks.

Nurse informaticists play a vital role in the successful planning, design, and implementation of information technology. However, to achieve that success, nurse informatics must have an in-depth knowledge of complex systems and strategies to manage its behavior.

REFERENCES

Arthur, B. (2009). *The nature of technology: What it is and how it evolves.* New York, NY: Simon and Schuster.

Bejan, A., & Zane, J. P. (2012). *Design in nature: How the constructal law governs evolution in biology, physics, technology, and social organization.* New York, NY: Doubleday.

Clancy, T. R. (2010). Technology and complexity: Trouble brewing? *Journal of Nursing Administration, 40*(6), 247–249.

Clancy, T. R., & Delaney, C. (2005). Complex nursing systems. *Journal of Nursing Management, 13*(3), 192–201.

Clancy, T. R., Effken, J., & Persut, D. (2008). Applications of complex systems theory in nursing education, research and practice. *Nursing Outlook, 56*(5), 248–256, e3.

Garg, A. X., Adhikari, N. K., McDonald, H., Rosas-Arellano, M.P., Devereaux, P. J., Beyene, J., ... Haynes, R. B. (2005). Effects of computerized clinical decision support systems on practitioner performance and patient outcomes: A systematic review. *Journal of the American Medical Association, 293*(10), 1223–1238.

Kendall, K. E., & Kendall, J. E. (2006). *Systems analysis and design* (6th ed.). Upper Saddle River, NJ: Pearson Prentice Hall.

Patel, V. L., Arocha, J. F., & Kaufman, D. R. (2001). A primer on aspects of cognition for medical informatics. *Journal*

of the American Medical Informatics Association: JAMIA,
8(4), 324–343.

Rittel, H., & Webber, M. (1973). Dilemmas in a general
theory of planning. Amsterdam, Elsevier Scientific
Publishing, *Policy Sciences, 4,* 155–169. [Reprinted in
Cross, N. (Ed.). (1984). *Developments in design methodol-*
ogy (pp. 135–144). Chichester: J. Wiley & Sons.]

Skyttner, L. (2001). *General systems theory: Ideas & applica-*
tions. Singapore: World Scientific.

Taleb, N. (2012). *Antifragile: Things that gain from disorder.*
New York, NY: Random House.

Weick, K. E., & Sutcliffe, K. M. (2001). *Managing the*
unexpected—Assuring high performance in an age of
complexity (pp. 10–17). San Francisco, CA: Jossey-Bass.

38

The Quality Spectrum in Informatics

Rosemary Kennedy / Heidi Bossley / Juliet Rubini / Beth B. Franklin

• OBJECTIVES

1. Describe what a quality measure is, the different types of measures, and the data from which they can be derived.
2. Discuss why it is important to measure the quality of care, who has historically been involved in measurement development, and the different uses of measures.
3. Describe the major government and other standards initiatives in quality measurement data infrastructure.
4. Discuss the role of standard terminologies in quality measurement.
5. Describe how clinical quality measures support Meaningful Use of electronic health records (EHRs) and quality management.
6. Describe the development of an eMeasure, its format, and its potential uses for quality improvement and nursing care.

• KEY WORDS

Quality management
Electronic clinical quality measures
Meaningful Use (MU)
Performance measurement
Performance improvement
Clinical decision support
Quality reporting
Electronic health records
Structured terminology
Standards organizations
Nursing quality reporting

INTRODUCTION

In this chapter the role of informatics in defining, measuring, and improving care quality will be described. The essential elements of quality measurement will be explored, including explaining the components of a quality measure, the different types of quality measures, the data from which they can be derived, why it is important to measure the quality of care, and for what uses. This will be followed with an overview of the major government initiatives and reporting programs in quality measurement including the data infrastructure required to ensure success in these programs. The chapter will conclude with an explanation of the life cycle of electronic quality measurement.

In the last decade, there has been a move toward capturing quality measurement information real time as patient care is provided, and subsequently aggregating and reporting the data to support longitudinal measurement. To achieve this goal, quality reporting has evolved from paper medical record chart abstraction to electronic quality reporting using the electronic health record (EHR).

DRIVERS OF QUALITY MEASUREMENT USING INFORMATICS

The Medicare and Medicaid EHR Incentive Programs provide financial incentives for continuously measuring and reporting of clinical quality measures to help ensure that the healthcare delivery system can deliver effective, safe, efficient, patient-centered, equitable, and timely care (Centers for Medicare & Medicaid Services, n.d.). The financial incentives are based on Meaningful Use of EHRs. This is guided by the National Quality Strategy (NQS) (AHRQ, n.d.), adopted by the Department of Health and Human Services, focused on three aims of better care and better health, at lower costs. Achieving the NQS requires a national infrastructure for electronic quality measurement.

Electronic clinical quality measures use a wide variety of data gathered as a by-product of patient care delivery. When data necessary for quality measurement are captured as a by-product of care delivery, and when those data are easily shared between health information technology (IT) systems, care can be better coordinated, and is safer, more efficient, and of higher quality.

Ideally, the nation will achieve the NQS by taking full advantage of the EHR to capture high-quality clinical data for quality reporting and performance improvement. For instance, using a diagnosis from an EHR problem list captured during care is a more valid source for quality measurement than administrative claims (Tang, Ralston, Arrigotti, Qureshi, & Graham, 2007).

QUALITY MEASUREMENT

The quality of care provided in healthcare is often defined as "the degree to which health care services for individuals and populations increase the likelihood of desired health outcomes and are consistent with current professional knowledge" (Institute of Medicine, 1990). One of the best ways to determine whether the care provided was effective in improving the desired health outcomes in an evidence-based manner is through measuring or quantifying the performance of an individual or organization. Performance measurement in healthcare is not a new concept as many

organizations have been developing and using measures to assess the quality of care for several decades. In recent years, the focus has evolved from improving the quality of care at the local level to determining and paying for the care provided based on the level of quality and cost. This evolution has led to increased rigor in the development and specification of performance measures and leveraging data that are collected at the point of care. These data can be aggregated easily, making the use of electronic data the obvious option.

Performance of the healthcare provider or institution is analyzed through the following constructs or types: structure, process, and outcomes (Donabedian, 1980). These constructs serve as a methodology by which clinical care can be examined to show where gaps in care may be.

Structure is defined as "the relatively stable characteristics of the providers of care, of the tools and resources they have at their disposal, and of the physical and organizational setting in which they work" (Donabedian, 1980, p. 81). Structural measures include nurse staffing ratios, the existence of systems such as the use of a registry, and other aspects that would be considered necessary components to ensure appropriate and high-quality care is delivered.

Process is "a set of activities that go on within and between practitioners and patients" (Donabedian, 1980, p. 79). These measures assess whether an action or step that is needed for patient care is provided. They are reliant on evidence-based guidelines or research and most often show what percentage of the time a provider or institution is compliant with an assessment or intervention.

Outcomes are "changes in a patient's current and future health status that can be attributed to antecedent health care" (Donabedian,1980, p. 83). Outcome measures are focused on the success or lack thereof to improving a patient's health status. These may either be short term (typically within the 12 months or less) or long term. This type of measure often requires risk adjustment to account for differences in patient characteristics that are outside of the control of the entity being measured (National Quality Measures Clearing House, n.d., Allowance for patient or population factors section, para. 6). These characteristics vary depending on the intent of the measure and can include items such as severity of illness or co-morbidities.

In order to develop a clearly defined, precisely specified measure, it is critical that the intent of the measure is well outlined. For example, defining the intent of the measure as the quality of care provided to patients with a diagnosis of diabetes would be too broad; rather, if the measure intent was to determine the number of patients with diabetes whose blood pressure is within acceptable targets, it lends itself to developing and specifying a measure.

Once the intent of the measure is clearly defined, the different components of the measure should then be specified. These components include:

- Initial patient population: defines the total population of interest; this may be focused on patients with a specific diagnosis or on procedures that are performed for example.

- Denominator: "The lower part of the fraction used to calculate a rate or ratio defining the total population of interest for a quality measure" (NQMC, n.d., Denominator section, para. 1); often the same as initial patient population but also may be a subset or more narrow focus.

- Numerator: "The upper part of the fraction used to calculate a rate or ratio defining the subset of the population of interest that meets a quality measure's criterion of quality" (NQMC, n.d., Numerator section, para. 1). This focuses on the structure, process, or outcome of interest.

- Exclusions (also called exceptions): "Characteristics defined during the delivery of care that would mean that care specified in the numerator was contraindicated, refused by the patient, or not possible for some other compelling and particular circumstance of this case" (NQMC, n.d., Exclusions/exceptions section, para. 1).

Within each of these components, specific definitions should be included such as who is being measured (patient population, diagnoses, age, gender if applicable, measurement period, or timeframe), what is being measured (the outcome, process, or structure of interest), and what patients, treatments, or other aspects are not appropriate to include.

Performance measures are usually calculated as counts ("the number of times the unit of analysis for a measure occurs"), ratios ("a score that may have a value of zero or greater that is derived by dividing a count of one type of data by a count of another type of data"), or rates/proportions ("A score derived by dividing the number of cases that meet a criterion for quality (the numerator) by the number of eligible cases within a given time frame (the denominator) where the numerator cases are a subset of the denominator cases") (NQMC, n.d., Scoring of the Measure section, para. 3–9).

Within performance measurement, there is an increasing push to design measures to be broadly applicable with the ability to drill down into specific age groups, conditions, etc., as desired. This type of measurement is more feasible using electronic data.

WHAT DO WE MEASURE?

Performance measures typically focus on one of the following areas:

- Patient experience: measures that capture how care was provided through the eyes of the patient and/or caregiver

- Quality of care delivered: measures that capture whether care was received in accordance with clinical evidence and guidelines; these measures typically look at overuse, inappropriate use/unnecessary care, or underuse

- Access: measures that examine whether a service or treatment was provided and available in a timely manner

- Cost: measures that examine the amount (usually in dollars) spent to provide services, procedures, treatments, etc.

While most measures look at one aspect of care such as overuse of services, more and more measures are developed that take an increasingly comprehensive view to reflect how patients truly receive care. These composites are groupings of two or more measures that include processes and/or outcomes of care into a single score. For example, a composite of the quality of care a patient with asthma might look at whether the patient is receiving the appropriate treatments as well as the number of emergency department visits he or she may have had over the last year. Composites can be weighted where the score of one or more measures is given priority over others or calculated as an all or none.

In light of performance measurement moving to better reflect the care a patient receives, developers, payers, and others continue to explore ways to combine more than one aspect of care. For example, there is a growing desire to measure the efficiency of the provider or entity by combining the quality of care received (preferably outcomes) with the resources and the associated cost used to provide that care. Developers, payers, and others have taken this concept a step further to measure value (Bankowitz, Bechtel, Corrigan, DeVore, Fisher, & Nelson, 2013). By combining quality (outcomes) and patient experience over the cost or expenditures to provide that care, it then allows patients, purchasers, employers, and others to make informed decisions on providers or institutions with whom they might want to partner or from whom they want to receive care.

WHO DO WE MEASURE?

Quality, cost, and other aspects of care are measured at specific levels of analysis and settings of care. In order to ensure that a measure can be precisely specified, the measure developer will determine which individual or entity to be measured. This decision is usually made based on the goal of the program or activity for which the measure will be used. Levels of analysis for measure specification include the individual level (e.g., nurse, physician), group (e.g., practice, clinic), entity (e.g. hospital, health plan) or the population level (e.g., measuring across a community or geographic region). Understanding what settings of care should be included is critical, particularly when one begins to specify the measure. Setting for which the measure is applicable is determined based on the evidence supporting the measure and the intended use of the measure. Settings of care vary from ambulatory (e.g., clinic, pharmacy, laboratory), inpatient (e.g., hospital, inpatient rehabilitation facility), and other locations including the patient's home.

HOW DO WE MEASURE?

Performance measures are derived from a variety of sources but are also related to the level of analysis and setting of care for which the measure is intended. For example, when measures were created two decades ago, paper medical records were the primary source of information in hospitals and practices. Most measures developed for those groups were specified using that data source. For measures that seek to look at the quality of care provided by a home health agency, the data source may well be the Outcome and Assessment Information Set (OASIS).

There are various data sources including clinical data (i.e., cost, procedures, pharmacy, lab, imaging), medical records (either paper or electronic), patient-reported data (i.e., surveys, portals), registry, and others. Medical records (either paper or electronic) have been considered the gold standard when measuring a provider's performance but this thinking is evolving, particularly when the patient's experience or perspective is desired, leading to the development of patient-reported data, primarily through surveys.

As patient care and quality activities continue to evolve, the emphasis is now on providing access to data that are real time, can be tracked longitudinally, and can be communicated across systems and providers to enhance the coordination of care for patients. This emphasis has driven much of the adoption and implementation of electronic data sources in healthcare. Given the increasing implementation of electronic health record systems in practices, hospitals, and other entities, measures must now be specified using this data source, requiring additional granularity in the specifications, coding, and other aspects, which are outlined further in this chapter.

WHO DEVELOPS MEASURES, WHY, AND IN WHAT ENVIRONMENTS?

Performance measurement has evolved over the last 10 years. Initial efforts to capture and use data to define the quality of care provided to patients included groups focused on a providers' quality of care such as The Joint Commission's (TJC) ORYX® program, the National Committee for Quality Assurance's Healthcare Effectiveness Data and Information Set (HEDIS®) program, the AMA-convened Physician Consortium for Performance Improvement (PCPI®) or on a specific condition or disease like the Diabetes Quality Improvement Program. These programs and associated measures were developed to enable providers and patients determine the quality of care that hospitals provided through the TJC program, the PCPI for physicians, and health plans with the HEDIS program. Within the nursing community, the American Nurses Association (ANA) established the National Database of Nursing Quality Indicators to enable comparison of valid and reliable nursing-sensitive indicators at the national, regional, and state level for comparison down to the unit level (Montalvo & Dunton, 2007).

Many of these measures were developed to enable quality improvement activities at the point of care—meaning real-time data and feedback to facilitate changes to the care provided to patients. As the focus shifted to use performance measures for accountability purposes (i.e., pay for reporting and/or performance, public reporting), the healthcare community identified the need for an entity to vet and endorse national standards, which then became the National Quality Forum (NQF). This shift created a focus on measures that were more rigorously specified and shown to be reliable and valid to enable patients, employers, purchasers, and others to make informed choices on which entity was provided the highest level of care. Performance measures are now actively used in federal and state programs to enable patients to identify who provides high-quality care and purchasers and employers to select and partner with them.

While these developers and programs were focused on public reporting and paying for performance, other smaller groups continued to develop measures for use in national, state, and private programs. Today, medical specialty societies or accreditors are no longer the primary developers of measures; rather, quality improvement collaboratives serve as a key contributor to measure development and federal agencies such as the Centers for Medicare and Medicaid Services (CMS) and the Office of the National Coordinator for Health Information Technology (ONC) are funding and encouraging groups such as regional collaboratives, and health systems to develop measures that can be derived from electronic sources (i.e., EHRs, registries) and are patient centered.

At the end of the day, we cannot improve without knowing where care is lacking. Performance measurement provides a method by which we can assess where we need to improve our processes that lead to improved patient outcomes. A goal of measurement is that it be a by-product of care delivery to the greatest extent possible to enable us to track improvement real time and longitudinally. By integrating these measures into electronic systems, we will be furthering that goal. The integration of quality measures within electronic systems requires use of data standards.

WHAT ARE THE QUALITY REPORTING PROGRAMS?

Quality reporting programs have been in existence in healthcare for over a century. Collecting and reporting quality data have become more organized and focused over the past 50 years with a major growth in the past 10–20 years. Organizations such as the Centers for Medicare and Medicaid Services (CMS), The Joint Commission, the American College of Surgeons, other professional organizations, and state and local quality initiatives have been major players in moving healthcare quality reporting programs to where we are today. Many point to the Institute of Medicine's sentinel report *To Err is Human* as a turning point for the rapid growth of quality reporting programs since 2000. Hospitals, physician offices, pharmacies, ambulatory centers, and others that provide healthcare services to consumers (e.g. laboratories) may be required to report quality data. Reporting programs have evolved over the past decade but the goal of these programs is to improve patient safety through the use of electronic health records. Nursing informatics professionals can support these efforts through data analytics, program knowledge, and a keen understanding of the data collection and storage in an EHR.

Historically, claims data have been used to track and monitor patient services. The data were used to reimburse providers for care. It also provided data to track quality of care as the information reflected the procedures completed for the patient. For example, if a claim was submitted for a patient for an influenza vaccine the provider would get reimbursed and the insurer could track patients who received the preventive service. A standard format for reporting claims data has made it easier to track quality data. However, claims data do not tell the full story

of the patient's visit, services provided, and outcomes to adequately describe the quality of clinical care. Using the example above, many consumers receive their influenza vaccine at the local pharmacy or grocery store, their church or a community-sponsored flu clinic. Most flu clinics, if not free, require a nominal cash payment and the service may not be reported to a provider or an insurer through the claims payment process. Although it may be relatively easy to report the number of doses administered we may not know the ages, gender, race, etc., of the population receiving the vaccine. This data could be collected in an EHR by providers who collect the data during a patient visit.

Informatics nurses (IN) and informatics nurse specialists (INS) must be aware of quality programs used at their facility/institution, particularly those programs that rely on clinical data that can be collected and retrieved from the EHR. INs and INSs must understand the intent of the quality programs, data requirements, reporting timelines, staff education requirements for data input (data collection) or timing of data input, querying the data, organizing and interpreting the data, and understanding what the results mean and how to apply it. The INs and INSs must work with organization staff and senior management to understand the results and to develop a strategy to improve or maintain the quality of care based on the quality programs results.

The sections below will discuss at a high level a few of the current federal quality initiatives, the role of The Joint Commission in quality, and the National Database for Nursing Quality Indicators (NDNQI). Each program has its own criteria. As EHRs mature and evolve and their use becomes more widespread, quality program criteria will change. However, the common goal of quality of care to ensure patient safety will remain steadfast.

Federal Programs to Support Quality Reporting

Since the early 2000s, and in conjunction with the growth of electronic health records in the inpatient and ambulatory care settings, there has been a movement to collect and report measures using clinical data. The process to convert was slow until incentive programs started by the federal government boosted the movement.

Included in the American Recovery and Reinvestment Act (ARRA) is the Health Information Technology for Economic and Clinical Health Act (HITECH). HITECH provisions incentive payments by the Centers for Medicare & Medicaid Services (CMS) for reporting of "meaningful use" of certified EHR technology by eligible professionals, hospitals, and critical access hospitals.

The Medicare and Medicaid EHR Incentive Program, more commonly known as Meaningful Use (MU), is the most notable of the current quality reporting programs. The MU program is open to eligible professionals (EPs) (e.g. individual physicians, nurse practitioners), eligible hospitals (e.g. acute care facilities but not children's hospitals), and critical access hospitals (CAH). Providers must demonstrate meaningful use of a certified electronic health system (EHR) while providing patient care.

The Medicare incentive program is administered by CMS, while the Medicaid incentive programs are administered voluntarily by states and territories. The Medicare MU program for EPs started in 2011 and continues through 2016 with 2014 being the last year for initial participation in the program. The Medicaid program runs through 2021 with 2016 being the final year to enroll. Providers with a certified EHR system can enroll and participate in either the Medicare or Medicaid MU program but not both.

Eligible hospitals can participate in the MU hospital incentive programs. Participation started in FY 2011 with payment incentives continuing until FY 2016.

CMS requires that providers participating in the MU program show they are using their EHR meaningfully. In other words, using an EHR is positively affecting the care they are providing. Providers show meaningful use by meeting all criteria established by CMS for each stage of the program.

Meaningful Use had three stages:

- Stage 1: Data capture and sharing data with patients or other healthcare providers
- Stage 2: Advance clinical processes
- Stage 3: Improved outcomes

Providers must satisfy Stage 1requirements to obtain financial incentives and move to Stage 2. Stage 1 of MU for eligible providers (e.g., individual physicians) requires reporting data for a consecutive 90-day period during a calendar year. Stage 1 serves as the foundation for Stages 2 and 3. Stage 2 requires providers to submit quality data for one consecutive year for core measures, menu measures, and clinical quality measures (CQM). These criteria have been defined as through federal regulations. As of the writing of this chapter, CMS in conjunction with the Office of the National Coordinator (ONC) have proposed extending the end of Stage 2 to 2016 and delaying the start of Stage 3. Federal rule will determine the revised start date. Notice of proposed rulemaking for revisions to Meaningful Use Stage 2 and 3 was issued in Fall 2014.

Hospitals enrolled in MU must also submit data on core and menu objectives as well as CQMs. The core and menu objectives and CQMs for hospitals vary from the EPs. For more information on the core and menu objectives it is suggested the reader visit the CMS Web site (www.cms.gov).

During each of these stages, providers must meet specific criteria set forth by the program. INs and INSs working at facilities enrolled in this program must be aware of the requirements and the timelines for data submission. For example, if data are being submitted for height, weight, (list them out) then the IN/INS should be aware of how the data are being entered, that the data are being correctly entered by end users and periodically during the reporting period querying the EHR to ensure the information is reportable. Any deviation from what is expected should trigger a discussion for a plan to correct how the end user is entering the data.

A second CMS quality program is the Physician Quality Reporting System, or PQRS, for eligible professionals. The PQRS program uses both financial incentive payments and payment adjustments to promote quality reporting. Information reported is for covered Physician Fee Schedule (PFS) services. Claims data and registry data are used to report quality measures for this program. PQRS participation is voluntary and open to individual providers and group practices. Participation in PQRS does not satisfy enrollment in CMS's MU program. Program requirement changes INs and INSs working with providers enrolled in PQRS are encouraged to follow program requirements and changes on the CMS Web site (www.cms.gov).

The Hospital Inpatient Quality Reporting (Hospital IQR formerly RHADAPU) program is also a CMS-sponsored quality program. RHADAPU is a Medicare run program. Measure data required by this program mirror common diagnoses seen among hospitalized Medicare patients. The program looks at clinical and claims data. It was developed with the goal of providing consumers with information about the quality of care at hospitals. With this comparison consumers can then make more informed decisions about where to seek care. Consumers can view this information on the Hospital Compare Web site. The Hospital IQR program reports and information about how the hospital compares to others facilities provide an opportunity to improve clinical care. Measure data collected for the Hospital IQR program can also be used for other quality reporting programs such as those of the Joint Commission.

National Database of Nursing Quality Indicators (NDNQI) is a quality improvement program of the American Nurses Association (ANA). The program focuses on nursing measures. It provides nurses and their leadership with data about where nursing is meeting standards and where it needs to improve patient outcomes. It also provides healthcare facilities with the ability to compare themselves to similar size and type facilities at the local, regional, and national levels (NDNQI, n.d.).

Unlike other quality reporting programs, the NDNQI uses unit level data. Information collected and reported quarterly at the unit level includes, but is not limited to, fall/injury fall rate, nursing hours per patient day, nursing skill mix, Peripheral IV infiltration rate, RN Education/Certification, nurse turnover orate, central-line-associated bloodstream infection rate, and pain assessment/intervention/reassessment cycles completed.

The Joint Commission accredits healthcare organizations including, but not limited to, hospitals, physician offices, nursing homes, ambulatory health centers, and home care. The Joint Commission's ORYX® program, according to their Web site, "…integrates outcomes and other performance measure data into the accreditation process." The Joint Commission believes performance measurement data are crucial to accreditation. They work in concert with the CMS to align measures common to both organizations quality programs in an effort to decrease the burden and cost of data collection and reporting for healthcare organizations. ORYX data are published by the Joint Commission on their Web site. The data provide data comparison at the state and national levels. In addition to using quality measures to accredit organizations, the Joint Commission develops quality measures and quality tools.

The Healthcare Effectiveness Data and Information Set (HEDIS®) is a tool providing measure performance data on care and services based on 80 measures across five domains. According to the National Committee on Quality Assurance (NCQA), which maintains the program/runs HEDIS, the information is used by 90% of America's health plans as it provides a picture of care provided. Examples of measure data collected for HEDIS include medication management for asthma, blood pressure control, breast cancer screening, and childhood and adolescent immunizations. As part of the HEDIS life cycle, measures are evaluated at least every three years to determine if they continue to benefit the program. Measures that are no longer of value are retired.

HEDIS data also allow employers and others who provide healthcare plans to analyze performance of the plans so they may select the plans deemed best for their employees. The *Quality Compass* tool, available through the NCQA Web site, allows employers to access information and makes comparisons of health plans. HEDIS data are available in the *State of Health Care Quality* report. This report provides a thorough, in-depth picture of the nation's healthcare system. HEDIS data are also used in the "report cards" of health plans found in the news media.

The Agency for Healthcare Research and Quality (AHRQ), part of the Department of Health and Human Services (DHHS), states on their Web site: "AHRQ's mission is to produce evidence to make healthcare safer, higher quality, more accessible, equitable, and affordable, and to work with the U.S. Department of Health and Human Services (HHS) and other partners to make sure that the evidence is understood and used." To this end, one aspect of AHRQ's work is in the area of quality. AHRQ supports many programs to improve quality in the inpatient and ambulatory settings. The AHRQ Quality Indicators (QIs) program uses hospital inpatient administrative data. Currently, AHRQ QI™ modules include Prevention Quality Indicators, Inpatient Quality Indicators, Patient safety Indicators, and Pediatric Quality Indicators.

AHRQ also has an extensive portfolio of quality tools to assist physicians, nurses, and other healthcare providers to improve quality of care. For example, through AHRQ's Comprehensive Unit-based Safety Programs (CUSP) hospitals can learn how to reduce the incidence of catheter-associated urinary tract infections (CAUTI), or central-line-associated blood stream infections (CABSI). Reduction in the incidence of both these infections will improve patient safety and quality of care. It is suggested that the reader refer to AHRQ's Web site for current information on quality programs currently in progress at the Agency.

AHRQ provides to the public multiple quality reports. Among those available on their Web site are the National Healthcare Quality report (NHQR) and the National Healthcare Disparities Report (NHDR). The reports, published annually, "…measure trends in effectiveness of care, patient safety, timeliness of care, patient centeredness, and efficiency of care" per the AHRQ Web site.

The National Quality Measures Clearinghouse (NQMC) is an AHRQ initiative. NQMC's mission is to "…provide practitioners, health care providers, health plans, integrated delivery systems, purchasers and others an accessible mechanism for obtaining detailed information on quality measures, and to further their dissemination, implementation, and use in order to inform health care decisions."

As quality reporting programs shift from reporting claims data to reporting clinical data to meet program requirements, INs and INSs must be knowledgeable about the local, state, and national programs their organization participates in. Keeping up with the rapid changes of each program can be a challenge. Working with your organizations quality department, checking program Web sites, participating in publically available Webinars and seminars, etc., will help keep you informed of the most current program requirements. As INs and INSs it may be your responsibility to ensure the data elements are in the EHR, the data are being entered in discrete fields in a timely manner, are extracted periodically to review, understand reporting program deadlines, being able to interpret the data, and recommend to management processes to improve quality of care and patient safety.

WHY ARE STANDARDS IMPORTANT?

Data collected in an EHR are often identified by local, idiosyncratic, and sometimes redundant and/or ambiguous names rather than unique, well-organized codes from standard code systems. Without standardized dialog boxes, drop-down lists, or other pre-defined menu options, there is no consistency in the content captured in free-text fields. As such, comparisons of entries across patients, providers, or other systems are exceedingly challenging and even with the use of sophisticated coding tools and analytics to interpret the underlying content may be inaccurate. Hospitals, clinics, and other healthcare entities must devote significant resources to document, abstract, and report these mandated performance measures. It is conservatively estimated that hospitals spend 22.2 minutes per heart failure case to abstract the data, which in aggregate amount to more than 400,000 person-hours spent each year by U.S. hospitals (Fonarow, Srikanthan, Costanzo, Cintron, Lopatin, 2007).

Retrieving data for quality measurement is challenging. The process is mostly retrospective. Data are stored in different sources in the EHR and there are different kinds of data that do not map. In essence, humans are creating the data after analyzing different terms and codes in the EHR. Data and information standards are needed to solve these problems.

Overview of Standards

Standards can be defined as any norm, convention, or requirement that is universally agreed upon by participating entities (Business Dictionary, 2013). Many of us are familiar with standards even though we may not realize it. Many may remember the days prior to the proliferation of information technology in banking: one had to plan ahead for an international trip and purchase travelers checks. Today, one can hop on a plane on a whim and be able to purchase dinner in Kiev on a credit card and withdraw cash from an ATM with a debit card—doing so securely and being assured a fair exchange rate. With standards that are applied across an industry, for instance, the use of SWIFT standards in banking, one can easily see the advantages to standardization (Infosys, 2013). The ability to access money in a checking account from India on Tuesday and Italy on Thursday is an excellent example. Information technology has been a huge catalyst that has both enabled and enforced this standardization within banking.

We are all familiar with areas, beyond healthcare, that are lacking in standardization. The simple act of purchasing shoes or clothing made outside of the United States can be a frustrating experience. If one does not know their European size or have access to a chart to convert from United States to other sizes, the deal may not go through. This simple example highlights the need for standardization. As we look to healthcare and its current struggle to standardized, it is easier to understand why this issue is so important. In our clothing example, the chances that someone may be injured or die as a result of a lack of standardization are highly unlikely. In healthcare, the risk is eminent. There are many organizations that seek to help with this standardization in healthcare. One of the most important standardization organizations in electronic quality measurement is Health Level 7 (HL7), which will be described in the next section.

Overview of Health Level 7 (HL7)

The Health Level 7 (commonly referred to as HL7) organization came into existence in 1987 to begin solving standards issues in healthcare. HL7 is a non-profit organization that includes both corporate and individual members from all domains of healthcare. It is an American National Standards Institute (ANSI) accredited standards developing organization that focuses on creating and maintaining a framework of related standards for the exchange, integration, sharing, and retrieval of electronic health information (Health Level 7, 2014).

HL7 operates through volunteer work groups of professionals and one such group, the Clinical Quality Information Workgroup, is working closely with ONC and CMS to create and maintain information technology standards in support of improving healthcare quality, including clinical care, and to foster collaboration between quality measurement, outcomes, and improvement stakeholders. To this end, several projects are currently underway to help streamline the quality measurement development process. There are three key projects:

1. *Harmonization of a common data model* (sourced from many of the current models in use like the Virtual Medical Record [vMR] and the Quality Data Model [QDM] for quality that can be used for quality measures and clinical decision support).

2. *Harmonization of an expression language* that will allow measure developers to express certain mathematical and time-related concepts that are important in measurement in a way that is easily understood and carried out by implementers.

3. *Development of a common set of meta-data* (with definitions) that can be used in measure development.

HL7 Source Data Standards

HL7 has several primary standards that have led to the development of data standards around quality measurement. The Reference Information Model (RIM) is the foundation of much of HL7's development work. The RIM is a large, pictorial representation of the HL7 clinical data domains and identifies the life cycle of information.

HL7 standards pertain to four key areas of health information exchange: conceptual standards like the RIM, document standards (e.g., HL7 Consolidated Document Architecture), application standards, and messaging standards (e.g., HL7 v2.x and v3.0). This section will focus on document and messaging standards as they pertain to quality measurement.

From the RIM, many of HL7's primary standards have been developed. Important among those are the Version 2 (v2) and Version 3 (v3) Product Suites. The v2-messaging standard is considered the most widely adopted and used standard in the HL7 product line. This standard is the foundation of electronic data exchange and has been widely implemented in 95% of U.S. healthcare organizations to date (Health Level 7, 2014).

With the release of v3, HL7 attempted to move toward a more standardized programming language with the use of extensible markup language (XML). This use of XML makes v3 more human readable while maintained machine readability with the same data set. Unfortunately, there is no backward compatibility between v2 and v3, which has created challenges as v2 has been widely adopted in the United States and v3 has been adopted internationally.

The Clinical Document Architecture (CDA®) is a document markup standard that specifies the structure and semantics of clinical documents for the purpose of exchange between healthcare providers and patients. CDA states that a clinical document must contain certain key characteristics:

1. Persistence
2. Stewardship
3. Potential for authentication
4. Context
5. Wholeness
6. Human readability

HL7 Data Standards in Quality Measurement

From these source standards within HL7, specifically CDA, two important document standards have been developed to enable quality measurement. The Health Quality Measure Format or HQMF is the document standard for coding and representing an eMeasure. The HQMF is used by measure developers to define a clinical quality measure that is consumable by both a computer and a human (Health Level 7, n.d.).

The Quality Reporting Document Architecture or QRDA is the document standard for reporting the data that are determined to have met the criteria of the eMeasure. The QRDA standard has three levels of reporting capability: category I, II, and III. QRDA Category I is a patient-level report that contains the clinical information specified in the measure for one patient. A QRDA level II will have multi-patient information across a defined population that may or may not identify individual patient data within the summary. And lastly, a QRDA level III report is an aggregate quality report with a result for a given population and period of time. One can think of the QRDA as the result of a clinical quality measure from the EHR. It is then generally submitted to CMS or any other requesting or reporting agency.

The QRDA standard is referenced in the certification criteria for EHRs set forth by ONC. As part of the meaningful use legislation, providers and hospitals must use EHR technology that is certified by the federal government to meet certain standards and criteria. The QRDA standard is one of many HL7 standards that are referenced in these criteria.

Value Sets and Value Set Authority Center

Value sets can be defined lists of specific values (terms and their codes) derived from single or multiple standard vocabularies used to define clinical concepts (e.g., patients with diabetes, clinical visit, reportable diseases) used in clinical quality measures and to support effective health information exchange (National Library of Medicine, 2014b). Some of the standard vocabularies (or terminologies) used to define these value sets will be discussed in the next section. Value sets are developed by measure developers and are ideally shared across developers. Each value set is represented by a unique object identifier (OID) that is registered on the HL7 Web site. Until October 2013, value sets were created and maintained in the Measure Authoring Tool (MAT). Since late October 2013, the value sets for the 2014 CQM's were migrated to the new Value Set Authority Center (VSAC), which can be accessed at www.vsac.nlm.nih.gov.

The Value Set Authority Center (VSAC) serves as the official repository of the value sets for the Meaningful Use 2014 Clinical Quality Measures (CQM's) and is maintained by the National Library of Medicine (NLM), in collaboration with the ONC and CMS. Search, retrieval, and download capabilities are provided through a Web interface and

APIs. The VSAC also provides authoring tools for users to create value sets related to quality measures.

Terminology Standards

There are many terminologies currently in wide use within healthcare to represent clinical aspects or data types. All of these terminologies require a common format or standard to ensure that communication and transmission of data in the electronic realm are as clear as possible due to the increasing focus on collecting and sharing data across systems and for quality improvement and accountability purposes. There are several terminologies that play key roles in the representation of clinical care within EHRs and there are many mappings across the various terminologies to enable data sharing and valid representations of these data across settings and providers.

The Systemized Nomenclature of Medicine (SNOMED) is comprehensive, multi-lingual healthcare terminology (International Health Terminology Standards Development Organizations, 2014). SNOMED is important in EHR development and use as it allows for the recording of clinical data in ways that enable meaning-based retrieval, is mapped to other code sets that may be used in specific healthcare settings (e.g., LOINC), and certification and other standard setting organizations are encouraging the use of this terminology in performance measures.

Other code systems that are frequently used in performance measures include:

- LOINC® or the Logical Observation Identifiers Names and Codes: a universal code system for identifying laboratory and clinical observations (Regenstrief Institute, 2014)
- RxNorm: pertains specifically to medications and acts as a normalized naming system for generic and branded drugs (National Library of Medicine, 2014a)
- International Classification of Diseases (ICD): the classification used to code and classify diseases and other health characteristics (World Health Organization, n.d., Centers for Disease Control, 2013)
- Current Procedural Terminology (CPT): a code system that reports procedures, office, emergency departments and other visits, and other services provided by healthcare professionals (American Medical Association, 2014)
- The International Classification of Diseases (ICD): a code system used to classify diseases and other

health problems for health records and other vital records. The structure enables storage and retrieval of diagnostic information for quality, clinical, and other purposes (World Health Organization, n.d.).

Quality Data Model (QDM)

Once a measure developer has determined the clinical concepts in a quality measure and has built the associated value sets, use of the Quality Data Model or QDM will enable expression of performance measurement data for electronic measurement. The QDM can be thought of as a backbone for representation of quality criteria used in clinical guidelines, quality measures, and clinical decision support (CDS) and is used by stakeholders involved in electronic quality measurement and reporting, such as measure developers, federal agencies, health IT vendors, standards organizations, informatics experts, providers, and researchers. The QDM also makes up the logical portion of the Measure Authoring Tool or MAT. The QDM is currently being harmonized, through efforts in HL7, with other logical models to enhance its capabilities and expressiveness.

eCQM Life Cycle (From Measurement to Improvement)

Medicare and Medicaid EHR Incentive Programs provide financial incentives for the "Meaningful Use" of certified EHR technology to improve patient care (Cipriano, Bowles, Dailey, Dykes, Lamb, & Naylor, 2013). Achieving meaningful use of EHRs for quality measurement, reporting, and improvement requires the use of standards to integrate quality measures within EHRs for real-time quality reporting. This involves a series of steps as depicted in the Quality Management Life Cycle in Fig. 38.1.

The steps in the Quality Management Life Cycle will be described by applying the data standards presented in this chapter to an eMeasure from the MU incentive program. The quality measure was developed by the Joint Commission and assesses "the number of patients diagnosed with confirmed VTE who received an overlap of Parenteral (intravenous [IV] or subcutaneous anticoagulation and warfarin therapy." This measure involves all members of the clinical team and has implications for nursing practice. The life cycle of a quality measure from standardized representation of measure concepts and logic to integration within the EHR and generation of quality reports will be described. This description will be extended to show how the EHR can leverage data

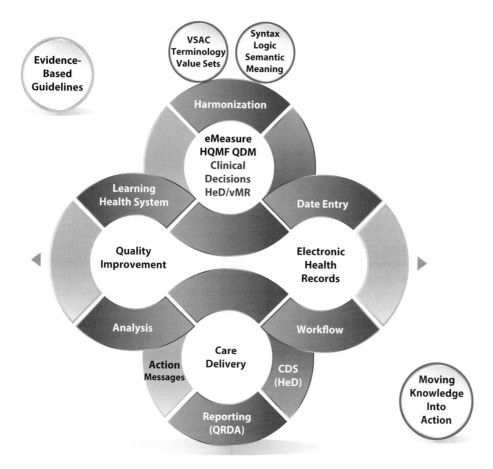

• **FIGURE 38.1.** Quality Management Life Cycle. (Reproduced, with permission, from Rosemary Kennedy. © Rosemary Kennedy, 2014.)

standards to support total quality management for venous thromboembolism care as it pertains to nursing practice.

The eMeasure life cycle includes the following steps:

Measure Title: Venous Thromboembolism Patients with Anti-coagulant Overlap Therapy, Steward: The Joint Commission

1. First, the intent of the measure is clearly and specifically defined as follows:

    a. "For patients who received less than five days of overlap therapy, they should be discharged on both medications or have a reason for discontinuation of overlap therapy. Overlap therapy should be administered for at least five days with an international normalized ratio (INR) greater than or equal to 2 prior to discontinuation of the parenteral anti-coagulation therapy, discharged on both medications or have a reason for discontinuation of overlap therapy." (http://cms.gov/Regulations-and-Guidance/Legislation/EHRIncentivePrograms/eCQM_Library.html).

2. Once the measure intent is defined, the different components of the measure are then specified—"who" is being measured and "what" is being measured. The components of this measure include the:

    a. Initial patient population of interest: Patients with a diagnosis code for venous thromboembolism (VTE) with a patient age greater than or equal to 18 years, and a length of stay less than or equal to 120 days

b. Denominator: Patients with confirmed VTE who received warfarin

c. Numerator: Patients who received overlap therapy (warfarin or parenteral anti-coagulation):

- Five or more days, with an INR greater than or equal to 2 prior to discontinuation or parenteral therapy, or

- Five or more days, with an INR less than 2 and discharged on overlap therapy, or

- Less than five days and discharged on overlap therapy, or

- With documentation of reason for discontinuation of overlap therapy, or

- With documentation of a reason for no overlap therapy

d. Denominator Exclusions:

- Patients less than 18 years of age

- Patients who have a length of stay greater than 120 days

- Patients with Comfort Measures Only documented

- Patients enrolled in clinical trials

- Patients discharged to a healthcare facility for hospice care

- Patients discharged to home for hospice care

- Patients who expired

- Patients who left against medical advice

- Patients discharged to another hospital

- Patients without warfarin therapy during hospitalization

- Patients without VTE confirmed by diagnostic testing

The level of granularity provides useful information for EHR designers, so they can start mapping quality measure concepts, such as "documentation of a reason for discontinuation of overlap therapy," to EHR functionality such as "addition of reason for discontinuation of overlap therapy." Furthermore, some of the measure components relate to nursing documentation such as "documentation of patients who are receiving comfort measures only."

3. After the measure is specified, indicating "who" is being measured and "what" is being measured, the measure needs to be further defined using standardized codes (QDM, SNOMED, LOINC, RxNorm, and CPT) for concepts contained within the measure (confirmed diagnosis of VTE, comfort measures, etc.), as well as standardized expression language (HTML and XML) to represent the logic contained within the measure (patients who received less than five days of overlap therapy should be discharged on both medications or have a reason for discontinuation of overlap therapy). This is accomplished with HQMF, which defines a representation of the quality measure that is consumable by both a human and computer. This expression can be described in three ways:

a. A human readable format (HTML) allows users to understand how the elements are defined and the underlying logic used to calculate the measure. This is useful when EHR designers, quality experts, clinicians, and the leadership team are making decisions about how the measures will be integrated within electronic systems. The human readable format provides a common language for all professionals involved in healthcare

b. A computer readable format (XML) enables the creation of automated queries against electronic systems for quality reporting (QRDA). Ideally electronic systems read the XML and will generate the QRDA for reporting

c. A list of the specific codes (SNOMED, QDM, RxNorm, ICD10, CPT) used by developers of electronic systems to ensure that accurate, valid, and reliable data capture can be supported (diagnoses, medications). The list of codes is referred to as "value sets." These value sets are contained within dictionaries (or concept repositories) of electronic health systems. The applications contained within electronic systems use the codes to process logic contained within the quality measures to generate quality reports (QRDA) necessary for MU

With this infrastructure, a vast array of healthcare data can be reported and analyzed, thereby turning data into knowledge that can be put to immediate use. This quality measurement infrastructure can help make advances toward becoming a learning health system.

In summary, the eMeasure supports quality reporting for MU but can also support real-time decision-making, performance improvement, and overall quality management. Two examples follow:

1. The eMeasure content can be used to guide clinical decision support through automatic alerts and reminders. For instance, this measure states that patients who receive less than five days of overlap therapy should be discharged on both medications or have a reason for discontinuation of overlap therapy. Electronic systems can use this content to alert the clinician at time of discharge to act in accordance with the measure.

2. EHR designers can integrate the measure rationale within EHRS to facilitate education and clinical decision support (CDS), please see box below. Clinicians can access the rationale from within the EHR. For this measure the rationale is as follows:

MEASURE RATIONALE

For patients who present with a confirmed acute VTE, parenteral anti-coagulation is the first line of therapy because of its rapid onset of action. Because the oral anti-coagulant warfarin has a very slow onset of action, it cannot be used as mono-therapy for acute VTE. Pretreatment with parenteral anti-coagulants prior to initiation of warfarin also avoids an early period of hypercoagulability that can result from the selective inhibition of proteins S and C (which have very short half-lives). Warfarin can be initiated on the first day of treatment after the first dose of a parenteral anti-coagulant has been given. Warfarin interferes with the synthesis of vitamin K–dependent pro-coagulant factors (factors II, VII, IX, and X) as well as some anti-coagulant factors (proteins S and C). It takes several days for warfarin to achieve its effect because time is required for normal coagulation factors to be cleared from plasma. The adequacy of warfarin therapy is monitored by measurement of the international normalized ratio (INR). The INR can sometimes appear prolonged (or "therapeutic") as soon as 24 hours after the institution of warfarin due to a reduction in factor VII levels, even while factor II levels are still high and the patient is not in fact therapeutically anti-coagulated. Because factor II has a half-life of 60–72 hours, a minimum of five days of parenteral anti-coagulation is recommended as "overlap therapy" while warfarin is being initiated. Parenteral therapy should also be continued until the INR is greater than or equal to 2.0, even if this takes longer than five days, so that patients are fully anti-coagulated during the period before warfarin takes its full effect.

This measure has implications for nursing practice. Some of the data necessary for calculation of the measure are derived from documentation performed by nurses. Nurses, in providing care to patients with VTE, document additional data related to the prevention and management of VTE. The infrastructure related to MU code sets, such as SNOMED (which includes recognized nursing terminologies), can be used to support coding of nursing data.

The clinical quality measures represent conditions reflective of nursing practice. For each of conditions contained within the clinical quality measures, nursing care is provided and frequently represented within the care plan. The care plan can be structured within the EHR using standardized terminology such as Clinical Care Classification (see Fig. 38.2). This shows how nursing practice and documentation supports reporting on conditions represented within the eCQM for MU.

The value of using the data infrastructure as described above includes:

a. Enhanced decision-making (use the above measure to alert a nurse that patients who receive less than five days of overlap therapy should be discharged on both medications or have a reason for discontinuation of overlap therapy). Once the medications are ordered, the electronic system can populate the patient care plan with interventions as depicted in Fig. 38.2.

b. Creation of nursing dashboards to answer such questions as: "How many patients received discharge education?" The electronic dashboards can be used for a total quality management program to enhance quality and safety.

c. Streamlined measurement and comprehensive exchange between systems so nursing impact on outcomes can be compared across settings, the nation, and internationally.

d. Generation of new knowledge to advance nursing practice.

e. Effective use of electronic health records to support both care delivery and performance improvement.

Diagnosis: Venous Thromboembolism **Nursing Diagnosis:**	**Medical/Nursing Orders / Treatments / Interventions:**
• Tissue Perfusion Alteration—S48.0 (Tissue Perfusion Component) • Acute Pain—Q63.1 (Sensory Component) • Knowledge Deficit of Disease—D08.3 (Cognitive/Neuro Component) • Knowledge Deficit of Dietary Regimen—D08.2 (Cognitive/Neuro) **Expected Outcomes/Goals of Care:** • Improve Tissue Perfusion Alteration—S48.0.1 • Improve Acute Pain—Q63.1.1 • Improve Knowledge Deficit of Disease Process—D08.3.1 • Improve Knowledge Deficit of Dietary Regimen—D08.2.1	• Assess level / Control of Pain—Q47.0.1 • Administer Pain Assessment Instrument—Q47.0.2) • Administer Demerol 100 mg / PRN/ Q4H—H24.4.2 • Administer Warfarin 100 mg OD—H24.4.2 • Monitor Warfarin IV to prevent site infection—F79.1.1 • Coordinate Daily Blood Test—K32.1 .4 • Assess Daily left leg Edem—S69.0.1 • Elevate Leg on two pillows—S69.0.2 • Teach information re Disease Treatment—G18.6.3 • Teach information regarding diet—G18.1.3

• **FIGURE 38.2.** Deep Vein Thrombosis Plan of Care Coded with CCC. (Permission from SabaCare Inc. February 10, 2014.)

SUMMARY

In this chapter, we have described what quality measurement is and the move from traditional paper-based abstraction of this information to the use of standards and terminologies to enable electronic capture of real-time data for quality improvement purposes. Standards and terminologies continue to evolve with the increased implementation and the potential uses for nursing care have not yet been fully realized. While many national programs currently focus on those individuals and entities that are paid based on the services provided (i.e., physicians, hospitals), there are many opportunities to leverage the data used for quality measurement to enhance the care provided by nurses today as outlined in the example provided at the end of this chapter.

REFERENCES

Agency for Healthcare Research and Quality. (n.d.). *National quality strategy*. Retrieved from http://www.ahrq.gov/workingforquality/. Accessed on January 23, 2014.

American Medical Association. (2014). *Current Procedural Terminology (CPT)*. Retrieved from http://www.ama-assn.org/go/cpt. Accessed on February 9, 2014.

Bankowitz, R., Bechtel, C., Corrigan, J., DeVore, S. D., Fisher, E., & Nelson, G. (2013, May 9). *Health affairs blog. A framework for accountable care measures*. Retrieved from http://healthaffairs.org/blog/2013/05/09/a-framework-for-accountable-care-measures/. Accessed on January 17, 2014.

Business Dictionary. (2013). *Business dictionary*. Retrieved from www.businessdictionary.com. Accessed on January 23, 2014.

Centers for Disease Control. (2013). *International classification of diseases*. ICD-9. Retrieved from http://www.cdc.gov/nchs/icd.htm. Accessed on January 23, 2014.

Centers for Medicare & Medicaid Services. (n.d.). *Clinical quality measures basics*. Retrieved from http://www.cms.gov/Regulations-and-Guidance/Legislation/EHRIncentivePrograms/ClinicalQualityMeasures.html. Accessed on February 1, 2014.

Cipriano, P., Bowles, K., Dailey, M., Dykes, P., Lamb, G., & Naylor, M. (2013). The importance of Health information technology in care coordination and transitional care. *Nursing Outlook, 61*(6), 475–488.

Donabedian, A. (1980). *Explorations in quality assessment and monitoring* (Vol. 1). Ann Arbor, MI: Health Administration Press.

Fonarow, G. C., Srikanthan, P., Costanzo, M. R., Cintron, G. B., Lopatin, M. (2007). ADHERE Scientific Advisory Committee and Investigators. An obesity paradox in acute heart failure: analysis of body mass index and inhospital mortality for 108927 patients in the acute decompensated heart failure national registry. *Am Heart J, 153*(1):74–81.

Health Level 7. (2014). *Health Level 7*. Retrieved from www.hl7.org. Accessed on February 9, 2014.

Health Level 7. (n.d.). *Health quality measure format (HQMF)*. Retrieved from http://www.hl7.org/special/committees/

projman/searchableprojectindex.cfm?action=edit&Project Number=756. Accessed on February 9, 2014.

Infosys. (2013). *Messaging standards in the financial industry*. Retrieved from http://www.infosys.com/finacle/solutions/thought-papers/Documents/messaging-standards-financial-industry.pdf. Accessed on January 23, 2014.

Institute of Medicine. Lohr, K. N. (Ed). (1990). *Medicare: A strategy for quality assurance* (Vol. 1). Washington, DC: National Academy Press. Accessed on February 9, 2014.

International Health Terminology Standards Development Organization. (2014). *SNOMED*. Retrieved from http://www.ihtsdo.org/snomed-ct/

Montalvo, I., & Dunton, N. (2007). *Transforming nursing data into quality care*. Silver Spring, MD: American Nurses Association.

National Database for Nursing Quality Indicators. *NDNQI™*. (n.d.). Retrieved from http://www.nursingquality.org/About-NDNQI; http://www.nursingquality.org/. Accessed on January 22, 2014.

National Library of Medicine. (2014a). *RxNorm*. Retrieved from http://www.nlm.nih.gov/research/umls/rxnorm/. Accessed on February 9, 2014.

National Library of Medicine. (2014b). *Value set authority center*. Retrieved from https://vsac.nlm.nih.gov/. Accessed on February 9, 2014.

National Quality Measures Clearinghouse. (n.d.). *Glossary*. Retrieved from http://www.qualitymeasures.ahrq.gov/about/glossary.aspx. Accessed on January 14, 2014.

Regenstrief Institute. (2014). *LOINC*. Retrieved from www.loinc.org. Accessed on February 9, 2014.

Tang, P. C., Ralston, M., Arrigotti, M. F., Qureshi, L., & Graham, J. (2007). Comparison of methodologies for calculating quality measures based on administrative data versus clinical data from an electronic health record system: Implications for performance measures. *Journal of the American Medical Informatics Association, 14*, 10–15.

World Health Organization. (n.d.). *International classification of diseases (ICD)*. Retrieved from http://www.who.int/classifications/icd/en/. Accessed on February 1, 2014.

39

Translation of Evidence into Nursing Practice

Lynn McQueen / Heather Carter-Templeton / Kathleen A. McCormick

• OBJECTIVES

1. Understand translational science and closely related terminology.
2. Identify tools supporting the translation of evidence at the data, information, knowledge, and wisdom meta-structure levels.
3. Describe evolution of evidence-based practice and evolving trends in the translation of evidence into practice.
4. Describe how informatics is used as a tool to promote and facilitate knowledge generation and translation in practice.
5. Describe models and frameworks connecting critical thinking to processes that support the use of evidence into nursing practice.
6. Discuss how informatics tools serve to promote use of evidence and the application of knowledge in practice.
7. Identify professional nursing groups and networks that help expand and improve resources to assist in translating evidence into nursing practice.
8. Discuss how professional nurses might engage in advancing the next steps and how informatics tools can be used to deliver evidence into nursing practice.

• KEY WORDS

Evidence
Knowledge generation
Clinical practice guidelines
Evidence-based practice tools
Meaningful use
Performance metrics
Quality and safety of patient care

INTRODUCTION

The nursing discipline has evolved from the days when research was left to those in academe. An increased emphasis on evidence-based practice (EBP) now requires nurses at all levels to engage in EBP (Phillips et al., 2006).

For a nurse practicing across inpatient, ambulatory, home, and other settings as well as education, administration, and research, it can be challenging to keep up with both the latest technology as well as new scientific publications. Yet staying current is central to safe and high quality care even though care based on evidence is not always the norm (Melnyk & Fineout-Overholt, 2012). Although nurses in different settings may consider different types of information to be "evidence," the profession is rapidly learning together how human and electronic information resources as well as print information resources contribute to improved outcomes (Carter-Templeton, 2013). Informatics facilitates this journey by strengthening the merger of evidence with technology in convenient, yet transformative, ways. This chapter focuses on the translation of evidence into practice and how translation intersects with technology.

DEFINING EVIDENCE, IMPLEMENTATION, AND TRANSLATIONAL SCIENCES

EBP adds action to the use of evidence. EBP provides processes for using evidence to generate knowledge. It is a widely used term that is easier to define than to operationalize. When defining EBP, Melnyk & Fineout-Overholt highlight the importance of using evidence to support decisions by saying that EBP is a "problem solving approach to clinical decision-making that involves the conscientious use of the best available evidence (including a systematic search for and critical appraisal of the most relevant evidence) to answer a clinical question with one's own clinical expertise along with patient values and preferences to improve outcomes for individuals, groups, communities and systems" (2011). EBP has many siblings and the distinctions can be confusing. *Implementation science is the study of methods to promote the integration of research findings and evidence into healthcare policy and practice* (National Institutes of Health Fogarty International Center, 2013). Implementation science is growing field that is both multi-faceted and complex. It is especially relevant to nurses and others who work directly with patients since it focuses on what is needed to improve outcomes.

EBP is also central to what Titler and Everett (2001) define as "translational research," which tests the effect of interventions to facilitate the rate and extent to which evidence-based practices are adopted (2001). Translational research and implementation science both capture the significance of key variables that influence EPB. These variables are part of the local environmental context that so often complicates the implementation of evidence, such as introducing a new intervention based on a current clinical practice guideline recommendation with the goal of assimilating the intervention into routine clinical practice (Harrison & Graham, 2012). Since there is no one standard international terminology that conclusively defines

translation, sorting out the definitions can be overwhelming. Yet understanding the commonly used terms associated with evidence-driven care is potentially valuable since adhering only to one way of thinking about evidence misses what these terms have in common. The collective actions associated with terms like EBP, implementation science, translational research, knowledge translation, and related terms share a goal to move science close to what makes a difference for patients and populations. These actions can be simplified into the term "translation." Although defined in different ways, translation emphasizes processes such as dissemination and implementation of empirical, patient-centered findings that have been rigorously tested in broad populations and sub-groups before deemed ready for implementation in clinical practice. Feedback and evaluation often follow implementation. As evidence moves through dissemination, implementation, evaluation, and other stages, evidence-driven care is fostered through iterative and interactive processes (Harrison & Graham, 2012). Although there is growing awareness of the importance of evidence uptake, we are in the early stages of knowing how to systematically operationalize translation and sustain improvements after safety and quality related interventions end. But much is being learned and technology offers momentum. Struggling with what it takes to apply evidence in ways that promote lasting, safe, cost-effective, and high quality care is gradually leading to measurable outcome improvements.

TOOLS USED FOR SUPPOTING TRANSLATION OF DATA TO INFORMATION TO KNOWLEDGE TO WISDOM

Nursing is an information-based discipline (Graves & Corcoran, 1989). Nursing informatics unites nursing science, computer science, and information science in ways that transform what this means. The evolution of nursing as an information-based discipline changes how data, information, and knowledge are managed in nursing practice (Staggers & Thompson, 2002). Figure 39.1 is inspired by Englebardt & Nelson's (2002) Relationship of Data, Information, Knowledge, and Wisdom and illustrates examples of tools facilitating translation at each informatics meta-structure level. The actions occurring as data are transformed into information, knowledge, and wisdom are dynamic and iterative. What is learned through research, evaluation, quality improvement, and safety activities contributes to wisdom. Once wisdom is achieved, feedback contributes to ongoing improvements and to generate new hypotheses.

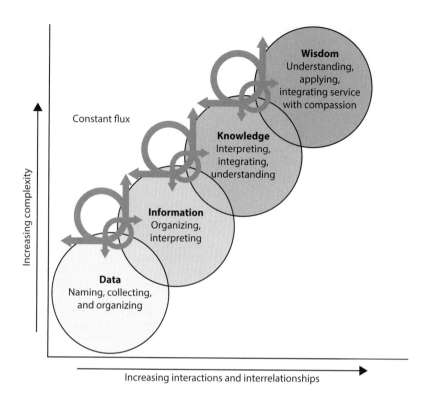

Increasing complexity

Constant flux

Wisdom
Understanding, applying, integrating service with compassion

Knowledge
Interpreting, integrating, understanding

Information
Organizing, interpreting

Data
Naming, collecting, and organizing

Increasing interactions and interrelationships

• **FIGURE 39.1.** Example of Tools Facilitating Translation at Each Informatics Meta-structure Level. Revised Data Information Knowledge Wisdom (DIKW) model–2013 version. (Copyright © 2013 Ramona Nelson, Ramona Nelson Consulting. All rights reserved. Reprinted with permission.)

In an evolving healthcare system, nurses' information needs are fluid and evolve. The development of knowledge accompanies the use of evidence. But only recently is the scientific knowledge base relevant to translational research and implementation science been strong enough to support use of specific evidence-based tools and strategies during translation as well as address how local factors, such as attitudes toward EBP, influence translation (Upton, Upton, & Scurlock-Evans, 2014). Measurement of the impact of using a specific evidence-based tool aids in ongoing understanding of the barriers and facilitators that influence sustained improvements. Peer-reviewed publications reporting the results of measuring impact adds to the relevance of the scientific knowledge base. Nurses are in the early stages of identifying best practices as well as gaps in the body of knowledge related to Health Information Technology (HIT) implementation (Abbott, Foster, Marin, & Dykes, 2013). As innovations spread, more will be known about how to tailor HIT tools to a local setting, including better understanding about how to adjust implementation strategies based on factors associated with the nursing interventions, patients, and resources.

EVOLUTION OF EVIDENCE

How Evidence Is Generated

Research results can be used to address important clinical questions after being accepted as part of the evidence base for a clinical question. Research results become part of the evidence base for a disease or condition only after going through rigorous and explicit processes designed to find, compare, and combine data. Reviews of research findings involve critical appraisal using explicit and objective inclusion and exclusion criteria. Such criteria identifies studies to be considered when trying to answer a clinical question, such as which nursing interventions for reducing pain are the most effective and scientifically grounded. An organized approach is used to identify valid and reliable peer reviewed publications to be considered further. Rigorous methods determine the efficacy of specific interventions and their effectiveness when used with real patients outside of tightly controlled conditions. Advanced statistical analysis, using Bayesian or other methods, helps understand how best to combine findings. Through these techniques, systematic reviews pull together what is known about the benefits and harms of the interventions surrounding a clinical question. Credible methodology helps reveal the trade-offs associated with key treatment, diagnostic, or prevention interventions. The cumulative findings associated with specific questions can then be reviewed and rated by unbiased experts. Typically, ratings are accomplished by a multi-disciplinary expert team. A team's systematic review often results in rated recommendations about what does and does not contribute to improved outcomes.

Evidence is rated by experts using one of several methods. Table 39.1 shows the U.S. Preventive Services Task Force's (USPSTF) widely used grading scheme (2008) applied to suggestions for practice. The methods used by USPSTF and other credible groups are revised over time as methods evolve. The USPSTF assigns an A, B, C, D, or I letter grade to signify the strength of each recommendation that comes from synthesizing research findings. Table 39.1 shows suggested practice for each letter grade. The graded recommendations produced through this process can be used as the basis for evidence-based tools, such as clinical practice guidelines. During 2012, the USPSTF updated its definition for grade C recommendations, which can be the most complex for clinicians to implement. The basic meaning of the C recommendation indicates that the net weight of benefits and harms is very close and needs to be considered within the context of conditions, circumstances, and preferences. While the statistical magnitude of net benefit for a C recommendation is considered small, it may or may not seem

small to an individual patient or family or in the eyes of the providers caring for the patient or to the community as a whole. Values can influence how a specific clinical choice is viewed. In these cases, the USPSTF recommends "selectively" providing the service—meaning that patient and community preferences, clinician input, and costs may rise in importance. In these instances, it is especially important to guard against the potential for bias. Bias arises from conflicts of interest or other avenues that risk the integrity of the processes involved with synthesizing evidence and using this evidence to create evidence-based tools. Bias can influence ultimate credibility of the final products and can occur at any point between the selection of research findings through translation and evaluation.

Suggestions for Practice Based on Recommendation Grades

The availability of evidence and evidence-based tools is only the beginning. The U.S. Centers for Disease Control and Prevention (CDC) provides a representation showing the convergence of evidence synthesis with expert judgment (Spencer et al., 2013). Figure 39.2 shows a conceptual framework nurses can use when planning and improving evidence-based practices. A nurse can apply this model by rating the quality/strength of evidence as weak, moderate, strong, or rigorous. This rating is associated with the potential impact of applying the evidence-based practice in a clinical setting. The quality of the evidence is

TABLE 39.1	Suggestions for Practice to Use Recommended Grades (USPSTF, 2008)	
Grade	**Definition**	**Suggestions for Practice**
A	The USPSTF recommends the service. There is high certainty that the net benefit is substantial.	Offer or provide this service.
B	The USPSTF recommends the service. There is high certainty that the net benefit is moderate or there is moderate certainty that the net benefit is moderate to substantial.	Offer or provide this service.
C	The USPSTF recommends selectively offering or providing this service to individual patients based on professional judgment and patient preferences. There is at least moderate certainty that the net benefit is small.	Offer or provide this service for selected patients depending on individual circumstances.
D	The USPSTF recommends against the service. There is moderate or high certainty that the service has no net benefit or that the harms outweigh the benefits.	Discourage the use of this service.
I Statement	The USPSTF concludes that the current evidence is insufficient to assess the balance of benefits and harms of the service. Evidence is lacking, of poor quality, or conflicting, and the balance of benefits and harms cannot be determined.	Read the clinical considerations section of USPSTF Recommendation Statement. If the service is offered, patients should understand the uncertainty about the balance of benefits and harms.

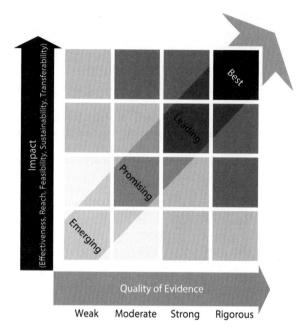

• **FIGURE 39.2.** A Conceptual Framework for Planning and Improving Evidence-Based Practices. (Reproduced from Spencer L.M. et al (2013). Found at http://www.cdc.gov/pcd/issues/2013/13_0186.htm.)

interpreted with consideration given to impact. Impact is quantified in terms of effectiveness, reach, feasibility, sustainability, and transferability. Within this framework, the term "impact" goes beyond traditional ideas of clinical significance or clinical importance, which focus on whether a nurse or other clinician would alter their practice based on the statistical significance of research findings. Frameworks of this kind make it easier to communicate about the potential use or rejection of the interventions identified as "best practices" when evidence and judgment are combined. The use of a framework and common terms aids accountability and transparency about how decisions were reached. Early in the application of a framework, such as CDC's conceptual framework, nurses may want to discuss how terms like "impact" and "clinical significance" are defined by members of the clinical team and by the patients and family members involved.

The Origins of Evidence-Based Practice

EBP employs a systematic approach to clinical decision-making using the best evidence (Sackett, Straus, Richardson, Rosenberg, & Hayes, 2000). Although nurses have long promoted rational choice based on current

research findings, the use of a systematic approach to finding and applying evidence as the basis for decisions has only been emphasized over the past 25 years.

Throughout the 1990s, ideas about how to find and use research results evolved. The term EBP became popular after 1992 when first used by Gordon Guyatt and a group he led at McMaster University (Guyatt, 2002). David L. Sackett described EBP as the best use of current best evidence in making decisions about the care of individual patients (Sackett, 2000). Over time, EBP came to describe a systematic approach to organizing, collecting, and using research findings in ways that contribute to the best possible outcomes. As this occurred, nursing roles were revitalized as informatics brought clinical decision support and other tools closer to the bedside.

As methods for synthesizing evidence improved, literature searches and reviews, meta-analysis, evidence reviews, and evidence-based tools proliferated. Such synthesized evidence in the form of review papers and similar formats are of growing relevance to nurses since multiple studies and multiple applications are included (Sales, 2013). But the methodological challenges are significant as we try to generalize evidence across groups and settings. Can recommendations from a guideline that applies to men automatically be used with women? Is an intervention more clinically significant than another if they are equal statistically yet one is preferred (over the other) strongly by patients? If an implementation strategy worked in an inpatient setting, can it be used in an ambulatory setting? Answers to these and a host of similar questions are sought as the knowledge base associated with EBP grows and reveals conditions that foster sustained improvement in specific settings. For example, Harden, Burke, Haile, and Estabrooks (2013) explored the degree to which specific interventions, identified within a systematic review, align in ways that facilitate translation of research into practice.

INFORMATICS TOOLS THAT PROMOTE AND FACILITATE KNOWLEDGE GENERATION OF EVIDENCE

Approximately 87% of adult Americans now have regular Internet access (Pew Research Center, 2014), evidence is often sought through Web-based resources. Nurses help themselves, their students, patients, professional nursing groups, and their clinical team understand whether the information commonly downloaded about a specific condition or disease is accurate (valid and reliable) while pointing out potential benefits and harms. Caution may be needed if information is being used without critical review. A nurse can generate (and regularly update) lists of credible online evidence-based resources to suggest to patients, families, and other providers. Because evidence becomes outdated, nurses can monitor to be sure that their teams and patients have current information, including understanding any legal and ethical concerns or privacy issues.

Criteria to evaluate health-related information found online has been developed and disseminated by several organizations including HON Code, American Medical Association, Internet Health Care Coalition, Hi-Ethics, and MedCertain (Berland, Elliott, & Morales, 2001). However, criteria developed by these groups vary in scope and scale and have not been shared in a systematic way. In addition, most of these criteria were designed for evaluating health and medical information, not necessarily nursing.

Youth, young adults, and increasingly the rest of us are using mobile and portable devices, including tablets, portable computers, and smart phones to seek the evidence and engage with actual automated interventions (such as online counselling). Web-based screening, prevention, outreach, and intervention tools help patients access valid and reliable evidence about fundamental public health issues, such as obesity, stress management, and tobacco cessation, while also helping patients track, reinforce, and manage healthy choices and gain online support.

E-mail, evidence, and twitter alert systems involve voluntary registration based on clinical interest in order to receive alerts or updates related to interventions. They are ideal for receiving information about new evidence or to send alerts about a safety concern, such as spreading information that a medication has been found dangerous. Alerts are often linked to resources that allow access to the scientific literature matched to a specific clinical interest. Alerts also deliver information that has already been rated. However, the credibility of the informant often needs to be appraised.

Assessments and interventions provided via a technology platform may occur without a provider. Some of these tools allow for tracking and feedback about the patient's use of the tool to a nurse or other clinician. Some of these tools are interactive and Web-based or may be run from a DVD, local computer, or flash-drive. Mobile tools, such as phones and tablets, are also used. Nurses help by addressing what is lost (in terms of non-verbal interactions, cues, and physical assistance) versus what is gained (through access and convenience) when a technology-based intervention works with other non-nursing clinicians. Nurses can then tailor these tools to the needs of specific patients.

MODELS AND THEORETICAL FRAMEWORKS CONNECTING CRITICAL THINKING TO PROCESSES THAT SUPPORT THE USE OF EVIDENCE IN NURSING PRACTICE

Models and frameworks help link critical thinking to step-wise processes that promote the use of evidence, including accounting for factors that lead to safe and lasting outcome and organizational improvements. Because translation involves implementing evidence and evidence-based tools outside tightly controlled situations, such as Randomized Controlled Trials (RCT), theories help nurses critically examine the contextual factors, assumptions, and influences surrounding implementation. Using models and frameworks helps nurses prepare a cogent plan for translation within complicated situations, such as the implementation of an EBP when change and disruption are anticipated.

Nursing leaders across countries have contributed to theories about translation and quality improvement. These theories include Donabedian's (1980) structure, process, and outcomes framework, which focus on problem solving. Other theories directly relevant to translation are found in Rogers' Diffusion of Innovations model, the Funk Model, the PRECEDE Model, the Chronic Care Model, the PARiHS Model, the Stetler Model, the Iowa Model and Translation Research Model, Russworm's and Larrabee's Model, the ARCC Model, Kitson's Framework, Melnyk and Fineout-Overholt's Model of EBP, the Lean Framework, the PICOT Model, the QUERI model, Rossworm and Larrabee's Model, and the Institute for Healthcare Improvement's breakthrough model. Some of these models are briefly described below.

Exploring how nurses conceptualize translation helps nurses learn from each other. Specific contributions include Roger's understanding of "attributes" (including complexity) and Alison Kitson's emphasis on understanding the environment, including the importance of a clearly articulated collaborative Knowledge Translation (KT) approach that can be embedded into the research design (Kitson, Powell, Hoon, Newbury, Wilson, & Beilby, 2013). The Promoting Action on Research Implementation in Health Services (PARIHS) framework helps define and measure key factors leading to successful implementation and has been widely used, including by Squires et al. (2012) who designed strategies to implement research-based policies and procedures. Dr. Marita Titler provided leadership for AHRQ's TRIP initiatives and has also studied the context in which EBPs are translated. Important influences found include: (1) the nature of the innovation (such as the strength of evidence) and (2) the manner it is communicated to nurses and physicians (Herr et al 2012; Titler 2010; Titler 2011). Dr. Carole Estabrooks described the importance of considering the significant needs found in complex care environments, such as nursing homes (Estabrooks et al., 2013). Dr. Cheryl Stetler evolved her practitioner-oriented Stetler Model of Evidence-Based Practice in ways that have shaped the evolution of EBP (Stetler, 2001; Stetler et al., 2006; Stetler & Caramanica, 2007; Stetler 2010) and also synthesized literature on use of the PARIHS framework, including development of a companion guide to assist researchers using PARIHS (Stetler, Damschroder, Helfrich, & Hagedorn, 2011). The PARIHS framework is widely used internationally, including Bergström, Peterson, Namusoko, Waiswa, and Wallin (2012) who used PARIHS as a framework for knowledge translation in Uganda.

As new technologies combine with novel approaches to measuring the complex factors affecting outcomes, theories and frameworks are being customized, including tailoring them to the workflow of nurses and the needs of developing nations (Dalheim, Harthug, Nilsen, & Nortvedt, 2012). Melnyk and Finout-Overholt adopted EBP competencies for nurses and advanced practice nurses (APNs) working in real-world clinical situations (Melnyk, Gallagher-Ford, Long, & Fineout-Overholt, 2014). Rycroft-Malone et al. (2012) and McCormack et al. (2013) described a new approach known as realist review and synthesis, which focuses on understanding the mechanisms by which an intervention works or does not work. Hynes, Whittier, and Owens (2013) used the QUERI model to demonstrate how HIT approaches could be characterized as facilitators or barriers to implementation. Three pathways were found to contribute to translation: (1) compliance and collaboration with information technology policies and procedures; (2) operating within organizational policies and building collaborations with end users, clinicians, and administrators; and (3) obtaining and maintaining research resources and approvals. Harrison, Graham, van den Hoek, Dogherty, Carley, and Angus (2013) emphasized the importance of planning support in development of a framework called CAN-IMPLEMENT. In Canada, The Queen's University Research Roadmap for Knowledge Implementation (QuRKI) is being used to highlight mutually supporting/interconnected cycles of research studies supporting implementation (Harrison & Graham, 2012). In Australia, multi-disciplinary Health Networks were used as a framework to collaboratively develop evidence-based policies and drive implementation (Briggs, Bragge, Slater, Chan, & Towler, 2012).

INFORMATICS TOOLS THAT PROMOTE THE USE OF EVIDENCE AND APPLY KNOWLEDGE TO PRACTICE

Adoption of evidence is now understood far beyond passively providing access to a single clinical practice guideline or Webinar. The attention has shifted to understanding the conditions that foster ongoing and lasting change once the evidence is found and introduced, often using multiple implementation strategies. Increasingly, not only is the intervention being tested based on the best available evidence but the implementation strategies being used to apply the evidence are also grounded in science. Boulet, Bourbeau, Skomro, and Gupta (2013) authored one of many studies focusing on the complex barriers that cross the patient, provider, and healthcare system boundaries and suggested innovative, multi-faceted approaches to implementation. Such studies provide local evidence about what will hopefully work when an EBP is translated. What will facilitate implementation and what will be the barriers? Under what conditions is successful implementation anticipated? Young, Foster, Silander, and Wakefield (2011) demonstrated how complicated such investigations can become. Although home telehealth programs can be tailored to facilitate older adults' access to care, collecting data was challenging during this study because the patients did not want to be critical. But sustained improvement depended upon understanding patient perspectives about the benefits and challenges of care coordination and home telehealth. Ultimately, it was documented that patients were frustrated by equipment problems, as well as slow response, and care coordinator inaccessibility. Understanding the influence of patient perceptions assured that expectations could be met. This facilitated translation.

The information explosion presents challenges to healthcare providers who seek new evidence on an ongoing basis. Evidence-based clinical or point-of-care resources, especially literature reviews, make it easier to access information. Easy access helps nurses avoid making decisions based on experience alone or on the advice of a colleague or teacher. Evidence-based tools help by organizing evidence and aiding cognition in evidence selection, interpretation, implementation, and evaluation. When coupled with technology, evidence-based tools become central to practice. Yet this occurs within a climate of constant change and new incentives. Although rapid advances in access, quality, and safety are possible, nurses are challenged to create, find, test, implement, and evaluate the right evidence-based tools. Such tools include complex technology new to some nurses, including innovative decision support using mobile health-based approaches (Hyun et al., 2013).

Decision support includes integrating experience with the evidence. Evidence-based tools are not "cookbooks." When implementing a clinical intervention using an automated evidence-based tool, clinical judgment is needed. Because translation and decision support overlap, each is inherently multi-disciplinary. Nursing joins public health, medicine, and other health disciplines in seeking better understanding of the conditions needed to successfully apply evidence to decision support in real situations, then measure the impact and feed data back after evaluation. As evidence brokers, computer-literate nurses bring to their teams knowledge of how to identify and then critically appraise the best available evidence or use the evidence-based tool(s) to support decisions. This includes knowing how to explain evidence to clinicians, families, and teams with varying degrees of scientific expertise and computer literacy. Explaining evidence includes understanding the "unintended consequences" that accompany translation and dealing with uncertainty when evidence is incomplete, misleading, or contradictory. For example, what happens when an automated clinical practice guideline recommends treatment for a specific clinical condition, such as cancer, but does not address priorities or contraindications with co-existing diagnoses, such as diabetes? Even the best evidence-based tool rarely applies to all patients without being tailored to sub-groups or accounting for the patients' preferences. For some patients or sub-groups, multiple evidence-based tools may need to be translated at the same time or specific interventions from different evidence-based tools tried together. Models help nurses create a cogent plan that pulls these interventions together.

Decision support now occurs within the context of change. Fueled by healthcare reform, HIT supports EBP by making it easier to access and use evidence and evidence-based tools, such as automated reminders. The U.S. Center for Medicaid and Medicare Services (CMS) defines the "meaningful use" provision in the Affordable Care Act (ACA) legislation in ways that promote the use of evidence to drive improved outcomes, quality, and safety. The implications and pace are staggering. Within this environment, there are incentives that promote automated systems facilitating advances in HIT. Such advances promote EBP but also reveal gaps in quality and safety as well as disparities. Carefully planned use of HIT contributes to new and restructured systems that address the over-use, under-use, and misuse of healthcare (Doebbling and Flanagan, 2011). Understanding the context in which HIT and EBP merge means studying what works and does not work during translation. This sometimes means feeding data back

as the intervention is being implemented using methods such as formative evaluation. Although nurses are in the early stages of investigating factors associated with organizational context, such as explaining variation in the use of HIT during translation (Doran et al., 2012), there are a growing number of studies seeking to understand what makes a difference. For example, Currie, Lockett, and El Enany (2013) studied policy influences on those translating evidence into practice, including factors related to social position.

The Use of Electronic Health Records (EHRs)

Automated tools are often linked to computerized health records, such as Electronic Health Record (EHR), which refers to patient records collected across settings, ideally to support care along the continuum of an individual's lifespan. As a result of the proliferation of electronic health data, clinical intelligence and other uses of aggregated data promote the conversion of meaningful information into knowledge (Harrington, 2011). EHRs can be especially powerful if the data are standardized and copied into data warehouses or datamarts where data can be easily exchanged for follow-up purposes.

Because EHR promotes meaningful use of technology and enhances information exchange, it plays a growing role in the translation of evidence into practice. EHR provides a vehicle to transmit evidence by embedding evidence-based tools into routine nursing functions. In doing so, EHR impacts quality and safety, hopefully in positive ways. For example, when EHR observations relevant to the implementation of a clinical practice guideline are pooled and analyzed, the data can then be shared, aggregated, and interpreted in ways that promote quality and safety. Later, these data may become part of the body of evidence used to update the next version of a clinical practice guideline. Poe, Abbott, and Pronovost (2011) used peer coaches to build and sustain competencies needed by nurses using EHR in clinical settings. Both satisfaction and confidence increased through the use of an evidence-based coach intervention. Nurses are cautioned, however, to actively participate in the development, monitoring, implementation, and use of their EHRs. Ongoing diligence is needed to assure the timeliness of updates, the accuracy of input, as well as the usefulness and safety of output.

Applying Evidence in Informatics to Improve Safety and Quality of Care

Nurses seeking to improve the safety and quality of care within their organizations can often find literature reviews, systematic reviews, meta-analyses, or evidence-based tools that address their specific goals or are relevant to their areas of practice (Tricco et al., 2012). Technology-based tools can be used within an organization in ways that make it easier and faster to implement evidence-based tools while also making it harder to harm a patient. Evidence-based tools such as electronically available clinical practice guidelines, clinical decision support, automated performance measures, and computerized reminders can be embedded into routines of care with feedback provided "just in time" to impact processes, intermediate outcomes, outcomes, and sometimes influence costs, patient and provider satisfaction, and even work force issues. Electronic tools used to promote quality and safety offer a promising approach, for example, by aggregating patients who might benefit from being screened for an intervention or identifying which patients are at risk of a medication or other error. The impact of electronic tools like these needs to be carefully evaluated prior to, during, and after implementation (Calloway Akilo, & Bierman, 2013). Such evaluations may reveal characteristics of the organization and staff that will promote lasting use of an evidence-based tool.

A dynamic high functioning quality and safety culture requires that nurses continually examine the conditions needed to foster ongoing learning. It is important that data resulting from quality and performance measures not be used to punitively punish providers when targets or goals are not reached. Ongoing improvements in performance, quality, and safety based on the best available evidence are aided through evidence-based tools combined with an open environment where the cause of errors or poor performance can be explored outside a climate of fear. Performance, quality, and safety do not come through the technology alone but are influenced by those who implement, monitor, and use the technology. Innovation and progress are impeded by fear. The tools associated with implementing bar-coded patient wrist bracelets that match automated records to prevent patients from receiving the wrong medication or surveillance systems designed to detect healthcare-acquired infections are only useful when safely implemented and maintained. It is difficult to build a performance-driven culture when fear of reprisal is the norm. For example, automated quality and safety tools used within operating rooms can reduce the risk of reading an x-ray backward, losing count of sponges and instruments, or operating on the wrong patient or the wrong side. This occurs systematically once local evidence about what works and does not work can be used to understand the complex factors that influence translation. Although this can seem overwhelming, simulation and similar tools increasingly are used to help understand and prepare nurses for complex procedures, especially when the margin for error is small and options for training are limited.

Evidence Embedded into Clinical Decision Support Tools (CDS)

Evidence is often embedded in Clinical Decision Support (CDS) tools. *CDS captures the* processes used to enhance health-related decisions and actions with pertinent, organized clinical knowledge and patient information, to improve health and healthcare delivery (HIMSS, 2011). CDS comes in many forms and interactive automated programs that assist clinicians with decisions, usually at the point of care. Decision analysis and CDS tie the probability of a specific clinical option to the likely results. The probability of alternative strategies can then be quantified. Many decision support tools are part of an EHR and promote the timeliness of a diagnosis or treatment intervention. CDS includes automated templates for orders and referrals that link to reminders or other forms of evidence.

Computerized pathways, flow charts, algorithms, and critical paths are CDS tools that facilitate implementation in ways that reduce errors and promote compliance. Checks and triggers are embedded to guide clinicians through diagnostic and treatment interventions based on guideline recommendations. Algorithm-based decision systems can be used, for example, to prompt clinicians about the correct interval for a laboratory test.

Automated reminders are a form of decision support used in "real time" or at the point of patient contact. For example, an automated system can analyze a patient's age and risk factors to generate a screen or audible reminder when an evidence-based intervention is appropriate but not performed.

Evidence Integrated into Care Coordination and Continuum of Care Mapping

Case management and care coordination are key roles for nurses who follow a panel of patients, including assuring that evidence-based diagnostic and treatment interventions are completed. Communication and information sharing are promoted electronically across providers throughout the flow of their work so that the patient benefits from coordinated care.

Cognitive Aids (Clinical Business Intelligence, Automated GIS, Big Data, Visual Analytics, Clinical Analytics) and Advanced Informatics to Support Evidence in Practice

Cognitive aids help nurses use data and link it to evidence by expanding the ability to quickly process, compare, and interpret large volumes of complex data. Automated tools that help make sense of the growing abundance of structured and unstructured data are growing in popularity and availability, and are sometimes now used at the point of care. These tools can be used to retrospectively look back using data to support performance measurement or to support population health. Cognitive aids can also be used prospectively by aggregating the data then using it to predict and offer guidance for future care.

Pathways can be developed to foster variance analysis, which compares patients to a group using aggregated data. Geographic Information Systems or Geographic Information Science (GIS) refers to Web sites or services that connect data from different sources in order to share, remix, repurpose, and reconnect them.

Clinical and Business Intelligence takes data from large healthcare databases in order to analyze and feed it back in ways that aid interpretation and inform decisions. Visualization of multiple datasets can be integrated using a common format that enhances how much information is needed to support a decision. Such tools are transformative in their ability to interactively engage nurses and patients as they combine data with experience as well as generate new hypotheses.

Trigger Tools, Bundles, and Rapid Cycle Testing

The Institute for Health Care Improvement (IHI) and other groups use many different automated tools that often work in tandem with quality and safety efforts. "Triggers" measure harm through retrospective review of records using clues about adverse events. A bundle is a group of three to five evidence-based practices linked together. A bundle is used to promote adoption of specific interventions. Impact can then be measured and the data fed back.

Automated Performance Measures

Quality and safety measurement is an efficient way to promote the use of evidence and move it quickly into practice. Clinical quality measures, as well as performance measures related to quality and safety, quantify differences in the care provided to individuals, organizations, plans, facilities, or networks. Performance measures and indicators are often based on clinical practice guidelines or other synthesized (credible) evidence.

A performance measure or indicator is derived using administrative or clinical data, often pulled from automated records. An example of an electronic measure (using an EHR) is the number of patients who appropriately received antibiotics for pneumonia within four hours of arriving at a care setting. The numerator is the number who received the intervention (antibiotics) divided by the

total number of patients eligible (patients who should have received them). Such measurement assesses provider and organizational performance, which is then available for benchmarking, quality improvement efforts, and financial decisions. Patient safety indicators (PSI) use abstracted administrative data to help providers identify risks. For example, when patients unexpectedly die or are identified after readmission (when not expected to be readmitted) within 30 days of discharge, patient safety tools, including Root Cause Analysis, can be used to understand and correct errors. Robust performance measures increasingly are developed, tested, and introduced, including composite (combined) and "tightly linked" measures for specific conditions. Poorly constructed measures can lead to bias or "gaming."

Emerging Technologies and Trends

Clinical analytics (previously described) holds exciting promise for advancing quality and safety, for example, when coupled with Lean, Six Sigma, or a similar framework. Using clinical analytics, high degrees of variation in outcomes can be identified at an early point that may promote prevention, safety, and clinical improvements. Automated tools used for EBP are evolving quickly. Nurses lead by implementing and evaluating these tools, especially new ones, during translation activities. For example, "ubicom" (also called ubicomp or pervasive computing) uses ambient intelligence (an intelligent environment) to embed human interactions into routine practices or activities. Sensors may be worn to unobtrusively collect cardiac data. As ambient intelligence becomes more common, nurses can measure and report not only the effectiveness of the tool itself but also the effectiveness of the implementation strategies used to apply the evidence. These reports and studies will help nurses address the implications for education, risk, compliance, and teamwork when new technologies appear.

Human Communication Principles Still Apply

Evidence is translated at the level understood by each patient and by the providers in a clinical team. When applying evidence, many factors associated with patients (and their families), as well as other providers, require attention, including culture and literacy. Consider the different approaches to diabetes education that might be needed when teaching a patient who routinely uses technology to talk, transmit, and text versus another patient who rarely (or never) sees a computer. Age, language, exposure, and comfort with technology often need to be considered before discussions about evidence and care can even begin with a patient. HIT interface designs need to support patient–clinician interactions and relationships. As patients increasingly bring their own information into healthcare decisions and articulate their preferences, the skills needed to foster the best possible choices expand. Fueled by technology, expectations are changing. Patients and families often facilitate use of evidence by challenging their providers to explain the options for care. Rather than push technology onto patients, it may help observe what the patient understands about their own documentation and work with the patient as a partner in adapting newer technologies. Communication about why a specific test or intervention is being suggested requires explaining the evidence. Email, texting, and other electronic media can facilitate such communication. Automated training materials can also be conveniently provided at a reasonable cost, by either sending materials electronically or providing them at the point of care. Patients may ask a nurse about evidence that does not exist. Even when evidence is strong, the factors related to its use in real settings are often limited. For example, it can be challenging when patients ask about what others with their same diagnosis choose or want to talk about costs or the trade-offs associated with their own personal values. Patient preferences are especially relevant when the condition is chronic and non-life-threatening, such as cataract extraction. In these instances, the patient's preferences become the focus of the decision.

PROFESSIONAL NURSING GROUPS AND NETWORKS THAT PROVIDE RESOURCES TO TRANSLATE EVIDENCE INTO NURSING PRACTICE

Nursing groups and networks help expand and improve resources by creating, promoting, and assisting expansion of the knowledge base surrounding EBP. Key groups include The Office of the National Coordinator for Health Information Technology (ONC), Healthcare Information and Management Systems Society (HIMSS), The Alliance for Nursing Informatics (ANI), The American Medical Informatics Association (AMIA), The American Nursing Informatics Association (ANIA), and ANIA's sister organization, The Capital Area Roundtable on Informatics in Nursing (CARING). The U.S. Agency for Healthcare Research and Quality also provides a wide array of resources, including interactive tools for patients, such as the U.S. Health Information Knowledgebase—which is a meta-data registry of data standards, and results from their Knowledge Transfer and Translating Research Into Practice (TRIP 1 and TRIP II) programs (www.ahrq.gov).

Sigma Theta Tau International sponsors conferences, research, and resources to support evidence-based information and implementation and translation into practice. They sponsor a scholarly journal entitled "Worldviews on Evidence-Based Nursing."

International Evidence Dissemination Through the Cochrane Collaboration and Joanna Briggs Institute

There is a growing list of notable International nursing, health services, and informatics groups that contribute to our knowledge based about EBP, including The Cochrane Collaboration (www.cochrane.org), which hosts a library of evidence reviews, and The Knowledge Translation+ (KT+) resources provided by McMaster University's Health Information Research Unit (http://plus.mcmaster.ca/np/). KT+ exemplifies the proliferating resources available to nurses seeking peer-reviewed articles, systematic reviews relevant to safety and quality improvement, professional education, automated clinical decision support, and patient resources. The Cochrane Collaboration includes a Nursing Care Field (CNCF) since so many nurses use the evidence available in nursing (http://www.cncf.cochrane.org). One of the nursing collaborators within the CNCF is the Joanna Briggs Institute. Within Nursing the Joanna Briggs collaborative includes over 70 entities globally to also engage in development, dissemination, implementation, and translation of evidence to improve care to patients delivered by nurses (http://joannabriggs.org). In the United States Joanna Briggs Collaborative Centers are located in Indiana, Louisiana, New Jersey, Oklahoma, Texas, and California. Canadian collaborative centers are in Ontario, Canada.

HOW PROFESSIONAL NURSES MIGHT ENGAGE IN ADVANCING EVIDENCE, INFORMATICS TOOLS, INTEGRATION, AND TRANSLATION INTO PRACTICE

Nurses lead in a number of important ways related to the use of technology in translation. Ideas for next steps as nursing moves forward include the need for nurses to:

- Promote evidence-driven care aided by theories, such as QuRKI, that help find solutions amid the interconnected cycles of research and translation. The Queen's Roadmap within QuRKI is one of the useful approaches nurses can use, study, and report about as they systematically improve quality and safety. Such roadmaps are useful in addressing the complexity associated with translation (Harrison & Graham, 2012). As QuRKI and other approaches are used, nurses can share what they learn about the context in which the evidence is used. This attention to context helps nurses identify and manage the facilitators and barriers needed to translate a clinical practice guideline recommendation or other external evidence. For example, nurses can more easily learn how to form strategic and collaborative relationships that naturally foster evidence-informed implementation and facilitate sustained buy-in.

- Clearly describe the choices and rationale surrounding implementation strategies. This rationale links the choice of implementation strategies to determinants of change and helps draw meaningful interpretations (van Achterberg, 2013).

- Create research-practice alliances and other collaborative relationships to use information about the local context in ways that help identify "best practices" that foster change (Harrison & Graham, 2012).

- Explicitly address the limitations surrounding translation efforts, such as difficulty generalizing findings, the need for more advanced methods, little information about costs, and the complexity of measuring disparities and involving patients.

- Explicitly address the limitations surrounding technology applied to healthcare, such as automating poor quality interventions that are not grounded in the best available evidence. Implementing the wrong information can easily lead to faulty automated processes that waste resources, cause frustration, and potentially harm patients.

- Pursue conceptual clarity such that meaningful evaluations and comparisons are possible. This may include use of existing classifications (van Achterberg, 2013).

- Identify security and privacy risks and help patients and others to address them.

- Collaborate across education, administration, clinical care, research, and policy boundaries to standardize terminology and expand the knowledge base about effective solutions to complex healthcare problems. Nurses can foster teamwork across silos in ways that address inconsistencies in terms such as "clinical significance." Many of the definitions relevant to EBP change over time and can be hard to measure. Nurses can help define and standardize key definitions while promoting consensus

about how to measure a patient's response to an intervention in ways that adhere to evidence-based standards or "best practices."

- Define clear goals for translation that capture the complex factors influencing nurses as they strive to apply evidence in real situations.

- Define methodological issues. For each one, explicitly define the state of the science, study design, and measurement complexities in ways that advance translational research (Newhouse, Bobay, Dykes, Stevens, & Titler, 2013).

- Build the skills needed to discuss evidence with patients who are computer literate as well as those who do not use technology to access research findings and use them as the basis for their questions.

- Promote the inclusion and active participation of nurses as part of the multi-disciplinary teams that synthesize research findings and translate evidence into evidence-based tools.

- Participate in the peer review of evidence-based tools and other expert review and feedback.

- Educate teams and organizations that performance and quality measurement are useful and valuable but can also be harmful. Negative results (such as not reaching a target) can be used to improve care and reduce risks but should only lead to punitive action when serious issues, such as patient safety, reveal risk.

- Explicitly address the risk of bias or other threats to the integrity of evidence-based tools. Conflicts of interest are possible at any point, including the selection of "experts" who rate the evidence or those who choose the recommendations to translate. Caution is needed so that bias does not lead to underestimating potential risk, ignoring resource or costs (unless they are intentionally ignored), or promoting overtreatment (Choe, Bernstein, Standiford, & Hayward, 2010; Kerr & Hayward, 2013).

- Promote active dialog within clinical teams and with patients to address recommendations that lack conclusive net weight of benefits and harms.

- Provide input from the beginning in the design and implementation of HIT projects and offer caution that HIT can both help and harm patients.

- Support patients to access accurate evidence by helping them use online tools believed to contribute to positive outcomes, such as an automated self check-in tool that encourages patients to tailor their behavior to their goal as they pursue change. The nurse may want to practice with the patient to help set up the automated messaging systems that accompany some tools.

- Provide expert advice or monitoring of text-based communication through e-mail, social media, listservs, networks, forums, or a mobile format. While online groups and chat rooms offer convenience, they also sometimes lead to exchange of misinformation. Nurses can help by monitoring or serving as a resource.

SUMMARY

Because the findings from an individual peer reviewed publication rarely make their way into the accepted standards of nursing care, few also lead directly to improved outcomes. But evidence synthesis combined with enabling technologies are transformative (Cullen, Titler, & Rempel, 2011). Nurses help the profession as well as patients, teams, and professional groups by identifying literature reviews, meta-analyses, and evidence-based tools that are ready for translation and a good fit for a specific patient group and setting. These tools are used at the intersection of technology and translation, where nurses reduce both the time it takes to bring evidence into practice as well as unexplained variation. The nurse accomplishes this in exciting new ways, including by combining CDS, clinical informatics, and other evidence-based tools that promote use of clinical protocols, including Meaningful Use Core Measures. Graphical displays at integrated workstations help track patients and prioritize care. The Queen's Roadmap (QuRKI) offers one approach that nurses can use as they systematically plan translation in ways that take into account complex factors that influence success. As nurses bring this vision into focus, HIT advances will no longer outpace the profession's ability to move evidence into practice and outcomes will improve.

REFERENCES

Abbott, P. A., Foster, J., Marin, H. F., & Dykes, P. C. (2013). Complexity and the science of implementation in health IT-knowledge gaps and future visions. *International Journal of Medical Informatics*. Retrieved from http://www.ijmijournal.com/article/S1386-5056(13)00227-X/fulltext. Accessed on January 21, 2014.

Bergström, A., Peterson, S., Namusoko, S., Waiswa, P., & Wallin, L. (2012). Knowledge translation in Uganda: A qualitative study of Ugandan midwives' and managers' perceived relevance of the sub-elements of the context cornerstone in the PARIHS framework. *Implementation Science, 7*, 117.

Berland, G., Elliott, M., & Morales, L. (2001). Health information on the Internet: Accessibility, quality, and readability in English and Spanish. *Journal of the Medical Association, 285*(20), 2612–2638.

Boulet, L. P., Bourbeau, J., Skomro, R., & Gupta S. (2013). Major care gaps in asthma, sleep and chronic obstructive pulmonary disease: A road map for knowledge translation. *Canadian Respiratory Journal: Journal of the Canadian Thoracic Society, 20*(4), 265–269.

Briggs, A. M., Bragge, P., Slater, H., Chan, M., & Towler, S. C. (2012). Applying a Health Network approach to translate evidence-informed policy into practice: A review and case study on musculoskeletal health. *BMC Health Services Research, 12*, 394.

Calloway, S., Akilo, H. A., & Bierman, K. (2013). Impact of a clinical decision support system on pharmacy clinical interventions, documentation efforts, and costs. *Hospital Pharmacy, 48*(9), 744–752.

Carter-Templeton, H. (2013). Nurses' information appraisal within the clinical setting. *CIN: Computers, Informatics, Nursing, 31*(4), 167–175.

Choe, H. M., Bernstein, S. J., Standiford, C. J., & Hayward, R. A. (2010). New diabetes HEDIS blood pressure quality measure: Potential for overtreatment. *The American Journal of Managed Care, 16*(1), 19–24.

Cullen, L., Titler, M. G., & Rempel, G. (2011). Enabling technologies promise to revitalize the role of nursing in an era of patient safety. *Western Journal of Nursing Research, 33*(3), 345–364.

Currie, G., Lockett, A., & El Enany, N. (2013). From what we know to what we do: lessons learned from the translational CLAHRC initiative in England. *Journal of Health Services and Research Policy, 18*(3), 27–39.

Dalheim, A., Harthug, S., Nilsen, R. M., & Nortvedt, M. W. (2012). Factors influencing the development of evidence-based practice among nurses: A self-report survey. *BMC Health Service Research, 12*, 367.

Doebbeling, B. N., Flanagan, M. E. (2011). Emerging perspectives on transforming the healthcare system: redesign strategies and a call for needed research. *Med Care.* 49 Suppl:S59–S64.

Donabedian, A. (1980). *Explorations in quality assessment and monitoring (*Vol. 1). Ann Arbor, MI: Health Administration Press.

Doran, D., Haynes, B. R., Estabrooks, C. A., Kushniruk, A., Dubrowski, A., Bajnok, I., … Bai, Y. Q. (2012). The role of organizational context and individual nurse characteristics in explaining variation in use of information technologies in evidence based practice. *Implementation Science, 7*, 122.

Estabrooks, C. A., Poss, J. W., Squires, J. E., Teare, G. F., Morgan, D. G., Stewart, N., … Norton, P. G. (2013). A profile of residents in prairie nursing homes. *Canadian Journal on Aging, 32*(2), 223–231.

Graves, J. R., & Corcoran, S. (1989). The study of nursing informatics. *Image, 21*(4), 227–231.

Guyatt, G. R. (2002). *Users' guide to the medical literature.* Chicago: AMA Press.

Harden, S. M., Burke, S. M., Haile, A. M., & Estabrooks, P. A. (2013). Generalizing the findings from group dynamics-based physical activity research to practice settings: What do we know? *Evaluation & the Health Professions.* May 28. doi:10.1177/0163278713488117.

Harrington, L. (2011). Clinical intelligence. *Journal of Nursing Administration, 2011*(41), 12.

Harrison M. B., & Graham I. D. (2012). Roadmap for a participatory research-practice partnership to implement evidence. *Worldviews on Evidence-Based Nursing*, Sigma Theta Tau International, 9(4), 193–255.

Harrison, M. B., Graham, I. D., van den Hoek, J., Dogherty, E. J., Carley, M. E., & Angus, V. (2013). Guideline adaptation and implementation planning: A prospective observational study. *Implementation Science, 8*(49). doi:10.1186/1748-5908-8-49.

Herr, K., Titler, M., Fine, P. G., Sanders, S., Cavanaugh, J. E., Swegle, J., … Forcucci, C. (2012). The effect of a translating research into practice (TRIP)--cancer intervention on cancer pain management in older adults in hospice. *Pain Medicine, 13*(8), 1004–1017.

HIMSS. (2011). *Improving outcomes with CDS: An implementer's guide.* Retrieved from https://www.himss.org/

Hyun, S., Hodorowski, J. K., Nirenberg, A., Perocchia, R. S., Staats, J. A., Velez, O., & Bakken, S. (2013). Mobile health-based approaches for smoking cessation resources. *Oncology Nursing Forum, 40*(4), E312–E319.

Hynes, D. M., Whittier, E. R., Owens, A. (2013, March). Health information technology and implementation science: partners in progress in the VHA. *Medical Care, 51*(3 Suppl. 1), S6–S12. doi:10.1097/MLR.0b013e3182884509.

Kerr, E. A., & Hayward, R. A. (2013). Patient-centered performance management: enhancing value for patients and health care systems. *Journal of the American Medical Association. 310*(2), 137–138. doi:10.1001/jama.2013.6828.

Kitson, A., Powell, K., Hoon, E., Newbury, J., Wilson, A., & Beilby, J. (2013). Knowledge translation within a population health study: How do you do it? *Implementation Science, 8*, 54.

McCormack, B., Rycroft-Malone, J., Decorby, K., Hutchinson, A. M., Bucknall, T., Kent, B., … Wilson, V. (2013). A realist review of interventions and strategies to promote evidence-informed healthcare: a focus on change agency. *Implementation Science, 8*, 107.

Melnyk, B. M., Fineout-Overholt, E. Gallagher-Ford, L., Kaplan, L. (2012) The state of evidence-based practice in US nurses. *The Journal of Nursing Administration, 42*(9), 410–417.

Melnyk, B. M., Gallagher-Ford, L., Long, L. E., & Fineout-Overholt, E. (2014, January 21.). The establishment of evidence-based practice competencies for practicing registered nurses and advanced practice nurses in real-world clinical settings: Proficiencies to improve healthcare quality, reliability, patient outcomes, and costs. *Worldviews on Evidence-Based Nursing.* doi: 10.1111/wvn.12021.

National Institutes of Health Fogarty International Center. (2013). *Frequently asked questions about implementation science.* Retrieved from http://www.fic.nih.gov/News/Events/implementation-science/Pages/faqs.aspx. Accessed on January 30, 2014.

Newhouse, R., Bobay, K., Dykes, P. C., Stevens, K. R., & Titler, M. (2013). Methodology issues in implementation science. *Medical Care, 51*, S32–S40.

Pew Research Center. (February , 2014). By Fox, S. and Rainie, L. *The Web at 25.* Available at: http://www.pewinternet.org/2014/02/25/the-web-at-25-in-the-u-s.

Phillips, J. M., Heitschmidt, M., Joyce, M. B., Staneva, I., Zemansky, P., Francisco, M. A., … Kranzer, S. F. (2006). Where's the evidence: An innovative approach to teaching staff about evidence-based practice. *Journal for Nurses in Staff Development, 22*(6), 296–301.

Poe, S. S., Abbott, P., & Pronovost, P. (2011). Building nursing intellectual capital for safe use of information technology: A before-after study to test an evidence-based peer coach intervention. *Journal of Nursing Care Quality, 26*(2), 110–119.

Rycroft-Malone, J., McCormack, B., Hutchinson, A. M., DeCorby, K., Bucknall, T. K., Kent, B., … Wilson, V. (2012). Realist synthesis: Illustrating the method for implementation research. *Implementation Science, 7*, 33.

Sackett, D. L., Straus, S. E., Richardson, W. S., Rosenberg, W., & Hayes, R. B. (2000). *Evidence-based medicine: How to practice and teach EBM.* London: Churchill Livingstone.

Sales, A. E. (2013). Reflections on the state of nursing implementation science. *International Journal of Nursing Studies, 50*(4), 443–444.

Spencer, L. M., Schooley, M. W., Anderson, L. A., Kochitzky, C. S., DeGroff, A. S., Delvin, H. M., & Mercer, S. L. (2013). Seeking best practices: A conceptual framework for planning and improving evidence-based practices. *Preventing Chronic Disease: Public Health Research, Practice, and Policy, 10*, e207.

Squires, J. E., Reay, T., Moralejo, D., Lefort, S. M., Hutchinson, A. M., & Estabrooks, C. A. (2012). Designing strategies to implement research-based policies and procedures: a set of recommendations for nurse leaders based on the PARiHS framework. *The Journal of Nursing Administration, 42*(5), 293–297.

Staggers, N., & Thompson, C. (2002). The evolution of definitions for nursing informatics: A critical analysis and revised definition. *Journal of the American Informatics Association, 9*, 255–261.

Stetler, C. (2001). Updating the Stetler Model of research utilization to facilitate evidence-based practice. *Nursing Outlook, 49*, 272–279.

Stetler, C. (2010). Stetler model. In J. Rycroft-Malone & T. Bucknall (Eds.), *Evidence-based practice series: Models and frameworks for implementing evidence-based practice: Linking evidence to action*. Oxford: Wiley-Blackwell.

Stetler, C., & Caramanica, L. (2007). Evaluation of an evidence-based practice initiative: Outcomes, strengths and limitations of a retrospective, conceptually-based approach. *Worldviews on Evidence-Based Nursing, 4*, 187–199.

Stetler, C., Legro, M., Wallace, C., Bowman, C., Guihan, M., Hagedorn, H., … Smith, J. L. (2006). The role of formative evaluation in implementation research and the QUERI experience. *Journal of General Internal Medicine, 21*, S1–S8.

Stetler, C. B., Damschroder, L. J., Helfrich, C. D., & Hagedorn, H. J. (2011). A guide for applying a revised version of the PARIHS framework for implementation. *Implementation Science, 6*, 99.

Titler, M. G. (2010). Translation science and context. *Research and Theory for Nursing Practice, 24*(1), 35–55.

Titler, M. G. (2011). Nursing science and evidence-based practice. *Western Journal of Nursing Research, 33*(3), 291–295.

Titler, M. G., & Everett, L. Q. (2001). Translating research into practice: Considerations for critical care investigators. *Critical Care Nursing Clinics of North America, 13*(4), 587–604.

Tricco, A. C., Ivers, N. M., Grimshaw, J. M., Moher, D., Turner, L., Galipeau, J., … Shojania, K. (2012). Effectiveness of quality improvement strategies on the management of diabetes: A systematic review and meta-analysis. *Lancet, 379*(9833), 2252–2261.

Upton, D., Upton, P., & Scurlock-Evans, L. (2014). The reach, transferability, and impact of the evidence-based practice questionnaire: A methodological and narrative literature review. *Worldviews on Evidence-Based Nursing, 11*(1), 46–54.

U.S. Preventive Services Task Force. (2008). *U.S. preventive services task force grade definitions*. Retrieved from http://www.uspreventiveservicestaskforce.org/Page/Name/grade-definitions. Accessed on January 30, 2014.

van Achterberg, T. (2013). Nursing implementation science: 10 ways forward. *International Journal of Nursing Studies, 50*(4), 445–447.

Young, L.B., Foster, L., Silander, A., & Wakefield, B. (2011). Home telehealth: Patient satisfaction, program functions, and challenges for the care coordinator. *Journal of Gerontological Nursing, 37*(11), 38–46.

40

Improving Healthcare Quality and Patient Outcomes Through the Integration of Evidence-Based Practice and Informatics

Joanne M. Seasholtz / Bernadette Mazurek Melnyk

• OBJECTIVES

1. Define evidence-based practice.
2. Discuss how evidence-based practice impacts healthcare quality, safety, and cost reduction.
3. Discuss barriers and facilitators for successful implementation of evidence-based practice in the clinical setting.
4. Discuss the evidence-based practice paradigm and process.
5. Identify technology tools in clinical practice which support evidence-based practice.
6. Discuss the role of clinical decision support systems in evidence-based practice.
7. Identify considerations for a successful Clinical Decision Support System.
8. Discuss integration of evidence-based practice in clinical areas.
9. Discuss a professional practice model which supports evidence-based practice.
10. Identify data types of standardized terminology.
11. Explain the differences between data, information, knowledge, and wisdom.
12. Discuss options available with vendors in support of evidence-based practice.
13. Identify regulatory and agency impacts on decision support.

• KEY WORDS

Evidence-based practice
Decision support
Clinical decision support
Evidence-based adaptive clinical decision support
PICOT
Data
Nursing informatics
Clinical terminology
Technology tools
Professional practice model
Quality measures

INTRODUCTION

There is mounting evidence that implementation of evidence-based practice (EBP) by nurses and other health professionals results in higher quality healthcare, improved patient outcomes, less variation in care, and reduced costs compared with care that is steeped in tradition or based on outdated policies and practices (McGinty & Anderson, 2008; Melnyk & Fineout-Overholt, 2011). In addition, findings from studies have supported that when nurses believe in the value of EBP and are able to implement evidence-based care, they have higher job satisfaction and better group cohesion, which are key determinants of job turnover guide best practices (Block, 2006; Krumholz, 2008). In contrast to research that generates new knowledge and evidence for practice, EBP translates evidence from research into clinical practice to improve healthcare quality and patient outcomes. (Maljanian, Caramanica, Taylor, et al., 2002; Melnyk, Fineout-Overholt, Giggleman, & Cruz, 2010). Because of the known positive outcomes associated with EBP, the Institute of Medicine set a goal that 90% of healthcare decisions will be evidence based by 2020 (McClellan, McGinnis, Nable, & Olsen, 2007). Despite its positive outcomes and recent mandates by leaders, professional organizations, and policy-makers to base and reimburse care on the best and latest evidence, EBP is not consistently implemented by numerous healthcare systems and clinicians across the United States (Bodenheimer, 2008; Melnyk & Fineout-Overholt, 2011).

There is no doubt that the use of technology with clinical decision support systems can enhance the delivery of evidence-based care. However, technology must be used by clinicians who implement the steps of EBP and healthcare organizations that cultivate system-wide cultures of EBP if high-quality evidence-based care is to be sustained.

In 2000, Sackett and colleagues defined EBP as the conscientious use of current best evidence in making decisions about patient care (Sackett et al., 2000). Since then, EBP has been broadened and described as a problem-solving approach to the delivery of care that integrates the best evidence from well-designed studies with a clinician's expertise and patient preferences and values in making clinical decisions (Melnyk & Fineout-Overholt, 2011). Both external evidence (i.e., findings from research) and internal evidence (i.e., evidence that is generated from outcomes management or quality improvement projects) should be used in evidence-based decision-making. When clinicians deliver EBP in a context of caring as well as an organizational culture and environment that supports EBP, the highest quality of care and best patient outcomes are achieved.

If healthcare systems are to be re-designed to improve the quality of care and patient outcomes as well as reduce costs, clinicians must translate internal and external evidence that is collected, analyzed, and critically appraised into useful information to guide best practices (Block, 2006; Krumholtz, 2008).

The Seven Steps of Evidence-Based Practice

There are seven steps in the EBP process (Melnyk & Fineout-Overholt, 2011) (Table 40.1). In the first step, which is step 0, a spirit of inquiry in clinicians and a culture of EBP must be cultivated in order to stimulate the asking of burning clinical questions to improve patient care. Once a clinical question is generated, step 1 in the EBP process involves formatting clinical questions into PICOT format (P = patient population, I = intervention or interest area, C = comparison intervention or group, O = outcome, and T = time). Formatting clinical questions in PICOT format is necessary to streamline the search for evidence to answer the question. An example of a PICOT question about a treatment is: In depressed adolescents (P), how does the delivery of cognitive behavior therapy in person (I) versus delivery of Web-based cognitive behavior therapy (C) affect depressive symptoms (O) three months after treatment (T)?

In Step 2 of the EBP process, a search for the evidence is conducted by entering each key word from the PICOT question into the database that is being searched (e.g., Medline, CINHAL) and then combining the search words together to reveal the studies that may answer the

TABLE 40.1	The Steps of the Evidence-Based Practice (EBP) Process

0. Cultivate a spirit of inquiry.
1. Ask the burning clinical question in PICOT format.
2. Search for and collect the most relevant best evidence.
3. Critically appraise the evidence (i.e., rapid critical appraisal, evaluation, and synthesis).
4. Integrate the best evidence with one's clinical expertise and patient preferences and values in making a practice decision or change.
5. Evaluate outcomes of the practice decision or change based on evidence.
6. Disseminate the outcomes of the EBP decision or change.

Reproduced, with permission, from Melnyk, B.M., & Fineout-Overholt, E. (2011). *Evidence-based practice in nursing & healthcare. A guide to best practice (2nd ed)*. Philadelphia: Wolters Kluwer/Lippincott Williams & Wilkins.

question. Reliable resources that should be used to find an answer to the PICOT question include systematic reviews, clinical practice guidelines, pre-appraised literature, and studies from peer-reviewed journals.

In Step 3 of EBP, a rapid critical appraisal of the studies from the search is conducted followed by an evaluation and synthesis of the research evidence.

In Step 4, evidence is integrated with the clinician's expertise and patient preferences and values to make a decision regarding whether a practice change should be made. Once a practice change is made based on the best evidence, outcomes should be measured to determine positive outcomes of the change (i.e., Step 5). Evaluation of outcomes is an essential step in EBP as it helps determine if the EBP practice change was successful, effective, equitable, timely, and needs to be modified or discarded (Gawlinski, 2007). The last step in the EBP process, Step 6, is disseminating the outcome of the practice change through presentation or publication so that others can benefit from the process.

Barriers and Facilitators of Evidence-Based Practice

There are multiple barriers to advancing EBP in healthcare systems, including (a) misperceptions by clinicians that it takes too much time, (b) lack of EBP knowledge and skills, (c) organizational cultures that do not support EBP, (d) lack of resources, including clinical decision support tools, (d) executive leaders and managers who do not model and/or support EBP, (e) lack of EBP mentors to work with point-of-care staff on implementing evidence-based care, (f) inadequate access to databases by clinicians in order to track patient and system outcomes, and (g) negative attitudes toward research (Fineout-Overholt, Melnyk, & Schultz, 2005; Hannes et al., 2007; McGinty & Anderson, 2008; Melnyk et al., 2004; Melnyk, Fineout-Overholt, Feinstein, Sadler, & Green-Hernandez, 2008; Melnyk, Fineout-Overholt, Gallagher-Ford, & Kaplan, 2012).

Findings from studies also have established key facilitators of EBP that include (a) strong beliefs about the value of EBP and the ability to implement it, (b) EBP knowledge and skills, (c) organizational cultures that support EBP, (d) EBP mentors who have in-depth knowledge and skills in evidence-based care as well as individual and organizational change, (e) administrative support, (f) clinical promotion systems that incorporate EBP competencies, and (g) EBP tools at the point of care, such as clinical decision support systems (Melnyk, 2007; Melnyk, Fineout-Overholt, & Mays, 2008; Melnyk et al., 2004; Newhouse, Dearholt, Poe, Pugh, & White, 2007).

Cultivating a Culture That Supports and Sustains Evidence-Based Practice

In order to cultivate a culture and environment that supports and sustains EBP, an organization must provide system-wide support for evidence-based care. This support begins with a vision, philosophy, and mission that incorporate EBP as a key component, which are made visible to all throughout the organization. High-level administration and nurse managers must not only "buy-in" to this vision, but also model EBP themselves as much of how clinicians perform is learned through observation of their key leaders and managers. Integrating EBP and the newly created EBP competencies for registered nurses and advanced practice nurses throughout the clinical ladder system if one exists also establishes the importance of evidence-based care for staff advancement (Melnyk, Gallagher-Ford, Long & Fineout-Overholt, 2014). Furthermore, ample resources and supports must be provided to clinicians that enhance their ability to provide evidence-based care. Examples of resources and supports are identified in Table 40.2.

TABLE 40.2	Supports and Resources for Clinicians to Enhance Ability to Provide Evidence-Based Care
Support and Resource	**Examples**
Regular EBP education and skills building sessions	
Tools at the point of care	EBP-designated computers
	Clinical Decision support tools
	Evidence-based policies and procedures
EBP journal clubs and fellowship opportunities	
EBP mentors	Advanced Practice Nurses
	Clinicians with excellent EBP skills
	Clinicians with knowledge in individual and organizational change strategies
Access to databases to track outcomes data	
Funding for EBP implementation and outcomes management projects	
Regular recognition of EBP accomplishments	Annual EBP poster or conference events

Data from Melnyk, Gallagher-Ford, Long & Fineout-Overholt (2014).

THE ROLE OF TECHNOLOGY IN SUPPORTING EVIDENCE-BASED PRACTICE

Technology Tools in Clinical Practice

Nurses, nurse practitioners, and healthcare providers today are very cognizant of the push for cost containment, improved patient safety, improved quality of care, and reduced variation in care throughout not only the United States but the world. It is readily observed there is a shift in healthcare choices being made based on quality and outcomes, not solely cost as reimbursement moves toward payments for quality.

Information technology (IT) has brought to healthcare a compendium of new tools which support EBP. As a consequence, IT has not only improved, but also complicated many currently existing processes. A goal of informatics is to use technology to bring critical and essential information to the point of care to increase efficiency, make healthcare safer and more effective, and improve quality and outcomes (National Quality Forum, 2008). Despite the advancement in information technology, the most effective, evidence-based care remains evasive for nurses (Anderson & Willson, 2008; Benoliel, 1996; Glaser, 1978).

Competencies

Nursing professionals range in age from their early 20s to their 60s with the average age of a registered nurse today in their early 50s. This range presents a significant range of learning skills and comfort with technology and evidence-based practice.

Nursing students today are very adept with using iPADs, iPhones, laptops, and other technology devices. They have been using them since childhood. In 2006, a National League of Nursing (NLN) study revealed 60% of nursing programs had a computer literacy requirement and 40% had an information literacy requirement. Less than 50% of the respondents stated informatics was integrated into the curriculum and experience with information systems provided during the clinical experiences (National League for Nursing, 2008). As an outcome of the study the NLN published a position statement recommending nursing schools require all nursing students graduate with knowledge and skills in each of three critical areas: computer literacy, information literacy, and informatics.

Pravikoff, Tanner, and Pierce (2005) found that nurses use experientially acquired information from interactions with peers, patients, colleagues, and physicians greater than scientific evidence from medical and research journals. This finding still exists today.

It is imperative for nurses today to have the skills required to engage in EBP. Preparing undergraduate nursing students in EBP and the use of the proper technology has significance for advancing EBP in nursing. Rush (2008) states, "the preparation of undergraduate nursing students for using evidence to guide practice is no longer optional. Evidence-based practice is imperative for insuring quality, cost-effective safe care and more predictable outcomes for healthcare consumers" (p. 190).

DECISION SUPPORT AND EVIDENCE-BASED PRACTICE

Decision Support Systems

Decision support systems (DSS) "are automated tools designed to support decision-making activities and improve the decision-making process and decision outcomes. Such systems are intended to use the enormous amounts of data that exist in information systems to facilitate decision processes" (Androwich & Kraft, 2011, p. 427).

Clinical decision support systems (CDSS) are systems designed "to support healthcare providers in making decisions about the delivery and management of patient care" (Androwich & Kraft, 2011, p.427). They have "the potential to improve the patient safety and outcomes for specific patient populations, as well as compliance with clinical guidelines and standards of practice and regulatory requirements" (p. 427).

Evidence-based adaptive clinical decision support systems are systems designed with multiple rules and access to multiple databases for information. They are complex systems and contain mechanisms to incorporate new findings and evidence (Sims et al., 2001).

Standardization of Terminology and Data

Clinical Terminology is a factor which plays a significant role in increasing the availability of evidence at the point of care. Clinical terminologies have not matured to a level to be used in clinical information systems (CIS). Standardized clinical terminology is necessary for evidence to be both computable and interoperable with multiple systems. The next step is to facilitate EBP by increasing the transparency to the healthcare provider.

To be efficient, the evidence for EBP must be incorporated into the everyday workflows and care processes used by nurses and other healthcare providers. The data must be integrated with the clinical systems used by the providers and provide readily accessible evidence-based knowledge for the end user at the point of care when needed. To be successful it is essential to link evidence to assessments, results, documentation, orders, and plans of care. Gugerty (2006) states, "It's in these forms- plans of care, order sets, standardized rules and alerts, and the like- that evidence will finally be widely, consistently, and reliably used at the point of care" (p. 23).

Standardized nursing terminology is required for quantifiable and retrievable data. It allows for coding of Nursing practice in the EHR. Information technology systems document and code nursing practice, aggregate and compare coded data across client settings, populations, and time, and develop core databases for data mining and meta-analysis. Terminology is also required for compliance with regulatory and payer requirements. Examples of Nursing Classifications used today are listed in Table 40.3.

What are the criteria for standardized nursing terminology? Cimino, Hripsak, Johnson, and Clayton (1989) identified criteria for the design of a controlled healthcare vocabulary. These criteria included: Domain completeness, Unambiguous terms, Nonredundancy, Synonyms, Multiple classifications of terms, Consistency of views, and Explicit relationships. Other criteria which have been identified in the literature include free, designed for computer based systems, and developed from evidence based practice.

Identification of Common Data Definitions. It is not uncommon for different departments, hospitals, and systems to have different definitions of the same data elements. Unless everyone is using the same set of data definitions there will be errors in data collection, analysis, and conclusions. This is one reason the Meaningful Use Core Measures and Quality Measures are explicitly defined for data collection and reporting. Travers & Mandelkerhr (2008) identified seven aspects which should be considered for identification of common data definitions. (Table 40.4). Each of these is also essential for Meaningful Use Core Measures and Quality Measures.

Tools for Managing Clinical Data. Tools can vary from Excel spreadsheets and Access databases to database programs.

Data quality. Inaccurate and incomplete data will impact the quality of the data upon which decisions will be made and impact quality. Data end users should understand how the data they are using are defined. Many computer programs contain features to prevent data entry errors by restricting the type of data which can be entered such as a date in numeric form or limiting the range.

System Selection Issues. Clinicians should participate in the selection process for clinical information systems and consider data requirements during the selection process. They should consider the quality and availability of the data for use on the back end to facilitate other uses of routinely collected health data such as benchmarking, quality improvement, research, and surveillance. Vendors should be questioned as to the types of reports available, ability to customize reports and create ad hoc reports, and the ability to export data for use with other applications. "Data consistency and completeness are critical to the scientific rigor or retrospective studies" (Hruby, McKiernan, Bakken, & Weng, 2013, p. 563). "Underestimating the importance of data management can hinder data quality, impair research results, misinform clinical practice, or generate invalid hypotheses for new clinical trials" (p. 563).

TABLE 40.3	Examples of Nursing Classification Systems

CCC (Clinical Care Classification)

NANDA (North American Nursing Diagnosis Association)

NIC (Nursing Intervention Classification)

NOC (Nursing Outcomes Classification)

ICNP (International Classification of Nursing Practice)

Examples of medical classifications include:

ICD-9, ICD-10

AMA CPT codes

NDC (National Drug Classification)

LOINC (Logical Observation Identified Names and Codes)

SNOMED-CT (Systemized Nomenclature of Combined Terminology)

TABLE 40.4	Aspects to Consider for Identification of Common Data Elements

Agreement on the definition of the data element

Data Elements. Sufficient data are required

Description

Numerator and denominator definitions for rates

Data storage format, i.e., text, numerical

Units of measure

Default values

Is the data element required?

Data from Travers & Mandelkehr (2008).

Considerations for Successful CDSS

Lee (2013) completed an extensive literature search to identify and organize the systems features of decision support technologies targeted at nursing practice into assessment, problem identification, care plans, implementation, and outcomes. Byrne and Lang (2013) examined nursing data elements from evidence-based recommendations for clinical decision support. The analysis provided a description of the representation of data elements and issues related to the availability of data for use in the future development of clinical decision support systems to prevent ICU delirium. They found the matched data elements were primarily text based, entered by RNs on flow sheets and care plans. "Even though there was a high number of potential data element matches, there was considerable variable data availability related to clinical, conceptual, and technical factors. The further development of valid and reliable data that accurately capture the interaction between nurse, patient, and family is necessary before embarking on electronic clinical decision support" (Byrne & Lang, 2013, p. 1). Byrne and Lang found the build of the CDSS could allow for multiple data sources to be analyzed but that did not address the practical implications of redundancy, ambiguity, and lack of conceptual clarity identified in the data sources. From their study they provide three recommendations for the capture of nursing care in a standardized format to be used in CDSS support. They were (1) improve the electronic capture of nursing phenomena and care processes, (2) promote use and integration of standardized nursing terminologies such as ICNP and SNOMED-CT, and (3) capitalize on data elements with high data availability.

Sittig (1999) identified five elements as pre-requisites for a clinical real-time point-of-care clinical decision support system. They include:

1. INTEGRATED, REAL-TIME PATIENT DATABASE: The database must be able to integrate data under a common patient identified. It stores and updates all data as soon as results are available, forming the basis of any real-time CDSS effort and ability to implement logic that involves patient-specific data from multiple data sources.

2. DATA-DRIVE MECHANISM: A data-drive mechanism enables a flag or trigger to be established and set so that a program can be activated when a particular type of data or data item (e.g., clinical laboratory results or a chest radiograph report) is stored in the database. These triggered events allow for the system to be automatic, real time, and asynchronous. Such systems are called real time in that they run as soon as the data are stored, instead of at a specified time of day (Sittig, 1999).

3. KNOWLEDGE ENGINEER: An informatics expert who is responsible for extracting and translating the clinical knowledge into machine executable logic.

4. TIME-DRIVE MECHANISM: This allows for programs to be executed automatically at a specific time in the future (e.g., 2 a.m.) or after a specific time interval has passed (24 hours after transfer). Logic can be used to remind clinicians to perform specific activities or to check that the appropriate action has been performed.

5. LONG-TERM CLINICAL DATA REPOSITORY: A long-term clinical data repository contains the patient-specific data from a variety of clinical sources collected over a period of several years. It allows for the development of reliable statistical predictors of specific events. For example, one could develop a logistic regression equation that identifies the pathogen most likely to be found in a particular specimen and recommends the least expensive antibiotic. The database could also be used to identify potential problem areas, such as the percentage of patients with diabetes who have not had an HBA1C test performed within the last six months. (Sittig 1999, accessed on June 25, 2010).

The functions of clinical decision support systems include alerting, reminding, critiquing, interpreting, predicting, diagnosing, interpreting, image recognition, assisting, and suggesting (Lyerla 2008). One of the benefits of clinical decision support systems is the evidence can be driven into practice in a timely manner. Garg et al. (2005) reported that 76% of reviewed studies indicated that clinician performance was improved through the use of reminders. Diagnostic aiding systems were found to be beneficial in 40%. Automatic prompts to the end user were more effective than the end user needing to activate a system with changes in physician performance 73% with auto prompts, and 47% when required to activate the system. The highest success function identified was the use of reminders and alerts.

Decision support systems are passive or active. A passive system would notify an individual of an event, such as an abnormal finding where an active system will offer suggestions or take actions such as place a specific order when specific criteria are met. Decision support systems always allow for the provider to have the option to ignore the alert, override the alert, or inactivate the alert after their synthesis of the information and suggested actions. It must always be remembered the clinician is the final decision-maker.

Clinical decision support systems allow for optimization of both the efficiency and effectiveness with which clinical decisions are made and care is delivered. The costs of clinical decision support systems can be high, however, the savings occur in the improved decision-making at the bedside, improved quality and outcomes, and reduction of errors. Mullett, Evans, Christenson, and Dean (2001) concluded at InterMountain Healthcare Primary Children's Medical Center in Utah the use of a pediatric anti-infective decision support tool in the Pediatric Intensive Care Unit (PICU) was beneficial to the patient and reduced the rates of erroneous drug orders, improved therapeutic dosage targets, and decreased anti-infective costs per patient.

Disparities have been documented by Medicare and other agencies in the treatment of diseases such as heart disease and congestive heart failure. This was one of the incentives behind the CORE measures to reduce variation in practices when evidence has proven the impact of procedures and medications. The goal is to reduce variations, cost and improve quality and this is being expanded in 2014 to include CORE measures and quality measures. CORE measures can be found on the CMS Website at www.cms.gov/Regulatons-and-Guidance/Legislation/EHRIncentivePrograms/index.html.

WHAT CAN OUTSIDE REFERENCE SOURCES (VENDORS) BRING TO THE TABLE?

The tools for evidence-based practice have evolved from paper and pencil to evidence-based practice embedded in the clinical information systems via links and decision support systems at the point of care. The utilization of technology has also moved the amount of evidence available at the point of care from low to high.

Not only have the methods for using evidence changed, but also the producers or originators of evidence-based practice have changed in the past 20 years. In the 1980s, Clinical Practice Guidelines were developed by individual hospitals and the responsibility was on the hospitals. That trend changed in the 2000s to eliminate healthcare delivery organizations from building their own to their use of commercial vendors for information and incorporation into practice. Healthcare organizations are no longer building their own evidence-based packages but instead partnering with governmental agencies (Medicare), professional societies, and companies such as Zynx, Wolters-Kluwer, Thomson, Clineguide, and Micromedex who are in the business of providing evidence-based packages. The vendor provides the evidence, however, they do not decide what evidence is chosen to incorporate into practice. With vendors maintaining the responsibility for reviewing the research and presenting the best practices to the facilities

the information can be incorporated into the bedside care in a more expedious manner.

Electronic health record (EHR) system vendors also provide various services. Their services can be categorized into three areas (Kawamoto, Hongsermeier, Wright, Lewis, Bell, & Middleton, 2013):

1. In-house CDS content. Vendors provide a variety of in-house CDS content such as alerts and reminders, order sets, documentation templates, drug–drug and allergy checking and flowsheets. This requires regular updates and client maintenance.

2. Third-party CDS content. Vendors use third-party CDS content.

3. Content knowledge sharing. The vendor provides a knowledge sharing environment. Options may include a vendor hosted portal where clients can access information provided by the vendor or by its clients on how to implement a specific CDS capability, or a vendor hosted environment where clients share resources such as rules and workflows, and shared benchmarking database with associated analytics.

INTEGRATION OF EBP TECHNOLOGY IN THE CLINICAL AREAS

Barriers to research implementation were identified three decades ago. Melnyk (2013) states "although progress has been made over the years, the same barriers to EBP identified decades ago (e.g., time, lack of knowledge and skills, peer resistance, lack of access to resources, and EBP mentors) continue to exist is healthcare systems. Most recently… new findings indicate that resistance from leaders and managers along with environments steeped in tradition were top barriers to provision of evidence based care" (Melnyk, 2013, p. 127).

Information Access

There are over 150,000 medical articles published each month (Matter, 2006). Table 40.5 provides several examples, along with their Web addresses, of sources for EBP available today. Most are free, however, some sites do have a subscription fee.

Data, Information, Knowledge, Wisdom, Healthcare Business Intelligence

Worthley (2000) defines data as the raw materials from which information is generated and information is the relevant, usable commodity needed by the end user. "Information is born when data are interpreted" (Bylone,

TABLE 40.5	Sources for Journals and Bibliographic Databases	
MEDLINE	Indexes over 5200 journals worldwide from 1966 to present.	www.nlm.nih.gov/medlineplus
CINAHL	Cumulative Index to Nursing and Allied Health Literature. Abstracts of journals, books, pamphlets, dissertations, software, and other forms of education for nursing and allied health professionals since 1982.	www.ebscohost.com/nursing/products/cinahl-databases
CRISP	Computer Retrieval of Information on Scientific Projects. A searchable database of federally funded biomedical research projects conducted at universities, hospitals, and other research institutions that have been supported by the Department of Health and Human Services since 1972.	
EMBASE	A bibliographic database which covers drug research including side effects and drug interactions.	
OVID	Provides access to a variety of resources including bibliographic databases (such as MEDLINE, EMBASE, and CINAHL); full-text journals; and other clinical information products such as Evidence-Based Medicine Reviews.	www.ovid.com
Cochrane Reviews	The Cochrane Collaboration prepares, maintains, and disseminates systematic reviews of healthcare interventions focusing primarily on systematic reviews of controlled trials of therapeutic interventions.	www.cochrane.org/cochrane-reviews
The Joanna Briggs Institute	An international collaborative of nursing, medical, and allied health researchers, clinicians, academics, and managers who provide best practice information sheets.	www.joannabriggs.org
BMG Clinical Evidence	Provide an annual edition of Clinical Evidence Concise which provides current comprehensive and user-friendly, evidence-based literature for clinicians.	http://clinical evidence.bmj
The Agency for Healthcare Research and Quality	AHRQ. A U.S. Government agency which focuses primarily on medical healthcare services.	www.ahrq.gov
National Quality Measures Clearinghouse	NQMC is sponsored by AHRQ to promote widespread access to quality measures by the healthcare community. It is a public resource for evidence-based clinical practice guidelines.	www.qualitymeasures.ahrq.gov
The National Institute of Nursing Research	One of 27 institutes at the National Institutes of Health (NIH). Supports research to establish the scientific knowledge for the care of individuals across the life span for nursing.	www.nln.nih.gov
The Sarah Cole Hirsh Institute for Best Nursing Practices Based on Evidence	The institute is affiliated with the Frances Payne Bolton School of Nursing at Case Western Reserve. Systematic reviews are published in the open access publication, *Online Journal of Issues in Nursing*.	

2010, p.130). In order for information to be useful it needs to be accurate, timely, complete, concise, and relevant (Worthley, 2000). Englebardt and Nelson (2002) explain the Nelson Data to Wisdom Continuum: Data is provided; data generate information; information generates knowledge and the interpretation, integration and understanding of knowledge lead to wisdom. Healthcare business intelligence requires a foundation that encompasses comprehensive data management of reporting, analytics, data warehousing, and dashboards. Successful business intelligence provides information knowledge at the clinician's

fingertips. Five tenets of successful healthcare business intelligence are data quality, sponsorship and leadership, technology and architecture, value, and culture change (Montalvo, 2013, p. 23).

Weiskopf and Weng (2013) found there is little consistency in the methods used to assess EHR quality data. Overhage, Ryan, Reich, Hartzema, and Stang (2012), and Weiskoph and Weng (2013) believe if the reuse of EHR data for clinical research is to become accepted, researchers and clinicians should adopt validated, systemic methods of EHR data quality assessment. They empirically derived five dimensions of data: (1) Completeness: accessibility, accuracy, availability, omission, presence, quality, validity, rate of recording. (2) Correctness: Is an element present in the EHR true? This dimension includes accuracy, corrections made, errors reported, validity tested. (3) Concordance: Is there agreement between the elements in the EHR, or between the EHR and other data sources? Other considerations are agreement, consistency, reliability, variation. (4) Plausibility: Does an element in the EHR make sense in light of other knowledge about what that element is measuring? Are the data accurate, believable, trustworthy, and valid. (5) Currency: Is an element in the EHR a relevant representation of the patient state at a given point in time? This is a dimension of timeliness (p. 145). "Although the five dimensions of data quality derived during our review were treated as mutually exclusive within the literature, we feel that only three can be considered fundamental: correctness, completeness, and currency. By this we mean that these dimensions are non-reducible and describe core concepts of data quality as it relates to EHR data reuse" (p. 148).

Bowles et al. (2013) found doing research across multiple institutions using electronic health records presents multiple issues even when working with sites with the same vendor. Contributing factors identified included differing versions of the EHR, customizations, variations in documentation of policies and procedures and quality, and user interfaces.

TECHNOLOGY IS ONLY A TOOL FOR EBP

Integration of Evidence Into Healthcare Decisions

The transition to EBP is a cultural change process. In 2008, Anderson and Willson completed a study on the use of CDSS in nursing. They found only six studies that involved CDSS to promote evidence-based practice in nursing. They concluded that nursing is lagging behind the progress made in other disciplines, however given the mandate for CDSS to qualify for federal incentives they propose an increase in CDSS use within nursing will occur.

Castillo & Kelemen (2013) identified 12 characteristics of successful clinical decision support systems. The twelve characteristics include (1) incorporate into existing systems, (2) integrate into the current workflow, (3) provide specificity, (4) incorporate user involvement, (5) provide education and training, (6) provide sufficient system support, (7) provide automated system prompts, (8) provide straightforward alerts, (9) have simple clinical decision support system displays, (10) prompt acknowledgment, (11) require minimal clinical decision support system data entry, and (12) have continuous clinical decision support system evaluation and monitoring.

Brokel, Shaw, and Nicholson (2006) found in implementing clinical rules to automate steps in delivering evidence-based care that to be successful there must be (1) the use of uniform coded terminologies, (2) a culture to transform care with the use of evidence-based practices, (3) processes in place to guide the organization and staff, and (4) inter-disciplinary involvement which is required to be successful (p. 203). The transformation from paper checklist requires an organizational culture to re-design workflow processes to improve the use of evidence-based practice guidelines rules in an electronic health record. The health system required an organizational culture to re-design workflow processes to improve the use of evidence-based guidelines. (Brokel et al., 2006)

Dogherty, Harrison, Graham, Vandyk, and Keeping-Burke (2013) identified factors associated with the success and failure of participants' efforts to facilitate evidence-based practice. Note their factors were not technology issues but process and culture such as engagement, resource deficits, lack of focus on an issue, development of strategic partnerships. Table 40.6 identifies the complete list of positive and negative factors.

Regulatory and Accreditation Agency Impacts

There are concerns that many documentation processes and requirements are heavily focused on payment and regulatory requirements rather than care delivery. Much of what is currently documented and contained in the health record is in response to medico-legal, reimbursement, and accreditation and regulatory requirements. Data capture is influenced by federal and state regulations. ARRA (American Recovery and Reconciliation Act) and Center for Medicare and Medicaid Services (CMS) meaningful use regulations published July 13, 2010 (Blumenthal &

TABLE 40.6	Culture and Process Factors Which Impact Participants' Efforts to Facilitate EBP	
Positive	**Negative**
A focus on a priority issue	Poor engagement or ownership
Relevant evidence	Resource deficits
Development of strategic Partnerships	Contextual issues
Use of multiple strategies to effect change	Lack of evaluation or sustainability
Facilitator characteristics and approach	

Data from Dogherty et al (2013).

Tavenner, 2010) have significantly altered the applications and functionality emphasized. These acts and regulations have deadlines and monetary incentives and penalties in place for healthcare providers and institutions. The Centers for Medicare and Medicaid Services (CMS) established 24 objectives for eligible hospitals seeking incentive benefits. For Stage 1 hospitals are required to meet 14 core objectives and select an additional five from the remaining nine objectives. One mandatory objective of Meaningful Use is the meaningful use of decision support systems. The CMS objective requires that eligible hospitals identify a high priority condition and then implement one clinical decision support rule related to that condition, along with a way to track compliance (CMS Federal Register, 2010). The Health Information Technology for Economic and Clinical Health (HITECH) Act was enacted in 2009 and seeks to improve patient care outcomes and healthcare delivery through major investments in health information technology. The goals are to improve quality, safety, and efficiency of patient care; engage patients and families; improve care coordination; and ensure adequate privacy and security for personal health information (Bowles et al., 2013). Meaningful Use (MU) establishes a set of standards which govern the use of electronic health records. MU stage 1 criteria focused on electronically capturing health information in a standard format and initiating the reporting of clinical quality measures and provider health information. Stage 2 criteria focused on health information exchanges, data interoperability, and electronic transmission of patient care summaries across multiple settings. Stage 3 to be launched in 2016 focuses on decision support for national high priority conditions, improving quality, safety, and efficiency, leading to improved health outcomes and access to comprehensive patient data through patient-centered health information exchanges. Additional documentation and data burdens are applied with the CMS requirements for incentive payments with meaningful use. These include the ability to report specific data elements from the EHRs, ability to report on specific quality measures, and data exchange between providers and systems for meaningful use objectives and clinical quality measures (Cusack et al., 2013, p. 135; Murphy, Wilson, & Newhouse, 2013).

Opportunities are present to empower nurses with information technology tools to leverage the vast clinical knowledge base to improve care, increase patient safety, and meet regulatory requirements.

Optimizing Existing Systems and Applications

The success of a CDS depends on many factors; one of which is end-user satisfaction. A system for which the end

user builds work-arounds does not provide any benefit. Three barriers have been identified. They are (1) excessive use of alerts and reminders, (2) outdated or inaccurate information in the system, and (3) inappropriate levels of the alerts. Lyerla (2008) explains "a reminder or alert that is too general may produce too many messages and result in clinician frustration, causing the reminder to be ignored, whereas a system that is too specific may not produce enough messages resulting in missed appropriate messages" (p. 229). The development of intelligent systems will depend on high-quality data derived from patient and clinical sources. The EHR will continue to be a major source of information along with data for a clinical data warehouse. One important challenge which remains is the high prevalence of narrative text in the electronic record. Currently there is work on natural language processing and information retrieval, however it has not been perfected to meet the criteria for standardized language.

It is imperative that technology assists in getting evidence to nurses at the point of care. Again, this can be accomplished via various methods such as embedded hyperlinks, text messages, and icons. Nurses need access to the information during their care provision, not three hours later. The integration of the evidence into daily workflows is essential so clinicians can move readily from task-based care to managing care and knowledge-based decisions. When this is achieved Matter (2006) explains the clinicians will be functioning at an elevated level of critical thinking and incorporate evidence-based practice into their daily work to improve efficiency, effectiveness, and patient outcomes.

The AMIA 2011 policy meeting stated, "The consensus of the meeting was that, in the move to technology-enabled healthcare environment, the main purpose of documentation should be to support patient care and improved outcomes for individuals and populations and that documentation for other purposes should be generated as a byproduct of care delivery." (Cusack et al., 2013, p. 134).

SUMMARY

Karlene Kerfoot (2009) states, "Nurses are either professional owners of their practice or merely renters" (p. 36). Nurses who own their practice are personally involved and care about their outcomes. They feel accountable for their practice and treat it like an owner would.

It is necessary to create transparency. Nurses who own their practice need information to take the appropriate actions and make the correct decisions. To support this model, nurses need access to real-time information they can use to intervene and analyze care. This includes information from both internal and external sources. They need to be able to use the power of information effectively with the help of information technology, decision support systems, and evidence-based practice to change their practice and be responsible for their outcomes.

Evidence-based practice is not just about connecting nurses with the evidence, it is also about transforming the structures and culture of healthcare organizations to enable staff nurses to use research evidence to make more effective decisions. The evidence does not make the decisions, people do and people work in environments which can encourage or discourage evidence-based practice approaches. Technology can readily support evidence-based practice, however, it is only a tool.

Florence Nightingale (1859) wrote "Let whoever is in charge keep this simple question in her head. Not how can I always do the right thing myself, but how can I provide for this right thing to always be done?" (p. 24).

The electronic health record and evidence-based practice have made great strides in the past 20 years. We are moving forward with providing evidence-based usable information at the point of care in a transparent format to not only meet regulatory, reimbursement, and government requirements, but also improve quality and outcomes and reduce costs and variations in care. The end result is to produce a more enhanced, transparent, and comprehensive system for individualized use by both patients and care providers.

REFERENCES

Anderson, J., & Willson, P. (2008, May/June). Clinical decision support systems in nursing. Synthesis of the science for evidence-based practice. *Computers, Informatics, Nursing*, 151–158.

Androwich, I., & Kraft, M. (2011). Incorporating evidence: Use of computer based clinical decision support systems for health professionals. In V. Saba & K. McCormick (Eds.), *Essentials of nursing informatics* (5th ed., p. 427). New York, NY: McGraw Hill.

Benoliel, J. (1996). Grounded theory and nursing knowledge. *Quality Health Research, 6*(3), 40.

Block, D. (2006). *Healthcare outcomes management: Strategies for planning and evaluation.* Sudbury, MA: Jones & Bartlett.

Blumenthal, D., & Tavenner, M. (2010). The "meaningful use" regulation for electronic health records. *The New England Journal of Medicine, 363*(6), 501–504.

Bodenheimer, T. (2008). Transforming practice. *The New England Journal of Medicine, 359*(20), 2086, 2089.

Bowles, K., Potashnik, S., Ratcliffe, S., Rosenberg, M., Shih, N., Topaz, M., … Naylor, M. (2013). Conducting research using the EHR across multihospital systems. Semantic harmonization implications for administrators. *Journal of Nursing Administration, 43*(6), 355–360.

Brokel, J., Shaw, M., & Nicholson, C. (2006). Expert clinical rules automate steps in delivering evidence-based care in the electronic health record. *CIN: Computers, Informatics, Nursing, 24*(4), 196–205.

Bylone, M. (2010). Effective decision making: Data, data, & more data! *AACN Advanced Critical Care, 21*(2), 130–132.

Byrne, M., & Lang, N. (2013, December). Examination of nursing data elements from evidence–based recommendations for clinical decision support. *Computers, Informatics, Nursing, 31*(12):605–614.

Castillo, R., & Kelemen, A. (2013, July). Considerations for a successful clinical decision support system. *Computers Informatics Nursing, 31*(7):319–326.

Cimino, J., Hripcsak, G., Johnson, S, & Clayton, P (1989). Designing an introspective, multipurpose, controlled, medical vocabulary. Columbia-Presbyterian Medical Center, NY: Center for Medical Informatics Columbia University.

CMS Website. Retrieved from www.cms.gov/Regulations-and-Guidance/Legislation/EHRIncentivePrograms/index.html

Cusack, C., Hripsak, G., Bloomrosen, M., Rosenbloom, S., Weaver, C., Wright, A., … Mamykina, L. (2013). The future state of clinical data capture and documentation: A report from AMIS's 2011 policy meeting. *Journal American Medical Informatics Association, 20,* 134–140.

Dogherty, E., Harrison, M., Graham, I., Vandyk, A., & Keeping-Burke, L. (2013). Turning knowledge into action at the point of care: The collective-based practice. *Worldview on Evidence-Based Nursing, 10*(3), 129–139.

Englebardt, S., & Nelson, R. (2002). *Health care informatics: An interdisciplinary approach* (p. 13). St. Louis, MO: Mosby Elsevier.

Fineout-Overholt, E., Melnyk, B., & Schultz, A. (2005). Transforming health care from the inside out: Advancing evidence-based practice in the 21st century. *Journal of Professional Nursing, 21*(6), 335–344.

Garg, G., Adhikari, N., McDonald, H., Rosas-Arellano, M., Devereaus, P., Beyene, J., … Haynes, R. (2005). Effects of computerized clinical decision support systems on practitioner performance and patient outcomes: A systematic review. *Journal of American Medical Association, 293*(10), 1223–1238.

Gawlinski, A. (2007). Evidence-based practice changes: Measuring the outcome. *AACN Advanced Critical Care, 18*(3), 320–322.

Glaser, B. (1978). *Theoretical sensitivity: Advances in the methodology of grounded theory.* Mill Valley, CA: Sociology Press.

Gugerty, B. (2006). The holy grail: Cost-effective healthcare evidence transparently and consistently used by clinicians. *Journal Healthcare Informatics Management, 20*(3), 21–24.

Hannes, K., Vandersmissen, J., DeBlaeser, L., Peeters, G., Goedhuys, J., & Aertgeerts, B. (2007). Barriers to evidence-based nursing: A focus group study. *Journal of Advanced Nursing, 60*(2), 162–171.

Hruby, G., McKiernan, J., Bakken, S. & Weng, C. (2013). A centralized research data repository enhances retrospective outcomes research capacity: A case report. *Journal American Medical Informatics Association, 20,* 563–567.

Kawamoto, K., Hongsermeier, T., Wright, A., Lewis, J., Bell, D., & Middleton, B. (2013). Key principles for a National Clinical Decision Support Knolwedge Sharing Framework: Synthesis of insights from leading subject matter experts. *Journal American Informatics Association, 20,* 199–206.

Kerfoot, K. (2009, October). The CNO's role in professional transformation at the point of care. *Nurse Leader, 7*(5), 35–38.

Krumholz, H.M. (2008). Outcomes research: Generating evidence for best practice and policies. *Circulation, 118,* 209–318.

Lee, S. (2013, October). Features of computerized CDSS supportive of nursing practice: A literature review. *CIN: Computers, Informatics, Nursing,* 477–495.

Lyerla, F. (2008). Design and implementation of a nursing clinical decision support system to promote guideline adherence. *CIN: Computers, Informatics, Nursing, 26*(4), 227–233.

McClellan, M. B., McGinnis,M., Nable, E. G., & Olsen, L. M. (2007). *Evidence based medicine and the changing nature of healthcare.* Washington, DC: National Academies Press.

McGinty, J., & Anderson, G. (2008). Predictors of physician compliance with American Heart Association Guidelines for acute myocardial infarction. *Critical Care Nursing Quarterly, 31*(2), 161–172.

Melnyk, B. M. (2007). The evidence-based practice mentor: A promising strategy for implementing and sustaining EBP in healthcare systems. *Worldviews on Evidence-Based Nursing, 4*(3), 123–125.

Melnyk, B. M. (2013). The future of evidence-based health care and worldviews: A worldwide vision and call for action to improve healthcare quality, reliability, and population health. *Worldviews on Evidence-Based Nursing, 10*(3), 127–128.

Melnyk, B. M., & Fineout-Overholt, E. (2011). *Evidence-based practice in nursing & healthcare: A guide to best practice* (2nd ed.). Philadelphia, PA: Wolters Kluwer/ Lippincott, Williams & Wilkins.

Melnyk, B. M., Fineout-Overholt, E., Feinstein, N. F., Li, H., Small, L., Wilcos, L., & Kraus, R. (2004). Nurses' perceived knowledge, beliefs, skills, and needs regarding evidence-based practice: Implications for accelerating the paradigm shift. *Worldviews on Evidence Based Nursing, 1*(3), 185–193.

Melnyk, B. M., Fineout-Overholt, E., Feinstein, N. F., Sadler, L. S., & Green-Hernandez, C. (2008). Nurse practitioner educators' perceived knowledge, beliefs, and teaching strategies. *Journal of Professional Nursing, 24*(1), 7–13.

Melnyk, B., Fineout-Overholt, E., Gallagher-Ford, L., & Kaplan, L. (2012). The state of evidence-based practice in US. nurses: Critical implications for nurse leaders and educators. *Journal of Nursing Administration, 42*(9), 410–417.

Melnyk, B. M., Fineout-Overholt, E., Giggleman, M., & Cruz, R. (2010). Correlates among cognitive beliefs, EBP implemenation, organizational culture, cohesion and job satisfatction in evidence-based practice mentors from a Community Hospital System. *Nursing Outlook, 58*(6), 301–308.

Melnyk, B. M., Fineout-Overholt, E., & Mays, M. (2008). The evidence-based practice beliefs and implementation scales: Psychometric properties of two new instruments. *Worldviews on Evidence Based Nursing, 5*(4), 208–216.

Melnyk, B. M., Gallagher-Ford, L., Long, L. E., & Fineout-Overholt, E. (2014). The establishment of evidence-based practice competencies for practicing registered nurses and advanced practice nurses in real world clinical settings: Proficiencies to improve healthcare quality, reliability, patient outcomes and costs. *Worldviews on Evidence-based Nursing, 11,* 5–15.

Montalvo, I. (2013, June). How smart are you data? *Nursing Management, 44*(6), 23–24.

Mullett, C., Evans, R., Christenson, J., & Dean, J. (2001). Development and impact of a computerized pediatric antiinfective decision support program. *Pediatrics, 108*(4), E75.

Murphy, L., Wilson, M., Newhouse, R. (2013). Data analytics. Making the most of input with strategic output. *Journal of Nursing Administration, 43*(7/8), 367–371.

National League for Nursing. (2008). *Position statement. Preparing the next generation of nurses to practice in a technology-rich environment: An informatics agenda.* Retrieved from www.nln.org.aboutnln/position Statements/informatics_052808.pdf. Accessed on June 23, 2008.

National Quality Forum. (2008). *Wired for quality: The intersection of health IT and healthcare quality.* Retrieved from www.quality forum.org/publications/2008/08/ Wired_for_Quality_The_Intersection_of_Health_IT_ and_Healthcare_Quality. Accessed on December 16, 2014.

Newhouse, R. P., Dearholt, S., Poe, S., Pugh, L., & White, K. M. (2007). Organizational change strategies for evidence-based practice. *Journal of Nursing Administration, 37*(12), 552–557.

Nightingale, F. (1859). *Notes on nursing: What it is and what it is not* (p. 24). London, UK: Harrison and Sons.

Overhage, J., Ryan, P., Reich, D., Hartzema, A., & Stang, P. (2012). Validation of a common data model for active safety surveillance research. *Journal American Medical Informatics Association, 19,* 54–60.

Pravikoff, D., Tanner, A., & Pierce, S. (2005). Readiness of US nurses for evidence-based practice. *American Journal Nursing, 105*(9), 40–51.

Rush, K. (2008). Connecting practice to evidence using laptop computers in the classroom. *CIN: Computers, Informatics, Nursing, 26*(4), 190–196.

Sackett, D., Straus, S., Richardson, W. S., Rosenberg, W., & Haynes, R. B. (2000). *Evidence-based medicine: How to practice and teach EBM*. London: Churchill Livingstone.

Sims, I., Gorman, P., Greenes, R., Haynes, B., Kaplan, B., Lehman, H., & Tong, P. (2001). Clinical decision support systems for the practice of evidence-based medicine. *Journal American Medical Informatics Association, 8*(6), 527–534.

Sittig, D. (1999). *Prerequisites for a real time clinical decision support system*. Retrieved from http://www.informatics-review.com/thought/prereqs.html. Accessed on June 25, 2010.

Travers, D., & Mandelkehr, L. (2008). The emerging field of informatics. *North Carolina Medical Journal, 69*(2), 127–131.

Weiskopf, N., & Weng, C. (2013). Methods and dimensions of electronic health record data quality assessment: Enabling reuse for clinical research. *Journal American Medical Informatics Association, 20*, 144–151.

Worthley, J. (2000). *Managing information in healthcare: Concepts and cases*. Chicago, IL: Health Administration Press.

41

Incorporating Evidence: Use of Computer-Based Clinical Decision Support Systems for Health Professionals

Margaret Ross Kraft / Ida M. Androwich

• OBJECTIVES

1. Describe computerized clinical decision support systems (CDSS), including types, characteristics, and the levels of responsibility implicit in the use of each type.
2. Describe effects of CDSS on clinician performance and patient outcomes in healthcare.
3. Understand the features, benefits, and limits of CDSS.
4. Discuss the relationship of DSS to electronic health records and meaningful use.
5. Develop a future vision for CDSS within nursing.

• KEY WORDS

Clinical decision support
Decision support systems
Information systems
Knowledge and cognition
Meaningful use

INTRODUCTION

Decision support systems (DSS) are automated tools designed to support decision-making activities and improve the decision-making process and decision outcomes. Such systems are intended to use the enormous amounts of data that exist in information systems to facilitate decision processes. A clinical decision support system (CDSS), designed to support healthcare providers in making decisions about the delivery and management of patient care, has the potential to improve patient safety and outcomes for specific patient populations, as well as compliance with clinical guidelines and standards of practice and regulatory requirements. Within the complexity of today's healthcare environment, there is an increasing need for accessible information that supports and improves the effectiveness of decision-making and promotes clinical accountability and the use of best practices. Clinical tasks to which CDSS may be applied include alerts and reminders, diagnostic assistance, therapy critiques and plans, medication orders, image recognition and interpretation, trend analysis, and information retrieval. The primary goal of clinical decision support systems is to optimize the efficiency and effectiveness with which clinical decisions are made in order to improve the manner in which care is delivered. Without the ability to recall and process all available complex information, decisions in healthcare often cannot be justified on the basis of available knowledge, costs, benefits, possible risks, and patient preferences (Weed & Weed, 1999).

Clinicians depend on timely, reliable, and accurate information to make clinical decisions. Availability of such information depends on how data are collected, stored, retrieved, and transformed into meaningful information. Computers have virtually unlimited capacity for processing and storage of data. Humans, on the other hand, have limited storage (memory) and processing power, but do have judgment, experience, and intuition. Decision support systems integrate and capitalize on the strengths of both. Improving the efficiency and effectiveness of nursing practice supports the demand for more and more professional accountability for practice. Consequently, CDSS tools that aid nurses in improving their effectiveness in care delivery, identifying appropriate interventions, determining areas in need of policy or protocol development, and supporting patient safety initiatives and quality improvement activities are increasingly needed. Accuracy, timeliness, availability, and reliability of information are just as important to nursing as they are to other healthcare providers. Nurses as knowledge workers need access to current knowledge where it is useful: in clinics, at the bedside, in homes, offices, and research that makes contributions to evidence-based nursing practice. Nursing, as a learning discipline, requires current practice information to inform future care.

A CDSS includes a set of knowledge-based tools that can be fully integrated with the clinical data embedded in the electronic health record (EHR) to assist providers by presenting information relevant to the healthcare problem(s) being faced. The ideal CDSS is available at the point of care with quick (real time) responses, requires minimal training, is easily integrated into the practice workflow, and is user friendly. It should have a powerful search function that can access useful and reliable information from existing knowledge sources. These may include electronic libraries, medical dictionaries, drug formularies, other databases, and expert opinion. A CDSS is only as effective and accurate as its underlying knowledge base. Knowledge sources can provide simple facts, relationships, evidence-based best practices, and the latest in clinical research. CDSS may focus on treatment, diagnosis, population health management, or specific patient information. Systems may be passive, requiring the clinician to access (pull) the advice or with a higher level of information processing, systems may be active, giving unsolicited advice (push).

The availability of reliable clinical information and the propagation and management of clinical knowledge within CDSS has the potential to transform healthcare delivery.

However, it is important to remember that the clinical user's experience, knowledge base, and understanding of the current context of care are not replaced by, but, rather, supported in the decision-making process. In no way does a CDSS usurp the clinician's decision-making role. Final decisions should always be made by clinicians who can accept or reject the CDSS information within the context of the existing healthcare situation. Implementation of CDSS requires the development of a strategy built on an understanding of available CDSS tools, clinician readiness to adopt and use CDSS, and areas within the organization that carry significant risks to patient safety. CDSS is a "tool" system, not a "rule" system. As decision-making is optimized, compliance with current, evidenced-based guidelines increases. Choices for diagnostics or treatment are increasingly supported by evidence. Consequently, chronic condition management and patient workups will be more focused in the future.

CDSS Definitions and Concepts

"Clinical Decision Support is a process for enhancing health-related decisions and actions with pertinent, organized clinical knowledge and patient information to improve health and healthcare delivery. Information recipients can include patients, clinicians and others involved in patient care delivery; information delivered can include general clinical knowledge and guidance, intelligently processed patient data, or a mixture of both; and information delivery formats can be drawn from a rich palette of options that includes data and order entry facilitators, filtered data displays, reference information, alerts and others." (CDS/PI, 2013) According to HIMSS (Health Information Management Systems Society), "clinical decision support is a process for enhancing health-related decisions and actions with pertinent, organized clinical knowledge and patient information to improve health and healthcare delivery" (HIMSS.org, 2011).

"Clinical decision support (CDS) provides clinicians, staff, patients or other individuals with knowledge and person-specific information, intelligently filtered or presented at appropriate times, to enhance health and healthcare. CDS encompasses a variety of tools to enhance decision-making in the clinical workflow. These tools include computerized alerts and reminders to care providers and patients; clinical guidelines; condition-specific order sets; focused patient data reports and summaries; documentation templates; diagnostic support, and contextually relevant reference information, among other tools" (healthIT.gov, 2014).

In 2007, the American Medical Informatics Association (AMIA) developed a roadmap for action on CDS (Osheroff, Teich, Middleton, Steen, Wright, & Detmer, 2007), which identified a framework of three pillars supporting the full benefits of CDS. These pillars were (1) best knowledge available when needed, (2) high adoption and effective use, and (3) continuous improvement of knowledge and CDS methods. The AMIA roadmap identified the tasks that would lead to widespread successful use of CDS. At that time, it was recognized that no public or private entity existed that could be responsible for a work plan. A relatively new initiative to promote action on the use of CDS is the CDS/PI Collaborative, a multi-stakeholder collaborative launched by TMIT Consulting, a firm founded by Dr. Jerome Osheroff in 2011. The CDS/PI Collaborative goal is "better use of clinical decision support to address healthcare imperatives for improvement in quality, patient safety, patient satisfaction and cost control." Products of this collaborative effort include the development of a CDS configuration template, a set of resources designed to improve care with CDS, identification of benefits of the use of CDS for providers, stakeholders, vendors, and the identification and explanation of the "five rights" of CDS (cpi/pi.org).

Nurses are familiar with the "five rights" related to medication administration and recently the concept has been applied to CDS as the "right information to the right people in the right intervention formats through the right channels at the right point in workflow" (CDS/PI Collaborative, 2013). The expectation of the application of the five rights of CDS is that healthcare-related decisions and patients outcomes will be improved.

CDSS software has a knowledge base designed for the clinician to aid in clinical decision-making related to patient care. The computer has virtually unlimited capacity for processing and storage of data. The human, on the other hand, has limited storage (memory) and processing power, but does have judgment, experience, and intuition. Decision support systems integrate and capitalize of the strengths of both. The three key purposes of a DSS are to assist in problem solving with semi-structured problems, support but not replace the judgment of a manager or clinician, and improve the effectiveness of the decision-making process. Highly structured or deterministic problems, which can be solved with existing facts, and completely unstructured problems, which are highly dependent on values and beliefs, are generally not well suited for decision support.

CDSS IMPACT ON CLINICIANS

There is growing pressure for clinicians including nurses to use knowledge at the point of care that is based on researched evidence. The use of CDSS to find and prevent errors related to gaps between optimal and actual practice can result in improved quality of care. Applications of CDSS

suggest the ability to lessen the incidence of adverse drug events, nosocomial infections, and the inappropriate use of antibiotics. Successful use of a CDSS requires integration with the user's normal workflow. Of significance to clinicians is the integration of CDSS within clinical workflow. If the use of a CDSS does not fit into the normal sequence of care delivery it will not be adopted for use. This means that user requirements must be translated into a system that supports workflow while incorporating evidence to improve practice. CDSS must be designed to support clinician requirements rather than dictate clinician workflow practices. The involvement of healthcare professionals in CDSS selection is essential to system acceptance. It is important to consider how a CDSS will affect organizational culture, practice, and personnel attitudes.

Nurses have begun development of CDSS specific for their practice as well as using existing CDSS. For instance, nurses may use MEWS (Modified Early Warning System), a bedside tool that uses vital signs to identify patients likely to deteriorate. At least one hospital has moved this tool to an electronic format providing for more speed in the decision process (Snyder, HIMSS 14, 2014) with a 50% reduction in code blue events. Bowles and colleagues (2012) implemented and tested an inter-disciplinary DSS tool to standardize and improve the discharge planning process. Skiba, Cleveland, Gilbert, and Dandreau (2012) have addressed the effectiveness of CDSS on the implementation of obesity prevention guidelines.

The move to the electronic health record (EHR) has led to an understanding of the dual nature of information needs for decision support. First, evidenced-based information (content) needs to be available at the point of care to inform the **present** patient encounter. Second, key data entered in the process of documentation need to be entered in a manner that they can be able to be aggregated to inform **future** patient encounters. New knowledge becomes a transparent by-product of care and moves from *"TRIP"—translating research into practice* to *"TPIR"—translating practice into research.* The lag of practice behind knowledge could be shortened if not eliminated by the availability of current knowledge to support the decision-making process.

Classic CDSS Content

Included in the field of healthcare decision support are systems that support organizational, executive/managerial, financial, and clinical decisions. Administrative systems, including those designed for finance or quality, generally support the business decision-making process. These systems encompass decision processes for other than direct patient care delivery, and even if clinical in nature, such as quality improvement systems, are mainly used for strategic planning, budgeting, financial analysis, quality management, continuous process improvement, and clinical benchmarking. In these systems, decisions occur at the strategic, tactical, population or aggregate, and operational levels, not at the individual level. The clinical decision support systems focus on real-time decision support, goal orientation, and intelligence gathering, and are designed to be used at the point of care by clinicians. Recently, healthcare agencies have begun to understand that combination systems offer optimal value to the organization. Such systems are able to support outcomes performance management by integrating operational data (the business side)—budgeting, executive decision-making, financial analysis, quality management, and strategic planning data—with clinical data (the clinical side)—clinical event tracking, results reporting, pharmaceutical ordering and dispensation, differential diagnoses, real-time clinical pathways, literature research, and clinical alerts. The goals of a CDSS implementation are variable but address the use of best clinical practices, patient safety, and patient empowerment as well as the financial well-being of the institution (Jenders & Sittig, 2007).

DSSs could be divided into data based (population based), model based (case based), knowledge based (rule based), and graphics based. In this view, a *data-based* system provides decision support with a population perspective and uses routinely collected, longitudinal, cohort, and cross-sectional databases. Population-based information is used to enhance clinical decision-making, and enhance medical practice. A *model-based* DSS is driven by access to and manipulation of statistical or financial data and optimization or simulation. The data in this instance are compared to various decision-making and analytic models. A model is a generalization that can be used to describe the relationships among a number of observations to represent a perception of how things fit together. The models may be pathophysiologic, statistical, or analytic. Some model-based examples are linear programming, such as scheduling nurses or physicians or resource allocation, simulation, such as emergency department or operating room scheduling or provider profiling.

A *knowledge-based* system relies on expert knowledge that is either embedded in the system or accessible from another source and uses some type of knowledge acquisition process to understand and capture the cognitive processes of healthcare providers. Much of what is considered evidence-based practice refers to knowledge-based decision support. Yet there are many issues with maintaining current evidence in DSS. Such issues include identifying the policy and research challenges in developing and maintaining practice evidence in machine readable repositories. The

DSS experts have coined a term "evidence-adaptable CDSS" to describe a new type of CDSS that has a knowledge base that is constantly updated with the most current evidence available and is viewed as both a goal and necessity.

The construction and upkeep of clinical protocols or guidelines are not easy. Often there are multiple authors, protocol selection is not always straightforward, multiple protocols may be available, or there is a situation that demands a departure from protocols assumptions. Some early expert systems were referred to as using the "Greek Oracle" approach, where the DSS provided a solution from "on high," but others have called for a "catalyst" approach, whereby the DSS serves as a catalyst and provides guidance, but the user remains in control.

In many ways, CDSS distinctions are somewhat artificial and are increasingly blurred. A very simplistic, broad view of DSS is a "push–pull" distinction mentioned earlier. In a "pull" system, the provider needs to take some action independent of the usual workflow to initiate a request for support or to query the system for additional information, whereas in a "push" system the system automatically generates the alert in response to a clinician action such as a medication order for which the patient has reported an allergy.

CDSS Development. CDSS development requires a team approach. The first step in the development process is identification of the information needs that leads to the question of whether a CDSS would be helpful. Next is the need to identify the stakeholders with interest in the topic. Stakeholders can include physicians, nurses, administrative staff, Quality and Safety Education in Nursing (QSEN) staff, and even patients. As a group, the stakeholders must address CDSS goals. It is important to synthesize and validate a unified working list of goals and objectives. As the specific clinical issue is addressed, determination of potential frequency of use is necessary to determine whether assignment of resources to a development project is justified. Is this a frequently encountered unstructured or semistructured problem? Is there sufficient evidence that justifies the assignment of necessary resources for development? Is the proposed CDSS to be built to address process and outcome data, departmental needs, the needs within the community of service, or a result of reporting and accreditation issues? Will the proposed system address a strategic target such as medication safety? If the decision is to move forward, an inventory of all available information systems such as laboratory, radiology, and pharmacy systems as well as the clinical record system, order systems, and administrative systems may be data and information sources. CDSS capabilities depend on availability of coded data, use of standard vocabularies, and the ability to aggregate data from multiple sources.

The knowledge base of the CDSS must be clearly defined and a system for knowledge update must be in place. After the system inventory, it is necessary to select CDSS interventions as part of the process of developing specifications for the system build. Building the CDSS requires an identification of when and how interventions are triggered, the data source and content of the intervention, how the information is delivered to the recipient, and also needs a feedback mechanism. After a CDSS is built, it must be tested and only then should it "go live." The system launch requires planning that addresses not just a date but all the necessary educational preparation of the end users. The final step of CDSS development is evaluation and system enhancement as needed. Ongoing assessment of intervention use and usability, evaluation of intervention performance against objectives, and continuous enhancement of CDSS provide value to users.

A successful CDSS emerges from and supports performance improvement initiatives (Osheroff et al., 2012). The choice of a CDSS target may be related to a patient benefit that outweighs any possibility of harm, practices supported by evidence, physician practice patterns, disease management, chronic care management, and national quality measures. Also considered is the gap that exists between what is ideal and what is real. The CDSS development looks at preventing errors, optimizing decision-making, and improving the care process.

CDSS governance involves executive leadership, management oversight, project managers, and the end users. Successful development and implementation depend on strong executive support for clinical quality improvement and belief in information technology (IT) as a tool to achieve desired quality. A history of previously successful IT projects has a positive impact. Communication with the stakeholders must be successful and the key end users must be involved in implementation.

Osheroff et al. (2012) identify a taxonomy of CDS interventions for data entry , data review, and the tasks of assessment and understanding as well as CDS that can be either time or data triggers (see Table 41.1).

KNOWLEDGE AND COGNITIVE PROCESSES

Knowledge engineering is the field concerned with knowledge acquisition (extracting or eliciting knowledge from experts) and the organization and structure of that knowledge within a computer system. Building a knowledge-based or expert system requires an understanding of the cognitive processes of healthcare providers and how they deal with complexity. Most DSS take advantage of the research on human reasoning and decision-making.

How do nurses solve problems? Or even determine that there is a problem? What information seeking behaviors do nurses use? Is "intuition" really a case of statistical pattern recognition? When an expert nurse claims that the patient "just didn't look right," is it intuition or do years of nursing experience that place that patient three standard deviations from the mean of all the patients cared for? Answering these questions requires an understanding of the decision-making process, human diagnostic reasoning, and critical thinking. Nurses recognize various types of knowledge such as declarative knowledge and procedural knowledge. Declarative knowledge can be considered the "know what" or descriptive knowledge, procedural knowledge is the "know how," and the processes of reasoning and inference produce the "know why."

A variety of methods have been used to elicit knowledge from expert clinicians. Some knowledge elicitation techniques require clinicians to "think aloud." The term surveillance is used to describe nurses' cognitive work in identifying and preventing patient complications. Rhudy and Androwich (2013) explored surveillance in

TABLE 41.1	CDS Type Taxonomy
CDS Tasks of Data Entry	
Smart Documentation Forms	
Order sets, Care Plans, Protocols	
Parameter Guidance	
Critiques and Warnings, i.e., "Immediate alerts"	
CDS Tasks of Data Review	
Relevant Data Summaries for a single patient	
Multi-patient Monitors	
Predictive and Retrospective Analytics	
CDS Tasks of Assessment and Understanding	
Filtered Reference Information	
Knowledge Resources	
Expert Workup	
Management Advisors	
CDS NOT Triggered by Tasks	
Data-Triggered Alerts	
Time-Triggered Alerts	

Reproduced, with permission, from Osheroff, J., Teich, J., Levick, D., Saldana, L., Velasco, F., Sittig, D., … Jenders, R. (2012). *Improving Outcomes with Clinical Decision Support: An Implementer's Guide*, 2nd ed. (p. 165). Chicago, IL: Healthcare Information and Management Systems Society (HIMSS).

the context of early recognition of patient complications. Their findings suggest that nurses do use surveillance and cues from change-of-shift handoff information to develop a mental image of the patient, which serves as a baseline for evaluating the patient's current state and making patient care decisions. Interviews with experts has been the most commonly used method of eliciting knowledge. The expert clinician is directly asked in a structured interview to describe a typical case and how aspects of the case influence care decisions. The advantages of this method are ease of use and the ability to draw out important information; however, a potential problem may be that the experts tend to say what they *think* that they do, but may be unaware of what they are actually doing or they may be unable to break down their thought processes into steps.

Cognitive Task Analysis (CTA) refers to a set of methods that capture the skills, knowledge, and processing ability of experts in dealing with complex tasks. The goal of CTA is to tap into "higher order" cognitive functions. This technique is beneficial in comparing the performance of an expert with the performance of someone less than expert. CTA attempts to identify pitfalls or trouble spots in the reasoning process of the beginner or intermediate level practitioner while comparing the reasoning process with that of the expert.

An important aspect of data presentation for ease of understanding and accuracy of decision-making is the manner with which the clinician is able to visualize patient data for decision-making. Edward Tufte (2001[1983]), in his seminal works on the visual display of data, demonstrated that the manner in which the data are displayed can lead to accurate or inaccurate decisions. He was able to demonstrate that had a "full" data picture been available, the "O ring" failure that led to the tragic crash of the Challenger Missile could have been avoided. Computer-based techniques which use interactive tools are also used to assess decision-making. These tools have the advantage of not needing to interact directly with the clinician but also tend to be overly simplistic for complex decision analysis. Rating and sorting methods, borrowed from the social sciences and protocol analysis, are also methods used. Each has advantages and disadvantages.

CDSS and Meaningful Use

The Center for Medicare and Medicaid Programs provides financial incentives for the "meaningful use" (MU) of certified EHR technology to improve the quality of patient care and "inform clinical decisions at the point of care" (healthit.hhs.gov). Incentives are based on how

providers show that they are "meaningfully using" their EHR data. The CDSS Taskforce of HIMSS worked on developing a link between CDS and specific Meaningful Use (MU). Implementation of MU takes place in three stages. Stage 1 focuses on the capture and sharing of data; stage 2 focuses on advancing clinical processes; and stage 3 addresses improved outcomes. Stage 1 achievement of meaningful use requires that at least one CDS rule be implemented and monitored for provider compliance. Stage 2 of the Meaningful use requires that clinical decision support be used to improve performance on high-priority health conditions. A CDSS could address the meaningful use objectives of drug, drug–drug, drug–allergy, and drug formulary checks, and support the maintenance of a medication allergy list. A CDSS deployed effectively can optimize its value in targeted clinical outcome measures and can assist in the management of chronic conditions. In 2010, Weingarten predicted that CDS would feature prominently in defining meaningful use. Beginning in 2014, all Medicare-eligible providers must electronically report their Clinical Quality Measures (CQM) data to CMS in order to demonstrate meaningful use. A CDSS deployed effectively can optimize its value in targeted clinical outcome measures.

Patient Decision Support

Another important area of decision support is patient decision support. Given the opportunity, patients may become more engaged in self-care when patients as well as clinicians have the information needed to make better decisions (Stevens, 2010). It can be difficult for patients to speak up during medical visits and they often struggle to communicate their needs and opinions to their providers. Online tools exist that can help the patient and family identify areas in which they may need help when making healthcare decisions (empoweredpatientsco alition.org, 2014; healthpartners.com, 2014). Patient Decision Support (PDS) tools assist patients in communicating with their providers and using medical evidence to make informed choices that are consistent with the patient's values while using evidence about consequences of medical alternatives. One systematic review of patient decision support literature has shown that PDS interventions increase patients' knowledge, produce more accurate expectations, and lead to more conservative approaches to treatment that are more congruent with patients' informed preferences (Walsh, Barr, Thompson, Ozanne, O'Neill, & Elwyn, 2014). Innovations in healthcare may be the key to the development of more personalized and effective patient decision support tools (Ng, Lee, Lee, & Abdullah, 2013).

RESPONSIBILITY OF USER: ETHICAL AND LEGAL ISSUES

The legal responsibility for treatment and advice given to a patient rests with the clinician regardless of whether a CDSS is used. Still unknown are the legal ramifications of not following CDSS advice. One must always consider the potential of adverse consequences but there seems to be no major adverse effect from the use of a CDSS; however, such systems must be developed with high standards of quality. There must be some way to provide a high degree of assurance that a CDSS has been developed according to quality and safety standards. CDSS will be expected to comply with a "duty of care" if CDSS is to become safely integrated into routine patient care. The knowledge base of a CDSS must be as reflective as possible of the current state of professional and scientific opinion and evidence and must draw upon traditional knowledge sources such as journals and textbooks to maintain currency. CDSS documentation should address the purpose of the system, the population for which the application is intended along with inclusion/exclusion criteria, the context for use, the expected user skill level, evidence source(s), and review and update methods. Keeping a CDSS current requires a commitment of technical, professional, and organizational dimensions. Any CDSS will be only as effective as the strength and accuracy of the underlying evidence base. The knowledge base of a CDSS must be as reflective as possible of the current state of professional and scientific opinion and evidence and must also draw upon traditional knowledge sources to maintain currency. CDSS documentation should address the purpose of the system, the population for which the application is intended along with inclusion/exclusion criteria, the context for use, the expected user skill level, evidence source(s), and review and update methods.

FUTURE OF CDSS

Despite the many challenges of developing and implementing CDSS, it is clear that the use of decision support will increase. Today's healthcare environment is complicated by diverse priorities, providers, and practice modes. The evidence needed for improved practice is in the patients' records. CDSS development has been promoted with the increased focus on and expanded implementation of EHRs, an improved understanding of the potential benefits of CDSS, and the incentives for meaningful use. Vendors are beginning to include CDSS in their products. Acceptance depends largely on organizational culture, leadership attitudes, and provider involvement.

SUMMARY

The development of CDSS requires a huge financial and intellectual investment but also represents the potential of reduction in care costs through improvement of the decision process at the point of care and a reduction in the possibility of costly errors. Current evidence indicates that CDSS can improve patient care quality, reduce medication errors, minimize variances in care, improve guideline compliance, and promote cost savings. Wider implementation of EHRs and the incentives for the use of CDSS are tied to the Meaningful Use initiative of CMS. Wider adoption of such tools will support clinical care decisions through the provision of additional and current information at the time and place of care delivery while final decision authority will remain with the clinician. Ease of use within existing workflow practice will determine the success of a CDSS. Although no one single CDSS is in widespread use, such systems, whether simple or complex, are becoming ubiquitous and research on the use of CDSS is growing.

REFERENCES

Bowles, K., Holland, D., & Potashnik, S. (2012). Implementation and testing of interdisciplinary decision support tools to standardize discharge planning. NI 2012. Montreal, Canada.

CDS/PI Collaborative. (2013). *Getting better faster–Together (SM)*. Retrieved from https://sites.google.com/site/cds for Piimpera tivespublic/cds. Accessed on October 9, 2013.

empoweredpatientscoalition.org. (2014). *Patient decision support*. Accessed on February 20, 2014.

healthIT.gov. (2014). *Definition of CDSS*. Accessed on January 31, 2014.

healthpartners.com. (2014). *Patient decision support*. Accessed on February 14, 2014.

HIMSS.org. (2011). *Definition of CDSS*. Accessed on January 31, 2014.

Jenders, R., & Sittig, D. (2007). Improving outcomes with clinical decision support. AMIA Conference. Washington, DC.

Stevens, M., (2010). *mHealth: Telemedicine delivers patient decision support*. Retrieved from www.clinical-innovation.com. Accessed on December 17, 2014.

Ng, C. J., Lee, Y. K., Lee, P. Y., & Abdullah, K. L. (2013). Health innovations in patient decision support: Bridging the gaps and challenges. *Australian Medical Journal, 6*(2), 95–99.

Osheroff, J., Teich, J., Levick, D., Saldana, L., Velasco, F., Sittig, D., ... Jenders, R. (2012). *Improving Outcomes with Clinical Decision Support: An Implementer's Guide* 2nd ed. (p. 165). Chicago, IL: Healthcare Information and Management Systems Society (HIMSS).

Osheroff, J., Teich, J., Middleton, B., Steen, E., Wright, A., & Detmer, D. (2007). A roadmap for national action on clinical decision support. *Journal of American Medical Informatics Association, 14*(2), 141–145.

Rhudy, L., & Androwich, I. (2013). Surveillance as an intervention in the care of stroke patients. *Journal of Neuroscience Nursing, 45*(5), 262–271.

Skiba, D., Cleveland, B., Gilbert, K., & Dandreau, D. (2012). Comparing the effectiveness of CDSS on provider's behaviors to implement obesity prevention guidelines. NI 2012, Montreal, Canada.

Snyder, M. (2014). Computerization of the MEWS tool. HIMSS14, Orlando, Florida.

Tufte, E. R. (2001 [1983]). *The visual display of quantitative information* (2nd ed.). Cheshire, CT: Graphics Press, ISBN 0-9613921-4-2.

Walsh, T., Barr, P., Thompson, E., Ozanne, C., O'Neill, C., & Elwyn, G. (2014, January 23). Undetermined impact of patient decision support interventions on healthcare costs and savings: Systematic review. *British Medical Journal, 348.*

Weed, L., & Weed, L. (1999). Opening the black box of clinical judgment—an overview. *British Medical Journal, 319,* 1–4.

Weingarten, S. (2010). *Clinical decision support and meaningful use. Perspectives from Zynx Health. Podcast interview.* Retrieved from www.healthbusinessblog.com. Accessed on August 2, 2010.

PART 7

Educational Applications

Diane J. Skiba

42

Nursing Curriculum Reform and Healthcare Information Technology

Eun-Shim Nahm / Marisa L. Wilson

• OBJECTIVES

1. Describe the background of and needs for curriculum reform in nursing education in the twenty-first century.
2. Discuss prior academic and other professional organizational efforts to transform nursing education with an emphasis on healthcare information technology.
3. List information technology competencies required by nurses with different levels of education.
4. Identify current national trends in nursing education associated with informatics.
5. Explain the content and process of the American Nurse Credentialing Center (ANCC) Nursing Informatics Certification examination.

• KEY WORDS

American Association of Colleges of Nursing (AACN) Essentials for Nursing
Electronic Health Records (EHR)
Healthcare Information Technology (HIT)
HITECH
Informatics competency
Knowledge, skills, and attitudes (KSA)
Nursing education curriculum
Nursing Informatics (NI)
Patient safety
Quality and Safety Education for Nurses (QSEN)
Technology Informatics Guiding Educational Reform (TIGER)

BACKGROUND: TRANSFORMATION OF HEALTHCARE USING INFORMATION TECHNOLOGY

Rapid advancement and policy driven change in healthcare information technologies (HIT) in the twenty-first century offers nurses a great opportunity to augment their ability to manage patient information, generate knowledge, and provide quality care. Since the Institute of Medicine (IOM)'s report, *To Err Is Human,* was released, a great deal of effort has been made to transform healthcare using information technologies (Committee on Quality of Health Care in America & Institute of Medicine, 2001; Newhouse, Dearholt, Poe, Pugh, & White, 2007). In fact, in the current digital era, hospitals cannot be sustained without HIT, which allows healthcare providers to deliver safer and efficient care. Healthcare ITs help clinicians manage a large volume of clinical data and access the most up-to-date evidence-based health information. They also allow secure data exchange between patients, care providers, and organizations. Credentialing organizations has also recognized the importance of HIT in healthcare organizations. In nursing, Magnet status recognition by the American Nurses Credentialing Center (ANCC) represents healthcare organizations' quality patient care, nursing excellence, and innovations in practice (American Nurses Credentialing Center [ANCC], 2014a). Hospitals can earn the recognition by meeting a set of standards for quality indicators and standards of nursing practice. A strong presence and effective utilization of HIT is an essential component in the Magnet recognition process.

Migration of paper-based health records to an electronic format has been a national priority for the current federal administration. In an effort to make HIT become available to the majority of healthcare providers, the Office of the National Coordinator (ONC) funded several information technology (IT) training programs and regional extension centers (U.S. Department of Health & Human Services, n.d.). Furthermore, Title XIII of the ARRA, Health Information Technology for Economic and Clinical Health Act (HITECH), authorized incentive payments through Medicare and Medicaid to clinicians and hospitals when they used electronic health records (EHRs) privately and securely to achieve specified improvements in care delivery Blumenthal, 2009; Blumenthal & Tavenner, 2010). Meaningful use (MU) is to (The Office of National Coordinator, n.d.-a):

- Improve quality, safety, efficiency, and reduce health disparities
- Engage patients and family
- Improve care coordination, and population and public healthMaintain privacy and security of patient health information

MU criteria and objectives are phased out in three stages over a five-year period (2011–2016). Stage I (2011–2012) focused on data capturing and sharing. Currently, Stage 2 (2014) highlights the advancement of clinical processes. This stage has a particular direct impact on patients and their caregivers as MU requires that providers give patients (>5% of those they see) access to their EHRs and use secure eMessaging to communicate with them. To meet MU requirements (Centers for Medicare & Medicaid Services, 2013), hospitals nationwide are implementing new information systems,

including "tethered personal health records" (PHRs), which allow patients to access their EHRs and are integrated into "patient portals," secure Web sites providing health tools such as eMessaging or prescription refills (Emani et al., 2012; Office of the National Coordinator for Health Information Technology, n.d.).

In order to provide optimal care in this rapidly changing and technology-laden healthcare environment, nurses must have a full understanding of the changes in healthcare and be properly prepared to use the available technological resources. This chapter will discuss:

1. The impact of healthcare information technology (IT) on current healthcare

2. Major efforts in nursing curriculum revisions

3. Nursing education reform in the current technology-rich environment

4. Major domains and attributes of HIT competencies needed for nursing students and practicing nurses in the current healthcare environment

5. Informatics competency for faculty members

THE IMPACT OF HEALTHCARE INFORMATION TECHNOLOGY ON CURRENT HEALTHCARE

Many years ago, healthcare teams used to bring a cart full of paper-based patient medical records during rounds. Physicians and nurses often furiously documented to-do lists on pieces of paper or in notebooks. Recent advancements of HIT and the national push for using EHRs have revolutionized and impacted every aspect of healthcare delivery. For instance, currently most patients gather a significant amount of health information about their health online even before they meet with healthcare providers. When the patient goes to a clinic or hospital, he/she is admitted to a registration (or an admission) system before the patient sees his/her care providers. The data in those systems then are forwarded to other clinical systems including electronic health records, laboratory and pharmacy systems, as well as other ancillary systems. Eventually the persons' health data in those systems are forwarded to finance systems and then sent to necessary insurance companies and other regulatory organizations (Borycki, Kushniruk, Joe, Armstrong, Otto, Hoe, et al, 2009). Clinicians in the current era make rounds with a portable workstation on wheels (WOW) (a.k.a computers on wheels [COWs]), which is connected to the hospitals' main EHR systems using a wireless connection. They look for the most up-to-date evidence-based clinical information needed for the patient right at the bedside using various portable systems (iPad, tablet computers, personal digital assistant [PDA] devices).

In addition, Meaningful Use (MU) requires that eligible professionals and hospitals must meet the specific requirements for using EHRs to receive incentives and avoid penalties from Medicare and Medicaid.

The current national HIT policies have had significant implications for healthcare providers, and the use of HIT systems in healthcare settings will continue to increase at a rapid pace. Current HIT has already transformed various aspects of healthcare delivery, including regulations related to healthcare data and information. For instance, the 1996 Health Insurance Portability and Accountability Act (HIPAA) was introduced to establish mechanisms to secure data stored in servers as well as during transmission to the other healthcare parties (Centers for Medicare and Medicaid Services, 2010; U.S. Department of Health & Human Services, 2010).

In recent years, much has changed in healthcare since HIPAA was enacted over 15 years ago. Thus, the HIPAA Omnibus Rule was introduced in 2013 to protect patient privacy and safeguard patients' health information in an ever-expanding digital age (U.S. Department of Health & Human Services, 2013). On the other hand, the demand for electronic health information exchange among care providers and care settings is growing along with national emphasis on the quality, safety, and efficiency of healthcare delivery (The Office of National Coordinator, n.d.-b).

At the systems' level, healthcare providers must ensure the accuracy and completeness of data, as well as appropriate interoperability between the systems. Implementation and maintenance of HIT are complex and dynamic processes and increasing numbers of HIT experts and clinicians are being involved in this process. An enormous challenge for both healthcare organizations and educational institutions is the preparation of competent healthcare informaticians and clinicians competent in the use of health information technologies.

With the national push, the adoption rates of these HIT technologies by clinicians and hospitals have been accelerated. To achieve the successful adoption of HIT in healthcare, it is also critical to ensure clinicians' competency to use healthcare IT. Nurses' competency for using HIT is particularly important because they are the largest group of direct healthcare providers in the United States, accounting for 19.6% of all healthcare workers in 2008 (approximately 3 million) (U.S. Bureau of Labor Statistics, 2010; U.S. DHHS Health Resources and Services Administration, 2010). In fact, nursing as a healthcare discipline has been ahead in terms of educating healthcare professionals who are specialized in healthcare IT. For instance, nursing informatics (NI) was created as an area of graduate specialization at the University of Maryland School of Nursing (UM SON) in 1988, and NI was officially recognized as a specialty practice area by the American Nurses Association (ANA) in 1992 (Gassert, 2000). Since then, informatics has become a core course for many baccalaureate programs, and many nursing schools have offered graduate degree programs focusing on nursing and healthcare informatics. Many nursing schools, however, struggle with the inclusion of informatics competencies at all levels since many faculty members are unfamiliar with the informatics content.

The advancement of available information communication technologies has also changed nursing education drastically. Nursing schools teach their students using innovative technologies emphasizing evidence-based practice and problem-solving abilities. Many nursing schools have high fidelity simulation labs allowing students more opportunities to learn about critical components of practical cases from school. Stakeholders expect nursing students to be competent in using HIT when they arrive in practice settings. Nursing as a profession has recognized the major reform of nursing education, and significant efforts are being made in many areas of the nursing domain, including revision of essentials for all levels of nursing education (American Association of Colleges of Nursing [AACN], 1994, 2008, 2011, 2014). With these changes, informatics is now essential for all levels of nursing education.

In addition to the reform in nursing education, the landmark document, *The Future of Nursing: Leading Change, Advancing Health*, by the Institute of Medicine examined the current nursing workforce and made critical recommendations to transform the nursing profession in an effort to improve the health of the U.S. population (Institute of Medicine, 2010). Those recommendations are focused on four areas, including an informatics field:

- Nurses should practice to the full extent of their education and training.

- Nurses should achieve higher levels of education and training through an improved educational system that promotes seamless academic progression.

- Nurses should be full partners, with physicians and other healthcare professionals, in re-designing healthcare in the United States.

- Effective workforce planning and policy-making require better data collection and an improved information infrastructure.

EFFORTS IN NURSING CURRICULUM REVISIONS

Background

An increased awareness of patient safety and the use of HIT in healthcare called for changes in the nursing curriculum. The IOM report, *Health Professions Education: A Bridge to Quality*, is a result of a 2002 summit followed by the IOM's report, *Crossing the Quality Chasm* (Committee on Quality of Health Care in America & Institute of Medicine, 2001). This inter-disciplinary summit was held to discuss reforming education for health professionals to enhance quality and patient safety (Institute of Medicine Committee on Health Education Profession Summit, 2002). The report proposed five core competencies for healthcare professionals (Committee on Quality of Health Care in America & Institute of Medicine, 2001; Institute of Medicine Committee on Health Education Profession Summit, 2002):

- *Provide patient-centered care – identify, respect and care about patients' differences, values, preferences, and expressed needs .... and continuously advocate disease prevention, wellness, and promotion of healthy lifestyles, including a focus on population health.*

- *Work in interdisciplinary teams – cooperate, collaborate, communicate, and integrate care in teams ....*

- *Employ evidence-based practice – integrate best research with clinical expertise and patient values for optimum care, and participate in learning and research activities to the extent feasible.*

- *Apply quality improvement – identify errors and hazards in care; understand and implement basic safety design principles ... design and test interventions to change processes and systems of care, with the objective of improving quality.*

- *Utilize informatics – communicate, manage knowledge, mitigate error, and support decision making using information technology.*

Since then, many efforts have been made by nursing professional organizations and the AACN to revise the nursing curriculum to be aligned with the IOM competencies.

Quality and Safety Education for Nurses (QSEN)

The overarching goal of the three phases of the QSEN project, which was supported by the Robert Wood Johnson Foundation (RWJF), is to address the competencies necessary to continuously improve the quality and safety of the healthcare systems in which they work (Cronenwett et al., 2007; Quality and Safety Education for Nurses [QSEN], 2010). Phase I of the project identified six competencies that needed to be developed during pre-licensure nursing education (Table 42.1). The group also proposed clarified competencies in the areas of knowledge, skills, and attitudes (KSAs).

Phase II work of QSEN was focused on competencies for graduate and advanced practice nurses (APNs). The QSEN faculty members collaborated with APNs who practiced in direct patient care and worked on the development of standards of practice, accreditation of educational programs, and certification (Cronenwett et al., 2009).

TABLE 42.1	QSEN Competencies
Patient-centered Care	Recognize the patient or designee as the source of control and full partner in providing compassionate and coordinated care based on respect for a patient's preferences, values, and needs.
Teamwork and Collaboration	Definition: Function effectively within nursing and inter-professional teams, fostering open communication, mutual respect, and shared decision-making to achieve quality patient care.
Evidence-based Practice (EBP)	Integrate best current evidence with clinical expertise and patient/family preferences and values for the delivery of optimal healthcare.
Quality Improvement (QI)	Definition: Use data to monitor the outcomes of care processes and use improvement methods to design and test changes to continuously improve the quality and safety of healthcare systems.
Safety	Minimize the risk of harm to patients and providers through both system effectiveness and individual performance.
Informatics	Use information and technology to communicate, manage knowledge, mitigate error, and support decision-making.

The workgroups that participated in Phase II generated KSAs for graduate-level education. Additionally, in Phase III, the AACN worked on developing the capacity of faculty engaged in pre-licensure nursing education to mentor their colleague faculty integration of the evidence-based content on the six QSEN competencies (QSEN, 2012).

Phase IV supports Institute of Medicine's recommendation increasing number of nurses with advanced degree. These efforts are being led by the Tri-Council for Nursing, consisting of the American Association of Colleges of Nursing, National League for Nursing, American Nurses Association, and the American Organization of Nurse Executives (AONE).

The IOM/QSEN competencies and the pre-licensure KSAs are embedded in the new AACN Essentials for nursing education (Cronenwett, Sherwood, & Gelmon, 2009; Cronenwett et al., 2009; Dycus & McKeon, 2009).

The American Association of Colleges of Nursing Essentials for Nursing

In response to the urgent calls to transform healthcare delivery and to better prepare today's nurses for professional practice, the AACN convened a task force on essential patient safety competencies in 2006 (AACN, 2006b). The taskforce recommended specific competencies that should be achieved by professional nurses to ensure high-quality and safe patient care. Those competencies were identified under the following areas: (1) critical thinking; (2) healthcare systems and policy; (3) communication; (4) Illness and Disease Management; (5) ethics; and (6) information and healthcare technologies. Since then, the AACN revised the Essentials of Baccalaureate Education for Professional Nursing Practice in 2008 (AACN, 2008).

In regard to the essentials for graduate programs, the AACN made a decision to migrate advanced practice nursing programs (APNs) from the master's level to the doctorate level (doctor of nursing practice [DNP] program) by the year 2015 (AACN, 2014). Under this decision, many master's programs that prepare advanced practice registered nurses (APRNs) have already transitioned or in the process of making transition. The Essentials of Doctoral Education for Advanced Nursing Practice were developed in 2006 (AACN, 2006a) and the informatics competency is one of the essentials for this education program. This has a major impact on education at the graduate level. Some non-APRN master's speciality programs (e.g., informatics, healthcare leadership and administration, and community-health nursing) still maintain master's program. The essentials for master's education were revised in 2011 (AACN, 2011).

Among various changes regarding essentials in nursing education since 2001, major emphasis has been on patient safety and healthcare IT. The major focus of this chapter is to discuss nursing curriculum from the context of HIT, and Table 42.2 focuses on AACN essentials in the area of information management and technology.

Technology Informatics Guiding Educational Reform (TIGER) Initiative

The recent Technology Informatics Guiding Educational Reform (TIGER) Initiative epitomizes nurses' efforts to translate high-level initiatives on nursing education reform to a practice level (Hebda & Calderone, 2010; TIGER, 2014a; TIGER, 2014b). TIGER's aim is to fully engage practicing nurses and nursing students in the electronic era of healthcare. TIGER's goal is to create and disseminate action plans that can be duplicated within nursing and other multi-disciplinary healthcare training and workplace settings. In Phase I of the TIGER summit, stakeholders from various fields, including nursing practice, education, vendors, and government agencies, participated in the discussions, and the TIGER team developed a 10-year vision and three-year action plan for transforming nursing practice and education (TIGER, 2014a). In Phase II, TIGER formalized cross-organizational activities/action steps into nine collaborative TIGER teams (TIGER, 2009).

1. Standards and Interoperability
2. Healthcare IT National Agenda/HIT Policy
3. Informatics Competencies
4. Education and Faculty Development
5. Staff Development/Continuing Education
6. Usability/Clinical Application Design
7. Virtual Demonstration Center
8. Leadership Development
9. Consumer Empowerment/Personal Health Record

Currently TIGER is working on Phase III that integrates the TIGER recommendations into the nursing community as well as other disciplines across the continuum of care.

Some of the important activities include the development and implementation of a Virtual Learning Environment Center (VLE) and developing another invitational summit (TIGER, 2014b). The VLE is an interactive Web-based learning environment where the learners can develop knowledge and skills in the area health information technology.

TABLE 42.2	Information Management and Technology-Related Essentials for Nursing Education	
Baccalaureate Education (2008). http://www.aacn. nche.edu/education/ pdf/BaccEssentials08.pdf (AACN, 2008)	Essential IV: Information Management and Application of Patient Care Technology: • Knowledge and skills in information management and patient care technology are critical in the delivery of quality patient care.	The baccalaureate program prepares the graduate to: 1. Demonstrate skills in using patient care technologies, information systems, and communication devices that support safe nursing practice. 2. Use telecommunication technologies to assist in effective communication in a variety of healthcare settings. 3. Apply safeguards and decision-making support tools embedded in patient care technologies and information systems to support a safe practice environment for both patients and healthcare workers. 4. Understand the use of CIS systems to document interventions related to achieving nurse sensitive outcomes. 5. Use standardized terminology in a care environment that reflects nursing's unique contribution to patient outcomes. 6. Evaluate data from all relevant sources, including technology, to inform the delivery of care. 7. Recognize the role of information technology in improving patient care outcomes and creating a safe care environment. 8. Uphold ethical standards related to data security, regulatory requirements, confidentiality, and clients' right to privacy. 9. Apply patient care technologies as appropriate to address the needs of a diverse patient population. 10. Advocate for the use of new patient care technologies for safe, quality care. 11. Recognize that re-design of workflow and care processes should precede implementation of care technology to facilitate nursing practice. 12. Participate in the evaluation of information systems in practice settings through policy and procedure development.
Master's Education (2011). Retrieved from http:// www.aacn.nche. edu/Education/pdf/ Master%27sEssentials11. pdf. (AACN, 2011)	Essential V: Informatics and Healthcare Technologies	The master's-degree program prepares the graduate to: 1. Analyze current and emerging technologies to support safe practice environments, and to optimize patient safety, cost-effectiveness, and health outcomes. 2. Evaluate outcome data using current communication technologies, information systems, and statistical principles to develop strategies to reduce risks and improve health outcomes. 3. Promote policies that incorporate ethical principles and standards for the use of health and information technologies. 4. Provide oversight and guidance in the integration of technologies to document patient care and improve patient outcomes. 5. Use information and communication technologies, resources, and principles of learning to teach patients and others. 6. Use current and emerging technologies in the care environment to support lifelong learning for self and others.

(continued)

TABLE 42.2	Information Management and Technology-Related Essentials for Nursing Education *(continued)*	
Doctoral Education for Advanced Nursing Practice (2006). http://www.aacn.nche.edu/DNP/pdf/Essentials.pdf. (AACN, 2006a)	IV. Information Systems/Technology and Patient Care Technology for the Improvement and Transformation of Healthcare	The DNP program prepares the graduate to: 1. Design, select, use, and evaluate programs that evaluate and monitor outcomes of care, care systems, and quality improvement including consumer use of healthcare information systems. 2. Analyze and communicate critical elements necessary to the selection, use, and evaluation of healthcare information systems and patient care technology. 3. Demonstrate the conceptual ability and technical skills to develop and execute an evaluation plan involving data extraction from practice information systems and databases. 4. Provide leadership in the evaluation and resolution of ethical and legal issues within healthcare systems relating to the use of information, information technology, communication networks, and patient care technology. 5. Evaluate consumer health information sources for accuracy, timeliness, and appropriateness.
Master's Education (2011). Retrieved from http://www.aacn.nche.edu/Education/pdf/Master%27sEssentials11.pdf. (AACN, 2011)	Essential V: Informatics and Healthcare Technologies	The master's-degree program prepares the graduate to: 1. Analyze current and emerging technologies to support safe practice environments, and to optimize patient safety, cost-effectiveness, and health outcomes. 2. Evaluate outcome data using current communication technologies, information systems, and statistical principles to develop strategies to reduce risks and improve health outcomes. 3. Promote policies that incorporate ethical principles and standards for the use of health and information technologies. 4. Provide oversight and guidance in the integration of technologies to document patient care and improve patient outcomes. 5. Use information and communication technologies, resources, and principles of learning to teach patients and others. 6. Use current and emerging technologies in the care environment to support lifelong learning for self and others.

INFORMATICS COMPETENCIES FOR PRACTICING CLINICIANS

The essentials and competencies recommended by the IOM, AACN, QSEN, and TIGER address essential competencies that need to be addressed in educational programs. A great deal of effort also has been made in developing more executable competency lists that can be used in practice settings.

American Nurses Association

Nursing Informatics. The Scope and Standard of Practice (ANA, 2008) addressed an NI-specific domain.

As discussed earlier, nursing informatics is an essential component for any nurse. The competencies contained in the NI Scope and Standards matrix were categorized into three overall areas: (1) computer literacy, (2) information literacy, and (3) professional development/leadership (ANA, 2008). Computer literacy addresses competencies in the area of the psychomotor use of computers and other technological equipment. Information literacy competencies are related to the ability to identify a need for information as well as the ability to find, evaluate, organize, and use the information effectively. Professional development and leadership competencies address ethical, procedural, safety, and management issues for informatics solutions in nursing practice, education, research, and administration.

The competency framework includes all nurses with different levels of NI education (e.g., nurses with and without graduate-level NI specialty education) and different NI functional areas (e.g., analysis, consultation). The categories of educational and functional roles within the competency matrix include:

- Beginning Nurse
- Experienced Nurse
- Informatics Specialist/Informatics Innovator
- Administration Analysis
- Compliance and Integrity Management
- Consultation
- Coordination
- Facilitation and Integration
- Development
- Educational and Professional Development
- Policy Development and Advocacy
- Research and Evaluation
- Integrated Areas

The ANA's Nursing Informatics Scope and Standards Revision Workgroup is working on the revision of the current Nursing Informatics Scope and Standard of Practice (ANA, 2014). The public comment period for the draft version closed on January 17, 2014.

TIGER Informatics Competencies Collaborative Recommendations

Upon extensive review of the literature, the TIGER Informatics Competency Collaborative (TICC) recommends specific informatics competencies for all practicing nurses and graduating nursing students (TIGER Informatics Competencies Collaborative, 2014c). The TIGER NI competencies model consists of the following three areas: (1) basic computer competencies; (2) information literacy; and (3) information management.

For the basic computer competencies, the TICC adopted the European Computer Driving License (ECDL) competencies and made its recommendations. The European Computer Driving License (ECDL)/International Computer Driving License (ICDL) is an internationally recognized Information and Communication Technology and digital literacy certification (The European Computer Driving Licence Foundation Ltd., 2014b). The ECDL certification program was developed through the Task Force of the Council of European Professional Informatics Societies in 1995. The new ECDL training program includes various

modules and the certificate program is run worldwide through a network of Accredited Test Centres (ATCs) (The European Computer Driving Licence Foundation Ltd., 2014a). The specific recommendations made by the TICC were based on the old ECDL/ICDL Syllabus 5.0.

eHealth Literacy

One area that needs further discussion in the competencies addressed by the AACN (American Nurses Association, 2008) and the TICC (TIGER Informatics Competencies Collaborative, 2014) is eHealth literacy. Norman and Skinner (2006a) defined eHealth literacy as "the ability to seek, find, understand, and appraise health information from electronic sources and apply the knowledge gained to addressing or solving a health problem" eHealth therefore requires combined literacy skills in several domains. Norman and Skinner (2006b) suggest six domains of eHealth literacy: traditional literacy, information literacy, media literacy, health literacy, computer literacy, and scientific literacy.

With the rapid growth in the use of eHealth at the global level, the concept of eHealth literacy has become more important than previous times (Chan & Kaufman, 2011; Norman & Skinner, 2006a). eHealth literacy is often discussed at the consumers' level because consumers in the current age can access a large amount of health information online and many of them may not be prepared to locate the information they need or evaluate the quality of the information found from different sources (Chan & Kaufman, 2011; Norman & Skinner, 2006b; Norman, 2011). Although nurses have much knowledge in general health than the public, eHealth literacy is also a concern for them. Unlike many younger generations, nurses who did not grow up with technologies may spend less time exploring online health information and may be less familiar with search functions. Considering the nurse's role as an educator for consumers and the heightened emphasis on evidence-based practice, nurses must be properly prepared to be eHealth literate.

NURSING INFORMATICS AS A SPECIALTY PROGRAM AT THE GRADUATE LEVEL

The ANA defines Nursing informatics (NI) as: *"a specialty that integrates nursing science, computer science, and information science to manage and communicate data, information, knowledge and wisdom in nursing practice. NI supports consumers, patients, nurses, and other providers in their decision-making in all roles and settings. This* support is accomplished through the use of information structures, information processes, and information technology" (ANA, 2008).

The NI Scope and Standards of Practice clearly differentiate between informatics nurse specialists (INSs) and informatics nurses (INs). The INSs are those formally prepared at the graduate level in informatics and INs are generalists who have gained on-the-job training in the field but do not have the educational preparation at the graduate level in an informatics-related area (ANA, 2008).

With the national emphasis on HIT education, various types of informatics-related educational programs are available at the graduate level, such as nursing informatics, healthcare informatics, bio-medical informatics, etc. Most informatics educational programs are moving toward online programs and/or hybrid (mainly online with some face-to-face classes) programs. The curriculum and credits vary a great deal depending on the program. The nursing informatics field also has unique characteristics. For instance, unlike other clinical nurses, the majority of the colleagues of the INSs are from other disciplines, such as computer science, information management, business (vendors), or administrators. The roles the INSs assume also vary (Sensmeier, 2007). In a 2009 Informatics Nurse Impact Survey (N = 432) conducted by the Healthcare Information and Management Systems Society (HIMSS), participants were asked to indicate the roles that nurses play with regard to IT (HIMSS, 2009).The findings showed the following results: user education (93%), system implementation (89%), user support (86%), workflow analysis (84%), getting buy-in from end users (80%), system design (79%), selection/placement of devices (70%), quality initiatives (69%), system optimization (62%), system selection (62%), database management/reporting (53%) (Note: only includes roles with greater than a 50% response rate). In a subsequent 2011 Nursing Informatics Workforce Survey (N = 660) (HIMSS, 2011), the majority of informaticians reported that their primarily work involves the area of systems implementation (57%) and systems development (53%), followed by Quality initiatives (31%).

Additionally, recent scientific discoveries in biomedical informatics and genomics, as well as the rapid growth in mHealth and eHealth, have made a significant impact on healthcare informatics and the roles of nursing informatics specialists. These changes led to the revision of the ANA's Nursing Informatics Scope and Standards of practice (ANA, 2014). The revision also addresses other recent trends in technology, such as knowledge representation, tools to manage public health concerns, and nanotechnologies.

Considering these varying roles and areas of practice, it is logical that each program may have a different emphasis or strength. Assurance of quality standards of each program, however, is particularly concerning considering that there is no regulatory body or speciality organization that could set standards for educational programs in nursing informatics.

CERTIFICATION IN NURSING INFORMATICS AND RELATED HIT

Currently the American Nurses Credentialing Center (ANCC), an accredited agency, offers the generalist nursing informatics certification (RN-BC) (ANCC, 2014b). The minimum academic degree required to take the examination for this certification is a bachelor's or higher degree in nursing or a bachelor's degree in a relevant field. The test content outline for the nursing informatics certification examination can be found on ANCC's Web site (http://www.nursecredentialing.org/InformaticsTCOs) (ANCC, 2014c). The main content as of October 2014 includes:

1. Foundations of Practice (71 items, 47.33%), which includes the Scope and Standards of Informatics Practice, ethics, privacy and confidentiality, regulation and policy, management of data, healthcare industry trends, team building, conflict management, computer science, information science, cognitive science, nursing science, testing and evaluation methodologies, workflow processing, and theories that support the NI practice.

2. System Design Life Cycle (SDLC) (39 items, 26.00%) which includes the phases and tasks contained within the SDLC process along with the NI leadership role in managing the process.

3. Data Management and Healthcare Technology (40 items, 26.67%), which includes the current evidence about data to knowledge, data mining, and management.

As discussed previously, nursing informaticians' primary responsibilities vary a great deal and their work environments also differ (e.g., hospitals, vendors, consulting firms). Each job or setting may require a different certificate, such as project manager, information administrator. Based on the 2011 HIMSS Nursing Informatics Workforce Survey, 19% of the respondents reported having a certificate in nursing informatics offered through the ANCC (HIMSS, 2011). Many survey participants reported having a certificate(s) in other areas such as Certified Professional in Healthcare Information & Management System (CPHIMS) offered by HIMSS (HIMSS, n.d.). Table 42.3 summarizes information for selected certifications relevant to nursing informatics.

TABLE 42.3	Selected Certifications Relevant to Nursing Informatics		
Certifications	Organization	Qualification	Requirements	URL
NI certificate	AACN	Hold a bachelor's or higher degree in nursing or a bachelor's degree in a relevant field.	1. Hold a current, active RN license within a state or territory of the United States or the professional, legally recognized equivalent in another country. International Applicants: Learn about additional requirements for candidates outside the United States. 2. Have practiced the equivalent of two years full time as a registered nurse. 3. Have completed 30 hours of continuing education in informatics nursing within the last three years. 4. Meet one of the following practice hour requirements: • Have practiced a minimum of 2000 hours in informatics nursing within the last 3 years. • Have practiced a minimum of 1000 hours in informatics nursing in the last three years and completed a minimum of 12 semester hours of academic credit in informatics courses that are part of a graduate-level informatics nursing program. • Have completed a graduate program in informatics nursing containing a minimum of 200 hours of faculty-supervised practicum in informatics nursing	http://www.nursecredentialing.org/Informatics-Eligibility.aspx
Certified Professional in Healthcare Information & Management Systems (CPHIMS)	HIMSS	Baccalaureate degree	Five years of associated information and management systems experience, three (3) of those years in healthcare.	http://www.himss.org/health-it-certification?navItemNumber=17564
		Graduate degree	Three years of associated information and management systems experience, two (2) of those years in healthcare.	

Certification	Organization	Degree	Requirements	URL
Registered Health Information Administrator (RHIA®)	AHIMA	Baccalaureate degree	Successfully complete the academic requirements, at the baccalaureate level, of an HIM program accredited by the Commission on Accreditation for Health Informatics and Information Management Education. Or Graduate from an HIM program approved by a foreign association with which AHIMA has a reciprocity agreement.	http://www.ahima.org/certification/RHIA
Physician board—clinical informatics (as a comparison to nursing discipline)	The American Board of Preventive Medicine	MD	1. Graduation from medical school that was accredited at the time of graduation, graduation from a school in Canada or outside the United States that has been deemed satisfactory to the board 2. Unrestricted and currently validated license 3. Clinical year of post-graduate clinical training 4. Coursework completion of courses required for a Master's of Public Health or equivalent Master's or Doctoral post-graduate Degree 5. Residency of no less than two years 6. Full-time training or in practice for at least one of the three years prior to application	http://www.theabpm.org/public/infobook.pdf
Project Management Certifications	PMI	A secondary degree (high school diploma, associate's degree, or the global equivalent) Or A four-year degree (bachelor's degree or the global equivalent)	1. At least five years of project management experience 2. 7500 hours leading and directing projects 3. 35 hours of project management education Or 1. At least three years of project management experience 2. 4500 hours leading and directing projects 3. 35 hours of project management education	http://www.pmi.org/en/Certification/Program-Management-Professional-PgMP.aspx
Project Management Professional (specific example)				

INFORMATICS COMPETENCIES FOR FACULTY MEMBERS

In the past few years, there have been significant changes in nursing education. (AACN, 2008, 2011). Informatics competency has been addressed as a vital component in those changes. IOM's Future of Nursing report also emphasized that efficient management of data and a robust informatics infrastructure are components in transforming the nursing profession (IOM, 2010). Additionally, the current emphasis on meaningful use of EHR demands that nurses be competent in managing health data and information. These changes also require nursing faculty member be competent in healthcare informatics. The majority of current nursing faculty members also face challenge in a way instruction is delivered. Previously, most nursing education was delivered via classroom face-to-face settings. However, with the exponentially growing information communication technologies, more instruction is being delivered using online format. Current popularity with social networking programs has added additional complexity to the current online learning environment.

To address these pressing needs, the National League for Nursing Issues call for Faculty Development and Curricular Initiatives in Informatics (National League for Nursing, 2008) The RWJ also supported QSEN Phase IV specifically focusing on the goal of building capacity for nursing faculty members who are competent in the six QSEN competencies and to serve as peer mentor for other faculty members (QSEN, 2012). The AACN also plays a major role in building this capacity. For example, in 2012, AACN sponsored the QSEN Nursing Informatics Deep Dive Workshop (DDW) in San Francisco Bay Area to build develop, pilot, and evaluate a curriculum to improve the informatics knowledge and competencies of nursing faculty and health system educators who provide informatics training (AACN, 2012). All materials are available for use in the classroom through the QSEN Web site.

Simulation-Based Learning

Use of high-fidelity simulation has become the gold standard in current nursing education (Burns, O'Donnell, & Artman, 2010; Schiavenato, 2009). The purpose of simulation in clinical settings is to replicate the important aspects of a clinical situation where students or clinicians can work to gain knowledge and experience (Jeffries & Rogers, 2007; Nehring, 2009). Most nursing schools have multiple high-tech simulation labs including high fidelity simulators. Those labs provide students with various simulated clinical settings. For instance, the University of Maryland School of Nursing has an entire simulated hospital in its school consisting of 24 labs including an operating suite, a community/home healthcare lab, and a diagnostic laboratory. To augment the simulation environment, some schools use an academic version of the EHR system (AllBusiness.com, 2009; Borycki et al., 2009; Joe et al., 2009; Otto & Kushniruk, 2009). Implementing the EHR in simulation labs allows students to have an opportunity to develop competencies in using HIT before they go into the clinical setting. In addition, most EHRs have decision support systems which could significantly augment students' learning. When schools implement these academic EHR systems, they must have a thorough plan and a multitude of resources. For instance, the school must have network infrastructures that can support the program, and have a designated project manager who is familiar with system deployment. There will be a great deal of work in developing use cases and building tables in the system, which also requires the clinical faculty members' participation. It will be necessary to educate faculty members about the system since they must be competent to teach classes using the EHR. Policies and procedures for using the system within the lab must be developed and clearly communicated to the students before the system is deployed. The project manager must also consider various human factors and ergonomic issues, as well as system characteristics (Cacciabue & Cacciabue, 2004; Nielsen, 1993).

Inter-disciplinary Collaboration

As emphasized by the NIH Roadmap initiative, the advancement of science can be made more effective by combining inter-disciplinary knowledge and skills (National Institutes of Health -Office of Portfolio Analysis and Strategic Initiatives, 2006). The recent NIH Clinical Translational Science Awards (CTSAs) have stimulated collaboration among disciplines and impacted both the clinicians' and researchers' paradigm in approaching research, practice, and education. Most of the changes have been mainly addressed in research and science fields thus far (Chesla, 2008; Sampselle, Pienta, & Markel, 2010; Woods & Magyary, 2010). However, nursing education must embrace this initiative and prepare both our students and clinicians. One example of an approach could involve EHRs. EHRs can be an excellent communication and collaboration tool among inter-professional care providers in healthcare settings. Class projects and papers that incorporate data and information from EHRs can provide students the opportunity to exercise skill sets required for inter-disciplinary collaboration which is an important competency within informatics. When a HIT system is implemented in a hospital setting, various professionals (e.g., IT professionals, clinicians, administrators, vendors, lawyers) have to work together as a team for a prolonged period, and the system often affects many departments and professionals concurrently. Upon the completion of system deployment, the systems will continue to require management and upgrades. Learning about inter-disciplinary collaboration is critical in nursing education, and is becoming more important as technology becomes more advanced and as healthcare becomes more complex.

Informatics Competencies for Faculty Members

Innovative technologies in teaching and learning can produce optimal outcomes only when the instructors are competent in using those technologies. Previously we discussed the essential educational components needed to ensure nursing students' and practicing nurses' competencies in using healthcare information technologies and managing information. Current students who grow up with technologies often outpace their faculty members in using technologies (Curran, Sheets, Kirkpatrick, & Bauldoff, 2007). When faculty members need to teach online class, they also have to learn about not only using technology but also re-orient themselves to a whole new way of teaching the content. For instance, the way that online students respond may be different from the students who take face-to-face classes. Faculty members must be properly supported to fully adopt the newest technologies (Griffin-Sobel et al., 2010). Some continuing education modalities for faculty members include half-day workshops, short refresher courses before the beginning of each semester, or online self-learning modules. If the school offers many online classes, a sufficient number of instructional design specialists should be a part of the staff.

Faculty members who teach informatics must have a specific expertise in the field. With the heightened awareness of IT in healthcare technologies and the revised essentials for the baccalaureate and the DNP curriculums, increasing numbers of informatics classes are being required as core courses in nursing programs. The AACN's decision to migrate the ANP programs to the DNP level further accelerates this need. However, there is a significant shortage of faculty members who have an expertise in healthcare informatics and who can teach students. More doctorally prepared informatics faculty members with a proper education/training are needed in NI education.

CONCLUSION

Information technology has revolutionized current healthcare. Consumers now can access enormous amounts of health information online even before they come to the hospital. Healthcare providers and students can access evidence-based health information right at the bedside. However, adoption of EHRs in healthcare has been slow, resulting in missed opportunities to provide safer and better quality care. Recently, the government has made significant efforts to implement EHRs nationwide to deliver safer care and improving the efficiency of healthcare delivery. These changes in healthcare delivery present multiple exciting opportunities for nursing education. In addition, with the advancement of information communication technology, face-to-face classes are being replaced by online classes, and high-tech and high-fidelity simulation-based nursing education has become a standard. New generations of nursing students are expected to be informatics competent. This chapter reviewed major HIT-related changes in our current healthcare system and efforts made by nursing organizations to reform the nursing curriculum. In the past decade, the nursing profession has made great advancements in transforming nursing practice, education, and research. Recent emphasis on inter-disciplinary collaboration will further accelerate its progress.

REFERENCES

AllBusiness.com. (2009). *University of Pennsylvania School of Nursing and Eclipsys Form Academic Partnership to bring HIT to nursing education curriculum.* Retrieved from http://www.businesswire.com/news/home/20090114005680/en/University-Pennsylvania-School-Nursing-Eclipsys-Form-Academic#. UupiOD1dXTo. Accessed on January 30, 2014.

American Association of Colleges of Nursing. (1994). *The essentials of master's education for advanced practice nursing.* Retrieved from http://www.aacn.nche.edu/education/mastessn.htm. Accessed on January 30, 2014.

American Association of Colleges of Nursing. (2006a). *The essentials of doctoral education for advanced nursing practice.* Retrieved from http://www.aacn.nche.edu/DNP/pdf/Essentials.pdf. Accessed on January 30, 2014.

American Association of Colleges of Nursing. (2006b). Hallmarks of quality and patient safety: Recommended baccalaureate competencies and curricular guidelines to ensure high-quality and safe patient care. *Journal of Professional Nursing, 22*(6), 329–330. doi:10.1016/j.profnurs.2006.10.005.

American Association of Colleges of Nursing. (2008). *The essentials of baccalaureate education for professional nursing practice.* Retrieved from http://www.aacn.nche.edu/education/pdf/BaccEssentials08.pdf. Accessed on January 30, 2014.

American Association of Colleges of Nursing. (2011). Task force on the essentials of master's education in nursing. Retrieved from http://www.aacn.nche.edu/members-only/meeting-highlights/2011/spring/MastersEssentials.pdf. Accessed on May 29, 2014.

American Association of Colleges of Nursing. (2012). *QSEN informatics initiative*. Retrieved from http://www.aacn.nche.edu/qsen-informatics. Accessed on May 29, 2014.

American Association of Colleges of Nursing. (2014). *The doctor of nursing practice (DNP)*. Retrieved from http://www.aacn.nche.edu/dnp. Accessed on January 30, 2014.

American Nurses Association. (2008). *Nursing informatics: Scope and standards of practice*. Silver Spring, MD: American Nurses Association.

American Nurses Association. (2014). *Nursing informatics: Scope and standards of practice* (2nd ed.). (draft). Retrieved from http://www.nursingworld.org/Comment-Nursing-Informatics. Accessed on January 30, 2014.

American Nurses Credentialing Center. (2014a). *The Magnet Recognition Program® overview*. Retrieved from http://www.nursecredentialing.org/Magnet/ProgramOverview.aspx. Accessed on January 30, 2014.

American Nurses Credentialing Center. (2014b). *Nurse credentialing: Informatics nursing*. Retrieved from http://www.nursecredentialing.org/InformaticsNursing. Accessed on January 30, 2014.

American Nurses Credentialing Center. (2014c). *Nursing informatics test content outlines*. Retrieved from http://www.nursecredentialing.org/InformaticsTCOs. Accessed on January 30, 2014.

Blumenthal, D. (2009). Stimulating the adoption of health information technology. *The New England Journal of Medicine, 360*(15), 1477–1479. doi:10.1056/NEJMp0901592.

Blumenthal, D., & Tavenner, M. (2010). The "meaningful use" regulation for electronic health records. *The New England Journal of Medicine, 363*(6), 501–504. doi:NEJMp1006114.

Borycki, E. M., Kushniruk, A. W., Joe, R., Armstrong, B., Otto, T., Ho, K., ... Frisch, N. (2009). The University of Victoria interdisciplinary electronic health record educational portal. *Studies in Health Technology and Informatics, 143*, 49–54. doi:10.3233/978-1-58603-979-0-49.

Burns, H. K., O'Donnell, J., & Artman, J. (2010). High-fidelity simulation in teaching problem solving to 1st-year nursing students: A novel use of the nursing process. *Clinical Simulation in Nursing, 6*(3), e87–e95. doi:10.1016/j.ecns.2009.07.005.

Cacciabue, P. C., & Cacciabue, C. (2004). *Guide to applying human factors methods*. London: Springer.

Centers for Medicare and Medicaid Services. (2010). *HIPAA - General information: Overview*. Retrieved from http://www.cms.hhs.gov/HIPAAGenInfo/01_Overview.asp. Accessed on January 30, 2014.

Centers for Medicare & Medicaid Services. (2013). *Meaningful use*. Retrieved from http://www.cms.gov/Regulations-and-Guidance/Legislation/EHRIncentivePrograms/Meaningful_Use.html. Accessed on October 7, 2013.

Chan, C. V., & Kaufman, D. R. (2011). A framework for characterizing eHealth literacy demands and barriers. *Journal of Medical Internet Research, 13*(4), e94. doi:10.2196/jmir.1750.

Chesla, C. A. (2008). Translational research: Essential contributions from interpretive nursing science. *Research in Nursing & Health, 31*(4), 381–390. doi:10.1002/nur.20267.

Committee on Quality of Health Care in America & Institute of Medicine. (2001). *Crossing the quality chasm: A new health system for the 21st century*. Washington, DC: National Academy Press.

Cronenwett, L., Sherwood, G., Barnsteiner, J., Disch, J., Johnson, J., Mitchell, P., ... Warren, J. (2007). Quality and safety education for nurses. *Nursing Outlook, 55*(3), 122–131. doi:10.1016/j.outlook.2007.02.006.

Cronenwett, L., Sherwood, G., & Gelmon, S. B. (2009). Improving quality and safety education: The QSEN learning collaborative. *Nursing Outlook, 57*(6), 304–312. doi:10.1016/j.outlook.2009.09.004.

Cronenwett, L., Sherwood, G., Pohl, J., Barnsteiner, J., Moore, S., Sullivan, D. T., ... Warren, J. (2009). Quality and safety education for advanced nursing practice. *Nursing Outlook, 57*(6), 338–348. doi:10.1016/j.outlook.2009.07.009.

Curran, C., Sheets, D., Kirkpatrick, B., & Bauldoff, G. S. (2007). Virtual patients support point-of-care nursing education. *Nursing Management, 38*(12), 27–33. doi:10.1097/01.NUMA.0000303868.95890.1e.

Dycus, P., & McKeon, L. (2009). Using QSEN to measure quality and safety knowledge, skills, and attitudes of experienced pediatric oncology nurses: An international study. *Quality Management in Health Care, 18*(3), 202–208. doi:10.1097/QMH.0b013e3181aea256.

Emani, S., Yamin, C. K., Peters, E., Karson, A. S., Lipsitz, S. R., Wald, J. S., ... Bates, D. W. (2012). Patient perceptions of a personal health record: A test of the diffusion of innovation model. *Journal of Medical Internet Research, 5; 14*(6): e150. doi:10.2196/jmir.2278.

Gassert, C. (2000). Academic preparation in nursing informatics. In M. J. Ball, K. J. Hannah, S. K. Newbold, & J. V. Douglas (Eds.), *Nursing informatics: Where caring and technology meet* (pp. 15–32). New York, NY: Springer.

Griffin-Sobel, J. P., Acee, A., Sharoff, L., Cobus-Kuo, L., Woodstock-Wallace, A., & Dornbaum, M. (2010). A transdisciplinary approach to faculty development in nursing education technology. *Nursing Education Perspectives, 31*(1), 41–43.

Healthcare Information and Management Systems Society (HIMSS). (2009). *HIMSS 2009 informatics nurse impact survey*. Retrieved from http://www.himss.org/files/HIMSSorg/content/files/HIMSS2009NursingInformaticsImpactSurveyFullResults.pdf. Accessed on January 30, 2014.

Healthcare Information and Management Systems Society (HIMSS). (2011). *2011 HIMSS nursing informatics workforce survey*. Retrieved from http://www.himss.org/files/HIMSSorg/content/files/2011HIMSSNursingInformaticsWorkforceSurvey.pdf. Accessed on January 30, 2014.

Healthcare Information and Management Systems Society (HIMSS). (n.d.). *Certified Professional in Healthcare Information & Management Systems (CPHIMS)*. Retrieved from http://www.himss.org/health-it-certification/cphims?navItemNumber=13647. Accessed on January 30, 2014.

Hebda, T., & Calderone, T. L. (2010). What nurse educators need to know about the TIGER Initiative. Technology Informatics Guiding Education Reform. *Nurse Educator, 35*(2), 56–60. doi:10.1097/NNE.0b013e3181ced83d.

Institute of Medicine. (2010). *The future of nursing: Leading Change, advancing health*. Washington, DC: The National Academies Press.

Institute of Medicine Committee on Health Education Profession Summit. (2002). *Health professions education: A bridge to quality*. Washington, DC: National Academy Press.

Jeffries, P., & Rogers, K. (2007). Theoretical frameworks for simulation design. In P. Jeffries (Ed.), *Simulation in nursing education: From conceptualization to evaluation* (pp. 21–33). New York, NY: National League of Nursing.

Joe, R. S., Kushniruk, A. W., Borycki, E. M., Armstrong, B., Otto, T., & Ho, K. (2009). Bringing electronic patient records into health professional education: Software architecture and implementation. *Studies in Health Technology and Informatics, 150*, 888–892.

National Institutes of Health. (2006). *NIH roadmap for medical research*. Retrieved from http://pubs.niaaa.nih.gov/publications/arh311/12-13.pdf.

National League for Nursing. (2008). *National League for Nursing issues call for faculty development and curricular initiatives in informatics*. Retrieved from http://www.nln.org/newsreleases/informatics_release_052908.htm. Accessed on January 30, 2014.

Nehring, W. M. (2009). History of simulation in nursing. In W. M. Nehring & F. R. Lashley (Eds.), *High-fidelity patient simulation in nursing education*. Sudbury, MA: Jones & Bartlett Publishers.

Newhouse, R. P., Dearholt, S. L., Poe, S. S., Pugh, L. C., & White, K. M. (2007). *Johns Hopkins nursing Evidence-based practice model and guidelines*. Indianapolis, IN: Sigma Theta Tau International.

Nielsen, J. (1993). *Usability engineering*. San Diego, CA: Morgan Kaufmann.

Norman, C. (2011). eHealth literacy 2.0: Problems and opportunities with an evolving concept. *Journal of Medical Internet Research, 13*(4), e125. doi:10.2196/jmir.2035.

Norman, C. D., & Skinner, H. A. (2006a). eHEALS: The eHealth Literacy Scale. *Journal of Medical Internet Research, 8*(4), e27. doi:10.2196/jmir.8.4.e27.

Norman, C. D., & Skinner, H. A. (2006b). eHealth literacy: Essential skills for consumer health in a networked world. *Journal of Medical Internet Research, 8*(2), e9. doi:10.2196/jmir.8.2.e9.

Office of the National Coordinator for Health Information Technology. (n.d.). *What is a patient portal?* Retrieved from http://www.healthit.gov/providers-professionals/faqs/what-patient-portal. Accessed on January 30, 2014.

Otto, A., & Kushniruk, A. (2009). Incorporation of medical informatics and information technology as core components of undergraduate medical education - time for change! *Studies in Health Technology and Informatics, 143*, 62–67. doi:10.3233/978-1-58603-979-0-62.

QSEN. (2012). *Graduate-level QSEN competencies: Knowledge, skills and attitudes*. Retrieved from http://www.aacn.nche.edu/faculty/qsen/competencies.pdf. Accessed on January 30, 2014.

Quality and Safety Education for Nurses (QSEN). (2010). *Quality and safety education for nurses*. Retrieved from http://www.qsen.org/. Accessed on January 30, 2014.

Sampselle, C. M., Pienta, K. J., & Markel, D. S. (2010). The CTSA mandate: Are we there yet? *Research and Theory for Nursing Practice, 24*(1), 64–73. doi:10.1891/1541-6577.24.1.64.

Schiavenato, M. (2009). Reevaluating simulation in nursing education: Beyond the human patient simulator. *Journal of Nursing Education, 48*(7), 388–394. doi:10.3928/01484834-20090615-06.

Sensmeier, J. (2007). Survey demonstrates importance of nurse informaticist role in health information technology design and implementation. *CIN: Computers, Informatics, Nursing, 25*, 180–182. doi:10.1097/01.NCN.0000270048.90776.bb.

Technology Informatics Guiding Education Reform. (2009). *Collaborating to integrate evidence and informatics into nursing practice and education: An executive summary*. Retrieved from http://www.tigersummit.com/uploads/TIGER_Collaborative_Exec_Summary_040509.pdf. Accessed on January 30, 2014.

Technology Informatics Guiding Educational Reform (TIGER). (2014a). *About TIGER*. Retrieved from http://www.tigersummit.com/About_Us.html. Accessed on January 30, 2014.

Technology Informatics Guiding Educational Reform (TIGER). (2014b). *TIGER Initiative working on Phase III*. Retrieved from http://www.tigersummit.com/. Accessed on January 30, 2014.

Technology Informatics Guiding Educational Reform (TIGER) Informatics Competencies Collaborative. (2014c). *Technology Informatics Guiding Educational Reform (TIGER) Informatics Competencies Collaborative (TICC): Final report*. Retrieved from http://tigercompetencies.pbworks.com/f/TICC_Final.pdf. Accessed on January 30, 2014.

The European Computer Driving Licence Foundation Ltd. (2014a). *ECDL: How we certify*. Retrieved from http://www.ecdl.org/programmes/index.jsp?p=102&n=2373. Accessed on January 30, 2014.

The European Computer Driving Licence Foundation Ltd. (2014b). *European Computer Driving License (ECDL)/*

International Computer Driving License (ICDL) Foundation. Retrieved from http://www.ecdl.org/programmes/ecdl_icdl. Accessed on January 30, 2014.

The Office of National Coordinator. (n.d.-a). *EHR incentives & certification*. Retrieved from http://www.healthit.gov/providers-professionals/meaningful-use-definition-objectives. Accessed on January 30, 2014.

The Office of National Coordinator. (n.d.-b). *Health information exchange (HIE)*. Retrieved from http://www.healthit.gov/HIE. Accessed on January 30, 2014.

University of Wisconsin Oshkosh. (2009). *Plane crash disaster triage UW Oshkosh accelerated nursing second life exercise*. Retrieved from http://www.youtube.com/watch?v=pDX6-52y-QE. Accessed on January 30, 2014.

U.S. Bureau of Labor Statistics. (2010). *Employment projections: Labor force (demographic) data*. Retrieved from http://www.bls.gov/emp/ep_data_labor_force.htm. Accessed on January 30, 2014.

U.S. Department of Health & Human Services. (2010). *Privacy and security standards*. Retrieved from http://www.cms.gov/Regulations-and-Guidance/HIPAA-Administrative-Simplification/HIPAAGenInfo/PrivacyandSecurityStandards.html. Accessed on January 30, 2014.

U.S. Department of Health & Human Services. (2013). *Omnibus HIPAA rulemaking*. Retrieved from http://www.hhs.gov/ocr/privacy/hipaa/administrative/omnibus/index.html. Accessed on January 30, 2014.

U.S. Department of Health & Human Services. (n.d.). *Workforce development programs*. Retrieved from http://www.healthit.gov//providers-professionals/health-it-education-opportunities. Accessed on January 30, 2014.

U.S. DHHS Health Resources and Services Administration. (2010). *The registered Nurse population: Findings from the 2008 National Sample Survey of Registered Nurses*. Retrieved from http://bhpr.hrsa.gov/healthworkforce/rnsurveys/rnsurveyfinal.pdf. Accessed on January 30, 2014.

Woods, N. F., & Magyary, D. L. (2010). Translational research: Why nursing's interdisciplinary collaboration is essential. *Research and Theory for Nursing Practice, 24*(1), 9–24. doi:10.1891/1541-6577.24.1.9.

43

The TIGER Initiative

Michelle R. Troseth

• OBJECTIVES

1. Discuss the TIGER Initiative agenda.
2. Describe the evolution of the TIGER Initiative.
3. Describe examples of how The TIGER Initiative has impacted practice and education reform by providing resources to advance the integration of technology into practice, education, and consumer engagement.

• KEY WORDS

Decade of healthcare technology
Grassroots effort
Technology Informatics Guiding Education Reform
Invitational summit
Collaborative Workgroups
Virtual Learning Environment
The TIGER Initiative Foundation

This chapter describes a wonderful story of what can occur when individuals committed to a common cause come together and take action. The best part is that this story has no ending ... the roots of the **TIGER (Technology Informatics Guiding Education Reform) Initiative** is already having a ripple effect across the healthcare industry and the work that is being accomplished through TIGER is now being cited, as it will continue to be in the future, as being a significant catalyst for change in addressing the call for healthcare transformation by the Institute of Medicine (Institute of Medicine, 2001, 2003). These two landmark reports addressed major changes needed for both practicing clinicians and educators. For practicing clinicians, the first report notes that, "The use of tools to organize and deliver care has lagged far behind biomedical and clinical knowledge. Carefully designed, evidence-based care processes, supported by automated clinical information and decision support systems, offer the greatest promise of achieving the best outcomes from care for chronic conditions. Systems must facilitate the application of scientific knowledge to practice and provide clinicians with the tools and supports necessary to deliver evidence-based care consistently and safely." (IOM, 2001, p. 12). For educators, the second report called for new ways for health professions to be educated and it identified five core competencies for all healthcare professionals: *provide patient-centered care, work in inter-disciplinary teams, employ evidence-based practice, apply quality improvement, and utilize informatics* (IOM, 2003, p. 3). Both of these reports, along with the federal efforts described below to address the need for widespread health information technology adoption, were the catalysts for the beginning of the TIGER Initiative, and its continued evolution.

THE DECADE OF HEALTHCARE TECHNOLOGY (2004)

National HIT Agenda

In early 2004, U.S. President George W. Bush declared the *Decade for Health Information Technology* and created the Office of the National Coordinator of Health Information Technology. In May 2004, Secretary of Health and Human Services, Tommy Thompson, appointed Dr. David Brailer as the first National Health Information Technology Coordinator. This was an exciting time for health professions committed to the transformational role health information could play in substantial improvements in safety, efficiency, and other health reform efforts. In July 2004, Brailer convened the first national health information technology summit in Washington, DC, and launched the strategy to give U.S. citizens the benefits of an electronic health record within a 10-year timeframe.

Where Is Nursing?

A very important observation was made at this first Office of the National Coordinator (ONC) event. The nation's 3 million nurses who comprise up to 55% of the workforce were not represented and/or clearly identified as an important integral part of achieving the ONC vision and strategy. It left many begging the question, "Where is nursing?" There was also a keen awareness that without nursing engagement not only was the National HIT Agenda at risk, but nursing would be at risk by not acting on a wonderful opportunity to significantly advance the agenda to transform practice and education with evidence and informatics. In his books, *Leading Change* (Kotter, 1996) and *A sense of urgency* (Kotter, 2008), the author describes the impact that having *a true sense of urgency* can have on large-scale effective change. When the sense of urgency is as high as possible and among as many people as possible, the greater the successes of leading transformational change efforts will be. Leaders in nursing realized the sense of urgency to begin a grassroots effort following this initial HIT summit and moved to birth a movement that would assure nursing was at the table and were key stakeholders/advocates as health information technologies were integrated into the nation's healthcare delivery systems and academic programs.

THE BIRTH OF THE TIGER INITIATIVE (2005)

Challenges and Opportunities Facing Nursing

The grassroots leadership efforts began to take action and network with others to determine first steps and gather key individuals to attend the first TIGER meeting. The first official TIGER gathering was held on January 14, 2005, hosted by Johns Hopkins University School of Nursing. A diverse group of nursing leaders across the country engaged in conversation about the skills and knowledge needed by the healthcare provider/nurse in the twenty-first Century. Trends and patterns on topics such as basic skills, critical thinking, change management, evidence-based practice, knowledge-workers, curriculum integration, professional practice, inter-disciplinary collaborative practice, leadership, global military systems, national standards, clinical documentation, public policy, and more emerged as current challenges and opportunities facing nurses during this informatics revolution. It was identified that the opportunity was more than just tackling "informatics"—the focus needed to be more on quality care and evidence-based care. There was a unique window of opportunity for TIGER to build on the successes of informatics and to connect more key stakeholders in an effort to move a bigger whole forward in guiding true transformation. Lastly, TIGER needed to tap the power of the 3 million nurses in the workforce by finding ways of getting many of them engaged to move the TIGER agenda forward. It was decided, at that time, to hold an invitational summit in an effort to bring together a diverse group of stakeholders (professional organizations, governmental organizations, technology vendors, informatics specialists, etc.) to further advance the sense of urgency and action needed to assure that nurses were able to provide safe, efficient, and patient-centered care to all. At that time, questions were raised concerning whether or not the summit should include all disciplines to help meet the IOM aims and competencies. While this was recognized as being very important, there was consensus that it was critical to begin with moving the nursing workforce forward first and then to expand out as recommendations were made from the summit.

Setting the Vision for TIGER

The following vision statement and expected outcomes were developed to guide the early stages of the TIGER Initiative:

TIGER Vision
- Allow informatics tools, principles, theories, and practices to be used by nurses to make healthcare safer, effective, efficient, patient-centered, timely, and equitable.

- Interweave enabling technologies transparently into nursing practice and education, making information technology the stethoscope for the twenty-first century.

TIGER Expected Outcomes

- Publish a Summit report, including Summit findings and exemplars of excellence.

- Establish guidelines for organizations to follow as they integrate informatics knowledge, skills, and abilities into academic and practice settings.

- Set an agenda whereby the nursing organizations specify what they plan to do to bridge the quality chasm via information technology strategies.

THE TIGER SUMMIT (2006)

See Fig. 43.1.

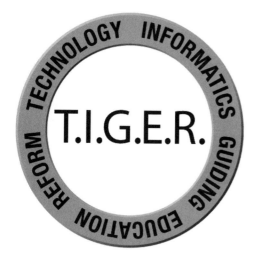

• **FIGURE 43.1.** TIGER Summit Logo. (Reproduced, with permission, from Healthcare Information and Management Systems Society [HIMSS].)

The Invitational Summit

To prepare for the invitational summit, a program committee was formed that planned for over a year for the event. A fundraising committee was also formed to secure funds to support the TIGER Summit and expected outcomes. Over 25 diverse sponsors made contributions to the summit and grants were received from the Agency for Healthcare Research and Quality (AHRQ), Robert Wood Johnson Foundation (RWJF), and the National Library of Medicine (NLM).

The invitational summit was held at the end of October in 2006 and was hosted by the Uniformed Services University of the Health Sciences in Bethesda, MD. Over 100 leaders from the nation's nursing administration, practice, education, informatics, technology organizations, governmental agencies, and other key stakeholders participated in the very interactive two-day summit. External facilitators from Bonfire Communications created an open-space experience that included small and large group dialogs; unique graphic art to capture the vision, outcomes of the dialogs and action plans; and the use of an audience response system (ARS) to capture current realities as well as gain consensus. To stimulate imagination and thinking, a Gallery Walk experience was done on Day One in which participants were able to "walk through" and review cutting-edge technology and clinical decision support systems being utilized in healthcare environments today. The TIGER Executive and Program Committee felt that it was important to build on some national exemplars in practice and education today. A total of seven national exemplars were shared with time for questions and answers from participants.

10-Year Vision and Three-Year Action Steps

The entire summit was focused on creating movement toward consensus on a 10-year vision and a three-year action plan. The 10-year vision was more clearly evolved by doing collective work around seven pillars and then content streaming the patterns and most salient points. With the seven pillars and rich content as its framework, a three-year action plan was identified to achieve the 10-year vision of evidence and informatics transforming practice and education. This required intense group work and collaboration amongst the participants.

The last Call for Action before participants left the summit was for each leader of a participating organization to identify definable action plan goals that they could take back to their organization. Each participant signed the "TIGER Commitment Wall" to show their commitment to the TIGER Vision and Action Plans as well as to continue to promote and engage others in the TIGER Initiative.

Following the TIGER Summit a Web site was established to record the several events and actions to the TIGER Summit as well as to post new information. In addition, the summit report *Evidence and Informatics Transforming Nursing: 3-Year Action Steps toward a 10-Year Vision* (2007) was developed and widely distributed via a published report as well as via a pdf download from the Web site (Technology Informatics Guiding Education Reform, 2007). The report provided a summary of the summit as well as recommendations for specific stakeholder groups: Professional Nursing Organizations, Academic Institutions, Information Technology, Government and

Policy Makers, Healthcare Delivery Organizations, Health Information Management Professionals/Health Science Libraries. Leaders from five major nursing organizations including the American Colleges of Nursing, American Nurses Association, American Organization of Nurse Executives, National League for Nursing, and Sigma Theta Tau International affirmed their commitment and need for the profession to continue to support the TIGER Initiative.

THE TIGER COLLABORATIVE WORKGROUPS (2007–2008)

Several months after the summit, and after several follow-up meetings with the TIGER Executive Steering Committee, it was decided to move into phase II of TIGER. Building off the summit pillar and action plans, nine key collaboratives were identified to dig deeper and tap a broader engagement from the nursing community to address the recommendations made at the summit. Each collaborative was assigned co-leaders to facilitate the workgroup as well as write a final report and share the workgroup final findings and recommendations. A summary of the purpose, outcomes, and access to the published reports can be found in Table 43.1.

THE TIGER INITIATIVE TODAY (2009–2014)

The TIGER Initiative Foundation

The past five years have continued to demonstrate continuous momentum toward the 10-year vision. The years 2009–2010 kept critical TIGER leader volunteers busy with sharing the collaborative reports as well as seeking new opportunities for further TIGER engagements with key stakeholder, nursing, and other inter-disciplinary professional organizations. During this time the foundation was being laid for building out a Virtual Learning Environment (VLE) including collaborating partners such as the National Library of Medicine and the Uniform Services University of the Health Sciences. In July 2011, the TIGER Initiative Foundation was formed as a 501(c)(3) organization operating for charitable, educational, and scientific purposes. This was a significant milestone for TIGER as it provided a structure to strategically grow TIGER including having a dedicated Senior Director and full Board of Directors. A new TIGER Web site, www.thetigerinitiative.org, was established that has been a central hub for connecting TIGERs and sharing the many TIGER activities that occur with the more than 1500 volunteers that have been engaged with the TIGER Initiative.

Refreshed TIGER Vision and Mission

The first priority of the new Board of Directors was to re-evaluate the TIGER vision and mission. The new TIGER Vision is *to enable nurses and interprofessional colleagues to use informatics and emerging technologies to make healthcare safer, more effective, efficient, patient-centered, timely and equitable by interweaving evidence and technology seamlessly into practice, education and research fostering a learning healthcare system* and the new TIGER Mission statement is *Advancing the integration of health informatics to transform practice, education and consumer engagement.* The board also focused on a strategic priority to launch the TIGER VLE. Committees were also formed to focus on Education, Foundation Development, and Inter-disciplinary & Consumer Engagement.

Virtual Learning Environment (VLE)

In February 2012, the TIGER Initiative Foundation VLE was officially launched. The VLE provides an interactive Web-based learning opportunity which includes information about HIT and related topics for healthcare professionals and consumers (Schlak, 2013). The Web-based format provides dynamic and real-time information on topics such as electronic health records, usability, clinical decision support, health information exchange, care coordination, meaningful use, standards and interoperability, consumer health information, mobile health, privacy and security, health IT and nursing practice, and many other related topics. It also provides the opportunity for sponsors to share their contributions of integrating health informatics to transform practice, education, and consumer engagement via white papers, demonstrations, videos, and other educational assets. The VLE enables users to download information into a virtual briefcase as well as utilize social media and chat rooms to engage with other TIGERs. Currently there are over 400 individuals across multiple countries that have active TIGER VLE memberships and two universities are using the VLE to augment classroom curriculum. There is great opportunity for interprofessional teams in practice and academia to leverage the TIGER VLE to learn and develop knowledge and skills regarding technology and informatics to better integrate into their daily work. A good case has been made for why faculty need access to the VLE (Skiba, 2013) with examples of how to find valuable resources and ways to engage with students using the Web-based platform.

TABLE 43.1	TIGER Phase II Collaborative Workgroups	
TIGER Collaborative	**Purpose**	**Outcome Summary**
Standards & Interoperability	To accelerate the following action steps identified at the Summit: • Integrate industry standards for health IT Interoperability with clinical standards for practice and education • Educate practice and education communities on health IT standards • Establish use of standards and set hard deadlines for adoption	Provides definitions and rationale for standardization and interoperability. Developed "Nursing Health IT Standards Catalog" and provided Web-based tutorials on benefits of interoperable systems and standard harmonization. For more detailed information: http://www.thetigerinitiative.org/docs/TigerReport_StandardsAndInteroperability_001.pdf
National Health IT Agenda	To identify the most relevant health IT agenda and policies that are important to the TIGER and nursing profession's mission and to assist in closing any representation gaps on policy issues.	Identified major national health IT organizations that need nursing engagement and participation. Developed tutorials to educate and encourage nurses to participate in HIT-related policy development, healthcare reform, and accelerate widespread HIT adoption. For more detailed information: http://www.thetigerinitiative.org/docs/TigerReport_NationalHITAgenda_001.pdf
Informatics Competencies	To establish the minimum set of informatics competencies for *all* practicing nurses and graduating nursing students.	Collected over 1000 informatics competencies than narrowed focus to describe the minimum set of competencies around: 1. Basic Computer Competencies 2. Information Literacy 3. Information Management (including use of an electronic health record) Several educational resources for each type were identified and provided. For more detailed information: http://www.thetigerinitiative.org/docs/TigerReport_InformaticsCompetencies_001.pdf
Education & Faculty Development	To engage key stakeholders to integrate informatics into curriculums and create resources and programs to implement and sustain changes. Collaborate with industry and service partners to support faculty creativity in the adoption of informatic tools within the curriculum.	Formed seven working groups to work with key stakeholders. Effective in influencing the accrediting agencies to include informatics education be incorporated into nursing curriculum. NLN position statement, titled *Preparing the Next Generation of Nurses to Practice in a Technology-Rich Environment: An Informatics Agenda*. AACN took the lead incorporating informatics as an essential element of Baccalaureate *and the Doctor of Nursing Practice Education*. Participation in surveys for ADN and State Boards related to informatics were done. HRSA collaboration that resulted in the Integrated Technology into Nursing Education and Practice Initiative (ITNEP). Webinars for educators on how schools can integrate informatics into curriculum and partnership examples to teach about the electronic health record and clinical documentation. For more detailed information: http://www.thetigerinitiative.org/docs/TigerReport_EducationFacultyDevelopment_001.pdf

(continued)

TABLE 43.1	TIGER Phase II Collaborative Workgroups *(continued)*	
TIGER Collaborative	**Purpose**	**Outcome Summary**
Leadership Development	To engage nursing leadership to develop revolutionary leadership that drives, empowers, and executes the transformation of healthcare.	Evaluated current nursing leadership development programs for the inclusion of informatics competencies. Built upon the American Organization of Nurse Executives (AONE) and developed a survey to identify most urgent program development needs. The survey provided insight into leadership competencies required. Aligned with the Magnet® Recognition Program to highlight how nurse leaders use major HIT implementations as an integral part of their Magnet journey and meeting the 14 forces of magnetism. Identified criteria for leadership development related to informatics. For more detailed information: http://www.thetigerinitiative.org/docs/TigerReport_Leadership_Collaborative_000.pdf
Usability & Clinical Application Design	To further define key concepts, patterns, trends, and recommendations to HIT vendors and practitioners to assure usable clinical systems at the point of care.	Synthesized a comprehensive literature review from nursing and other disciplines and analyzed in the areas of Determining clinical information requirements, safe and usable clinical design, usability evaluations, and human factor foundations. Collected case studies that illustrated usability/clinical application design that are good examples to follow and bad examples to avoid. Reviewed the AAN Technology Drill Down (TD2) Project findings. Developed recommendations for HIT vendors and practitioners to adopt sound principles of usability and clinical design for healthcare technology. For more detailed information: http://www.thetigerinitiative.org/docs/TigerReport_Usability_000.pdf
Virtual Demonstration Center	To explore the creation of a virtual "Gallery Walk" to all nurses, nursing faculty, and nursing students via a Web access to technology applications.	Provided visibility to the vision of IT-enabled practice and education. Demonstrated future IT resources. Demonstrated collaboration between industry, healthcare organizations, academic institutions, and professional organizations to create educational modules for nurses that are based upon informatics competencies. Used practice examples from different practice environments to demonstrate best practices, results of research, case studies, and lessons learned by partnering with professional nursing organizations. For more detailed information: http://www.thetigerinitiative.org/docs/TigerReport_VirtualLearningCenter_001.pdf
Consumer Empowerment & Personal Health Records (PHRs)	To make information available to nurses about PHRs and to engage inclusion of this content into nursing curricula and practice.	Identified several ways that nurses can impact the adoption and use of the consumer empowerment strategies such as the PHR. For more detailed information: http://www.thetigerinitiative.org/docs/TigerReport_ConsumerEmpowermentAndPHR_001.pdf

A new component being added to the Faculty Development Learning Community is a series of curriculum guides (Skiba, 2013) that tie Outcome Competencies, Content, Learning Activities/Resources, and Teaching Strategies for specific topics such as Use of Technology to Support Safety and Quality Care Delivery, Clinical Decision-making, Communication and documentation of inter-professional care, and Consumer Engagement. The last one is related to Involvement with Systems Development Life Cycle. All of the curriculum guides are crosswalked to the AACN's Essentials of Baccalaureate Education for Professional Nursing, TIGER Competencies, QSEN, and the Canadian's Nursing Informatics Entry-into-Practice Competencies for Registered Nurses. The TIGER VLE can be accessed via the Web site www.thetigerinitiative. com to become a member and get access to the plethora of great learning materials and interactive learning venues (Fig. 43.2).

International and Interprofessional Expansion

Two strategic priorities the TIGER Initiative Foundation is focused on for the next few years is in increasing the TIGER vision/mission across international borders and to engage interprofessional colleagues in education and practice. The first step at international expansion was at the NI2012 Conference in Montreal, Canada, where the International Committee was officially launched with five countries including Brazil, United Kingdom, Taiwan, Germany, and Canada. The TIGER International Committee led a TIGER session at MedInfo 2013 in Copenhagen which generated much interest from other countries to become engaged. Recently 28 new countries have been invited to join the TIGER International Committee to share learning needs, synergies and engage in the VLE. There is a growing momentum in healthcare today on creating true interprofessional education and practice environments (Christopherson & Troseth, 2013) and it is critical that leaders in informatics to be aware of this momentum. The TIGER Initiative Foundation has committed to transitioning to an Interprofessional Board of Directors in the future and to include other healthcare professions in TIGER activities and the TIGER VLE learning environment.

The Leadership Imperative Report

At the writing of this chapter, The TIGER Initiative Foundation is preparing to launch another Collaborative

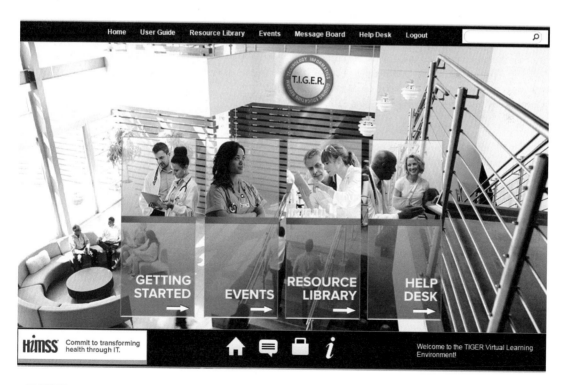

• **FIGURE 43.2.** TIGER Virtual Learning Environment (VLE). (Reproduced, with permission, from Healthcare Information and Management Systems Society [HIMSS].)

Report. It was recognized at the TIGER Summit the significance of leadership to be engaged and support the vision and mission of TIGER which resulted in the TIGER Revolutionary Leadership Report. The new leadership collaborative report *The Leadership Imperative: TIGER's Recommendations for Integrating Technology to Transform Practice and Education (2014)* resulted from the continued recognition of how critical leadership is to fulfill the TIGER vision and mission and to *lead the way* by providing transformational leadership that drives and executes the transformation of healthcare (Technology Informatics Guiding Education Reform, 2014). The report addresses the need to focus on both practice and technology as well as provides valuable information, tools, and resources for leaders to access and utilize as they integrate technology into practice and education. The report will be launched at the TIGER Institute at HIMSS 2014 and will be available on the TIGER Web site.

ONCE A TIGER ALWAYS A TIGER

Brief Summary and Conclusion

The sign of significant changes to come was palpable back in 2004 as our nation began to address healthcare reform by announcing this would be the decade for healthcare technology. A great sense of urgency to set a vision and course of action for nurses to lead and, in turn, engage *all* nurses was the beginning of Technology Informatics Guiding Education Reform; The TIGER acronym was perfect as hundreds of nurses launched into action. The grass roots effort took root and emerged into an innovative social disruption that continues to grow. Many TIGERs have shared that the sense of collaboration and teamwork has been an amazing experience. The number of volunteer hours has been simply astounding! Today TIGER has also expanded its presence on social media with a TIGER Facebook and TIGER Twitter@AboutTIGER. The timing of TIGER is even more significant now with the passing of the 2009 American Recovery and Reinvestment Act (ARRA) and the phased mandate for "Meaningful Use" of the electronic health records. The development of the TIGER Initiative Foundation has provided a solid home

for TIGER that has resulted in the launching of an exciting TIGER VLE that helps provide tools and resources that are support many of the ANA Certification topics such as human factors, information technology, information management, professional practice, models and theories, and management and leadership. Expanding TIGER beyond international boundaries and interprofessional silos will also help spread the vision and take the actions necessary to integrate evidence and technology informatics into our daily work to make healthcare safer, effective, efficient, patient-centered, timely, and equitable.

REFERENCES

Christopherson, T., & Troseth, M. (2013, October). Interprofessional education and practice: A 40-year-old new trend experiencing rapid growth. *CIN: Computers, Informatics, Nursing. 31*(10), 463–464. doi:10.1097/CIN.0000000000000022.

Institute of Medicine. (2001). *Crossing the quality chasm: A new health system for the 21st century*. Washington, DC: The National Academy Press.

Institute of Medicine. (2003). *Health profession education: A bridge to quality*. Washington, DC: The National Academy Press.

Kotter, J. (1996). *Leading change*. Boston, MA: Harvard Business Press.

Kotter, J. (2008). *A sense of urgency*. Boston, MA: Harvard Business Press.

Schlak, S., Anderson, C. & Sensmeier, J. (2013, February). The TIGER has jumped into the virtual learning environment! *CIN: Computers, Informatics, Nursing, 31*(2), 57–58. doi:10.1097/NXN.0b013e318289c7a6.

Skiba, D. (2013). Back to school: TIGER and the VLE. Why faculty need to access this site. *Nursing Education Perspectives, 34*(5), 356–359.

Technology Informatics Guiding Education Reform. (2007). *The TIGER initiative: Evidence and informatics transforming nursing: 3 Year action steps toward a 10 year vision*. Retrieved from http://www.tigersummit.com/Summit

Technology Informatics Guiding Education Reform. (2014). *The Leadership Imperative: Recommendations for Integrating Technology to Transform Practice and Education*. Retrieved from: http://www.thetigerinitiative.org/docs/TIGERReportTheLeadershipImperative.pdf

44

Initiation and Management of Accessible, Effective Online Learning

Patricia E. Allen / Khadija Bakrim / Darlene Lacy / Enola Boyd / Myrna L. Armstrong

• OBJECTIVES

1. Explore the past and present perspectives of distance education.
2. Compare and contrast important interactive electronic tools that support online learning.
3. Examine essential strategies and types of support required for the online learner and faculty.
4. Recognize future trends in online education.

• KEY WORDS

Distance education
Faculty workload
Online learning
Faculty development

DEFINITIONS

The literature still tends to use a variety of terms such as distance education, Web-based or online learning, and online education to reflect this type of non-traditional education, which in educational reality is becoming a mainstream approach to learning. Some definitions include "institution-based, formal education where the learning group is separated, and where interactive telecommunications systems are used to connect learners, resources, and instructors" (Simonson, Smaldino, Albright, & Zvacek, 2009, p. 12). The concept is now associated with learner accessibility, since online learning is experienced locally or globally, at home, a dormitory, or in the work place, regardless of a rural or urban setting, across state lines, and even internationally. The American Association of Colleges of Nursing (AACN, 2008) continues to use Reinert and Fryback's (1997) and Russell's (1998) definitions to further

clarify this type of learning as "a set of teaching/learning strategies to meet the learning needs of students that are separate from the traditional classroom setting and the traditional role of faculty." Today with the use of the Internet, the terms *online education* and *online learning* (which will be used interchangeably in this chapter) are being used to reflect the broader view of these educational experiences.

GOALS FOR THIS CHAPTER

Following a brief historic review of distance education, this chapter focuses on today's high-quality, cost-effective, learner-centered approach to online education, examining it from both the student and faculty perspectives. This includes the importance of applicable educational principles needed to promote interactivity; legal, ethical, and copyright issues; active learning; and effective learner and student support, as well as some of the major academic and pedagogic issues impacting faculty developing creative courses.

THE HISTORICAL EVOLUTION

This type of education has always experienced bumps and surges of acceptance. Even the term *distance education* denotes remoteness or isolation to call attention to the differences from the traditional classroom education. While distance education has been available in the United States since before the turn of the nineteenth century, schools and educators have often required a reason to develop and conduct education for students beyond the traditional classroom setting. Initial development centered primarily on vocational training.

Historically, educational regulatory agencies have not been very supportive; approval for off-campus or extension sites was needed when the sites were separated from the originating school or when geographical barriers existed, even when the same faculty were teaching both types of courses. Some states even defined the number of miles for approval. Another approach to distance education, depending on the school's technological resources, could also mean that the faculty drove "the distance" to the off-campus sites, then provided face-to-face (F2F) instruction.

Use of Technology

The advent of print, audio, television, and the computer has assisted distance education strategies, and eventually led to online learning. In the United States, the distance education movement began with the Boston-based Society to Encourage Studies at Home in 1873, followed in 1885 by the University of Wisconsin developing "short courses" and Farmer's Institutes. By 1920, a Pennsylvania commercial school for correspondence studies had enrollments of more than 2,000,000. Unfortunately, dropout rates averaged around 65%. In 1919, radio was the first technology used for distance education, later followed by telephone service. Wisconsin again became a pioneer by using audio conferencing equipment with telephone handsets, speaker phones, and an audio bridge to connect multiple phone lines for the first two-way interactive distance education for physicians and nurses (Armstrong, 2003; Schlosser & Anderson, 1994). Next came television, so that complex and abstract concepts could be illustrated through motion and visual simulation. Satellite technology for distance education in the United States was implemented in the early 1980s. As these methodologies grew in sophistication and complexity, distance education students began to experience greater transparency of the technology, which enhanced the educational experience. Computer technology came slowly to the forefront of distance education with computer-based education (CBE), computer-assisted instruction (CAI), and computer-managed instruction, and then its use exploded. Yet, it has been the combination of the various interactive Web-based technologies that have really provided the force for creative educational strategies, as well as innovative ideas from faculty that have provided the momentum and impact of online education.

EXAMINING TECHNOLOGIES USED IN ONLINE LEARNING

A number of technologies are employed in the delivery of online learning, yet not all online programs use all of the technologies described.

Learning Management Systems

A Learning Management System (LMS) is a software product that was first designed for corporate and government training divisions as a tool to assess workers' skills for job positions, and then provide specific training, either individually or in groups. Learning management systems are also commonly used for K–12 education and the higher education level to track student achievement in outcomes-based educational programs (Waterhouse, 2005). Another term for LMS that is used more frequently in academic settings is Course Management System (e.g., Blackboard and Desire2Learn). They provide the same functionality as an LMS. The general functions for LMS software includes distribution of course content, communication among the users, interaction with course resources, testing, grading, and tracking records.

LMS becomes significantly more powerful by incorporating third-party applications such as Turnitin, Respondus, Lockdown Browser, and provides an array of sophisticated features. The major functionalities and tools of LMS are summarized in Table 44.1.

Content Management Systems

A content management system is a database of learning objects, which may include many items developed for instructional use. A content management system allows course developers to develop learning objects such as videos, modules, assessments, or any other materials used for online learning. It provides version tracking so that

TABLE 44.1	LMS Features	
LMS Features	**Tools**	**Functionality**
Synchronous Communication	Chat Whiteboard Video conference	• Virtual office hours • Online tutoring and training sessions • Real-time communication • Student-led meeting • Visual presentation of concepts • Guest speakers
Asynchronous Communication	Discussion Forum E-mail Journal	• Read and reply to others • Peer interaction • Self- or group reflections
Collaborative Projects Development	Wiki Blog	• Group collaboration • Sharing information • Self-reflections
Testing and Grading	Online tests Self-assessments Survey Polls	• Formative and summative assessment • Informal test questions • Vote on issues
Social Media Integration	Twitter Facebook YouTube RSS feeds	• Social connections • Collaboration • Building community

changes to these learning objects can be implemented without losing previous versions of the items. Another benefit to such systems is the ability of developers to share learning objects. They can be used as previously developed or modified to fit the need of the current course. Finally, content management systems are designed to integrate with course management systems. This allows the development of materials to take place outside the course itself. Then, building the course becomes as simple as selecting learning objects and placing them into the course. Course management systems such as *Blackboard* offer a content management system that is designed to fully integrate with their system.

Emergence of Massive Open Online Courses

A massive open online course (MOOC) is a model for delivering free learning content. Many MOOCs do not require pre-requisites other than Internet access and interest. Recently, MOOCs are beginning to offer academic credit. The concept of MOOCs originated in 2008 among the open educational resources (OER) movement. MOOCs provide participants with course materials that are normally used in a conventional education setting—such as examples, lectures, videos, study materials, and problem sets. MOOCs are typically provided by higher education institutions, often in partnership with "organizers" such as Coursera, edX, and Udacity, though some MOOCs are being offered directly by a college or university.

MOBILE COMPUTING

The rapid changes in new technologies and access to content anywhere and anytime allow learners to experience learning in a variety of settings and not just in schools (Prensky, 2004). Mobile computing devices are playing an increasingly important role in our personal, professional, and educational life. There are many different mobile devices including personal digital assistants (PDAs), smart phones, tablet PCs, and laptop computers. The recent advances in mobile devices make online learning possible through the powerful computing capability built into their conveniently small sizes, Internet connectivity, and the availability of many types of mobile software applications (apps) (Johnson, Levine, Smith, & Stone, 2010). Because of the mobility and strong Internet connectivity, learning becomes ubiquitous and seamless (Liu, Tan, & Chu, 2009). Learners who are taking online courses can use mobile devices anywhere to access the course content, complete learning activities, communicate with classmates, and work on group projects.

Mobile devices become usable and functional enough to produce an impact on the education software industry, including LMS software. The number of applications for mobile devices has increased dramatically. For example, Google Docs for mobile allows accessing, editing, and sharing documents. Books have also gone digital and for many people e-books are now more desirable than books. Readers have the freedom to read e-books using e-raiders like Kindle or Nook, tablets, and smart phones.

Although the integration of functional mobile computing devices is no longer the real challenge, the focus becomes mainly on how this technology should be used to fulfil the core mission of learning (Cain, Bird, & Jones, 2008). Swan, Hooft, and Kratcoski (2005) found that the effective use of the mobile device increases the quality and quantity of student work.

FACULTY SUPPORT

With the number of online courses increasing, the American Association of State Colleges and Universities emphasizes the critical need for faculty well experienced in teaching online (Orr, Williams, & Pennington, 2009). In order to assist in successful online education, faculty must receive appropriate support, technical expertise, and online infrastructure. The role of the online instructor has developed into that of a facilitator rather than a knowledge distributor. This is achieved by monitoring and guiding students to learn critical concepts, principles, and to develop skills, rather than just lecture material (Easton, 2003).

Faculty Development

Faculty development is a critical component to the success of any online education, especially as colleges and universities are using numerous Adjunct Faculty to assist with the increased student enrollments and teaching responsibilities (Allen, Arnold, & Armstrong, 2006). Academic institutions are taking a proactive approach to faculty support. Numerous workshops and one-to-one support in course development and technical issues are the most common types of training faculty receive. The faculty development activities are designed to assist and improve faculty teaching at all levels of the educational programs. Workshops, seminars, Webinars, and peer coaching are among services available for faculty development. The focus of these services should not be limited to technical skills development, but must include pedagogical issues. For example, strategies to create active learning activities, engage online learners, or motivate online students are topics that, if explored in depth, would help faculty be more effective online teachers (Lahaie, 2007).

Disaggregated Faculty

According to Allen, Keough, and Armstrong (2013) a new disaggregated model for faculty content delivery has emerged and is designed for consistency of content delivery as programs respond to large numbers of students. This model segregates design, teaching, and assessment of student learning into a team approach to course delivery (Rosenbloom, 2011).

Robison (2013) indicates the disaggregated model helps build a network of student support while the student is learning. This model also provides access to a variety of perspectives due to the availability of different faculty in areas of knowledge providing learning enhancement (Robison, 2013).

Support for Course Development

Developing and delivering an effective online course requires pedagogical and technological expertise. Instructors new to online teaching are not likely to have such skills. An example used at our university is the Jumpstart Program. Hixon (2007) defined Jumpstart as a series of workshops that may take more than a week. These workshops include a team of support professionals, including instructional designers, librarians, and media production specialists, who help faculty increase their knowledge, productivity, and teaching experience with technology. Evaluation findings document that this Jumpstart program significantly influences the faculty members in their online course development process.

Allen, Bakrim, Lacy, Boyd, and Armstrong (2006) note that online course development requires a team involving instructional designers, technical support staff, and content experts. The content expert offers an outline of topics that should be covered. The instructional designer provides help in course structure organization and functionality, and the technical support provides assistance with integration of technology tools. This model of team course development is common in most non-academic settings and has been adopted by a number of academic organizations. However, course development carried out by the instructors who will be teaching the course is still a common practice in many colleges and universities that offer online learning.

Technological tools for online learning are constantly being developed and improved, with the aim to make online learning more interesting and more effective (Moar, 2003). Regardless of faculty teaching experience, technology support is critical in online teaching. Appropriate training on using new technologies, routine technical support, and instructional guidance are the common support that faculty receive (Gopalakrishnan, 2006).

Faculty Workload

Faculty workload refers to the number of courses taught by an instructor (Boyer, Butner, & Smith, 2007). The allocation of faculty time in Higher Education usually includes teaching, scholarship activities, and community service. Because teaching online is thought to require more time and effort compared with traditional face-to-face teaching, workload adjustment is usually used by institutions to promote faculty involvement in non-teaching activities.

Actual research into the assumption of increased development time has been limited. Freeman's (2008) research findings suggest that the time spent with online course development seems to be proportional to classroom teaching. As with traditional classroom development, usually the extra time devoted to making the course effective and applicable then produces a significant reduction of faculty time after first-time delivery. Freeman (2008) offers four Lessons for Distance Education Administration:

1. "Make sure faculty understand that they are starting something new."
2. "Teach your faculty to think about their course in a different way, to be ready to do things differently."
3. "Use your instructional designers. As the faculty member is developing the course with the instructional designer, the designer should be on the lookout for time-consuming approaches."
4. "The more an administrator knows about the process of course development, the better he/she can manage [the faculty workload issue]." (para. 9)

COURSE DEVELOPMENT

The use of the Web for courses can be divided into three categories: hybrid courses, Web-enhanced face-to-face courses, and fully online courses. The selection of approach depends on the needs of the organization, the nature of the content, and the faculty as summarized in Table 44.2.

Learner Assessment in Online Courses

Assessment is an important aspect in the learning process. *Assessment* is defined as a means to test and evaluate student performance and ensure that students meet the outcomes designed for the course (Waterhouse, 2005). The assessment may take different forms, such as:

- Online quizzes and exams.
- Self-assessment: Students assess their own learning as they progress through the course.

- Online discussion: Students respond to questions, reply to peers messages, and discuss course materials.
- Papers: Students submit research papers, or essays. Posting papers to the online discussion forum can spark discussion. Rubrics provide guidelines and a method for self-evaluation.
- Individual or collaborative projects: Students develop a project individually or as members of a group by using clear directions and guidelines.
- Presentations: Synchronous communication systems can be used to make presentations or even have debates. A student can use a whiteboard or show a Web site they would like everyone to view while holding a live discussion.
- ePortfolio: It is an online application for collecting the student's work that demonstrates meaningful documentation of individual abilities. Electronic portfolios can serve as a means to assess student's ability over time, and if the student has met each objective or learning outcome as determined by the instructor or the academic program.

STUDENT SUPPORT

One of the most critical factors in a student's success with online learning is student support. Moore and Kearsley (2005) noted that the absence of student support could drastically affect student retention, and tends to increase student frustration and feelings of inadequacy, which in turn leads to the student dropping out of the program. Several investigators have proposed a wide range of student support services that should help students be successful. These services include precourse orientation (Nash, 2005), free tutoring services (Raphael, 2006), and online technical support (Moore & Kearsley, 2002). These academic services allow students to be familiar with the technology and improve student-to-instructor and student-to-student communication. The main goal is to increase students' ease with the cyber environment and encourage constant connection with their peers. In addition to academic support, services that focus on students' affairs are also important to success and retention. Services such as online library resources (Gaide, 2004; Raphael, 2006), online advising (Herbert, 2006; Osika, 2006), and a common course management system (Osika, 2006) could be part of an integrated student support system aimed at making online learning exciting and successful.

TABLE 44.2	Advantages and Disadvantages of Each Type of Course Delivery Mode (Aydogdu & Tanrikulu, 2013; Dell, Low, & Wilker, 2010; Herman & Banister, 2007; Weber & Lennon, 2007)		
Course Delivery Mode	**Description**	**Advantages**	**Disadvantages**
Hybrid	A portion of the course is delivered online and a portion is delivered on site	• Moderate level of real-time social interaction • Building learning community prior to moving to the online environment • Broadening communication using technology and face-to-face meeting • Accommodate a variety of learning styles • Flexibility with reduced meeting times	• Keep up with face-to-face and online components • Having scheduled sessions on campus may be less flexible • Require basic computer skills • Possibility of incompatible technology and Internet connection with that of the institution • Requires much upfront time and effort for the instructor
Web-Enhanced	Face-to-face courses use Web-based technology to facilitate self-studying	• Extensive level of real-time social interaction • Supplement in-class materials with various multimedia tools as well as be the main source of information needed for in-class discussions	• Lecture-oriented class • Technical difficulty if technologies are not used correctly
Fully Online	All of content and communication are conducted entirely online and no face-to-face component	• 24/7 access, time to digest and reflect on content • Cost—flexibility, convenience, savings of travel time • Students perform assignments and take tests online • Activities are student centered rather than instructor centered • Convenience, accessibility, ability to spend time on course content and class discussions before responding • Student attendance and content consumption can be tracked online • Discussion Grading—Discussion participation can be tracked and graded	• Lack of rich, contextual cues from face-to-face interaction, potential feeling of separation from class, instructor, classmates, difficulty in using technologies • Lack of rich, contextual cues from face-to-face interaction, potential feeling of separation from classmates and instructor • Writing is often intensive • Required mastered basic computer skills • Academic Dishonesty—No proctored exams tend to entail cheating • Speed and mediation of discussion—The flow of the discussion is slower

Orientation to the Online Environment

Orientation programs designed to introduce new students to the online environment are crucial to assure a smooth transition, especially for students without prior experience in online learning. The goals of orientations and tutorials are to ensure that students are familiar with the online environment and are aware of expectations. Free tutorials are also helpful, especially with difficult or challenging tasks such as navigating the Web course space, using new software packages and/or equipment, or performing technical procedures (e.g., uploading a file to a Web site).

Communication and Flexibility

There are two basic types of Web-based communication:

- Asynchronous communication tools such as e-mail, discussion boards, and blogs. Course participants use these tools when they are online; however, the person to whom they communicate may not be online. They serve as a messaging interface between communicators.

- Synchronous communication tools require participants to be online to communicate at the same time. These tools include chat, whiteboard, desktop conferencing, and video conferencing such as Skype.

To ensure effective communication, instructors must select the most appropriate tool for the class. This will depend on accessibility to the technology and the levels of students' skills. Communication is strongly affected by course flexibility (due dates and/or assignment submission). Building flexibility in the course structure allows the faculty to compensate for unexpected technological problems, as well as provides opportunities to respond to student feedback.

Accessibility in Online Learning

To avoid creating barriers in online learning, federal and state laws, and local guidelines and policies for online learning such as Americans with Disabilities Act (ADA) and Rehabilitation Act, require that the online learning should be accessible to the broadest range of possible learners. Accessibility of content becomes a legal requirement in many situations. It is important to present instructional content in a format that accommodates the diverse needs and learning styles. Some elements for accessibility include alternative text for images, appropriate color and contrast, accessible and consistent navigation, closed captioning for audio/video materials.

Accessibility also applies to online testing. Students with disabilities can have many different types of limitations that affect their abilities to take tests. These individuals who are protected by disability legislation can ask for alternative format and extra time to take tests. Students must apply for an "accommodation" through the university's student services for accommodations to be made by the school.

LEGAL, ETHICAL, AND COPYRIGHT ISSUES

The faculty is accountable for educational content they teach. However, accountability is even more at the forefront of education at this time. Eaton (2011) defines accountability as the "how and the extent to which higher education and accreditation accept responsibility for the quality and results of their work and are openly responsive to constituents and the public" (p. 8).

The Higher Education Act, reauthorized in 2008, made additional demands on accreditors to be more accountable and subsequent creation of rules during 2009 and 2010 expanding accountability expectations even more (Eaton, 2011).

Legal concerns relate to established laws associated with telecommunication technologies, whereas ethical concerns relate to the rights and wrongs stemming from the values and beliefs of the various users of the distance education system. Three major areas that are of concern regarding legal issues include copyright protection, interstate commerce, and intellectual property. Privacy, confidentiality, censorship, freedom of speech, and concern for control of personal information continue to be as relevant today as in 1998 when Bachman and Panzarine (1998) identified these cyber ethical issues.

Copyright Protection

Copyright is a category of intellectual property and refers to creations of the mind (World Intellectual Property Organization, n.d.). According to the World Intellectual Property Organization (WIPO) Web site (www.wipo.int/policy/ed/sccr/) The Standing Committee on Copyright and Related Rights (SCCR) is currently engaged in discussion of:

- Limitations and Exceptions
- Broadcasting Organizations

This protection for Copyright is based on the Copyright Act of 1976, and was last amended November, 1995 (World Intellectual Property Organization, n.d.). Copyright law protects "works of authorship," giving developers and publishers the right to control unauthorized exploitation of their work (Radcliff & Brinson, 1999). Although there have been no new federal laws since 1976 to address educational multimedia concerns, the Consortium of College and University Media Centers has published the Fair Use Guidelines for Educational Multimedia (Dalziel, 1996). When combining content such as text, music, graphics, illustrations, photographs, and software it is important to avoid copyright infringement (Radcliff & Brinson, 1999). Additionally, the Digital Millennium Copyright Act was passed in October 1998. The UCLA Online Institute for Cyberspace Law and Policy lists the highlights of the Digital Millennium Copyright Act at gseis.ucla.edu/iclp/dmca1.htm and the U.S. Copyright Office Summary can be located at www.copyright.gov/legislation/dmca.pdf. As noted by the dates of citations here, regulations and legislative guidance seem to lag from the technological changes incorporated within the online educational arena.

Intellectual Property

A common question by faculty is, "Who owns the course?" According to Kranch (2008) there is a great deal of controversy over who owns academic coursework materials.

U.S. copyright law is intended to provide ownership and control of what an individual has produced. However, its relationship to faculty-produced work is not as clear. Although faculty may own the materials they have developed for use in their online courses, it is always good to have a memo of understanding documenting the specific use of the materials as well as the accrued benefits (Billings & Halstead, 2009).

The issue of "work made for hire" is the point of controversy. According to the 2003 U.S. Copyright Office document, as indicated by Kranch (2008), a "work made for hire" is defined in the following ways:

1. A work prepared by an employee within the scope of his or her employment
2. A work specially ordered or commissioned for use as a contribution to a collective work

The bottom line of this section is that faculty should know their employer's policy pertaining to intellectual property rights. Over the last several years, universities, government, and private organizations have noted the need to clearly delineate their policies in this area. For example, our school has an established university-wide committee providing advisory opinions to the Provost on matters related to patentable discoveries and inventions, and/or copyrightable material, which had been developed by University employees.

MIT Open Courseware (2010) is a free and open digital publication of educational material (http://ocw.mit.edu/index.htm). However, there are specific guidelines and requirements for the use of Open Courseware. Although Open Courseware is available to anyone, material used in education from any Open Courseware participant is consistent with materials from any university and/or faculty. Additional information on Open Courseware can be found at http://ocw.mit.edu/help/.

Extensive resources on intellectual property law and rights can be found at the following sites:

- Indiana University Information Policy Office (informationpolicy.iu.edu)
- Office of Technology Transfer and Intellectual Property at Texas Tech University Copyright (www.ttuhsc.edu/HSC/OP/OP57/op5702.pdf); Intellectual Property (www.ttuhsc.edu/hsc/op/op52/op5206.pdf)
- Legislative initiatives regulating intellectual property and copyright are found in the Technology, Education and Copyright (TEACH) Act (www.arl.org/pp/ppcopyright/index.shtml)
- The Berkeley Digital Library at Sunsite is an excellent resource for national perspectives on intellectual property (sunsite.berkeley.edu/Copyright)
- The Creative Commons Web site (creativecommons.org/about/what-is-cc) is a non-profit organization that works to increase the amount of creativity in the body of work available to the public for free and legal sharing, use, repurposing, and remixing.

Ethical behavior in the nursing profession has been established by groups such as the American Nurses Association (ANA) in the Code of Ethics (ANA, 2001) and the American Association of Colleges of Nursing's (AACN, 2008) competencies for baccalaureate nursing education. These nursing values and ethics are fundamental in practice decisions and are just as applicable in nursing education, whether education be face to face or online. Mpofu (n.d.) regards ethical considerations in online teaching as performing your work within the context of professional practice and the confines of institutional regulations. However, over and above professional and institutional ethics, nurse educators must contend with legal and ethical issues that take on a new dimension when applied to online education. While issues such as copyright, privacy, licensing, fair and acceptable use, and plagiarism are certainly not unique to online education, they assume new dimensions and different proportions. Another source for consideration with ethics issues can be found in *Best Practice Strategies to Promote Academic Integrity in Online Education* (Version 2.0, June 2009) (wiche.edu/attachment_library/Student_Authentication/BestPractices.pdf).

EFFECTIVENESS OF ONLINE EDUCATION

Online learning for nursing courses is exploding. Advertisements about "new online education for working professionals" certainly have appeal, capturing the attention of many people seeking to fit further education into their busy schedules. Yet, there are still some traditional students who do not pay attention to online education, there are still some faculty who avoid the concept by raising questions of quality rather than exploring the educational principles used in online learning, and there are still some who believe the only "gold standard" of education continues to be the traditional classroom setting (Allen, Arnold, & Armstrong, 2006). Additionally, questions emerge concerning the validity of the courses: Is it really possible to earn a degree while at home or in the work setting without driving long distances and sitting in tedious lecture classes? Is the interaction with the faculty equal to the same interaction that occurs in the classroom? Is this really applicable to clinical nursing?

Overall, market-driven demands of educational reform and creative, visionary faculty have moved online learning, transforming both academic and continuing nursing education, by capturing new types of educational experiences and innovative kinds of pedagogy (Allen & Seaman, 2010; Allen, Arnold, & Armstrong, 2006). The outcomes have been an empowerment of the nursing student and working professional to have numerous important educational choices. Now, in addition to quality, the educational decisions are often based on accessibility and the amount of time needed to complete the course or program.

Online learning offers more alternatives to accommodate individual circumstances and educational needs. Now, it is becoming a commonly accepted instructional method in higher education institutions, and the numbers of online courses are constantly increasing to accommodate the large number of students enrolling. For the past six years, online enrollment has grown at a greater rate than the total higher education enrollment (Allen & Seaman, 2010). According to the Sloan Consortium Report (2013), overall online enrollment increased to 7.1 million in 2013, with the majority of doctoral-granting universities (80%) offering online courses or programs.

In order to purport quality, educational outcomes must be similar for both the on-campus and online learning students; countless studies over at least three decades have documented this (Dede, 1990; Mahan & Armstrong, 2003; Schlosser & Anderson, 1994). Findings reflect that regardless of the delivery method, online learning students receive the same grades or do better than those students receiving traditional instruction. Overall, student evaluations are good to very good following online education activities. In essence, good online education theory and good education theory are actually the same; the education just transcends the barriers of time and space.

PROGRAM EVALUATION AND ACCREDITATION

Program evaluation is an ongoing process in online education and requires a framework for evaluation to be adopted by the faculty, standards, and outcomes to be defined, as well as a timeline for measurement of outcomes. Program evaluation focuses on review and improvement. The need for curriculum revision, resources, and faculty and staff may become apparent during this ongoing review process. Program evaluation allows educators to facilitate meaningful change, while providing feedback. All program evaluation gathers evidence for measurement against predetermined outcomes. The framework will provide the steps to outcome attainment. With systematic program evaluation, revision decisions are based on the evidence from findings rather than assumptions. To obtain this evaluative data, program surveys by faculty, students, and administrators should be completed and analyzed annually. Additionally, course surveys should be completed by students at the end of each course.

Regional accreditation agencies assist in guiding programs for maintaining standards in program delivery, and regional credentials are sought after by major colleges and universities. Regional accreditation is a continuous improvement process involving the entire university or college. Many of the regional accrediting agencies, such as the Southern Association of Colleges and Schools (SACS), engage the college or university to pursue a continuous improvement process of self-evaluation, reflection, and improvement for not only face-to-face learning but distance learning as well (Southern Association of Colleges and Schools, 2010). Other regional accrediting agencies providing excellent resources for online program assessment and evaluation include Western Interstate Commission on Higher Education (WICHE) and WICHE Cooperative for Educational Technologies (WCET), a division of WICHE, providing good practices and policies to ensure the effective adoption and appropriate use of technologies in teaching and learning online (wcet.wiche.edu/advance).

Accreditation agencies require that each facet of the online program be critically and logically appraised to reflect the quality of the programmatic goals and outcomes designated within the program. There is no one type of accreditation applied to online education. In fact, there are several types of accreditations for different institutional statuses, and they are categorized into regional, national, and professional accreditations (see Table 44.3).

STANDARDS FOR QUALITY IN ONLINE EDUCATION

To ensure the quality of online education, various organizations (Table 44.4) have recently developed standards for this type of education. The main purpose of these standards is to guide the development and evaluation of online learning programs offered through colleges and universities.

TABLE 44.3	Regional, Professional, and National Accreditation
Regional Accreditation Organizations	**Professional Accreditation**
There are six regional accreditation agencies. These agencies accredit both public and private schools, and two-year or four-year institutions by reviewing their program and delivery methods based on established standards and requirements. The online programs are expected to meet the general institution standards as well as other criteria specific to online setting such as faculty support, faculty qualification, student support, and the necessary infrastructure to develop and deliver effective online education. For more information, see www.neasc.org.	Professional accreditation varies by discipline and is a key to defining a quality unit or discipline within a community college, college, and/or university. For nursing, two widely sought professional accrediting agencies are the Accreditation Commission for Nursing Education (ACEN) and Commission on Collegiate Nursing Education (CCNE). Both ACEN and CCNE are recognized by the U.S. Department of Education. The CCNE agency accredits only baccalaureate and higher degree programs in nursing. ACEN offers accreditation to vocational and practical nursing programs, associate's, diploma, bachelor's, master's, and doctoral programs within nursing schools and/or departments. Both require online education offerings to be equivalent to site-based offerings and may have specific standards to be addressed by the school in the accreditation process.

TABLE 44.4	Organizations With Standards Supporting Quality Online Education	
Quality Matters	**The Online Learning Consortium**	**Teaching, Learning, and Technology Group**
Quality Matters (QM) is another evaluative process that employs a set of standards based on best practices in instructional design developed to verify the quality of online or hybrid courses. It is based on faculty-oriented peer review and provides tools for the review process while focusing on course design more than content or delivery method (Pollacia & McCallister, 2009). For more information visit www.qualitymatters.org.	The Online Learning Consortium (2013) is dedicated to making online learning a mainstream higher education delivery methodology, and this international consortium provides tools, best practices, and directions for educators. The Sloan Best practice model can be viewed at http://olc.onlinelearningconsortium.org/conference/2014/ALN/welcome.	The Teaching, Learning, and Technology Group (TLT) is an important not-for-profit group providing excellent resources related to online learning and the effective evaluation and assessment of online programs. The group provides technology updates to help college and university faculty improve online learning methodologies through the use of the latest technology. Many resources for educators can be found on the TLT Group's Web site (www.tltgroup.org/about.htm). A major project of interest by the TLT Group has been the Flashlight Program. This program is an inexpensive Web 2.0 tool for program evaluation and evaluation research opportunities. This rich online resource for educators provides evaluation measures, validated surveys, rubrics, model questions, and survey matrices for use by institutions. Visit their Web site for additional information about this helpful evaluation and assessment tool (www.tltgroup.org/Flashlight/flashlightonline.htm).

FUTURE TRENDS

The future trends in online learning will be defined by student empowerment and technological advancements. The population and student enrollments have grown extensively during the last six years (Allen & Seaman, 2010) and it is anticipated that the field of online education will witness a tremendous growth both in terms of quantity as well as quality. For example, Hodgins (2007) predicts that learning content will be customized for each learner, rather than mass produced. In the future, data analytics will be used to identify individual student learning needs and the role of faculty as mentors will be strengthened (Johnson et al., 2013). Huge data sets will allow advisors to see academic risks in real time and intervene with the student. By focusing on processes of actual cognitive development Stanford University is researching new forms of assessment in order to measure twenty-first century skills (Skiba, 2013). Additionally, immersive virtual learning environments tailored to the learner's desired competency set will emerge. Here the student will enter an immersive virtual environment which transcend real world time and there be paired with virtual teammates designed to enable the student to meet identified competencies (Dede, 2013).

The next apparent trend changing online learning is the advancement of technologies. Gaming, learning analytics, and mobile applications are now the norm as well as tablet computing and use of ebooks (Skiba, 2013). We now expect are tools to have geo-everything and gesture-based computing through a tap or a swipe, but the future may bring technology that allows computing through subtle body gestures with wearable computing (Skiba, 2013). Along with the wearable technology, 3D printing will become commonplace (Hidalgo, 2013). Futurists have been predicting the rise of the *ubiquitous computing device* for years (Bull & Garofalo, 2006; Swan, Van 'T Hooft, Kratcoski, & Schenker, 2007; Weiser, 1991). A ubiquitous device is one to which users have become so accustomed, they no longer notice the device itself when they are using it. Instead, users tend to focus on what they get from the device. One example of this in our life is the refrigerator. We may open the door of the refrigerator, but often are thinking of the food we get from the device, rather than the device itself. Some authors go even farther, defining the ubiquitous device as a single device or service that takes care of all of our computing needs (Pendyala & Shim, 2009). These computing devices will continue to be part of an exciting new world for online learning opportunities.

The 2013 Horizon Report by the New Media Consortium described six technologies that universities will likely mainstream within the next five years. One of these technologies is gesture-based computing, which is also called Gesture Recognition. This refers to technology that recognizes and interprets the motions and movements of its users. Instead of using the mouse or keyboard, the users employ natural body movements to control the device, such as shaking, rotating, tilting, touching, or moving the device in space. It is expected that in four to five years this type of technology will emerge in educational settings and have a considerable impact on teaching and learning (www.nmc.org/horizon).

There will be more technologies that offer live interactive instruction. With all the growth in online education, the need for effective course management systems will be ever more crucial. Furthermore, technological advancements will also increase the need for developing effective teaching strategies that exploit the capabilities of technology. Massively Open Online Courses (MOOCs) will continue to explode as noted in the latest NMC Horizon Report (Johnson et al., 2013). And the movement on the horizon is for MOOCs to determine mechanisms for awarding credit (Kolowich, 2013).

Skiba (2014) recently noted students of the future will use mobile devices more, but will also still value a mix of online and face-to-face learning environments and although technology will enhance achievement of their learning goals students will continue to value privacy. There is a limit to connectivity and students will continue to keep academic and social lives in separate silos (Skiba, 2014).

REFERENCES

Allen, I. E., & Seaman, J. (2010). *Going the distance: Online education in the United States, 2011*. Retrieved from http://www.onlinelearningsurvey.com/. Accessed on January 20, 2014.

Allen, P.E., Arnold, J., & Armstrong, M. L. (2006). Accessible effective distance education, anytime, anyplace. In V.K. Saba & K. A. McCormick (Eds.), *Essentials of Nursing Informatics*, 4th ed. (pp. 533–548). New York, NY: McGraw-Hill.

Allen, P., Keough, V., & Armstrong, M. (2013). Creating innovative programs for the future. *Journal of Nursing Education, 52*(9), 486–491. doi: 10.3928/01484834-20130819-05. Epub 2013 Aug 19.

Allen, P. E., Bakrim, K., Lacy, D., Boyd, E., & Armstrong, M. L. (2006). Initiation and management of accessible, effective online learning. In V. K. Saba & K. A. McCormick (Eds.), *Essentials of nursing informatics*. (4th ed., pp. 545–557). New York, NY: McGraw-Hill.

American Association of College of Nursing. (2008). *The essentials of baccalaureate education for professional nursing practice*. Washington, DC: Author.

American Nurses Association. (2001). *Code of ethics for nurses with interpretive statements*. Washington, DC: Author.

Armstrong, M. L. (2003). Distance education: Using technology to learn. In V. K. Saba & K. A. McCormick (Eds.), *Essentials of computers for nurses: Informatics for the new millennium* (3rd ed., pp. 413–425). New York, NY: McGraw-Hill.

Aydogdu, Y., & Tanrikulu, Z. (2013). Corporate e-learning success model development by using data mining methodologies. *Education and Science, 30*(170), 95–111.

Bachman, J. A., & Panzarine, S. (1998). Enabling student nurses to use the information superhighway. *Journal of Nursing Education, 37*(4), 155–161.

Billings, D. M., & Halstead, J. A. (2009). *Teaching in nursing: A guide for faculty.* St. Louis, MO: Saunders Elsevier.

Boyer, P. G., Butner, B. K., & Smith, D. (2007). A portrait of remedial instruction: Faculty workload and assessment techniques. *Higher Education, 54,* 605–613.

Bull, G., & Garofalo, J. (2006). Commentary: Ubiquitous computing revisited—A new perspective. *Contemporary Issues in Technology & Teacher Education,* 271–274.

Cain, J., Bird, E. R., & Jones, M. (2008). Mobile computing initiatives within pharmacy education. *American Journal of Pharmaceutical Education, 72*(4), 1–7.

Dalziel, C. (1996). *Fair use guidelines for educational multimedia.* Retrieved from http://www.libraries.psu.edu/mtss.fairuse/dalziel.html

Dede, C. (2013). Connecting the dots: New technology-based models for postsecondary learning. *EDUCAUSE Review, 46*(5). Retrieved from http://www.educause.edu/ero/article/connecting-dots-new-technology-based-models-postsecondary-learning

Dede, C. J. (1990). The evolution of distance learning: Technology-mediated interactive learning. *Journal of Research in Computing in Education, 22*(3), 247–264.

Dell, C. A., Low, C., & Wilker, J. F. (2010). Comparing student achievement in online and face-to-face class formats. *Journal of Online Learning and Teaching, 6*(1), 30–42

Eaton, J. S. (2011). U.S. accreditation: Meeting the challenges of accountability and student achievement. *Evaluation in Higher Education, 5*(1), 20.

Easton, S. S. (2003). Clarifying the instructor's role in online distance learning. *Communication Education, 52*(2), 87–105.

Gaide, S. (2004). Best practices for helping students complete online degree programs. *Communication Education, 52*(2), 87–105.

Gopalakrishnan, A. (2006). Supporting technology integration in adult education. Critical issues and models of basic education. *Adult Basic Education, 16*(1), 39–56.

Herbert, M. (2006). Staying the course: A study in online student satisfaction and retention. *Online Journal of Distance Learning Administration.* Retrieved from http://www.westga.edu/~distance/ojdla/winter94/herbert94.htm

Herman, T., & Banister, S. (2007). Face-to face versus online coursework: A comparison of costs and learning outcomes. *Contemporary Issues in Technology Education, 7*(4), 318–326.

Hidalgo, J. (2013*). The future of higher education: Reshaping universities through 3D printing.* Retrieved from http://www.engadget.com/2012/10/19/refreshing-universities-through-3d-printing/

Hixon, E. (2007). *Working as a team: Collaborative online course development.* 23rd Annual Conference on Distance Teaching & Learning. Retrieved from http://www.uwex.edu/disted/conference/Resource_library/proceedings/07_5084.pdf

Hodgins, W. (2007). Distance education but beyond: "meLearning"—What if the impossible isn't? *Journal of Veterinary Medical Education, 34*(3), 325–329.

Johnson, L., Adams Beccker, S., Cummins, M., Estrada,V., Freeman, A., & Ludgate, H. (2013). *NMC Horizon Report: 2013 Higher Education Edition.* Austin, TX: The News Media Consortium.

Johnson, L., Levine, A., Smith, R., & Stone, S. (2010). *The 2010 Horizon Report.* Austin, TX: The New Media Consortium.

Kolowich, S. (2013, February, 7). American Council on Education recommends 5 MOOCs for credit. *Chronicle of Higher Education.* Retrieved from http://chronicle.com/article/American-Council-on-Education/137155

Kranch, D. A. (2008). Who owns online course intellectual property? *Quarterly Review of Distance Education Research That Guides Practice, 9*(4), 350.

Lahaie, U. (2007). Web-based instruction: Getting faculty onboard. *Journal of Professional Nursing, 23*(6), 335–342.

Liu, T. Y., Tan, T. H., & Chu, Y. L. (2009). Outdoor natural science learning with an RFID-supported immersive ubiquitous learning environment. *Educational Technology & Society, 12*(4), 161–175.

Mahan, K., & Armstrong, M. L. (2003). Distance education: What was, what's here, and preparation for the future. In M. Armstrong & S. Fuchs (Eds.), *Providing successful distance education and telehealth* (pp. 19–37). New York, NY: Springer.

MIT Open Courseware Consortium. (2010). *Information about the consortium.* Retrieved from http://ocw.mit.edu./index.htm

Moar, D. (2003). The teacher's role in developing interaction and reflection in an online learning community. *Education Media International, 40,* 127–128.

Moore, M. G., & Kearsley, G. (2002, 2005). *Distance education: A systems view* (2nd ed.). Belmont, CA: Wadsworth.

Mpofu, S. (n.d.). *Ethics and legal issues in online teaching.* Retrieved from http://www.col.org/pcf2/papers/mpofu.pdf

Nash, R. (2005). Course completion rates among distance learners: Identifying possible methods to improve retention. *Online Journal of Distance Education Learning Administration, 8*(4). Retrieved from http://www.westga.edu/~distance/ojdla/winter84/nash84.htm

Online Learning Consortium (2013). *Going the distance: Online education in the United States.* Retrieved from http://olc.onlinelearningconsortium.org/conference/2014/ALN/welcome

Orr, R., Williams, M., & Pennington, K. (2009). Institutional efforts to support faculty in online teaching. *Innovation Higher Education, 34,* 257–268.

Osika, E. (2006). The concentric support model: How administrators can plan and support effective distance learning programs. *Distance Education Report, 10*(21), 1–6.

Pendyala, V. S., & Shim, S. S. Y. (2009). The Web as the ubiquitous computer. *Computer, 42*(9), 90–92.

Prensky, M. (2004) What can you learn from a cell phone? Almost anything! *Journal of Online Education Innovate, 1*(5).

Radcliff, C. F., & Brinson, R. P. (1999). *Copyright Law* (1999). Retrieved from http://library.findlaw.com/1999/Jan/1/241476.html

Raphael, A. (2006). A needs assessment: A study of perceived need for student services by distance learners. *Online Journal of Distance Education Learning Administration.* Retrieved from http://www.westga.edu/~distance/ojdla/summer92/raphael92.htm

Reinert, B., & Fryback, P. (1997). Distance learning and nursing education. *Journal of Nursing Education, 36*(9), 421.

Robison, J. (2013). *A new role for faculty in the virtual classroom.* Retrieved from http://www.evollution.com/distance_online_learning/a-new-role-for-faculty-in-thevirtual-classroom/

Rosenbloom, B. (2011). *Envisioning online learning: The disaggregated professor.* Retrieved from http://onlinelearning.commons.gc.cuny.edu/author/brucelr

Russell, T. L. (1998). *The no significant difference phenomenon.* Retrieved from http://cuda.teleeducation.nb.ca/nosignificantdifference

Schlosser, C. A., & Anderson, M. L. (1994). *Distance education: Review of the literature.* Washington, DC: Association for Educational Communications & Technology.

Skiba, D. J. (2013). On the horizon: The year of the MOOCs. *Nursing Education Perspectives, 34*(2), 136–138.

Skiba, D. J. (2014). The connected age: Implications for 2014. *Nursing Education Perspectives, 35*(1), 63–65.

Simonson, M., Smaldino, S., Albright, M., & Zvacek, S. (2009). *Teaching and learning at a distance: Foundations of distance education* (4th ed.). Boston, MA: Allyn & Bacon & Pearson.

Southern Association of Colleges and Schools (SACS). (2010). *Standards and accreditation process for schools.* Retrieved from http://www.sacscoc.org/principles.asp

Swan, K., Hooft, M., & Kratcoski, A. (2005). Uses and effects of mobile computing devices in K–8 classrooms. *Journal of Research on Technology in Education, 38*(1), 99–112.

Swan, K., Van 'T Hooft, M., Kratcoski, A., & Schenker, J. (2007). Ubiquitous computing and changing pedagogical possibilities: Representations, conceptualizations and uses of knowledge. *Journal of Educational Computing Research, 36*(4), 481–515.

Waterhouse, S. (2005). *The power of eLearning: The essential guide for teaching in the digital age.* Boston, MA: Pearson Education, Inc.

Weber, J. M., & Lennon, R. (2007). Multi-course comparison of traditional versus web-based course delivery systems. *The Journal of Educators Online, 4*(2), 1–19.

Weiser, M. (1991). The computer for the 21st century. *Scientific American, 265*(3), 94.

World Intellectual Property Organization. (n.d.). *What is intellectual property?* Retrieved from http://www.wipo.int/about-ip/en

45

Social Media in the Connected Age: Impact on Healthcare Education and Practice

Diane J. Skiba / Sarah Knapfel / Chanmi Lee

• OBJECTIVES

1. Describe the evolution of the Internet and the movement toward the Connected age.
2. Describe the use of social media and mobile tools in healthcare education and practice.
3. Identify the challenges and issues related to the use of social media in healthcare education and practice.

• KEY WORDS

Connected Age
Digital tools
Social networking
Social media
Mobile apps

INTRODUCTION

The Internet has revolutionized the computer and communications world like nothing before. The Internet is at once a world-wide broadcasting capability, a mechanism for information dissemination, and a medium for collaboration and interaction between individuals and their computers without regard for geographic location (Leiner et al., 1997, p. 102).

There is no doubt the Internet provided the necessary infrastructure to revolutionize the way scientists and researchers from the worlds of academia, business, and government could share data, interact, and collaborate with each other. But it was not until the introduction of the World Wide Web that "everyday people" without computer programming skills were enabled to reap the benefits of this revolution. The Web not only changed how governments and businesses operate, it has impacted every facet of society—how we work, learn, play, and now, even how we manage our health.

In this chapter, there is a brief history of the evolution of the Internet to the Web and now to the Connected Age. There is a specific focus on the use of social media digital tools, and its impact on healthcare and education. This is particularly true as we evolve from the Web 2.0 era to the Connected Age where it is not only access and interactions but about establishing relationships. As Sarasohn-Kahn (2008, p. 2) noted, "the use of social media on the Internet are empowering, engaging and educating consumers and providers in healthcare." In the Connected Age, everything and everyone is interconnected that ultimately will have an impact on how we learn as well as how we receive healthcare. The benefits and challenges related to the growing use of these tools are also discussed.

HISTORICAL PERSPECTIVE

Internet

As early as the 1960s, computer scientists began to write about the creation of a network of interconnected computers where scientists could share and analyze data by interacting across the network (Leiner et al., 1997). According to Cerf (1995), "the name 'Internet' refers to the global seamless interconnection of networks made possible by the protocols devised in the 1970s through DARPA-sponsored research." The Internet is defined as "a computer network consisting of a worldwide network of computer networks that use the TCP/IP network protocols to facilitate data transmission and exchange" (http://wordnetweb.princeton.edu/perl/webwn). Over the next decade, various government agencies and companies conducted considerable research to support the advancement of the Internet. It was not until 1985 that a broader community, in particular the academic community beyond the computer scientists, was given access to the Internet. NSF funding for the Internet continued for almost a decade before the Internet was redistributed to regional networks with the eventual move toward interconnecting networks across the globe.

As the Internet came to expand, Tim Berners-Lee wrote his seminal paper *Information Management: A proposal* that circulated throughout the European Council for Nuclear Research (CERN) organization. The paper explicated his ideas that using a hypertext system that would allow for storage and retrieval of information in a "web of notes with links (like references) between them is far more useful than a fixed hierarchical system" (Berners-Lee, 1989). In 1990, Berners-Lee's paper was recirculated and he began development of a global hypertext system that would eventually become the World Wide Web (WWW). As the WWW concept evolved, Marc Andreessen and Eric Bina at the University of Illinois developed a browser called Mosaic that provided a graphical interface for users. This browser is credited with popularizing the Web.

World Wide Web

It is important to note that although many use the terms *Internet* and *Web* synonymously, there are differences between them. Whereas the Internet is the network of interconnected computers across globe, the Web is an application that supports a system of interlinked, hypertexted documents. One uses the Internet to connect to the Web. A Web browser allows the user to view Web pages that contain text, images, and other multimedia.

Web 1.0. The Web in its first iteration (Web 1.0) allowed users to access information and knowledge housed on Web pages complete with text, images, and even some multimedia. It was considered a dissemination vehicle that democratized access to information and knowledge. Many in the field designate the time period between 1991 and 2004 as Web 1.0. This was an important era and, as noted by Friedman (2005), the world suddenly became flat—his metaphor for the leveling of the global playing field. The convergence of the personal computer with the world of the Internet and all its services facilitated the flattening. The flattening was particularly powerful in the world of commerce but also exploded in higher education, making it easier for students to access knowledge beyond their own academic campus. For healthcare, it was a time when consumers could now have access to health information and knowledge that was not locked in an academic library or in a distant place.

Web 2.0. O'Reilly and Doughtery introduced the term *Web 2.0* at a 2004 conference brainstorming session (http://oreilly.com/web2/archive/what-is-web-20.html) about the failures of the dot-com industry. It was apparent that despite the demise of the dot-com industry, "the web was more important than ever, with exciting new applications and sites popping up with surprising regularity" (O'Reilly, 2005). There were several key concepts that formed the definition of Web 2.0. First, the Web is viewed as a platform rather than an application. Second, the power of the Web is achieved by harnessing the collective intelligence of the users. A third important principle was that the Web provided rich user experiences.

The introduction of Web 2.0 embodies the long history of community spirit of the Internet conceived by its originators. As Leiner and colleagues (1997, p. 206) noted, "the Internet is as much a collection of communities as a collection of technologies, and its success is largely attributable to satisfying basic community needs as well as utilizing the community effectively to push the infrastructure forward."

The transition from an information dissemination platform to an engaging, customizable, social and media-rich environment epitomizes this next generation of the Web. As Downes (2005) stated, "the Web was shifting from being a medium, in which information was transmitted and consumed, into being a platform, in which content was created, shared, remixed, repurposed, and passed along." Another important feature was the idea of users interacting and sharing information, ideas, and content. Owen, Grant, Sayers, and Facer (2006) aptly described the transition of the Web, "we have witnessed a renaissance of this idea in the emergence of tools, resources and practices that are seen by many as returning the web to its early potential to facilitate collaboration and social interaction."

Although some have predicted (Berners-Lee, Hendler, & Lassila, 2001) that there will be Web 3.0, known as the Semantic Web, this never materialized as projected. There have been more recent references to such terms as the Internet of Things (IOT) and the Connected Age. Both are fairly similar but there are some distinctions. Ashton (2009) first described the IOT as "describe a system where the Internet is connected to the physical world via ubiquitous sensors." In the 2012 Horizon Report (Johnson, Adams, & Cummins, 2012, p. 30), IOT "is the latest evolution of network-aware smart objects that connect the physical world with information." Skiba (2013, p. 63) noted, "Several attributes are associated with these smart objects; they are small, easy to attach and unobtrusive, contain a unique identifier and data or information, and can connect with an external device on demand (e.g., your smartphone or tablet)."

CONNECTED AGE

More recently, Oblinger (2013) introduced the concept of the Connected Age in higher education. Abel, Brown, and Suess (2013) describe the Connected Age as an environment that "offers new ways to connect things that were previously considered disparate and 'un-connectable': people, resources, experiences, diverse content, and communities, as well as experts and novices, formal and informal modes, mentors and advisors." Oblinger (2013, p. 4) further noted, "Connecting is about reaching out and bringing in, about building synergies to create a whole that is greater than the sum of its parts. Connecting is a powerful metaphor. Everyone and everything—people, resources, data, ideas—are interconnected: linked and tagged, tweeted and texted, followed and friended. Anyone can participate." As noted by Skiba (2014, p. 63), "In higher education, we can think of these as learning pathways, created by the individual or guided by other students or faculty. The bottom line is that learning pathways are about connecting the dots—in the classroom, online, or even with people and places outside the traditional academic environment."

In healthcare, Caulfield & Donnelly (2013) offered a model of Connected Health that "encompasses terms such as wireless, digital, electronic, mobile, and tele-health and refers to a conceptual model for health management where devices, services or interventions are designed around the patient's needs, and health related data is shared, in such a way that the patient can receive care in the most proactive and efficient manner possible. In this model, patients, caretakers, and providers are 'connected' by means of timely sharing and presentation of accurate and pertinent information regarding patient status through smarter use of data, devices, communication platforms and people." Iglehart (2014, p. 2) concurred that Connected health is "an umbrella term to lessen the confusion over definitions of telemedicine, telehealth and mHealth." Iglehart (2014) as considered connected health as an emerging disruptive technologies that has the potential to transform the healthcare delivery system.

Although both terms, IOT and Connected Age, speak to connections to everything and everyone, IOT focuses on those connections with physical objects whereas the Connected Age refers to more virtual connections especially with people, resources, and ideas. It is within the context of the Connected Age, that we examine the digital tools being used to transform education and healthcare practice.

In the Connected Age, digital tools are primarily associated within the broad context of social media and mobile applications. The Pew Research Internet Project has witnessed three technology revolutions since it began studying the Internet. The three revolutions include broadband, mobile connectivity, and the rise in social media and social networking in everyday life (http://www.pewinternet.org/three-technology-revolutions/). The three revolutions are primary driving forces behind the Connected Age. According to Fox and Rainie (2014), the World Wide Web turned 25 on March 14, 2014, and has reached 87% penetration in terms of adult usage in the United States. There is also considerable growth of cell phones from 53% in 2000 to now 90% and also smartphones has increased to 58%. When participants were asked about the impact on their lives, 90% claimed the Internet was a positive influence. Users noted that being online was essential for not only job-related responsibilities but for a many other facets of their lives such as learning, health, politics, family, friends, and community interactions. It is interesting to note that 67% of users indicated that online communications were positive and strengthened relationships with family and friends.

Facebook

In a 2013 update specific to social media, Duggan and Smith (2013) found that although 73% use social networking sites, Facebook being the most prevalent, there are 42% who are also exploring other social networking platforms. On a daily basis, most users check both their

Facebook and their instagram accounts. There is a growing use of Pinterest, LinkedIn, and Twitter.

In terms of mobile devices, the Pew Internet Research Mobile Fact Sheet (http://www.pewinternet.org/fact-sheets/mobile-technology-fact-sheet/) indicated as of January 2014, 90% of American adults have cell phones of which 78% have smart phones (Pew Internet Research Mobile Fact Sheet, 2014). There are also 52% of American adults with tablet computer devices and 32% with e-reader devices. It is also interesting to note that 70% of teens (13 to 17 years old) and 79% of young adults (aged 18–24) are owners of smart phones (Nielsen Corporation, 2013).

According to Nielsen's Digital Consumer Report (Nielsen Corporation, 2014), social media is well integrated into the fabric of everyday life. The Digital Consumer Report documented that 64% of social media users log in at least once a day and almost 50% log into their social network on their smart phone on a daily basis. "Mobile devices are certainly driving the growth in social media, as social media app usage increased 37 percent in 2013 compared to last year" (http://www.nielsen.com/us/en/newswire/2014/whats-empowering-the-new-digital-consumer.html).

DIGITAL TOOLS IN EDUCATION AND PRACTICE

To better understand the tools being used in the Connected Age, it is important to define social media. In some cases, social media is used as the broad category that encompasses all of the Web 2.0 tools. Anthony Bradley (2010) in his blog (blogs.gartner.com/anthony_bradley/2010/01/07/a-new-definition-of-social-media) offered a new definition, "social media is a set of technologies and channels targeted at forming and enabling a potentially massive community of participants to productively collaborate.... enable collaboration on a much grander scale and support tapping the power of the collective in ways previously unachievable." According to Bradley (2010), there are six defining characteristics that distinguish social media from other collaboration and communication IT tools. These characteristics are Participation, Collective, Transparency, Independence, Persistence, and Emergence. Participation echoes the "wisdom of the crowds" concept, but note that there is no wisdom if the crowd does not participate. The term *collective* refers to the idea that people collect or congregate around content to contribute, rather than the way individuals create and distribute content in the Web 1.0 world. Transparency refers to the fact that everyone can see who is contributing and what contributions are made. Independence refers to the anytime, anyplace concept; people can participate regardless of geography

or time. Persistence refers to the notion that information or content being exchanged is captured and not lost as in a synchronous chat room. Lastly, "the emergence principle embodies the recognition that you can't predict, model, design and control all human collaborative interactions and optimize them as you would a fixed business process" (Bradley, 2010). Taken together these characteristics define the new world of social media.

Blogs

In the Connected Age, social writing and communication are important concepts for sharing resources and ideas as well as for making connections with people similar to you. Social writing can take many forms and include, but are not limited to, wikis, blogs, and microblogging. Blogs, short for Web logs, are considered to be personal Web sites where content is displayed for visitors to review and comment upon (Adams, 2008). A top listing of health-related blogs is available at the following Web site: http://labs.ebuzzing.com/top-blogs/health. The Health Care Social Media List, maintained by the Mayo Clinic's Social Media Health Network, documents the types of social media being used by hospitals across the United States. There statistics demonstrate although blogs were once very popular, there are fewer blogs being maintained by hospitals. Of the 1544 hospitals (http://network.socialmedia.mayoclinic.org/hcsml-grid/0), only 209 have blogs.

Wikis are coined after the Hawaiian work for fast, and are a means to establish an easily and quickly accessed consumer-driven knowledge base (Meister, 2008); they are essentially collaborative tools that are "based on social regulation rather than technical safeguards" (Digital Library Federation, 2008). Wikis, as a form of social writing, are also prevalent in healthcare. CliniWiki (www.informatics-review.com/wiki/index.php/Main_Page) is a popular wiki targeted toward clinical informatics topics. This wiki contains information on a variety of topics in such areas as clinical decision support systems, unintended consequences of technology, federal initiatives, and usability. Professional organizations, such as HIMSS, also maintain a Decision Support Wiki (http://himssclinicaldecisionsupportwiki.pbworks.com/w/page/18288587/FrontPage). An interesting educational Web site in informatics is the University of Edinburgh's Informatics wiki (https://www.wiki.ed.ac.uk/display/Informatics/Home) that is focused primarily on educational opportunities, student projects, discussions, and resources. Another important wiki is of course the ever-popular Wikipedia (http://en.wikipedia.org/wiki/Main_Page) that maintains over 4 million articles.

Microblogging, the combination of texting and blogging, adds a new dimension to communication and social writing and is growing in popularity. Historically, electronic mail (e-mail), instant messaging, and text messaging have been less public forms of communication. These forms have been seen as one-to-one communication. Microblogging, using such tools like Twitter, now allows consumers to post content to a Web site, which then automatically distributes the content to others who have "subscribed" to the individual's site; this creates short bursts of communication among any number of individuals (Hawn, 2009). These microblogging sites allow social communication to come directly to consumers, rather than requiring that consumers go and seek it out themselves. These short bursts of communication, known as Tweets, are limited to a specific number of characters (140). In education, twitter is being used in various ways. One example is when conference participants tweet information being presented at the conferences to their students (McKendrick, Cumming, & Lee, 2012). Educators are also using Twitter in the classroom to encourage student engagement.

In healthcare, there is a rise in the use of microblogging especially in the public health arena. According to Eysenbach (2009), "Infodemiology can be defined as the science of distribution and determinants of information in an electronic medium, specifically the Internet, or in a population, with the ultimate aim to inform public health and public policy." The electronic medium can be supply driven, such as the information being published in blogs, microblogs, and discussion groups, or it can be demand driven that includes Web searching and navigation. Some examples of the use of Twitter include its use in tracking trends in health behaviors: physical activity (Zhang et al., 2013); dietary (Hingle et al., 2013); smoking (Myslín, Zhu, Chapman, & Conway, 2013); and prescription drug abuse (Hanson, Cannon, Burton, & Giraud-Carrier, 2013). Other uses include dissemination of vital information during disasters and documentation of the extent of crisis such as the H1N1 or SARS viruses.

SOCIAL NETWORKING

Social networking embraces many of the defining characteristics of the Connected Age and is a major component of connected learning and connected health. First, participation and collaboration were two of the principal themes in Web 2.0 (Eysenbach, 2008) and are the driving forces behind the social media movement with continued relevance in the Connected Age. Eysenbach (2008) further noted, "Social networking …involves the explicit modeling of connections between people, forming a complex network of relations, which in turn enables and facilitates collaboration and collaborative filtering processes."

Another aspect of social networking is the ability to share user-generated content in the form of videos, stories, or photographs. In addition to adding and viewing content, consumers can also post comments to media someone else has contributed, thus adding another level of communication to these sites (Skiba, 2007).

Of the available digital tools, social networking offers the most opportunity for peer support and consumer engagement. Users can make connections with people that they already know in person or may connect with others through associations that they create (Boyd & Ellison, 2007). Essentially, the social networking site serves as a powerful tool to engage and motivate consumers to share personal information, establish relationships, and communicate with others.

This is definitely exemplified in the phenomenal growth of social networks such as Facebook. Facebook celebrated its tenth anniversary in 2014 and is considered the dominant social networking site where 57% of adults and 73 % of teens (12–17 years old) used Facebook. According to a recent Pew Research Center study, despite the growing number of adults using Facebook on a daily basis, the younger generation "are not abandoning the site" (Smith, 2014). Here are some additional facts about Facebook. Although users dislike some aspects of Facebook (sharing too much personal information and posting photos without permission), the users do not want to miss out on social activities. Second, 47% like the ability to share photos and videos with friends as well as sharing with many people at the same time. They also like updates from their friends and humorous content. Third, 50% of adult users have over 200 friends on Facebook. Fourth, younger rather than older users have "unfriended" a person. Fifth, although most users do not change their status on Facebook, they do like to comment on friend's postings. Lastly, those that do not use Facebook are still familiar with Facebook through their family members.

Higher education, including healthcare professional education, is taking full advantage of the collaborative features of social networks and mobile access to create dynamic and collaborative learning experiences. The dynamic nature of collaboration via the Internet offers learners the opportunities to share working knowledge, provide professional support, and create communities of learning. Social media complements and supports e-learning opportunities where students are able to have more control over the pace, sequence, and timing of their learning experience (Ruiz, Mintzer, & Leipzig, 2006). These new digital learning environments aim at deepening the level of engagement for the student experience (Boulos, Maramba, & Wheeler, 2006) and also allows students to connect to a vast array of accessible resources, knowledge, expertise, and social connections (Alliance for Excellent Education, 2014).

In the field of informatics, Skiba & Barton (2009) described the use of social networking tools at the University of Colorado College of Nursing. In this graduate program, they have embraced the use of social media to engage and retain online learners but also to attract potential students to the program. The program incorporates various social media, such as social networking and virtual worlds, as part of the online learning environment. Another example is the University of Oregon Biomedical Informatics program that includes the use of blogs to connect students and faculty within their programs. More recent applications of social networks are appearing as universities and specific programs form LinkedIn groups of their graduates or current students. In nursing education, one of the best known social networks was Meet Stella Bellman (Skiba, 2010), a mannequin in a simulation lab at Mesa Community College (https://www.facebook.com/stella.bellman) and was used to connect and communicate with nursing students.

Healthcare institutions and consumers have already begun to capitalize on the limitless utility of social networking. Numerous hospitals and healthcare-related organizations have social networking sites where patients and visitors can explore details about the facility, learn more about available services, and find information about diseases and/or treatments (Sarasohn-Kahn, 2008). Of the available social networking sites, Facebook stands out as one of the more popular, as it has proven useful for resource sharing, communication, and collaboration (Mazman & Usluel, 2010). According to the Mayo Clinic's Center for Social Media List, of the 1544 hospitals using social media, there are 1292 hospitals that have Facebook social networks and 651 that have LinkedIn groups. To learn more about the top hospitals that are social media friendly, you can visit the rankings of hospitals conducted by MHdegree.org (http://mhadegree.org/top-50-most-social-media-friendly-hospitals-2013/). At the top of the list are Mayo Clinic, Cleveland Clinic, University of Texas MD Anderson Cancer Center, Mt Sinai Medical Center, and the University of Michigan Hospitals and Health Centers.

Social Network

One of the first social networks in healthcare was Matthew Zackery's i2y social network (I am too young for this Cancer Foundation). At one of the first Health 2.0 conferences, Zackery presented his experiences in creating the social network targeted for young adults with cancer. To learn more, you can visit the following Web site: http://stupidcancer.org/

The Centers for Disease Control (CDC) has embraced the use of social media and was used extensively in their H1N1 campaign. The CDC site (www.cdc.gov/h1n1flu) not only connects people to the CDC, but also to other social networks such as Facebook, My Space, and Daily Strength. It provides videos, podcasts, e-cards, widgets, RSS feeds, and the ability to get text messages and join their Twitter subscription. Their Web site (http://www.cdc.gov/socialmedia/) contains a variety of resources that are used such as current campaigns as well as a Social Media Toolkit to help people create their own social media campaigns.

Perhaps one of the most interesting and well-researched social networking sites is PatientsLikeMe (www.patientslikeme.com). Through this social network, patients from all over the world convene and share their experiences while dealing with chronic conditions such as Multiple Sclerosis (Sarasohn-Kahn, 2008). The creators' brother, who was living with amyotrophic lateral sclerosis (ALS), was the inspiration for the network. Two brothers and a friend, all Massachusetts Institute of Technology engineers, created this network with the following goals in mind: (1) share health data, (2) find patients with similar conditions, and (3) learn from each other. Patients are asked to share data in the hope of improving the lives of all diagnosed with that particular disease. The site currently supports over 250,000 members, over 2000 health conditions, over 40 published research studies, and over 1 million treatment and symptom reports (http://www.patientslikeme.com/).

The site does not have any fees and is kept free from advertising through revenues stemming from research awareness programs, market surveys, and the sale of processed anonymized data (Brownstein, Brownstein, Williams, Wicks, & Heywood, 2009). Members use aliases rather than real names and can openly share details about their healthcare experiences, drug regimens, and treatment side effects (Hansen, Neal, Frost, & Massagli, 2008; Sarasohn-Kahn, 2008). The primary motives behind such sharing are to ask or offer advice and to build a relationship with others in similar situations (Hansen et al., 2008). "Rather than disseminating medical advice, PatientslikeMe serves as a platform for peers to interact with one another in a data-driven context" (Brownstein et al., 2009, p. 889). Patients have actually taken information they have learned from PatientsLikeMe to their own healthcare providers to request to be put on specific treatments (Goetz, 2008). More recently, PatientsLikeMe has launched a Data for the Good Campaign to encourage patients to share their health data to advance healthcare research (http://news.patientslikeme.com/press-release/patientslikeme-launches-data-good-campaign-encourage-health-data-sharing-advance-medic).

A recent report by the eHealth Initiative with funding from the California Healthcare Foundation examined the use of social media to prevent behavioral risk factors associated with chronic disease. According to this report (eHealth Initiative Report, 2014, p. 7), "By seeking and sharing information online, health consumers (or "ePatients") are using social media to become more equipped, enabled, empowered, and engaged in managing their health, care, and wellness." Although healthcare providers continue to play a primary role in the provision of health information, "more Americans than ever value social networks (e.g. friends, family members, and fellow patients) for emotional support and advice on everyday health issues" (eHealth Initiative Report, 2014, p. 7). Healthcare is in essence becoming more social (Sarasohn-Kahn, 2008; Fox & Jones, 2009, HIMSS Social Media Work Group, 2012). Fox (2011) summarized it as "Peer-to-peer health care is a way for people to do what they have always done – lend a hand, lend an ear, lend advice – but at internet speed and at internet scale."

The eHealth Initiative Report (2014) developed a specific taxonomy to classify social media tools for chronic diseases. This taxonomy includes such tools as Internet support groups, media sharing, messaging boards/discussions, microblogs, social networking general and specific to a particular disease, Weblogs, and social games and challenges.

Grajales, Sheps, Ho, Novak-Lauscher, & Eysenbach (2014) conducted a narrative review of social media and its use in healthcare. They reviewed 76 articles, 44 Web sites, and 11 policy reports to derive 10 categories of social media: blogs, microblogs, social networking sites, professional networking sites, thematic networking sites, wikis, mashups, collaborative filtering sites, media sharing sites, and virtual worlds. They found that social media was fairly extensive, there was a need to begin to address challenges related to governance, ethics, professionalism, privacy, confidentiality, and information quality.

MOBILE HEALTH

As new tools are introduced in healthcare, it is not only changing the delivery of care but it is changing the dynamics of healthcare and the interactions between consumers and their providers. This is particularly true as one explores the growing of mobile devices and apps that allow for Connected Health interactions. World Health Organization (2011) defines mobile health or mHealth as "medical and public health practice supported by mobile devices, such as mobile phones, patient monitoring devices, personal digital assistants (PDAs), and other wireless devices. mHealth involves the use of voice and short messaging service (SMS) as well as more complex functionalities such as 3G systems, global positioning systems (GPS), and Bluetooth technology."

The use of smart phones has greatly impacted the mHealth arena. Smart phones allow consumer and patients to use mobile health applications. Most mobile apps are available through mobile store platforms like Apple App Store, Google Play for the Android. There are also more than 100 apps approved by the FDA for use in healthcare (Aitken & Gauntlett, 2013). In a Pew Internet and American Life Study of Mobile health (Fox & Duggan, 2012), they found that 52% of smartphone users accessed health information from their phones. This was particularly true for adults who were Latino, African American, between the ages of 18 and 49. Users with a college degree or being a caregiver especially for someone who had a recent medical crisis were also good indicators of accessing health information through their smartphones. The study also found although there were many healthcare apps available, only about 18% of smart phones users use these apps to track or manage their health. The most frequently used health apps were for exercise, diet, or weight apps.

A more recent study conducted by the IMS Institute for Healthcare Informatics (Aitken & Gauntlett, 2013) analyzed healthcare apps to assess their value. Over 40,000+ healthcare apps from the Apple iTunes app store were downloaded. After several iterations of exclusions, a total of 14,243 apps related to consumer health. These apps were classified according to the patient's journey: prevention/healthy lifestyles, symptoms or self-diagnosis, finding a healthcare provider or facility, education post-diagnosis, filling prescriptions, and compliance. The majority of apps were in the overall wellness category (prevention and healthy lifestyles) with diet and exercise being the dominant apps. In terms of functionality, most apps were limited in their functions, with most providing just information. According to the report (Aitken & Gauntlett, 2013, p. 8), "there is a subset of apps with impressive functionality (e.g. electrocardiogram (ECG) readers, blood pressure monitors, blood glucose monitors)." In addition, only one-fifth track or capture consumer-initiated data. Most of the apps have fewer than 500 downloads and five apps account for 15% of all health app downloads. Although there are some apps that cover the total patient's journey and can be therapy or demographic specific, there is a disconnect between apps available and the population of older adults and seniors who have the most healthcare needs. As smartphone users increase in these age groups so may the apps available to them.

Another source of free healthcare apps is the Department of Health & Human Services Digital Strategy for Mobile apps site (http://www.hhs.gov/digitalstrategy/

mobile/mobile-apps.html). Here you can find a variety of apps from the CDC, National Institutes of Health, National Cancer Institute, and the National Library of Medicine. These apps are available for multiple operating systems and across multiple devices like smart phone or tablets.

In addition to consumer available apps, there is also a group of medical apps that are approved by the FDA. According to the FDA, there are several types of mobile apps that required to be regulated. The first category is mobile apps that transform a mobile platform into a regulated medical device (light, vibrations, camera, or other similar sources to perform medical device functions and are used by a licensed practitioner to diagnose or treat a disease). The second category is apps that connect to an existing device type for purposes of controlling its operation, function, or energy source (such as implantable or body worn medical devices). The last category refers to apps that display, transfer, store, or convert patient-specific medical device data from a connected device. To read more, go to http://www.fda.gov/MedicalDevices/ProductsandMedicalProcedures/ConnectedHealth/MobileMedicalApplications/ucm368743.htm. To review a list of mobile medical apps approved by the FDA, go to http://www.fda.gov/MedicalDevices/ProductsandMedicalProcedures/ConnectedHealth/MobileMedicalApplications/ucm368784.htm

BENEFITS OF SOCIAL MEDIA

To understand the benefits of social media, it is important to examine the growing number of studies over time. In the past, most studies were descriptive. In a review by Skiba, Guillory, and Dickson (2014), there are three general areas of research in social media. The first focused primarily on the content being shared on social media, in particular social networks and Twitter. The second area was the specific use of social media by patient populations such as diabetics or cancer patients. The final area was related to the use of social media for recruitment of patients for research studies and the collection of data from social media could be used as an additional form of research data. Some interesting findings were that Facebook, YouTube, and Twitter were the most common social media platform and PatientsLikeMe was the most studied network to date (Skiba et al., 2014).

More recently, there have many more research studies, including clinical trials that have examined the impact of social media tools on patient care. The growth of these studies has generated several systematic reviews to provide evidence for the use of these tools in promoting and managing various patient populations. Here is a sampling of some systematics studies. Moorhead et al. (2013)

completed a systematic review to examine the uses, benefits, and limitations of social media for health communications. Capurro et al. (2014) conducted a systematic review of social networking sites for Public Health practice and research. Chang, Chopra, Zhang, and Woolford (2013) analyzed studies in the role of social media in online weight management. Maher et al. (2014) conducted a systematic review of the effectiveness of behavior change interventions through social networks. Most found promising results but there was a need for additional studies.

The eHealth Initiative Report (2014) concluded that social media provides a multitude of benefits to patients by "enabling health education and enhancing behavior by:

- Breaking down the walls of patient-provider communication
- Improving access to health information
- Providing a new channel for peer-to-peer communications
- Developing meaningful relationships
- Establishing communities of patients, caregivers, and family members
- Engaging and empowering people"

The development and continuing research in the use of social media will expand and more studies will continue to provide additional evidence of their effectiveness. There is little doubt that the social life of healthcare (Fox & Jones, 2009) will continue. Despite their prospects, digital tools in the Connected Age do not come without certain limitations and risks. Like any element of our digital environment, they pose concerns for privacy, security, and legal issues.

CHALLENGES OF SOCIAL MEDIA

According to the eHealth Initiative Report (2014), there are several key challenges affecting the widespread adoption of social media in healthcare. First, there are concerns about privacy and HIPAA compliance. There are also concerns about the balance of transparency and anonymity associated with the sharing of personal information online. The quality, validity, reliability, and authenticity of information are an issue especially when there is user-generated information. There is also the challenge of the digital divide specifically with differing populations such as the elderly, minorities, the disabled, those living in rural areas, and those in poor or undeserved areas without access to broadband. The final challenge in this report also mentions the lack of theoretical and evaluation models for social media given the paucity of effectiveness data. Grajales et al. (2014) also echo many of the same challenges, "The potential violation of ethical standards, patient privacy, confidentiality, and professional codes of practice, along with the misrepresentation of information, are the most common contributors to individual and institutional fear against the use of social media in medicine and health care."

The Connected Age places unique circumstances around the sharing of protected health information, as it is generally patient, student, or consumer driven. That is, the consumer voluntarily divulges his or her information. In such cases the HIPAA regulations do not apply, however, healthcare institutions' attempts to abide by the law may hinder their adoption of Web 2.0 applications (Hawn, 2009). The sharing of personal information is also an issue with the use of social media by students. It is not just the sharing by healthcare professional students of their own information in social networks but also the potential of them sharing personal health information of their patients on social networks. Such was the case of nursing students posting a picture of a patient's placenta (Skiba, 2011).

There are also concerns about privacy and confidentiality. Their concerns are not unfounded since the rates of identity theft are on the rise and Internet security cannot ever be fully ensured (Acoca, 2008; LaRose & Rifon, 2006). Social media applications promote information sharing and the open display of personal information, such as age, gender, and location. Posting this and other content creates digital footprints or lingering information that can be connected back to the consumer who provided it (Madden, Fox, Smith, & Vitak, 2007); these bits of information can then be found and coalesced to form a more complete picture of the individual, thus negating the apparent transparency supposed by Web 2.0 applications (Madden et al., 2007). A recent study conducted by Grajales et al. (2013) found there are worries about sharing data, many U.S. adults (94%) are willing to share their health data to improve care and believe that data sharing can help other patients as well as themselves. Users of social media are at risk for social threats as well (Nosko, Wood, & Molema, 2010). Characterized as stigmatizing and bullying, social threats can pose significant dangers to consumers and those with whom they are affiliated (Nosko et al., 2010).

In addition, there may be legal issues related to risk management and liabilities. It has long been known that Internet content is not regulated and may be unreliable (Eysenbach & Diepgen, 1998; Powel, Darvell, & Gray, 2003). Healthcare and educational organizations in the Connected Age must also be cognizant of the legal implications. Not only will they have to monitor the content being shared on their site for appropriateness, reliability, and quality of their information, they will also need to be

sure there are no copyright infringements (Lawry, 2001). Healthcare practice licenses are also an issue considering that in the Connected Age, there are no real geographic boundaries (Grajales et al., 2014).

The digital divide, or gap in usability, exists for some consumers who either lack physical access to the Internet or do not have knowledge or skills to navigate the myriad information on the Internet safely and effectively (Baur & Kanaan, 2006; Cashen, Dykes, & Gerber, 2004). Physical access limitations can be described as lack of resources to obtain the hardware or software to utilize these tools (Baur & Kanaan, 2006; Cashen et al., 2004). Lack of experience describes the knowledge and skill deficit that hinders a consumer's ability to navigate tools effectively and safely. Some have also found that ethnic disparities do exist in regard to Internet access but, surprisingly, not in regard to social media use (Chou, Hunt, Beckjord, Moser, & Hesse, 2009).

As with most innovations, these challenges can be partially addressed through the development and implementation of social media policies by organizations, including user-generated networks. This is particularly important given that most healthcare agencies are risk adverse regarding patient care. Professional organizations, such as American Nurses Association, American Medical Association, and the National Council of State Boards of Nursing, have provided guidance and social media policies (Skiba et al., 2014). Barton and Skiba (2012) also present social media policy recommendations for educational institutions. The Mayo Clinic Center for Social Media provides resources related to social media policies (http://network.socialmedia.mayoclinic.org/).

SUMMARY

There is no doubt that digital tools have transformed the world around us. By providing digital tools to students, healthcare professionals, and consumers, we are transforming healthcare education and practice. The addition of mobile devices facilitates the continuous use of social media tools in every aspect of our lives. In the Connected Age, learners can create their own learning pathways (Oblinger, 2013) as they seek knowledge and skills in either formal higher educational degree programs or professional development. For consumers, patients, and their families, the Connected Age provides opportunities for them to become more engaged in their healthcare decisions by expanding their connections from just family and friends to a cadre of other patients/consumers who are like them as well as a community of healthcare professionals who are experts in their particular health or disease conditions.

REFERENCES

Abel, R., Brown, M., & Suess, J. (2013). A new architecture for learning. *EDUCAUSE Review, 48*(5), 88, 90, 92, 96, 98, 100, 102.

Acoca, B. (2008). *Scoping paper on online identity theft.* Retrieved from http://www.oecd.org/dataoecd/35/24/40644196.pdf

Adams, S. A. (2008). Blog-based applications and health information: Two case studies that illustrate important questions for Consumer Health Informatics (CHI) research. *International Journal of Medical Informatics, 79*(6), e89–e96.

Aitken, M., & Gauntlett, C. (2013, October). *Patient apps for improved care: From novelty to mainstream.* IMS Institute for Healthcare Informatics. Retrieved from http://www.imshealth.com/deployedfiles/imshealth/Global/Content/Corporate/IMS%20Health%20Institute/Reports/Patient_Apps/IIHI_Patient_Apps_Report.pdf

Alliance for Excellent Education. (2014, March). *Connected learning: Harnessing the information age to make learning more powerful.* Retrieved from http://all4ed.org/reports-factsheets/connected-learning/

Ashton, K. (2009, June). That 'Internet of things' thing. *RFID Journal.* Retrieved from http://www.rfidjournal.com/article/view/4986.

Barton, A., & Skiba, D. (2012). Creating social media policies for education and practice. In P. A. Abbott, C. Hullin, C. Ramirez, C. Newbold, & L. Nagle (Eds). Studies in informatics: Advancing global health through informatics. *Proceedings of the NI2012. The 11th International Congress of Nursing Informatics* (pp. 16–20). Bethesda, MD: American Medical Informatics Association.

Baur, C., & Kanaan, S. (2006, June). *Expanding the reach and impact of consumer e-health tools.* Washington, DC: US Department of Health and Human Services Office of Disease Prevention and Health Promotion Health Communication Activities. Retrieved from http://www.health.gov/communication/ehealth/ehealthTools/default.htm

Berners-Lee, T. (1989). *Information management: A proposal.* CERN. Retrieved from http://www.w3.org/History/1989/proposal.html

Berners-Lee, T., Hendler, J., & Lassila, O. (2001). The semantic web. *Scientific American, 290*(4), 35–43.

Boulos, M. N. K., Maramba, I., & Wheeler, S. (2006). Wikis, blogs and podcasts: A new generation of Web-virtual collaborative clinical practice and education. *BMC Medical Education, 6*, 41.

Boyd, D. M., & Ellison, N. B. (2007). Social network sites: Definition, history, and scholarship. *Journal of Computer-Mediated Communication, 13*(1), Article 11. Retrieved from http://jcmc.indiana.edu/vol13/issue1/boyd.ellison.html

Bradley, A. (2010, January 7). A new definition of social media. *Gartner blog.* Retrieved from http://blogs.gartner.com/anthony_bradley/2010/01/07/a-new-definition-of-social-media

Brownstein, C. A., Brownstein, J. S., Williams, D. S., Wick, P., & Heywood, J. A. (2009). The power of social networking in medicine. *Nature Biotechnology, 27*(10), 888–890.

Capurro, D., Cole, K., Echavarría, M. I., Joe, J., Neogi, T., & Turner, A. (2014). The use of social networking sites for public health practice and research: A systematic review. *Journal of Medical Internet Research, 16*(3), e79. Retrieved from http://www.jmir.org/2014/3/e79/

Cashen, M. S., Dykes, P., & Gerber, B. (2004). eHealth technology and internet resources: Barriers for vulnerable populations. *Journal of Cardiovascular Nursing, 19*(3), 209–214.

Caulfield, B., & Donnelly, S. (2013). What is connected health and why will it change your practice? *QJM: An International Journal of Medicine, 106*(8), 703–707.

Cerf, V. (1995). *Computer networking: Global infrastructure for the 21st century.* Computer Research Association. Retrieved from http://www.cs.washington.edu/homes/lazowska/cra/networks.html

Chang, T., Chopra, V., Zhang, C., & Woolford, S. J. (2013). The role of social media in online weight management: Systematic review. *Journal of Medical Internet Research, 5*(11), e262. Retrieved from http://www.jmir.org/2013/11/e262/

Chou, W. S., Hunt, Y. M., Beckjord, E. B., Moser, R. P., & Hesse, B. W. (2009). Social media use in the United States: Implications for health communication. *Journal of Medical Internet Research, 11*(4), e48. Retrieved from http://www.jmir.org/2009/4/e48

Digital Library Federation. (2008). *A quick guide to wiki.* Retrieved from http://www.diglib.org/pubs/execsumm/wikiexecsumm.htm

Downes, S. (2005, October 17). E-learning 2.0. *eLearn Magazine.* Retrieved from http://www.elearnmag.org/subpage.cfm?section=articles&article=29-1

Duggan, M., & Smith, A. (2013, December). *Social media update.* Pew Research Center. Retrieved from http://www.pewinternet.org/2013/12/30/social-media-update-2013/

eHealth Initiative Report. (2014). *A report on the use of social media to prevent behavioral risk factors associated with chronic disease.* California Health Foundation. Retrieved from http://www.ehidc.org/resource-center/reports/view_document/365-report-a-report-on-the-use-of-social-media-to-prevent-behavioral-risk-factors-associated-with-chronic-disease

Eysenbach, G. (2008). Medicine 2.0: Social networking, collaboration, participation, apomediation, and openness. *Journal of Medical Internet Research, 10*(3), e22.

Eysenbach, G. (2009). Infodemiology and infoveillance: Framework for an emerging set of public health informatics Methods to analyze search, communication and publication behavior on the Internet. *Journal of Medical Internet Research, 11*(1), e11. doi:10.2196/jmir.1157. Retrieved from http://www.jmir.org/2009/1/e11

Eysenbach, G., & Diepgen, T. L. (1998). Towards quality management of medical information on the internet: Evaluation, labeling, and filtering of information. *British Medical Journal, 317,* 1496–1502.

Fox, S. (2011). *Medicine 2.0: Peer-to-peer health care.* Speech September 11, 2011. Pew Internet Studies. Retrieved from http://pewinternet.org/Reports/2011/Medicine-20.aspx

Fox, S., & Duggan, M. (2012, November). *Mobile Health 2012.* Pew Internet and American Life Project. Retrieved from http://www.pewinternet.org/2012/11/08/mobile-health-2012/

Fox, S., & Jones, S. (2009). *The social life of health information. California Health Foundation and Pew Internet and American Life Project.* Retrieved from http://www.pewinternet.org/Reports/2009/8-The-Social-Life-of-Health-Information.aspx

Fox, S., & Rainie, L. (2014, February). *The Web at 25.* Pew Research Center. Retrieved from http://www.pewinternet.org/2014/02/27/the-web-at-25-in-the-u-s/

Friedman, T. (2005). *The world is flat: A brief history of the 21st century.* New York, NY: Farrar, Straus & Giroux Publishers.

Goetz, T. (2008, March 23). Practicing patients. *New York Times.* Retrieved from http://www.nytimes.com/2008/03/23/magazine/23patientst.html

Grajales, F., Clifford, D., Loupos, P., Okun, S., Quattrone, S., Simon, M., … Henderson, D. (2013, January). *Social networking sites and the continuously Learning Health System: A survey.* Washington, DC: Institute of Medicine Roundtable on Value & Science-Driven Health Care. Retrieved from http://www.iom.edu/Global/Perspectives/2014/SharingHealthData.aspx

Grajales, F., Sheps, S., Ho, K., Novak-Lauscher, H., & Eysenbach, G. (2014). Social media: A review and tutorial of applications in medicine and health care. *Journal of Medical Internet Research, 16*(2), e13. Retrieved from http://www.jmir.org/2014/2/e13/

Hansen, D., Neal, L., Frost, J. H., & Massagli, M. P. (2008). Social uses of personal health information within Patientslikeme, an online patient community: What can happen when patients have access to one another's data. *Journal of Medical Internet Research, 10*(3), e15. Retrieved from http://www.ncbi.nlm.nih.gov/pmc/articles/PMC2553248

Hanson, C. L., Cannon, B., Burton, S., & Giraud-Carrier, C. (2013). An exploration of social circles and prescription drug abuse through Twitter. *Journal of Medical Internet Research, 15*(9), e189. Retrieved from http://www.jmir.org/2013/9/e189/

Hawn, C. (2009). Take two aspirin and Tweet me in the morning: How Twitter, Facebook, and other social media are reshaping healthcare. *Health Affairs, 28*(2), 361–368.

HIMSS Social Media Work Group. (2012, February 10). *HIMSS White Paper: Health care "Friending" Social Media: What Is It, How Is It Used, and What Should I Do?* Retrieved from http://www.himss.org/files/HIMSSorg/content/files/HealthcareFriendingSocialMediav15(4).pdf

Hingle, M., Yoon, D., Fowler, J., Kobourov, S., Schneider, M. L., Falk, D., & Burd, R. (2013). *Collection and visualization of dietary behavior and reasons for eating using Twitter, 15*(6), e125. Retrieved from http://www.jmir.org/2013/6/e125/

Iglehart, J. (2014, February). Connected health: Emerging disruptive technologies. *Health Affairs, 33*(2), 190. doi:10.1377/hlthaff.2014.0042.

Johnson, L., Adams, S., & Cummins, M. (2012). *The NMC Horizon Report: 2012 higher education edition.* Austin, TX: The New Media Consortium. Retrieved from http://www.nmc.org/publications/horizon-report-2012-higher-ed-edition

LaRose, R., & Rifon, N. (2006). Your privacy is assured—of being invaded: Websites with and without privacy seals. *New Media and Society, 8,* 1009–1029.

Lawry, T. C. (2001). Recognizing and managing website risks. *Health Progress, 82*(6), 12–13, 74.

Leiner, B., Cerf, V., Clark, D., Kahn, R., Kleinrock, L., Lynch, D., … Postel, J. (1997). The past and future history of the Internet. *Communications of the Association of Computing Machinery, 40*(2), 102–108.

Madden, M., Fox, S., Smith, A., & Vitak, J. (2007). *Digital footprints: Online identity management and search in the age of transparency.* Washington, DC: Pew Internet and American Life Project.

Maher, C. A., Lewis, L. K., Ferrar, K., Marshall, S., De Bourdeaudhuij, I., & Vandelanotte, C. (2014). Are health behavior change interventions that use online social networks effective? A systematic review. *Journal of Medical Internet Research, 16*(2), e40. Retrieved from http://www.jmir.org/2014/2/e40/

Mazman, S. G., & Usluel, Y. K. (2010). Modeling educational usage of Facebook. *Computers & Education, 55*(2010), 444–453.

McKendrick, D., Cumming, G., & Lee A. (2012). Increased use of Twitter at a medical conference: A report and a review of the educational opportunities. *Journal of Medical Internet Research, 14*(6), e176. doi:10.2196/jmir.2144. Retrieved from http://www.jmir.org/2012/6/e176/

Meister, J. C. (2008, February). *Wikis at work: Benefits and practices.* Chief Learning Officer. Retrieved from http://www.clomedia.com/in-conclusion/jeanne-c-meister/2008/February/2064/index.php

Moorhead, S. A., Hazlett, D. E., Harrison, L., Carroll, J. K., Irwin, A., & Hoving, C. (2013). A new dimension of health care: Systematic review of the uses, benefits, and limitations of social media for health communication. *Journal of Medical Internet Research, 15*(4), e85. Retrieved from http://www.jmir.org/2013/4/e85/

Myslín, M., Zhu, S. H., Chapman, W., & Conway, M. (2013). Using Twitter to examine smoking behavior and perceptions of emerging tobacco products. *Journal of Medical Internet Research, 15*(8), e174. Retrieved from http://www.jmir.org/2013/8/e174/

Nielsen Corporation. (2013, October). *Ring the bells: More smartphones in students' hands ahead of back-to-school season*. Retrieved from http://www.nielsen.com/us/en/newswire/2013/ring-the-bells-more-smartphones-in-students-hands-ahead-of-back.html

Nielsen Corporation. (2014, February). *Digital consumer report*. Retrieved from http://www.nielsen.com/us/en/newswire/2014/whats-empowering-the-new-digital-consumer.html

Nosko, A., Wood, E., & Molema, S. (2010). All about me: Disclosure in online social networking profiles: The case of FACEBOOK. *Computers in Human Behavior, 26*, 406–418.

O'Reilly, T. (2005, September 30). *What is Web 2.0?* Sebastopol, CA: O'Reilly Media, Inc. Retrieved from http://oreilly.com/web2/archive/what-is-web-20.html

Oblinger, D. G. (2013). The connected age for higher education is here. Are we ready for the future? *EDUCAUSE Review, 48*(5), 4–5. Retrieved from https://net.educause.edu/ir/library/pdf/ERM1356.pdf

Owen, M., Grant, L., Sayers, S., & Facer, K. (2006). *Social software and learning. Bristol, United Kingdom.* FutureLabs. Retrieved from http://www.futurelab.org.uk/research/opening_education.htm

Pew Internet and Family Mobile Technology Fact Sheet. (2014, January). Pew Research Center. Retrieved from http://www.pewinternet.org/fact-sheets/mobile-technology-fact-sheet/

Powel, J. A., Darvell, M., & Gray, J. A. (2003). The doctor, the patient and the World Wide Web: How the Internet is changing healthcare. *Journal of the Royal Society of Medicine, 96*, 74–76.

Ruiz, J. G., Mintzer, M. J., & Leipzig, R. M. (2006). The impact of e-learning in medical education. *Academic Medicine, 81*(3), 207–212.

Sarasohn-Kahn, J. (2008, April). *The wisdom of patients: Healthcare meets online social media.* Oakland, CA: California HealthCare Foundation. Retrieved from http://www.chcf.org/topics/chronicdisease/index.cfm?itemID=133631

Skiba, D. (2007). Nursing education 2.0: YouTube. *Nursing Education Perspectives, 28*(2), 100–102.

Skiba, D. (2010). Nursing Education 2.0: Social networking and the WOTY. *Nursing Education Perspectives, 31*(1), 44–46.

Skiba, D. (2011). Nursing Education 2.0: The need for social media policies for schools of nursing. *Nursing Education Perspectives, 32*(2), 126–127.

Skiba, D. (2013). The Internet of things (IOT). *Nursing Education Perspectives, 34*(1), 63–64.

Skiba, D. (2014). The connected age: Implications for 2014. *Nursing Education Perspectives, 35*(1), 63–65. doi:10.5480/1536-5026-35.1.63.

Skiba, D., & Barton, A. (2009). Using social software to transform informatics education. In K. Saranto, P. Brennan, H. Park, M. Tallberg, & A. Ensio (Eds.), *Connecting Health & Humans: Proceedings of NI2009. The 10th International Congress of Nursing Informatics* (pp. 608–612). Amsterdam, The Netherlands: IOS Press.

Skiba, D., Guillory, P., & Dickson, E. (2014). Social media in health care. In N. Staggers & R. Nelson (Eds.), *Health informatics: An interprofessional approach.* St. Louis, MO: Elsevier.

Smith, A. (2014, February). *6 New facts about Facebook.* Pew Research Center. Retrieved from http://www.pewresearch.org/fact-tank/2014/02/03/6-new-facts-about-facebook/

World Health Organization. (2011). *mHealth: New horizons for health through mobile technologies.* Global Observatory for eHealth Series. Volume 3. Retrieved from http://www.who.int/goe/publications/goe_mhealth_web.pdf

Zhang, N. I., Campo, S., Janz, K. F., Eckler, P., Yang, J., Snetselaar, L. G., & Signorini, A. (2013). Electronic word of mouth on Twitter about physical activity in the United States: Exploratory Infodemiology Study. *Journal of Medical Internet Research, 15*(11), e261. Retrieved from http://www.jmir.org/2013/11/e261/

46

A Paradigm Shift in Simulation: Experiential Learning in Virtual Worlds

Helen R. Connors / Judith J. Warren

• OBJECTIVES

1. Describe the use of Virtual Worlds (VW) such as Second Life (SL) as simulated learning.
2. Discuss the pedagogy that drives teaching and learning in the VW.
3. Create a supportive learning environment for educational innovation in VW.
4. Describe common applications to enhance learning in the VW.
5. Discuss future trends for learning in the VW.

• KEY WORDS

Virtual Worlds (VW)
Second Life (SL)
Simulation
Online education
Informatics education
Health professional education
Virtual worlds
User computer interface

INTRODUCTION

Hundreds of leading schools and universities across the globe use virtual worlds (VW) such as Second Life (SL) as an innovative part of their educational courses and programs. Online virtual worlds have multiple uses for teaching and learning. This environment enhances student engagement with course content and develops a sense of community among and between students and faculty. This virtual environment creates a powerful platform for interactive experiences that brings new dimensions to support best practices for learning. In this virtual environment, students and faculty can work together from anywhere in the world, giving education a global perspective and an expanded reach.

The major challenge for online education is student engagement and the evaluation of skill attainment. Virtual worlds provide an online, virtual laboratory that addresses this challenge. Faculty and student avatars can interact with each other, physically and verbally, in real time, thus facilitating simulations where students engage in demonstrating skill acquisition. Faculty are able to coach the skill development, as they now control the environment and can see what the student is doing. This type of evaluation in a real or simulated environment was previously unattainable in an online course. Furthermore, the virtual environment provides a forum for student presentations and interactions with a live audience. Field trips to other virtual environments create opportunities to hone skills in information searching and observation of activities and settings that can be viewed by the faculty and other students. This virtual learning environment can adapt and grow to meet different user needs and is limited only by one's imagination and creativity.

This chapter discusses educational application of virtual worlds with particular emphasis on Second Life. Second Life (www.secondlife.com), a three-dimensional (3D) virtual world, developed by Linden Lab and uniquely imagined and created by its residents was launched in 2003. SL is considered the largest virtual world with tens of millions of square meters of virtual land and more than 36 million registered users. Currently, SL is the most mature and popular virtual world platform being used in education; however, there are several dozen virtual worlds giving SL serious competition, though most are still small and even the largest does not come close to matching Second Life's massive land and user base. Over the past decade, a large number of colleges and universities have established a presence in SL (Knapfel, Moore, & Skiba, 2014; Michels, 2008). These efforts are largely for teaching courses, but also include recruitment activities for prospective students, fund raising, and research endeavors. Today, disenchanted with commercial virtual worlds but still convinced of their educational value, some institutions have started to build their own environment, where they have more control over the learning space (Young, 2010).

TEACHING AND LEARNING IN VIRTUAL WORLDS

The use of virtual worlds expands teaching and learning opportunities for campus-based and online classes. Teaching in a virtual world differs from teaching a traditional online course due to the 3D setting, the use of avatars to represent the participants, and the sense of presence. The degree of immersion and interactivity available in virtual worlds allows for a greater sense of presence which is believed to contribute to meaningful learning, especially when the course is online (Johnson, 2009; Calongne, 2008; Richardson & Swan, 2003). Virtual worlds such as SL facilitate real-time interaction between faculty and students when they are geographically apart. Furthermore, the environment can be controlled or simulated to create a learning experiences designed by the faculty member to achieve pedagogical goals. These planned learning environments previously had to be in one physical place (e.g., learning laboratories, clinical facilities). Second Life supports online education by moving the geography to a virtual space, thus creating a sense of presence for the faculty and students. The sense of presence is important for learner engagement, regardless of whether the experience is real or virtual. *Presence* is defined as "the subjective experience of being in one place or environment, even when one is physically situated in another" (Witmer & Singer, 1998). When in-world, the students feel as if they are actually in the virtual environment. A sense of immersion is also necessary for learning. *Immersion* is the sense of being enveloped by and interacting with the environment. While *involvement* is "a psychological state experienced as a consequence of focusing one's energies and attention on a coherent set of stimuli or meaningfully related activities and events" (Witmer & Singer, 1998). Second Life activities and simulations create presence and immersion for faculty and students, whether they are in traditional classes or online classes. The lack of a sense of presence has always been a major critique of online education. Now there is a tool that minimizes the sense of isolation and distance.

Faculty use virtual worlds for learning activities that require students to exercise higher order thinking. Students can create, apply, analyze, synthesize, and problem-solve using course content and previous knowledge. Teaching strategies include role-play, gaming, simulation of social and clinical skills, collaboration, social networking, and participation in live events such as lectures, conferences, and celebrations. Faculty are finding that they can stage clinical simulations, guide students through the inside of cell structures, or present other imaginative teaching exercises that cannot be done in "real life" due to cost, scheduling, location, or safety issues. The truth is we do not know all the possibilities of what we can and cannot do with this tool for education yet. There are active educational special interest groups, conferences, and listservs enabling faculty to share pedagogical strategies, ideas, and simulations. As Knapfel et al. (2014) recommend continued research is needed to explore best practices for use of VWs in education and practice.

THE PEDAGOGY OF TEACHING IN THE VIRTUAL WORLD

Although it is not the purpose of this chapter to discuss learning theory in detail, it is important to know there are several learning theories that support teaching and learning in virtual worlds. Technology for teaching and learning should always be selected to fit with the pedagogy. First consider the goals for the course and then select the technology tools and strategies that will help meet the proposed outcomes.

To begin with, learners in SL are adults and, therefore, Malcom Knowles' (1984) theory of andragogy provides an overarching framework for designing learning activities for adult learners. Andragogy is based on the following assumptions about adult learners: (1) adults are self-directed, goal oriented, and need to know why they are required to learn something; (2) they approach learning as problem centered rather than content centered; (3) they need to recognize the value of learning and how to incorporate that learning into their jobs or personal lives; and (4) they learn best through experiential learning that incorporates their diverse life experiences in the development of new knowledge. Since adult learners take a great deal of responsibility for their own learning, this greatly alters the role of the faculty in learning environments in general but especially in virtual worlds such as SL. It also should be noted that environments like SL are well suited to applying the assumptions of adult learning theory; however, teachers and learners must adapt to this paradigm shift and to this new environment.

Other learning theories utilizing the principles of andragogy that educators most frequently apply to SL are experiential learning theory, social learning theory, constructivism, connectivism, and collaborative learning theory (Bandura, 1977; Bruner, 1966; Bruner, 1996; Siemens, 2004; Kolb, Boyatzis, & Mainemelis, 2000; Smith & MacGregor, 1992). Many of these theories have overlapping principles that can be mixed and matched to enhance best practices in education (Chickering & Gamson, 1987). Technology advancement and social networking tools such as SL provide rich learning environments for developing and facilitating learning activities that promote the use of these theories. In the authors' opinions, no one model fits best as it will depend upon the goals of the course as well as the teaching and learning style of the faculty and students. Also, some components of a particular theory may not be satisfied in a virtual world like SL. Today, although explosive, only the tip of the iceberg is being seen by colleges, universities, and training programs using VWs. As the trend continues to grow in popularity, educators and researchers will realize the expansion of current theories as well as new theories and patterns of learning will be developed.

Designing the Learning Space

Working in virtual worlds is not always intuitive. Faculty need to rethink how the course material is structured and delivered. They need technical assistance to help with

complex instructional design decisions that are congruent with the pedagogy, teaching strategies, and outcomes. Faculty should not be expected to be the technology experts; rather, they should team up with an IT professional for design and delivery support associated with technical training and technical issues. As a team they will work together to adopt and integrate this technology as an innovative practice for teaching, learning, and research. The challenge that faculty faces is determining the various nuances of their audience, understanding the content, determining the best approach to deliver the content, and developing a comfort level with the technology (Hodges & Collins, 2010).

Commonly, the virtual world learning space is designed to replicate the traditional learning space. Areas are developed to support broadly defined educational activities. These virtual areas typically include a large lecture hall or auditorium for presentations, smaller classrooms for discussion, an exhibition hall for displaying student work, and faculty office space for meeting with students. However, this real-world approach to virtual world learning space brings with it similar constraints on the types of teaching and learning that can happen in those spaces (Gerald & Antonacci, 2009). For example, large lecture halls, whether in the real world or the virtual world, are based on objectivist approach to course design, and such spaces do little to support more collaborative and constructivist learning approaches. Gerald and Antonacci (2009) suggest that in addition to designing spaces to meet traditional learning needs, the majority of the learning space can be designed to meet specifications for course projects. These spaces might include a home to practice assessing and remediating disability issues, a community living center as the context for database development, an operating room simulation for learning complex medical procedures, a health clinic for interacting with simulated patients and inter-professional team members, or perhaps a grocery store, restaurant, and exercise facility for teaching learners healthy living skills. Let the course or project goals and your creativity guide the design. Here are some things to consider in designing the learning space.

Orientation

Calongne (2008) points out that although it is tempting to begin a virtual world class with an orientation to the software and the virtual world itself, students need action and excitement to help them envision how the technology will enrich their learning experience. She recommends that faculty sell the benefits first and then discuss how it works. Begin with exciting examples from other classes or research projects to make the experience real, personal, and engaging; then, provide a brief introduction demonstrating how to use the tool effectively. Keep in mind that in higher education, not all students are created equally. Creating an avatar and figuring out how to move, look around, and interact with others may be a challenge for some students, but not all. Getting everyone to the in-world class site may require extra time initially, so plan for it, and you may want to provide alternative communication support for added assistance, if needed. Finally, if some students are hesitant, mitigate any fears or risks associated with using the technology and create a safe learning environment.

Orienting students to virtual worlds should follow the precepts of experiential learning. The SL Web site has very clear directions for downloading the portal to the environment and then leads the individual through creating an avatar. Encourage students to engage in this experience of downloading software and creating an avatar by letting them know they are developing health informatics competencies. An orientation to participating in SL also is needed. Within directions for this exercise, a possible statement to achieve this purpose may be:

> Second Life is an immersive virtual environment. An avatar is a user's self-representation in the form of a 3-dimensional model. In Second Life, creating your avatar is part of how you will interact with other residents. Some people design their avatar as a life-like representation of self. As the popularity of Second Life grows, many professional meetings occur in this virtual world; please dress you avatar in casual or professional clothes. The user controls the avatar through the use of the mouse or keyboard to walk, fly, and sit. An avatar can interact with other avatars through instant messages or the audio function (using a headset).

Once the avatar is created there are several video tutorials to teach students how to navigate their avatars in SL, see Table 46.1 for suggestions. Upon completion of the tutorials, the faculty and student avatars should be ready to enter SL. Students need to feel competent enough with the technology to carry out required task and to meet the learning objectives. Basically, they should be able to move, look around, customize avatars, and interact with each other. During the first SL activity, a support person, knowledgeable in SL technology, should be available to troubleshoot problems with software and microphone use. After the first SL experience, students are ready to engage in more activities and openly share their enthusiasm for this type of interaction. As faculty begin to envision more activities, they will need additional support to make these happen without having to take time to become experts in using and building in SL.

TABLE 46.1	Resources for Orienting New Second Life Users
Resources for Orienting New SL Users	**URLs and SL URLs**
Virtual Ability, http://www.virtualability.org/	If you have an SL account, teleport to http://maps.secondlife.com/secondlife/Virtual%20Ability/127/127/23
YouTube videos created by Virtual Ability	Part One: www.youtube.com/watch?v=XAjG4Tv6LvU
	Part Two: www.youtube.com/watch?v=AVzyi0MOsJM&feature=related
	Part Three: www.youtube.com/watch?v=Cnyt6rASfo0&feature=related
Getting Started in Second Life	http://wiki.secondlife.com/wiki/Getting_started_with_Second_Life
	http://community.secondlife.com/t5/English-Knowledge-Base/Second-Life-Quickstart/ta-p/1087919
Getting Started in Second Life by Savin-Bade, Tombs, White, Poulton, Kavia, and Woodham	www.jisc.ac.uk/publications/generalpublications/2009/gettingstartedsecondlife.aspx

Course Design

Virtual worlds use a mix of media-rich course materials selected to correspond to the learning activities and the students' learning needs. Learning activities are experiential and can be designed to be synchronous or asynchronous, allowing students to interact with the subject matter to study, discuss, create, and express their views of the content under the supervision of the faculty member. The faculty's role shifts from the authoritative expert to that of the dominant expert who stimulates and supervises exploration while providing structure, guidance, feedback, and assessment (Calongne, 2008). Virtual worlds provide immense opportunities for innovation and cultivate new ways to meet higher order learning. Rather than lecture, the class activity may involve teams of students taking a virtual field trip, gathering information, and later submitting their assignment through an SL group chat space or by collaboratively creating a presentation, a project management plan, or some other scholarly product to illustrate application, analyses, synthesis, or evaluation of the learning. The exemplars that follow describe one institution's design principles and learning activities.

EXEMPLARS OF LEARNING IN SECOND LIFE

The University of Kansas Experience

The University of Kansas Medical Center (KUMC) is organized into three major schools: Medicine, Nursing, and Health Professionals. These schools are supported by the Department of Teaching and Learning Technology (TLT) located within the Division of Information Resources. TLT's mission is to provide leadership and support for the successful integration of new and existing educational technologies across KUMC learning environments. One of these technologies is Second Life, which KUMC faculty use for communication, presentations, immersive learning activities including simulation and role-playing, and research projects. The staff in the TLT department began exploring and researching the Second Life virtual world in 2004, just after it was released from beta. Struck by the educational potential of this new learning space, TLT staff began working with interested faculty to connect real-world course content with virtual world learning activities. Because of the interest expressed by faculty in the nursing informatics, nursing anesthesia, as well as the physical and occupational therapy programs, KUMC administrators in 2007 decided to purchase its own island or private space and named it KUMC isle. An island or private region allows for restricted access and other levels of control not available on the virtual mainland. Faculty worked closely with TLT to establish goals and objectives for teaching in SL and to get started by building the necessary learning space. Collaboration among the campus academic programs helps set standards and creates academic environments that are efficient and effective as well as model the real-world academic environment. Building on the success experienced in health informatics, physical therapy, and nurse anesthesia, other KUMC programs began to use SL to enhance learning and conduct research studies.

Graduate Health Informatics Program

Learning to be a health informaticist requires developing skills identifying use cases and workflows in clinical environments. These are experiential skills and are difficult to master in an online environment. Simulations and clinical experiences are the traditional approaches for teaching these skills, yet are not feasible in online courses where students reside in multiple states and time zones.

Virtual reality environments, like SL, provided the online platform for simulations to experience and practice informatics skills. Second Life was selected as the simulation environment for our online health informatics graduate program. These simulations facilitate the development of informatics competencies for future work environments.

The curriculum, among other skills, teaches information system design and database development. An SL simulation was constructed to facilitate learning these skills. The faculty designed the Jayhawk Community Living Center (JCLC), an assisted living facility, for the simulation. The JCLC was designed to include rooms for six residents, a day room, dining room, clinic room, nurses' station, medical records room, medication room, director's office, and conference room. Landscaping, including a deck over the water surrounding KUMC Island, was built to enhance the reality of the simulation (Fig. 46.1). Cues and artefact concerning information system requirements were placed in various locations within the JCLC so that students learned to observe the environment. Some of these cues were multiple telephones for residents, computer locations for staff, and floor plans for workflows. Faculty played the roles of Director of Nursing and staff nurse.

The purpose of one particular simulation is to design a fall-risk management information system for the JCLC. This would be the first electronic health record for the JCLC. Students are given a Request for Proposal (RFP) and information about falls: evidence-based protocols, workflows, and policies for the management of fall risk, and resident data concerning fall risk. Their first task is to meet with the Director of Nursing in the JCLC conference room to clarify the requirements for the information system. This meeting is conducted through text messaging within SL so that a transcript of the meeting is available for analysis (Fig. 46.2).

Next the students are taken on a tour of the JCLC, as they would be in real life, to observe and ask questions to clarify the requirements for the fall-risk information system. Students must design the entire system—architecture, software, Internet access, security and confidentiality constraints, and other relevant system functions. The deliverables for the design are storyboards, use cases, use-case diagrams, workflow diagrams, and activity diagrams for both current and future states.

In the database theory course, the students return to the JCLC to design and build an access database for the fall-risk management assessments. They must work with the staff again to determine database table structures (conceptual, logical, and physical data models), data entry forms, standard data queries, required reports, and training needs. This time the cues are very important, as the students must realize that each resident has two telephones

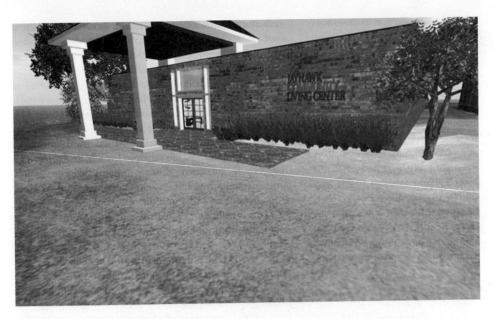

• **FIGURE 46.1.** The Jayhawk Community Living Center (JCLC).

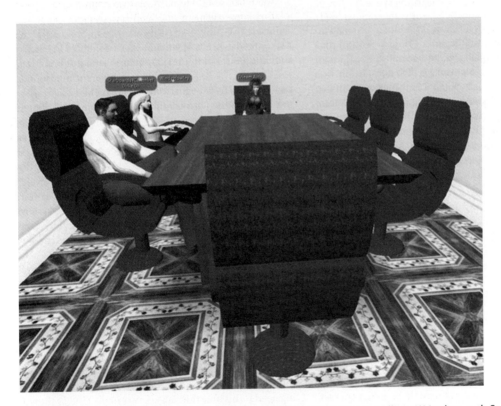

• **FIGURE 46.2.** Conference Room of the Director of Nursing With Director Ellipse Wrigglesworth Seated.

that must be in the database as well as other physical cues regarding data collection and input. This is a common problem in database design. Information concerning each resident is posted on a "Touch Me" card outside the resident's room (Fig. 46.3). The database produced by the students must contain all the information and address each design challenge embedded in the simulation.

Students enjoy the experience, request more class time in SL, and successfully develop informatics projects. SL is a great way to simulate a facility so students can learn to elicit user requirements for information systems. The challenges are scheduling meeting times, managing group interactions, practicing etiquette in group interactions, and learning to use the technology of SL.

Students present posters in SL as a way to demonstrate learning. Many of the presentations are about usability and design issues, system security approaches, federal regulations impacting the discipline of informatics, database management systems, and so forth. The simulation helps them learn to put together a poster and answer questions of attendees at the poster session. A poster pavilion module was created with six poster boards (Fig. 46.4). This module can be recreated to host as many presenters as is required.

Course Evaluations

A serendipitous finding in using SL was using The Beach on KUMC Isle as a place to celebrate the end of a course and for students to share with faculty what worked and what did not work. Early on, students suggested adjourning to the beach after the last class. Faculty facilitated the meeting and engaged the students in informal discussions about the use of SL. Students shared their enthusiasm for SL and then began to share perspectives on the course. The informal environment, outside the course, encouraged very productive discussions that lead faculty to change several course strategies. Now after every course, a Beach Party is conducted to debrief the course. Students continue to be very professional in their desire to help the courses evolve into highly successful experiences. The Beach is shown in Fig. 46.5.

Use of Second Life in Doctoral Nursing Courses

During the first semester, all doctoral students enroll in a technology and informatics course. This course is designed to assist the student in developing skills to complete an online doctoral program. Second Life is one of several Web 2.0 programs introduced to the students. Formal presentations of team projects are required. Students use instant messaging and SL to meet as a team to organize the work of their projects, thus enhancing their informatics skills. The presentations are conducted in the amphitheater, using microphones and speakers. Students are able to see the audience, pace the presentation, and answer questions just as they would in the real world. These students also enjoy the Beach Party at the end of the course and have helped make this course very popular (Figs. 46.6, 46.7, and 46.8).

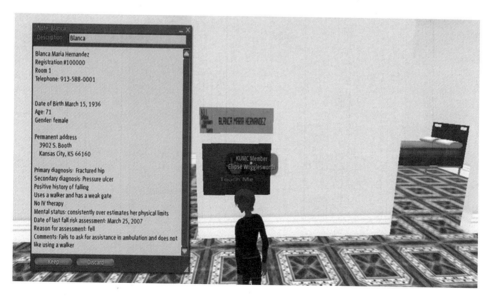

• **FIGURE 46.3.** "Touch Me" Cards With Resident Information to Be Placed in the Database.

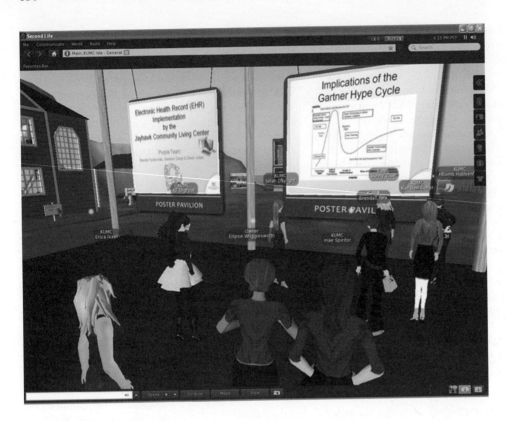

• **FIGURE 46.4.** Poster Pavilion.

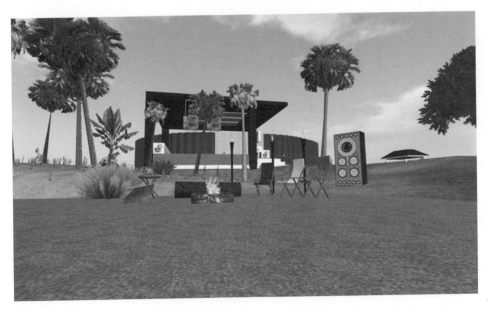

• **FIGURE 46.5.** The Beach, Complete With Palm Trees, Fire Pit, Places to Sit, and Tiki Torches.

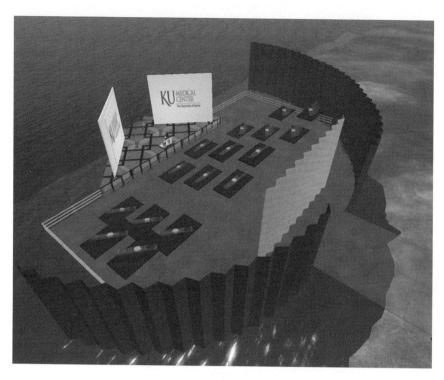

• **FIGURE 46.6.** The Amphitheater Used for Formal Presentations.

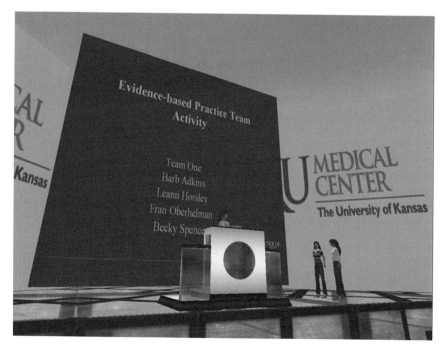

• **FIGURE 46.7.** Students Giving the Presentation and Using Slides.

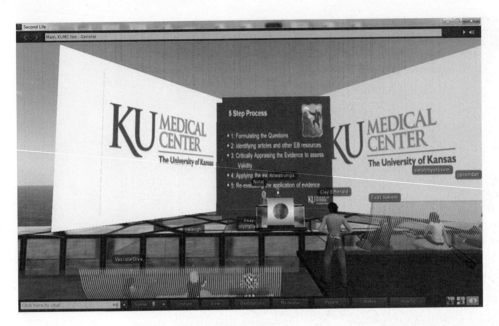

• **FIGURE 46.8.** Students Interacting With the Audience.

Nurse Anesthesia Program

TLT staff in collaboration with faculty in the Nurse Anesthesia program developed a virtual world operating room simulation to assist first-year Nurse Anesthesia students with learning the basic induction procedure. Nurse Anesthesia faculty members were already experienced with physical patient simulators, such as SimMan; however, they were especially interested in virtual simulations, since a large amount of their program trains students in different processes and procedures. The objectives for this project is to learn how the operating room is organized, to navigate the environment, to learn workflow and organizational skills, and to practice the basic induction procedure before stepping foot in the real-life operating room. The SL operating room is designed to look exactly like the operating room at KU Hospital (Fig. 46.9). The clocks and the tables and the other objects are in the same locations as they are in the real operating room. This creates the ability for students to be exposed to the layout of the operating room before they experience the real environment. Some of the equipment in the SL space is designed to be interactive so the students can manipulate them and gain confidence. To view how the student progresses through the learning activity and how the objects interact with each other, view the video tutorial of the Second Life Operating Room (http://www.youtube.com/watch?v=70CkcswfDe4).

Physical and Occupational Therapy Program

The physical and occupational therapy faculty partnered with TLT staff to develop virtual home environments in Second Life (Figs. 46.10 and 46.11). The home environment is a critical part of everyday life and participation in activities of daily living and instrumental activities of daily living. The homes were designed with a focus on objects within the home to assist students to identify environmental barriers and support, and to make critical decisions regarding environmental and task modification for clients. The student learning outcomes include inter-professional collaboration, patient-centered decision-making, and appreciation of the environmental and social context of functional mobility and occupational performance.

Physical and occupational therapy students working in teams use SL to evaluate the home of a disabled client. There are a series of three homes with different hazards to be identified. Students are given a patient record with information concerning the patient's abilities and disabilities. They then conduct a walk through and make recommendations for creating a safer home environment. Faculty control the visual cues and hazards, and so know when the students make accurate assessments. Once students make the recommendation, the TLT staff modified the home according to the recommendations and faculty and peers evaluate the modifications based on levels of support,

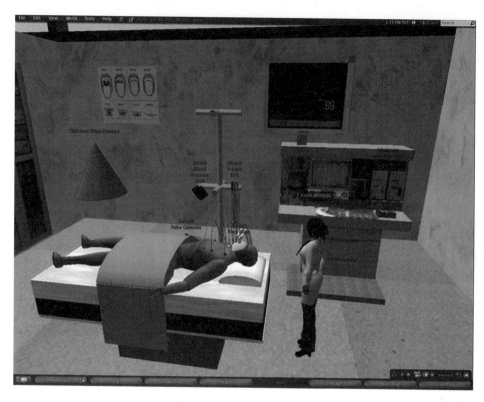

• **FIGURE 46.9.** Operating Room.

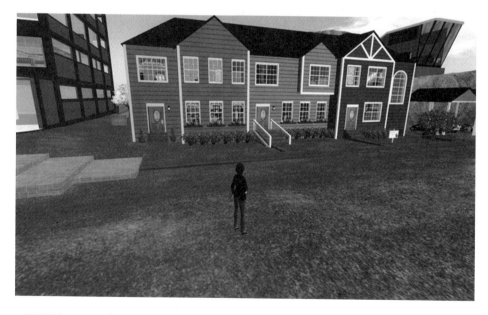

• **FIGURE 46.10.** The Row Houses for Home Evaluations.

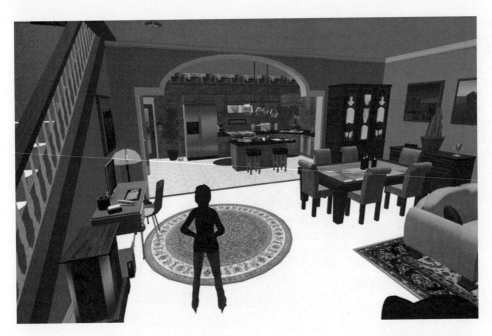

• **FIGURE 46.11.** Living Room and Kitchen of One of the Row Houses, Showing Safety Hazards.

unintended challenges, and client preferences. Seeing the outcomes of their recommendations is a step that is usually not able to be accomplished in the real-world because students are not always able to see their modifications carried out (Sabus, Sabata, & Antonacci, 2011).

Dietetics and Nutrition Weight Management Program

A faculty researcher in the Department of Dietetics and Nutrition saw a presentation by a faculty member in occupational therapy who was teaching a class in Second Life, and immediate thought this would be a good environment to use for weight management (Sullivan et al., 2013). Sullivan's research team studied 20 overweight and obese people in a program that involved either real-life or virtual reality meetings every week for three months. At the end of that period, all the subjects took part in a weight-maintenance program using Second Life. Sullivan found that while virtual reality compares favorably with face-to-face interactions in controlling weight loss, its true benefits were more readily apparent in weight maintenance. In the study, participants created avatars that could interact with the other cyber-dwellers in the group. Training and education took place on KUMC isle. Participants used headsets and microphones to communicate with others within the group. Since SL can automatically work with Web sites

like YouTube to pull in content to use within the simulation, during meetings of the avatars in a virtual conference room, group leaders could show videos or present other materials.

KUMC's original island environment included a conference room, house, gymnasium (Figs. 46.12 and 46.13), grocery store (Fig. 46.14), restaurant, and buffet. Each space provided the avatars with a setting to interact with each other as well as to check on calorie counts in food items, calories burned during exercise, and other helpful information. By using SL participants can simulate real-life situations without many of the consequences and repercussions that occur in real life. For example, the avatars can practice meal planning complete with calorie counts for items in the grocery store, dining out, or attending holiday parties, all in the anonymity of cyberspace. The goal of the simulation is to create a friendly environment where people can spend time researching healthier lifestyles without the fear of being judged.

As a result of Sullivan's preliminary research, she and her team received a grant from the National Institutes of Health to continue the research. Through this grant KUMC created a new island KUMC Healthy U. The new island expands opportunities for the participants. On KUMC Healthy U, avatars will be able to take advantage of restaurants with cashiers that total the amount of calories on customers' trays as they check out. A kiosk,

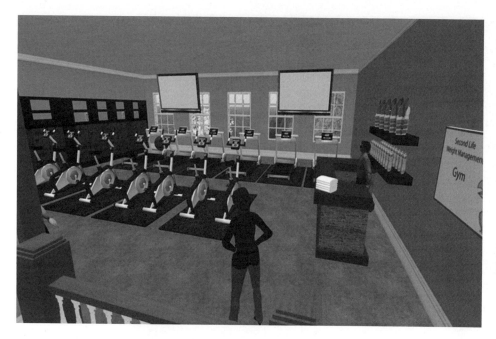

• **FIGURE 46.12.** Gymnasium for Weight Management Program.

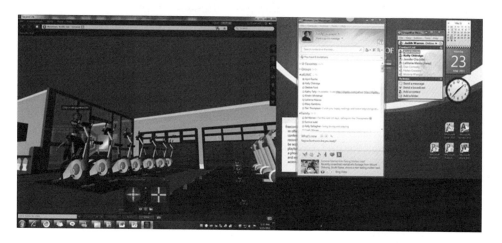

• **FIGURE 46.13.** Gymnasium for Weight Management Program.

known as Fast Food Frenzy, links avatars to the Web sites of various restaurants, which allows them to calculate the calories in their meals. The new island also includes a more elaborate gymnasium, complete with a swimming pool where avatars can register the calories burned as they swim, tread water, or take part in activities in the water. Trainers in the gym are able to help the research subjects by answering basic fitness questions. Avatars can also access fitness videos while doing their simulated running on treadmills. One of the highlights of the new island is trails where avatars can walk, run, or bike while Second Life keeps tabs on the calories burned. All participants in this study will receive the same weight-loss program for six months and then either be randomized to virtual reality or remain with a traditional method for 12 months of weight-loss maintenance. The overall aim

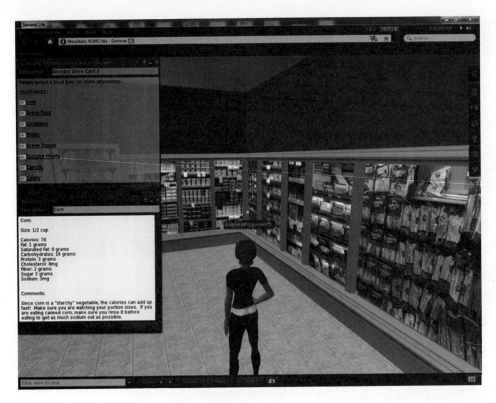

• **FIGURE 46.14.** Grocery Store With Note Cards.

is to compare the difference in weight-loss maintenance between the two groups. The resources developed in SL for this research project also are used by other faculty to meet their course objectives. For example, informatics students have developed smart phone apps that can be used for weight loss and maintenance. Undergraduate students can be assigned to shop in the virtual grocery store or dine in the many restaurants to learn about healthy food choices. Virtual worlds are valuable new research tools to study human behavior. Researchers can inexpensively prototype models and explore data visualization in unique ways.

Administrative Considerations: Creating a Supportive Environment

Educational innovation is a process of bringing new teaching strategies to satisfied learners and future knowledge workers. It is a conversion of new knowledge into value-added outcomes enhanced by novel teaching strategies. Innovation in education involves not only technological advances, but also pedagogical approaches.

Most innovative educators are recognizing and experimenting with the educational possibilities of virtual worlds. Also, student enthusiasm for these learning formats is strong, creating uniquely powerful interactive and compelling educational possibilities. At the same time, for many faculty members, teaching in SL can be daunting. Learning the new technology, meeting the needs of the technologically diverse students, understanding virtual reality pedagogy, and managing workload and time are some of the challenges. It is up to academic administrators to provide the support and resources to encourage faculty to use new technologies such as Second life and other emerging technologies. The goal is to minimize organizational barriers to student and faculty success. Challenges at the organizational level need to be anticipated and policies, procedures, and guidelines should be in place to help mitigate their impact on faculty and students. Faculty who desire to use SL need to be heard to feel supported, and to have an infrastructure in place that not only supports the present, but allows for growth and rewards faculty's efforts. Creating a supportive environment for successful adaptation of innovative teaching strategies requires resources, but, more importantly, it requires a cultural shift for many academic institutions.

A Culture of Innovation

As technology advances, today's learning environment needs to convey a culture of innovation and strategically plan to meet the challenge of change. Every academic organization has a culture; the issue is whether and how that organization supports innovation. A culture of innovation gives you a competitive edge because it makes you more nimble with an increased ability to respond to change. To be successful, a culture of innovation should reflect a balance between an openness to allow ideas to flow, and the creation of controls and supports around those ideas.

Academia is steeped in a tradition of hierarchical beliefs where research and scholarship is rewarded and educational innovation is not. To fully integrate a culture of innovation within the organization, key concepts of innovation need to be reflected in the organization's mission, vision, leadership, core values, hiring practices, metrics, rewards, and compensation. The concepts call for new interactions and partnerships involving a team approach to teaching, learning, and research. Also, success requires clear communication from leadership that describes how the institution understands educational innovation and that understanding should be built into the organizational behavior and modeled by the leader. Faculty and staff should feel comfortable and supported to take risks without fear of failure or retribution. As Melnyk and Davidson (2009) point out, "success in an innovative culture is viewed as going from one failure to the next with enthusiasm" (p. 2).

Strategic Planning and Support for Innovation

In the early 1990s, the University of Kansas Medical Center (KUMC) Division of Information Resources, in collaboration with the Schools of Medicine, Nursing and Allied Health, and the Division of Continuing Education, embarked on a strategic planning process to position the academic environment for the new wave of technology-based education. This planning process resulted in the formation of a re-envisioned academic support department—the Department of Teaching and Learning Technologies (TLT). The department is housed within the KUMC Information Resource Division. Central to its mission, the department has evolved over time to support new and diverse technologies, providing cutting edge technology tools for faculty and students. KUMC faculty, staff, students, and community have dependable access to core teaching and learning technologies as well as the

knowledge, skills, and support to be successful with these tools. They also are aware of promising new technologies, and have both the technical and pedagogical support to explore and evaluate the educational possibilities of these tools. As technologies mature, those with the greatest potential to enhance teaching and learning are integrated into our core technologies, establishing a pattern of innovation and success. This infrastructure, which includes four instructional designers and three technology specialists, has served the Medical Center campus well over the ensuing years as educational technologies advanced and became more affordable and acceptable. Key to KUMC's success is the partnership between faculty and the TLT staff to design, develop, and implement courses using enhanced technologies and to work collaboratively across KUMC academic programs to develop a community of technology educators who share ideas and challenge each other.

School of Nursing Administrative Support

The School of Nursing (SON) administration fully supports teaching in SL and serves as a liaison between the faculty and the TLT administrator to assure academic innovation and maintain quality and integrity of academic programs. Clear communication about faculty's pedagogical needs is essential to good outcomes and assures faculty the support they need. Faculty who are champions in this new learning environment need to be encouraged to take risks and should be rewarded for their efforts. To demonstrate its commitment to innovation, the SON revised its appointment, promotion, and tenure criteria, using Boyer's model of scholarship, to reflect the value of innovation in education, practice, and research. Boyer (1997) proposed an expanded definition of *scholarship* within the professoriate based on four functions: discovery, integration, application, and teaching. He argues that all forms of scholarship should be recognized and rewarded, and that this will lead to more personalized and flexible criteria for gaining tenure. Boyer proposes using "creativity contracts" that emphasize quality and innovation in teaching, while fostering professional growth that supports individuals and their passions. A balanced focus on all forms of scholarship is critical to meet the challenges in creating and sustaining innovative academic programs. Using this model, faculty are encouraged, supported, and rewarded for risk taking, pilot testing, and design thinking in their teaching practices.

The technology service support in the SON is another example of administration's support for the use of SL and other technology-supported practices. These services include an advanced technology environment for all faculty and staff, coordinated with all of the services at the

KUMC campus level. The SON supports two dedicated professionals who exclusively serve the technology needs of the school. The lead person is a network engineer who manages the school's file servers and other advanced technologies and is assisted by a person who provides local desktop assistance, database programming, and video-conferencing assistance to assist faculty teaching with a wide variety of technologies. The school's support staff also provides services such as notebook computer support for faculty and staff, assistance in purchasing hardware and software to support research and educational innovation, and assistance with mobile computing devices. Teaching in SL requires a computer with hefty specs to run

properly. Through these technology services and futuristic planning, the SON assures that faculty have what it takes to successfully teach in SL (see Table 46.2 for resources).

Faculty are the most important factor in the overall success of using SL and innovative teaching strategies. If faculty feel well supported (technology, design, administrative) and have a voice in determining policies and procedures for fostering innovative environments, they will be more willing to move in-world with SL. Specifically, faculty need training, professional development, and release time for initial increased workload and design issues. Since faculty work collaboratively with instructional design and technology specialists, recognize that

TABLE 46.2	Faculty Resources for Learning More About Second Life
Articles	Wiecha, J., Heyden, R., Sternthal, E., & Merialdi, M. (2010). Learning in a virtual world: Experience with using second life for medical education. *Journal of Medical Internet Research. 12*(1). Published online January 23, 2010. Retrieved from http://www.ncbi.nlm.gov./pmc/articles/PMC2821584/.
	Innovate (innovateonline.info/?view=issue) contains several articles on Second Life and the use of virtual worlds in education. Check out the June/July 2009 and the August/September 2009 issues.
	Oaks, S. (2011). Real learning in a virtual world. *The International HETL Review. 1*(3). Retrieved from https://www.hetl.org/feature-articles/real-learning-in-a-virtual-world/
	Davis, A., Khazanchi, D., Murphy, J., Zigurs, I., & Owens, D. (2009). Avatars, people, and virtual worlds: Foundations for research in metaverses. *Journal of the Association for Information Systems, 10*(2), 90–117.
	Harrison, D. (2009, February 18). Real-life teaching in a virtual world. *Campus Technology*. Retrieved from http://campustechnology.com/Articles/2009/02/18/Real-Life-Teaching-in-a-Virtual-World.aspx
	Ongley, J. (2009, October). *Education by avatar at the University of Hawaii*. Retrieved from http://www.hawaii.edu/malamalama/2009/10/second-life
	Antonacci, D., DiBartolo, S., Edwards, N., Fritch, K., McMullen, B., & Murch-Shafer, R. (2009). *The power of virtual worlds: A second life primer and resource for exploring the potential of virtual worlds to impact teaching and learning. Angel Learning White Paper*. Retrieved from http://www.angellearning.com/products/secondlife/downloads/The%20Power%20of%20Virtual%20Worlds%20in%20Education_0708.pdf
	Skiba, D. (2009). Nursing education 2.0: A second look at Second Life. *Nursing Education Perspectives, 30*(2), 129–131.
	Journal of Virtual Worlds Research. Retrieved from http://jvwresearch.org/index.php?_cms=default,3,0
Book	Boellstorff, T. (2010). *Coming of age in second life: An anthropologist explores the virtually human*. Princeton, NJ: Princeton University Press.
	Krotoski, A., Cezanne, P., Rymaszewski, M., Rossignol, J., Wagner., & Au, J. (2008). *Second Life: The official guide* (2nd ed.). New York, NY: John Wiley & Sons.
	Robbins, S., & Bell, Mike (2011). *Second life for dummies*. New York, NY: John Wiley & Sons.
	Bruns, A. (2008). *Blogs, Wikipedia, Second Life, and beyond: From production to produsage*. New York, NY: Peter Lang Pub Inc.
	Weber, A., Rufer-Bach, K., Platel, R. (2007). *Creating your world: The official guide to advanced content creation for Second Life*. New York, NY: John Wiley & Sons.
	Wankel, C., & Kingsley, J. (2009). Higher education in virtual worlds: Teaching and learning in second life. Bingley, UK: Emerald Group Publishing Limited.
	Percival, S. (2008). *Second Life: In-world travel guide*. Indianapolis, IN: Que Publishing.
Web sites	Examples of Education and Non-profits in SL: http://secondlife.com/destinations/learning
	Second Life Education Wiki: http://wiki.secondlife.com/wiki/Second_Life_Education

training needs shift from training faculty on software to training them on new teaching approaches, instructional design strategies, and workload management topics. Keep in mind that virtual worlds may not be for everyone; work with your champions and let them be the driver and set the standard. Celebrate your successes by having your champions showcase their work at faculty meetings and professional development sessions.

FUTURE TRENDS AND CONCLUSION

Virtual Worlds are environments that can provide valuable educational experiences for nursing and other health professions. The degree of immersion and interactivity available provides a greater sense of presence and engagement, contributing to better learning outcomes in both in-person and online courses. Faculty and staff are able to exercise their creativity to provide dynamic simulations for students in a novel, virtual world. The outcomes are well worth the effort and resources required to produce high-quality learning experiences. Virtual environments have extended the reach of educators into worlds without boundaries. These worlds are free from self-imposed constraints and opened to new ways of thinking, imagining, expressing, and building. Virtual Worlds can provide many unique learning opportunities; however, it is important to use VWs not for the sake of using the tool, but for how the tool can facilitate learning. Knapfel et al. (2014) provide an excellent overview of the history of VWs and give examples of how several schools and organizations are using SL to support education and practice.

As computer power and networking speeds are evolving virtual spaces for learning will continue to advance. The question is, are most educators ready to enter this space? Many faculty and administrators are not imaginatively equipped for what the technology can do or how to use it to enhance learning. However, this may change as the "gamer" generation becomes more mature and able to recognize the value of immersive learning from their past experiences.

Although this chapter focused on the use of SL, it is estimated that there are over 450 VWs. Some educational institutions, disenchanted with SL's pricing and policy change, have switched to other platforms such as OpenSim, ReactionGrid, OSgrid, and Active Worlds, to name a few. These are evolving open source virtual reality online platforms. However, as previously mentioned most are still small and even the largest does not come close to matching Second Life's massive land and user base. Each virtual world will have advantages and disadvantages. When selecting a VW platform it is important to consider

institutional needs, affordability, availability, usability, maintenance, and vendor stability. SL has a large following of educators who share ideas, content, teaching strategies and collaborate across learning spaces. It would be a shame to lose that cohesiveness as institutions become more scattered in their choice of virtual spaces. As these other options for virtual space mature, it is important to advocate for interoperability to enable avatars as well as content to be transported from one virtual space to another. Also, as these technologies continue to evolve and expand in use, it will be essential to conduct research to identify best practices for VW education and collaboration.

REFERENCES

Bandura, A. (1977). *Social learning theory*. New York, NY: General Learning Press.

Boyer, E. L. (1997). *Scholarship reconsidered: Priorities of the professoriate*. San Francisco, CA: Jossey-Bass.

Bruner, J. (1966). *Towards a theory of instruction*. Cambridge, MA: Harvard University Press.

Bruner, J. (1996). *The culture of education*. Cambridge, MA: Harvard University Press.

Calongne, C. M. (2008). Educational frontiers: Learning in a virtual world. *Educause Review, 43*(5), 36–42.

Chickering, A. E., & Gamson, Z. F. (1987). Seven principles for good practice in undergraduate education. *AAHE Bulletin, 39*(7), 3–6.

Gerald, S. P., & Antonacci, D. M. (2009). Virtual world learning spaces: Developing a Second Life operating room simulation. *EDUCAUSE Quarterly, 32*(1). Retrieved from http://www.educause.edu/ero/article/virtual-world-learning-spaces-developing-second-life-operating-room-simulation.

Hodges, E. M., & Collins, S. (2010). Collaborative teaching and learning in virtual worlds. *Educause Review, 45*(3), 62–63.

Johnson, C. M. (2009). Virtual worlds in healthcare higher education. *Journal of Virtual Worlds Research, 2*(2), 3–12.

Knapfel, S., Moore, G., & Skiba, D. J. (2014). Second Life and other virtual emerging simulations. In P. R. Jeffries (Ed.), *Clinical simulations in nursing education: Advanced concepts, trends, and opportunities* (pp. 90–100). Philadelphia, PA: J.B. Lippincott, Williams, and Wilkins.

Knowles, M. (1984). *The adult learner: A neglected species* (3rd ed.). Houston, TX: Gulf Publishing.

Kolb, D., Boyatzis, R., & Mainemelis, C. (2000). Experiential learning theory: Previous research and new directions. In R. J. Sternberg & L. F. Zhang (Eds.), *Perspectives on cognitive, learning and thinking styles*. Mahwah, NJ: Lawrence Erlbaum.

Melnyk, B. M., & Davidson, S. (2009). Creating a culture of innovation in nursing education through shared vision, leadership, interdisciplinary partnerships, and positive deviance. *Nursing Administration Quarterly, 33*(4), 288–295.

Michels, P. (2008, February 26). *Universities use Second Life to teach complex concepts*. Government Technology. Retrieved from http://www.govtech.com/gt/252550?topic=118264

Richardson, J. C., & Swan, K. (2003). Examining social presence in online courses in relation to students' perceived learning and satisfaction. *Journal of Asynchronous Learning, 7*(1), 68–88.

Sabus, C., Sabata, D., & Antonacci, D. M. (2011). Use of a virtual environment to facilitate instruction of an interprofessional home assessment. *Journal of Allied Health, 40*(4), 199–205.

Siemens, G. (2004, December 12). Connectivism: A learning theory for the digital age. *Elearnspace*. Retrieved from http://www.elearnspace.org/Articles/connectivism.htm

Smith, B. L., & MacGregor, J. T. (1992). *What is collaborative learning?* Retrieved from https://umdrive.memphis.edu/ggholson/public/collab.pdf

Sullivan, D. K., Goetz, J. R., Gibson, C. A., Washburn, R. A., Smith, B. K., Lee, J., ... Donnelly, J. E. (2013). Improving weight maintenance using virtual reality (Second Life). *Journal of Nutrition Education and Behavior, 45*(3), 264–268.

Witmer, B. G., & Singer, M. J. (1998). Measuring presence in virtual environments: A presence questionnaire. *Presence, 7*(3), 229–240.

Young, J. R. (2010, February 14). After frustration in second life colleges look to new virtual worlds. *The Chronicle of Higher Education*. Retrieved from http://chronicle.com/article/After-Frustrations-in-Second/64137/

PART 8

Research Applications

Virginia K. Saba

47

Computer Use in Nursing Research

Veronica D. Feeg / Theresa A. Rienzo

• OBJECTIVES

1. Describe general data and computer applications related to research in nursing, including proposal development and project implementation in both quantitative and qualitative research (*computer use in research*).
2. Summarize a range of computer-based, Web innovations, tablet and mobile applications that facilitate or support the steps of the research process, including data collection, data management and coding, data analysis, and results reporting.
3. Compare and contrast select computer software applications that can be used in quantitative and qualitative research data analysis related to the steps of the research process.
4. Describe specific research studies in the literature that exemplify quantitative and qualitative methodologies on computer applications in healthcare.
5. Describe general categories of research that focuses on computer use in healthcare, from clinical applications and informatics integration to health and wellness (*nursing research on computer use*).
6. Introduce the new emphasis on "big data" and the growing interest in analysis of existing data to answer research questions on populations.
7. Describe the drivers for promoting informatics research and computer applications today for improving safety and quality of healthcare in the future (*research on nursing informatics*).

• KEY WORDS

Nursing informatics research
Research process
Research methodology
"Big Data"
Quantitative
Qualitative
Data collection
Data mining

Data management
Data analysis
Research applications
Computer applications
Internet research
Secondary analysis
Meta-analysis

INTRODUCTION

Nursing research involves a plethora of tools and resources that researchers employ throughout the research process. From the individual or collaborative project initiation, through refinement of the idea, selection of approaches, development of methods, capturing the data, analyzing the results, and disseminating the findings, computer applications are an indispensable resource for the researcher. The investigators must be well prepared in a variety of computerized techniques for research activities as they are employed in the domain of knowledge that will be investigated. Without the power of technology, contemporary research would not reach the levels of sophistication required to discover and understand health and illness today.

In addition to the traditional approaches of the scientific method, researchers today have new avenues to explore in the development of knowledge. New opportunities to mine existing data for evaluation and discovery are forming a bridge between the process of conducting research and the products of discovery. New tools for automatic capture and analysis are changing the methods textbooks. New online strategies and apps are being implemented as the process of researching health and the product of researched interventions in health. From mobile applications that are downloadable to smart phones for researchers or patients or both, to tools for exploring large data sets that have been already captured, computer use in nursing has exploded concomitantly with computers in healthcare.

What is also of importance for computer use in nursing is the research on computerized applications and nursing informatics, which is revolutionizing how health information is documented in the Electronic Health Record (EHR) and producing pools of searchable secondary data waiting to be tapped. The context for nursing informatics research has proliferated since the National Institute of Nursing Research (NINR) published an agenda outlining the need for nursing informatics research in the Nursing Informatics Research Agenda (NINR, 1993). Other reports called for organizing priorities (Brennan, Zielstorff, Ozbolt, & Strombom, 1998) and constructing models to develop a context connecting nursing and informatics that would provide the basis for studying the practice of nursing informatics (Effken, 2003). Today, hospital-wide information technology (IT) is the spine of all healthcare delivery, which is tied to reimbursement, and which inevitably forms the data engine that health systems put to work to research improvement and outcomes-driven questions. It is therefore imperative to understand the underlying terminologies and sources of

data, communication of those connected pieces of information, and the elements in the nursing environments through informatics research if one is to understand how computers and nursing research co-exist.

Outside the EHR and computerized health systems, in the rapidly changing world of Internet technologies, information management and computer-enhanced intervention research on the use of computers have produced a new body of science that will continue to grow. Blending the focus of computer use in research (tools and process) and research on computer use (informatics research) calls for an understanding of process and products. This chapter will provide an overview of the research process for two separate and fundamentally different research approaches—quantitative and qualitative—and discuss select computer applications and uses relative to these approaches. The discussion will be supplemented by examples of current science and the trajectory of research on the impact of informatics, electronic records, treatments, and integrated technologies using the computer as a tool.

The computer has been a tool for researchers in many aspects of the research process and has gone beyond its historic application once limited to number crunching and business transactions. Field-notes binders, ring tablets, index cards, and paper logs have all but disappeared in the researchers' world. Personal computers, laptops, PC-tablets and iPads, and handheld devices have become part of the researcher's necessary resources in mounting a research project or study. Wireless technologies are ubiquitous and connect people to people as well as researchers to devices. Cloud computing today connects diverse enterprises with stable sources of software and data that can be shared or used by anyone, at any time or any place. Numerous enhancements have been added to the well-known text processing software products that reduce time and effort in every research office. In addition, a wide range of new technologies for database management of subjects, contacts, or logistics have emerged in the research product marketplace. Nurse researchers use a range of hardware and software applications that are generic to research development operations in addition to the tools and devices that are specific to research data collection, analysis, results reporting, and dissemination. New apps appear continuously, customized to the data collection, management, or analysis process.

In today's electronic healthcare environment, numerous advances have been made with the sources of data collection relative to general clinical applications in nursing, health, and health services. System implementations for large clinical enterprises have also provided opportunities for nurses and health service researchers to identify and extract information from existing computer-based resources. In an era when the federal government is calling for comparative effectiveness research (CER) to address the rising costs of healthcare (Congressional Budget Office [CBO], 2007; Sox & Greenfield, 2009), the richness of capturing nursing data that can be managed and mined for advanced analyses should be recognized in the development of electronic health records (EHRs) and other sources.

In addition, the era of Web-based applications has produced a wide range of innovative means of entering data and, subsequently, automating data collection in ways that were not possible before. With the advancements in clinical systems, acceptable terminology and vocabularies to support nursing assessment, interventions, and evaluation, computers are increasingly being used for clinical and patient care research. Although research is a complex cognitive process, certain aspects of carrying out research can be aided by software applications. For example, examination of nursing care/patient outcomes and the effect of interventions would have been prohibitive in the past, but with the aid of computers and access to large data sets, many health outcomes can be analyzed quantitatively and qualitatively. It is noteworthy when hospital systems today can use analytics across institutions with large samples of existing data to compare and predict best outcomes with select interventions, for example, examining pre-operative procedures that minimize post-operative complications. In one hospital example, a procedure was changed with results from a rapid analysis of system-wide data, reducing mortality and morbidity related to post-op complications. They went from asking the research question to implementing the procedural change in less than six months (Englebright, 2013)—change that in the past would have taken 17 years in randomized trials as has been reported.

With a wider view of computer use in nursing research, the objective of this chapter is fourfold: (1) to provide an overview of general computer and software applications related to the stages of the research process; (2) to describe how computers facilitate the work of the researcher in both quantitative and qualitative aspects; (3) to highlight research on computer use in healthcare; and (4) to give attention to the explosion of research in categories delineating clinical and nursing informatics research. These will serve as a snapshot of the research on computer use for the future with contextual influences.

To begin, the chapter will focus on some of the considerations related to the logistics and preparation of the research proposal, project planning, and budgeting, followed by the implementation of the proposal with data capture, data management, data analysis, and information presentation. The general steps of proposal development,

preparation, and implementation are applicable to both quantitative and qualitative approaches. However, no discussion about computer use in research could be complete without acknowledging the range of research now appearing in the literature that examines the trajectory of new technologies and computer use in patient care. With increasing emphasis on cost and quality of healthcare, the computer-sources-of-data and computer-as-intervention must be part of understanding computer use in nursing research today.

PROPOSAL DEVELOPMENT, PREPARATION, AND IMPLEMENTATION

All research begins with a good idea. The idea is typically based on the nurse researcher's identification of a problem that is amenable to study using a philosophical and theoretical orientation. The philosophical aspect sets the stage for selecting one's approach to investigating the problem or developing the idea. Good clinical ideas often come from personal experiences, based on the researcher's foundation of knowledge that aids in drawing inferences from real clinical situations. These unfold by way of iterative consideration of problem and process—leading the investigator to evolve an approach to the problem, and subsequently a theoretical paradigm to address the problem. Because the theoretical paradigm emerges from these iterative considerations, and because the theoretical perspective will subsequently drive the organization of the research study, it is important to distinguish between these two distinct approaches. Each theoretical paradigm directs how the problem for study will unfold. The researcher uses a selected theoretical approach and operationalizes each step of the research process that will become the research design and methodology, either qualitative, quantitative, or some combination of both in mixed methods (Creswell, 2014). Each approach can be facilitated at different points along the proposal process with select computer applications. These will be described as they relate to the methodology.

Quantitative or Qualitative Methodology

The important distinction to be made between the quantitative and qualitative approaches is that for a quantitative study to be successful, the researcher is obliged to fully develop each aspect of the research proposal before collecting any data, i.e., a priori, whereas, for a qualitative study to be successful, the researcher is obligated to allow the data collected to determine the subsequent steps as it unfolds in the process and/or the analysis. Quantitative research is derived from the philosophical orientations of empiricism and logical positivism with multiple steps bound together by precision in quantification (Polit & Beck, 2011). The requirements of a hypothesis-driven or numerically descriptive approach are logical consequences of, or correspond to, a specific theory and its related tenets. The hypothesis can be tested statistically to support or refute the prediction made in advance. Statistics packages are the mainstay of the quantitative methodologist, but are not the only connection to computers for the researcher.

The qualitative approaches offer different research traditions (e.g., phenomenology, hermeneutics, ethnography, and grounded theory, to name a few) that share a common view of reality, which consists of the meanings ascribed to the data such as a person's lived experiences (Creswell, 2012). With this view, theory is not tested, but rather, perspectives and meaning from the subject's point of view are described and analyzed. For nursing studies, knowledge development is generated from the participant's experiences and responses to health, illness, and treatments. The requirements of the qualitative approach are a function of the philosophical frames through which the data unfold and evolve into meaningful interpretations by the researcher. A variety of software applications assist the qualitative methodologist to enter, organize, frame, code, reorder, and synthesize text, audio, video, and sometimes numeric data (Polit & Beck, 2011).

General Considerations in Proposal Preparation

Several computer applications have become indispensable in the development of the research proposal and generally in planning for the activities that will take place when implementing the study. These include broad categories of office programs including word processing, spreadsheet, and database management applications. According to Forrester Research, an independent research firm, Microsoft Office products currently capture 80% of users with 64% of enterprises using Office 2007 (Montalbano, 2009). Office 365 is the new release from Microsoft, programs with cloud capability that continue to offer improved clerical tools to manage the text from numerous sources and assemble them in a cogent and organized package. The cloud connectivity gives researchers access to all programs and data virtually from anywhere. PC, Mac, and Droid tablets and smart phones extend the reach of all connectivity with a range of text processing and data management standard tools.

Microsoft Office products provide capabilities and a platform into which other off-the-shelf applications can

be integrated. Tables, charts, and images can be inserted, edited, and moved as the proposal takes shape, with final products in publishable forms. Personal computer applications that allow inserting simple graphic designs give the researcher a powerful means of expressing concepts through art. Line art and scanned images using Adobe industry standards such as Illustrator CC (www.adobe.com) or Photoshop CC (www.photoshop.com), now with cloud capability, can be integrated into the document for clear visual effects. These offer the researcher and grant managers tools to generate proposals, reports, and manuscripts that can be submitted electronically directly or following conversion to portable document formats (pdf) using Adobe Acrobat or other available conversion products.

There are a variety of reference management software products available as add-ons to word processing, with ranging prices and functionalities. For example, unique template add-ons give Microsoft Word additional power to produce documents in formatted styles. Bibliographic management applications emerge frequently and librarians often help sort out best ways to keep reference materials in order. Common programs such as Reference Manager, Procite, and Endnote are products of the Thomson Corporation (2009) (www.refman.com/rmcopyright.asp), the industry standard software tools for publishing and managing bibliographies on the Windows and Macintosh desktops. RefWorks adds another option for reference management from a centrally hosted Web site (www.refworks.com). Searching online is one function of these applications, and then working between the reference database and the text of the proposal document is efficient and easy, calling out citations when needed with "cite as you write" capability into the finished document. Output style sheets can be selected to match publication or proposal guidelines.

Research applications and calls for proposals are often downloadable from the Internet into an interactive form where individual fields are editable and the documents can be saved in a portable format such as Adobe Acrobat, printed, or submitted from the Web. The Web also allows the researcher to explore numerous opportunities for designing a proposal tailored to potential foundations for consideration of funding. Calls for proposals, contests, and competitive grants may provide links from Web sites that give the researcher a depth of understanding of what is expected in the proposal. There are more and more home grown submission procedures today for grants and journal manuscripts with Web-based instructions. These often convert the documents automatically to portable formats (pdf) for submission with key data fields organized and sorted for easier review procedures. Instructions are customized for the user.

Research Study Implementation

A funded research study becomes a logistical challenge for most researchers in managing the steps of the process. Numerous demands for information management require the researcher to maintain the fidelity of the procedures, manage the subject information and paper flow, and keep the data confidential and secure. These processes require researchers to use a database management system (DBMS) that is reliable. Several DBMS software applications exist and have evolved to assist the researcher in the overall process of study implementation. These applications are operations oriented, used in non-research programs and projects as well, but can assist the researcher in management of time, personnel, money, products, and ultimately dissemination, with reporting capability for reviews and audits.

The ubiquitous Microsoft Office suite includes programs that manage data in a relational database (Microsoft Access) and number crunch in a flat database (Microsoft Excel) available to every researcher. Proprietary database applications and new customized, more sophisticated, integrated, and proprietary database management applications from companies such as Oracle and Lotus provide the researcher with ways to operationalize the personnel, subjects, forms, interviews, dates, times, and/or tracking systems over the course of the project. Most of these applications require specially designed screens that are unique to the project if the research warrants complicated connections such as reminders, but simple mailing lists and zip codes of subjects' addresses and contact information in a generic form can also be extremely useful for the researcher. Some of these applications are beginning to include add-ons to increase application portability with devices such as the smartphones and tablets, and mini-tablets.

Several other generic computer programs can aid the researcher in daily operations and project management. Spreadsheet applications are invaluable for budgeting and budget planning, from proposal development through project completion. One multi-purpose Microsoft Office application is Microsoft Excel. Universally understood and easy-to-use Excel allows the researcher to manage costs and calculate expenses over the course of the project period, producing a self-documenting plan by categories to track actual spending and money left. Templates can be developed for repetitive tasks. Scheduling and project planning software is also available from Microsoft including Microsoft Project that allows the project director to organize the work efficiently and track schedules and deadlines using Gantt charts over the lifetime of the project. In more sophisticated research offices, customized

tracking and data capture devices, programs and systems have been launched, including the exemplar of data management tools from the recent U.S. Census that have captured and made data available to researchers with data tools (http://www.census.gov/main/www/access.html).

One other important consideration related to research proposal implementation for the seasoned researcher or the novice, doctoral dissertation investigator is the essential step of submitting the proposal to the Institutional Review Board (IRB). Home institutions that have IRBs will have specific procedures and forms for the researcher who can benefit from the proposal development electronically. In some institutions, the IRB document management has been done through contracts with outside Internet organizations providing mechanisms for posting IRB materials, managing the online certifications required, and communicating with the principle investigators. One such example is IRBNet.org, hosting services for organizations to manage IRB and other administrative documents associated with the research enterprise (Research Dataware, LLC, 2014).

In summary, the general considerations of developing and conducting a research study are based on philosophical approaches and will dictate which methodology the researcher will use to develop the study. Although this will subsequently influence the research and computer applications to be used in carrying out the project, the steps of proposal preparation are less specific, and the computer applications are useful in both quantitative and qualitative studies. After identifying the research problem, however, the researcher must proceed through the steps of the process, where computers play an important role that is unique to each of the methodologies.

THE QUANTITATIVE APPROACH

Data Capture and Data Collection

Data capture and data collection are processes that are viewed differently from the quantitative and qualitative perspectives. Nurses may already be familiar with data collection that is focused on the management of patient care. Patient monitoring, patient care documentation, and interview data are collected by nurses, although not always for research purposes. Data collection can take a number of forms depending on the type of research and variables of interest. Computers are used in data collection for paper-and-pencil surveys and questionnaires as well as to capture physiologic and clinical nursing information in quantitative or descriptive patient care research. There are also unique automated data capturing applications that have been developed recently that facilitate large group data capture in single contacts or allow paper versions of questionnaires to be scanned directly into a database ready for analysis or provided online with Web-based survey tools.

Paper and Pencil Questionnaires. Paper and booklet surveys do still exist today in data collection, but new enhancements aid the researcher in time-saving activities. Surveys and questionnaires can be scanned or programmed into a computer application either in a microcomputer or on a Web site accessed through the Internet. Computers are being used for direct data entry in studies where subjects enter their own responses via a computer, and simultaneous coding of response to questions and time "online" can be captured or Web surveys can be distributed widely. These online survey tools can provide a wide range of applications, including paper or portable versions, and range in price and functionality.

The use of notebook microcomputers, tablets, and mini-tablets have gained popularity in recent years for allowing the user to enter the data directly into the computer program at the time of the interview with a subject, with innovations emerging in touch screens, screen pens, and even wireless data entry with smartphones (Moss & Saba, 2011). Responses to questions can be entered by the respondent or a surrogate directly into the computer or Web site through Internet access. There are several research study examples where patients with chronic conditions used a computer application or the Internet as the intervention as well as the data capture device; patients or caregivers responded to questions directly and the data were processed with the same system (Berry et al., 2010; Mullen, Berry, & Zierler, 2004). Other examples of unique data capture in research include individual devices such as the "Smart Cap" used to measure patient compliance with medications. The Medication Event Monitoring System (MEMS®6) (Fig. 47.1) automates digitized data that can be downloaded for analysis in research such as patient adherence studies (Figge, 2010; Rolley et al., 2008).

A variety of online survey tools also provide researchers the power to collect data from a distance, without postage, using the Internet. These applications can present questionnaire data in graphically desirable formats, depending on the price and functionality of the software, to subjects delivered via e-mail, Web sites, blogs, and even social networking sites such as Facebook or Twitter if desirable. Social media mechanisms such as blogs and tweets are often providing sources of data analyses, albeit questionably scientific, that have sometimes been harnessed to extract meaning for researchers. Web surveys, although often criticized for yielding poorer response rates than traditional mail (Granello & Wheaton, 2004), are becoming

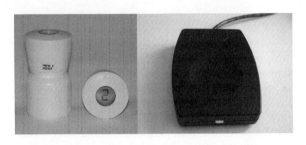

• **FIGURE 47.1.** MEMS (Medication Event Monitoring System) SmartCap Contains an LCD Screen; MEMS Reader Transfers Encrypted Data From the MEMS Monitor to the Web Portal. (Published with permission of MWV Healthcare/Aardex Group, www.aardexgroup.com.)

increasingly popular for their cost and logistical benefits. The data from the Internet can be downloaded for analysis and several applications provide instant summary statistics that can be monitored over the data collection period. Several of these programs are available for free with limited use; others yield advanced products that can be incorporated into the research, giving mobility (e.g., smartphones) and flexibility (e.g., scanning or online entry) to the data capture procedures. Several of these applications include (1) Survey Monkey (www.surveymonkey.com); (2) E-Surveys Pro (www.esurveyspro.com); (3) Survey System (www.surveysystem.com); (4) Qualtrics (www.qualtrics.com); and (5) SNAP Survey software (www.snapsurveys.com). Many of these products continue to enhance functionality and delivery modes as well as integration with statistical analysis programs and qualitative narrative exportability. An example of screen flexibility and scanning output in SNAP is shown in Fig. 47.2.

Several special applications have been used in nursing research that can facilitate large group data capture. Group use applications in specially designed facilities have been developed to engage an audience in simultaneous activity, recording their impressions through electronic keypads located proximal to the users, and capturing that information for display or later analysis. One type of application, Expert Choice 11.5 (Expert Choice, 2014) uses the analytic hierarchy process (AHP), a mathematical technique, with handheld keypad technology to elicit group responses and automatically score, analyze, prioritize, and present information back to the group graphically. AHP has been used as the multiple criteria decision-making analysis technique in nursing research studies (Kimiafar, Sadoughi, Sheikhtaheri & Sarbaz, 2014; Kodadek & Feeg, 2002), and the Expert Choice software allows for group data entry. This kind of groupware for collaborative decision-making

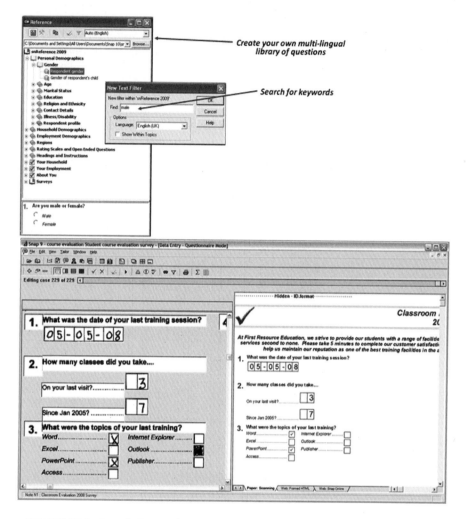

Create your own multi-lingual library of questions

Search for keywords

• **FIGURE 47.2.** Sample Screens for SNAP Survey Software. (Reproduced, with permission, from Snap Surveys, www.snapsurveys.com.)

can supplement data collection from a focus group to add a quantitative component to the subjective question as it elicits and captures opinion via pairwise comparisons (www.expertchoice.com).

Software packages also exist that can be integrated with the researcher's scanner to optically scan a specially designed questionnaire and produce the subjects' responses in a database ready for analysis. OmniPage 18 (Nuance Imaging, 2014) is a top-rated optical character recognition (OCR) program that converts a scanned page into plain text. Programs such as SNAP Survey software (www.snapsurveys.com) and Remark Office OMR 8 (Gravic Inc., 2014) can facilitate scanning large numbers of questionnaires with speed and accuracy. These

products, enhanced even more with Web-based products such as Remark Web Survey (Gravic Inc., 2014), increase the accuracy of data entry with very low risk of errors, thereby improving the efficiency of the data capture, collection, and entry processes.

Physiologic Data. The collection of patient physiologic parameters has long been used in physiologic research. Some of these parameters can be measured directly from patient devices such as cardiac monitoring of heart rhythm, rate, and fluid or electrolytes and be captured in the patient care records of the hospital systems. For example, hospitals have developed mechanisms to use information from intensive care unit (ICU) data to calculate benchmarks for mortality and resource use. Now that many measurements taken from various types of imaging (e.g., neurologic, cardiovascular, and cellular) have become digitized, they can also be entered directly from the patient into computer programs for analysis. Each of these applications is unique to the measures, such as systems to capture cardiac functioning and/or pulmonary capacity, devices that can relay contractions, or monitors that pick up electronic signals remotely. Numerous measurements of intensity, amplitude, patterns, and shapes can be characterized by computer programs and used in research. For example, the APACHE system in its multiple versions has been tested in benchmarking hospital mortality and outcomes from captured physiologic data in several groups of patients in the ICU (Paul, Bailey, Van Lint, & Pilchers, 2012; Zimmerman, Kramer, McNair, & Malila, 2006). Each of these measurement systems has evolved with the unfolding of research specific to their questions, and within each community of scholars, issues about the functionality, accuracy, and reliability of electronic data extracted from these physiologic devices are debated.

Along with the proliferation of clinical diagnostic measurement systems, there has been a rapid expansion of unique computer applications that have emerged for the data analysis aspects of these clinical systems, physiologic and record sources. Millions of gigabytes of data are stored in machines that can be tapped for multiple studies on the existing data. Data mining is a powerful tool in the knowledge discovery process that can now be done with a number of commercial and open-source software packages (Berger & Berger, 2004). Data mining and the evolving "big data" initiatives to make patient care data available introduce new ways to manipulate existing information systems.

With increased attention to comparative effectiveness research (CER), several government and private organizations are encouraging researchers to hone the techniques to extract valid and reliable information from these large data sets (Sox & Greenfield, 2009). Data mining is a mechanism of exploration and analysis of large quantities of data in order to discover meaningful patterns and rules, applied to large physiologic data sets as well as clinical sources of data. The nature of the data and the research question determine the tool selection (i.e., data-mining algorithm or technique). Tools and consultants exist to help researchers unfamiliar with data mining algorithms use data mining for analysis, prediction, and reporting purposes (MSDN Library, 2000). Many of the first commercial applications of data mining were in customer profiling and marketing analyses. Today, many special technologies can be applied, for example, to predict physiologic phenomena such as genetic patterns in tumors that might respond to therapy based on classification of primary tumor gene expression

or tissue rejection post-heart transplantation from blood samples and biopsies (Berger & Berger, 2004).

The National Institutes of Health (NIH) is undertaking several initiatives to address the challenges and opportunities associated with big data. As one component of the NIH-wide strategy, the Common Fund in cooperation with all NIH Institutes and Centers is supporting the Big Data to Knowledge (BD2K) initiative, which aims to facilitate broad use of biomedical big data, develop and disseminate analysis methods and software, enhance training for disciplines relevant for large-scale data analysis, and establish centers of excellence for biomedical big data (NIH, 2012).

Unique Nursing Care Data in Research. Scientists and technologists from a variety of disciplines are working hard to identify the domain of data and information that is transferable across situations, sites, or circumstances that can be captured electronically for a wide array of analyses to learn how the health system impacts the patients it serves. The American Nurses Association (ANA) has supported the need to standardize nursing care terms for computer-based patient care systems. The clinical and economic importance of structured recording to represent nursing care was recognized by the acceptance of the nursing minimum data set (NMDS) (Werley, Lang, & Westlake, 1986). The ANA has accepted seven systems of terminology for the description of nursing practice: the North American Nursing Diagnosis Association (NANDA) taxonomy of nursing diagnosis, (Clinical Care Classification [CCC] System) (McCormick, Lang, & Zielstorff, 1994; Saba, 1997, 2007; Zielstorff, Lang, & Saba, 1995), Nursing Interventions Classification (Bulechek & McCloskey, 1997), Nursing Outcomes Classification (Daly, Maas, & Johnson, 1997), patient care data set (Ozbolt, 1999), Omaha Home Healthcare (Martin & Norris, 1996), and the International Classification of Nursing Practice (Saba, 1997, 2007; Zielstorff et al., 1995). The Clinical Care Classification System (sabacare.com) nursing terminology has been accepted by the U.S. Department of Health and Human Services (HHS) as a named standard within the Healthcare Information Technology Standards Panel (HITSP) Interoperability Specification for Electronic Health Records, Biosurveillance and Consumer Empowerment as presented to a meeting of the American Health Information Community (AHIC), a federal advisory group on health information technology (DHHS, 2007). (See Appendix A for a full discussion of the CCC System.)

Although none of the above has emerged as a single standard, national efforts (Dykes, 2013) and collaborative efforts with the International Classification of Nursing Practice (ICNP) from the International Council of Nursing (ICN) are underway to "harmonize" the data elements in the NMDS and SNOMED CT (Systematized Nomenclature of Medicine Clinical Terms) (Coenen & Jansen, 2013). With a structured coding system to record patient care problems that are amenable to nursing actions, the actual nursing actions implemented in the care of patients, and the evaluation of the effectiveness of these actions, researchers can analyze large nursing data (Bakken, 2013; Byrne & Lang, 2013; Englebright, Aldrich, & Taylor, 2014). Outcomes research and quality indicators extracted from health information systems (HIS) have become the data end points that can justify healthcare services (Nahm, Vaydia, Ho, Scharf, & Seagull, 2007). The American Recovery and Reinvestment Act (ARRA) of 2009 (Public Law 111-5) called for increased development, certification, and wide-range "meaningful use" of EHRs across healthcare. The federal government has incentivized development of cross-platform compatibility and collaboration. Research on outcomes of care is one of the centerpieces of this massive policy that has begun to show an impact on integrated information technologies in healthcare that can transform practice. Nursing research on nursing practice captured from standardized terminology will be essential to document outcomes of nursing care.

Data Coding

In most quantitative studies, the data for the variables of interest are collected in a numerical form. These numerical values are entered into designated fields in the process of coding. Coding may be inherent in software programs for the physiologic data and many of the electronic surveys. The coding may be generated by a computer program from measurements directly obtained through imaging or physiologic monitoring, or entered into a computer by a patient or researcher from a printout or a questionnaire or survey into a database program. Most statistical programs contain data editors that permit the entry of data by a researcher as part of the statistical application. In such a situation, fields are designated and numerical values can also be entered into the appropriate fields without the use of an extra program. For mechanisms that translate and transfer source data to prepare it for analysis, generic programs such as Microsoft Excel serve multiple needs. In addition to allowing simple transfers of data from source to a statistical analysis package, Excel has its own powerful, but simple, analysis capabilities and exceptionally easy-to-use graphic translators that can turn statistics into visual graphs and charts.

Coding data is a precise operation that needs careful consideration and presents the researcher with challenges that warrant technical or cognitive applications. Coding data is a combination of cognitive decisions and mechanical clerical recording of responses in a numerical form with numerous places for error to occur. There are several ways of reviewing and "cleaning" the data prior to analysis. Some computer programs allow for the same data to be entered twice called double-data entry or two-pass verification. This is done preferably by different people to check for errors, with the premise that if the double entry does not match, one entry is wrong. One also must check for missing data and take them into consideration in the coding and analyses. New versions of advanced statistical software help in these activities. Reviewing data for values outside of those allowable is another way of examining the data for errors. It can best be done by examining the multiple printouts produced by the statistical software packages or procedures invoked in the statistical application and by carefully perusing for outliers or artifacts.

Another type of data coding can be described in the example of the process of translating data from documentation of patient care using coding strategies. Current research on coding nursing data using standardized nursing terminology from standardized codes is evident in several research studies in the literature (Englebright et al., 2014). For example, using precisely coded data from a standardized terminology can produce data that can be aggregated and statistically analyzed into meaningful information. In several studies by Saba and Taylor (2007), Moss and Saba (2011), and Saba and Arnold (2004), researchers have discussed mechanisms of aggregating nursing action types, e.g., assess, perform, teach, or manage, into aggregated information on the amount of time or effort a nurse spends in a day and concomitant costs associated. Another application of coding data occurs with mapping concept codes from one terminology to another. For example, coding data for a nursing diagnosis can be mapped between terminologies for interoperability, e.g., mapping the CCC Nursing Diagnosis concept of pain to a SNOMED-CT code for the same concept (CCC Acute Pain—Q63.1 mapped to SNOMED Acute Pain—274663001). These translations of codes support the ever-evolving interoperable computer systems that produce nursing data reports which can cross platforms or institutions.

Data Analysis

Data analysis in a quantitative study combines a variety of techniques that apply statistical procedures with the researcher's cognitive organization of research questions, results, and visual or textual information, translated into tables, charts, and graphs to make the data meaningful.

It translates the numeric and conceptual elements of the inquiry into meaningful representations of information. In general, the statistical analyses are ordered by the conceptual arrangement of hypotheses, variables, measurements, and relationships, and ultimately answer the research questions. There are many ways to consider data analysis. The presentation below is organized around the broad types of research of interest in nursing and general research goals or questions. The researcher may use different types of analyses depending on the goal of research. These goals may require different statistical examinations: descriptive and/or exploratory analyses, hypothesis testing, estimation of confidence intervals, model building through multivariate analysis, and structural equation model building. Various types of nursing research may contain a number of these goals. For example, to test an intervention using an experimental or quasi-experimental design, one may first perform descriptive or exploratory analyses followed by tests of the hypotheses. Quality improvement, patient outcome, and survival analysis studies may likewise contain a number of different types of analyses depending on the specific research questions.

In general, the statistical analysis steps of the research process rely heavily on the functions specific to a variety of statistical software applications. Two of the most popular programs in use today are the IBM SPSS Statistics 22 (formerly Statistical Package for Social Sciences) (IBM SPSS Statistics, 2014) and Statistical Analysis Services (SAS Version 9.2), however a variety of other packages and programs exist, such as STATA or Minitab 17 (Minitab, Inc., 2014) unique to particular scientific disciplines. Which package one selects depends on the user's personal preference, particular strengths, and limits of the applications including number of variables, options for analyses, and ease of use. These packages have given the user the power to manipulate large data sets with relative ease and test out statistical combinations that have exponentially improved the analyses possible in a fraction of time that it once took.

The different types of analyses required by the goals of the research will be addressed further. This description will be followed by examples of types of nursing research that incorporate some of these types of analyses.

Descriptive and Exploratory Analysis. The researcher may first explore the data means, modes, distribution pattern, and standard deviations, and examine graphic representations such as scatter plots or bar graphs. Tests of association or significant differences may be explored through chi-squares, correlations, and various univariate, bivariate, and trivariate analyses, and an examination of quartiles. During this analysis process, the researcher may recode or transform data by mathematically multiplying or

dividing scores by certain log or factor values. Combining several existing variables can also create new variables. These transformations or "re-expressions" or "dummy-coding" allow the researcher to analyze the data in appropriate and interpretable scales. The researcher can then easily identify patterns with respect to variables as well as groups of study subjects of interest. Both commercial statistical packages provide the ability to calculate these tests and graphically display the results in a variety of ways.

IBM SPSS Statistics 22 provides the user with a broad range of capabilities for the entire analytical process. SPSS is a modular, tightly integrated, and full-featured software comprised of the SPSS base and a range of add-on modules. With SPSS, the researcher can generate decision-making information quickly using a variety of powerful statistics, understand and effectively present the results with high-quality tabular and graphical output, and share the results with others using various reporting methods, including secure Web publishing. SAS 9.2 provides the researcher with tools that can help code data in a reliable framework, extract data for quality assurance, exploration, or analysis, perform descriptive and inferential data analyses, maintain databases to track, and report on administrative activities like data collection, subject enrollment, or grant payments, and deliver content for reports in the appropriate format. SAS allows for creating unique programming within the variable manipulations and is often the format for large publicly available data sets for secondary analysis. Stata 13 and SYSTAT 13 are also fully integrated statistical packages with full database management capabilities and a range of sophisticated statistical tests particularly useful for epidemiologists and physical scientists. All of these statistical packages have evolved to provide an integrated collection of tools that assist in aspects of research study management—from planning to dissemination—in addition to the reputable statistical analyses and data manipulation capabilities that they have provided for many years.

As part of exploratory analysis, simple, binary, and multiple regression analyses can be used to examine the relationships between selected variables and a dependent measure of interest. Certain models can be developed to determine which collection of variables provides the best prediction of the dependent measure. Printouts of correlation matrices, extensive internal tests of data assumptions on the sample, and regression analysis tables provide the researcher with condensed, readable statistical information about the relationships in question.

Hypothesis Testing or Confirmatory Analyses. Hypothesis testing or confirmatory analyses are based on an interest in relationships and describing what would occur if a hypothesis were true. The analysis of data allows us to compare the actual outcomes with the hypothesized outcomes. Inherent in hypothesis testing is the probability (P value) of an event occurring given a certain relationship. These are conditional relationships based on the variables selected for study, and the typical mathematical tables and software for determining P values are accurate only insofar as the assumptions of the test are met (Polit & Beck, 2011). Certain statistical concepts such as statistical power, type II error, selecting alpha values to balance type II errors, and sampling distribution are decisions that the researcher must make regardless of the type of computer software. These concepts are covered in greater detail in research methodology courses and are outside the scope of the present discussion. An example, Power and Precision (Version 2), is a computer program for statistical power analysis and confidence intervals (Biostat, 2014).

Model Building. An application used for a confirmatory hypothesis testing approach to multivariate analysis is structural equation modeling (SEM) (Byrne, 1984). Byrne describes this procedure as consisting of two aspects: (1) the causal processes under study are represented by a series of structural (i.e., regression) equations and (2) these structural relations can be modeled pictorially to enable a clearer conceptualization of the theory under study. The model can be tested statistically in a simultaneous analysis of the entire system of variables to determine the extent to which it is consistent with the data. If goodness of fit is adequate, the model argues for the plausibility of postulated relationships among variables (Byrne, 1984). Most researchers may wish to consult a statistician to discuss the underlying assumptions of the data and plans for testing the model. Traditionally, different types of modeling programs, such as LISREL (Joreskog & Sorbom, 1978) (see www.ssicentral.com) or EQS (Byrne, 1984) (see Multivariate Software, www.mvsoft.com), are commercially available. The researcher will identify latent (unobservable) variables of interest (e.g., emotions) and link them to those that are observable (direct measurement) and plan with the statistician to specify and examine the impact of one latent construct on another in the modeling of causal direction.

IBM SPSS 22 offers Amos 22, a powerful SEM and path analysis add-on to create more realistic models than if using standard multivariate methods or regression alone. Amos is a program for visual SEM and path analysis. User-friendly features, such as drawing tools, configurable toolbars, and drag-and-drop capabilities, help the researcher build structural equation models. After fitting the model, the Amos path diagram shows the strength of the relationship between variables. Amos builds models that realistically reflect complex relationships because any variable,

whether observed (such as survey data) or latent (such as satisfaction or loyalty), can be used to predict any other variable.

Meta-Analysis. Meta-analysis is a technique that allows researchers to combine data across studies to achieve more focused estimates of population parameters and examine effects of a phenomenon or intervention across multiple studies. It uses the effect size as a common metric of study effectiveness and deals with the statistical problems inherent in using individual significance tests in a number of different studies. It weights study outcomes in proportion to their sample size and focuses on the size of the outcomes rather than on whether they are significant.

Although the computations can be done with the aid of a reliable commercial statistical package such as Meta-Analysis (Borenstein, Hedges, Higgins, & Rothstein, 2009), the researcher needs to consider the following specific issues in performing the meta-analysis (Polit & Beck, 2011): (1) justify which studies are comparable and which are not, (2) rely on knowledge of the substantive area to identify relevant study characteristics, (3) evaluate and account for differences in study quality, and (4) assess the generalizability of the results from fields with little empirical data. Each of these issues must be addressed with a critical review prior to performing the meta-analysis.

Meta-analysis offers a way to examine results of a number of quantitative research that meet meta-analysis researchers' criteria. Meta-analysis overcomes problems encountered in studies using different sample sizes and instruments. The software application Meta-Analysis provides the user with a variety of tools to examine these studies. It can create a database of studies, import the abstracts or the full text of the original papers, or enter the researcher's own notes. The meta-analysis is displayed using a schematic that may be modified extensively, as the user can specify which variables to display and in what sequence. The studies can be sorted by any variable including effect size, the year of publication, the weight assigned to the study, the sample size, or any user-defined variables to facilitate the critical review done by the researcher (Fig. 47.3).

Graphical Data Display and Analysis. There are occasions when data need to be displayed graphically as part of the analysis and interpretation of the information or for more fundamental communication of the results of computations and analyses. Visualization software is becoming even more useful as the science of visualization in combination with new considerations of large data from the "Fourth Paradigm" unfolds (Hey, Tansley, & Tolle, 2009). These ideas begin with the premise that meaningful interpretation of data intensive discoveries needs

· **FIGURE 47.3.** Comprehensive Meta-Analysis (CMA) User Interface. (www.meta-analysis.com/pages/features/spreadsheet.html. Published with permission of Biostat, Inc.)

visualizations that facilitate understanding and unfolding of new patterns. Nurses are currently discovering new ways to present information in meaningful ways through these visualization techniques (Delaney, Westra, Monsen, Gillis, & Docherty, 2013).

Most statistical packages including SPSS, SAS, and STATA, and even spreadsheets such as Excel provide the user with tools for simple to complex graphical translations of numeric information, thus allowing the researcher to display, store, and communicate aggregated data in meaningful ways. Special tools for spatial representations exist, such as mapping and geographic displays, so that the researcher can visualize and interpret patterns inherent in the data. Geographic information system (GIS) technology is evolving beyond the traditional GIS community and becoming an integral part of the information infrastructure of visualization tools for researchers. For example, GIS can assist an epidemiologist with mapping data collected on disease outbreaks or help a health services researcher graphically communicate areas of nursing shortages. GIS technology illustrates relationships, connections, and patterns that are not necessarily obvious in any one data set, enabling the researcher to see overall relevant factors. ArcGIS 10 system is a GIS for management, analysis, and display of geographic knowledge, which is represented using a series of information sets.

The information sets include maps and globes with three-dimensional capabilities to describe networks, topologies, terrains, surveys, and attributes.

In summary, the major emphasis of this section has provided a brief discussion about the range of traditions, statistical considerations, and computer applications that aid the researcher in quantitative data analysis. As computers have continued to integrate data management functions with traditional statistical computational power, the researchers have been able to develop more extensive and sophisticated projects with data collected. Gone are the days of the calculator or punch cards, as the computing power now sits on the researchers' desktops or laptops, with speed and functionality at their fingertips.

THE QUALITATIVE APPROACH

Data Capture and Data Collection

The qualitative approach focuses on activities in the steps of the research process that differ greatly from the quantitative methods in fundamental sources of data, collection techniques, coding, analysis, and interpretation. Thus, the computer becomes a different kind of tool for the researcher in most aspects of the research beginning with the capture and recording of narrative or textual data.

In terms of qualitative research requiring narrative content analysis, the computer can be used to record the observations, narrative statements of subjects, and memos of the researcher in initial word processing applications for future coding. Software applications that aid researchers in transcription tasks include text scanners, such as OmniPage 18 (Nuance Imaging, 2014). Other devices include vocal recorders or speech recognition software such as consumer priced Dragon Naturally Speaking 12 (Nuance Dragon Solutions, 2014), where the researcher can input the information into text documents by speaking into a microphone without typing. New digital recorders are also on the market that use sophisticated and higher cost voice recognition software. From these technologies, researchers or transcriptionists can easily manipulate the recording and type the data verbatim. Even iPhones and smartphones have high-quality recording applications that aid the qualitative research capture narrative statements. These narrative statements, like the quantitative surveys, can be either programmed for use in other applications or subjects' responses can be entered directly into the computer.

Qualitative Data Collection. Audiotaping is often used for interviews in qualitative studies, whereby the content is transcribed into a word processing program for analysis. The narrative statements are stored for subsequent coding and sorting according to one's theoretical framework. Through analysis, categories from the data emerge as interpreted by the researcher. It is important to point out that for both quantitative and qualitative data, the computer application program is only a mechanical, clerical tool to aid the researcher in manipulating the data. Using the Internet for indirect and direct data collection in qualitative studies can also provide a vehicle for data analysis that yields a quantitative component as well as the qualitative analysis. Computers are not only able to record the subject's responses to the questions but can record the number of minutes the subject was online and the number of times they logged in. Many new online technologies are providing functionality for qualitative studies: for example, Audacity (audacity.sourceforge.net), an open source free audio recording package, can edit captured voice and export audio data to be analyzed; conversely, online survey packages such as SurveyMonkey (surveymonkey.com) can now export participants' free text data into qualitative software packages.

Data Coding and Data Analysis

Historically, qualitative researchers have relied on narrative notes, often first recorded as audio and later transcribed by a typist. Coding qualitative text data was a time-consuming task, often involving thousands of pages of typewritten notes and the use of scissors and tape for the development of coding and categories. With the advent of computer packages, the mechanical aspects of the coding and sorting have been reduced. The researcher must decide on which text may be of interest and can use a word processing program to search for words, phrases, or other markers within a text file. However, this process is cumbersome and time consuming, with limited ways to aggregate text into meaningful combinations for identifying themes from the narrative.

Some specific software packages developed for qualitative data analysis (QDA) interface directly with the most popular word processing software packages. The early application program Ethnograph (Seidel & Clark, 1984; Seidel, Friese, & Lenard, 1994) was one of the first packages developed specifically for the purpose of managing some of the mechanical tasks of qualitative data analysis. Ethnograph 6.0 gave users a project management interface with functions to code, edit, and search data. The older non-numerical unstructured data indexing, searching, and theorizing (NUD-IST) software was another qualitative package commonly used, now absorbed in other QDA products. This program assisted the researcher to establish an index of data codes and seek relationships among the coding categories. The ease with which researchers can code and recode large amounts of data with the aid of computerized programs encourages the researcher to experiment with different ways of thinking about data and re-categorizing them. Retrieval of categories or elements of data is facilitated by computer storage. Newer technologies have evolved from Ethnograph and NUD-IST with improved user interfaces, including the latest versions of NVivo 10, MAXQDA 11 (MAXQDA: The Art of Data Analysis, 2012), and ATLAS.ti 7 (ATLAS.ti 7, 2014).

Qualitative research, like quantitative research, is not a single entity, but a set of related yet individual traditions, aims, and methods. Some individual traditions within qualitative research are ethnography, grounded theory, phenomenology, and hermeneutics. The distinguishing feature of qualitative research is that the goal is to understand the qualities or essence of phenomena and/or focus on the meaning of these events to the participants or respondents in the study. The forms of data are usually the words of the respondents or informants rather than numbers. Computerization is especially helpful to the researcher in handling large amounts of data. However, it must be stressed that the computer applications aid the analysis as a management tool rather than an analytical one. Synthesis of the data is still the interpretive work of the researcher.

Computer Application Programs. A number of general-purpose or specific software packages can be used in qualitative analysis: one package is a free text retrieval program such as that available in a word processing program; another is any number of standard database management or indexing programs; third is a program specifically developed for the purpose of qualitative analysis.

General Purpose Software. Word processing programs offer a number of features useful to the qualitative researcher in the early stages of analysis. The ability to search for certain key words allows the researcher to tag the categories of interest. In addition, such features as cut and paste; linking texts; insertion of pictures, tables, and charts; and the inclusion of video and audio data enhance the application. Add-on applications specific to integrating multiple elements help the researcher organize a range of data and materials for analysis. These files can then be incorporated into more sophisticated programs. A comprehensive program is ATLAS.ti (Version 7.0), a powerful workbench for the qualitative analysis of large bodies of textual, graphical, audio, and video data. It offers a variety of tools for accomplishing the tasks associated with any systematic approach to "soft" data, such as material that cannot be analyzed by formal and statistical approaches in meaningful ways (ATLAS.ti 7, 2014).

Special Purpose Software. Several software products have evolved and improved for the specific purpose of analyzing qualitative data. Ethnograph from Qualis Research (2008) is one such older program, which is used after the data have been entered with a word processing program and converted to an ASCII file. Each file can be designated by its context and identifying features using markers provided by the computer program. The researcher can have the program to produce a file that numbers each line of the narrative data. From this line file, the researcher can begin to assign each line or paragraph a category. The researcher keeps track of the category definitions and is alert to dimensions that emerge. Recoding can be done to provide for inductive thinking and iterative comparisons. Through the use of a search command, the computer program can be made to search for data segments by categories throughout the typed document.

NVivo 10 and XSight from QSR provide a new generation of software tools with multiple advantages for researchers. Because qualitative research takes many forms, these two applications can be selected based on the user's specific methodologic goals, the nature and scale of the study, and the computer equipment. While NVivo 10 supports fluid, rich data, detailed text analysis, and theory

building, it also can manage documents, audio and video files as categories, attributes, or nodes in visual displays that show the structure and properties of the document (Fig. 47.4). The latest version of NVivo 10 also allows researchers to import exported data from other applications such as the online survey tool, Survey Monkey, as well as bibliographic management programs, Facebook and Twitter. New analysis tools provide the research ways to cluster, map, and visualize text and images in meaningful ways to aid the interpretive process in the qualitative analysis.

Conceptual Network Systems. A system known as concept diagrams, semantic nets, or conceptual networks is one in which information is represented in a graphic manner. The objects in one's conceptual system (e.g., age and experiences) are coded and represented by a box diagram (node). The objects are linked (by arcs) to other objects to show relationships. Like rule-based systems, semantic nets have been widely used in artificial intelligence work. In order to view the relationships of an object in the system, the researcher examines the node in the graph and follows the arcs to and from it. Semantic network applications may be useful in model building and providing a pictorial overview. Decision Explorer (Banxia, 2014) offers the user a powerful set of mapping tools to aid in the decision-making process for audience response activities. Ideas can be mapped and the resulting cognitive map can be further analyzed (Fig. 47.5). The software has many practical uses, such as gathering and structuring interview data and as an aid in the strategy formulation process. The software is primarily described as being a recording and facilitation tool for the elicitation of ideas, as well as a tool to structure and communicate qualitative data. It allows the user to gather and analyze qualitative data and thus make sense of many pieces of qualitative data in order to achieve a coherent picture of a given issue or problem (Banxia, 2014).

Data Analysis for Qualitative Data. Qualitative data analyses often occur on an ongoing basis with data collection in a reflexive and iterative fashion. There is no clear demarcation of when data collection should end and analysis should begin. The process of obtaining observations, interviews, and other data over a period of time results in a vast body of narrative that may include hundreds or thousands of pages of field notes and researcher memos. Although computer applications can aid considerably in organizing and sorting this mass of data, the theoretical and analytical aspects of decision-making about concepts and themes must be made by the researcher. Researchers can only use the tools to help in creating composites

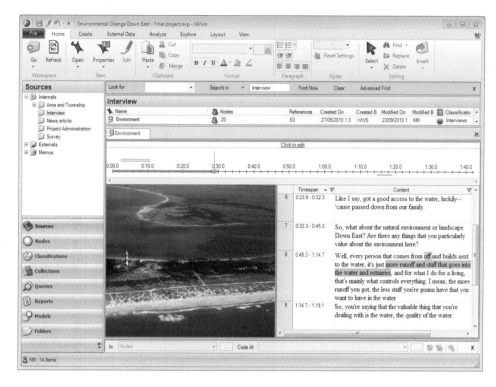

• **FIGURE 47.4.** Screenshot of NVivo9 Main Window. (www.qsrinternational.com. Published with permission from QSR International.)

described by methodologists in coding levels and categorical clusters (Polit & Beck, 2011).

As an example, some of the tasks the computer can facilitate in data analysis using grounded theory (one approach to qualitative research) are as follows. Once a researcher has determined which parts of the interviews and observations can be tagged as categories, certain properties or dimensions can be determined and coded up through levels. The researcher may engage in "constant comparison," comparing the meanings of all incidents that have been similarly categorized. This process should continue until the researcher determines that the categories are internally consistent, fit with the data, and are saturated. Saturation is achieved when the researcher can find no more properties for a category and new data are redundant with the old (Creswell, 2012).

Classic qualitative methods experts Strauss and Corbin (1990) suggested that in the later stages of research, the researcher may engage in axial coding. In this stage, the researcher elaborates and explains key categories, considering the conditions under which the event occurs, the processes that take place, and possible consequences. Another well-known methodologist, Glaser

(1978) indicated that the researcher may engage in theoretical sampling, which is a deliberate search for episodes in incidents that enlarge the variances of properties and place boundaries around categories. Using software, these cognitive processes are applied by the researcher in data analysis of narrative interviews, field notes, and supplementary data.

Uses and Caution. Software programs exist for qualitative research that save researcher time doing file management, reducing the manual labor of cutting, pasting, sorting, and manual filing. They may also encourage the researcher to examine the data from different perspectives, recoding and reorganizing the data in different frameworks. However, one must be mindful that qualitative analysis is a cognitive process, not a mechanical one. The essence of qualitative research is the meaning and interpretation of the data within context. The ability of software enhancements to generate quasi-frequency distributions and cross-tabulations tend to further increase the investigator's confidence in believing such findings and relationships, when in fact these may be an artifact of the way in which the data are manipulated. While computer programs

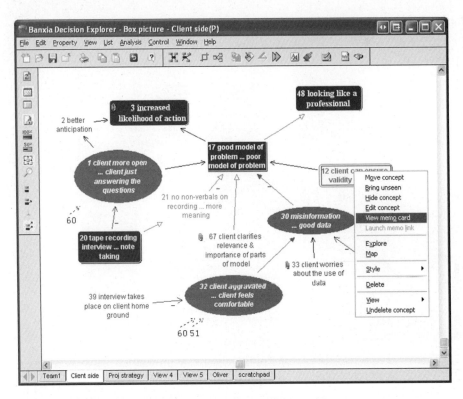

• **FIGURE 47.5.** Example of Cognitive Mapping Analysis. (Published, with permission, of BANXIA® Software Ltd., www.banxia.com/dexplore/pictures.html.)

facilitate coding, organization of data, and preparation of the data for interpretation, they cannot replace the thinking and decision-making that is at the heart of qualitative analysis. As in all research, the burden of analysis and interpretation rests with the researchers (Polit & Beck, 2011).

Dissemination of Results

While dissemination of results continues to occur by traditional means such as presentations at professional meetings and publication in journals and monographs, online reporting is becoming increasingly common. Some Web sites frequented by nurses are peer-reviewed journals such as Online Journal of Nursing Informatics (www.cisnet.com) and selected nursing articles on various Web sites such as that of the ANA (www.nursing-world.org). Nursing forums sponsored by various professional nursing organizations (e.g., American Journal of Nursing, Sigma Theta Tau, and National League for Nursing) often allow participants to chat online with presenters or authors of certain articles on designated dates during scheduled

times. Nearly all organizations have their own Web sites. Some examples are the Alzheimer's Disease Education and Referral Center (www.alzheimers.org), American Heart Association (www.americanheart.org), American Medical Informatics Association (www.amia.org), and RAND Corporation (www.rand.org). The Cochrane Collection has numerous centers all over the world through the Cochrane Collaborative (www.cochrane.org). As with all publications, online as well as hardcopy, the information accessed must be evaluated by the users regarding appropriateness for the purpose for which it was retrieved.

Reports to most government and some non-government agencies require the researcher to submit a converted document online. Grant proposals submitted to the federal government currently require online submission with conversion to PDF. National Institutes of Health (NIH) applicants are directed to a page with downloadable programs to convert the documents before submitting them (www.grants.gov/help/download_software.jsp). In fact, there is a trend for all manuscripts to be submitted online for print, online, or both. Online journals continue to grow.

In addition, there has been a rise in the number of open access journals that give researchers more options for dissemination. Online journals have been discussed in the nursing and academic community with mixed reception; while it allows the researcher-consumer of articles the ability to search wider publicly available science, other stakeholders in the publishing and academic worlds have been concerned on the ramifications of this disruptive innovation (Broome, 2014). Regardless of the method of submission and medium for publication, the published article may be incorporated into one or several online bibliographic retrieval systems. The researcher is not finished until the work is disseminated.

This chapter has summarized the processes of quantitative and qualitative research and described select computerized tools that can assist the researcher in proposal preparation, data collection, data coding, data analysis, and dissemination for both types of research. The following section highlights examples for three categories of research on computer use and nursing informatics in (1) electronic data such as data mining large electronic data sets and electronic nursing documentation; (2) Web-based interventions; and (3) specialized computer applications in clinical practice. The examples include both quantitative and qualitative studies in which the nurse researchers inevitably used a variety of software tools in the proposal development, data collection, measurement of variables, analysis, and dissemination activities.

EXAMPLES OF RESEARCH STUDIES

Computers are inextricably tied to the process of conducting research, but there are also good examples of research on computer use in the nursing literature. Several of the following examples also describe computerized processes for conducting quantitative and qualitative research approaches. These examples provide focus on nursing research related to computer use and informatics as well as using computers in the process of doing the research.

Clinical Interventions With Computers

Over the past 10 years, Internet applications have been introduced into practice and tested in a variety of clinical trials aimed to improve conditions for patients. For example, a team of researchers developed the Personal Patient Profile-Prostate (P3P), a Web-decision support system for men newly diagnosed with prostate cancer that assesses patients' preferences prior to clinic visit and gives providers' and patients' information to aid decision-making among choices of treatment. The studies showed

that decision support was feasible with the technology support (Berry et al., 2010). Decision regret was significantly influenced by personal characteristics and post-treatment symptoms, although the P3P was not itself significant on the outcomes measured in the study (Berry, Wang, Halpenny, & Hong, 2012). In another Web-based intervention, caregivers were randomly assigned to one of two types of online support groups and compared to non-active participants on their depressive symptoms, caregiver burden, and quality of life. In this study, both types of online support groups reduced depressive symptoms and improved quality of life over non-active participants (Klemm, Hayes, Diefenbeck, & Milcarek, 2014).

Technology, Electronic Data, and Electronic Documentation Research

There are several different studies that highlight using electronic data and electronic health records in data mining or care documentation.

Secondary Analysis of Large Data Sets. Large public data sets are becoming more available to nurse researchers to explore health-related questions. The sites provide tutorials and assistance, making them more accessible for secondary analyses. For example, the Agency for Healthcare Research and Quality (AHRQ) provides health services investigators with the tools and data sources for a variety of health-related systems. One data source is the Medical Expenditures Panel (MEPS) database, a multi-year set of large-scale surveys of families and individuals, their medical providers, and employers across the United States (meps.ahrq.gov). MEPS is the most complete source of data on the cost and use of healthcare and health insurance coverage (AHRQ, 2011). Another collection used by a variety of nurse researchers is the HCUP data from AHRQ. HCUP databases bring together the data collection efforts of State data organizations, hospital associations, private data organizations, and the Federal government to create a national information resource of encounter-level healthcare data. It includes the largest collection of longitudinal hospital care data that enable research on a broad range of health policy issues, including cost and quality of health services, medical practice patterns, access to healthcare programs, and outcomes of treatments at the national, State, and local market levels (hcup-us.ahrq.gov) (AHRQ, 2014).

The electronic health records (EHRs) today are frequently providing source data for studies. These hospital systems have been used in the literature. For example, EHRs were used in a study done by Almasalha and colleagues (2012). They examined 596 episodes of care that included pain as a problem on a patient's care plan using statistical and data mining tools to identify hidden patterns in the information on end-of-life (EOL) hospitalized patients. Findings suggested new understanding about patient care, for example, EOL patients with hospital stays less than three days were less likely to meet the pain relief goals than those with longer hospital stays. Westra and colleagues (2011) studied urinary and bowel incontinence for home health patients using electronic health record data to predict improvements. In these cases, the EHR served as the data sources.

Figar and colleagues (2011) used a private health information system (HIS) clinical documentation system to study whether captured data could predict influenza outbreaks. They used a local interface terminology server which provides support through data auto-coding of clinical records and analyzed specific data sets to compare the burden of influenza in epidemiological weeks identified among 150,000 Health Maintenance Organization members in Argentina. The HIS detected the outbreak two weeks before the health department gave a national alert and was useful in assessing morbidity and mortality during the 2009 influenza epidemic H1N1 outbreak.

Computerized Documentation of Nursing Care Plans.

Moss and Saba (2011) studied the utility of costing out nursing care with the CCC terminology on five most commonly executed interventions. Using an observation study of nurses performing routine care on an acute-care unit, investigators collected data with a specialized data collection program entered directly into the PC database. A total of 251 interventions were observed, coded, and analyzed. From the analysis of time spent on each entered intervention, researchers could describe the four action types by average cost and percent of activity. The study demonstrated the feasibility of valuating the nursing care given to patients based on the standardized CCC terminology.

In a randomized trial on electronic documentation of nursing care plans, Feeg, Saba, and Feeg (2008) tested the quality of nursing student care planning on a bedside personal computer (PC) using a standardized nursing terminology in a specially designed Microsoft Access database program (Clinical Care Classification System) compared with an open-text format type-in application with the same terminology. Students were randomly assigned to one of the two versions of electronic nursing documentation formats and interviewed two simulated patients who served for all of the participants. The simulated patients were interviewed about their symptoms: one presented with congestive heart failure, the other with pneumonia. Students were instructed to document the care immediately following the interview on a laptop stationed at the patient's bedside. Measures were developed to assess the quality of the care plans and the participants' evaluation of using the system. Data were analyzed revealing a statistically significant difference (p = .05) for the Microsoft Access care plans completed by students and a statistically significant difference in the students' reports on using the system (p = .025). In a follow-up field study, the system was implemented on 49 students over three semesters who documented care for each patient they were assigned to in their clinical rotations. Students were assessed on their care plan documentation and they reported usability and satisfaction with the computer-based documentation system. Results continued to show that the coded language and PC care planning method was efficient and effective (Mannino & Feeg, 2011).

Web-Based Tools and Interventions.

A significant body of research has been conducted on using the Internet as a tool for conducting research, as well as studies on Web-designed interventions for clinical problems. For example, Yen and Bakken (2009) tested the usability of a Web-based tool for managing open shifts on nursing units. Using observational and interview approaches, they evaluated a Web communication tool (BidShift) designed to allow managers to announce open work shifts to solicit staff to request their own work shifts. They used specialized software to capture screens and vocal utterances as participants were asked to think aloud as they completed three subtasks associated with the open-shift management process. After task completion, they were asked about the process and their responses were recorded. Their data were managed and coded using Morae, specialized software developed for usability testing (www.techsmith.com/morae.asp). This example of qualitative research reported participants' patterns of use and themes related to their perceptions of usability of the communication tool.

In another qualitative study on electronic encounters using Web-based videoconferencing, Nystrom and Ohrling (2008) created a series of e-meetings for new fathers of children under one year old to "meet" in parental support groups. The technology allowed both one-on-one and group encounters. The fathers were interviewed using a narrative approach and content analysis was applied to the interview data. The researchers identified three categories from the transcripts: (1) being unfamiliar and insecure talking about fatherhood, (2) sharing experiences and being confirmed, and (3) being supported and limited by the electronic encounters.

Andersen and Ruland (2009) studied an Internet-based online patient–nurse communication (OPNC) service to support patients with prostate and breast cancers. Using qualitative content analysis, they examined 276 messages in a tailored Internet support intervention over 15 months. Two main themes emerged: (1) concerns about physical symptoms and treatment side effects and (2) worries and questions about treatment and follow-up. They concluded that the OPNC service can meet patients' needs for advice and information, thus improving the quality of care.

In a qualitative study by Lichenstein, McDonough, and Matura (2013), 98 participants who self-identified as caregivers for a person with pulmonary hypertension (PH) engaged in an online discussion board posted by the Pulmonary Hypertension Association over an 18-month period. Clinical variables collected were medications and oxygen use, and years since diagnosis. Thematic analysis yielded four themes: fear and frustration, questions and concerns, someone to listen to, and moving on with life. Results showed that caregivers of people with pulmonary hypertension may be ill equipped to care for their loved one because of lack of knowledge or psychological distress.

In a review of Web-based cognitive behavioral interventions for chronic pain, researchers conducted a systematic review and meta-analysis to quantify the intervention efficacy for treatment of patients with chronic pain. Using 11 studies from MEDLINE and other data sources, the investigators found that Web-based interventions for chronic pain resulted in small pain reductions in the intervention groups compared with waiting-list control groups (Macea, Gajos, Calil, & Fregni, 2010).

Specialized Computer Applications in Clinical Care. Computer-based administration of assessment is a reliable means of collecting patient assessment data as demonstrated by the report by Wilkie and colleagues (2009) who evaluated the feasibility and acceptability of a pentablet-based software program that assesses patients' cancer-related symptoms, the PAIN*ReportIt®*. In the study, 131 patients were able to use the computerized tool and reported high acceptability scores.

Vawdrey and colleagues (2011) pilot tested a tablet computer application for patients to participate in their hospital care. A prototype application was developed for a tablet computer using EHR queries and updates in real time. Patients were invited to participate in the study after consultation between the patient's providers and the investigator, an attending cardiologist. They were given an iPad device and encouraged to use the application. Structured interviews were used to test the patient engagement and the tablet usefulness of having access to patient's own medication and hospital history.

Mobile technologies have also proliferated in health-related applications today. For example, systems that support medication management of patients with SMS texting and Web-based interface programs have emerged using simple cell phones and sophisticated smartphones. The MyMediHealth (MMH) is a medication management system that includes a medication scheduler, a medication administration reminder engine and sends text messages to patient phones (Stenner, Johnson, & Denny, 2012).

In a review done by Schroeder (2009), a variety of studies used computerized telephone technologies as an assessment tool specifically for the collection of daily, self-reports of HIV risk behaviors. The review presented advantages of applications of interactive voice response technology (IVR) to HIV risk behavior research, including feasibility studies, assessment mode comparisons between IVR and alternative self-reporting methods, and unique findings derived from event-level data analyses illuminating risk factors for unprotected intercourse on within-person level. The author concluded that these specialized interactive, computerized voice systems are highly promising tools for various research and healthcare applications that should be considered more frequently for use in HIV-risk populations.

Some studies that incorporate remote technologies in special applications have been described in the literature. Mahoney (2011) reported on several mixed methods studies that describe innovative monitoring intervention research with older adults and their informal and/or formal caregivers. The studies were conducted in "real world" homes and focused on improved ways to monitor elders, taking into account the goal of independence and privacy, to alert caregivers on elders' activities and safety issues. In another collection of case studies, Rantz and colleagues (2010) describe instances of technology-enhanced monitoring capabilities, using sensors, alarms, and environmentally embedded devices, that wirelessly communicate with programmed systems for the purpose of detecting potential problems.

These and other innovations that connect computer technology with nursing practice have emerged with research to support their functionality, ease of adoption, and efficacy. The range of innovation has been astounding as the technologies have increasingly become less expensive, smaller, wireless, and now interconnected with cloud computing. Nursing research and computers today are inseparable in both areas of using computers for the research and studying the impact of computers on patient care.

SUMMARY

This chapter has reviewed two research paradigms and philosophical orientations—qualitative and quantitative methods—that specify different underlying approaches to research and the use of computers in various stages of the research process. It also highlighted examples of research on computer use with these quantitative and qualitative approaches. A variety of computer applications are available via commercialized packages that serve the nurse researcher in conducting research. With the advancements in applications development and delivered wirelessly and the wide use of smaller devices such as smartphone technologies, the potential for innovation and research on health abounds. Prompted by large consortia that foster technology innovation such as Health Datapalooza (healthdatapalooza.org), an annual conference for researchers and entrepreneurs, one can expect the emergence of many evidence-based interventions aided by smartphones, tablets, and minis in the near future. With the federal government emphasis on big data, the enhancements made to aid researchers to tackle existing data sets, and the cloud to house and connect researchers and subjects from distances, one can expect a proliferation of research techniques and acceptable evidence using secondary data. In addition, research on computer applications and informatics is a growing body of science that will continue to appear in the literature with a renewed purpose of collecting and storing meaningful data for multiple uses.

Carrington and Tiase (2013) state, "Health information technology (HIT), and more specifically, nursing informatics, is the driving force for the transformation of health care in the United States…Nurses'…role in the use of technology [has evolved]" (p. 136). Nursing informatics research has been influential in shaping health. In a review of literature published in one year, Carrington and Tiase describe topics ranging from EHR, monitoring, and human–computer interaction to bar code administration. The studies were 31% qualitative, 54% quantitative, and 15% mixed methods.

Conclude that the design, implementation, and evaluation of nursing technologies show promise in nursing efficiencies that affect patient safety and healthcare cost, the two driving forces of policies that shape healthcare.

The contextual influences on nursing research are discussed by Bakken and colleagues (2008). The nursing informatics research agenda for the next 10 years must expand users of interest to include inter-disciplinary researchers; build upon the knowledge gained in genomic and environmental data; guide the re-engineering of nursing practice; harness new technologies to empower patients and their caregivers in collaborative knowledge development, particularly related to the social network technologies; and evaluate innovative methodologies that recognize human–computer interface factors.

REFERENCES

Agency for Healthcare Research and Quality. (2011). *Medical Expenditure Panel Survey.* Rockville, MD: Agency for Healthcare Research and Quality. Retrieved from www.meps.ahrq.gov/mepsweb/

Agency for Healthcare Research and Quality (AHRQ). (2014, January). HCUP Home. *Healthcare Cost and Utilization Project (HCUP).* Agency for Healthcare Research and Quality, Rockville, MD. Retrieved from www.hcup-us.ahrq.gov/home.jsp

Almasalha, F., Xu, D., Keenan, G., Khokhar, A., Yao, Y., Chen, Y., … Wilkie, D. (2012). Data mining nursing care plans of end-of-life patients: A study to improve healthcare decision making. *International Journal of Nursing Knowledge, 24*(1), 15–24.

Andersen, T., & Ruland, C. (2009). Cancer patients' questions and concerns expressed in an online nurse-delivered mail service: Preliminary results. In K. Saranto M. Tallberg, A. Ensio, P. Flatley, & H. Park. (Eds.), *Connecting health and humans.* Fairfax, VA: IOS Press.

ATLAS.ti 7. (2014). Thousand Oaks, London: SAGE. Retrieved from http://www.atlasti.com

Bakken, S. (2013, December 3). Why a nursing terminology? *Presentation at the CCC Workshop,* Nashville, TN.

Bakken, S., Stone, P., & Larson, E. (2008). A nursing informatics research agenda for 2008–2018: Contextual influences and key components. *Nursing Outlook, 56,* 206–214.

Banxia. (2014). Decision Explorer. Banxia Software Ltd, Kendal, Cumbria, UK. Retrieved from http://www.banxia.com/dexplore

Berger, A. M., & Berger, C. R. (2004). Data mining as a tool for research and knowledge development in nursing. *Computers, Informatics, Nursing, 22*(3), 123–131.

Berry, D. L., Halpenny, B., Wolpin, S., Davison, J., Ellis, W., Lober, W. B., … Wulff, J. (2010). Development and evaluation of the personal patient profile-prostate (P3P), a web-based decision support system for ment newly diagnosed with localized prostate cancer. *Journal of Medicine Internet Research, 12*(4), e67.

Berry, D. L., Wang, Q., Halpenny, B., & Hong, F. (2012). Decision preparation, satisfaction and regret in a multcenter sample of men with newly diagnosed localized prostate cancer. *Patient Education Counseling, 88*(22), 262–267.

Biostat. (2014). *Power and precision.* Englewood, New Jersey. Retrieved from http://www.power-analysis.com/home.htm

Borenstein, M., Hedges, L., Higgins, J., & Rothstein, H. (2009). *Introduction to metaanalysis.* Chichester, UK: John Wiley & Sons. Retrieved from http://www.meta-analysis.com

Brennan, P. F., Zielstorff, R. D., Ozbolt, J. G., & Strombom, I. (1998). Setting a national research agenda in nursing informatics. *Medinfo, 9,* 1188–1191.

Broome, M. (2014). Open access publishing: A disruptive innovation. *Nursing Outlook, 62*(2), 125–127.

Bulechek, G. M., & McCloskey, J. (1997). All user s of NIC encouraged to submit new interventions, suggest revisions. Iowa Intervention Project Research Team. *Image: The Journal of Nursing Scholarship, 1*, 10–20.

Byrne, B. M. (1984). *Structural equation modeling with EQS and EQS/Windows: Basic concepts, applications, and programming.* Thousand Oaks, CA: Sage.

Byrne, M., & Lang, N. (2013). Examination of nursing data elements from evidence-based recommendations for clinical decision support. *CIN: Computers, Informatics, Nursing, 31*(12), 605–614.

Carrington, J., & Tiase, V. (2013). Nursing informatics year in review. *Nursing Administration Quarterly, 37*(2), 136–143.

Coenen, A., & Jansen, K. (2013, December 3). Harmonising ICNP and the CCC – International Council of Nursing. *Presentation at the CCC Workshop,* Nashville, TN.

Congressional Budget Office (CBO). (2007, December). *Research on the comparative effectiveness of medical treatments: Issues and options for an expanded federal role.* Washington, DC: CBO Report.

Creswell, J. W. (2012). *Qualitative inquiry and research design: Choosing among five approaches.* Thousand Oaks, CA: Sage.

Creswell, J. W. (2014). *Research design: Qualitative, quantitative, and mixed methods approaches* (4th ed.). Thousand Oaks, CA: Sage.

Daly, J. M., Maas, M. L., & Johnson, M. (1997). Nursing outcomes classification: An essential element in data sets for nursing and healthcare effectiveness. *Computers in Nursing, 15*, S82–S86.

Delaney, C., Westra, B., Monsen, K., Gillis, C., & Docherty, S. (2013, November 6). Big data 4th paradigm nursing research: Informatics exemplars. *Presentation at the CTSA Nurse Scientists SIG Meeting.*

Department of Health and Human Services (DHHS). (2007, January). *Breaking news: Nationwide health information technology standard for nursing.* Washington, DC: Department of Health and Human Services.

Dykes, P. (2013, December 3). Coding Clinical care Classification System Research Model. *Presentation at the CCC Workshop,* Nashville, TN.

Effken, J. A. (2003). An organizing framework for nursing informatics research. *Computers, Informatics, Nursing, 21*, 316–323.

Englebright, J. (2013, December 3). Who is adopting the CCC? Nurse executives. *Presentation at the CCC Workshop,* Nashville, TN.

Englebright, J., Aldrich, K., & Taylor, C. (2014). Defining and incorporating basic nursing care actions into the electronic health record. *Journal of Nursing Scholarship, 46*(1), 50–57.

Expert Choice, Inc. (2014). *Expert Choice® 11.5.* Arlington, VA. Retrieved from http://www.expertchoice.com

Feeg, V. D., Saba, V., & Feeg, A. (2008). Testing a bedside personal computer clinical care classification system for nursing students using Microsoft Access®. *Computers, Informatics, Nursing, 26*(6), 339–349.

Figar, S., Aliperti, V., Salazar, E., Otero, C., Schpilberg, M., Taliercio, V., ... de Quiros, F. (2011). Healthcare information systems to assess influenza outbreaks. *Applied Clinical Informatics, 2*, 75–85.

Figge, H. (2010). Electronic tools to measure and enhance medication adherence, *U.S. Pharmacist 36*(4), (Compliance and Adherence suppl.) 6–10.

Glaser, B. G. (1978). *Theoretical sensitivity.* Mill Valley, CA: Sociological Press.

Granello, D., & Wheaton, J. (2004). Online data collection: Strategies for research. *Journal of Counseling and Development, 82*, 387–393.

Gravic, Inc. (2014). *Remark Office®, Remark Classic®, Remark Web Survey®.* Retrieved from http://www.gravic.com/remark

Hey, H., Tansley, S., & Tolle, K. (2009). *The fourth paradigm: Data-intensive scientific discovery.* Seattle, WA: Microsoft Corporation.

IBM SPSS Statistics. (2014). *Statistical package for social sciences (SPSS).* Chicago, IL. Retrieved from http://www.spss.com/statistics

Joreskog, K. G., & Sorbom, D. (1978). *LISREL IV's user's guide.* Chicago, IL: National Educational Resources.

Kimiafar, K., Sadoughi, F., Sheikhtaheri, A., & Sarbaz, M. (2014). Prioritizing factors influencing nurses' satisfaction with hospital information systems: A fuzzy analytic hierarchy process approach. *CIN: Computers, Informatics, Nursing, 32*(4), 174–181.

Klemm, P., Hayes, E., Diefenbeck, C., & Milcarek, B. (2014). Online support for employed informal caregivers: psychosocial outcomes. *CIN: Computers, Informatics, Nursing, 32*(1), 10–20.

Kodadek, M., & Feeg, V. (2002). Using vignettes to explore how parents approach end-of-life decision making for terminally ill infants, *Pediatric Nursing, 28*(4), 333–340, 343.

Lichenstein, S., McDonough, A., & Matura, L. (2013). Cyber support: Describing concerns of caregivers of people with pulmonary hypertension. *CIN: Computers, Informatics, Nursing, 31*(12), 581–588.

Macea, D., Gajos, K., Calil, Y., & Fregni, F. (2010). The efficacy of web-based cognitive behavioral interventions for chronic pain: A systematic review and meta-analysis. *Journal of Pain, 11*(10), 917–929.

Mahoney, D. (2011). An evidence-based adoption of technology model for remote monitoring of elders' daily activities. *Ageing International, 36*, 66–81.

Mannino, J., & Feeg, V. (2011). Field-testing a PC electronic documentation system using the CCC with nursing students. *Journal of Healthcare Engineering, 2*(2), 223–240.

Martin, K. S., & Norris, J. (1996). The Omaha system: A model for describing practice. *Holistic Nursing Practice, 11*, 75–83.

MAXQDA: The Art of Data Analysis. (2012). *VERBI GmbH Software*. Berlin, Germany. Retrieved from http://maxqda.com

McCormick, K. A., Lang, N., Zielstorff, R., Milholland, D. K., Saba, V., Jacox, A. (1994). Toward standard classification schemes for nursing language: Recommendations of the American Nurses Association Steering Committee on databases to support clinical nursing practice. *Journal of the American Medical Informatics Association, 1*, 421–427.

Minitab, Inc. (2014). *Minitab 17: Learn more*. State College, PA.

Montalbano, E. (2009, June 4). *Forrester: Microsoft Office in no danger from competitors. PC World*. Retrieved from http://www.pcworld.com/businesscenter/article/166123/forrester_microsoft_office_in_no_danger_from_competitors.html

Moss, J., & Saba, V. (2011). Costing nursing care: Using the Clinical Care Classification System to value nursing intervention in an acute-care setting. *CIN: Computers, Informatics, Nursing, 29*(8), 455–460.

MSDN Library. (2000). *Building and using data mining models*. Microsoft Corporation. Retrieved from http://msdn.microsoft.com/library/default.asp?url=/library/en-us/olapdmad/agdatamining_686r.asp

Mullen, K., Berry, D., & Zierler, B. (2004). Computerized symptom and quality-of-life assessment for patients with cancer. Part II: Acceptability and usability. *Oncology Nursing Forum, 31*(5), E84–E89.

Nahm, E., Vaydia, V., Ho, D., Scharf, B., & Seagull, J. (2007). Outcomes assessment of clinical information system implementation: A practical guide. *Nursing Outlook, 55*, 282–288.

NIH Big Data to Knowledge (BD2K). (2012). *About BD2K*. Bethesda, MD: U.S. Department of Health and Human Services, National Institutes of Health.

NINR Priority Expert Panel on Nursing Informatics. (1993). *Nursing informatics: Enhancing patient care*. Bethesda, MD: U.S. Department of Health and Human Services, U.S. Public Health Service, National Institutes of Health.

Nuance Dragon Solutions. (2014). *Dragon Naturally Speaking®10*. Burlington, MA. Retrieved from http://www.nuance.com/naturallyspeaking

Nuance Imaging. (2014). *OmniPage Pro® 17*. Burlington, MA. Retrieved from http://www.nuance.com/imaging

Nystrom, K., & Ohrling, K. (2008). Electronic encounters: Fathers' experiences of parental support. *Journal of Telemedicine and Telecare, 14*, 71–74.

Ozbolt, J. G. (1999). Testimony to the NCVHS hearings on medical terminology and code development. School of Nursing and Division of Biomedical Informatics, School of Medicine, Vanderbilt University.

Paul, E., Bailey, M., Van Lint, A., & Pilcher, D. (2012). Performance of APACHE III over time in Australia and New Zealand: a retrospective cohort study. *Anaesthesia Intensive Care, 40*, 980–994.

Polit, D. F., & Beck, C. T. (2011). *Nursing research: Generating and assessing evidence for nursing practice*

(9th ed.). Philadelphia, PA: Wolters Kluwer/Lippincott, Williams & Wilkins.

Qualis Research. (2008). Ethnograph 6.0. Colorado Springs, CO. Retrieved from http://www.qualisresearch.com/default.htm

Rantz, M., Skubic, M., Alexander, G., AUd, M., Wakefield, B., Galambos, C., … Miller, S. (2010). Improving nurse care coordination with technology. *CIN: Computers, Informatics, Nursing, 28*(6), 325–332.

Research Dataware, LLC. (2014). IRBNet. *Innovative solutions for compliance and research management*. Retrieved from http://www.irbnet.org

Rolley, J., Davidson, P., Dennison, C., Ong, A., Everett, B., & Salamonson, Y. (2008). Medication adherence self-report instruments: Implications for practice and research. *Journal of Cardiovascular Nursing, 23*(6), 497–505.

Saba, V., & Arnold, J. (2004). Clinical care costing method for the Clinical Care Classification System. *International Journal of Nursing Terminology Classification, 15*(3), 69–77.

Saba, V. K. (1997). Why the home healthcare classification is a recognized nursing nomenclature. *Computers in Nursing, 15*, S69–S76.

Saba, V. K. (2007). *Clinical Care Classification (CCC) System manual: A guide to nursing documentation*. New York, NY: Springer Pub.

Saba, V., & Taylor, S. (2007). Moving past theory: Use of a standardized, coded nursing terminology to enhance nursing visibility. *CIN: Computers, Informatics, Nursing, 25*(6), 324–331.

Schroeder, K. (2009). Interactive voice response technology to measure HIV-related behavior. *Current HIV/AIDS Reports, 6*(4), 210.

Seidel, J., & Clark, J. (1984). The ethnograph: A computer program for the analysis of qualitative data. *Qualitative Sociology, 7*(12), 110–125.

Seidel, J., Friese, S., & Lenard, C. (1994). *Ethnograph (version 4.0)*. Amherst, MA: Qualis Research Associates.

Sox, H. C., & Greenfield, S. (2009). Comparative effectiveness research: A report from the Institute of Medicine, *Annals of Internal Medicine, 151*, 203–205.

Stenner, S., Johnson, K., & Denny, J. (2012). PASTE: Patient-centered SMS text tagging in a medication management system. *Journal of the American Medical Informatics Association, 19*, 368–374.

Strauss, A., & Corbin, J. M. (1990). *Basics of qualitative research: Grounded theory procedures and techniques*. Newbury Park, CA: Sage.

The Thomson Corporation. (2009). Reference Manager (Version 8). Carlsbad, CA: Thomson ISI ResearchSoft. Retrieved from http://www.refman.com/pr-rm11.asp

Vawdrey, D., Wilcox, M., Collins, S., Bakken, S., Feiner, S., Boyer, A., & Restaino, S. (2011). A tablet computer application for patients to participate in their hospital care. *AMIA Annual Symposium Proceedings*, 1428–1435. Retrieved from http://www.ncbi.nlm.nih.gov/pmc/articles/PMC3243172

Werley, H. H., Lang, N. M., & Westlake, S. K. (1986). The nursing minimum data set conference: Executive summary. *Journal of Professional Nursing, 2,* 217–224.

Westra, B., Savik, K., Oancea, C., Chormanski, L., Holmes, J., & Bliss, D. (2011). Predicting improvements in urinary and bowel incontinence for home health patients using electronic health record data. *Journal of Wound, Ostomy and Continence Nursing, 38*(1), 77–87.

Wilkie, D., Kim, Y. O., Suarez, M., Dauw, C., Stapleton, S., Gorman, G., … Zhao, Z. (2009). Extending computer technology to hospice research: Interactive pentablet measurement of symptoms by hospice cancer patients in their homes. *Journal of Palliative Medicine, 12*(7), 599–602.

Yen, P., & Bakken, S. (2009). Usability testing of a Web-based tool for managing open shifts on nursing units. In K. Saranto, M. Tallberg, A. Ensio, P. Flatley & H. Park. (Eds.), *Connecting health and humans.* Fairfax, VA: IOS Press.

Zielstorff, R. D., Lang, N. M., Saba, V. K., McCormick, K. A., Milholland, D. K. (1995). Toward a uniform language for nursing in the US: Work of the American Nurses Association Steering Committee on databases to support clinical practice. *Medinfo, 8*(2), 1362–1366.

Zimmerman, J., Kramer, A., McNair, D., & Malila, F. (2006). Acute physiology and chronic health evaluation (APACHE) IV: Hospital mortality assessment for today's critically ill patients. *Critical Care Medicine, 34*(5), 1297–1310.

Information Literacy and Computerized Information Resources

Diane S. Pravikoff / June Levy

• OBJECTIVES

1. Define information literacy.
2. Identify steps in choosing appropriate databases.
3. Identify steps in planning a computer search for information.
4. Identify sources of information for practicing nurses.
5. Identify the difference between essential and supportive computerized resources.

• KEY WORDS

Information literacy
Information retrieval
Information resources
Health reference databases

INTRODUCTION

This chapter presents information about electronic resources that are easily available and accessible and can assist nurses in maintaining and enhancing their professional practices. These resources aid in keeping current with the published literature, in developing a list of sources for practice, research, and/or education, and in collaborating with colleagues.

As is evidenced in earlier chapters, nurses use computers for many purposes. In the past, most of the focus has been on computerized patient records, acuity systems, and physician ordering systems. One of the major purposes for which computers can be used, however, is searching for information. Many resources are available by computer, and the information retrieved can be used to accomplish different ends. Computers also are available in various sizes, improving portability and availability wherever a

nurse is practicing. Many of the resources described in the following sections will be available via mobile devices.

To maintain professional credibility, nursing professionals must (1) keep current with the published literature, (2) develop and maintain a list of bibliographic and other sources on specific topics of interest for practice, research, and/or education, and (3) collaborate and network with colleagues regarding specifics of professional practice. Electronic resources are available to meet each of these needs. This chapter addresses each of these requirements for professional credibility and discusses both essential and supportive computerized resources available to meet them. *Essential* computerized resources are defined as those resources that are vital and necessary to the practitioner to accomplish the specific goal. In the case of maintaining currency, for example, these resources include bibliographic retrieval systems such as MEDLINE or the CINAHL database, current awareness services, review services, or point-of-care tools and may be accessible on the World Wide Web. *Supportive* computerized resources are those that are helpful and interesting and supply good information but are not necessarily essential for professional practice. In meeting the requirement of maintaining currency, supportive computerized resources include document delivery services, electronic publishers, and meta-sites on the World Wide Web. There are many resources available to meet each of the above requirements for professional credibility. For the purposes of this chapter, selective resources are identified and discussed as examples of the types of information available. Web site URLs of the various resources are included as well. It is important that the nursing professional determine her or his exact requirements before beginning the search. Planning the search will be stressed throughout this chapter.

INFORMATION SEEKING BEHAVIOR OF REGISTERED NURSES

Multiple practice standards organizations (Institute of Medicine [IOM], Agency for Healthcare Research and Quality [AHRQ], American Nurse Credentialing Center [ANCC]'s Magnet Recognition Program, American Association of Colleges of Nursing [AACN], National League for Nursing [NLN], The Joint Commission [TJC]) insist that nursing care be based on information derived from best practice evidence. To identify best evidence and apply it in the care of the patient, the nurse must apply the information literacy process (Association of College and Research Libraries, 2000):

1. Recognize the need for evidence.

2. Know how to search and find relevant information.

3. Access, utilize, and evaluate such information within the practice environment.

Information literacy is identified as a competency for the basic nurse (American Nurses Association, 2008). The American Library Association describes the "information literate" person as one who can "recognize when information is needed and have the ability to locate, evaluate, and use effectively the needed information" and identifies it as a basic competency for higher education (American Library Association, 1989, p.1).

While the importance of maintaining currency with published literature is stressed, research has indicated that nurses often do not access the tools needed to do so. Neither do they have the ability to utilize these tools, if available, within their work setting. A national study (Pravikoff, Pierce, & Tanner, 2005) of 3000 nurses licensed

to practice in the United States was conducted in 2004 to better understand the readiness of nurses to utilize evidence-based nursing practice, based on their information literacy knowledge and competency.

This landmark study demonstrated that many nurses were not aware that they needed information; once they recognized a need, online resources available for them to use were inadequate and respondents had not been taught how to use online databases to search for the information they needed. Additionally, they did not value research as a basis on which to formulate and implement patient care.

Since these findings were published, many subsequent studies have been conducted in various specialty areas and countries with similar results (Majid et al., 2011; O'Leary & Mhaolrunaigh, 2011; Ross, 2010; Yadav & Fealy, 2012). Melnyk, Fineout-Overholt, Gallagher-Ford & Kaplan (2012) surveyed randomly selected members of the American Nurses Association and found that over 70% of respondents either needed or strongly needed (1) tools to implement evidence-based practice, (2) online education and skills-building modules in evidence-based practice, and (3) an "online resource center where best EBPs for patients are housed and experts are available for consultation" (p. 412). Melnyk, et al. (2012) determined that nurses valued and were ready to practice nursing based on evidence but need several things to be able to do so: more time, knowledge, skills, access, and a supportive organizational culture.

The rate of expansion in health information technology (e.g., electronic health records) is phenomenal; additionally, clinical knowledge is multiplying exponentially and dissemination methods are changing to include scholarly databases and social networking. Despite the demands for EBP, nurses continue to have difficulty finding information they need for practice and prefer colleagues as their primary source (Marshall, West, & Aitken, 2011).

Nurses—students, clinicians, educators, and managers—must develop efficient and effective search strategies that embrace information literacy as a framework to search the myriad of information resources available for evidence. According to recent efforts, education is embracing the change by embedding well-designed courses that offer opportunities to develop these skills throughout program curricula (Moreton, 2013; Powell & Ginier, 2013; Stombaugh et al., 2013). Results indicate that such courses are indeed effective in improving the nurse's skills and confidence in searching for evidence (Boden, Neilson, & Seaton, 2013; Clapp, Johnson, Schwieder, & Craig, 2013). Change in practice culture is needed to infuse information literacy throughout the workplace.

The resources and search strategy introduced in this chapter provide the reader with tools that will become the basis of life-long learning for the nurse—tools for evidence-based practice.

MAINTAINING CURRENCY WITH THE PUBLISHED LITERATURE

It is obvious that one of the most important obligations a nurse must meet is to maintain currency in her or his field of practice. With the extreme demands in the clinical environment—both in time and amount of work—nurses need easily accessible resources to answer practice-related questions and ensure that they are practicing with the latest and most evidence-based information. Information is needed about current treatments, trends, medications, safety issues, business practices, and new health issues, among other topics.

The purpose of the information retrieved from the sources listed below is to enable nurses to keep abreast of the latest and most evidence-based information in their selected field. Both quantity *and* quality must be considered. When using a resource, check that:

1. The resource covers the required specialty/field
2. The primary journals and peripheral material in the field are included
3. The resource is updated regularly and is current
4. The resource covers the appropriate period
5. The resource covers material published in different countries and languages
6. There is some form of peer review, reference checking, or other means of evaluation

Essential Computerized Resources

Essential computerized resources for maintaining currency include bibliographic retrieval systems for the journal literature, current awareness services, review services of the journal literature, point-of-care tools, and currently published books. All of these assist the nurse in gathering the most current and reliable information.

Bibliographic Retrieval Systems

One of the most useful resources for accessing information about current practice is the journal literature. Although there may be a delay between the writing and publishing of an article, this time period is seldom more than a few months. The best way to peruse this literature is through a bibliographic retrieval system, since there is far too much literature published to read it all. Bibliographic retrieval systems also allow filtering and sorting of this vast amount of published material.

A bibliographic retrieval system database allows the nurse to retrieve a list of citations containing bibliographic details of the material indexed, subject headings, and author abstracts. The nurse can search these systems using specific subject headings or key words. Most bibliographic retrieval systems have a controlled vocabulary, also known as a thesaurus or subject heading list, to make electronic subject searching much easier. For this reason, the vocabulary is geared toward the specific content of the database. These controlled vocabularies are made available online as part of the database. Key word searching is necessary when there are no subject headings to cover the concepts being searched. The nurse can also search by specific fields including author, author affiliation, journal title, journal serial number (ISSN), grant name or number, or publication type. In bibliographic retrieval systems, most fields in the records are word-indexed and can be searched individually to retrieve specific information.

Previously available as print indexes, these systems are now available electronically through online services, or via the World Wide Web. To access them, a computer with a modem and/or Internet access is required.

Since each of these bibliographic retrieval systems has its own specific content, a nurse may have to search several systems to retrieve a comprehensive list of citations on a particular topic. Directories of descriptions of bibliographic retrieval systems can be found at many sites on the World Wide Web, e.g., universities (University of California, San Francisco [www.library.ucsf.edu]), medical centers (University of Kansas Medical Center A. R. Dykes Library [http://library.kumc.edu/database-descriptions.xml]), and government agencies (National Library of Medicine [http://wwwcf2.nlm.nih.gov/nlm_eresources/eresources/search_database.cfm]).

The main bibliographic retrieval systems that should first be considered are MEDLINE/PubMed, the CINAHL database, Mosby's Index, ERIC, PsycINFO, the SocialSciences Citation Index, and SocIndex.

MEDLINE/PubMed. The NLM provides free access to many online resources (Table 48.1). One of these, MEDLINE, covers 5600 journals in 39 languages with over 20 million references from 1946 to the present in the fields of medicine, nursing, preclinical sciences, healthcare systems, veterinary medicine, and dentistry. The nursing subset in MEDLINE covers 189 nursing journals. The database is updated weekly on the World Wide Web (U.S. National Library of Medicine, 2013a, 2013b). The NLM's databases use a controlled vocabulary (thesaurus) called MeSH (Medical Subject Headings)

TABLE 48.1	Selected Online Databases		
Database	**URL**	**Subject**	**Type**
General databases			
AIDSinfo	http://aidsinfo.nih.gov	HIV/AIDS clinical trials; prevention, medical practice guidelines	Factual and referral
ClinicalTrials.gov	http://clinicaltrials.gov	Patient studies for drugs and treatment	Factual and referral
Health Hotlines	http://healthhotlines.nlm.nih.gov	Directory of organizations providing specialized information services	Factual and referral
HSRProj (Health Services Research Projects in progress)	http://wwwcf.nlm.nih.gov/hsr_project/home_proj.cfm	Ongoing grants and contracts in health services research	Research project descriptions
HSRR (Health Services and Sciences Research Resources)	http://wwwcf.nlm.nih.gov/hsrr_search/index.cfm	Research datasets and instruments used in health services research	Factual
HSTAT (Health Services Technology Assessment Texts)	http://www.ncbi.nlm.nih.gov/books/NBK16710/	Clinical practice guidelines, technology assessments, and health information	Full text
Locator Plus	http://locatorplus.gov	Catalogs of books, audiovisuals, and journal articles held at National Library of Medicine	Bibliographic citations
MEDLINE/PubMed	http://www.ncbi.nlm.nih.gov/pubmed	Biomedicine. Abstracts to articles in thousands of biomedical journals	Bibliographic citations
MedlinePlus	http://www.nlm.nih.gov/medlineplus/	Health information	Factual, bibliographic citations
MeSH Vocabulary File	http://www.ncbi.nlm.nih.gov/mesh	Thesaurus of biomedicine-related terms	Factual
OLDMEDLINE	http://www.nlm.nih.gov/databases/databases_oldmedline.html	Biomedicine articles 1947–1965	Bibliographic citations
Women's Health Resources	http://www.womenshealthresources.nlm.nih.gov/	Health topics and research initiatives for women's health	Factual
TOXNET databases (Toxicology Data Network)			
CCRIS (Chemical Carcinogenesis Research Information Systems)	http://toxnet.nlm.nih.gov/cgi-bin/sis/htmlgen?CCRIS	Chemical carcinogens, mutagens, tumor promoters, and tumor inhibitors	Factual
ChemIDplus	http://chem.sis.nlm.nih.gov/chemidplus/chemidlite.jsp	Identification of chemical substances	Factual
DART (Developmental and Reproductive Toxicology Database)	http://toxnet.nlm.nih.gov/newtoxnet/dart.htm	Test results Developmental and reproductive toxicology	Bibliographic citations
GENE-TOX (genetic toxicology)	http://toxnet.nlm.nih.gov/cgi-bin/sis/htmlgen?GENETOX	Genetic toxicology test results on chemicals	Factual
Haz-Map	http://hazmap.nlm.nih.gov/index.php	Effects of exposure to chemicals. Links jobs and hazardous tasks with occupational diseases	Factual

(continued)

TABLE 48.1	Selected Online Databases *(continued)*		
Database	**URL**	**Subject**	**Type**
HSDB (hazardous substances data bank)	http://toxnet.nlm.nih.gov/cgi-bin/sis/htmlgen?HSDB	Hazardous chemical toxic effects, environmental fate, safety, and handling	Factual
IRIS (Integrated Risk Information Systems)	http://toxnet.nlm.nih.gov/cgi-bin/sis/htmlgen?IRIS	Potentially toxic chemicals	Factual
ITER (international toxicity estimates for risk)	http://toxnet.nlm.nih.gov/cgi-bin/sis/htmlgen?iter	Data of human health risk assessment	Factual
TOXLINE (toxicology Literature online)	http://toxnet.nlm.nih.gov/cgi-bin/sis/htmlgen?TOXLINE	References from toxicology literature	Bibliographic citations
TRI (toxics release inventory)	http://toxnet.nlm.nih.gov/cgi-bin/sis/htmlgen?TRI	Annual releases of over 600 toxic chemicals to the environment, amounts transferred to waste sites, and source reduction and recycling data	Numeric

Source: US National Library of Medicine. (2013). *NLM databases, resources & APIs*. Retrieved from http://wwwcf2.nlm.nih.gov/nlm_eresources/eresources/search_database.cfm. Accessed on January 17, 2014.

(MeSH: http://www.ncbi.nlm.nih.gov/mesh). These index terms facilitate subject searching within the databases.

MEDLINE and the nursing subset are available free over the World Wide Web through the NLM's home page at http://www.nlm.nih.gov. There are two ways to search this database: PubMed and the NLM Gateway. The NLM Gateway is a Web-based system that allows users to search multiple NLM retrieval systems simultaneously. The database is also available through the commercial vendors mentioned below. All of these options allow the nurse to search by subject, key word, author, title, or a combination of these. An example of different searches with a display using the EBSCOhost interface is shown in Figs. 48.1 and 48.2.

Loansome Doc allows the nurse to place an order for a copy of an article from a medical library through PubMed or the NLM Gateway (https://docline.gov/loansome/login.cfm). The full text of articles for some journals is available via a link to the publisher's Web site from the PubMed abstract or record display. Some of the full text is available free of charge. The links indicating free full-text display on the Loansome Doc order page prior to order placement and on the Loansome Doc Order Sent page immediately after the order is finalized. NLM has a fact sheet for Loansome doc users covering the registration process, how to place an order, order confirmation, check order status, and updating account information (http://www.nlm.nih.gov/loansomedoc/loansome_home.html).

CINAHL. The CINAHL database, produced by Cinahl Information Systems, a division of EBSCO Information Services (EBSCO), provides comprehensive coverage of the literature in nursing and allied health from 1982 to the present. CINAHL has expanded to offer five databases including three full-text versions. The database covers chiropractic, podiatry, health promotion and education, health services administration, biomedicine, optometry, women's health, consumer health, and alternative therapy (EBSCO, 2014). More than 4900 journals as well as books, pamphlets, dissertations, and proceedings are indexed. Some journals covered are published in other countries. It is updated weekly.

The CINAHL database also uses a controlled vocabulary for effective subject searching. The CINAHL *Subject Heading List* uses the NLM's MeSH terms as the standard vocabulary for disease, drug, anatomic, and physiologic concepts. There are approximately 12,714 unique CINAHL terms for nursing and the allied health disciplines. Specific field searching and quality filters are available in the CINAHL database and are similar to those found in MEDLINE. An example of different searches with a display using the EBSCOhost interface is shown in Figs. 48.3 and 48.4.

An essential part of research papers is the list of references pointing to prior publications. Cited references for more than 1300 nursing and allied health journals are searchable in the CINAHL database.

Mosby's Index. Content from over 3150 peer-reviewed journals, trade publications, and electronic titles, and provides access to over 3 million records, as far back as 1974,

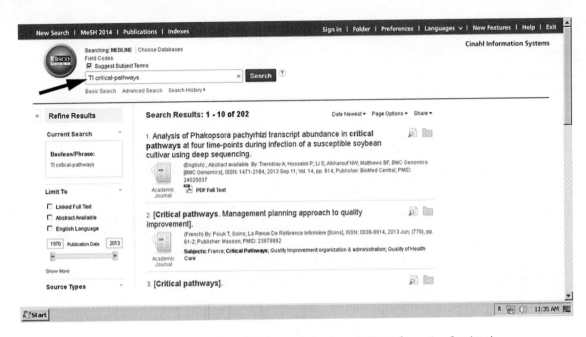

· **FIGURE 48.1.** MEDLINE Search. (Reproduced with permission from EBSCO Information Services.)

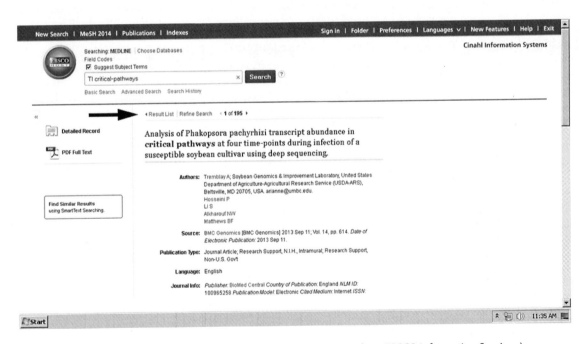

· **FIGURE 48.2.** MEDLINE Search Result. (Reproduced with permission from EBSCO Information Services.)

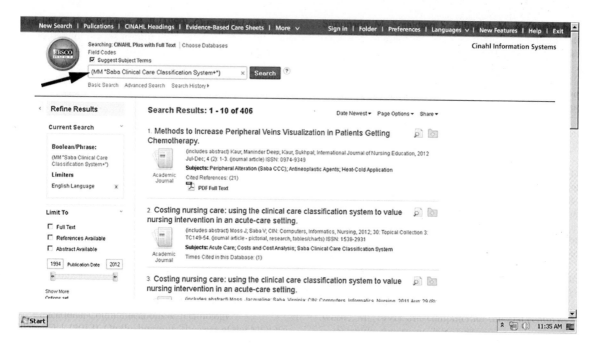

• **FIGURE 48.3.** CINAHL Search. (Reproduced with permission from EBSCO Information Services.)

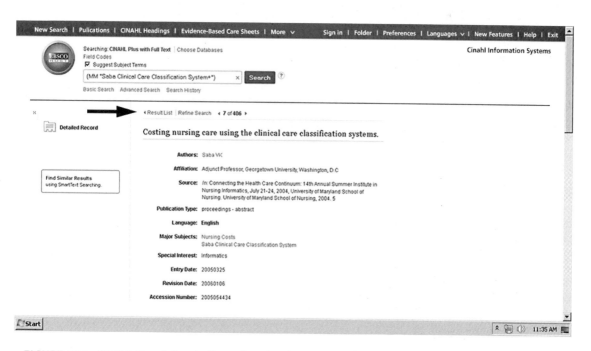

• **FIGURE 48.4.** CINAHL Search Result. (Reproduced with permission from EBSCO Information Services.)

is indexed in this database. It uses the EMTREE Thesaurus, a hierarchically structured, biomedical thesaurus, which has been enhanced for nursing. Both the thesaurus and the index are published by Elsevier B.V. (Elsevier, 2014).

ERIC. The ERIC (Educational Resources Information Center) database is sponsored by the Institute of Education Sciences (IES) of the U.S. Department of Education and contains more than 1,400,000 citations covering education-related literature (Educational Resources Information Center, 2013). It covers virtually all types of print materials, published and unpublished, from 1966 to the present day. Currently more than 650 journal titles are indexed in ERIC. It is updated monthly. This database gives the nurse a more comprehensive coverage of education than any other bibliographic retrieval system. The *Thesaurus of Eric Descriptors*, a controlled vocabulary, assists with computer searches of this database on the Internet through the World Wide Web (ERIC). As with the other two bibliographic databases mentioned, nurses are able to access all of the data in each record on ERIC by searching, using subject headings or key words or by searching for a word(s) in a specific field.

PsycINFO. The PsycINFO database, produced by the American Psychological Association, provides access to psychologically relevant literature from more than 2543 journals, dissertations, reports, scholarly documents, books, and book chapters with more than 3 million references from the 1880s to the present. Updated weekly, most of the records have abstracts or content summaries from material published in over 49 countries. Using the *Thesaurus of Psychological Index Terms* of more than 8400 controlled terms and cross references, the nurse can search for specific concepts effectively. Key word and specific field searching are also available (American Psychological Association, 2014).

Social Sciences Citation Index. This database can be accessed via Web of Science for a fee. Web of Science includes a broad range of databases offering "multidisciplinary coverage from more than 12,000 high impact research journals worldwide" (Thomson Reuters, 2014). This particular index was developed by the Institute for Scientific Information and is a multi-disciplinary citation index which covers more than 3000 journals in the social, behavioral, and related sciences. The nurse can search the cited references as in the citation index in the CINAHL database.

Google Scholar. Google Scholar (GS) offers a version of the Google search engine with which most nurses are

familiar. In fact, approximately 67% of the more than 170 billion Internet searches each month are conducted using Google (Sullivan, 2013). Like PubMed, GS is free to access and use and links to some full text articles. It offers broad search capability across many disciplines and types of literature including articles from scholarly journals, theses, books, Web sites, and court opinions. This capability may be useful in an initial search on a topic to get an overview, but may not be precise enough for a specific search. Limited advance search capability is available but a searcher cannot limit to a specific resource type (e.g., research, clinical trial) or discipline. Good analytical and evaluative skills are essential (Badke, 2013). GS is not a replacement for the above-described academic databases but one to be used in conjunction with them. It may also be particularly useful for nurses who do not have easy access to a hospital or academic library where such databases are typically housed.

Of particular note when searching GS are the "Cited by" and "Related articles" options with each citation. It is possible to examine the development and direction of a concept, idea, or innovation by seeing citations of other authors referring to a given article. Authors can also easily find where their work has been cited.

A few other bibliographic retrieval systems to keep in mind are databases such as the database AgeLine (http://www.ebscohost.com/academic/ageline) owned by EBSCO; the Excerpta Medica database EMBASE (http://www.elsevier.com/online-tools/embase), the National Technical Information Service NTIS database (http://www.ntis.gov/); and the UMI Proquest Digital Dissertations (http://www.umi.com/en-US/products/dissertations/individuals.shtml).

Current Awareness Services

Most bibliographic retrieval systems are updated weekly or monthly. In addition to the delay between the writing and publishing of the material that is indexed in the database, there is also a delay between the receipt of material, the indexing, and finally the inclusion of the citations for the indexed material in the database. To obtain access to more current material than that available in a bibliographic database, the nurse should use a current awareness service.

Current awareness services are helpful when used in addition to bibliographic retrieval systems. These services provide access to tables of contents of journals and allow individuals to request articles of interest. They may include not only journal articles but also proceedings from conferences, workshops, symposia, and other meetings. Often, hospital or university librarians may provide these services as well. Unlike the bibliographic databases, where subject searching using controlled vocabulary is available, only key word searching for the subject, author, title, or journal is available in current awareness services or databases.

Some current awareness services or databases are Current Contents Connect, the in-process database for MEDLINE (formerly PREMEDLINE), and the PreCINAHL records on EBSCOHost. Current Contents Connect from Thomson Reuters (http://thomsonreuters.com/current-contents-connect/) provides a Web-friendly current awareness service to table of contents, abstracts, and bibliographic information from the most recently published scholarly journals as well as from more than 7000 relevant, evaluated Web sites (Current Contents Connect, 2014). PubMed's in-process records (formerly PREMED-LINE) provide basic information and abstracts before the citations are indexed and are found as part of a topic search.

The PreCINAHL records offered by Cinahl Information Systems, a division of EBSCO, publishers of the CINAHL database, are available on EBSCOHost and provide a method to access basic information, abstracts, and sometimes full text before the citations are formally indexed. The records are retrieved as part of a topic search. They can also be excluded from a topic search.

The second type of current awareness provided by Cinahl Information Systems is within the bibliographic database itself, where the searcher is able to choose from a group of 36 specific or special interest categories, which actually function as "virtual" databases. Possibilities include such areas as advanced nursing practice, case management, home healthcare, or military/uniformed services. By selecting one of these categories, documents are retrieved that are either in specific journals in the field or have been selected by indexers as being of interest to those in that field. The results can be limited by any of the available limits on the database, e.g., publication type such as research, journal subset such as blind peer reviewed, and presence of full text. A nurse with limited time can peruse the latest literature in one of these fields in this way (Fig. 48.5).

Review Services

Although the bibliographic retrieval systems and the current awareness services and databases act as filters to the ever-exploding volume of literature, sometimes the information retrieved needs to be evaluated to determine whether or not it is appropriate. For example, a monthly literature search might be done on a bibliographic and current awareness database and then a review service checked for commentaries on the sources retrieved. Supportive computerized

resources that synthesize the literature include the Joanna Briggs Institute for Best Practice (joannabriggs.org), Clinical Evidence (BMJ Publishing at http://clinical evidence.bmj.com/x/index.html), or the Cochrane Library Database of Systematic Reviews (http://www.cochrane.org/cochrane-reviews). Review services such as Doody's Review Service (http://www.doody.com/drs/) or reviews noted in bibliographic databases or review journals, such as *Evidence-Based Nursing, Evidence-Based Practice, Best Practice,* and *ACP Journal Club* can also be used to evaluate sources. Review services provide information to searchers about recently published books, journal articles, audiovisuals, and software. These reviews may also include ratings, opinions, or commentaries about the material.

Doody's Review Service is a service in which members develop a profile and a weekly bulletin is e-mailed describing books and software that meet the parameters of the profile. According to the Web site, the service currently contains over "130,000 book, eBook, and software titles in 140 specialties". The searcher can use author names, title, specialty, publisher, and key words to find books of interest. The results show price, ISBN, and publisher as well as a rating, when available. Materials are rated using a star system and a questionnaire that assesses the extent to which objectives are met and the appropriateness of the work's readability, among other criteria. The information presented allows serious consideration of the book along with information to assist in making choices.

It is well known that books are generally long in the development stage and are not as current as journal articles or documents on the World Wide Web; however, the *depth* of material presented in books must be considered. An in-depth discussion of *all* aspects of cardiac rehabilitation, for example, may be valuable in planning care and would probably not be included in a journal article where space is a consideration. Yet it would still be necessary for maintaining currency in the field.

Point-of-Care Resources

Point-of-care resources are resources that support patient care at the bedside. Lists of these resources are available from http://library.upstate.edu/evidence/pointofcare, and from http://nnlm.gov/training/nursing/sampler.html#evid.

Mosby's Nursing Suite. Mosby's Nursing Suite from Elsevier (www.confidenceconnected.com) includes Mosby's Nursing Consult, Mosby's Nursing Skills, and Mosby's Index (discussed earlier). Mosby's Nursing Consult provides information to help nurses with patient care. The database includes evidence-based nursing monographs, nursing

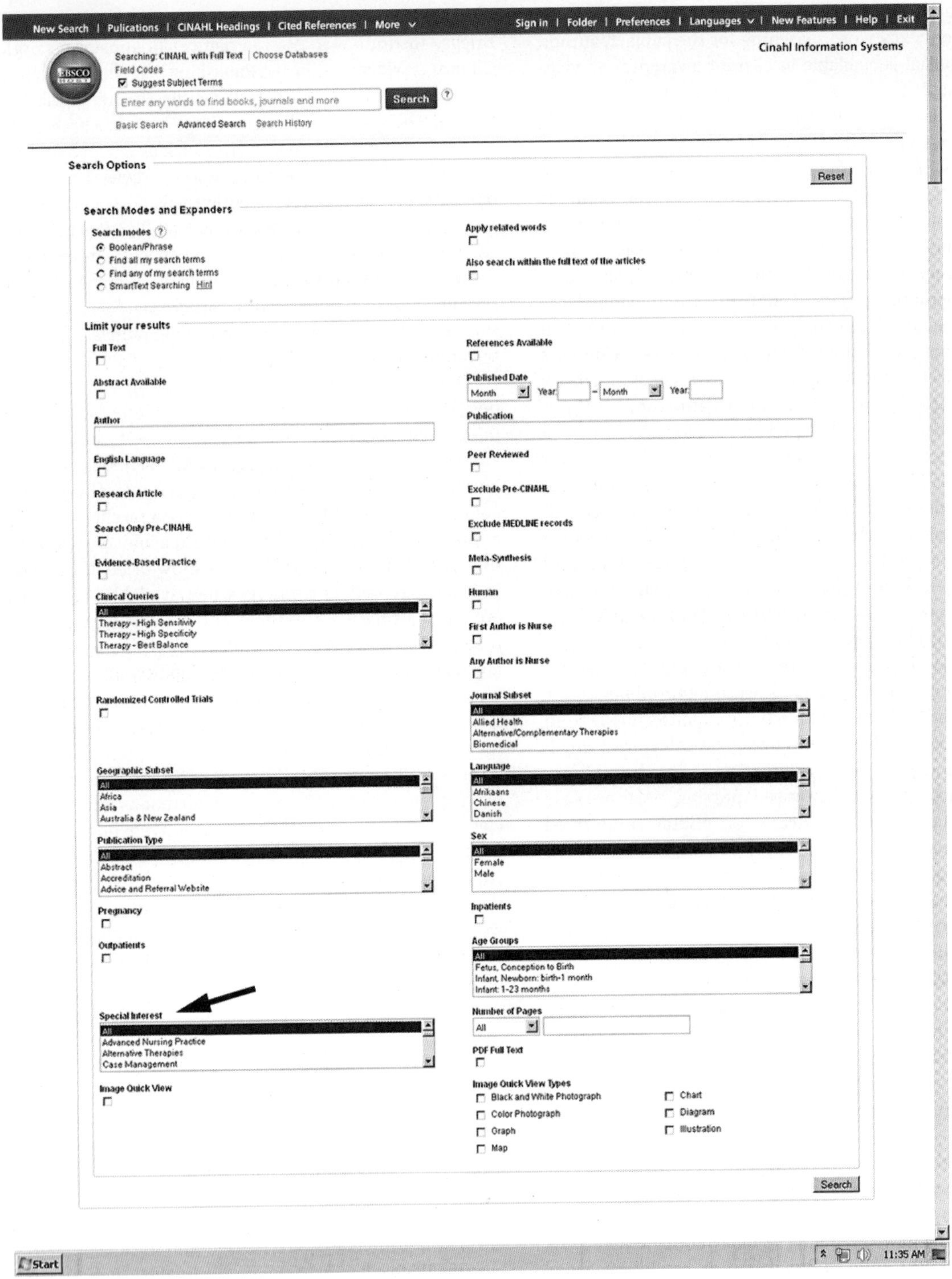

• **FIGURE 48.5.** Search for Special Interest Categories. (Reproduced with permission from EBSCO Information Services.)

journals and clinics, nursing and medical reference texts, practice guidelines, images, drug information, and several thousand customizable patient handouts. Mosby's Nursing Skills is an online skills reference and competency management resource from Elsevier. There are over 1300 nursing skills that use a learning management system (LMS) which allows nurse managers and educators to assign, track, and manage skills and test hospital staff (Elsevier, 2014).

Nursing Reference Center. Nursing Reference Center (NRC), published by EBSCO, is a point-of-care tool designed to provide relevant clinical resources to nurses and other healthcare professionals. The database offers staff nurses, nurse administrators, nursing students, nurse faculty, and hospital librarians the best available and most recent clinical evidence from thousands of full-text documents. Nursing Reference Center contains over 3600 Quick Lessons and Evidence-Based Care Sheets covering conditions and diseases, cultural competencies, patient education resources, drug information, continuing education, lab and diagnosis detail, legal cases, research instruments, and best practice guidelines. Quick Lessons are clinically organized nursing overviews of diseases and conditions. They represent the best available evidence and are designed to match the nursing work flow. They provide nurses with information the nurses need about diseases, including a description of the disease; its signs and symptoms; typical tests the clinician will order to diagnose it, or measure progress in treating it; the interventions nurses will likely be involved in while the patient is in their care; and information necessary to share with the patient/patient's family.

Evidence-Based Care Sheets provide evidence about aspects of a disease or a condition in terms of what we know about it and what we can do about it. The evidence is coded as to its strength so the user can evaluate it and determine its applicability to their practice.

In the database, there are nearly 1200 nursing skills and procedures, providing access to clinical papers detailing the necessary steps to achieve proficiency in a specific nursing task. Skill Competency Checklists are provided with these documents. Many papers are also available that define key considerations to providing culturally competent care to specific population groups.

Point-of-care reference books include *Davis's Comprehensive Handbook of Laboratory & Diagnostic Tests with Nursing Implications*; *Taber's Cyclopedic Medical Dictionary*; *Davis's Drug Guide for Nurses*; *AHFS Drug Essentials*; *Diseases and Disorders: A Nursing Therapeutics Manual*, and more.

There are more than 3600 evidence-based customizable patient handouts (English and Spanish) together with thousands of detailed medical illustrations. Nearly 1400 continuing education modules are also available. These modules are accredited through the American Nurses Credentialing Center (ANCC) and the International Association for Continuing Education and Training (IACET). Over 30 CE modules have been accredited by the Commission for Case Manager Certification.

Users can search NRC by entering keywords in the Find field and then clicking on the Search button. NRC will display a Result List that is sorted by source type—for example, Quick Lessons, Skills, Evidence-Based Care Sheets, Drugs, etc. Users can search the database using the standard nursing process ADPIE (assessment, diagnosis, planning, implementation, evaluation). Nursing process limiters are used to clarify a search in NRC. Users can select one or multiple nursing process limiters to rapidly target applicable content.

Users can launch a *CINAHL*-type search, and limit searches by document types, full-text, publication date, or source. They can also browse CINAHL headings or indexes and other EBSCOhost databases that may be subscribed to by the institution.

Users can store search results, persistent links to articles, images, saved searches, alerts, and Web pages to pull in the latest information needed on the floor and to create department-specific patient education packets.

A Nursing Reference Center "app" is available for the iPhone, iPad, and iPod Touch for nurses who wish to access it via those devices.

Supportive Computerized Resources

Supportive computerized resources that assist the nurse in maintaining currency provide additional information and enhance the value of the essential computerized resources described previously.

Obtaining a bibliographic list of citations is only the first step in obtaining information on a particular topic. After carefully evaluating the citations, either from the title and/or the abstracts, or after using one of the review processes described previously, the nurse will need to get the full text of the sources retrieved. Many articles are available in full text directly through the bibliographic databases searched. If not, a local library or academic institution would be a place to go to locate the items retrieved in a search.

Document Delivery Services. Publishers of journals or books, database vendors, and providers (NLM, American Psychological Association, Ovid Technologies, EBSCO, Proquest Information and Learning), and document delivery services are secondary sources through which full text of items can be obtained for a fee. Fees differ depending on the service, the urgency of the request, and the publisher's charges. Copy is usually sent via fax, mail, or electronic delivery. Many libraries provide document delivery for each other through services such as DocLine, an automated interlibrary loan (ILL) request routing and referral system provided through the National Library of Medicine.

Electronic Publishers. Many publications are now being published electronically, either as an "e-journal" only or as a print journal with electronic supplements. There are several advantages to this form of publication such as speed, ease of availability, and space required for publication. Searching for information in these journals is relatively easy. The *Morbidity and Mortality Weekly Report (MMWR)*, published by the Centers for Disease Control and Prevention, is one such electronic publication that can be subscribed to and provided by e-mail. The credibility and accuracy of the source of electronically published material must always be considered just as it is in print publications. The criteria mentioned along with additional criteria discussed later can be useful in evaluating this material. Two examples of electronic-only nursing journals are the *Online Journal of Issues in Nursing*, published by the American Nurses Association, and the *Online Journal of Nursing Informatics*, published in Pennsylvania. Other journals such as *Nursing Standard Online* have print counterparts but may have portions that are only electronic.

Nursing publishers and organizations have their own Web sites, which have details about new publications, sometimes full text of some of the latest journal articles, official position statements of organizations, and/or practice guidelines. To identify the Web sites of nursing publishers and organizations, search Web site indexes such as Yahoo! (www.yahoo.com) or Google (www.google.com), or browse Web site lists on Web sites such as that of the University of Buffalo Library (http://library.buffalo.edu) or the Allnurses.com site (http://allnurses.com) have been provided. On a Web site index such as Yahoo! or Google, do a general search for "nursing and publishers," "nursing and organizations," or "nursing and associations" or under the specific names of the publishers and organizations (e.g., Sage, Sigma Theta Tau). Advanced search options are also available.

Lippincott Williams & Wilkins (www.nursingcenter.com) has placed over 60 journals including the *AJN, American Journal of Nursing*; *Nursing Research*; *CIN: Computers, Informatics, Nursing*; and *JONA: Journal of Nursing Administration*, among others, on their journals page with issues from January 1996 to the present. The site has search capability that allows key word searching of the contents of the journals on the site. There are both free and fee-based articles available on the site.

Many nursing organizations provide a significant amount of support to practicing nurses. They publish journals and provide these as a member benefit. They also provide access to the full text of their position statements and/or practicing guidelines. Some of these resources are the American Nurses Association's Web site NursingWorld (www.nursingworld.org) and the Web sites of the American Academy of Nurse Practitioners (www.aanp.org), American College of Nurse Practitioners (www.acnp.enpnetwork.com), the Association of Pediatric Hematology/Oncology Nursing (www.aphon.org), and many others. Details regarding new publications and ordering items can be found on the Web sites of most publishers.

Meta-sites on the World Wide Web. Since there is so much information on the World Wide Web, identification and evaluation of Web sites is very important to determine which provide valid information. One of the ways to identify Web sites is to consult a meta-site. There are several Web sites that can be classified as meta-sites concerning the same specific topic. The Hardin Meta Directory of Internet Health Sources, sponsored by the Hardin Library for the Health Sciences at the University of Iowa (http://guides.lib.uiowa.edu/nursing), is one of these as is the National Information Center on Health Services Research & Healthcare Technology (NICHSR) (http://www.nlm.nih.gov/hsrinfo/index.html), a government site. These sites basically function as lists of lists that provide links to other subject-specific Web sites.

Once the Web sites have been identified, it is very important to evaluate them. At minimum, the nurse should consider the following: (1) Who created the site? (2) Is its purpose and intention clear? (3) Is the information accurate and current? (4) Is the site well designed and stable? (5) How frequently is it updated? Additionally, who sponsors or benefits from the site? Is there a fee involved? Is its foundation evidence based?

There are also Web sites that can be used to evaluate other Web sites. HON (Health on the Net Foundation) (www.hon.ch) is an international initiative funded by the various European entities to promote effective Internet development and use in the areas of medicine and health. Other Web sites that critically evaluate sites are National Council Against Health Fraud (www.ncahf.org), a voluntary health agency that focuses on health fraud, and Quack Watch (www.quackwatch.org), founded out of concern about health-related frauds, myths, and misconduct. Additionally, Web sites providing information or discussions concerning specific diseases should be evaluated in this way (e.g., the Web sites of the American Diabetes Association [www.diabetes.org], American Heart Association [www.heart.org], and the Multiple Sclerosis Foundation [www.msfacts.org]).

DEVELOPING AND MAINTAINING A LIST OF SOURCES FOR RESEARCH/PRACTICE/EDUCATION

Essential Computerized Resources

The purpose of the information retrieved from these information resources is to enable nurses to answer specific questions that relate to research, practice, and/or education. For example:

- A staff nurse needs to find information to share with her or his colleagues on oral care and the prevention of pneumonia.
- A nursing student has to finish a term paper and needs to find five nursing research studies on caring for a Hispanic patient with a myocardial infarction.
- A nurse manager needs to find research studies and anecdotal material showing the best way to prevent patient falls in her or his health facility.

Bibliographic Retrieval Systems. Resources essential in answering these types of questions again include bibliographic databases as well as various Web sites. Once again, the resources need to be carefully evaluated for coverage and currency. Once a resource has been selected, the nurse breaks down her or his needs into a search statement such as, "I need information on oral care and prevention of pneumonia." The information on this topic would best be found in a bibliographic database. On such a database, the best method of searching is to do a subject search using a controlled vocabulary (MeSH headings in MEDLINE, CINAHL subject headings in the CINAHL database, and so forth).

Search Strategies. One of the most important aspects of searching the literature is formulating the exact strategy to obtain the information from a resource, whether from a bibliographic retrieval system or a Web site. There are six steps in planning the search strategy.

1. Plan the search strategy ahead of time.
2. Break down the search topic into components. To find information on oral care and the prevention of pneumonia, remember to include synonyms or related terms. The components of the above search would be oral hygiene or mouth care and prevention of pneumonia. Sometimes the terms for the search will be subject headings in the database's subject heading list (often called a thesaurus); in other cases, they will not be (Fig. 48.6).
3. Check for terms in a subject heading list, if available. If the concept is new and there are no subject headings, a text word or key word search is necessary. For example, before the term *critical path* or *critical pathways* was added to the CINAHL or MeSH Subject Heading List, respectively, it was necessary to do a text word search for this concept. A search using the broad term *case management* would have retrieved many articles that would not necessarily discuss or include critical paths. Combining the two concepts results in a more specific result: articles on case management that include critical paths.
4. Select *operators*, which are words used to connect different or synonymous components of the search. The AND operator, for example, makes the search narrower or more specific as the results of the search for two different terms will only result in records that include *both* terms as subject headings (Fig. 48.7)

   The OR operator can be used to connect synonymous or related terms, which broadens the search (Fig. 48.8). An example combining subject headings using OR and AND operators is shown in Fig. 48.9.

   The NOT operator can be used to exclude terms (Fig. 48.10).
5. Run the search. For the search on oral care and pneumonia, select the option *explode* for the subject headings oral hygiene and mouth care. This would ensure the retrieval of articles on the broad heading and the more specific headings. For example, the specific headings under oral hygiene are "dental devices, home care" and "toothbrushing."
6. View the results.

Practice Guidelines and Position Statements. Organization-specific practice guidelines, position statements, and standards of practice can often be accessed and obtained from the Web site of an individual's professional organization. These are extremely useful documents that present information on scope of practice, qualifications, and education among other important details. Additionally, Cinahl Information Systems currently includes nurse practice acts as one of its publication types in the CINAHL database. These appear in full text and can be read online or printed.

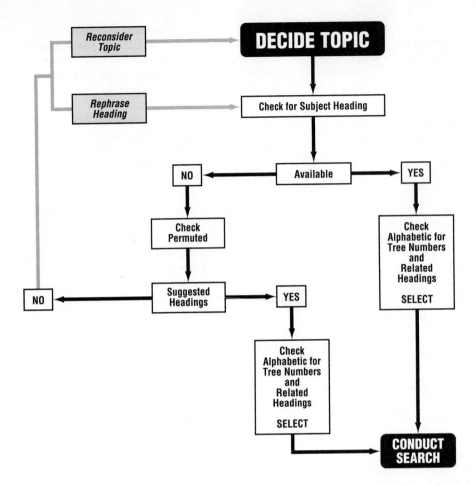

• **FIGURE 48.6.** Strategy for a Successful Literature Search. (Reproduced with permission from EBSCO Information Services.)

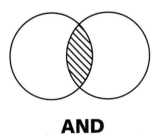

AND

Concept 1 "AND" Concept 2 = This means that only articles with both concept 1 and concept 2 are searched for.

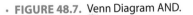

• **FIGURE 48.7.** Venn Diagram AND.

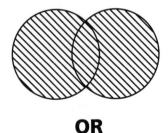

OR

Concept 1 "OR" Concept 2 = This means that articles with either concept 1 or concept 2 are searched for.

• **FIGURE 48.8.** Venn Diagram OR.

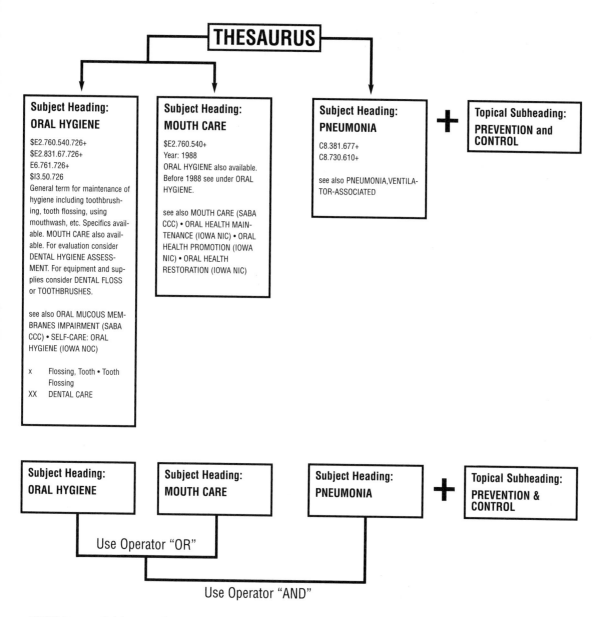

THESAURUS

Subject Heading:
ORAL HYGIENE

$E2.760.540.726+
$E2.831.67.726+
E6.761.726+
$I3.50.726
General term for maintenance of hygiene including toothbrushing, tooth flossing, using mouthwash, etc. Specifics available. MOUTH CARE also available. For evaluation consider DENTAL HYGIENE ASSESSMENT. For equipment and supplies consider DENTAL FLOSS or TOOTHBRUSHES.

see also ORAL MUCOUS MEMBRANES IMPAIRMENT (SABA CCC) • SELF-CARE: ORAL HYGIENE (IOWA NOC)

x   Flossing, Tooth • Tooth
     Flossing
XX   DENTAL CARE

Subject Heading:
MOUTH CARE

$E2.760.540+
Year: 1988
ORAL HYGIENE also available. Before 1988 see under ORAL HYGIENE.

see also MOUTH CARE (SABA CCC) • ORAL HEALTH MAINTENANCE (IOWA NIC) • ORAL HEALTH PROMOTION (IOWA NIC) • ORAL HEALTH RESTORATION (IOWA NIC)

Subject Heading:
PNEUMONIA

C8.381.677+
C8.730.610+

see also PNEUMONIA, VENTILATOR-ASSOCIATED

+

Topical Subheading:
PREVENTION and CONTROL

Subject Heading:
ORAL HYGIENE

Subject Heading:
MOUTH CARE

Subject Heading:
PNEUMONIA

+

Topical Subheading:
PREVENTION & CONTROL

Use Operator "OR"

Use Operator "AND"

• **FIGURE 48.9.** Subject Headings Using OR and AND Operators. (Reproduced with permission from EBSCO Information Services.)

Continuing Education and Computer-Assisted Learning. Many nurses do not have the time or money to attend conferences and workshops to keep abreast of the latest information in their specialties or to complete the necessary units or credits for continuing education (CE) for relicensure or recertification. The World Wide Web is a wonderful source for nurses that can be used to satisfy

their requirements for CE. To identify CE Web sites visit the Nursefriendly National Consumer Health Directories (http://www.nursefriendly.com/ceu/), or use one of several search engines, Google at www.google.com, Yahoo! at www.yahoo.com, or Ask at www.ask.com to obtain CE nursing sites. There are many nursing sites or point-of-care resources that offer online CE and CEU certificates, such

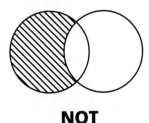

NOT

Concept 1 "NOT" Concept 2 = This means that articles with concept 1 that do not include concept 2 are searched for.

• FIGURE 48.10. Venn Diagram NOT.

as Nursing Reference Center through EBSCO, RnCeus.com, and the CE Connection at Lippincott Williams & Wilkins site at http://www.nursingcenter.com/lnc/CEConnection. A directory of free online continuing education opportunities for nurses can be found at nurseCEU.com.

As mentioned at the beginning of this chapter, nurses use computers for many purposes. Computer-assisted instruction (CAI), computer-assisted learning (CAL), and interactive videodisc (IVD) provide easy learning experiences using a computer.

Supportive Computerized Resources

Supportive computerized resources that assist in practice, research, and education contain all types of health information including drug and treatment information, anatomy, and physiology. Specific products such as the *Merck Manual of Diagnosis and Therapy* (www.merck.com) or the *Physician's Desk Reference* available as *PDRhealth* (http://www.pdrhealth.com/drugs) are also available on the World Wide Web. The Visible Human Project (www.nlm.nih.gov/research/visible/) includes complete, anatomically detailed, three-dimensional representations of the male and female human bodies. The National Library of Medicine itself claims to be the "largest health science library in the world."

Other Web sites of particular interest in this category include the Nursing Theory Page (http://www.sandiego.edu/nursing/research/nursing_theory_research.php) and the Virginia Henderson Global Nursing e-Repository (http://www.nursinglibrary.org/vhl/pages/aboutus.html) as well as the Interagency Council on Information Resources in Nursing (ICIRN) (http://icirn.org). ICIRN prepares a list of "Essential Nursing Resources" which are available online only at www.icirn.org.

COLLABORATION AND NETWORKING REGARDING ISSUES OF PROFESSIONAL PRACTICE

Nurses frequently gather information from their personal networks—either at the worksite or at professional meetings. The increased availability of computers makes contact with other professionals much easier, resulting in networking and collaboration possibilities heretofore impossible. Information retrieved by this method enables nurses to learn from their colleagues' experiences. When considering with whom to network, the specialty of the person should be evaluated along with experience, the material they have published in their field, and the research undertaken by the institution with which they are affiliated. Most of this information is not published and would be unavailable through traditional information resources.

Computerized resources for collaboration and networking vary in several technical details (e.g., their focus, the presence or absence of a moderator to monitor messages, the number of participants, and their level of interactivity).

Essential Computerized Resources

Electronic Mail and Listservs. An important fundamental computerized resource for collaboration and networking is e-mail, which is at the core of almost any electronic communication. Necessary components for e-mail are access to Internet services (often provided by cable television and local telephone companies) and e-mail viewing software, such as Internet Explorer or Firefox. E-mail allows one-to-one communication between individuals and can provide immediate response to practice-related questions.

A second essential computerized resource for collaboration is an electronic discussion group or "listserv." Listservs allow individuals to subscribe free of charge and to read and respond to messages via e-mail. Since the messages are posted to all of the members, the listserv allows sharing and dissemination of information with colleagues. Some listservs have a closed membership for a specific group (e.g., librarians or specific nursing groups), and some are moderated. In a moderated group, an individual or group of individuals reads the messages prior to distribution to the group. Subject-specific listservs include NURSENET (general nursing), Nursing-L (nursing informatics), NRSED (education issues/faculty), and NurseRes (research). Specialty listservs are very helpful in increasing dialog between individuals within the same specialty.

Supportive Computerized Resources

Electronic Bulletin Boards, Forums, Newsgroups, Blogs, Chat Rooms, and Social Networking Sites. Bulletin boards, forums, newsgroups, and chat rooms are examples of supportive computerized resources. Similar to a traditional bulletin board, the electronic version has an administrator who sends the discussion to various Web sites, where nurses visit to read and participate in the discussion. This format for electronic networking has almost entirely been replaced by forums and newsgroups, which have become more and more sophisticated in their interactivity and design. The premise behind each of them is similar. An individual posts a message concerning a topic (known as a thread) for others to read and respond to. Allnurses.com has a "Break Room," a general topic area in which nurses are invited to discuss anything of particular interest to them. Newsgroups operate in much the same way. Nursezone.com is an online news magazine that offers blogs, a job center, and various nurse-related information. All of these resources are interactive but on a delayed basis. An individual may respond to a message immediately or wait several days. Chat rooms, on the other hand, are interactive in real time. Conversations in chat rooms can be compared to telephone conversations. "Nursing Chat Room" in Linkedin is an example focused especially on psychiatric nursing.

Each of these methods of collaboration and networking provides an option for nurses to contact and build relationships with other professionals concerning issues important to them. Newer social networking sites such as Linkedin, Facebook, and Twitter offer great potential for sharing experiences and ideas about practice issues. Using features of Smartphones such as texting also enhance communication opportunities.

All of the above sites offer end users the ability to disseminate information about practice and/or products that they have found useful. By "liking" a particular site, an end-user can be included in any notifications about new information on that site. For example, a commercial entity that produces an insulin pump can create a Facebook account, post information about its operations or products, and promote itself to other account holders.

SUMMARY

While these three categories of information needs have been discussed as if they were independent of one another, a nurse might often find that she or he has needs that transcend all three categories or that fall under a different category each time, depending on the task. For example, a staff nurse may need to investigate the best methods to assess and manage pain. The process of retrieving appropriate information would be to first search for research studies and anecdotal material on the topic of pain measurement and pain management. This would involve a search for pain measurement or pain with therapy, drug therapy, and diagnosis using essential computerized resources such as bibliographic retrieval systems like MEDLINE or the CINAHL database. The nurse would also consult a point-of-care tool such as Mosby's Nursing Consult or Nursing Reference Center to locate the latest evidence on a particular patient care topic.

Networking with other professionals facing the same task would be an additional step in this process. The nursing listservs mentioned under the "Collaboration and Networking Regarding Issues of Professional Practice" section would be an important and essential resource, while e-mailing or texting colleagues who are specialists in the field of pain would be a supportive resource. To locate specialists, a bibliographic retrieval system could be searched for research studies on pain measurement or management. The author affiliation field in the records retrieved would help track the institution with which the author is affiliated. Social networking sites can be useful in identifying and reviewing specialists in a given area of practice.

Making sure to keep current on any new material published on pain measurement and pain management, by using current awareness services or Web sites, would also be vital in locating information on this topic. Bibliographic retrieval systems, already used as an essential resource, could be searched each month to assess what new material had been published on the topic. Supportive computerized resources might include a similar search for papers on the Cochrane Library's Database of Systematic Reviews.

An important part of identifying and using these essential and supportive computerized resources is the evaluation of each of them to assess whether or not they contain the information needed. Therefore, the nurse must determine what she or he is looking for, identify the most appropriate resources to locate the information needed, and, using the criteria discussed throughout this chapter, evaluate the resources to assess if they are valid, current, and accurate.

Finally, it is important to realize that computerized information resources are like a "moving target," in that technology is changing so quickly that resources used today may be gone, unavailable, or outdated tomorrow. The use of bibliographic retrieval systems, search engines, and meta-sites encourages searching by *subject* or *concept*, which is the most reliable way to cope with the ever-changing nature of technology. This is vital to maintaining currency with the published literature, developing and maintaining a list of sources of topics of interest for practice, research, and/or education, and collaboration and networking with colleagues regarding issues of professional practice.

REFERENCES

American Library Association. (1989). *Presidential Committee on Information Literacy: Final report.* Retrieved from http://www.ala.org/ala/mgrps/divs/acrl/publications/whitepapers/presidential.cfm

American Nurses Association. (2008). *Nursing informatics: Scope and standards of practice.* Silver Spring, MD: Nursebooks.org.

American Psychological Association. (2014). *PsychInfo.* Retrieved from http://www.apa.org/pubs/databases/psycinfo/index.aspx

Association of College and Research Libraries of the American Library Association. (2000). *Information literacy competency standards for higher education.* Retrieved from http://www.ala.org/acrl/standards/informationliteracycompetency

Badke, W. (2013). Coming back to Google Scholar. *Online Searcher, 37,* 65–67.

Boden, C., Neilson, C. J., & Seaton, J. X. (2013). Efficacy of screen-capture tutorials in literature search training: A pilot study of a research method. *Medical Reference Services Quarterly, 32,* 314–327. doi:10.1080/02763869.2013.806863.

Clapp, M. J., Johnson, M., Schwieder, D., & Craig, C. L. (2013). Innovation in the Academy: creating an online information literacy course. *Journal of Library & Information Services in Distance Learning, 7,* 247–263. doi:10.1080/1533290X.2013.805663.

Current Contents Connect. (2014). *Description.* Retrieved from http://thomsonreuters.com/current-contents-connect/.

EBSCO Information Services. (2014). *The CINAHL database.* Retrieved from http://www.ebscohost.com/biomedical-libraries/the-cinahl-database

Educational Resources Information Center. (2013). *About the ERIC program.* Retrieved from http://www2.ed.gov/programs/eric/index.html

Elsevier, B. V. (2014). *Mosby's Suite—Mosby's Index.* Retrieved from http://confidenceconnected.com/

Majid, S., Foo, S., Luyt, B., Zhang, X., Theng, Y-L., & Mokhtar, I. A. (2011). Adopting evidence-based practice in clinical decision making: Nurses' perceptions, knowledge, and barriers. *Journal of the Medical Library Association, 99,* 229–236. doi:10.3163/1536-5050.99.3.010.

Marshall, A. P., West, S. H., & Aitken, L. M. (2011). Preferred information sources for clinical decision making: Critical care nurses' perceptions of information accessibility and usefulness. *Worldviews on Evidence-Based Nursing, 8,* 224–235. doi:10.1111/j.1741-6787.2011.00221.x.

Melnyk, B. M., Fineout-Overholt, E., Gallagher-Ford, L., & Kaplan, L. (2012). The state of evidence-based practice in US nurses: Critical implications for nurse leaders and educators. *Journal of Nursing Administration, 42,* 410–417. doi:10.1097/NNA.0b013e3182664e0a.

Moreton, E. (2013). Embedding information literacy into evidence-based practice. *Nursing and Allied Health Resources Section (NAHRS) Newsletter, 33*(2), 5–6.

O'Leary, D. F., & Mhaolrunaigh, S. N. (2011). Information-seeking behaviour of nurses: Where is information sought and what processes are followed? *Journal of Advanced Nursing, 68,* 379–390. doi:10.1111/j.1365-2648.2011.05750.x.

Powell, C. A., & Ginier, E. C. (2013). Lessons learned: Year-by-year improvement of a required information competency course. *Medical Reference Services Quarterly, 32,* 290–313. doi:10.1080/02763869.2013.806862.

Pravikoff, D. S., Pierce, S. T., & Tanner, A. B. (2005). Readiness of U.S. nurses for evidence-based practice. *American Journal of Nursing, 105*(9), 40–52.

Ross, J. (2010). Information literacy for evidence-based practice in perianesthesia nurses: Readiness for evidence-based practice. *Journal of PeriAnesthesia Nursing, 25*(2), 64–70. doi:10.1016/j.jopan.2010.01.007.

Stombaugh, A., Sperstad, R., Van Wormer, A., Jennings, E., Kishel, H., & Vogh, B. (2013). Using lesson study to integrate information literacy throughout the curriculum. *Nurse Educator, 38,* 173–177. doi:10.1097/NNE.0b013e318296db56.

Sullivan, D. (2013). *Google still world's most popular search engine by far, but share of unique searchers dips slightly.* Retrieved from http://searchengineland.com/google-worlds-most-popular-search-engine-148089

Thomson Reuters. (2014). *Social sciences citation index.* Retrieved from http://thomsonreuters.com/social-sciences-citation-index

U.S. National Library of Medicine. (2013a). *Databases, resources & APIs.* Retrieved from http://wwwcf2.nlm.nih.gov/nlm_eresources/eresources/search_database.cfm

U.S. National Library of Medicine. (2013b). *Number of titles currently indexed for Index Medicus® and MEDLINE® on PubMed®.* Retrieved from http://www.nlm.nih.gov/bsd/num_titles.html

Yadav, B. L., & Fealy, G. M. (2012). Irish psychiatric nurses' self-reported barriers, facilitators and skills for developing evidence-based practice. *Journal of Psychiatric & Mental Health Nursing, 19,* 116–122. doi:10.1111/j.1365-2850.2011.01763.x.

PART 9

Big Data Initiatives

Kathleen A. McCormick

49

Genomics and Information Technology for Personalized Health

Kathleen A. McCormick / Kathleen A. Calzone

• OBJECTIVES

1. Explain the basics and current status of genetic and genomics in healthcare so as to understand the continuum of care areas where genomics and Information Technology (IT) are known to facilitate risk identification, diagnosis, and establish prognosis and symptom management.
2. Define why genetics and genomics require Big Data Analysis and how it relates to Personalized Health.
3. Describe the implications for genetic and genomic information for nursing informatics.
4. Identify toolkits that are available in learning about genomics and applying bioinformatics in clinical practice.
5. Understand the ethical, legal, social issues (ELSI), and HHS regulations.
6. Identify genetic and genomic resources that are available for nurses.
7. Summarize The Blueprint for Nursing Research in Genomic Applications.

• KEY WORDS

Genome sequencing
Genetics
Genomics
Comparative genomics
Understanding genome function
Bioinformatics
Big Data and analytics
Human genome and human disease
Nursing applications in genomics
Genomic ethical, legal, and social issues
Translational bioinformatics
Educational competencies

INTRODUCTION

This is an extraordinary time in healthcare, where genomic discoveries are rapidly being translated into practice to improve health outcomes. In fact, progress over the last few years has resulted in a transition from genetics, the study of single gene variations into genomics which encompasses all genetic variation coupled with other influences such as the environment and personal factors (Green, Guyer, & National Human Genome Research Institute, 2011; Guttmacher & Collins, 2002). Genomics changes the healthcare implications from what was predominately specialty care associated with rare Mendelian disorders such as Huntington's disease (genetics) into the use of genomic information and technologies as part of the healthcare for common complex conditions such as cancer, heart disease, and diabetes (genomics).

The rapidity in which genomic information is becoming clinically relevant is directly correlated to the reduction in costs of genomic technologies. Within reach is the capacity to perform whole genome sequencing on an individual for $1000 or less, considered within range of other healthcare expenses facilitating clinical use (Calzone, 2013). In fact, as of April 2013, the cost for whole genome sequencing had fallen to below $6000, a cost reduction of more than $10,000 in just two years (Wetterstrand, 2014). Not surprisingly, the capacity to effectively study, store, utilize, and track the rapidly evolving genomic information evidence base is not just a function of preparing the healthcare workforce in the science of genomics, but relies heavily on the design and implementation of the informatics infrastructure needed to support clinical genomic research and translation (McCarthy, McLeod, & Ginsburg, 2013).

The interface between genomics and informatics is extensive and extends into areas beyond traditional discovery and building the evidence base for analytic validity, clinical validity, and clinical utility of genomic information. For genomic healthcare applications to achieve their optimal benefit, informatics becomes essential to facilitate effective translation into practice such as evidence curation, point-of-care provider decision support, electronic health record capacity for data storage and retrieval when indicated, and the ability to establish and track quality metrics on genome technologies and the impact of genomics on health outcomes (Ginsburg, Staples, & Abernethy, 2011; McCarthy et al., 2013). The genomic technology cost reduction and resulting expansion of genomic clinical applications have resulted in a new visioning in the informatics community. This has resulted in an interface between bio-informatics and clinical informatics termed bio-medical informatics, an essential component of genomic translation (Overby & Tarczy-Hornoch, 2013).

The importance of this interface is also highlighted in the draft Second Edition of the *Nursing Informatics: Scope and Standards of Practice*, which has included an entire section on genetics and genomics (American Nurses Association Nursing Informatics Scope and Standards Revision Workgroup, 2014). This chapter will provide an update on the intersection between genomics, informatics and translation of genomics from research into practice.

INTERFACE OF GENOMICS IN THE HEALTHCARE CONTINUUM

While oncology has the largest scope of genomic healthcare applications, routine common health conditions are also benefiting from the use of genomic information. Indeed, genomics influences the entire healthcare continuum (Fig. 49.1) beginning before birth through end of life.

Preconception and Prenatal

The preconception and prenatal period has an established platform for genomic applications in clinical care. The American College of Obstetricians and Gynecologists, the American College of Medical Genetics and Genomics, as well as others maintain a series of clinical practice guidelines which cover preconception/prenatal genetic

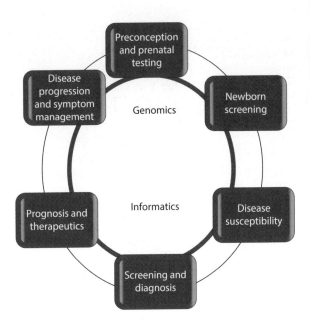

· **FIGURE 49.1.** Genomic Influences on the Healthcare Continuum. (Adapted from Calzone K.A. et al. [2013]).

care (The American College of Medical Genetics and Genomics, 2014; The American College of Obstetricians and Gynecologists, 2014). Family history assessment is a critical element for identification of conditions for which clinical practice guidelines exist which may include referral to a genetic specialist and/or further evaluation possibly including genetic testing (Lin et al., 2013). These can include conditions which can impact the health of the mother, for example, thrombophilia; the outcome of the pregnancy, for example, recurrent pregnancy loss or preterm birth; or conditions that can affect the fetus such as cystic fibrosis, or neural tube defects (Lin et al., 2013). Even in the absence of a prior history in the family of a given health condition, other indications for referral to genetics that may include genetic testing exist. These include advanced maternal age where, for example, the risk for fetal chromosomal abnormalities can be increased as well as parents of specific ethnic backgrounds who are at risk for diseases that are more prevalent in that ethnic group, for example, Tay-Sachs and Ashkenazi Jewish heritage (Lin et al., 2013).

Newborn Screening

Newborn screening (NBS) represents one of the largest public health applications of genomic information. A dried blood spot obtained from a heel prick of a newborn is used to perform analyses that can help identify conditions in which early diagnosis could improve outcomes and the harms of population-based screening are outweighed by the benefits (DeLuca, Zanni, Bonhomme, & Kemper, 2013). The Discretionary Advisory Committee on Heritable Disorders in Newborns and Children (DACHDNC) provides national guidance about which health conditions should be included as part of NBS (U.S. Department of Health and Human Services, 2013). This committee was previously known as the Secretary's Advisory Committee on Heritable Disorders in Newborns and Children. The committee considers several factors in making recommendations as to what disorders should be screened for. These include evidence that screening in the newborn improves health outcomes; screening will cause minimal harm to those unaffected; and the feasibility and readiness of states to implement the screening (Kemper et al., 2013). Currently the Uniform Screening Panel for NBS includes 31 core disorders and 26 secondary disorders (U.S. Department of Health and Human Services, 2013). However, NBS varies across states as individual states can choose which conditions from the Uniform Screening Panel to include and states can also opt to include conditions not recommended as part of the Uniform Screening Panel. For most of the conditions included in the NBS

Uniform Screening Panel, abnormal results do not constitute a definitive diagnosis of a condition but serve as a screening tool that requires additional evaluation of the newborn. As such, NBS can produce false positives, false negatives, and ambiguous results.

In general, NBS is mandatory in most states with specific consent or opt out policies defined by the state (Blout et al., 2014). Dried blood spot cards are kept for a minimum of two years but beyond that states can opt to retain the specimens for longer. Retained specimens are being used for quality control purposes, refinement and development of new tests, as well as public health and research purposes (Benkendorf, Goodspeed, & Watson, 2010). Consent for future use of the dried blood spot also varies by state, with not all states requiring consent for future use (Therrell et al., 2011). The National Society of Genetic Counselors (Blout) recently published their position that parents should be educated and informed about the scope of NBS by a qualified healthcare provider and informed about retention of specimens for future use (Blout et al., 2014).

Next steps aimed at expanding and improving NBS include the consideration of next generation genome technologies such as whole genome or exome sequencing. In September 2013, the National Human Genome Research Institute funded several institutions to explore the use of next generation sequencing in the newborn. The ethical, legal, and social issues (ELSI) surrounding the use of these technologies in the newborn is a component of each study funded. The challenges that will be evaluated as part of these studies include management of potential findings, the changing evidence base of genetic variations identified, tracking genetic variations that may not have immediate health implications, the management of incidental findings, and the interface between the public health and clinical care services (National Human Genome Research Institute, E. K. S. N. I. o. C. H. a. H. D., 2013).

Disease Susceptibility

The evidence associated with the genetic basis of an inherited susceptibility to disease has continued to expand with an escalating number of commercially available genetic tests with established analytic validity, clinical validity, and clinical utility. Genetic testing for mutations in genes associated with inherited cancer susceptibility is well established with more than 55 cancer syndromes identified to date (Lindor, McMaster, Lindor, & Greene, 2008). However, genetic testing for disease susceptibility is increasingly occurring in other common complex conditions such as heart disease (Wung, Hickey, Taylor, & Gallek, 2013).

The identification of a germline susceptibility gene mutation is relevant both to individuals diagnosed with a given health condition whose management may be altered as a result of this information, as well as for individuals with no evidence of disease who could benefit from mutation-specific risk management to reduce risk or identify disease early. Additionally, once the genetic basis for a disease is established in a family, based on the gene mutations established Mendelian pattern of transmission, who else in the family is also at risk and should be tested can be readily identified.

Evidence-based guidelines are available to guide when these tests should be considered. Family history remains a cornerstone of guidelines for consideration of germline genetic testing where early onset disease and multiple affected family members can often be detected (Berg et al., 2009). As evidence about inherited susceptibility to disease accumulates, other indicators for testing have emerged such as tumor features (de la Cruz et al., 2012; Hampel & de la Chapelle, 2013; Hampel et al., 2008).

Developments in the risk assessment arm of the healthcare continuum include the transition into multiplex testing, which involves testing for mutations in multiple genes in one comprehensive test. This remains controversial given the complexity of the genetic counseling and the interpretation and management decisions based on the findings (Domchek, Bradbury, Garber, Offit, & Robson, 2013). However, this is the first step toward a future that involves whole genome or exome analysis that will ultimately become less expensive than single gene or multiple gene testing (Wetterstrand, 2014).

Screening and Diagnosis

Genetic information, which may include a genetic test, has long been used to establish and/or confirm a diagnosis of a genetic condition, which can inform therapeutic decision-making. However, expansion of the use of genomic information in the screening and diagnostic arena continue to emerge. An example includes efforts to further increase the specificity of risk calculation models by integrating genomic information such as single nucleotide polymorphisms (SNP), a common type of genetic variation. SNPs, single DNA base pair changes, can impact risk for diseases as well as metabolism of medications (National Human Genome Research Institute, 2012). SNPs are common in the general population so the number of people impacted can be significant. However, most SNPs result in risk elevation only slightly above that of the general population (i.e., OR <1.5) (Ku, Loy, Pawitan, & Chia, 2010). Integrating one or more SNPs into established risk prediction models such as the Breast Cancer Risk Assessment Tool

(http://www.cancer.gov/bcrisktool/) have been studied to determine if the accuracy of the calculation can be increased (Wacholder et al., 2010). However, thus far this work has not achieved evidence of clinical utility. Nonetheless, improving the discriminatory accuracy of established disease risk assessment models as well as developing new risk models using genomic information are important aims and SNP selections as well as large sample sizes for study are critical factors (Wu, Pfeiffer, & Gail, 2013).

The inclusion of genomic information in screening and/or diagnostic tests has also been gaining momentum. Some of the focus has been on the development of screening and/or diagnostic tests which are sensitive, specific, and less invasive than standard screening tests using molecular markers collected from blood, urine, or stool (Ahlquist, 2010). Screening for colorectal cancer has been one area of considerable study in part given the challenges associated with adherence to screening colonoscopy in the general population. As technology has advanced, the sensitivity and specificity of this kind of colon screening has progressed to the point where a stool DNA test has been found to detect cancer as well as precursor adenomas with high rates of sensitivity (Berger & Ahlquist, 2012). Larger studies are already underway to evaluate the feasibility, sensitivity, and specificity of this type of test in a screening environment, a necessary step on the pathway to new colorectal screening options (Berger & Ahlquist, 2012).

Prognosis and Therapeutics

There are many ways in which genomics is being used to inform prognosis and therapeutics. This is perhaps best illustrated looking at the role of cancer tumor genomic profiling in cancer care. Genetic variation is at the heart of cancer, a disease in which genetic changes are directly associated with the disease. These changes can vary based on disease as well as type of genetic change (i.e., Copy number changes, mutations, chromosomal translocation) (McDermott, Downing, & Stratton, 2011). Understanding the scope of genetic variation in cancer is informing prognosis, therapeutic decision-making, as well as therapeutic targets. Several large-scale tumor initiatives have helped inform this field such as The Cancer Genome Atlas (TCGA) that involves in part genomic characterization of specific tumor types; therapeutically applicable research to generate effective treatments (target) which is a similar effort focused on childhood malignancies, and most recently the pan-cancer project which builds on TCGA with further study and analysis of tumor genomes (Cancer Genome Atlas Research Network, 2013; The Cancer Genome Atlas, 2014; Therapeutically Applicable Research to Generate Effective Treatments, 2014).

The elucidation of the cancer tumor genome has several clinically relevant applications; some of which have already been translated into practice. First, some inherited cancer syndromes confer cancers, which have distinct tumor phenotypes. Lynch syndrome which is associated with colon, endometrial, ovarian, as well as other cancers is associated with germline mismatch repair gene mutations resulting in evidence of microsatellite instability in colon and endometrial tumors (Hampel et al., 2006). There are many limitations of family history for instance provider time and capacity to complete and analyze the history; missing information; and small uninformative families. Additionally, the reliance on traditional family history indicators for consideration of genetic testing may not fully reflect the full spectrum of patients with inherited gene mutations. Therefore, tumor features consistent with a given cancer syndrome, in this case evidence of microsatellite instability, provide a mechanism for identifying patients who would be candidates for further evaluation by genetic specialists (Hampel & de la Chapelle, 2013).

Tumor gene expression profiling for different cancers including common malignancies such as breast, colon, and lymphoma have helped identify prognostic sub-types that extend beyond traditional pathologic and staging criteria which then impacts therapeutic decision-making (McDermott et al., 2011). One very significant use of tumor specific information is the identification of novel therapeutic targets, which serve as the platform for the development of new targeted treatments. This is perhaps one of the most remarkable areas of growth in cancer care in the past decade with the development of multiple agents for a variety of tumor types (i.e., Lung cancer, breast cancer, chronic myeloid leukemia) targeting a vast array of genetic variations (Arteaga & Baselga, 2012; McDermott et al., 2011).

Pharmacogenomics

Another area of progress in therapeutics is pharmacogenomics. Progress in the genomics of drug metabolism including pharmacodynamics, pharmacokinetics, efficacy, and the illumination of pathway/drug-specific inducers and inhibitors is rapidly progressing. Consider that many people will at some point in their life be prescribed a medication whose dose, inhibitors, and/or inducers already are or may be in the future optimized based on genomic information. Pharmacogenomic applications already in practice encompass common health conditions including drugs treating cardiovascular disease, cancer, and infectious diseases (Wang, McLeod, & Weinshilboum, 2011). Currently, the U.S. Food and Drug Administration (FDA) has more than 150 medications that have pharmacogenomic

biomarkers included in the drug label (U.S. Food and Drug Administration, 2013).

Inhibitors and inducers based on the pharmacogenomics of a drug are also critical and extend the agents potential contraindications. Inhibitors decrease or inactivate a specific metabolizing enzyme while inducers do the opposite, increase the enzyme. Both effects can alter drug metabolism, response, and potential adverse effects (Ma, Lee, & Kuo, 2012).

Disease Progression and Symptom Management

Monitoring for cancer disease progression is a novel and expanding area of genomic application. In the hematologic malignancies, assays have been developed to measure specific genetic variations that can be indicative of therapy response, resistance, or disease progression (McDermott et al., 2011). Research is ongoing evaluating how similar strategies could be applied to the monitoring of patients with solid tumors (McDermott et al., 2011).

Pharmacogenomics has implications in more than one arm of the healthcare continuum. In this aspect, the area of symptom management is a primary application, use of drugs to manage/treat symptoms of a health condition (i.e., pain control), and the same concepts described above are relevant in terms of efficacy and drug metabolism. Similarly, the concurrent use of over-the-counter medications or prescribed medications may serve as inhibitors or inducers of a primary prescribed agent to treat a condition. A good example to illustrate this importance of this is the over-the-counter herbal supplement St. John's wort used to treat depression, which induces *CYP3A4* (Goey, Mooiman, Beijnen, Schellens, & Meijerman, 2013). *CYP3A4* is part of a large family of cytochrome P450 enzymes involved in drug metabolism. *CYP3A4* is involved in the metabolism of a number of cancer therapeutics, for example, the taxanes (Krens, McLeod, & Hertz, 2013).

INFORMATICS, GENOMICS, AND THE HEALTHCARE CONTINUUM

To realize the benefits of genomics to healthcare outcomes, genomic information has to be effectively translated into practice. Some of the major challenges associated with the translation of genomics into practice include the availability of clinical practice guidelines which necessitate data derived from large studies; the limited healthcare workforce genomic knowledgebase which will require novel strategies for education given the current fiscal climate; and the infrastructure needed to integrate genomics into healthcare delivery systems such as the electronic health record (EHR), and point-of-care decision support (McCarthy et al., 2013). At the cusp of the $1000 genome, managing the breadth of genomic health information that will continue to evolve over time is a remarkable undertaking, yet it has the opportunity to truly improve and personalize healthcare. Informatics plays a vital role in every phase of the application of genomics to the healthcare continuum and as such emerges as the keystone of effective genomic clinical translation.

WHY GENETICS AND GENOMICS REQUIRE BIG DATA ANALYSIS

Since the last chapter was written in Essentials of Informatics, Version 5, the concepts of genomics and bioinformatics have meshed with the concept of Big Data. That is because when one adds genomics to the phenotype data of the electronic health record, and adds additional information from laboratory data and tissue repositories, one has petabytes of data for patients with a specific health condition. Big Data is also considered in need of architecture and platforms that support the insurance industry and pharmaceutical agent development. This chapter will describe the new concepts in Big Data for personalized health and genomic data.

For genomic data to be used in personalized health, molecular pathways involved in disease susceptibility, disease manifestation, and/or progression can be activated by genomic changes described above. For example, in cancer, several major tumors have multiple genomic alterations that lead to abnormal proliferation or survival of cells. In order to target the abnormal tissue exactly, pharmaceutical agents are matched to the correct genomic pathway of cell proliferation or survival that has become abnormal.

The technologies used to find out what pathway is abnormal in the genomic profile have been previously described (Quackenbush, 2002). The human genome is 3 gigabytes and a laboratory might produce 40 gigabytes of data per day and the technologies for sequencing are producing in any research or laboratory environment about 300 gigabytes per eight days (Garraway, 2012).

Needs of the Infrastructure to Support Personalized Care

Because of the volume of genomic information and clinical data within an Electronic Health Record (EHR) and/or Clinical Trials Databases, a blueprint for informatics has been proposed by the Data and Informatics Working Group (DIWG) to the Director, NIH, to support personalized healthcare (DIWG Report, 2012). Included in the blueprint are facilities to store data that not only facilitates research and outcomes, but also includes the documentation of the clinical care and potential safety issues. First, the systems need to facilitate cross-generational sharing of genomic data from family and laboratory data. Secondly, the systems should be able to manage, analyze, and interpret the data with decision logic to report to the clinicians and patients making decisions. Thirdly, the system requires a common terminology or taxonomy of terms in both the genomic and clinical and/or research databases. And finally, the formatting of the data storage for exchange with larger groups of people needs to be structured so that it supports queries from multiple sources.

A Nine-Step Process From Patient's Genetic/ Genomics Profile to Treatment Efficacy Requiring Bioinformatics and Informatics Support

The interaction between the genomic, molecular pathways for a patient, and the specific drug response involves data from multiple sources. A multi-step process is described that has been adapted from Garraway, 2013. The steps include (1) the patient encounter, (2) imaging data, (3) tissue biopsy, (4) genomics/molecular/proteomic profiling, (5) data interpretation after identifying the somatic and germline alterations, listing potentially actionable and consequential variants, and prioritizing events for evaluating response, (6) decision support for treatment decision, (7) description of the clinical response (including the potential toxicities (adverse events and safety) of the treatment management to the patient in addition to outcomes such as a decrease in the tumor response (i.e., treatment effectiveness, clinical condition, survival, exacerbation, or mortality), (8) determination of the tissue to drug management resistance, and (9) re-assessment of a new therapeutic approach.

Step 5 of the process is the interpretation of what the genomic alteration might be matched to a specific targeted treatment where the Big Data findings are occurring. There are multiple public and private databases that require analysis of the genes and pathways involved in the abnormality prior to an actionable treatment course being selected. Both the clinical actions and the biologic actions need to determine the relevance to the treatment. These involve heuristic tools, curated and annotated databases, genomic tumor databases, and other knowledgebases that include outcome databases, genomic registries, integrative analysis tools, and machine learning systems. And in many cases these are several possible treatment alternatives to a particular abnormality. There may be standard treatments that have known outcomes, clinical trials, or experimental therapies, and some with no known clinical or treatment evidence.

Additional Nursing Data Needs Requiring Informatics

Some additional data generated during this nine-step process include (1) informed consent, (2) family history (pedigree), (3) signs and symptoms prior to treatment, (4) genetic counseling, (5) quality of life, (6) pain and functional activities assessment, (7) symptom observations such as sleep, fatigue, nausea/vomiting, (8) side effect observations such as anemia, bone marrow hypocellular, disseminated intravascular coagulation, febrile neutropenia, hemolyisis, hemolytic uremia, leukocytosis, lymph node pain, spleen disorder, thrombotic thrombocytopenic purpura; and (9) communication management to the patient and the clinical diagnosis and treatment team.

When patients enter clinical trials where groups of patients' tissues are sequenced and treatment is begun to determine effectiveness, from 100 to 200 patients may be entered into the protocols. The volume of data in the process and additional data are magnified by 100 to 200 times. The types of clinical trials are either adaptive or basket types.

In adaptive trials, all of the possible treatments matched to the genome are tried. In the basket type all the patients with a specific gene mutation are given a specific drug, and all the patients with another mutation are given another drug.

Bioinformatics Defined

Through all the steps in these processes, informatics tools are the essential component of diagnosis and interpreting data to select patient treatments and measure potential outcomes. Another way to simplify the understanding of the informatics infrastructure is to look at how we collect, store, access, analyze, exchange data, and integrate research and clinical data to facilitate personalized medicine. Biomedical informatics has been defined as the "science that develops methods, techniques, and theories regarding how to use data, information and knowledge to support and improve biomedical research, human health, and the delivery of healthcare services" (AMIA, 2014). In this chapter, bioinformatics is separated from healthcare information technology in that bioinformatics supports the use of computer and databases to analyze genes, genomes, and proteins from varying tissue sources.

TOOLKITS THAT ARE AVAILABLE IN LEARNING ABOUT GENOMICS AND APPLYING BIOINFORMATICS IN CLINICAL PRACTICE

In a 2012 report of the Institute of Medicine, where bioinformatics tools going forward were described, the panel recommended:

- Utilizing standardized, open source databases with professional annotation, analytics, and curations
- Integrating research and clinical data
- Supporting open source platforms for the development of software
- Considering secondary uses of IT infrastructure as a way to reduce overall costs (Institute of Medicine [IOM], 2012a, p. 3)

The process of personalized health is often called clinical translational research process when the benefits of research are translated into clinical practice. The IOM panel in 2012 recommended:

- Standardizing clinical data similar to high-quality research data
- Developing new statistical methods and study designs for use with clinical trials
- Developing better data mining and filtering approaches to sort through massive datasets
- Connecting genomic and molecular data with clinical data
- Structuring clinical data to support the research data
- Integrating data that are already in the public domain to generate new hypotheses for testing
- Ensuring processes are guided with a research framework
- Using a systems view of disease, which postulates that disease is a result of perturbations of one or more biological networks that lead to altered expressions of information (IOM, 2012a, p. 3)

Managing the Large Volume and Scale

The large volume of data and scale is a result of a dynamic environment where discoveries are occurring with incredible speed, patient populations are more dynamic and even global, and patients may come with pre-existing conditions that require sub-group analysis, and the ability to data mine large amounts of data. In addition many areas are using open source networks and multiple communities. One new model is for groups to utilize the advances of cloud computing in bioinformatics.

Cloud computing is a model that increases the storage, computation, and collaboration capacity in personalized health while reducing the time needed for data mapping and analysis. The cloud can be a shared resource that can be accessed over the Internet to do the complex integration of databases and analysis tools to make informed interpretations of the data. NIST provides guidance on assuring Cloud storage security and authentication similar to any other large database (National Institute of Standards, 2014). Further research is needed to identify security, reliability of using clouds, handling and sharing intellectual property on clouds, and maintaining regulatory compliance.

What Is the Hoopla About HADOOP

Apache Hadoop is a large-scale open source distributed processing framework platform that allows big data to be brought into existing data warehouses. The architectural framework allows data management, and analytics for processing, storage, and using data. It is the data processing that has worked well in large Web-based enterprises as Google and Yahoo! It can be used to move large-scale data to a Cloud. Associated with it have been related technologies such as Hive, Hadapt, Impala, Sqrrl, HBase, Know, and Pig. Recently released was YARN (yet another resource negotiator) with version 2. Users are describing it as a new style of programming that is helpful in this big data environment (Hadoop, 2014).

Public Databases Available

With the vast number of siloed databases from molecular, clinical, and epidemiological data that already reside in databases, one can quickly visualize that an integrated data warehouse or repository in the public domain can allow not only for (1) hypothesis-driven studies, but also for (2) hypothesis-generated diagnosis and treatment, (3) potential regimes that allow for discovery of new hypothesis of potential diagnostic biomarkers, and (4) treatment regimes matched to improve health.

One of the large data repositories is the National Center for Biotechnology Information (NCBI) Gene Expression Omnibus (GEO). This repository holds more than 1 million publicly available microarray datasets and support MIAME standards (NCBI/MIAME, 2014). Another repository called COSMIC (Catalogue of Somatic Mutations in Cancer) is a European repository with more

than 1 million somatic mutations identified for human cancers (COSMIC, 2014). Data and consultation can also be purchased from Assay Depot, an online marketplace for scientific and pharmaceutical research services. This includes the purchase of assays, animal models, and services from vendors.

The Broad Institute developed a Connectivity Map (cmap) that is a repository of genome-wide transcriptional expression data from human cell lines created with responses from different drugs at varying doses. It currently includes 7000 expression profiles representing 1309 compounds. This links the gene expression data with the drug gene expression data (Broad Institute, 2014). Discovery lies within these databanks.

A CASE FOR INTEGRATION INTO NURSING INFORMATICS

In modern Healthcare Information Technology most of the data currently exist in silos and the analysis and interpretation requires the integration of data from various systems, or access to data in distributed systems. Integrated data are more accessible and available to broader networks through exchanges. The data are definitely decentralized, but the analytics and decision support and interpretation require centrality of data, and accessibility at the point of care. The transition from siloed data to integrated data requires standards in data and validity assurance of data, normalization of data (or data cleansing), and policies of data sharing. In order for data to be analyzed, the integration of clinical and genomic data requires that data quality start at the point of care.

Managing the Standards

There are many areas where standards are needed in developing the biomedical informatics supports for personalized health. Inherent in the collection of data from disparate databases is the theoretical framework of the data, and adherence to standardized terminology in order to make the systems and data interoperable. Currently under discussion related to standards, are the standards to describe how the genomic data are being collected. In another Institute of Medicine Report on Precision Medicine, the panel recommended standards in genetic and genomic terminology (IOM, 2012b). Without it and the standards in clinical medicine, the integration of multiple databases will not result in meaningful interpretation. The precision of standards requires a considerable commitment to data harmonization and curation.

Validating Data for Analysis in Bioinformatics

A cautionary message is coming from the research scientists and the public genetic industry that not all data stored in databases from academic and public labs can be replicated by industry for new drug target validation prior to submission to the FDA. (Ioannidis & Panagiotou, 2011). It is because of these discrepancies that the FDA is reviewing validation issues for the clinical use of genome sequencing.

Data Sharing

To translate patient care information into discovery and positive outcomes of patient care requires data from multiple sources. The value of data sharing is that the best practices of diagnosis and treatment can be leveraged to many patients with a condition and to many healthcare providers. Data come from Electronic Health Records, doctors' and other healthcare providers' office and clinic records, personal health records from patients, research center data and networks, genomic and annotation services, and the patient themselves.

Policies and procedures for sharing these data are required. Governance policies and structures need to be put into the enterprise architectures. Since the patient needs to be available for a lifetime, their data need to be used and reused by many people, and treatments may change in the future that better match the patient being seen today, a static one time informed consent may be obsolete. As we look at more breaches occurring to our privacy and security in the financial sector, our most valuable asset of identity and health is our genetic structure. New cybersecurity infrastructures will have to be developed with new types of algorithms to encrypt data will have to be developed.

No Better Advocate for Personalized Health Than the Consumer/Patient

Consumers are more informed, use more common databases, and utilize more social networks in genetics, diagnosis, treatment, and outcomes. A significant amount of traffic on government Web sites involves patients. Because so many of the tools and databases are Web based, and the consumer has so much access to open information, they have the potential of being the biggest disruptive innovators. The consumer is also using mobile technology through telecommunications networks to access these databases. It is the patient/consumer who is knowledgeable about what is available, who has the potential to drive the implementation of genomics into healthcare.

Moving to the Future in Bioinformatics

Models of the next generation health IT system are able to comprehensively capture the genetic, genomic, biological, behavioral, social, environmental, and ecological factors relevant to disease susceptibility, risk, progression, and outcome of treatments. The look to the future reinforces that the systems we build today must be standardized and include validated data. Big data in the future will require new types of visualization and summary data that can be integrated into routine clinical care by multiple healthcare professionals. There will be new requirements for certifications in bioinformatics to prepare the kind of workforce needed for this expanding area of clinical practice and scientific research. There are models throughout the country that have supported research to link clinical and research data. We are learning from their innovations and move forward with optimism toward the totally integrated bioinformatics system in the future.

ETHICAL, LEGAL, AND SOCIAL ISSUES

As genomic discoveries continued to translate into clinical practice, there are several ethical, legal, and social issues that emerge including regulation of genetic and genomic tests, and other incidental findings. A brief description of each area follows.

Regulation of Genetic and Genomic Tests

The regulations associated with genetic testing have not kept pace with the current environment. As such discoveries in the laboratory can progress directly to clinical testing including directly to consumer marketing and/or testing despite insufficient evidence of analytic and clinical validity (Javitt & Hudson, 2006). To address this gap, the Centers for Disease Control (CDC) Office of Public Health Genomics established the Evaluation of Genomic Applications in Practice and Prevention (EGAPP), which conducts systematic evidence reviews on the validity and utility of genetic tests (Evaluation of Genomic Applications in Practice and Prevention, 2010). Unfortunately, the evidence reports have not been able to keep pace with the genetic tests that are being introduced clinically.

There are also gaps in regulating the laboratories themselves. The Clinical Laboratory Improvement Act (CLIA) designates qualifications of laboratory personnel, standards for quality assurance, and documentation of tests and procedures for tests that produce clinical information (Schwartz, 1999). Genetic and genomic tests are classified as high complexity tests and as such CLIA mandates laboratory proficiency testing to confirm a laboratories capacity to perform and interpret these tests (Javitt & Hudson, 2006). To date proficiency laboratory evaluations for genetic and genomic tests are not mandated by CLIA (Hudson et al., 2006) Furthermore, proficiency testing for the continued development of new testing techniques is still required (Kalman et al., 2013).

Another avenue of regulation of genetic and genomic tests is through the Food and Drug Administration (FDA). Test kits produced for use by more than one laboratory are regulated by the FDA. However, most genetic and genomic tests are developed within individual laboratories, are not marketed to other laboratories as a kit, and as such fall outside the oversight of the FDA. This represents the majority of genetic and genomic tests currently available (Javitt & Hudson, 2006). Related to this regulatory gap, direct to consumer genetic and genomic tests that provide medical as well as other information but require no healthcare provider input or oversight prior to ordering the test have been developed and sold directly to the consumer (Hogarth, Javitt, & Melzer, 2008). As this market has continued to expand and expert panels called for additional oversight, the FDA in 2010 initiated a series of reviews and actions aimed at the genetic and genomic laboratory developed testing regulatory environment (Kuehn, 2010; National Human Genome Research Institute, 2014).

In the intervening period while the gaps in regulations are being addressed, the healthcare provider must assume the responsibility for not just when to consider a genetic or genomic test and what test to order now that multiplex testing is available, but selecting the laboratory that is capable of performing the test. To address this challenge, the CDC developed a framework (Office of Surveillance) for assessing analytic and clinical validity, clinical utility and ethical, legal, and social implications of genetic and genomic tests (Haddow & Palomaki, 2003). See Fig. 49.2 for an overview of the elements of the ACCE Model (Office of Surveillance, Epidemiology, and Laboratory Services, Public Health Genomics, & Centers for Disease Control and Prevention, 2010). ACCE does not incorporate personal utility into the model which is associated with potential indirect outcomes of testing such as understanding of genetics of a given disease and the influence of this information on personal decision-making (Foster, Mulvihill, & Sharp, 2009).

Additionally, the National Institutes of Health has established the Genetic Testing Registry http://www.ncbi.nlm.nih.gov/gtr/, which is a voluntary detailed listing of genetic tests available from the laboratories performing those tests as well as details about test techniques, ordering, and performance (Registry, 2014). As the complexity and volume of genetic and genomic tests continues to expand, provider decision support tools will continue to play an important role in the translation of this into routine clinical practice.

Incidental Findings

As the cost for whole genome analysis continues to decline, the application of these technologies in clinical and research settings continues to expand. With that comes the reality of how to best handle incidental findings. Incidental findings are defined as, "A finding concerning an individual research participant that has potential health or reproductive importance and is discovered in the course of conducting research but is beyond the aims of the study" (Wolf et al., 2008). This is not a phenomenon unique to genomics but has long been a component of healthcare. However, the sheer scope of the potential findings and the ever-changing evidence base of what meets the criteria for a clinically actionable finding create several challenges, resulting in an ongoing debate in the literature about how best to address this in both clinical and research settings.

Existing laws and federal regulations for human subjects research inadequate to no guidance and thus far legal cases have yet to emerge (Wolf, 2012). Consider the following, 45 CFR 46 Protection Of Human Subjects 46.102 states, *"Human subject* means a living individual about whom an investigator (whether professional or student) conducting research obtains: (1) Data obtained through intervention or interaction with the individual, (2) Identifiable private information" (Department of Health and Human Services, 2014). Yet identification through research analysis performed after death that reveals a germline mutation in which there is well-established analytic and clinical validity as well as clinical utility (i.e. *BRCA1* or *BRCA2* mutation associated with breast, ovarian, and other cancers) does have implications for living family members. As such, this discovery meets the criteria for an incidental finding. But what finding actually meets the threshold for meeting analytic and clinical validity as well as clinical utility standards? Several groups have grappled with this challenge. The National Heart, Lung, and Blood Institute (NHLBI) Working Group on Reporting Genetic Results in Research studies developed and then updated their recommendations which specify the following criteria:

- "The genetic finding has important health implications for the participant, and the associated risks are established and substantial.

- The genetic finding is actionable, that is, there are established therapeutic or preventive interventions

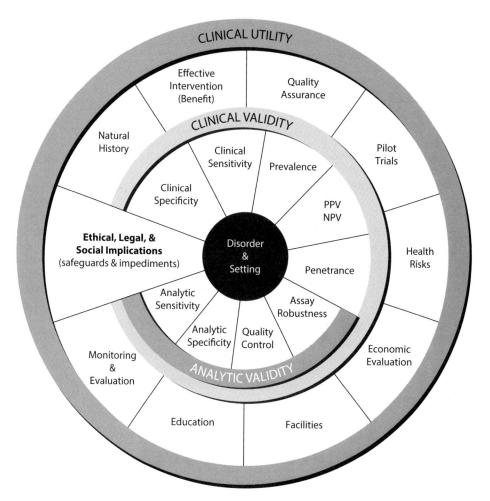

· **FIGURE 49.2.** ACCE Model (**A**nalytic Validity, **C**linical Validity, **C**linical Utility, and **E**thical, Legal, and Social Implications). (Reproduced from Office of Surveillance Epidemiology, and Laboratory Services, Public Health Genomics, & Centers for Disease Control and Prevention [2010], http://www.cdc.gov/genomics/gtesting/ACCE/index.htm.)

or other available actions that have the potential to change the clinical course of the disease.

- The test is analytically valid, and the disclosure plan complies with all applicable laws.
- During the informed consent process or subsequently, the study participant has opted to receive his or her individual genetic results" (National Heart, Lung and Blood Institute Working Group et al., 2010).

In 2013, the American College of Medical Genetics and Genomics (ACMG) published their policy statement on reporting of incidental findings from clinical exome and genome sequencing. An important distinction

between these two statements is that the ACMG policy statement is specific to clinical application of these technologies whereas the criteria established by NHLBI refer to research use of these technologies. ACMG specifically reviewed the existing evidence and specify that laboratories should interrogate the genome for a list of specific genes associated with specific phenotype/syndromes. This differs from classic incidental findings, which do not involve deliberate interrogation of the genome for abnormalities. The selection of conditions included in ACMG list was based on high prevalence and where interventions exist. Additionally, in contrast to NHLBI which defers to the patient agreeing to receive this information at the time of consent, ACMG's position is that the duty to warn surpasses patient autonomy and that the decision to disclose these results should not be restricted to the age of majority but encompass disclosure of results including adult onset disorders to the parents of children (Green et al., 2013).

As the genetic healthcare community has continued to grapple with how best to address the challenge of incidental findings, the Presidential Commission on the Study of Bioethical Issues also looked closely at this issue and published their report in December 2013 (Presidential Commission for the Study of Bioethical Issues, 2013). The Commission made several recommendations that can be classified into five major areas:

- Communication of results: Individuals should be provided with information about the potential for incidental findings and the methods that will be used for notification.

- Evidence-based guideline development: Professional organizations should strive to develop evidence-based guidelines for the management of potential findings from these techniques.

- Expand the evidence base: Funding agencies should continue to offer funding for research focused on incidental findings encompassing everything from discovery to disclosure considerations.

- Education: Education materials need to be developed for all key stakeholders, including healthcare providers, institutional review boards, and potential recipients of this information, that cover ethical, practical, and legal issues associated with incidental findings.

- Justice and fairness: All persons would have access to the information, guidance, and support required to make informed decisions about testing and management of outcomes (Presidential Commission for the Study of Bioethical Issues, 2013).

The intersection of informatics and challenge of managing incidental findings is clearly evident. First are the effective strategies for interrogating the genome, identifying and classifying the variations identified into buckets associated with clinical relevance, and tracking evidence changes that effect classification (Bemmels, Wolf, & Van Ness, 2012; Berg et al., 2013). Second is the need for a healthcare infrastructure that has the capacity to effectively integrate this information into workflow informatics systems such as the EHR (McCarthy, 2013). Third is the infrastructure to track individual genomic information as an individual moves through the healthcare continuum from birth to death and pull in the relevant information to guide healthcare when needed. For example, when a child is found to harbor a genetic predisposition to an adult onset disorder that would necessitate a change in management beginning at a particular age. Additionally, novel strategies for healthcare provider education in genomics and point-of-care decision support are critical.

EDUCATIONAL RESOURCES FOR NURSING IN GENOMICS AND INFORMATICS

Table 49.1 provides additional educational resources for nursing in genomics and informatics. Students reading this chapter should understand that the science of genetics and genomics and bioinformatics are evolving so fast that there are many sites to constantly monitor. Another useful reference is McCormick (2011) that cites many learning resources. Another excellent resource is *The Journal of Nursing Scholarship Genomic Nursing Webinar Series* 2013 Genomics Special Issue. Several authors describe the special issue and the importance in the delivery of care by all healthcare professionals, including nurses in every healthcare setting (Calzone, et al., 2013). Another resource with many Webinars and educational resources, including recommendations of curricula for genetic competencies is Genome.Gov (Genome.gov, 2014).

THE BLUEPRINT FOR GENOMIC NURSING SCIENCE

In 2012, the National Institutes of Health convened an inter-disciplinary panel to establish a Blueprint for genomic nursing science that could be used to focus research efforts to fill identified evidence gaps. The panel consisted of multiple government agencies, genomic experts, and representatives from key stakeholder groups. The Blueprint was established through an analysis of existing evidence, expert evaluation of the current state of the science, and then solicitation from the public for comments on the draft document, which were then incorporated into the final Blueprint (Genomic Nursing State of the Science Advisory Panel, 2013).

The Blueprint (Table 49.2) is mapped to the major focus areas of the National Institutes of Nursing Research Strategic Plan: health promotion and disease prevention; advancing the quality of life; innovation; and training. Cross-cutting themes that need to be considered with any of the research priorities included in the Blueprint were health disparities, cost, policy, and public education. The Blueprint focuses on two primary areas: the client, defined broadly as person, family, community, and/or population; and the context, which encompasses capacity building

TABLE 49.1	Selected Web sites Resources for Genomics and Informatics
Title	**Web site**
Electronic Medical Records and Genomics (eMERGE) Network	http://www.genome.gov/27540473
Essential Genetic and Genomic Competencies for Nurses with Graduate Degrees	http://www.nursingworld.org/MainMenuCategories/ EthicsStandards/Genetics-1/Essential-Genetic-and-Genomic-Competencies-for-Nurses-With-Graduate-Degrees.pdf
Genetics/Genomics Competency Center for Education (G2C2)	http://www.g-2-c-2.org
Genetic and Genomic Nursing: Competencies, Curricula Guidelines and Outcome Indicators, 2nd Edition	http://www.genome.gov/27527634
Genetics and Genomics for Health Professionals	http://www.genome.gov/27527599
Genetics and Your Practice	http://www.marchofdimes.com/gyponline/index.bm2
Genetics Home Reference	http://ghr.nlm.nih.gov
GeneTests/Gene Reviews	http://www.genetests.org
Genetics is Relevant Now: Nurses' Views and Patient Stories	http://www.cincinnatichildrens.org/ed/clinical/gpnf/resources/ curriculum/relevant-genetics.htm
Genomics and Disease Prevention	http://www.cdc.gov/genomics/
Genetics, Health, and Society	http://oba.od.nih.gov/SACGHS/sacghs_home.html
Global Genetics and Genomics Community (G3C)	http://www.g-3-c.org
International Society of Nurses in Genetics	http://www.isong.org
National Institute of Nursing Research Summer Genetics Institute	http://www.ninr.nih.gov/Training/TrainingOpportunitiesIntramural/ SummerGeneticsInstitute/
Pharmacogenomics Education Program	http://pharmacogenomics.ucsd.edu/
Teaching Genetics	http://teach.genetics.utah.edu/
Genetic Science Learning Center	
U.S. Surgeon General's Family History Initiative	http://www.hhs.gov/familyhistory/

Reproduced, with permission, from Genomic Nursing State of the Science Advisory Panel, Calzone K.A., Jenkins J., et al. (2013). A Blueprint for Genomic Nursing Science. Journal of Nursing Scholarship, 45(1), 96–104.

TABLE 49.2	Nursing Genomic Science Blueprint Mapped to NINR Strategic Plan Areas (Genomic Nursing State of the Science Advisory Panel, 2013)

NINR Strategic Plan Areas	Specific Nursing Research Categories	Advisory Panel Genomic Nursing Research Topic Areas[a]
Health Promotion and Disease Prevention	**Risk Assessment**	a. Biologic plausibility (e.g., pathways, mechanisms, biomarkers, epigenetics, genotoxicity) b. Comprehensive screening opportunities (e.g., family history, identify risk level [population based average and elevated]) c. Components of risk assessment (e.g., biomarkers, family history) d. Risk-specific healthcare decision-making
	Communication	a. Risk communication (e.g., interpretation, timing, risk reports to the health-care provider and client[b]) b. Informed consent c. Direct to consumer marketing and testing (e.g., uptake, utilization, dissemination)
	Decision Support	a. Informed consent b. Match of values/preferences with decision made c. Risk perception/risk accuracy d. Effect of decision support on decision quality (e.g., knowledge, personal utility)

(continued)

TABLE 49.2	Nursing Genomic Science Blueprint Mapped to NINR Strategic Plan Areas (Genomic Nursing State of the Science Advisory Panel, 2013) *(continued)*	
NINR Strategic Plan Areas	**Specific Nursing Research Categories**	**Advisory Panel Genomic Nursing Research Topic Areas[a]**
Advancing the Quality of Life	**Family**	a. Family context (e.g., family functioning, and structure, family relationships and communication) b. Ethical issues c. Healthcare provider communication with families
	Symptom Management	a. Biologic plausibility (e.g., pathways, mechanisms, biomarkers, epigenetics) b. Clinical utility c. Personal utility d. Pharmacogenomics (e.g., therapy selection, medication titration) e. Decision-making f. Evidence-based effectiveness of approaches
	Disease States (encompassing acute, common complex, and chronic)	a. Genomic-based interventions that reduce morbidity and mortality b. Gene/environment interactions (e.g., epigenetics, genotoxicity) c. Pharmacogenomics d. Evidence-based effectiveness of treatments/support
	Client Self-Management	a. Collecting and conveying information that informs self-management (e.g., family history) b. Lifestyle behaviors c. Environmental exposure and protection (e.g., occupational) d. Synergy of client and provider expectations (e.g., client/family-centered care) e. Personal utility

Innovation	**Technology Development**	a. Incorporation of new technologies (e.g., whole genome sequencing)
		b. Ethics
		c. Policy and guidelines to support applications
		d. Applications (e.g., clinical and analytic validity, and clinical utility)
		e. Genomic bioinformatics
		f. Translation, Dissemination, Implementation
		  i. Use of technology in information delivery
		  ii. Performance improvement by provider (e.g., point-of-care support)
		  iii. Resources that support genomic research (e.g., registries of tools, best practices, nursing outcomes)

	Informatics Support Systems	a. Data storage and use to facilitate research process and outcomes b. Facilitate cross-generational sharing of genomic data (e.g., family history, laboratory analyses) c. Managing, analyzing, and interpreting genomic information (e.g., sequencing data) d. Point-of-care decision support for client and healthcare provider e. Common terminology and taxonomy f. Common formats for data storage/exchange and queries
	Environmental Influences (encompassing physical, social environments, and policy context)	a. Evidence-based guidelines b. Healthcare reform c. Economics (e.g., cost-effectiveness) d. Regulatory gaps and/or variability

(continued)

TABLE 49.2	Nursing Genomic Science Blueprint Mapped to NINR Strategic Plan Areas (Genomic Nursing State of the Science Advisory Panel, 2013) *(continued)*	
NINR Strategic Plan Areas	**Specific Nursing Research Categories**	**Advisory Panel Genomic Nursing Research Topic Areas[a]**
Training	**Capacity Building**	a. Training future nursing scientists in genomics b. Preparing nursing faculty in genomics c. Education of current and future workforce in genomics (e.g., research nurse coordinators, advanced practice nurses, other healthcare professionals) d. Preparation of nurse scientists to lead inter-professional teams e. Preparation of clinical and administrative leaders to advance appropriate genomics/genetics integration into practice f. Innovative uses of bio-repositories (e.g., informed consent, result interpretation) g. Bioethics
	Education	a. Optimal methods to train the existing nursing workforce in genomics b. Optimal methods to train the nursing leadership in genomics to support genomic translation, research, and practice c. Optimal methods to integrate nursing genomic competencies in basic/pre-licensure and post-licensure in academic programs
Cross-Cutting Themes	**Health Disparities**	a. Racial, ethnic, socioeconomic, and cultural influences on disease occurrence and response to disease and treatment b. Genomic health equity (e.g., access) c. Diseases that disproportionately affect specific groups (e.g., minorities) d. Targeted therapeutics e. Overcoming misinformation and genomic "Myths"
	Cost	a. Cost-effectiveness b. Comparative effectiveness c. Value
	Policy	a. Policy as context of science b. Research to inform policy
	Public Education	a. Health literacy b. Genomic literacy

[a]The nursing science blueprint serves as a platform for potential inter-professional collaborations that can include but are not limited to any healthcare discipline; basic and behavioral scientists; ethicists; business; and/or informatic professionals.
[b]Clients refers to persons, families, communities, and/or population.

and informatics infrastructure support (Genomic Nursing State of the Science Advisory Panel, 2013).

Informatics figures prominently throughout the Blueprint. As discussed above, to address many of the client-based research priorities described in the Blueprint, large studies relying on massive data warehouses and big data analytics and interpretation are needed. Discoveries that are found to have clinical utility will be translated into practice more readily with informatics that facilitates work flow such as collection of documentation and interpretation of genomic information (i.e., family history);

ease of test selection and ordering; point-of-care decision support; and capacity to store, track, and retrieve genomic information while maintaining patient privacy in the electronic health record (Ullman-Cullere & Mathew, 2011).

Consider a specific example, pharmacogenomics, to elucidate the interface between informatics and the Blueprint. Pharmacogenomics is the use of genomic variation (inherited and acquired) in drug development and drug response including selection, efficacy, pharmacokinetics, pharmacodynamics, and toxicity. Drugs are used throughout the healthcare continuum, not just to treat common complex health disorders but also to reduce risk (i.e., chemoprevention) and ameliorate symptoms (i.e. pain control) (Wang, McLeod, & Weinshilboum, 2011). Biologic plausibility studies, which increasingly are performed, using big data, can encompass genomic pathway identification, which can identify targets for pharmaceuticals interventions, which are then followed by phenotype/drug-specific response assessments again relying heavily on informatics. Once the data are sufficient to establish analytic validity, and clinical validity and utility, translation into practice begins. To facilitate pharmacogenomic translation, the capacity of the healthcare workforce in genomics needs to be expanded (Phimister, Feero, & Guttmacher, 2012). In this era of cost containment, online education interventions are critical, but that is not sufficient.

Outcome assessments from any capacity building initiative must be incorporated as preliminary evidence indicates that traditional methods of continuing healthcare provider education may be insufficient given the complexity of this information (Badzek, Calzone, Jenkins, Culp, & Smith, 2013). Given the broad diversity, size, and interprofessional nature of the practicing healthcare workforce, most of which have no foundation in genomics, this is an especially complex undertaking.

As translation penetrates the practice environment, development of useful point-of-care decision support as drug selection is being considered. Some of these decisions needed at the point of care may include (a) for a given agent, should a genetic test be considered, (b) if so, what test, (c) where in the electronic health record can you readily access whether this has been performed before and, (d) if so, how do you retrieve those results, (e) if not performed before, how to order the test, retrieve the results, and (f) how to use that information to inform drug selection, dosing, and (g) whether any of the patients' existing medications serve as a genomic pathway inhibitor and inducer.

Given the rapidly evolving complexity and evidence base of pharmacogenomics, and the overlap of specific genetic variations with a wide range of drugs, informatics support systems become paramount. To develop these infrastructures, informatics policies that assure patient privacy to minimize harm need to be established (Ullman-Cullere & Mathew, 2011). Then comes one of the last phases of this example, the cost/benefit analysis and if benefits outweigh the costs, establishment of the infrastructure needed to assess quality indicators to assure patient outcomes are optimized.

Nursing research in genomics will help establish the evidence base needed to facilitate translation of genomics into practice to improve health outcomes. The Blueprint for Genomic Nursing Science provides the platform to accelerate nursing research addressing identified critical gaps. The science outlined in the Blueprint intersects with informatics on two primary platforms, research performed utilizing informatics, and research to develop informatics support systems needed to facilitate genomic translation (Genomic Nursing State of the Science Advisory Panel, 2013).

SUMMARY

Advancing technology and new knowledge about genomics underlies an increasing component of healthcare and has influences on the entire wellness to illness continuum. Therefore, genomics impacts the entire healthcare workforce and the translation of those discoveries into healthcare is rapidly progressing. Informatics plays a central role in the evidence generation and capacity building for translation into practice to realize the benefits of genomics.

REFERENCES

Ahlquist, D. A. (2010). Molecular detection of colorectal neoplasia. *Gastroenterology, 138*(6), 2127–2139.

American Medical Informatics Association (AMIA). (2014). Retrieved from http://www.amia.org/glossary. Accessed on February 28, 2014.

American Nurses Association Nursing Informatics Scope and Standards Revision Workgroup. (2014). *Call for public comment - Nursing informatics: Scope and standards of practice.* Retrieved from http://www.nursingworld.org/Comment-Nursing-Informatics. Accessed on January 3, 2014.

Arteaga, C. L., & Baselga, J. (2012). Impact of genomics on personalized cancer medicine. *Clinical Cancer Research, 18*(3), 612–618.

Badzek, L., Calzone, K. A., Jenkins, J., Culp, S., & Smith, S. (2013). *Evaluation of the Integration of Genetics and Genomics into Nursing Practice.* Paper presented at the 2013 ANCC National Magnet Conference®, Orlando, FL.

Bemmels, H. R., Wolf, S. M., & Van Ness, B. (2012). Mapping the inputs, analyses, and outputs of biobank research systems to identify sources of incidental findings and individual research results for potential return to participants. *Genetics in Medicine, 14*(4), 385–392.

Benkendorf, J., Goodspeed, T., & Watson, M. S. (2010). Newborn screening residual dried blood spot use for newborn screening quality improvement. *Genetics in Medicine, 12*(12 Suppl.), S269–S272.

Berg, J. S., Adams, M., Nassar, N., Bizon, C., Lee, K., Schmitt, C. P., ... Evans, J. P. (2013). An informatics approach to analyzing the incidentalome. *Genetics in Medicine, 15*(1), 36–44.

Berg, A. O., Baird, M. A., Botkin, J. R., Driscoll, D. A., Fishman, P. A., Guarino, P. D., ... Williams, J. K. (2009). National Institutes of Health State-of-the-Science Conference statement: Family history and improving health. *Annals of Internal Medicine, 151*(12), 872–877.

Berger, B. M., & Ahlquist, D. A. (2012). Stool DNA screening for colorectal neoplasia: Biological and technical basis for high detection rates. *Pathology, 44*(2), 80–88.

Blout, C., Walsh Vockley, C., Gaviglio, A., Fox, M., Croke, B., Williamson Dean, L., The Newborn Screening Task Force on behalf of the NSGC Public Policy Committee. (2014). Newborn screening: Education, consent, and the residual blood spot. The position of the National Society of Genetic Counselors. *Journal of Genetic Counseling, 23*(1), 16–19.

Broad Institute. (2014). Retrieved from http://www.broadinstitute.org/cmap/. Accessed on January 7, 2014.

Calzone, K. A., Jenkins, J., Nicol, N., Skirton, H., Feero, W. G., Green, E. D. (2013). Relevance of genomics to healthcare and nursing practice. *Journal of Nursing Scholarship, 45*(1), 1–2.

Cancer Genome Atlas Research Network, Weinstein, J. N., Collisson, E. A., Mills, G. B., Shaw, K. R., Ozenberger, B. A., ... Stuart, J. M. (2013). The Cancer Genome Atlas Pan-Cancer analysis project. *Nature Genetics, 45*(10), 1113–1120.

Catalogue of Somatic Mutations in Cancer (COSMIC). (2014). *What is COSMIC?* Retrieved from http://cancer.sanger.ac.uk/cancergenome/projects/cosmic/about. Accessed on January 7, 2014.

Data and Informatics Working Group (DIWG). (2012). *Draft report to the advisory committee to the director.* Retrieved from http://acd.od.nih.gov/Data%20and%20Informatics%20Working%20Group%20Report.pdf. Accessed on January 6, 2014.

de la Cruz, J., Andre, F., Harrell, R. K., Bassett, R. L., Arun, B., Mathieu, M. C., ... Gilcrease, M. Z. (2012). Tissue-based predictors of germ-line BRCA1 mutations: implications for triaging of genetic testing. *Human Pathology, 43*(11), 1932–1939.

DeLuca, J., Zanni, K. L., Bonhomme, N., Kemper, A. R. (2013). Implications of newborn screening for nurses. *Journal of Nursing Scholarship, 45*(1), 25–33.

Department of Health and Human Services. (2014). *Code of Federal Regulations.* Retrieved from http://www.hhs.gov/ohrp/humansubjects/guidance/45cfr46.html. Accessed on January 27, 2014.

Domchek, S. M., Bradbury, A., Garber, J. E., Offit, K., & Robson, M. E. (2013). Multiplex genetic testing for cancer susceptibility: out on the high wire without a net? *Journal of Clinical Oncology, 31*(10), 1267–1279.

Evaluation of Genomic Applications in Practice and Prevention. (2010, February 10). *Evaluation of genomic applications in practice and prevention.* Retrieved from http://www.egappreviews.org/. Accessed on February 17, 2010.

Foster, M. W., Mulvihill, J. J., & Sharp, R. R. (2009). Evaluating the utility of personal genomic information. *Genetics in Medicine, 11*(8), 570–574.

Garraway, L. (2012). *Molecular genetics of cancer.* Retrieved from http://isites.harvard.edu/fs/docs/icb.topic1128938.files/Molecular%20Genetics%20of%20Cancer.pdf. Accessed on December 19,2014.

Garraway, L. (2013). Genomic-driven oncology: Framework for an emerging paradigm. *Journal of Clinical Oncology, 31*(15), 1806-182-14.

Genome.gov. (2014). *Essentials of genetic and genomic nursing: Competencies, curricula guidelines, and outcome indicators* (2nd ed.). Retrieved from http://www.genome.gov/Pages/Careers/HealthProfessionalEducation/geneticscompetency.pdf. Accessed on January 7, 2014.

Genomic Nursing State of the Science Advisory Panel, Calzone, K. A., Jenkins, J., Bakos, A. D., Cashion, A. K., Donaldson, N., ... Webb, J. A. (2013). A blueprint for genomic nursing science. *Journal of Nursing Scholarship, 45*(1), 96–104.

Ginsburg, G. S., Staples, J., & Abernethy, A. P. (2011). Academic medical centers: Ripe for rapid-learning personalized health care. *Science Translational Medicine, 3*(101), 101cm127.

Goey, A. K., Mooiman, K. D., Beijnen, J. H., Schellens, J. H., & Meijerman, I. (2013). Relevance of in vitro and clinical data for predicting CYP3A4-mediated herb-drug interactions in cancer patients. *Cancer Treatment Reviews, 39*(7), 773–783.

Green, R. C., Berg, J. S., Grody, W. W., Kalia, S. S., Korf, B. R., Martin, C. L., ... Biesecker, L. G. (2013). ACMG recommendations for reporting of incidental findings in clinical exome and genome sequencing. *Genetics in Medicine, 15*(7), 565–574.

Green, E. D., Guyer, M. S., & National Human Genome Research Institute. (2011). Charting a course for genomic medicine from base pairs to bedside. *Nature, 470*(7333), 204–213.

Guttmacher, A., & Collins, F. S. (2002). Genomic medicine: A primer. The *New England Journal of Medicine, 347*(19), 1512–1520.

Haddow, J. E., & Palomaki, G. E. (2003). ACCE: A model process for evaluating data on emerging genetic tests. In M. Khoury, J. Little, & W. Burke (Eds.), *Human genome epidemiology: A scientific foundation for using genetic information to improve health and prevent disease* (pp. 217–233). New York, NY: Oxford University Press.

Hadoop. (2014). *Welcome to Apache™ Hadoop®!* Retrieved from http://hadoop.apache.org/. Accessed on February 28, 2014.

Hampel, H., de la Chapelle, A. (2013). How do we approach the goal of identifying everybody with Lynch syndrome? *Familial Cancer, 12*(2), 313–317.

Hampel, H., Frankel, W., Panescu, J., Lockman, J., Sotamaa, K., Fix, D., ... de la Chapelle, A. (2006). Screening for Lynch syndrome (hereditary nonpolyposis colorectal cancer) among endometrial cancer patients. *Cancer Research, 66*(15), 7810–7817.

Hampel, H., Frankel, W. L., Martin, E., Arnold, M., Khanduja, K., Kuebler, P., ... de la Chapelle, A. (2008). Feasibility of screening for Lynch syndrome among patients with colorectal cancer. *Journal of Clinical Oncology, 26*(35), 5783–5788.

Hogarth, S., Javitt, G., & Melzer, D. (2008). The current landscape for direct-to-consumer genetic testing: Legal, ethical, and policy issues. *Annual Review of Genomics and Human Genetics, 9,* 161–182.

Hudson, K. L., Murphy, J. A., Kaufman, D. J., Javitt, G. H., Katsanis, S. H., Scott, J. (2006). Oversight of US genetic testing laboratories. *Nature Biotechnology, 24,* 1083–1090.

Institute of Medicine. (2012a). *Informatics needs and challenges in cancer research: Workshop summary.* Washington, DC: National Academies Press.

Institute of Medicine. (2012b). *Toward precision medicine: Building a knowledge network for biomedical research and a new taxonomy of disease.* Washington, DC: National Academies Press.

Ioannidis, J. P., & Panagiotou, O. A. (2011). Comparison of effect sizes associated with biomarked reported in highly cited articles and in subsequent meta-analyses. *Journal of the American Medical Association, 305*(21), 2200–2210.

Javitt, G. J., & Hudson, K. (2006). Federal neglect: Regulation of genetic testing. *Issues in Science and Technology, 22,* 58–66.

Kalman, L. V., Lubin, I. M., Barker, S., du Sart, D., Elles, R., Grody, W. W., ... Zehnbauer, B. (2013). Current landscape and new paradigms of proficiency testing and external quality assessment for molecular genetics. *Archives of Pathology & Laboratory Medicine, 137*(7), 983–988.

Kemper, A. R., Green, N. S., Calonge, N., Lam, W. K., Comeau, A. M., Goldenberg, A. J., ... Bocchini Jr., J. A. (2014). Decision-making process for conditions nominated to the Recommended Uniform Screening Panel: statement of the US Department of Health and Human Services Secretary's Advisory Committee on Heritable Disorders in Newborns and Children. *Genetics in Medicine, 16*(2), 183–187.

Krens, S. D., McLeod, H. L., & Hertz, D. L. (2013). Pharmacogenetics, enzyme probes and therapeutic drug monitoring as potential tools for individualizing taxane therapy. *Pharmacogenetics, 14*(5), 555–574.

Ku, C. S., Loy, E. Y., Pawitan, Y., Chia, K. S. (2010). The pursuit of genome-wide association studies: where are we now? *Journal of Human Genetics, 55*(4), 195–206.

Kuehn, B. M. (2010). FDA: Gene tests need premarket approval. *Journal of the American Medical Association, 304*(2), 145.

Lin, B. K., Edelman, E., McInerney, J. D., O'Leary, J., Edelson, V., Hughes, K. S., ... Dolan, S. M. (2013). Personalizing prenatal care using family health history: Identifying a panel of conditions for a novel electronic genetic screening tool. *Personalized Medicine, 10*(3), 307–318.

Lindor, N. M., McMaster, M. L., Lindor, C. J., & Greene, M. H. (2008). Concise handbook of familial cancer susceptibility syndromes - second edition. *Journal of the National Cancer Institute Monographs, 38,* 1–93.

Ma, J. D., Lee, K. C., & Kuo, G. M. (2012). Clinical application of pharmacogenomics. *Journal of Pharmacy Practice, 25*(4), 417–427.

McCarthy, J. J., McLeod, H. L., Ginsburg, G. S. (2013). Genomic medicine: A decade of successes, challenges, and opportunities. *Science Translational Medicine, 5*(189), 189sr184.

McCormick, K. A. (2011). The future. In V. K. Saba & K. A. McCormick (Eds.), *Essentials of nursing informatics, version 5.* New York, NY: McGraw-Hill.

McDermott, U., Downing, J. R., & Stratton, M. R. (2011). Genomics and the continuum of cancer care. *New England Journal of Medicine, 364*(4), 340–350.

National Center for Biotechnology Information (NCBI)/ MIAME. (2014). *Gene Expression Omnibus.* Retrieved from http://www.ncbi.nlm.nih.gov/geo/. Accessed on January 07, 2014.

National Heart Lung and Blood Institute Working Group, Fabsitz, R. R., McGuire, A., Sharp, R. R., Puggal, M., Beskow, L. M., ... Burke, G. L. (2010). Ethical and practical guidelines for reporting genetic research results to study participants: updated guidelines from a National Heart, Lung, and Blood Institute working group. *Circulation, Cardiovascular Genetics, 3*(6), 574–580.

National Human Genome Research Institute. (2012). *Talking glossary of genetic terms.* Retrieved from http://www.genome.gov/glossary/index.cfm?id=185. Accessed on January 6, 2012.

National Human Genome Research Institute. (2014). *Regulation of genetic tests.* Retrieved from http://www.genome.gov/10002335. Accessed on January 17, 2014.

National Human Genome Research Institute & E. K. S. N. I. o. C. H. a. H. D. (2013). *NIH program explores the use of genomic sequencing in newborn healthcare.* Retrieved from http://www.genome.gov/27554919. Accessed on January 8, 2014.

National Institute of Standards. (2012). NIST cloud computing standards roadmap. http://www.nist.gov/itl/cloud/upload/NIST_SP-500-291_Version-2_2013_June18_FINAL.pdf. Accessed December 19, 2014.

Office of Surveillance, Epidemiology, and Laboratory Services, Public Health Genomics, & Centers for Disease Control and Prevention. (2010, December 12). *ACCE model list of 44 targeted questions aimed at a comprehensive review of genetic testing.* Retrieved from http://www.cdc.gov/genomics/gtesting/ACCE/acce_proj.htm. Accessed on February 1, 2011.

Overby, C. L., & Tarczy-Hornoch, P. (2013). Personalized medicine: Challenges and opportunites for translational bioinformatics. *Personalized Medicine, 10*(5), 453–462.

Phimister, E. G., Feero, W. G., & Guttmacher, A. E. (2012). Realizing genomic medicine. The *New England Journal of Medicine, 366*(8), 757–759.

Presidential Commission for the Study of Bioethical Issues. (2013). *Anticipate and communicate: Ethical management of incidental and secondary findings in the clinical, research, and direct-to-consumer contexts.* Bioethics.

gov: Presidential Commission for the Study of Bioethical Issues. Retrieved from http://bioethics.gov/sites/default/files/FINALAnticipateCommunicate_PCSBI_0.pdf

Quackenbush, J. (2002). Microarray data normalization and transformation. *Nature Genetics Supplement, 32*, 496–501.

Registry. (2014). *Genetic Testing Registry*. Retrieved from http://www.ncbi.nlm.nih.gov/gtr/. Accessed January 28, 2014.

Schwartz, M. K. (1999). Genetic testing and the clinical laboratory improvement amendments of 1988: Present and future. *Clinical Chemistry, 45*, 739–745.

The American College of Medical Genetics and Genomics. (2014). *American College of Medical Genetics and Genomics Practice Guidelines*. Retrieved from https://www.acmg.net/ACMG/Publications/Practice_Guidelines/ACMG/Publications/Practice_Guidelines.aspx. Accessed on January 10, 2014.

The American College of Obstetricians and Gynecologists. (2014). *Practice bulletin: Clinical pracitce guidelines for obstetricians-gynecologists*. Retrieved from http://www.acog.org/~/media/List%20of%20Titles/PBListOfTitles.pdf. Accessed on January 10, 2014.

The Cancer Genome Atlas. (2014). *TCGA program overview*. Retrieved from http://cancergenome.nih.gov/abouttcga/overview. Accessed on January 15, 2014.

Therapeutically Applicable Research to Generate Effective Treatments. (2014). *TARGET: Therapeutically Applicable Research to Generate Effective Treatments*. Retrieved from http://ocg.cancer.gov/programs/target. Accessed on January 15, 2014.

Therrell, B. L., Hannon, W. H., Bailey, D. B., Goldman, E. B., Monaco, J., Norgaard-Pedersen, B., ... Howell, R. R. (2011). Committee report: Considerations and recommendations for national guidance regarding the retention and use of residual dried blood spot specimens after newborn screening. *Genetics in Medicine, 13*(7), 621–624.

Ullman-Cullere, M. H., & Mathew, J. P. (2011). Emerging landscape of genomics in the electronic health record for personalized medicine. *Human Mutation, 32*(5), 512–516.

U.S. Department of Health and Human Services. (2013). *Discretionary Advisory Committee on Heritable Disorders in Newborns and Children*. Retrieved from http://www.hrsa.gov/advisorycommittees/mchbadvisory/heritabledisorders/. Accessed on January 7, 2014.

U.S. Food and Drug Administration. (2013, June 19). *Table of pharmacogenomic biomarkers in drug labels*. Retrieved from http://www.fda.gov/Drugs/ScienceResearch/ResearchAreas/Pharmacogenetics/ucm083378.htm. Accessed on September 17, 2013.

Wacholder, S., Hartge, P., Prentice, R., Garcia-Closas, M., Feigelson, H. S., Diver, W. R., ... Hunter, D. J. (2010). Performance of common genetic variants in breast-cancer risk models. *The New England Journal of Medicine, 362*(11), 986–993.

Wang, L., McLeod, H. L., & Weinshilboum, R. M. (2011). Genomics and drug response. *The New England Journal of Medicine, 364*(12), 1144–1153.

Wetterstrand, K. A. (2014). *DNA sequencing costs: Data from the NHGRI Genome Sequencing Program (GSP)*. Retrieved from http://www.genome.gov/sequencingcosts. Accessed on January 2, 2014.

Wolf, S. M. (2012). The role of law in the debate over return of research results and incidental findings: The challenge of developing law for translational science. *Minnesota Journal of Law, Science, and Technology, 13*(2), 1–9.

Wolf, S. M., Lawrenz, F. P., Nelson, C. A., Kahn, J. P., Cho, M. K., Clayton, E. W., ... Wilfond, B. S. (2008). Managing incidental findings in human subjects research: analysis and recommendations. *The Journal of Law, Medicine, and Ethics, 36*(2), 219–248.

Wu, J., Pfeiffer, R. M., & Gail, M. H. (2013). Strategies for developing prediction models from genome-wide association studies. *Genetic Epidemiology, 37*(8), 768–777.

Wung, S. F., Hickey, K. T., Taylor, J. Y., & Gallek, M. J. (2013). Cardiovascular genomics. *Journal of Nursing Scholarship, 45*(1), 60–68.

50

Global eHealth and Informatics

Amy Coenen / Claudia C. Bartz / Martha K. Badger

• OBJECTIVES

1. Describe international organizations and their roles in advancing global eHealth and informatics.
2. Discuss nursing's contributions to international health informatics initiatives.
3. Discuss applications of eHealth in the global health environment.
4. Explore current issues and trends for their effects on global eHealth and nursing.

• KEY WORDS

eHealth
Global health
mHealth
Nursing informatics
Telehealth nursing

Nurses are major stakeholder in the global healthcare community. As a profession, nursing has championed and contributed to a number of international health informatics and eHealth initiatives (Abbott & Coenen, 2008; Coenen, Marin, Park, & Bakken, 2001; Saba, Hovenga, Coenen, McCormick, & Bakken, 2003). While nursing and healthcare informatics are often described as sciences in the literature (Nelson & Staggers, 2014), eHealth is generally defined as a set of activities, processes, or means for the delivery of health services using information and communication technologies (ICT) at both the macro and the micro levels. More specifically, eHealth is defined as the use of ICT for health. Examples include using ICT for treating patients, conducting research, educating the health workforce, tracking diseases, and monitoring public health (World Health Organization [WHO], n.d.-a).

eHealth has been further described by the World Health Organization (WHO) as the transfer of health resources and healthcare by electronic means, encompassing three main areas (WHO, n.d.-b):

- The delivery of health information, for health professionals and health consumers, through the Internet and telecommunications.
- Using the power of IT and e-commerce to improve public health services, e.g., through the education and training of health workers.
- The use of e-commerce and e-business practices in health systems management.

The purpose of this chapter is to inform nurses about international eHealth initiatives and to describe the influence of nurses on these initiatives as well as how these initiatives will continue to influence the profession of nursing. eHealth policy and applications can be influenced by nurses in care delivery, education, administration, and research. This chapter includes a description of the roles of international health organizations in global eHealth and informatics, a discussion of eHealth applications in the global health environment with particular emphasis on the relevance to nursing, and an exploration of healthcare issues and trends in relation to global eHealth and nurses worldwide.

INTERNATIONAL ORGANIZATIONS INFLUENCING eHEALTH AND NURSING

With advances in healthcare technology, international health-related organizations have focused their efforts on exploiting the potential of eHealth for improvements in healthcare delivery and infrastructure. New programs and organizations are being established to respond to the development and growth of eHealth policy and applications internationally (Table 50.1).

International Council of Nurses

Founded in 1899, the International Council of Nurses (ICN) is the world's first and widest reaching international organization for health professionals. ICN is a federation of more than 130 national nurses associations, and represents more than 16 million nurses worldwide. The three goals of the ICN are to bring nursing together worldwide,

to advance nurses and nursing, and to influence health policy. The ICN is involved in initiatives related to professional nursing practice, nursing regulation, and socio-economic welfare for nurses. ICN promotes quality nursing care for all, with and through a competent and satisfied nursing workforce. ICN supports the advancement of experiential- and research-based nursing knowledge, which are hallmarks of a respected nursing profession (International Council of Nurses [ICN], 2013).

ICN represents the profession of nursing in a number of international venues, including the United Nations, World Health Organization, World Health Professions Alliance, other organizations discussed below. As the international voice for nursing, ICN recently added a new program with a focus on eHealth.

ICN eHealth Programme. The ICN eHealth Programme was launched in 2011 in response to the growing needs for professional participation in eHealth policies at the national and international levels. The ICN eHealth Programme encompasses three major initiatives:

- *International Classification for Nursing Practice (ICNP®)*, which is a terminology for nursing that provides an international standard for facilitating the description and comparison of nursing practice locally, regionally, nationally, and internationally

TABLE 50.1	List of International Organizations Influencing Nursing and eHealth	
Acronym	**Organization Name**	**Web Address**
HIMSS	Healthcare Information Management Systems Society	www.himss.org
	HIMSS Nursing Informatics Community	www.himss.org/get-involved/committees/nursing-informatics
HL7	Health Level Seven International	www.hl7.org
ICN	International Council of Nurses	www.icn.ch
	ICN eHealth Programme	www.icn.ch/pillarsprograms/ehealth
IHE	Integrating the Healthcare Enterprise	www.iheusa.org
IHTSDO	International Health Terminology Standards Development Organisation	www.ihtsdo.org
	IHTSDO Nursing Special Interest Group	csfe.aceworkspace.net/sf/projects/nursing_sig
IMIA	International Medical Informatics Association	www.imia-medinfo.org
IMIA-NI SIG	IMIA Nursing Informatics Special Interest Group	www.imia-medinfo.org/ni
ISfTeH	International Society for Telemedicine and eHealth	www.isfteh.org
ISO	Organization for International Standards	www.iso.org
WHO	World Health Organization	www.who.int
	WHO eHealth Unit	www.who.int/ehealth

- *ICN Telenursing Network,* which aims to involve and support nurses in the development and application of telehealth technologies

- *Connecting Nurses* initiative, which provides an online forum for nurses worldwide to share ideas, advice, and innovations

- Explore and support initiatives and programs internal to ICN adding ICT knowledge and capabilities as appropriate

The ICN eHealth Programme is based on the understanding that the visionary application of ICT can transform nursing and healthcare. The Programme aims to support eHealth practice, to be recognized as an authority on eHealth, and to position nurses as experts in the eHealth international community.

World Health Organization

The World Health Organization (WHO) is the authority for directing and coordinating health within the United Nations system. WHO provides leadership on global health matters such as shaping the health research agenda, setting norms and standards, articulating evidence-based policy options, providing technical support to countries, and monitoring and assessing health trends (http://www. who.int/about/en/).

Each year, WHO holds the World Health Assembly (WHA) in Geneva, Switzerland. The WHA is the decision-making body of WHO. ICN is a member of WHO, representing the profession of nursing. This past year (2013), eHealth was on the WHA agenda. A resolution (WHA66.24) on eHealth standardization and interoperability was approved and the importance of health data standardization as part of health systems and services was noted. (WHO, 2013).

World Health Organization Family of International Classifications. WHO has long maintained and used the International Classification of Diseases (ICD) for national and international reporting of morbidity and mortality statistics. In addition to ICD, WHO has developed the International Classification of Functioning (ICF) for documentation and reporting of functional abilities and health. A new endeavor under the leadership of World Health Organization Family of International Classifications (WHO FIC) is the development of the International Classification of Health Interventions (ICHI) which is a classification of interventions for use across all health professions.

International Medical Informatics Association

Established in 1989, the International Medical Informatics Association (IMIA) is an independent, non-governmental organization made up of national medical informatics associations, institutional (Academic and Corporate) and Affiliate Members, and Honorary Fellows. IMIA plays a global role in the application of information science and technology in the fields of health and biomedical informatics (International Medical Informatics Association [IMIA], 2013a).

International Medical Informatics Association-Nursing Informatics Special Interest Group (IMIA-SIG). IMIA has a Special Interest Group (SIG) that focuses on nursing informatics. Membership includes over 25 society (formerly country) representatives and several observer members. The SIG meets regularly at related informatics conferences (IMIA, 2013b). IMIA-NI aims to foster collaboration among nurses and other healthcare professionals to advance the development of nursing informatics. The Nursing Informatics SIG hosts an international conference every two years to promote the dissemination of new knowledge and research in the field of nursing informatics.

International Organization for Standardization

The International Organization for Standardization (ISO) is the world's largest developer of voluntary international standards. ISO standards provide state-of-the art specifications for products, services, and best practices, in an effort to make industry more efficient and effective. ISO was founded in 1947, and since then has published more than 19,500 standards and reports that address almost all aspects of technology and business, including health (http://www.iso.org/iso/home/about.htm).

ISO Technical Committee 215: Healthcare Informatics. ISO Technical Committee (TC) 215 for Healthcare Informatics has as its scope the standardization of health information resources, including health information and communications technology (ICT). The aim of the Committee is to promote interoperability between independent systems, to enable compatibility and consistency of health information and data and to reduce duplication of effort and redundancy (International Organization for Standardization, n.d.).

ISO TC 215 is also the body that is responsible for new standards that involve nursing informatics and telehealth nursing in the areas of terminology, telehealth, messaging, and a range of other topics related to eHealth. ISO

Technical Committees are composed of a set of different countries' Technical Advisory Groups (TAGs). The TAGs for TC 215 include individuals from standards development organizations, professional, governmental, or commercial organizations, as well as individuals representing themselves.

The recent approval of the new International Standard 18104 (Health Informatics, Categorical structures for representation of nursing diagnoses and nursing actions in terminological systems) is an example of a nursing-specific standard formalized by ISO. The new standard replaced ISO 18104:2003 Health Informatics—Integration of a Reference Terminology for Nursing (see Chapter 8). The purpose of Standard 18104 is to promote interoperability in healthcare systems. This ISO standard has been used to evaluate and support ongoing develop of nursing terminologies, especially in supporting the definition of high-level schemata in developing logic-based compositional terminologies such as ICNP (Hardiker & Coenen, 2007; Marin, Peres, & Dal Sasso, 2013).

International Health Terminology Standards Development Organisation

The International Health Terminology Standards Development Organisation (IHTSDO) is a not-for-profit organization based in Denmark. Its main purpose is to develop and maintain the Systematized Nomenclature of Medicine—Clinical Terms (SNOMED CT). SNOMED CT applications serve as an international, inter-disciplinary healthcare terminology. The organization focuses on supporting the implementation of interoperable, semantically accurate health record documentation (International Health Terminology Standards Development Organisation, n.d.).

As the voice for nursing internationally and as the developer of the ICNP, ICN is aware of the need to collaborate with IHTSDO to assure nursing domain content is available to nurses in IHTSDO member countries. In 2010, ICN announced a collaborative agreement with the IHTSDO to advance terminology harmonization and foster interoperability in health information systems (ICN, 2010).

ICN eHealth team members actively participate in the IHTSDO Nursing Special Interest Group with the aim of providing nurses with the resources needed to implement terminology to represent nursing practice in EHRs. The current focus of this participation is to harmonize ICNP and SNOMED CT. Results of these harmonization efforts include an equivalency table of ICNP nursing diagnosis and outcome concepts and SNOMED CT concepts. This table is available for download from the ICN Web site. The equivalency table is an early product of the ICN-IHTSDO collaboration. Nurses are invited to join ICN and the

IHTSDO Nursing Special Interest Group in this effort to advance the use of nursing terminologies in practice, administration, education, and research.

International Society for Telemedicine and eHealth

The International Society for Telemedicine and eHealth (ISfTeH) is a non-profit organization with close ties to WHO and ICN, as well as other international organizations. Its mission is to facilitate the international dissemination of knowledge and experience, as well as to support developing countries in the fields of telemedicine and eHealth. The ISfTeH is primarily an umbrella organization for national telemedicine and eHealth organizations and for individuals and academic centers working to integrate telehealth strategies and applications in healthcare. It promotes and supports telemedicine and eHealth activities worldwide, supports developing countries in the field of telemedicine and eHealth, and assists the start-up of new national organizations. The ISfTeH offers a variety of membership categories, including one for nurses.

The ISfTeH Telenursing Working Group is open to all interested nurses and other healthcare providers. Its mission is to provide a forum for exchange of knowledge and experiences of nurses and others who are working with or supporting nurses' use of eHealth applications (International Society for Telemedicine and eHealth, n.d.). The objective of the ISfTeH Telenursing Working Group is to support technology, business, and professional actions for telehealth nursing. These actions include advocating for increased use and evaluation of telehealth services by nurses; stimulating innovative ideas and promoting initiatives for further development of eHealth; supporting inter-disciplinary telehealth collaboration for improved healthcare delivery and outcomes; advancing nurses' knowledge and skills in telehealth through dissemination of research findings, education programs, and practice guidelines; and advocating for the ethical use of telehealth services. Nurses from around the world are active participants in the annual ISfTeH conference, Med-e-Tel, describing their work and research in eHealth, telehealth, and nursing.

Healthcare Information and Management Systems Society

Healthcare Information and Management Systems Society (HIMSS) is a global, not-for-profit organization focused on better health through ICT. HIMSS leads collaboratives and conferences to promote the positive use of ICT in healthcare. The HIMSS conferences in the USA, Europe, and Asia showcase exhibitors that represent commercial and non-commercial interests in the health ICT industry (Healthcare Information and Management Systems Society [HIMSS], n.d.-a).

In 2003, the HIMSS Nursing Informatics Community was founded in response to the increased recognition of the role of the nurses in health informatics. This new HIMSS community was intended to reach out to all nurses and promote involvement of those working in nursing informatics. The HIMSS Nursing Informatics Community provides domain expertise, leadership, and guidance to the organizations activities, initiatives, and collaborations with the global nursing informatics and eHealth communities. Nurses are invited to become members of HIMSS and the nursing informatics community (HIMSS, n.d.-b).

Health Level Seven International

Health Level Seven International (HL7) is a not-for-profit, standards development organization dedicated to providing a comprehensive framework and related standards for the exchange, integration, sharing, and retrieval of electronic health information that supports clinical practice and the management, delivery, and evaluation of health services. "Level Seven" refers to the seventh level of the International Organization for Standardization (ISO) seven-layer communications model for Open Systems Interconnection (OSI) at the application level. The vision of HL7 is to create the best and most widely used standards in healthcare in order to improve care delivery, optimize workflow, reduce ambiguity, and enhance knowledge transfer among all stakeholders, including healthcare providers, government agencies, the vendor community, fellow standards development organizations, and patients (Health Level Seven International [HL7], n.d.).

HL7 Nurses Group. The HL7 Nurses Group was started in 2009 during an HL7 International Working Group meeting. The goals of the HL7 Nurses Group are to explore how nurses can become more involved in the HL7 community, to exchange information, and to ensure that nursing practice and nurses are included in uses cases and criteria for the HL7 standards. Nurses are invited to join the HL7 Nurses Group List Service and to become involved in the group's efforts (HL7, 2014).

APPLICATIONS IN GLOBAL eHEALTH AND INFORMATICS

With new technologies, the collection, storage, and transmission of health data and information are changing the methods by which healthcare is delivered. Professional

nurses are leaders in this dynamic revolution to advance eHealth worldwide for health promotion, disease prevention, illness or injury care, and supporting a comfortable death. In this section, select applications for eHealth are discussed to provide an understanding of current nursing research, education, and practice in this area. Specifically, examples of innovations in the advancement of the Electronic Health Record (EHR) and Telehealth are described.

Electronic Health Record

The Electronic Health Record (EHR) is a longitudinal electronic record of patient health information generated by one or more encounters across care delivery setting. Optimally, the EHR supports and enhances quality of care with content appropriate to the healthcare setting and processes that enable decision support, outcomes reporting, and ease of use. As one of the major innovations in healthcare, the EHR has brought both challenges and hope for improved healthcare delivery systems and better health outcomes for people worldwide.

The EHRs developed in Denmark, New Zealand, and Sweden have been described as exemplars for EHR development in other countries looking to adopt national EHR solutions (Gray, Bowden, Johansen, & Koch, 2011). These three countries possess an advantage, in that their health authorities have strongly supported and promoted standardization, interoperability, and information sharing among healthcare providers.

The ability to document healthcare using standardized, interoperable system applications is recognized as essential to unleash the tremendous capacity offered by information sharing through the EHR. Electronic capture, storage, and retrieval of comparable health data across providers, settings, and specialties are the basis for meaningful use of the EHR. The development of the ICNP was based on understanding this need for a standardized, interoperable international nursing terminology.

Recent initiatives by international groups of nursing informatics experts include the following efforts to promote resources and tools for interoperable systems:

- ICN: An international unifying framework for nursing terminology, ICNP, has great potential for describing nursing practice, facilitating care transitions, and using consistent and accurate data for decision-making and policy development. It is only through its use in the EHR that the potential of ICNP will be realized. In addition to commercial software vendors and healthcare organizations being early adopters, a number of countries have endorsed ICNP as a national standard for nursing. ICN is developing resources to facilitate implementation of ICNP, such as ICNP Catalogs. Catalogs are subsets of ICNP content for use with select populations or in nursing specialty areas. Some examples of partnerships to create ICNP Catalogs are listed here:

- Clinical Care Classification (CCC): CCC is a nursing terminology representing nursing problems, interventions, and patient outcomes (Saba, 2012). In an effort to promote the use of nursing standards in the EHR, ICN partnered with SabaCare (developer of CCC) to harmonize nursing content and provide resources for nurses and EHR application developers. Finland has supported the national implementation of CCC. The ICNP-CCC catalog can facilitate re-use of these national data, as well as local data and information captured using CCC, at the international level.

- Community Nursing Data Set: The National Health Service (NHS) in Scotland has enabled community nursing teams to facilitate meeting the needs of people where they live and work. To maximize the healthcare records to enable person-centered, safe, and effective care and provide data for quality improvement, resource allocation, and workforce planning a minimum data set for community nursing was commissioned by the NHS. ICN and NHS in Scotland partnership facilitate the development of an ICN Catalog for community nursing that is available for nurses worldwide.

- Canadian-Health Outcomes for Better Information and Care (C-HOBIC): A suite of standardized clinical concepts that reflect nursing practice and are used to document and measure patient outcomes in EHRs was approved as a national standard by Canadian Health Infoway in 2012. Canadian Nurses Association (CAN), ICN, and IHTSDO work together to harmonize the concepts in C-HOBIC to help facilitating sharing data as in the EHR as patients transition across the various sectors of the health system.

- IHTSDO: For countries implementing SNOMED CT as an inter-disciplinary terminology for healthcare, nurses need to be involved and engaged in assuring the representation of the nursing domain content. As noted earlier in this chapter, ICN is partnering with IHTSDO to facilitate the harmonization of ICNP and SNOMED CT concepts

- WHO: With its worldwide influence, WHO has an opportunity to advance the reporting of health and illness globally through partnering with other professional organizations such as ICN in the achievement of standardization and interoperability. WHO-ICN collaborations have focused on harmonizing ICNP and ICF (Kim & Coenen, 2011) and on the development of an International Classification for Health Interventions (ICHI).

In addition to the potential of interoperable data and information, the EHR has the potential to change the relationship between the provider and the consumer. Imagine, as a nurse, that the clients you interact with in healthcare episodes, be they individuals, families, or communities, can access their health data and information in real time electronically. As the EHR evolves, nurses will use this new technology to support the shift from a provider-centered health system to a consumer-centric model of healthcare. Various EHR applications will facilitate nurses' access to their patients and the patients' access to their health providers.

Telehealth and mHealth in the eHealth Environment

Given the broad scope of eHealth and the use of ICT for health, the vast majority of nurses already use telehealth applications in their work. Telehealth nursing extends the capability and reach of nurses and aims to improve access and quality, while managing healthcare costs. While the use of technology changes the care delivery medium, and may necessitate new competencies, the nursing process and scope of practice are not significantly different in telenursing, whether in direct care nursing, education, or management (Schlachta-Fairchild, 2007).

From its establishment in 2009 to early 2014, about 300 members representing 64 countries have joined the ICN Telenursing Network. The membership represents nurses interested in or working in many different capacities. These include clinical practice (e.g., cardiovascular disease, pulmonary disease, intensive care, pediatric care, women's health, and mental health), education (both educators and nurses advancing their education), videoconferencing, tele-simulation, tele-counseling, tele-triage, telenursing standards and competencies development, rural and remote telehealth, community health, and industrial nursing.

Research reports involving eHealth applications can be found online and in print in almost all major journals related to healthcare and there are an increasing number of journals dedicated to telehealth research. Unfortunately, not all publications list researchers' credentials, making it somewhat difficult to identify nurse-led research, but careful scrutiny reveals nurses' involvement in almost every environment of telehealth care delivery and research.

The wide range of research known to be led by nurses or to include nurses among the research team reflects nursing's impact throughout healthcare. Examples include studies of nurses themselves (Farquharson et al., 2012; Kowitlawakul, 2011), nursing students (Chaung, Cheng, Yang, Fang, & Chen 2010; Glinkowski, Pawlowska, & Kozlowska, 2013), eICU (Rincon & Bourke, 2011), surgery (Inman, Maxson, Johnson, Myers, & Holland 2011), orthopedics (Jones, Duffy, & Flanagan 2011), neurology (Young-Hughes & Simbartl, 2011), communicable diseases (Côté et al., 2011), non-communicable diseases (Baldonado et al., 2013; Wakefield et al., 2012), and mental health (Badger, Segrin, Pasvogel, & Lopez, 2012; Sands, Elsom, Marangu, Keppich-Arnold, & Henderson, 2013). Nurses are essential in building the body of knowledge about telehealth applications and technologies in furthering healthcare access, quality, and cost management.

GLOBAL TRENDS SUPPORTED BY AND DRIVING eHEALTH

eHealth has influenced many changes in the health arena internationally. Three trends are discussed in this section: nurse care coordination, self-management, and health equity.

Nurse Care Coordination

Global trends are beginning to reflect the change in expectations of partnership among healthcare providers across various healthcare settings, the individual patient, family members, and community groups. Based on evidence (American Nurses Association, 2012) policy-makers at the local, national, and international levels are recognizing the importance of continuity of care to decrease costs and increase quality. With the increase in multiple health providers involved in one person's care and population mobility of both patients and health providers, countries are looking for solutions to reduce fragmentation of healthcare. In addition to increasing communication by using the EHR, another proposed solution is care coordination programs.

The American Academy of Nursing (Cipriano et al., 2013) offered a set of recommendations to guide the development of the EHR to support care coordination across the continuum of health service delivery. Along with the infrastructure needs, nurses' participation in identifying data and information needs for care coordination across settings and services will be essential. One committee in Integrating the Healthcare Enterprise (IHE), a non-profit initiative to engage healthcare professionals and industry to improve interoperability, is focused on patient care coordination (Integrating the Healthcare Enterprise, 2013). IHE has published a patient care coordination technical framework for testing that includes a patient plan of care profile based on data elements of the Nursing Process.

Huber and colleagues (Hübner, Kinnunen, Sensmeier, & Bartz, 2013) have promoted the work of IHE in coordination with their research in eNursing Summary profiles to advance exchange of nursing data and promote care coordination. Researchers in Germany (Hübner et al., 2012) and Finland (Häyrinen, Lammintakanen, & Saranto, 2010) have developed candidate models for an eNursing Summary. Both models include components of the Nursing Process. Understanding that context and environment impact local and nation implementation of standards, the question arises on whether there could be a universal concept or shared model of an international eNursing Summary. In an effort to engage more nurses around the globe, the researchers have proposed ongoing collaboration with IHE, ICN, and IMIA-NI to continue work toward an international eNursing Summary framework.

Clearly, care coordination is centered on the patient. A major focus of care coordination is to empower the patient as a partner in care. Promoting self-management has become an important component of nursing practice, especially in care of our aging population, persons with chronic illness, and those with known risks for health problems.

Self-Management

Concepts such as person-centered care (Bernabeo & Holmboe, 2013; Daley, 2012), person-centered medicine (Miles & Mezzich, 2011a; Miles & Mezzich, 2011b), patient-centered care (Bartz, 2013), and personalized medicine (Swan, 2012) are topics in today's healthcare literature in large part due to the recognition that the digital revolution has encouraged people to become more involved with their own health and wellness. An outcome of this involvement is the movement toward self-management, often supplemented with ICT in the person's home or other environments.

Literacy is one of many identified components included in the Individual and Family Self-Management Theory

(Ryan & Sawin, 2009). Further discussion about health literacy and digital literacy in the context of nursing and eHealth follows.

Health Literacy. The Health Promotion Glossary of the World Health Organization (WHO) states that, "Health literacy represents the cognitive and social skills which determine the motivation and ability of individuals to gain access to, understand, and use information in ways to promote and maintain good health" (WHO, 1998, p. 10). The word "use" distinguishes health literacy from health knowledge, wherein a health consumer may know a lot about health promotion and disease prevention, but is either unwilling or unable to translate this knowledge into action.

Baur (2011) purported that, of all the clinical disciplines, "nursing has a unique relationship to health literacy because nurses are responsible for the majority of patient, caregiver, and community health education and communication" (p. 63). Speros (2005) added that nurses are invested in increasing healthcare consumers' health literacy whose positive consequences include improved self-reported health status, lower healthcare costs, increased health knowledge, shorter hospitalizations, and decreased use of health services. Negative consequences of low health literacy include increased healthcare costs, poor adherence, medical and medication treatment errors, and "lack of skills needed to successfully negotiate the healthcare system" (Mancuso, 2008, p. 250).

A review of the literature revealed few publications by nurse researchers and practitioners about interventions to improve patients' health literacy. One study of a nurse-delivered, though not nurse-developed, health literacy intervention showed an increase in adherence to anti-retroviral medications among patients with limited reading ability (Kalichman, Cherry, & Cain, 2005). A second study of a nurse-tailored health literacy intervention regarding HIV medication adherence among African Americans resulted in no statistically significant difference between the control and intervention groups (Holzemer et al., 2006). Despite the lack of published intervention studies, the relationship between patients' and families' access to health information and their engaged in their own care has been supported (Schnipper et al., 2012). The importance of health literacy as a factor in promoting self-management will become more important with implementation of EHR and Telehealth. Nurses can take a lead in examining interventions in promoting health literacy across their multiple specialty areas (Fig. 50.1).

Schaefer (2008) concluded that health literacy interventions can be categorized into various types by mode of delivery, which include personal contact, computer, and written materials, as well as any combination of these

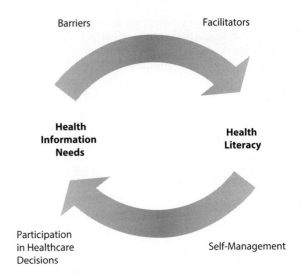

Barriers   Facilitators

Health Information Needs   Health Literacy

Participation in Healthcare Decisions   Self-Management

• **FIGURE 50.1.** Health Literacy Process.

types. Further, Speros (2011) suggested the following strategies to promote health literacy: creating a shame-free environment, using clear and purposeful communication, communicating in a patient-centered manner, reinforcing the spoken word, and verifying understanding.

Digital Literacy. The Internet has become one of the most ubiquitous sources of healthcare information. Digital literacy, therefore, has become an important component of health literacy for patients and healthcare providers alike. Gilster (1997) defines digital literacy as "the ability to understand and use information in multiple formats from a wide variety of sources when it is presented via computers" (p.19).

The Institute of Medicine (2011), in their report recommendations from their "Future of Nursing: Leading Change, Advancing Health" stressed the importance of digital literacy for nurses and other healthcare providers. Specifically, the IOM recommended healthcare organizations engage nurses and other frontline healthcare workers in the design, development, purchase, implementation, and evaluation of medical devices and electronic health record software. Early involvement allows nurses to ensure that new technology enhances, rather than hinders, their workflow and that nursing-based content is included in documentation software.

Digital literacy has the potential to enhance many aspects of human existence. According to the Bill and Melinda Gates Foundation (2013) access to information and knowledge is a great equalizer. It enriches lives, informs choices, and prepares people for meaningful employment and contribution to their communities. As part of the Gates funded initiative, a number of countries have benefited. In Chile, a national digital literacy campaign trained hundreds of thousands of people in basic technology skills, largely via a network of more than 300 public libraries. In Mexico, public libraries provide the only Internet access for nearly two-thirds of rural communities. In rural Botswana, public libraries serve as small business owners' offices, helping people make their businesses more sophisticated and competitive. In Ukraine, one community has used library Internet access to collect information about farming techniques, fundamentally changing the way they grow tomatoes and substantially increasing their crop quality and yield.

The European Computer Driving License (ECDL) Foundation (2013), which is known as the International Computer Driving License (ICDL) Foundation outside of Europe, recognizes the worldwide importance of developing a digitally literate society. However, digital literacy is not solely a matter of supplying hardware and software; it is also necessary to ensure that people have the requisite skills to use the technology effectively. In acknowledgment of this fact, a number of governments, education authorities, and not-for-profit organizations have launched initiatives aimed at raising the levels of digital literacy through training and certification. With health information systems expected to become increasingly important in enabling national health systems operate efficiently, the ECDL Health Information Systems Usage certification was designed for both health professionals and auxiliary staff, and has been introduced in the Middle East, the UK, Finland, Portugal, Italy, and Zambia. Professionals in the Pacific Islands are also benefitting from international digital skills training and certification, thanks to a new agreement with ICDL Asia.

Another effort to improve digital literacy is the Non-Roman Script Initiative (Non-Roman Script Initiative, 2013). The NRSI mission is to reduce barriers to using computers among language communities that do not use Roman script (e.g., Arabic, Khmer, and Chinese). NRSI's goal is to provide assistance, research and development for SIL International and its partners to support the use of non-Roman and complex scripts in language development.

PROMOTING HEALTH EQUITY THROUGH eHEALTH

Electronic commerce, commonly known as e-commerce, is the production, distribution, marketing, sale or delivery of goods, and services over the Internet or other electronic networks (World Trade Organization, 2014). The increased amount and velocity of exchanging products and information available are creating a revolution in the way that business is conducted. Access to the required technology to participate in exchange of products and information is an issue for eHealth. The population of the African continent is approximately 800 million, but only 4 million of them use e-mail (compared to 513 million globally) and of these, 2 million are based in South Africa (WHO, n.d.-b). Mobile broadband subscriptions across the world are increasing, while many people do not yet own a mobile phone.

In a 2014 position statement, ICN (2014) recognized that wealth influences readiness for ICT, with a clear demarcation between high-income countries and low-income countries. Nurses can demonstrate leadership in promoting policies at the global, regional, national, and local levels to provide the infrastructure and skills needed to make ICT a reality across all members of society, including both those receiving and those proving healthcare.

Nurses work with individuals, families, and communities to promote health, to prevent illness, to restore health, and to alleviate suffering (ICN, 2012). eHealth has the potential to transform both nursing and healthcare. eHealth is not just about the ICT, it is about using technology to collaborate, to communicate, and to advocate. At the same time, unless there is equity in access to technology sources of health information and knowledge, eHealth could serve to disenfranchise a large proportion of the world's population and a significant number of nurses and health providers in poor, disadvantaged areas of the world.

SUMMARY

Nursing informatics and global eHealth are inextricably linked. Several international organizations are committed to advancing global eHealth and informatics. Nurses are actively involved in these organizations and are making substantial contributions to international health informatics initiatives. These organizations include the International Council of Nurses, the World Health Organization, the International Medical Informatics Association, the International Organization for Standardization, the International Healthcare Terminology Standards Development Organisation, the International Society for Telemedicine and eHealth, the Healthcare Information Management Systems Society, and Health Level Seven International.

Nurses are also instrumental in the development and implementation of applications of eHealth in the global health environment, most notably through the electronic health record as well as telehealth and mHealth in the eHealth environment. Nurses are the driving force behind global trends that are supported by and driving eHealth, such as health literacy, nurse care coordination and self-management. One of the ultimate goals of eHealth is to promote global health equity.

REFERENCES

Abbott, P. A., & Coenen, A. (2008). Globalization and advances in information and communication technologies: Impact on nursing and health. *Nursing Outlook, 56*(5), 238–246.

American Nurses Association. (2012). *The value of nursing care coordination – A white paper.* Retrieved from http://www.nursingworld.org/care-coordination

Badger, T., Segrin, C., Pasvogel, A., & Lopez, A. M. (2012). The effect of psychosocial interventions delivered by telephone and videophone on quality of life in early-stage breast cancer survivors and their supportive partners. *Journal of Telemedicine and Telecare, 19*(5), 260–265.

Baldonado, A., Rodriquez, L., Renfro, D., Sheridan, S. B., McElrath, M., & Chardos, J. (2013). A home telehealth heart failure management program for veterans through care transitions. *Dimensions of Critical Care Nursing, 32*(4), 162–165.

Bartz, C. C. (2013). Evidence for person-centeredness in telehealth research. *Journal of the International Society for Telemedicine and eHealth, 1*(3), 86–92.

Baur, C. (2011). Calling the nation to act: Implementing the national action plan to improve health literacy. *Nursing Outlook, 59*, 63–69.

Bernabeo, E., & Holmboe, E. S. (2013). Patients, providers, and systems need to acquire a specific set of competencies to achieve truly patient-centered care. *Health Affairs, 32*(2), 250–258.

Bill and Melinda Gates Foundation. (2013). *What we do: Global libraries strategy overview.* Retrieved from http://www.gatesfoundation.org/What-We-Do/Global-Development/Global-Libraries

Chaung, Y. H., Cheng, H. R., Yang, Y. S., Fang, M. C., & Chen, Y. P. (2010). The effects of a web-based supplementary program for facilitating nursing students' basic nursing skills. *CIN: Computers, Informatics, Nursing, 28*, 305–310.

Cipriano, P. F., Bowles, K., Dailey, M., Dykes, P., Lamb, G., & Nayor, M. (2013). The importance of health information technology in care coordination and transitional care. *Nursing Outlook, 61*(6), 475–489.

Coenen, A., Marin, J. F., Park, H., & Bakken, S. (2001). Collaborative efforts for representing nursing concepts for computer-based systems: International perspectives. *Journal of American Medical Informatics Association, 8*(3), 202–211.

Côté, J., Ramirez-Garcia, P., Rouleau, G., Saulnier, D., Guéhéneuc, Y. G., Hernandez, A., & Godin, G. (2011). A nursing virtual intervention: real-time support for managing antiretroviral therapy. *CIN: Computers, Informatics, Nursing, 29*(1), 43–51.

Daley, K. A. (2012). Person-centered care – what does it actually mean? *The American Nurse, 44*(6), 3.

European Computer Driving License (ECDL) Foundation. (2013). *International digital agendas.* Retrieved from http://www.ecdl.org/index.jsp?p=2275&n=2749.

Farquharson, B., Allan, J. L., Johnston, D., Johnston, M., Choudhary, C., & Jones, M. (2012). Stress amongst nurses working in a healthcare telephone-advice service: relationship with job satisfaction, intention to leave, sickness absence and performance. *Journal of Advanced Nursing, 68*(7), 1624–1635.

Gilster, P. (1997). *Digital literacy.* New York, NY: Wiley.

Glinkowski, W., Pawlowska, K., & Kozlowska, L. (2013). Telehealth and telenursing perception and knowledge among university students in Poland. *Telemedicine and e-Health, 19*(7), 523–529.

Gray, B. H., Bowden, T., Johansen, I. B., & Koch, S. (2011). Electronic health records: An international perspective on "meaningful use". *Commonwealth Fund, 28*, 1–18. Retrieved from http://www.commonwealthfund.org/~/media/Files/Publications/Issue%20Brief/2011/Nov/1565_Gray_electronic_med_records_meaningful_use_intl_brief.pdf

Hardiker, N. R., & Coenen, A. (2007). Interpretation of an international terminology standard in the development of a logic-based compositional terminology. *International Journal of Medical Informatics, 76*(Suppl. 2), 274–280.

Häyrinen, K., Lammintakanen, J., & Saranto, K. (2010). Evaluation of electronic nursing documentation - Nursing process model and standardized terminologies as keys to visible and transparent nursing. *International Journal of Medical Informatics, 79*(8), 554–564.

Health Level Seven International. (2014). *HL7 Nurse Group.* Retrieved from http://wiki.hl7.org/index.php?title=HL7_Nurse_Group

Health Level Seven International. (n.d.). *About HL7.* Retrieved from http://www.hl7.org/about/index.cfm?ref=nav

Healthcare Information and Management Systems Society. (n.d.-a). *HIMSS.* Retrieved from http://www.himss.org/Index.aspx

Healthcare Information and Management Systems Society. (n.d.-b). *Nursing Informatics Committee.* Retrieved from http://www.himss.org/get-involved/committees/nursing-informatics?navItemNumber=17321

Holzemer, W. L., Bakken, S., Portillo, C. J., Grimes, R., Welch, J., Wantland, D., & Mullen, J. T. (2006). Testing a nurse tailored HIV medication adherence intervention. *Nursing Research, 55*, 189–197.

Hübner, U., Cruel, E., Gök, M., Garthaus, M., Zimansky, M., Remmers, H., & Rienhoff, O. (2012). Requirements engineering for cross-sectional information chain models. *Proceedings of the 11th International Nursing Informatics Conference NI2012*, Montreal, Canada.

Hübner, U., Kinnunen, U. M., Sensmeier, J., & Bartz, C. (2013). eNursing Summary - Where global standardisation and regional practice meet. *Proceedings of Medinfo 2013*, Copenhagen, Denmark.

Inman, D. M., Maxson, P. M., Johnson, K. M., Myers, R. P., & Holland, D. E. (2011). The impact of follow-up educational telephone calls on patients after radical prostatectomy: Finding value in low-margin activities. *Urologic Nursing, 31*, 83–91.

Institute of Medicine. (2011). *The future of nursing: Leading change, advancing health.* Washington, DC: The National Academies Press.

Integrating the Healthcare Enterprise. (2013). *IHE patient care coordination.* Retrieved from http://www.ihe.net/Patient_Care_Coordination/

International Council of Nurses. (2010). *ICN and IHTSDO team-up to ensure a common health terminology.* Retrieved from http://www.icn.ch/images/stories/documents/news/press_releases/2010_PR_04_AC-ICNP_IHTSDO.pdf

International Council of Nurses. (2012). *The ICN Code of Ethics for Nurses.* Geneva, Switzerland.

International Council of Nurses. (2013). http://www.icn.ch/about-icn/about-icn/

International Council of Nurses. (2014). *Position Statement International Council of Nursing. The right to connect via information and communication technology.* Retrieved from http://www.icn.ch/images/stories/documents/publications/position_statements/E12a_Right_Connect_Information_Communication_Technology.pdf

International Health Terminology Standards Development Organisation. (n.d.). *About IHTSDO.* Retrieved from http://www.ihtsdo.org/about-ihtsdo/

International Medical Informatics Association. (2013a). *Welcome to IMIA.* Retrieved from http://www.imia-medinfo.org/new2/node/1

International Medical Informatics Association. (2013b). *SIG NI nursing informatics.* Retrieved from http://www.imia-medinfo.org/new2/node/151

International Organization for Standardization. (n.d.). *ISO Technical Committee (TC) 215 for healthcare informatics.* Retrieved from http://www.iso.org/iso/iso_technical_committee?commid=54960

International Society for Telemedicine and eHealth. (n.d.). *About the ISfTeH.* Retrieved from http://www.isfteh.org/about

Jones, D., Duffy, M. E., & Flanagan, J. (2011). Randomized clinical trial testing efficacy of a nurse-coached intervention in arthroscopy patients. *Nursing Research, 60*(2), 92–99.

Kalichman, S. C., Cherry, J., & Cain, D. (2005). Nurse delivered antiretroviral treatment adherence intervention for people with low literacy skills and living with HIV/AIDS. *JANAC: Journal of the Association of Nurses in AIDS Care, 16*, 3–15.

Kim, T. Y., & Coenen, A. (2011). Toward harmonizing WHO international classifications: A nursing perspective. *Informatics for Health and Social Care, 36*(1), 35–49.

Kowitlawakul, Y. (2011). The Technology Acceptance Model: Predicting nurses' intention to use telemedicine technology (eICU). *CIN: Computers, Informatics, Nursing, 29*, 411–418.

Mancuso, J. M. (2008). Health literacy: A concept/dimensional analysis. *Nursing and Health Sciences, 10*, 248–255.

Marin, H. F., Peres, H. H. C., & Dal Sasso, G. R. M. (2013). Categorical structure analysis of ISO 18104 standard in nursing documentation. *Acta Paulista de Enfermagem, 26*(3), 299–306.

Miles, A., & Mezzich, J. E. (2011a). The care of the patient and the soul of the clinic: person-centered medicine as an emergent model of modern clinical practice. *The International Journal of Person Centered Medicine, 1*(2), 207–222.

Miles, A., & Mezzich, J. E. (2011b). The patient, the illness, the doctor, the decision: Negotiating a 'new way' through person-centered medicine. *The International Journal of Person Centered Medicine, 1*(4), 637–640.

Nelson, R., & Staggers, N. (2014). *Health informatics: An Interprofessional approach.* St. Louis, MO: Mosby.

Non-Roman Script Initiative. (2013). *NRSI: computers and writing systems.* Retrieved from http://scripts.sil.org/cms/scripts/page.php?site_id=nrsi&id=

Rincon, T. A., & Bourke, G. (2011). Standardizing sepsis screen and management via a tele-ICU program improves patient care. *Telemedicine Journal and E-Health, 17*, 560–564.

Ryan, P., & Sawin, K. J. (2009). The individual and family self-management theory: Background and perspectives on context, process, and outcomes. *Nursing Outlook, 57*, 217–225.

Saba, V. (2012). *Clinical Care Classification (CCC) System version 2.5* (2nd ed.). New York, NY: Springer Publishing Company.

Saba, V., Hovenga, E., Coenen, A., McCormick, K., & Bakken, S. (2003, September). Nursing language: Terminology models for nurses. *International Organization for Standardization (ISO) Bulletin*, 16–18.

Sands, N., Elsom, S., Marangu, E., Keppich-Arnold, S., & Henderson, K. (2013). Mental health telephone triage: Managing psychiatric crisis and emergency. *Perspectives in Psychiatric care, 49*, 65–72.

Schaefer, C. T. (2008). Integrated review of health literacy interventions. *Orthopaedic Nursing, 27*, 302–317.

Schlachta-Fairchild, L. (2007). *International competencies for telenursing.* Geneva, Switzerland: International Council of Nurses.

Schnipper, J. L., Gandhi, T. K., Wald, J. S., Grant, R. W., Poon, E. G., Volk, L. A., ... Middleton, B. (2012). Effects of an online personal health record on medication accuracy and safety: a cluster-randomized trial. *Journal of the American Medical Informatics Association, 19*, 728–734.

Speros, C. I. (2005). Health literacy: Concept analysis. *Journal of Advanced Nursing, 50*, 633–640.

Speros, C. I. (2011). Promoting nurse literacy: A nursing imperative. *Nursing Clinics of North America, 46*, 321–333.

Swan, M. (2012). Health 2050: The realization of personalized medicine through crowdsourcing, the quantified self, and the participatory biocitizen. *Journal of Personalized Medicine, 2*, 93–118.

Wakefield, J. B., Holman, J. E., Ray, A., Scherubel, M., Adams, M. R., Hills, S. L., & Rosenthal, G. E. (2012). Outcomes of a home telehealth intervention for patients with diabetes and hypertension. *Telemedicine and e-Health, 18*(8), 575–579.

World Health Organization. (1998). *Health promotion glossary*. Geneva, Switzerland: *World Health Organization*.

World Health Organization. (2013). *eHealth standardization and interoperability*. Retrieved from http://apps.who.int/gb/ebwha/pdf_files/WHA66/A66_R24-en.pdf

World Health Organization. (n.d.-a). WHO definition of ehealth. Retrieved from http://www.who.int/topics/ehealth/en/

World Health Organization. (n.d.-b). *Trade, foreign policy, diplomacy and health: eHealth*. Retrieved from http://www.who.int/trade/glossary/story021/en/

World Trade Organization. (2014). *Electronic commerce*. Retrieved from http://www.wto.org/english/thewto_e/whatis_e/tif_e/bey4_e.htm

Young-Hughes, S., & Simbartl, L. A. (2011). Spinal cord injury/disorder teleconsultation outcome study. *Rehabilitation Nursing, 36*(4), 153–172.

PART 10

International Perspectives

Susan K. Newbold

51

Nursing Informatics in Canada

Lynn M. Nagle / Kathryn J. Hannah / Margaret Ann Kennedy

• OBJECTIVES

1. Describe key drivers advancing Canadian nurses' use of information and communications technology.
2. Describe key organizations supporting the advancement of health and nursing information management in Canada.
3. Describe key nursing informatics initiatives currently underway in Canada.

• KEY WORDS

Health information
Nursing data standards
Nursing outcomes
Information and knowledge management

INTRODUCTION

Registered nurses should advocate for and lead efforts toward the collection, storage, retrieval and use of nursing care data to generate information on nursing outcomes.... These data are essential to expand knowledge, to evaluate the quality and impact of nursing care, to promote patient safety and to support integrated health human resources planning.

—Canadian Nurses Association (CNA), 2006a

Nursing's role in the management of information has long been considered to include the information necessary to manage client care and the information necessary for managing clinical operations. Over the years, client care and nursing management decision-making has become increasingly underpinned by the use of evidence. Like nurses in many other developed countries, Canadian nurses integrate information from a variety of sources to inform practice and improve the quality and safety of care delivery. Moreover, having ready access to information about practice outcomes equips the profession with evidence to demonstrate the essential contribution of nurses.

Substantial investments in information and communication technology (ICT) have been made in all sectors of Canadian healthcare. Acute care, long-term care, primary care, public health, and community-based nursing settings have all begun to realize the benefits of using ICT to support clinical care and administrative activities. Nonetheless, in a majority of Canadian care environments, information management activities continue to require clinicians to use a combination of electronic and paper records. Much work remains to be done to achieve a fully functional Electronic Health Record (EHR) in many settings. In this regard, nurses' documentation of care plans, interventions, and outcomes is to a large extent still lacking standardization of data capture methodology and standardized clinical terminology that can be readily coded for use in information systems. In many organizations nursing documentation is not yet part of the EHR. Additionally, while likely not a unique situation, Canada's existing health information repositories do not include comprehensive information about the impacts of nursing practice.

741

The Canadian Nurses Association (CNA) has taken the position that registered nurses and other stakeholders in healthcare delivery require information on nursing practice and its relationship to client outcomes (CNA, 2006a). The creation of a coordinated system to collect, store, and retrieve nursing data in Canada is essential for health human resource planning, and to expand knowledge and research on determinants of quality nursing care. Across Canada, the engagement of nurses to effectively achieve this vision is being supported by a variety of initiatives. Several professional nursing organizations including the CNA and its provincial and territorial affiliates, the Academy of Canadian Executive Nurses (ACEN), the Canadian Association of Schools of Nursing (CASN), the Canadian Nursing Informatics Association (CNIA), and other nursing informatics interest groups across Canada have been instrumental in advancing and supporting nurses' involvement in health informatics. Their collective efforts have included the (a) active dissemination of relevant information, (b) provision of opportunities for informatics education, (c) development of entry to practice competencies, (d) promotion and deployment of nursing data standards, and (e) development of a national nursing report. In this chapter, we describe these activities in further detail and highlight some of the ongoing challenges faced by the nursing informatics community in Canada.

KEY FACTORS DRIVING NURSES' USE OF INFORMATION AND COMMUNICATION TECHNOLOGY

Canadians have a healthcare system that is the envy of many countries. One of the things that make the Canadian healthcare system unique is the belief in health as a right rather than a privilege or an economic commodity. This philosophy is reflected in the principles upon which the provincial and territorial health systems in Canada are based, and it is legislated through the *Canada Health Act* (Government of Canada, Minister of Justice, 1985) by which all Canadian jurisdictions abide. These principles include universality, portability, accessibility, comprehensiveness, and public administration. In addition, health is a provincial and territorial responsibility in Canada, not a federal one. Conformity on health matters between provinces, territories, and the federal government is by mutual consent and agreement, not legislation. The publicly funded health system in Canada provides about 70% of healthcare, the other 30% is paid for out of pocket or by health insurance companies. Despite the philosophical and financial underpinnings of Canadian healthcare, in the interest of

future sustainability, it has been identified as needing substantial reform (Kirby, 2002; Romanow, 2002). A common outcome of health system reviews conducted throughout the first decade of the twenty-first century was the recognition of information systems being key enablers (and lack of quality information as a key barrier) to health sector reform. Specifically, Kirby's (2002) report cited the significance of improving health information management in Canada:

> *EHR solutions will enable the creation, analysis and dissemination of the best possible evidence from across Canada and around the world as a basis for more informed decisions by patients, citizens and caregivers; by health professionals and providers; and by health managers and policymakers. They will also help maximize the return on ICT investments through alignment, and drive the development of common standards and interoperability* (p. 176).

As a consequence of such recommendations, federal and jurisdictional investments in ICT were accelerated across Canada during the last decade, resulting in information management and supporting technologies being central to the delivery of health services.

In addition, an aging demographic and ever-escalating costs associated with chronic disease management have driven an increase in the use of ICT such as telemedicine and telehomecare. These cost-effective approaches used to remotely diagnose, manage, and monitor disease have been successful in keeping Canadians in their homes and local communities as well as supporting nursing practice. Indeed the essential coordination role of nurses in telehomecare is unfolding at a rapid pace in some regions of the country (Ontario Telemedicine Network, 2014). With a greater emphasis on primary care and the local delivery of health services, care is being increasingly deinstitutionalized. Furthermore, in response to increasing demands for care, changes are occurring in the scope of medical and nursing practice including a greater role for nurse practitioners. Based upon the growth reported in 2011, the number of nurse practitioners has more than tripled over the last decade (Canadian Institute for Health Information, 2011). In summary, nursing remains a central player in evolving mechanisms of care delivery, impacting the health of Canadians more than ever before.

There is also an increasing trend toward consumerism in which self-help groups, disease-specific groups, and other special interest groups expect to be involved in their own care and the management of their health information. The power differential between caregivers and patients is equilibrating such that with the advent of the Internet consumers now have ubiquitous access to information about disease management, treatment options, and provider performance. Citizens are now utilizing ICT to communicate with clinicians and exchange information about their health. The face of healthcare delivery will be forever transformed through these changes and the Canadian nursing community is recognizing the need to respond.

These are but a few of the factors influencing the drive toward identifying the essential data needs of nurses. In Canada, initiatives by healthcare organizations to develop or acquire automated information systems have historically focused on the utilization of data for the purposes of resource allocation, patient-specific costing, and health outcomes monitoring. In this regard, nurses have been using tools like workload measurement systems for many years without a substantive impact on practice or care. However, with the implementation of EHRs Canadian nursing has an unprecedented opportunity to advance the adoption of standardized clinical terminology and begin the realization of data repositories that include a representation of nursing practice. Nurses' use of information systems in practice, administration, education, and research has become pervasive and this is reason enough to ensure that these systems optimally serve the profession.

SUPPORT FOR THE ADVANCEMENT OF EFFECTIVE NURSING INFORMATION MANAGEMENT

Key National Organizations

Canadian Institute for Health Information. Created in 1992, the Canadian Institute for Health Information (CIHI) is an independent, pan-Canadian, not-for-profit organization, established jointly by federal, provincial, and territorial ministers of health that provides essential data and analysis on Canada's health system and the health of Canadians. Information is derived from many sources including hospitals, regional health authorities, medical practitioners, and governments. This information is further supplemented from other sources to support CIHI's analysis and the generation of reports that focus on (Canadian Institute for Health Information, 2012):

- Healthcare services
- Health spending
- Health human resources
- Population health

In existence for more than two decades, CIHI has become an acknowledged and trusted source of quality,

reliable, and timely aggregated health information for use in understanding and improving the management of the Canadian health systems and the health of Canadians.

Canada Health Infoway. As CIHI and its various aggregated databases evolved and matured, the focus was on health indicators and population health as well as information to manage the healthcare system. The healthcare community came to realize that there was still limited information available to caregivers for use in supporting decision-making related to the clinical care of individuals and groups of patients or clients of the health systems. In October 2000, the federal government committed initial funding to support the development and coordination of pan-Canadian health information systems necessary to achieve an electronic health record (EHR). This funding was recognition, by federal, provincial, and territorial governments, of the potential of ICT to improve the efficiency, cost-effectiveness, access, quality, and safety of health services in Canada. The Federal/Provincial/Territorial Advisory Committee on Health Infostructure (Advisory Committee on Health Infostructure, 2001) set its top priority as the development of EHR and telehealth. The committee identified an immediate need to begin putting building blocks in place for the next stages of EHR development.

Incorporated in January 2001, Canada Health Infoway (Infoway) is an independent, not-for-profit organization funded by the federal government. Infoway jointly invests with every province and territory to accelerate the development and adoption of EHR projects in Canada. Strategic investments have been directed to each of the provinces and territories in support of initiatives that provide the foundation for an interoperable pan-Canadian EHR.

Most Canadian jurisdictions have the beginnings of a basic infrastructure in place to support an interoperable EHR including (1) client registries, (2) provider registries, (3) drug information systems, (4) laboratory information systems, (5) diagnostic imaging information systems, (6) telehealth systems, and (7) public health surveillance systems. These foundational systems are providing the basis for provincial and territorial EHRs. However, there continues to be considerable regional/local variation in terms of adoption between organization and clinical professions, e.g., some institutions are still using paper and some health professionals lag behind in terms of adopting technology. Beyond the data from the foundational systems, other key data elements to be included in the national and jurisdictional EHRs have yet to be confirmed. Canadian nurses have been working to ensure that jurisdictional EHRs include patient-centered information and clinical outcomes data. Presently, there is also substantial investment being directed to the deployment of primary care electronic medical records (EMR) to support physician practice and a growing nurse practitioner practice across the country (Canada Health Infoway, 2008).

Through Infoway's leadership, Canada became a charter member of the International Health Information Standards Development Organization (IHTSDO) in 2006. The development and deployment of health data and technical standards are germane to the evolution of an interoperable EHR, and Infoway recognizes the centrality of this work in the achievement of their mission. The emerging EHR will ultimately incorporate data related to patient assessment and interventions contributing to patient outcomes and providers' patterns of practice. As the single largest group of healthcare providers, it is imperative that nurses' contributions to care are captured in the EHR.

Canadian Nurses Association. The Canadian Nurses Association first established its eNursing Strategy in 2006. The eNursing Strategy was based on three principles: nurses' access, competence, and participation in the use of ICT in healthcare (CNA, 2006b). These principles have served CNA well in guiding its activities related to informatics. CNA has actively led, participated in, and/or provided a nursing perspective on numerous national health informatics initiatives such as the EHR and data standards, NurseONE, The Canadian Health Outcomes for Better Information and Care (C-HOBIC), NNQR, CASN's Competency Development activities, and Canada Health Infoway's National Nursing Reference Group. Each of these efforts will be further elaborated in the sections that follow.

Canadian Nursing Informatics Association. Although the cadre of Canadian nurses working in informatics roles continues to grow, it is clear that efforts are needed to increase awareness among all nurses about the relevance of informatics to the profession. In particular, nurse leaders in practice and education need to embrace and actively advance the health informatics agenda and assure that nurses are engaged. Across Canada, provincial nursing informatics interest groups emerged during the 1990s in various parts of the country; some have continued to grow and expand while others languished.

In 2002, the Canadian Nursing Informatics Association (CNIA) was established with the goal of engaging nurses in all sectors and in all roles. In 2004, the scope and growth of the CNIA's national membership and compliance with the CNA criteria, afforded the CNIA "Associate Group" status within the CNA. This status brings further acknowledgment and recognition to the CNIA, as they collaborate with CNA to review and influence relevant national nursing policy and strategic planning related to informatics.

The CNIA also has a formal alliance with Canada's Health Informatics Organization, COACH, which has facilitated the appointment of the Canadian nurse nominee to the International Medical Informatics Association Special Interest Group Nursing Informatics (IMIA SIG-NI). The IMIA SIG-NI provides an opportunity to engage with international nursing informatics colleagues and share our knowledge beyond national borders. Opportunities to further leverage respective expertise and experiences are under discussion with colleagues in the United States, Europe, South America, and Australia. CNIA also maintains close relationships with several international colleagues who are trying to generate communities of interest in their own countries or to launch NI groups. Several international director roles have been established on the CNIA Board to enable mentoring and to share lessons learned from the Canadian experience.

The need to harness existing nursing informatics expertise, address the required informatics competencies of all nurses, and extend the profession's understanding of the significance of health informatics are key priorities for the CNIA. The overall objectives include the following:

- To provide nursing leadership for the development of nursing and health informatics in Canada
- To establish national networking opportunities for nurse informaticists
- To facilitate informatics educational opportunities for all nurses in Canada
- To engage in international nursing informatics initiatives
- To act as a nursing advisory group in matters of nursing and health informatics
- To expand awareness of nursing informatics to all nurses and the healthcare community

These objectives are being operationalized through a number of initiatives including biannual national conferences, a Web site, and a newly emerging informatics journal.

National Nursing Reference Group. In 2009, in partnership with the CNA, the Canada Health Infoway Clinical Adoption group established a nursing reference group (NRG) that includes practicing nurses, national nursing associations, and other provincial nursing leaders and informatics experts. The purpose of the NRG is to provide national nursing leadership, engagement, expertise, and input to inform Infoway's nursing strategy and plans to accelerate nursing's adoption and realization of the benefits of EHRs. The objectives of the NRG are to:

- Provide strategic-level advice and input on policies, priorities, and strategic plans aligned with Infoway's Clinical Adoption business strategy and clinical engagement
- Review and provide feedback on products, services, and projects under consideration, or being implemented where appropriate
- Provide strategic input on the needs and engagement of nurses in practice, education, policy, administration, and research
- Provide ongoing oversight and input into the established six key nursing strategic directions and tactical plans and associated working groups
- Act as liaisons and promote a coordinated approach of activities and strategies within their organizations and across partners

In May 2009, six strategic goals were developed and preliminary action plans were established to accelerate nursing engagement and EHR adoption:

1. Identification of nursing key business and functional requirements
2. Development of a structure and strategy for collaboration
3. Development of an education strategy
4. Development of a communications strategy
5. Advancing and leveraging the C-HOBIC implementation
6. Advancing and leveraging the NurseONE portal

In March 2010, the NRG met to review the previously identified nursing components of health information and to validate that these were still relevant and appropriate for inclusion in EHRs. The group overwhelmingly endorsed the elements as being relevant and worthy of continued development for capture within EHRs. Furthermore, the NRG supported the continued deployment and development of C-HOBIC and the need to secure additional funding to support this work. The NRG continues to meet annually.

Key National Initiatives Advancing Informatics in Nursing

NurseONE (www.nurseone.ca). NurseOne is an innovative, Web-based portal created and maintained by the Canadian Nurses Association (CNA) as a service for its members to assist them in "keeping current, credible,

competent, and connected" (CNA, 2014). Through this Web-based health information service, nurses and nursing students across the county can connect with each other through communities of practice and to credible, up-to-date electronic resources that support patient care and tools for lifelong learning such as, e-books, e-learning courses, specialty libraries, databases, Webliographies, continuing education Webinars.

Entry to Practice Informatics Competencies for Nurses. Among the issues related to the realization of effective information management among nurses in Canada is need for the inclusion of nursing informatics competencies in basic nursing education programs. At the time of writing, there is still a limited number of nursing education programs in Canada offering an informatics course or content about the use of ICT, and information management techniques and strategies related to nursing. Ideally such courses would also introduce concepts and provide hands-on experience related to the use of ICT in practice.

In 2011, the Canadian Association of Schools of Nursing (CASN) secured funding from Canada Health Infoway to develop entry-to-practice nursing informatics competencies and a toolkit to support faculty delivering the essential content. The competencies were created using consensus-based, iterative process, involving key stakeholders from across Canada. When the process concluded one over-arching competency statement reflective of the three competency domains and their associated indicators were identified as inclusive of the requisite knowledge and skills for nurses (see Table 51.1) (CASN, 2012). The published competency document also includes an articulation of the expectation that prior to admission, students will likely have already acquired a number of basic computer literacy competencies related to device and application use.

The informatics teaching toolkit was developed as a companion document to the competencies. The toolkit provides strategies and methods (e.g., relevant content, examples of integration within existing courses, downloadable slide presentations) to support faculty with the assimilation of informatics content into undergraduate curricula (CASN, 2013).

As nursing practice is increasingly enabled by technology, it is essential that basic nursing programs embrace nursing informatics. The national development of entry-level nursing informatics competencies has been a key step to ensuring that this occurs. In conjunction with nursing faculty members' use of the supporting resource toolkit, there is an expectation that these competencies will have an impact on nursing curricula across Canada.

TABLE 51.1   Nursing Informatics Entry-to-Practice Competencies for Registered Nurses (2012)

Over-arching competency: Uses information and communication technologies to support information synthesis in accordance with professional and regulatory standards in the delivery of patient/client care.

Information and Knowledge Management

Competency: Uses relevant information and knowledge to support the delivery of evidence-informed patient/client care.

Indicators:

- Performs search and critical appraisal of online literature and resources (e.g., scholarly articles, Web sites, and other appropriate resources) to support clinical judgment, and evidence-informed decision-making.
- Analyzes, interprets, and documents pertinent nursing data and patient data using standardized nursing and other clinical terminologies (e.g., ICNP, C-HOBIC, and SNOMED-CT, etc.) to support clinical decision-making and nursing practice improvements.
- Assists patients and their families to access, review, and evaluate information they retrieve using ICTs (i.e., current, credible, and relevant) and with leveraging ICTs to manage their health (e.g., social media sites, smart phone applications, online support groups, etc.).
- Describes the processes of data gathering, recording, and retrieval, in hybrid or homogenous health records (electronic or paper), and identifies informational risks, gaps, and inconsistencies across the healthcare system.
- Articulates the significance of information standards (i.e., messaging standards and standardized clinical terminologies) necessary for interoperable electronic health records across the healthcare system.
- Articulates the importance of standardized nursing data to reflect nursing practice, to advance nursing knowledge, and to contribute to the value and understanding of nursing.
- Critically evaluates data and information from a variety of sources (including experts, clinical applications, databases, practice guidelines, relevant Web sites, etc.) to inform the delivery of nursing care.

Professional and Regulatory Accountability

Competency: Uses ICTs in accordance with professional and regulatory standards and workplace policies.

Indicators:

- Complies with legal and regulatory requirements, ethical standards, and organizational policies and procedures (e.g., protection of health information, privacy, and security).
- Advocates for the use of current and innovative information and communication technologies that support the delivery of safe, quality care.
- Identifies and reports system process and functional issues (e.g., error messages, misdirections, device malfunctions, etc.) according to organizational policies and procedures.
- Maintains effective nursing practice and patient safety during any period of system unavailability by following organizational downtime and recovery policies and procedures.
- Demonstrates that professional judgment must prevail in the presence of technologies designed to support clinical assessments, interventions, and evaluation (e.g., monitoring devices, decision support tools, etc.).
- Recognizes the importance of nurses' involvement in the design, selection, implementation, and evaluation of applications and systems in healthcare.

Information and Communication Technologies

Competency: Uses information and communication technologies in the delivery of patient/client care.

Indicators:

- Identifies and demonstrates appropriate use of a variety of information and communication technologies (e.g., point-of-care systems, EHR, EMR, capillary blood glucose, hemodynamic monitoring, telehomecare, fetal heart monitoring devices, etc.) to deliver safe nursing care to diverse populations in a variety of settings.
- Uses decision support tools (e.g., clinical alerts and reminders, critical pathways, Web-based clinical practice guidelines, etc.) to assist clinical judgment and safe patient care.
- Uses ICTs in a manner that supports (i.e., does not interfere with) the nurse–patient relationship.
- Describes the various components of health information systems (e.g., results reporting, computerized provider order entry, clinical documentation, electronic Medication Administration Records, etc.).
- Describes the various types of electronic records used across the continuum of care (e.g., EHR, EMR, PHR, etc.) and their clinical and administrative uses.
- Describes the benefits of informatics to improve health systems, and the quality of inter-professional patient care.

Reproduced, with permission, from Nursing Informatics Entry-to-Practice Competencies for Registered Nurses. © 2012 Canadian Association of Schools of Nursing.

DEVELOPING THE NURSING COMPONENTS OF HEALTH INFORMATION FOR USE IN CANADA

In Canada, nurses are in the fortunate position of recognizing the need for nursing data elements at a time when the status of national health information was under review. The challenge for nurses continues to be how to capitalize on this timing and define those data elements required by nurses in Canada. To prevent losing control of nursing data, Canadian nurses are taking a proactive stance and mobilizing resources to ensure the development and implementation of a national health database that is congruent with the needs of nurses in all practice settings in Canada. Some initiatives intended to promote the vision of a national health database becoming a reality in Canada are in progress.

Health Information: Nursing Components

During the 1990s, the work of individual nurse leaders and the Canadian Nurses Association led to the 1997 consensus on five data elements: client status, nursing interventions, client outcome, nursing intensity, and primary nurse identifier.

- *Client status* is broadly defined as a label for the set of indicators that reflect the phenomena for which nurses provide care, relative to the health status of clients (McGee, 1993). Although client status is similar to nursing diagnosis, the term client status was preferred because it represents a broader spectrum of health and illness. The common label client status is inclusive of input from all disciplines. The summative statements referring to the phenomena for which nurses provide care (i.e., nursing diagnosis) are merely one aspect of client status at a point in time, in the same way as medical diagnosis.

- *Nursing interventions* refer to purposeful and deliberate health-affecting interventions (direct and indirect) based on assessment of client status, which are designed to bring about results that benefit clients (AARN, 1994).

- *Client outcome* is defined as a "clients' status at a defined point(s) following healthcare [–affecting] intervention" (Marek & Lang, 1993). It is influenced to varying degrees by the interventions of all care providers.

- *Nursing intensity* "refers to the amount and type of nursing resource used to [provide] care" (O'Brien-Pallas & Giovannetti, 1993).

- *Primary nurse identifier* is a single unique lifetime identification number for each individual nurse. This identifier is independent of geographic location (province or territory), practice sector (e.g., acute care, community care, and public health), or employer.

Identifying those data elements that represent the most important aspects of nursing clinical documentation for patient care is only the first step. Beyond their definition, there is the ongoing work of promoting and further developing the data elements and ensuring that they become integrated into an inter-professional, client-centred, pan-Canadian EHR. With every new government agency or initiative it is important to advocate for nursing data to be part of the inter-professional clinical data set.

In 2009, a nursing informatics think tank was hosted by the CNA and Infoway. It resulted in a renewed partnership with national nursing organizations representing nursing education, unions, nurse administrators, as well as professional colleges and associations that identified key strategies to advance nursing informatics in Canada (see National Nursing Reference Group previously in this chapter). The first strategy area is the identification of nursing requirements for the pan-Canadian EHR, including both required functionality for nursing and the nursing core data. Just over a year later, another forum attended by an even larger group of nursing leaders had moved the issue of nursing data forward to a renewed 2010 consensus that nurses in Canada require data on client assessment, nursing interventions, client outcomes, nursing intensity, and a unique nurse identifier. The forum also supported the position of the CNA, in advocating the International Classification of Nursing Practice® (ICNP®):

> The adoption of a single clinical terminology that… facilitates communication across all health settings, spoken languages and geographic regions, that has the capacity to represent client health data and the clinical practice of all healthcare providers…For a clinical terminology to adequately represent the practice of registered nurses across all regions and settings it, must be developed in collaboration with the International Council of Nurses…. The International Classification of Nursing Practice (ICNP®) which is compliant with international standards in a manner consistent with other disciplines. (CNA, 2006a)

The Canadian Health Outcomes for Better Information and Care (C-HOBIC) Project

Infoway has made an investment to support the early efforts to capture the "outcomes" dimension of patient care using nursing data. In the fall of 2006, the CNA partnered with the Ministries of Health in three Canadian provinces to undertake the inclusion of 32 nursing-sensitive patient outcomes measures in four categories in EHRs. Infoway provided funding for this work, launched as the Canadian Health Outcomes for Better Information and Care (C-HOBIC) project. This project supports the advancement and use of standardized patient assessments and related documentation. Further, these assessments enable the provision of feedback to nurses about patient outcomes and the ability to compare outcomes over time. Of additional value is that C-HOBIC provides an EHR adoption lever, providing information of use to nursing practice.

The C-HOBIC project builds upon work originating in the province of Ontario. A detailed history of this work is chronicled elsewhere (Nagle, White, & Pringle, 2007; Nagle, White, & Pringle, 2010; White & Pringle, 2005). The 32 C-HOBIC measures were derived from evidence in the nursing literature and are in four categories: functional status, symptoms, safety, and readiness for discharge. The measures are constituted by 32 data elements that are being collected in four sectors of the healthcare system: (1) acute care, (2) long-term care, (3) home care, and (4) complex continuing care. Each of the measures has a concept definition and an associated valid and reliable measurement instrument. As part of the C-HOBIC project, the concepts originally identified in Ontario were mapped to the International Classification of Nursing Practice®. The specific details of this mapping are reported elsewhere (Kennedy, 2008). Hannah, White, Nagle, and Pringle (2009) have provided more details about the C-HOBIC initiative in another publication. Experience with C-HOBIC to date indicates that these outcome measures can be collected using standardized tools across the healthcare system. Moreover, the nurses using the measures are deriving value in addressing clinical care issues and quality improvement for their patients and clients.

In Canada, nurses have come to recognize the need to incorporate nursing data into the national health information infostructure (i.e., national databases and EHR) as federal, provincial, and territorial health information systems are being restructured. To ensure that nursing data are incorporated into the national health infostructure, nurses must participate in the design, standards development, and pilot studies to ensure the capture of data that are essential to reflect nursing's contribution to healthcare in Canada.

As nurses in Canada pursue the development of core nursing data for inter-professional clinical information systems, several issues are germane. The first need is to ensure that data are available, reliable, valid, and comparable (i.e., data standards are established). To this end,

the CNA has endorsed the ICNP® for use in Canada. It is also important to define the scope of the compiled data set to ensure that only those essential data elements are collected and to avoid proliferation of data, i.e., C-HOBIC data. In addition, it is essential to promote the concept to ensure widespread use and educate the nurses to ensure the quality of the data that are collected.

National Nursing Quality Report-Canadian

Conceived in 2010 under the leadership of the Academy of Canadian Executive Nurses (ACEN) and the Canadian Nurses Association (CNA), the National Nursing Quality Report-Canadian (NNQR-C) is a pilot project to determine the feasibility of using outcomes and productivity indicators to establish a monitoring system for health professionals, utilizing existing databases (HOBIC/C-HOBIC, Resident Assessment Instrument—interRAI, Discharge Abstract Database-DAD, Management Information Systems-MIS) (VanDeVelde-Coke et al., 2012) The goals are to:

- Implement a national nursing quality report (NNQR-C)
- Evaluate the feasibility and costs associated with producing the indicators for healthcare organizations
- Evaluate the potential of these indicators to impact organizational quality improvement and quality outcomes

The NNQR is envisioned as a minimum set of input, process, and outcome indicators that can be collected nationally across the continuum of care; can be readily available through dashboard applications in healthcare institutions; and can be used as benchmarks to influence policy directions for nursing to improve client outcomes in all care settings. There are 15 indicators in the three categories of structure, process, and outcome. There are 10 pilot sites from acute care, long-term care, and inpatient mental health, representing the provinces of Manitoba, Ontario, New Brunswick, and Nova Scotia. The initiative has received a funding contribution from Canada Health Infoway as well as support from the sponsoring and participating organizations.

INFLUENCING NURSING INFORMATICS GLOBALLY: C-HOBIC, ICNP®, AND SNOMED-CT

In keeping with the progression toward systematically representing nursing data, CNA formally endorsed the International Classification for Nursing Practice (ICNP®)

in 2001 for use in Canada "as a foundational classification system for nursing practice in Canada" (CNA, 2001). This endorsement was renewed in 2006 as CNA continued to promote accurate and timely capture of nursing data (CNA, 2006a). The International Council of Nurses (ICN) goals of increasing the visibility of nursing contributions in healthcare, standardization of nursing data to support inter-sectoral comparability and analysis, as well as supporting evidence-based practice were highly aligned to the nursing goals in Canada, and Canada has actively contributed to the progression of ICNP® through research (Lowen, 1999; Kennedy, 2005; Kennedy & Hannah, 2007; Imam, 2009) and other professional contributions (Frisch, 2009; Stanton, 2006).

As the C-HOBIC work progressed, extensive collaboration led to the development and approval of the ICNP® Catalogue, Nursing Outcomes Indicators (available: http://www.icn.ch/pillarsprograms/icnpr-catalogues/). This was the first formally approved and accepted Canadian catalogue or subset of ICNP® available for international use.

Although Canada Health Infoway, in consultation with various stakeholder groups, adopted the Systematized Nomenclature of Medicine—Clinical Terms (SNOMED CT®) as the terminology for the pan-Canadian electronic health record, ICNP® remained the preferred terminology for nursing.

In March 2010, ICN and the International Health Terminology Standards Development Organization (IHTSDO) agreed to collaborate to harmonize terms in their two resources, further supporting interoperability (IHTSDO, 2010). Through this process, extensive efforts to cross-map and harmonize terms have improved both ICNP® and SNOMED CT®, resulting in numerous change requests for refinement of terms and new terms. The Nursing Outcome Indicators catalogue has been used as a demonstration project for this purpose and has been cross-mapped to SNOMED CT. On January 20, 2014, the International Council of Nurses (ICN) and the International Health Terminology Standards Development Organisation (IHTSDO) announced an equivalency table between the International Classification for Nursing Practice (ICNP®) concepts and SNOMED CT concepts (ICN, 2014). The table contains ICNP® Diagnosis and Outcomes Statements that have semantic equivalencies with SNOMED CT concepts.

CONCLUSION

It is clear that a continued priority for nursing in Canada is the deployment of solutions that support the capture and retrieval of essential nursing data. Further, Canadian nursing leaders are actively pursuing the vision to include these as core elements in a national health information database. There is no question that progress has been made during the last decade, but nursing leaders must continue to respond to the challenge to further advance this agenda. Early experience with the collection and use of the C-HOBIC measures demonstrates the great potential of a common clinical data set utilized across care settings. Establishing a standardized set of nursing components for health information has the potential to provide nurses with the data required to transform nursing into a profession prepared to respond to the health needs of Canadians in the twenty-first century; however, the window of opportunity to have nursing data elements included in a national data set is narrowing. We must continue our efforts to ensure that the vision of nursing components in our national health information system becomes a reality for nursing in Canada.

REFERENCES

Advisory Committee on Health Infostructure. (2001). *Tactical plan for a pan-canadian health infostructure: 2001 update.* Ottawa, Canada: Office of Health and the Information Highway, Health Canada.

Alberta Association of Registered Nurses (AARN). (1994). *Client status, nursing intervention and client outcome taxonomies: A background paper.* Edmonton, Canada: Author.

Government of Canada, Minister of Justice (1985). Canada Health Act. Retrieved from: http://laws-lois.justice.gc.ca, December 12, 2014.

Canada Health Infoway. (2008). *Infoway's investment programs.* Retrieved from http://www.infoway-inforoute.ca/lang-en/about-infoway/approach/investment-programs. Accessed on March 18, 2014.

Canadian Association of Schools of Nursing (CASN). (2012). *Nursing informatics entry to practice competencies for registered nurses.* Retrieved from http://casn.ca/vm/newvisual/attachments/856/Media/NursingInformaticsEntryToPractice CompetenciesFINALENG.pdf. Accessed on March 18, 2014.

Canadian Association of Schools of Nursing (CASN). (2013). *Nursing informatics teaching toolkit.* Retrieved from http://casn.ca/vm/newvisual/attachments/856/Media/2013ENNursingInformaticsTeachingToolkit.pdf. Accessed on March 18, 2014.

Canadian Institute for Health Information. (2011). *Canada's health care providers – 2011 provincial profiles: A look at 27 health professions.* Retrieved from https://secure.cihi.ca/estore/productFamily.htm?locale=en&pf=PFC2160. Accessed on March 18, 2014.

Canadian Institute for Health Information. (2012). *Canadian Institute for Health Information 2012-2017 strategic plan.*

Retrieved from https://secure.cihi.ca/estore/product Series.htm?pc=PCC287. Accessed on March 18, 2014.

Canadian Nurses Association. (2001, November). *Position statement: Collecting data to reflect the impact of nursing practice.* Ottawa, Canada: Author.

Canadian Nurses Association. (2006a). *Nursing information and knowledge management.* Ottawa, Canada: Author.

Canadian Nurses Association. (2006b). *E-nursing strategy for Canada.* Ottawa, Canada: Author. Retrieved from http://www.cna-aiic.ca. Accessed on March 18, 2014.

Canadian Nurses Association. (2014). NurseONE. Retrieved from http://www.cna-aiic.ca. Accessed on March 18, 2014.

Frisch, N. (2009). *Teaching ICNP® at the University of Victoria in BC, Canada.* University of Victoria, British Columbia, Canada. Retrieved from http://www.icn.ch/details/2/35.html. Accessed on March 18, 2014.

Hannah, K., White, P., Nagle, L. M., & Pringle, D. (2009). Standardizing nursing information for inclusion in electronic health records: C-HOBIC. *Journal of the American Medical Informatics Association, 16,* 524–530.

Imam, F. (2009). *Paraconsistency in healthcare ontologies.* Unpublished Master's Thesis. St. Francis Xavier University, Antigonish, NS, Canada.

International Council of Nurses (ICN). (2014, January 20). Press Release. *International Council of Nurses (ICN) and International Health Terminology Standards Development Organization (IHTSDO) partner to provide a new Informatics Resources for nurses.* Geneva, Switzerland, Copenhagen, Denmark. Retrieved from http://www.icn.ch/images/stories/documents/news/press_releases/2014_PR_02_ICNP_SNOMED.pdf. Accessed on March 18, 2014.

International Health Terminology Standards Development Organization (IHTSDO). (2010). *The International Council of Nurses and IHTSDO.* Retrieved from http://www.ihtsdo.org/about-ihtsdo/partnerships/icn. Accessed on December 12, 2014.

Kennedy, M. A. (2005). *Packaging nursing as politically potent: A Critical reflexive cultural studies approach to nursing informatics.* (Unpublished doctoral dissertation). University of South Australia, Adelaide, Australia.

Kennedy, M. A. (2008). *Mapping Canadian clinical outcomes in ICNP.* Retrieved from http://c-hobic.cna-aiic.ca/documents/pdf/ICNP_Mapping_2008_e.pdf. Accessed on March 18, 2014.

Kennedy, M. A., & Hannah, K. (2007). Representing nursing practice: Evaluating the effectiveness of a nursing

classification system. *Canadian Journal of Nursing Research, 39*(7), 58–79.

Kirby, M. J. L. (2002). *The health of Canadians – The federal role. Final report on the state of the health care system in Canada.* Retrieved from http://www.parl.gc.ca/content/sen/committee/372/soci/rep/repoct02vol6-e.htm. Accessed on March 18, 2014.

Lowen, E. (1999). *The use of the International Classification for Nursing Practice® for capturing community-based nursing practice.* Unpublished Master's Thesis. University of Manitoba, Winnipeg, MB, Canada.

Marek, K., & Lang, N. (1993). Nursing sensitive outcomes. *Papers From the Nursing Minimum Data Set Conference* (pp. 100–120). Ottawa, Canada: Canadian Nurses Association.

McGee, M. (1993). Response to V. Saba's paper on Nursing Diagnostic Schemes. *Papers From the Nursing Minimum Data Set Conference* (pp. 64–67). Ottawa, Canada: Canadian Nurses Association.

Nagle, L. M., White, P., & Pringle, D. (2007). Collecting outcomes in spite of our systems. *Canadian Journal of Nursing Informatics, 2*(3), 4–8.

Nagle, L. M., White, P., & Pringle, D. (2010). Realizing the benefits of standardized measures of clinical outcomes. *Electronic Healthcare, 9*(2), e3–e9.

O'Brien-Pallas, L., & Giovannetti, P. (1993). Nursing intensity. *Papers From the Nursing Minimum Data Set Conference* (pp. 68–76). Ottawa, Canada: Canadian Nurses Association.

Ontario Telemedicine Network. (2014). *Improving the lives of those with chronic disease through telehomecare.* Retrieved from http://www.otn.ca/en/programs/telehomecare. Accessed on March 18, 2014.

Romanow, R. (2002). *Building on values – The future of health care in Canada.* Ottawa, Canada: Government of Canada.

Stanton, S. (2006). *First Nations and Inuit Health Branch (FNIHB) of Health Canada Nursing Documentation System.* Ottawa, Canada: Author. Retrieved from http://www.icn.ch/details/2/32.html. Accessed on March 18, 2014.

VanDeVelde-Coke, S., Doran, D., Grinspun, D., Hayes, L., Boal, A.S., Velji, K., ... Hannah, K. (2012). Measuring outcomes of nursing care, improving the health of Canadians: NNQR (C), C-HOBIC and NQuiRE. *Nursing Leadership. 25*(2), 26–37.

White, P., & Pringle, D. (2005). Collecting patient outcomes for real: The Nursing and Health Outcomes Project. *Canadian Journal of Nursing Leadership, 18*(1), 26–33.

52

Nursing Informatics in Europe

Kaija Saranto / Virpi Jylhä / Ulla-Mari Kinnunen / Eija Kivekäs

• OBJECTIVES

1. Describe elements of the European Union eHealth initiatives.
2. Describe nursing terminology work in Europe.
3. Give examples of nursing informatics education in Europe.
4. Give examples of nursing informatics cooperation in Europe.
5. Describe possibilities of meaningful use of structured data.
6. Describe a national model for documenting nursing and implementing an electronic nursing care plan.
7. Give examples of future developments.

• KEY WORDS

Europe
Education
eHealth
Electronic health records
Health and nursing informatics
Nursing documentation
Terminologies
Standards

INTRODUCTION

The number of sovereign states in Europe is 50. This is not surprising for a continent, but when considering that the European Union has 28 member states and recognizes 24 official languages (European Union, 2012), the complexity of this geographical area becomes evident. The role of the European Union in both healthcare policy and practice has become increasingly important due to directives launched by the European Union Council. These initiatives, focused on specific developments and actions, have strengthened equality, quality, and safety among healthcare services for citizens in every country in the European Union.

The European Union plays an integral part in supporting research and development activities through various initiatives and programs that have created advances in both education and health. Concerning nursing, there are many formal and informal communities working toward joint efforts at the European level. Whether discussing education, practice, management, or research, the combining factor seems to be enthusiasm. This chapter focuses on the important subject of eHealth initiatives from the perspectives of patient safety, nursing language, education, management, and practice. Finally, the national Finnish nursing documentation project is described as an example of implementing a standardized nursing terminology into an electronic health record (EHR) system.

NURSING INFORMATICS AS PART OF THE eHEALTH STRATEGIES

In 2010, Europe had 738 million inhabitants that constituted 10.7% of the world's population. The European Union includes most of Europe, with 28 member countries and a population of beyond half a billion. This is over 50% larger than the population of the United States, although the European Union is less than half its geographic area (European Union, 2012). However, the European Union's population is not spread evenly across the continent; some countries are more densely populated than others. For example, Malta has about 1300 inhabitants/km², whereas Finland has 15 inhabitants/km² (European Union, 2012). This creates challenges for health services. National health services are delivered in different ways throughout the European Union. Thus, the numbers of registered nurses (RNs) and physicians differ from country to country. Table 52.1 identifies the numbers of registered nurses and physicians in each member state as of 2008 (WHO, 2013).

TABLE 52.1	Number of Nurses and Physicians (Physical Persons, PP) and Nurses and Physicians (PP) per 100,000, Year 2011			
	RN (PP)	**Physician (PP)**	**RN (PP) per 100,000**	**Physician (PP) per 100,000**
Austria	66,586	40,634	79,072	48,254
Belgium	n/a	32,182	n/a	29,961
Bulgaria	34,879	28,384	47,464	38,626
Croatia	25,485	12,490	57,884	28,368
Cyprus	n/a	2,553	n/a	29,617
Czech Republic	88,807	38,171	84,605	36,365
Denmark	n/a	n/a	n/a	n/a
Estonia	8,664	4,372	6,466	32,629
Finland	57,496*	n/a	1,07,202*	n/a
France	587,080	199,920	90,161	30,703
Germany	944,000	312,695	1,15,433	38,236
Greece	n/a	69,435	n/a	61,447
Hungary	63,661	29,500	63,841	29,584
Ireland	55,600	12,215	1,21,533	267
Italy	399,835	248,723	65,886	40,985
Latvia	10,611	6,456	51,555	31,367
Lithuania	23,713	12,407	73,593	38,505
Luxemburg	6,031	1,429	11,635	27,568
Malta	2,951	1,348	70,997	32,431
The Netherlands	n/a	49,242[a]	n/a	29,636[a]
Poland	223,563	84,221	5,803	21,861
Portugal	66,857	42,054	6,333	39,835
Romania	118,129	51,153	55,084	23,853
Slovakia	33,880	n/a	61,933	n/a
Slovenia	17,214	5,121	83,869	2,495
Spain	252,813	184,000	5,481	39,891
Sweden	n/a	n/a	n/a	n/a
United Kingdom	560,233	173,420	89,724	27,774

Data from WHO (2013)
*2010

Some of the differences can be explained through skill-mix issues; in other words, the roles of nurses are varied from country to country.

Although the European Union includes many different cultures, and the ways that healthcare is organized differ substantially from country to country, the national health systems face similar sets of challenges. Population growth has decreased and life expectancy has increased within the European Union during recent years, causing a transition toward an older population. By 2060, almost one-third of the European Union's population will be over 65 years old (17.4% in 2010) (European Union, 2012). Due to the aging population, the demand for health and social services is increasing. Further, the demand for health professionals is increasing, and many countries have already reported shortages of skilled nursing personnel. In the future it will be a challenge to balance supply and demand of nurses in the workforce. In addition to an aging population, higher income and educational level have some effect on the increased demand for services. Also, the expectations of citizens have increased; people are more conscious of their health and want the best care available (Commission of the European Communities, 2004). As use of the Internet has become more popular among citizens, it has also had an effect on the delivery of healthcare services. Thus, the traditional office visit model used in healthcare fails to meet citizens' diverse needs. Consequently, new ways of accessing health services and information should be introduced. European countries have to be able to fulfill citizens' needs and, at the same time, cut the increasing costs of healthcare services.

eHealth in European Union Policy Frameworks

Health informatics can offer solutions for these challenges. To promote the use of information and communication technology, the European Commission has produced several strategy initiatives, including the use of eHealth tools, to improve healthcare services. According to the eHealth Action Plan published in 2004 (Commission of the European Communities, 2004):

> eHealth is today's tool for substantial productivity gains, while providing tomorrow's instrument for restructured, citizen-centered health care systems and, at the same time, respecting the diversity of Europe's multi-cultural, multi-lingual health care traditions. There are many examples of successful eHealth developments including health information networks, electronic health records, telemedicine services, wearable and portable monitoring systems, and health portals. (p. 4)

More briefly, eHealth has been defined as health services and information delivered or enhanced through the Internet and related technologies (Eysenbach, 2001).

The European Commission introduced the eEurope initiative in 2000 (Commission of the European Communities, 2000). The purpose of this policy framework was to enable an information society for all Europeans and to ensure that the European Union was ready for the development of the information society, with the aim of creating fully integrated, interoperable, and modernized health systems using digital technologies. To achieve this, the European Commission published the eEurope 2002 Action Plan in 2000 (Commission of the European Communities, 2000). The aims of this plan, namely extending Internet connectivity and helping the member states adopt an existing legal framework, were achieved by 2002. Later in 2002, the eEurope 2005 Action Plan was released, focusing on utilization of broadband technologies, electronic health services, and improvement of the quality and cost-effectiveness of public services (Commission of the European Communities, 2002).

Europe's eHealth Action Plan

In tandem with the eEurope strategy initiatives, the European Commission introduced an Action Plan for a European eHealth Area in 2004 (Commission of the European Communities, 2004). The central points of the first eHealth Action Plan were information transfer, health and patient information, patient identifiers, mobility of patients and health professionals, infrastructure and health information networks, as well as monitoring the effects of new interventions.

The eHealth Action Plan included recommendations for disseminating best practices and experiences regarding eHealth applications across the European Union. The progress of eHealth application implementation was measured every two years during the period of 2004 to 2010. In addition, the Monitoring National eHealth Strategies study has analyzed the results obtained by European Union member states through 2009 (Empirica, 2009) and the eHealth Benchmarking study, funded by the European commission, aimed to analyze existing benchmarking sources. Based on the results of the benchmarking study, a European Union–level recommendation for eHealth benchmarking activities, including definition of indicators, data collection, and conclusions, was produced in 2009 (Meyer, Hüsing, Didero, & Korte, 2009).

In 2008, the European Commission published a recommendation on cross-border interoperability of EHR systems to support the goals of the eHealth Action Plan (Commission of the European Communities, 2008).

According to the recommendation, existing and future challenges of healthcare systems can be at least partly solved through implementation of eHealth applications. EHRs are a fundamental part of eHealth systems, and interoperability between information systems needs to be achieved in order to fully utilize the benefits of EHRs. The guidelines set minimum requirements for activities conducted by member states to ensure that EHR systems can work together across the European Union. In addition, the issues of evaluation and monitoring as well as education and awareness were introduced. The guidelines presented the following objectives (Commission of the European Communities, 2008):

- Establish elements of EHRs that should be exchangeable between systems.
- Enable health data to be shared among different healthcare systems.
- Build appropriate networked systems and services covering all healthcare areas.

Work to achieve interoperability continued in 2012 when the European Commission aimed to develop an eHealth European Interoperability Framework (EIF). The eHealth EIF is based on a generic European Interoperability Framework and it is meant to be an operational toolkit for stakeholders who participate to the deployment of eHealth systems. It should be noted that interoperability between information systems is not only a technical issue. Health data are always sensitive and trustworthy, thus, patient confidentiality and security are important. In addition, legal, ethical, economic, organizational, and cultural aspects need to be considered. The components of the eHealth EIF are as follows: governance, principles, agreements, the four levels of interoperability—legal, organizational, semantic, and technical—and the high-level use cases (European Commission, 2013).

Interoperability issues are one of the key aims of eHealth network. The network was established under the Directive on the application of patients' rights in cross-border healthcare (Klazinga, Fischer, & ten Asbroek, 2011). eHealth network is group of voluntary network of national authorities responsible for eHealth in European Union member states. The purpose of the network is to make guidelines in the area of eHealth in order to enable continuity of care and to ensure access to safe and quality healthcare (European Commission, 2014a).

National Roadmaps for eHealth

The eHealth Action Plan included a requirement for each member state to develop a national eHealth strategy in order to identify their current state and map a plan

for future development (Commission of the European Communities, 2004). National strategies focused on implementing eHealth systems, interoperability, utilizing EHRs, reimbursing eHealth services, and other related issues. Evaluation of national strategies conducted in 2008 showed that 25 out of 27 member states had formulated a national eHealth strategy (Hämäläinen, Doupi, & Hyppönen, 2008). Many of these strategies had links to national information society programs as well as to eEurope and i2010 information society programs. The Monitoring National eHealth Strategies study, published in 2010, showed that almost all European Union member states have detailed documents concerning eHealth goals, implementation, and achievements (Stroetmann, Artmann, & Stroetmann, 2011).

Finland introduced its eHealth strategy in 2007 (Ministry of Social Affairs and Health, 2007). It is based on the Finnish national information society strategy work started in the mid-1990s. The Finnish eHealth strategy has two main objectives: (1) to secure the access to information for those involved in care regardless of time or place and (2) to enable the involvement of citizens and patients, increasing the citizens' access to information and offering a high-quality of health information. The interoperability of information systems in healthcare is the starting point for information accessibility, and national-level legislation, recommendations, and specifications have been produced. The first aim is to attain interoperability between public and private service providers and then later between health and social welfare systems (Ministry of Social Affairs and Health, 2007). Electronic patient records already have a nationally defined structure, and the specification has been implemented in the information systems. In addition, several classifications and codes, such as the Finnish Classification on Nursing Diagnosis and Interventions, have been agreed upon. Finnish legislation supports availability of health information for citizens and Finland has already conducted implementation activities and plans. The core patient data are stored in the national electronic archive. The e-archive enables citizens to access their health data and e-prescriptions online. In addition, some regional Internet-based health services were introduced in Finland. The Hyvis portal, for example, is a free service District that complements regional health services and promotes the welfare of inhabitants by offering reliable information about health and healthcare services. The portal also includes the ability to make appointments for some healthcare services and to communicate with healthcare professionals. At the beginning of 2014, electronic services are under development and more possibilities are coming in the near future (Hyvis, 2013).

The role of health informatics, and certainly nursing informatics, has become increasingly prominent within the United Kingdom over the course of 2010. The U.K. Government is investing billions of pounds in developing information and communications technology (ICT) within the National Health Services to ensure that modernization and utilization of eHealth becomes a reality. All four countries now have national programs for ICT. In England, it is called NHS Connecting for Health; the Wales program is Informing Healthcare; Scotland has the eHealth program; and Northern Ireland's program is called HPSS ICT. A comprehensive list of the activities of each of these programs is beyond the scope of this chapter; see the Web sites below for additional information:

England: www.connectingforhealth.nhs.uk. Last updated 31 March 2013.

Wales: http://www.healthcarealliances.co.uk/Public/documents/AM0309IHC2.pdf

Scotland: http://www.ehealth.scot.nhs.uk/

Northern Ireland: www.dhsspsni.gov.uk (2013)

Toward eHealth Action Plan 2012–2020

In 2005, European Union introduced a new strategic framework for the information society and media called as i2010. eHealth had an important role in i2010, which focused on accessible eHealth services and the participation and inclusion of Europe's citizens in healthcare provision through electronic tools. Concurrent with policy framework, a sub-group on eHealth was established (European Commission, 2014b). The main objectives of the sub-group were to improve quality and accessibility of healthcare services, while supporting the cost-effectiveness of eHealth systems and services. One of the main tasks of the sub-group was to facilitate and contribute the implementation of the previously mentioned eHealth Action Plan.

The i2010 framework was followed by a new policy framework, the Digital Agenda for Europe, which focused on the utilization of the economic and social potential of Internet technologies in all fields of society (European Commission, 2010). In healthcare, the emphasis was on ambient assisted living (AAL) technologies, which makes ICT-based services accessible for all. To support these strategic plans, the European Union launched the AAL Joint Program for conducting research on and development of eHealth applications. The program aims to enhance the quality of life of older people by extending the time people can live in their homes, supporting functional capability of the elderly, and increasing the efficiency and productivity of used resources (Ambient Assisted Living Joint Programme, 2012). From the viewpoint of nursing informatics, AAL technologies offer the means to care for older patients who remain in their own homes and enables health information management at the point of care. In addition to AAL activities, the following actions will be included in the Digital Agenda during the coming years: secure online access for Europeans to their medical health data, widespread deployment of telemedicine services, and definition of a common minimum set of patient data for interoperability of electronic patient records (European Commission, 2010).

Despite of successful implementation of eHealth initiatives in the region, many barriers still exist for the wider deployment of eHealth services. In order to find solutions to tackle existing barriers, European Commission has launched a new eHealth Action Plan 2012–2020 (eHAP) aiming to innovative healthcare for the twenty-first century. It addresses the barriers and aims to fulfil the following objectives (European Commission, 2012, p. 6):

- Achieving wider interoperability of eHealth services

- Supporting research, development, and innovation in eHealth and well-being to address the lack of availability of user-friendly tools and services

- Facilitating uptake and ensuring wider deployment

- Promoting policy dialog and international cooperation on eHealth at global level

With these targets, the ultimate goal of the actions is to provide smarter, safer, and patient-centered health services in the European Union. A recent directive on the application of patients' rights in cross-border healthcare (Klazinga et al., 2011) enables citizens of European Union to seek health services from other EU country (Directives, 2011). To guarantee the continuity and safety of care, the cross-border exchange of health data is needed. The eHAP emphasizes the importance of data protection mentioning that it is a vital element of trust in eHealth. It also notifies the technological development and thus one part of it focuses on mobile health (mHealth). That means the utilization of mobile devices such as tablets and smartphones in health services (European Commission, 2012).

As stated in the eHAP the European Commission will work together with member states in order to facilitate wider deployment of eHealth services. Patient empowerment and skills to use eHealth services are essential for the uptake of eHealth. Not only patients need more information, but also health professionals' awareness of eHealth opportunities needs to be increased. The European Commission will support the development of evidence-based clinical practice guidelines for telemedicine services especially in the field of nursing. It is also important to measure the added value of eHealth services. For that purpose the Commission will launch sets of common indicators for the measurement of the added value and benefit of the eHealth. In addition Health Technology Assessment methodologies will be utilized in the evaluation of the costs and productivity of eHealth services in the period 2013–2016. In the near future research and innovation relating to eHealth tools and services will be supported under the Horizon 2020 program. (European Commission, 2012).

Cross-Border Activities in eHealth

The Directive on the application of patients' rights in cross-border healthcare (Klazinga et al., 2011) enables EU citizens a cross-border access to healthcare services in the European Union member states (Directives, 2011). The implementation of the directive has required the change of national legislation and national authorities have created guidelines for the citizens. Safe health information transfer is a basic principle of the cross-border healthcare. The Smart Open Services for European Patients (epSOS) pilot (2008–2014) attempts to achieve cross-border interoperability between electronic health record systems in Europe (epSOS, 2014). The aim of this pilot is to enable seamless patient health information exchange and improve the quality and safety of healthcare when people move between European countries. Totally 23 countries have participated on the pilot and are developing together a practical eHealth framework and infrastructure that makes possible to transfer patient health information between different healthcare systems in Europe. In the first phase the pilot focuses on two areas: access to important medical data for patient treatment (patient summary) and cross-border use of electronic prescriptions (e-Prescription). Patient summary includes the most important clinical date required to ensure safe and secure healthcare. It is mainly intended to be used in emergency situations, but also in the scheduled healthcare situations it is useful. e-Prescription includes medication prescription and dispensing. Medication is prescribed in the patient's home country with patient's consent. When travelling abroad, a patient has possibility to retrieve the prescribed medication. At the moment information transfer in both cases is in use only in certain epSOS countries. The project extension started in 2011 and it analyzes and tests the following services: the patient access to their data, the Medication-Related Overview, the Healthcare Encounter Report, the integration of the 112 emergency services, and the integration of the European Health Insurance Card (EpSOS, 2014).

eHealth Applications

In 2008, the Finnish National Institute for Health and Welfare (previously referred to as STAKES) in cooperation with the eHealth ERA project evaluated the implementation of eHealth policies and the deployment of eHealth applications in the European Union. According to the report (Hämäläinen et al., 2008), the main eHealth applications are EHRs, patient identifiers, health portals for informing patients and professionals on health issues and disease prevention, citizen card activities, and telemedicine. The Monitoring National eHealth Strategies study provided an update on the progress of eHealth activities in Europe (Stroetmann et al., 2011). Country Reports are available at http://www.ehealth-strategies.eu/database/database.html. The analysis of progress published in 2008 combined with the total number of reported activities in 2010 is presented in Table 52.2 (Hämäläinen et al., 2008; Stroetmann et al., 2011). The table presents an overview of the situation, but is not conclusive due to differences in the features and functions of eHealth applications in different countries, and deployment can be present only in primary or secondary care. In addition, deployment can be partly national, regional, or local (Hämäläinen et al., 2008).

The 2008 report shows that Finland was the only country to report activities in all 14 areas. Additionally, 11 countries (Austria, Belgium, Denmark, Germany, Greece, Hungary, Italy, Poland, Slovakia, Sweden, and the United Kingdom) have reported activities in more than 10 areas. All countries have reported activities on the EHR, but it is unknown whether these developments concern primary care, secondary, or both (Hämäläinen et al., 2008). More specific activities regarding the development of the EHR in 2008 are not conducted often: patient summary ($n = 10$), data definition/coding ($n = 15$), standards ($n = 20$), semantic interoperability ($n = 14$). In 2010, patient summary and EHR-like projects were in the routine use in 7 European countries. In two countries piloting of the system was going and 5 countries were at implementation phase. Surprisingly 20 European countries were at the planning stage (Stroetmann et al., 2011).

EHR deployment in the European Union has mainly progressed well, but there are interesting differences in the deployment status of other eHealth applications. In 2010, e-prescription activities (eCapture, eTransfer, eDispensation) were reported in 22 countries (21 countries in 2008), but eCapture was in use in 15 countries, eTransfer in 9 countries, and eDispensation in only 7 countries (Stroetmann et al., 2011). In 2010, the citizen health card is used in almost all countries ($n = 25$), but activities regarding professional cards are reported by a smaller number of countries ($n = 18$). However, in 2008

TABLE 52.2   Deployment Status of Various eHealth Applications

	Total 2010 Study[a]	Total (n = 27)	United Kingdom	Sweden	Spain	Slovenia	Slovakia	Romania	Portugal	Poland	The Netherlands	Malta	Luxemburg	Lithuania	Latvia	Italy	Ireland	Hungary	Greece	Germany	France	Finland	Estonia	Denmark	Czech Republic	Cyprus	Bulgaria	Belgium
EHR	27	27	1	1	1	1	1	1	1	1	1	1	1	1	1	1	1	1	1	1	1	1	1	1	1	1	1	1
Patient Summary	n/a	10	1	1				1			1					1			1			1	1	1		1		1
Data Definition/Coding	n/a	15	1	1			1	1		1	1			1				1	1	1		1		1				1
Standards	27	20	1	1	1	1		1		1	1			1		1		1	1	1	1	1		1		1		1
Semantic Interoperability	n/a	14	1	1	1	1				1	1				1	1		1	1	1		1		1	1	1		1
e-Prescription	22	21	1	1	1				1		1					1		1	1	1	1	1	1		1	2	2	1
Citizen Health Card	25	22			1	1	1	1	1	1	1	1	1	1	2	1		1		1	1	1	1			1	1	1
Professional Card	18	7		1		1		1								1		1			1	1		1				
Patient ID	26	24	1		1		1		1	1	1	1	1	1	1	1		1	1	1	1	1	1		1		1	1
Professional ID	22	16	1	1	1	1		1		1	1					1		1			1	1		1		1	1	1
Citizen Health Portals	n/a	23	1	1	1		1	1	1	1		1	1	1		1	1	1	1	1	1	1	1	1	1		1	1
Professional Health Portals	n/a	16	1	1	1	1	1						1	1	1		1	1	1	1		1	1	1	1			1
Telemedicine	27	24	1	1	1	1		1	1	1			1	1	1	1		1	1	1		1	1	1	1	1	1	1
Safety and Quality Activities	n/a	7	1	1		1	1			1					2				1	2		1						1

1: Reported activities (actual planning, development, use)
2: Reported no activities
Empty: Reported no activities
n/a: data not available

[a]Hämäläinen et al., 2008, p. 44; Stroetmann et al., 2011.

only 7 countries reported professional card activities, so the progress has been good (Hämäläinen et al., 2008). Different functions are included in citizens' health cards in different countries; the most common were patient ID and national health insurance coverage. In many countries, health cards and identification issues are closely related to each other. Almost all countries ($n = 26$) reported patient ID activities in 2010, while 22 countries reported professional ID activities. The type of identification method differs between countries. In general, there are two methods: healthcare-specific identifiers and national identification numbers. Based on the 2008 report (Hämäläinen et al., 2008), health portals for citizens (23 countries) are introduced more often than health portals for professionals (16 countries). Typically, citizens' health portals include information about general health and service systems. In accordance with the European Union's strategic goals, telemedicine applications are reported in all countries. The most common types of applications were teleconsultation and teleradiology including picture archiving communication systems (Hämäläinen et al., 2008).

Improvements in patient safety and quality of care are identified as a major benefit of eHealth, and the European Union has included them in the eHealth Action Plan as part of the i2010 strategic framework. In addition, the European Commission introduced in 2006 the eHealth for Safety study which aimed to identify key issues, topics, and challenges where ICT applications might improve patient safety and recommendation for future research topics (Empirica, 2007). These activities indicate the importance of patient safety issues in Europe, but surprisingly only 7 countries (Belgium, the Czech Republic, Finland, Greece, Slovakia, Sweden, and the United Kingdom) reported some activities in this field. Germany and Latvia reported no activities, and the data for the remaining 18 countries were missing (Hämäläinen et al., 2008).

European Union has adopted patient safety as a key goal in the development of nursing informatics applications and healthcare systems. At present, the EU-funded European Network for Patient Safety (EUNetPaS) project is coordinating national efforts. Also WHO has launched programs on a global scale that include the inventories of ongoing researches. Many European countries have executed studies to assess the magnitude of adverse events in their respective countries, mostly based on detailed audits of medical records or primarily involved in a running adverse event reporting programs (Klazinga et al., 2011).

A new EU-funded joint project concerning eHealth applications and activities was begun in the beginning of 2014. ENS4Care is a Thematic Network involving 24 partners coordinated by European Federation of Nurses Associations (EFN) (ENS4Care, 2014). During two-year period ENS4Care network aims to develop evidence-based ICT guidelines for the implementation of eHealth services in nursing and social care. The guidelines are based on best practices which have achieved major benefits in cost-effectiveness and better self-management of care. The project is targeted on the following key areas of care: healthy lifestyle and prevention, early intervention and clinical practice in integrated care, skills development for advanced roles, and nurse e-Prescribing. The ENS4Care will collect existing guidelines and good practices from participating organizations and their networks. Patient safety is one of the key drivers of the project and the project creates more understanding how ICT tools might improve safety in healthcare (ENS4Care, 2014).

NURSING TERMINOLOGY DEVELOPMENT IN EUROPE

In Europe, the first effort to have standardized nursing data took the form of a multi-national study from 1976 through 1985 called People's Needs for Nursing Care, which included participation by 11 European countries and was sponsored by the World Health Organization (WHO, 1977). In this study, the nursing process model was used as a framework. Since then the model has served as a standard for nursing documentation in many countries; nurses have mainly adopted four of its phases: assessment of nursing needs, planning of care, implementation of nursing actions, and assessment of nursing outcomes. In the early 1980s, there was considerably discussion and debate about whether nurses should use the nursing diagnosis as the second phase of the process. However, in many European countries nurses decided not to use the term *nursing diagnosis* and instead named the important conclusion after the assessment phase *nursing needs* or *nursing problems*. Nowadays, the nursing process model with three or seven phases is used as the basis for structuring nursing documentation in various electronic nursing information systems in Europe (Saranto et al., 2013).

The European Union has played an important role in supporting research and development activities with various initiatives and programs since the 1980s. Although these activities did not include nursing practice in the beginning, with the inception of the third framework program the European Union launched the Concerted Action on Nursing and delegates from member countries were invited to present proposals. The Danish Institute for Health and Nursing Research was elected to coordinate the Concerted Action on Telematics for Nursing: European Classification on Nursing Practice with regard to patient's problems, nursing interventions, and patient outcomes, including educational measures. The Concerted Action was later renamed the TELENURSING consortium and was funded by the European Union from 1991 through 1994. It brought together 15 member states.

At the same time, the International Council of Nursing (ICN) had started the development of the International Classification for Nursing Practice (ICNP), and since 1991 these two nursing classification projects worked together to support the development of the ICNP. Following the TELENURSING project, the consortium was successful in gaining further European Union funding to start the TELENURSE project (1995 to 1998) and no European countries were involved in the three phases of the project in seven work packages. The central focus of the project was on clinical nursing's aim to offer advanced ways of handling both nursing classifications of problems, interventions, and results as part of the registration of clinical data and collecting the information necessary to enhance the quality of clinical practice in nursing (Clark, 2003; Danish Institute for Health and Nursing Research, 1995). The outcomes of these projects had a crucial impact on nursing terminology development; in 1999, the ICNP alpha version was launched by the ICN with joint international efforts. As is well known, the ICNP elements—nursing phenomena (nursing diagnoses), nursing actions, and nursing outcomes—have been published in the ICNP Version 2 launched in 2009. The latest ICNP version has been launched in 2013 (ICN, 2013; ICNP, 2013).

Use of Nursing Terminologies in Europe

Consisting of various countries with their own national languages, the use of nursing terminologies in Europe involves a considerable amount of translation and cultural validation, particularly regarding a terminology originally written in English. Based on the results of a 2010–2011 survey, the use of nursing terminologies is not very common in European countries. However, the usage has extended since 2008 (Thoroddsen et al., 2009; Thoroddsen, Ehrenberg, Sermeus, & Saranto, 2012). Also, the results of the survey should be interpreted conditionally. Only 20 country members out of 30 European key informants replied to the electronic survey and countries like, e.g., Greece, the Netherlands, and Poland are not included in the results (Thoroddsen et al., 2012).

The NANDA International classification has been translated into many European languages, such as Dutch, French, German, Icelandic, Italian, Norwegian, Portuguese, and Spanish, but is still not in active use in nursing documentation (NANDA International, 2014). Seemingly, the countries that adopted the NANDA-I Classification have also translated the Nursing Interventions Classification (NIC) and Nursing Outcomes Classification (NOC). Some European countries have expressed a need to validate terminologies based on cultural differences in their healthcare service system.

Many European countries have followed the development work of the International Council of Nursing (ICN) and especially the terminology International Classification of Nursing Practice (ICNP). Translations have been accomplished in Brazilian Portuguese, Chinese (Simple), Chinese (Traditional), English, Farsi (Persian), French, German, Icelandic, Indonesian, Italian, Japanese, Korean, Norwegian, Polish, Portuguese, Romanian, Slovak, Spanish, Swedish. The translation has often been supported by the national nursing organizations. ICNP offers also translation guidelines (ICNP, 2013). The active use of the ICNP in healthcare settings is still in its infancy in many European countries, mainly due to differences in nursing documentation legislation, policies, or electronic information systems. However, many nursing schools are using the terminology in teaching nursing documentation (Thoroddsen et al., 2012).

The VIPS model (acronym for the Swedish spelling well-being, integrity, prevention, and safety) developed in Sweden by Professor Margareta Ehnfors and her associates is widely used in the Nordic countries. The VIPS model conceptualizes the essential elements of nursing care, clarifying and facilitating systems thinking and nursing recording. The focus of the model is on patients' functioning in daily-life activities rather than on pathophysiologic problems (Ehnfors, Ehrenberg, & Thorell-Ekstrand, 2002; Ehrenberg, Ehnfors, & Thorell-Ekstrand, 1996). A significant amount of research on the VIPS model has been conducted, showing that the model has good content validity in different areas of nursing care. The model has proven useful in different nursing specialties and is fully computerized in information systems (Saranto et al., 2013; Saranto & Kinnunen, 2009; Ehnfors, Ehrenberg, & Thorell-Ekstrand, 2013).

Many European countries have also used the International Classification of Functioning, Disability and Health (ICF, formerly known as the ICIDH, International Classification of Impairments, Disabilities, and Handicaps) launched in 2001 by WHO (ICF, 2013). The ICF highlights the terms "health" and "disability," meaning that every human being can experience a decrement in health and thereby experience some degree of disability. The ICF has been used in nursing as well as in rehabilitation context and several countries have started the process of streamlining ICF in their health and social information standards, e.g., Finland, Ireland, Italy, the Netherlands, and Sweden. Translations have been conducted in Chinese, English, French, Russian, and Spanish. Also a version for children and youth in English exists (ICF, 2013).

The National Health Service in England and other countries of the United Kingdom decided in the early 2000s to use a single, multi-disciplinary terminology across healthcare. This work evolved, combining with efforts in the United States and other countries, to become the Systematized Nomenclature of Medicine—Clinical Terms (SNOMED-CT). This terminology has maps to other classifications that have different but essential purposes. Nurses have been involved in the crucial task of ensuring that nursing content is adequately represented in this large, multi-disciplinary terminology (Casey, 2003; Dykes et al., 2011; Imel & Campbell, 2003; Ingenerf & Pöppl, 2007). Since this terminology is of English language origin, there is a major translation challenge for European countries adopting and implementing it into electronic information systems. At the moment, translations in European countries, such as Danish, Swedish, and Spanish, already exist. In 2013, translations for Lithuan and Slovak Republic were in process (The International Health Terminology Standards Development Organisation [IHTSDO], 2014).

Possibilities for Meaningful Use of Nursing Data

According to the study by Thoroddsen and colleagues (Thoroddsen et al., 2009; Thoroddsen et al., 2012), the use of standardized nursing terminologies in Europe is still quite rare which makes access to nursing data an obstacle. Though, as mentioned before, the usage has increased. In more than 60% of the institutions in the countries that replied 2008 (Thoroddsen et al., 2009), nursing data were not stored and could, therefore, not be retrieved. In the study 2010–2011 in less than half of the institutions in the countries that replied, nursing data were not stored. For the results, it is worrying that only 30 key informants out of 53 European countries could only be identified, and those who responded did not always have the knowledge or overview of the situation in their country in terms of nursing terminology and standardization work (Thoroddsen et al., 2012). Clinical patient data can answer a variety of questions presented by managers, researchers, or policy-makers when it is collected and used appropriately. Documentation developments, such as the increased standardization of patient records and the use of classifications, make healthcare data more reliable and useful for practice development, management, and research.

There are various local terminologies in nursing practice in addition to the international nursing classifications. This partly reflects the language differences, but also the differences in healthcare service systems. In many countries nurses have devoted their activities to making nursing visible. The nursing information reference model (NIRM)

developed in the Netherlands by Goossen, Epping, and Dassen (1997) has also been used widely in other countries to accommodate both the information needs of nurses at the clinical level and for aggregating data at higher levels (Goossen et al., 1997). The model has also been exploited in Finland in the national nursing documentation project.

Along with the NIRM, nursing minimum data sets have been used to indicate nurses' contribution in healthcare from administrative and economic perspectives. The use of the Belgian nursing minimum data set (B-NMDS) was the first attempt among European nurses to show a nursing contribution since 1988. The B-NMDS consists of 23 nursing interventions, medical diagnoses, patient demographics, nurse variables, and institutional characteristics. The data were collected four times per year (Sermeus, Delesie, Van Landuyt, Wuyts, Vandenboer, & Manna, 1994; Sermeus & Deleise, 1997). The B-NMDS has been revised into B-NMDS-II based on the Nursing Intervention Classification (Sermeus et al., 2005; van den Heede, Michiels, Thonon, Sermeus, 2009).

In Ireland, the need to improve understanding of how to use nursing resources most effectively has also emerged (MacNeela, Scott, Treacy, Hyde, 2006). The development of the Irish Nursing Minimum Data Set (I-NMDS) for general nursing and the I-NMDS for mental health nursing has advanced data collection for multiple purposes. There is a need to analyze and provide information on nursing trends; illustrate service provider trends and patterns in nursing and client care; inform hospital budgeting, nurse staffing levels, and consequently patient safety; as well as inform developments in nursing education. Further, there is a need for integrating the data used to forecast the supply and demand of nurses and mid-wives with specific knowledge, skills, and competencies into the electronic patient record to facilitate access to nursing information and decision-making (National Council for the Professional Development of Nursing and Midwifery, 2006; Morris et al., 2010). There have only been a few additional initiatives on NMDS in Europe, e.g., in Switzerland CH-NMDS (Berthou & Junger, 2003) and Finland.

In Finland, the nationally defined core nursing data (FiNMDS) includes nursing diagnoses, nursing interventions, nursing outcomes, patient care intensity, and nursing summary. The nursing summary consists of the four former items. At the national level, it has been decided that nursing summary will be among the first nursing representatives stored in the National Archive of Health Information in autumn 2014 (KanTa, 2013a).

Over the years, data collection and analysis has largely focused on indirect aspects of nursing service such as waiting times, length of stay, and operative procedures. Addressing the international challenge of expanding the nursing workforce with qualified nurses is of crucial importance and requires cooperation to accomplish. Researchers from 12 different European countries collaborated in one of the largest nursing workforce studies in Europe—the RN4CAST study (2009 to 2011). Through nurse, patient, and organizational surveys and administrative data, the RN4CAST study aimed to provide innovative forecasting methods by addressing not only volume, but also quality of nursing and patient care. Simultaneously to these research activities, the project entailed dissemination and stakeholder activities aimed toward achieving the study's objectives. Strategic collaboration was maintained with a stakeholder panel consisting of 13 healthcare—and nursing administration—related organizations to raise awareness of the project. The ambition of the RN4CAST project was to produce a policy breakthrough commensurate with the scientific strength of the project's findings and the accumulated evidence in the sector. This included producing both technical and scientific publications, as well as liaising with mass media. The study found that improved work environments were associated with better quality of care and patient satisfaction. According to study results deficits in hospital care were common in Europe (Sermeus et al., 2011; Aiken et al., 2012).

Patient safety research is a part of healthcare quality research. Patient safety research has focused on "non-traditional" areas, as the recognition of the interaction between human action and health systems has developed the idea of identifying the elements of healthcare procedures and creating "packages" of care that can be more readily defined, trained-for, and monitored. In Europe, patient safety research is based on national research programs, and it is also on European Commission Directorates' (Health and Consumer Protection, and Research) agenda (European Commission 2014c). A growing body of knowledge has been created on studying safety culture, the implementation of safety systems, and implementation of programs for specific projects on topics such as medication errors and reducing hospital infections (Klazinga et al., 2011).

DEVELOPMENTS IN NURSING INFORMATICS EDUCATION

In 1999, the ministers responsible for higher education in European countries signed the Bologna Declaration (named after the city in Italy where the meeting was held). They agreed on objectives for the development of a coherent and cohesive European Higher Education Area by 2010. The Bologna Process aimed to increase competitiveness and strengthen social and gender cohesion and reduce social inequalities both at the national and European levels. The member countries will promote effective quality assurance

systems, increase effective use of the system based on two cycles (first cycle degrees [bachelor level] should give access to second cycle programs, and second cycle degrees should give access to doctoral programs), and improve the recognition system of degrees and periods of studies. Further, the process includes the following important objectives: promotion of student and academic and administrative staff mobility, application of a system of easily readable and comparable degrees, active participation of all partners especially student involvement in the process, ensuring a substantial period of study abroad, developing scholarship programs for students from developing nations, and making lifelong learning a reality (Mantas, 2004).

Nursing informatics education has been a central topic among countries in the European Union. Parallel to the development of the Bologna Process within the fourth European Union framework program, the NIGHTINGALE project (1998 to 2002) aimed to create support for nursing informatics (NI) education and a means to describe state-of-the-art NI education, NI curriculum development, and educational material and validation of the products in the educators' group. Before NIGHTINGALE, there had already been active development work in health informatics education through the EDUCTRA (Education and Training in Health Informatics) project (1992 to 1994) and its successor, the IT-EDUCTRA project (1996 to 1998), both funded by the European Union, where the focus was not only on medical education but also on nursing IT competencies. Evident in the results of these projects, health and NI education varied greatly among and within the countries, providing a great challenge to develop course material for education. Since the NIGHTINGALE project, the structure and material for NI courses has been used as an example for enhancing NI curricula (Mantas, 1998).

During the 1990s, the European Union also funded the European Summer School in Nursing Informatics (ESSONI) consortium. Over the years, eight summer schools were organized in various European countries by the consortium. Based on changes in the European Union funding mechanism, the consortium was not able to continue and the tradition of effective and enthusiastic collaboration ended. However, the networks built up during the ESSONI years have created an atmosphere of flexible cooperation among participants and have advanced the development of NI education and research. Based on the ESSONI model, German partners have still from time to time carried out the educational tradition successfully.

Since the implementation of the Bologna Process first cycle degrees (i.e., at the bachelor's level), various in NI have been integrated into the nursing curricula in many countries. The topics have focused on health information systems, confidentiality and data protection, aspects of information technology, and the organizational impact in healthcare. Some nursing schools offer a special track in nursing or health informatics.

European universities have mainly included health informatics education in their programs. In some universities, at the University of Eastern Finland (UEF), for example, a Health Informatics program is offered as a specialty within the health and human services informatics master's degree program. However, the degree itself is multi-disciplinary and students may have a bachelor's degree in nursing or other health sciences, computer science, or business sciences when entering the program (University of Eastern Finland, 2014).

The UEF's master's degree program in health and human services informatics became 2012 the first master's degree program in the world to be certified by the International Medical Informatics Association. The association has almost 50 academic institutional members around the world. Audits for the new certification were launched in 2012, with the UEF's degree program one of four study programs to be audited. In addition to the UEF, only one other program was certified, a polytechnic-level study program in Chile. The audit practice that was used is to become the association's standard practice with the current criteria. The awarded certificate is valid for the next five years.

The University of Eastern Finland's degree program in HHSI is the only one of its kind in Finland and there are only a few similar programs in other European universities. The study program focuses on the planning, management, implementation, and evaluation of the use of social and healthcare information resources, as well as the development and evaluation of information technology and information systems from the point of view of the social and healthcare sector. Originally launched in Eastern Finland in 2000, the study program became a regular degree program, following an evaluation by the Ministry of Education and Culture in 2006. The degree program is based on IMIA's education recommendations from 1999 and their new version from 2009 (Mantas et al., 2010). The program has been adapted to the needs of Finnish social and healthcare service systems and the education is planned in accordance with the constantly changing needs of the field.

In Europe, nursing informatics is still quite often studied as integrated to clinical studies. In the United Kingdom, a master's degree in health informatics has existed since 1990, with programs open to nurses and other healthcare professionals. As a joint initiative of the University College London and the Whittington Hospital NHS Trust, health informatics courses are offered as multi-professional education. The Lancashire School of Health and Post-Graduate Medicine at the University of Central Lancashire provides a wide range of relevant and effective educational courses. All together in 16 European universities belonging to IMIA undergraduate and postgraduate programs also include health informatics education (International Medical Informatics Association [IMIA], 2014).

In Greece, the Health Informatics Laboratory, which is connected to the Faculty of Nursing of the University of Athens, serves the undergraduate and postgraduate studies of most of the Schools of Health Sciences of the university. In the Netherlands, the Institute of Health Policy and Management, as part of Erasmus Medical Center, offers three undergraduate English master's and two postgraduate English master's programs, which focus on different aspects of healthcare including health information management. In Denmark, Aalborg University offers a three-year master's degree in health informatics attended by more than 120 mid-career students per year from Scandinavia, Iceland, and Greenland.

Besides the degree programs, ICT competencies can be achieved by obtaining a driving license for computer use, especially for nurses working in hospitals or other healthcare organizations. One example is the European Computer Driving License (ECDL), which is a relevant and internationally recognized qualification for all computer users, not only nurses in healthcare. The ECDL is designed to improve understanding and to render the use of computers more effective among employees. It is designed for both novice and intermediate computer users. To enhance computer literacy, several countries have adopted this model for their in-service training in hospitals. Recently the model has been developed for citizens as well. EqualSkills and especially e-Citizen program explains how to use the Internet effectively to communicate with individuals and groups, retrieve information, and access products and services (European Computer Driving License, 2014).

NURSING INFORMATICS–RELATED COOPERATION IN EUROPE

The NI cooperation in Europe is based on the national nurses associations (NNAs) and other nursing-related organizations, working groups, and networks. At the European level, NNAs have worked together toward development in quality assurance, nursing workforce, and competencies. In many countries, NNAs have nursing informatics working groups, as well as NI-track sessions during their annual seminars, which have been very popular. These regular events have been mainly informal, discussing meaning of the discipline. More specific and formal efforts are needed in many European countries concerning NI education and practice development, and especially for the recognition of NI as a specialty in nursing.

At a national level, the NNAs play a central role in bringing ICT use into nursing practice. The most recent initiative has been focused on eHealth, highlighting the European Commission's eHealth Action Plan. In this huge endeavor, cooperation with other member countries is crucial. The role of the European Federation of Nurses Associations (EFN), established in 1971, is integral for establishing this cooperation. The EFN is the independent voice of the profession in Europe and consists of NNAs from 28 European Union member states and six associations which are from countries in membership of the European Union and/or of the Council of Europe. EFN is working for the benefit of 6 million nurses throughout Europe.

The mission of the EFN is to strengthen the status and practice of the nursing profession for the benefit of both citizens' health and the interests of nurses in the European Union and the rest of Europe (EFN, 2014). Concerning the eHealth initiatives in European Union member states, the EFN has encouraged nurses to focus on three targets: (1) the expected benefits of the eHealth movement such as optimization of services and continuity of care; (2) National enursing advancements like electronic documentation, patient and health professional cards, and telenursing; and (3) the barriers faced during implementation. According to the EFN, eHealth has enormous potential for enabling continuity of care, especially for individuals with long-term conditions, and improving the accessibility of health services leading to optimized and efficient care. The EFN has acknowledged the importance of eHealth developments on its political agenda and it actively participates on large-scale EU-funded projects in the field (ENS4Care, 2014).

Although the use of ICT in healthcare is highly advanced in Europe, there are still many developments, such as EHRs, e-prescribing, and patient and health professional cards that urgently need to be implemented in various countries. Some countries like Finland, Ireland, Portugal, and Sweden already have successful examples of nurses' involvement in prescribing medicines. However, changes are needed, especially in legislation, to make advances in e-prescriptions. Thus, the primary obstacle to eHealth adoption is national legislation, which often needs to be developed or revised. In some countries like Austria, Finland, Germany, Slovenia, and Sweden, there are legal initiatives regarding the extent to which various professionals or citizens should have access to electronic patient information (EFN, 2014).

It is essential to developing effective indicators and measures that assess quality, performance, and cost regarding nursing's contribution to patient outcomes and public health on a national and international level. The Nordic Nurses Federation (SSN, acronym for the Swedish words Nurses Cooperation in Nordic countries) has focused on quality indicators and nursing terminology issues during recent years. Nurses from NNAs in Denmark, Finland, Iceland, Norway, and Sweden have worked together, aiming to define quality indicators for nutrition, pain, pressure ulcers, falls, and terminologies as well as workforce measures. This work reflects various development activities in the Nordic countries, and the results are shared in seminars and panels during annual meetings (SSN, 2010).

At the moment, patient safety is a central principle of quality in healthcare and has high priority on the research agenda in most countries. Patient safety has become a priority issue on the European policy-makers agenda since the early 2000s. Many countries in the WHO European Region have adopted laws and regulations in which patients are described. Patient safety has been synthesized in four categories: initiatives at national level, initiatives at hospital level, initiatives involving professionals, and initiatives involving patients. The instrument used to enhance initiatives is a legislative measure at national level. The government issued a specific legislation in order to define which rules the healthcare providers have to respect when implementing patient safety strategy tools. In Denmark and Finland, Patient Safety Acts outlined the framework for patient involvement within the national organizations (HOPE, 2013, p. 6).

Consisting of numerous countries and their languages, Europe needs many forums to share and benchmark its developments in nursing. The Association for Common European Nursing Diagnoses, Interventions and Outcomes (ACENDIO) is a membership organization established in 1995 to promote the development of nursing's professional language and to provide a network across Europe for nurses interested in the development of a common language that describes the practice of nursing. The establishment of ACENDIO was heavily connected to the TELENURSING project (1992 to 1994). During that time and still today, there is a huge need for nurses throughout Europe to be able to share and compare information in order to research and improve care, manage nursing resources effectively, and ensure that nursing is visible in local, national, and European policy (ACENDIO, 2013).

Nurses in some European countries are developing their own terminologies to meet the need for a nursing language in their country. Others have adapted or translated terminologies and classifications developed in other countries or by other disciplines, but there is no overall coordination of these developments among countries. ACENDIO offers a discussion forum for European nurses, and also for nurses from outside Europe, to enable active participation in the development work in their own countries. Through bi-annual conferences and several national workshops the association tries to encourage its members to improve the status of nursing terminology, inform policy decisions, and strengthen or make visible the nursing contribution to health and patient care (ACENDIO, 2013).

The Association for Nomenclature, Taxonomy, and Nursing Diagnoses (the Spanish acronym AENTDE stands for Asociación Española de Nomenclatura, Taxonomía y Diagnósticos de Enfermeros) was created in 1996 by a group of Spanish nurses envisioning the future of the profession. The aims of the association are to contribute to the development of a nursing terminology able to identify the contribution of nursing care to the population's health and to improve and foster the knowledge and use of nursing terminologies among nurses in Spain, and further to collaborate with National and International organizations in the promotion of research and sharing of knowledge and experiences on the use of nursing diagnoses and other nursing terminologies. The association welcomes the participation of all nurses working with standardized nursing languages in clinical nursing, education, research, or administration (AENTDE, 2013).

The main activities carried out by the AENTDE are a biennial international symposium on Nursing Diagnoses and Terminologies and a biennial workshop. Since 1996 when the first international symposium was held, several international symposia and workshops have been organized by AENTDE, with the participation of both national and international nurses. Symposia have been held also jointly, e.g., in Madrid in 2010, together with NANDA-International. It was the first time that NANDA-International celebrated its congress outside the USA. Around 1000 nurses from all over the world joined the event, demonstrating the interest and importance of the development of nursing languages for the future of the profession. The workshops are more local, where about 200 Spanish nurses meet every other year somewhere in Spain to share and advance knowledge in the use of nursing terminologies. The Spanish health system is quite advanced in the use of electronic systems, and this is one of the reasons why the use of standardized nursing languages is so common in Spain (AENTDE, 2013).

The European Federation for Medical Informatics (EFMI) was established in 1976, and the nursing working group, now known as NURSIE, EFMI WG NURSIE

Nursing Informatics in Europe, formed in 1988. From the 32 member countries of EFMI, 18 country members and seven associate members belong to the NURSIE. The first chair of the working group was Dr. Marianne Tallberg, an active nurse from Finland, although the EFMI working group rules stated that, "A working group consists of experts selected and assigned in a special area" not necessarily meaning nursing. From the beginning, the aims of the working group have been constant, focusing on support for nurses and nursing organizations in the European countries with information and contacts, and to offer nurses opportunities to build contact networks within the field of informatics. This has been accomplished by arranging sessions, workshops, and tutorials in connection with the Medical Informatics European (MIE) conferences. The working group aims to support the education of nurses with respect to informatics and computing as well as to support research and development work in the field and to promote publishing of achieved results (EFMI, 2012). Many NURSIE members are also members of the International Medical Informatics Association's Special Interest Group for Nursing Informatics (SIGNI) (IMIA, 2014).

A recent survey among representatives of the 32 national member associations of EFMI presented challenges that European countries have faced in the further development of eHealth services (Moen et al., 2012). According to the study it is important to ensure that the development of eHealth services support sociable services and innovations in healthcare. Also the results emphasized the shift from ICT-based implementation to a comprehensive approach of healthcare development where eHealth with other important aspects have notified. In Europe a capacity building arena should be created. There is a need for a forum where experiences and new initiatives can be shared in order to enhance eHealth deployment (Moen et al., 2012).

Another development that built on the TELENURSE initiative was the development of a European standard for nursing terminology. This brought together nurses across Europe with the objective of including nursing in the efforts of the health informatics committee of the European Standard Organisation (CEN). The work progressed well and was adopted by the International Standards Organisation (ISO) under a cooperation agreement between the two standards organizations (the Vienna agreement). The resulting international standard focused on the conceptual structures that are represented in a reference terminology model for nursing, supporting mapping among terminologies and harmonization with terminology and information model standards outside the domain of nursing (Hämäläinen et al., 2013).

NURSING DOCUMENTATION IN FINLAND

The following paragraphs provide an example of how a standardized nursing terminology has been implemented in an EHR system. In Finland, the somewhat unified paper-based health record has been widely used for more than 30 years. Over the years, nursing documentation has been based on narrative text. Thus, it has been difficult to retrieve and reuse the information contained in care plans and nursing notes. Electronic information systems including some platforms for care documentation have been used for more than 10 years, but their structures have not been unified. This kind of development has not been given high priority in the nursing profession in the past. However, today all public and nearly all private healthcare providers already deploy electronic health records (Hämäläinen et al., 2013).

During the past decade in Finland, there has been considerable activity toward developing the EHR. In Finland, the Ministry of Social Affairs and Health launched a large project for improving health services from 2003 to 2007. The purpose of the project was to unify information systems, national data archives, and data security solutions. For the first time, nursing was recognized in the national project. As a part of the national project, the Nursing Documentation Project started in May 2005 and ended in October 2009. In 2010–2013 nursing is heavily involved in the development of National Archive of Health Information (KanTa, 2013a).

In Finland, nurses are the largest group of healthcare professionals and constitute the most active users of patient data in hospitals 24 hours per day, 7 days per week. This necessitates that tools and models adopted for daily practice support nursing from philosophical, ethical, and practical perspectives.

The Development of a National EHR System

The development of a nationally interoperable EHR started already in 2002 with requirements that public healthcare organizations should join the national patient record archive. The Ministry of Social Affairs and Health is in charge of the implementation of this decision and the specification of the EHR solution. The National Archive of Health Information (KanTa) (Fig. 52.1) (KanTa, 2013b) is the name of the national data system services for healthcare services, pharmacies, and citizens. The services include the electronic prescription, Pharmaceutical Database, My Kanta pages, and Patient Data Repository. The services are deployed in phases throughout Finland. The electronic prescription has been launched to the public sector and the private healthcare units are in progress.

After that the deployments of the Patient Data Repository service will start. The guidance and advice in matters related to deployment of the Kanta Services are provided by the National Institute for Health and Welfare of Finland (THL) OPER Unit (KanTa, 2013a). The timeline of Finnish healthcare ICT standardization for interoperability has been planned till 2016 (KanTa, 2013b).

In 2004, the core data elements of the EHR were introduced as part of the national EHR project. A national consensus on the data elements was reached at two special consensus seminars and working group meetings of healthcare professionals and software developers from IT suppliers. The definitions were also publicly available for comment on the Internet. *Core data* means health-related information required for data exchange between health information systems in a standardized format. The core data are defined as the data that can be standardized. Documentation of the core data requires the use of vocabulary, terminology, and classifications (Häyrinen, Saranto, & Nykänen, 2008). The updated term of core data according to the newest national guidelines is *essential patient record structures* (Lehtovirta & Vuokko, 2014).

The core data are the most significant information in the patient care process throughout different healthcare sectors, describing the patient's state of health or disease. The core information accumulates chronologically during patient care by different professionals. The aim of the core data is to give a holistic description of the patient's health and disease history, and of the care and guidance provided. The information is used in present and future care.

Development and Implementation of the National Nursing Documentation Model

The national nursing documentation model was adopted to describe nursing care in the EHR system. The nursing documentation model was based on the nursing decision-making process introduced by WHO in the late 1970s. The international model comprises four main phases: (1) assessment and naming the nursing needs (nursing diagnoses), (2) planning and describing the outcomes of care, (3) description of interventions performed, and (4) assessment of nursing outcomes (WHO, 1977; Ashworth et al., 1987).

The Nursing Minimum Data Set (NMDS) is a part of the core data elements including information on nursing diagnosis and needs, nursing interventions, nursing outcomes, nursing (discharge) summary, and patient care intensity. The national nursing documentation model is based on the defined nursing core data (NMDS), the process model

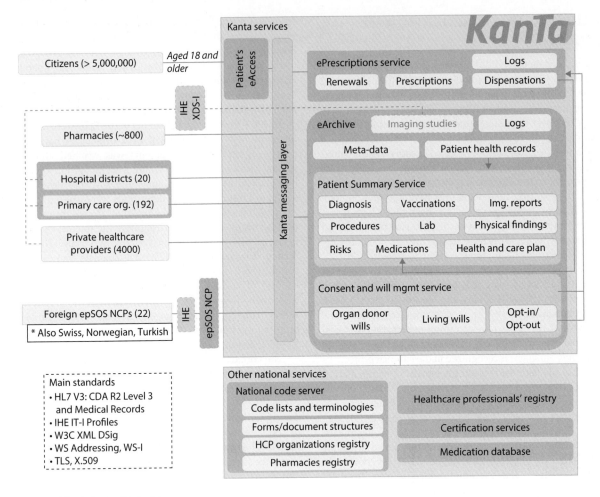

• **FIGURE 52.1.** KanTa-Architecture.

in decision-making, and the FinCC (Fig. 52.2). The documentation has been changed more in structured form and it gives several possibilities to meaningful use of the nursing documents. The national nursing documentation model and the Finnish Care Classification (FinCC) were developed in the National Nursing Documentation Project from 2005 to 2009. The aims in the nursing documentation project were to unify and standardize nursing documentation nationally and to connect it with the interdisciplinary core documentation of the patient history, national code server, and national data archive (Ikonen et al., 2007; Tanttu & Rusi, 2007).

The FinCC is a translation of the Clinical Care Classification (CCC) System (www.sabacare.com), and it was implemented after a cultural validation (Saba, 1992; Ensio, 2001). The CCC System is approved by the American Nurses Association (ANA) and is cross-mapped to the International Classification for Nursing Practice by the International Council of Nursing (ICN) and to the Unified Medical Language System (UMLS). The CCC System is also part of the international SNOMED-CT classification, and it can be used together with ICD-10. Clinical LOINC (Logical Observations, Identifiers, Names, and Codes) has integrated the CCC System of Nursing Diagnoses Outcomes in its clinical application. ABC Codes for Complimentary and Alternative Medicine (CAM) has adapted and selected the CCC System of Nursing Interventions for billing codes (Saba, 2007, 2012).

FinCC includes the Finnish Classification of Nursing Diagnosis (FiCND), Finnish Classification of Nursing Interventions (FiCNI), and Finnish Classification of Nursing Outcomes (FiCNO). FiCND and FiCNI have similar hierarchical structures (component, main category, and subcategory levels). The component level is the most abstract.

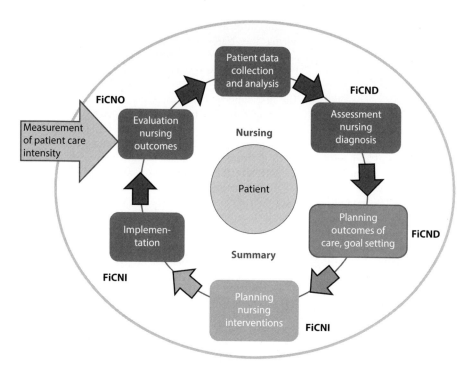

The most concrete main categories and sub-categories of the FiCND and FiCNI have been aggregated under the components, and they are actually used in nursing documentation (Ensio, Saranto, Ikonen, Iivari, 2006). The latest version 3.0 was launched in 2012. The number of main categories and sub-categories under each component varies. FiCND has 88 main categories and 150 sub-categories, while FiCNI has 127 main categories and 180 sub-categories. In all, there are 215 main categories and 330 sub-categories, totaling 545 (Liljamo, Kinnunen, & Ensio, 2012). The care components represent the functional, health behavioral, physiologic, and psychologic patterns of a patient. FiCNO can be described using three qualifiers: improved, stabilized, or deteriorated. When comparing nursing diagnoses and outcomes of nursing care, it is possible to evaluate the care process and measure the care outcomes.

The national nursing documentation model is used in all kinds of wards and units (e.g., primary care, special care, elderly care). The FinCC is utilized to:

- Document integrated patient care processes
- Perform multi-professional searches for information and knowledge to aid the decision-making process
- Analyze patient profiles and populations
- Predict care needs, resources, and costs

- Classify and track clinical care
- Develop evidence-based practice models
- Develop clinical plans of care, clinical pathways, and guidelines as well as for research and educational purposes
- Develop reports for nursing management, planning, education, research, and quality assessment.

Accurate and uniform standardized nursing documentation facilitates also the assessment of patient care intensity.

The Oulu Patient Classification (OPC) is used to measure patient care intensity. The OPC is based on the Roper, Logan, and Tierney model for nursing and the Oulu University Hospital's quality assurance program and value basis, which is characterized by a humanistic approach and current research results concerning patients' expectations of good care (Kaustinen, 1995; Onnela & Svenström, 1998; Rauhala & Fagerström, 2004).

The OPC has been built on the following areas of need, sub-sections:

- Planning and coordination of nursing care
- Breathing, blood circulation, and symptoms of illness

- Nutrition and medication
- Hygiene and secretion
- Activity, functioning, sleep, and rest
- Teaching and guiding of care/continued care, emotional support

In each of these sub-sections, the nurse classifies from $A = 1$ point to $D = 4$ points once a day. The care intensity of a patient can be scored between 6 and 24 points. The higher the score, the higher is the care intensity of the patient. The end product in the project was a cross-mapped classification material (FiCND, FiCNI, and OPC) in the national code server. The databases enable evaluation, analysis, and utilization of data for administrative and research purposes. (Rauhala & Fagerström, 2004; Fagerström, Rainio, Rauhala, Nojonen, 2000).

The FinCC and the OPC has been cross-mapped twice during the National Nursing Documentation Project (2005–2009) by expert nurses in various hospitals in Finland. All the main categories and sub-categories of the FiCNI have been cross-mapped to all OPC sub-sections. The first sub-section of the OPC, planning and coordination of care, has been cross-mapped to all the main categories and sub-categories of the FiCND (Liljamo & Kaakinen, 2009). The latest cross-mapping between the FinCC 3.0 and the OPC has been made during 2013 in a Delphi study (Liljamo & Saranto, 2012) (Fig. 52.3).

The measurement of patient care intensity is a part of the evaluation of nursing outcomes. The value of cross-mapping daily documentation of patient care and patient care intensity can be seen in reliability improvement of intensity data used in nursing management (Liljamo & Saranto, 2012). It facilitates also the aggregation of nursing summary.

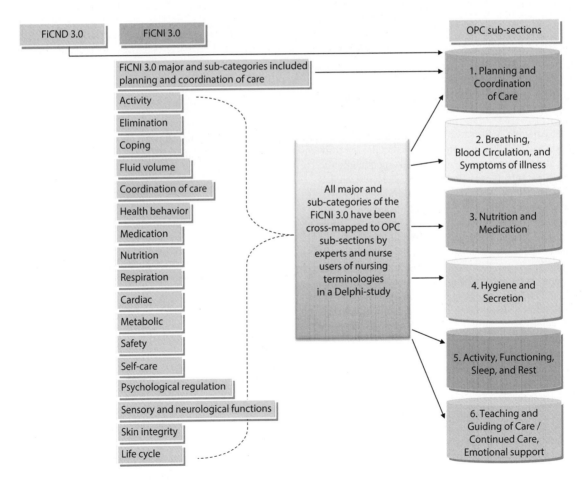

• **FIGURE 52.3.** FinCC 3.0 and OPC Cross-Mapping.

As already mentioned above, nursing diagnoses, nursing interventions, nursing outcomes, and patient care intensity form the structure of the nursing summary, also called nursing discharge summary. Nursing summary improves the continuity of care and patient safety, when the patient is discharged or transferred to another hospital. To some extent nursing summaries are sent electronically (eNursing summary) from one EPR to another. According to users, eNursing summary supplements or even improves the medical care summary. The feedback from the follow-up care has been very positive; it is clear and easy to read including comprehensive patient information. Nursing summary can easily be picked up from the National Archive of Health Information in case of new patient admission (KanTa, 2013a) (Fig. 52.4).

An education model and an e-education environment were also developed to support the implementation. Education was first launched to nurses in clinical settings, both in primary and specialized care. Education was built primarily on the content of classification and the theoretical assumptions of need theory. Surprisingly, having been in use for almost 30 years as a paper-based system,

the nursing process model also required discussion and review.

Continuous Validation of the FinCC

The development and maintenance of the FinCC have been organized at the University of Eastern Finland, at the department of Health and Social Management. The 10-member expert group of the terminology, comprising members from different Finnish healthcare organizations, supervises the terminology development, network with the users and researchers, and continuing evaluation of the FinCC. The national evaluation of the FinCC has been carried out in 2004, 2007, and 2010 by questionnaires to end users. The documentation model is included in the nursing curriculum at the Universities of Applied Sciences (Ensio, Saranto, Ikonen, et al., 2006; Liljamo, Kaakinen, & Ensio, 2008; Rajalahti & Saranto, 2009; Ora-Hyytiäinen et al., 2010; Kinnunen, Ensio, & Liljamo, 2011).

During the national eNNI-project 2008–2012 the national documentation model was implemented in cooperation with nursing teachers and students of the

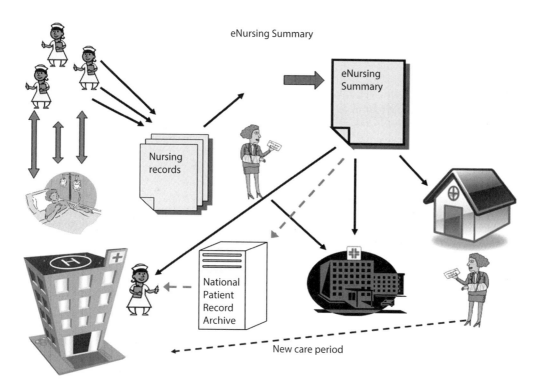

eNursing Summary

eNursing Summary

Nursing records

National Patient Record Archive

New care period

• **FIGURE 52.4.** eNursing Summary From Hospital to National Archive and Back. (Reproduced, with permission, from Minna Mykkänen and Henna Huovinen, Kuopio University Hospital, Finland.)

Universities of Applied Sciences ($n = 19$) and hospitals. eNNi acronym is for electronic-Documentation of Nursing Care—the Research and Development Project for the Creation of Nursing Informatics Competence in cooperation with those in education and nursing practice (Rajalahti & Saranto 2009; Ora-Hyytiäinen, Ikonen, Ahonen, Rajalahti, & Saranto, 2010).

According to the latest evaluation and the feedback of the FinCC users (Kinnunen, Ensio & Liljamo, 2011) the implementation of the National Documentation Model has been extended and proceeded quite well. The content of the components Coping, Role Relationship, and Life Cycle need to be developed and clarified, whereas components Medication, Secretion, and Skin Integrity had a high agreement among respondents. All in all, the expert group of the FinCC has a laborious process in the continuing development of the terminology. However, additionally also electronic patient records need to be evolved to better support and facilitate nursing documentation, and reuse of data.

The users have begun to see the benefits of structured nursing documentation and use of the EHR. The national nursing documentation including the FinCC has helped nurses structure the whole patient care process better. It has also guided the development of patient care. Statistics and reports of nursing process by systematic documentation benefit nursing management, planning, education, research, and quality assessment. The obstacles to be overcome are mainly technical problems (e.g., failures and problems in different EHRs), learning and accepting the new documentation model, which takes time approximately three months to become routine, and maintaining organization-wide commitment. EHRs must be developed to support nursing daily documentation so that the FinCC acts as a language in the nursing documentation, not the structure that needs to be followed.

FUTURE DEVELOPMENTS IN EUROPE

European nurses have been eager to adopt a standardized nursing language. Activities have focused on translations, validations, and implementations of classifications and data sets into practice. In addition, the history of international cooperation in the development of the ICNP is promising. However, we need to have new beginnings, especially regarding the implementation of terminologies into electronic information systems, to be able to build databases for nursing. These databases will enable evaluation, analysis, and utilization of data for administrative and research purposes, in addition to clinical use of data.

The European Commission has stated in its recommendation (Commission of the European Communities, 2008), it is highly important that those systems implemented should be interoperable with other systems not only within organizations and nationally, but also internationally. This ensures that the health information of European Union citizens would be accessible safely and securely. Thus, data transfer will benefit patients' and professionals' mobility in the region of the European Union. This vision challenges nurses to guarantee that nursing data are transferable (i.e., standardized).

Concerns for the effects on the nurse–patient relationship are often important to those considering the advanced use of technology in healthcare. Although information and communication technology can enhance the nurse–patient relationship, it cannot entirely replace it. Based on studies, information gained through ICT applications empower users by encouraging active participation and increasing patient satisfaction. Thus, the use of ICT in nursing can be seen as a means to provide good quality care as well as to strengthen patient safety consistent with the aims in the European Commission's eHealth Action Plans.

Like in the United States, it may not be taken for granted that nurses have an informatics career pathway in Europe. Despite the active work among eHealth initiatives and IT capacity in healthcare settings, nurses often participate in development work in addition to their daily duties. A number of nursing professionals have already developed expertise or degrees in health or nursing informatics, yet, their knowledge and skills are not sufficiently recognized or used to deliver benefits to patients and colleagues. This deficiency reflects the lack of health or nursing informatics expert positions in healthcare organizations, partly due to the fact that NNAs are not recognized for IT expertise because most do not have nursing informatics as a recognized specialty in Europe.

National nursing development work is very demanding and cannot be regarded only as an implementation project. The Finnish nursing documentation model has now been introduced to nurses all over the country, and nurses have adopted the model mostly with satisfaction. An expert group has been established to take care of the updates to the FinCC, as well as to organize continuous assessments. There are also visions of how to implement clinical pathways and guidelines into the documentation model to be able to support evidence-based nursing. From the technological progress point of view, nurses would also like to have decision support actions including alarms added to the systems. As always, a considerably amount of development work is still needed to enhance usability of the information systems.

Information sharing from the databases is still in its infancy, and nurse managers mostly use frequencies from the databases. Thus, more sophisticated data acquisition, statistical analysis, and tools for reporting are in the development process to be used in benchmarking at the organizational, regional, and national levels (and hopefully at the European and international levels soon!).

ACKNOWLEDGMENTS

The authors would like to end this chapter with a very important reminder from their distinguished mentor, and a living legend, Dr. Virginia K. Saba: "Only coded data can be reused!" It is important to keep that in mind.

In addition, the authors want to acknowledge Adjunct Professor Dr. Marianne Tallberg and Director of Research Anneli Ensio for their important contributions to this chapter.

REFERENCES

ACENDIO. (2013). *Association for common European nursing diagnoses, interventions and outcomes.* Retrieved from http://www.acendio.net. Accessed on March 22, 2014.

AENTDE. (2013). *Asociación Española de Nomenclatura, Taxonomía y Diagnósticos de Enfermeros.* Retrieved from http://www.aentde.com

Aiken, L. H., Sermeus, W., Van den Heede, K., Sloane, D. M., Busse, R., McKee, M., ... Kutney-Lee, A. (2012). Patient safety, satisfaction, and quality of hospital care: cross sectional surveys of nurses and patients in 12 countries in Europe and the United States. *British Medical Journal,* Mar 20;344:e1717. doi:10.1136/bmj.e1717.

Ambient Assisted Living Joint Programme. (2012). *Objectives.* Retrieved from http://www.aal-europe.eu/about/objectives/. Accessed on March 14, 2014.

Ashworth, P., Bjørn, A., Déchanoz, G., et al. (1987). People's needs for nursing care. A European study. A study of nursing care needs and of the planning, implementation and evaluation of care provided by nurses in two selected groups of people in the European Region. World Health Organization, Regional Office for Europe, Copenhagen, Denmark.

Berthou, A., & Junger, A. (2003). Nursing data- Developing a national nursing information system, in Naming nursing. In J. Clark (Ed), *Proceedings of the First ACENDIO Ireland/UK Conference* (pp. 197–207). Bern, Switzerland: Hans Huber.

Casey, A. (2003). Naming nursing in the UK. Goals and challenges, in naming nursing. In J. Clark (Ed.), *Proceedings of the First ACENDIO Ireland/UK Conference* (pp. 215–223). Bern, Switzerland: Hans Huber.

Clark, J. (Ed.). (2003). *Naming nursing. Proceedings of the First ACENDIO Ireland/UK Conference.* Bern, Switzerland: Hans Huber.

Commission of the European Communities. (2000). *eEurope2002. An information society for all. Action plan.* Retrieved from http://ec.europa.eu/information_society/eeurope/2002/documents/archiv_eEurope2002/action plan_en.pdf. Accessed on March 22, 2014.

Commission of the European Communities. (2002). *eEurope 2005: An information society for all.* Retrieved from http://ec.europa.eu/information_society/eeurope/2002/news_library/documents/eeurope2005/eeurope2005_en.pdf. Accessed on March 22, 2014.

Commission of the European Communities. (2004). *e-Health – making healthcare better for European citizens: An action plan for a European e-Health Area.* Retrieved from http://eurlex.europa.eu/LexUriServ/LexUriServ.do?uri=COM:2004:0356:FIN:EN:PDF

Commission of the European Communities. (2008). *Commission recommendation of 2 July 2008 on cross-border interoperability of electronic health record systems.* 2008/594/EC. Retrieved from http://eur-lex.europa.eu/LexUriServ/LexUriServ.do?uri=OJ:L:2008:190:0037:0043:EN:PDF. Accessed on March 22, 2014.

Danish Institute for Health and Nursing Research (DIHNR). (1995). The nursing research potential of electronic health care records and the role of nursing research centres in Europe. Copenhagen: DIHNR eHealth Strategies 2010. About the study. Retrieved from http://www.ehealth-strategies.eu/about/about.html. Accessed on March 22, 2014.

Directives. (2011). *Directive 2011/24/Eu of the European Parliament and of the Council of 9 March 2011 on the application of patients' rights in cross-border healthcare.* Retrieved from http://eur-lex.europa.eu/LexUriServ/LexUriServ.do?uri=OJ:L:2011:088:0045:0065:EN:PDF. Accessed on March 22, 2014.

Dykes, P. C., DaDamio, R. R., Goldsmith, D., Kim, H., Ohashi, K., & Saba, V. K. (2011). Leveraging standards to support patient-centric interdisciplinary plans of care. *AMIA ... Annual Symposium Proceedings* (pp. 356–363). Retrieved from http://www.ncbi.nlm.nih.gov/pmc/articles/PMC3243254/. Accessed on March 22, 2014.

EFMI. (2012). *About EFMI.* European Federation for Medical Informatics. Retrieved from http://www.helmholtz-muenchen.de/ibmi/efmi/index.php?option=com_content&task=view&id=11&Itemid=62. Accessed on March 22, 2014.

EFN. (2014). European Federation of Nurses Associations. Retrieved from http://www.efnweb.org/. Accessed on March 22, 2014.

Ehnfors, M., Ehrenberg, A., & Thorell-Ekstrand, I. (2002). The development and use of the VIPS-model in Nordic countries, in ACENDIO 2002. In N. Oud (Ed.), *Proceedings of the Special Conference of the Association of*

Common European Nursing Diagnoses, Interventions and Outcomes, in Vienna (pp. 139–168). Bern, Switzerland: Hans Huber.

Ehnfors, M., Ehrenberg, A., & Thorell-Ekstrand, I. (2013). Nya VIPS-boken. Studentlitteratur AB, Sverige.

Ehrenberg, A., Ehnfors, M., & Thorell-Ekstrand, I. (1996). Nursing documentation in patient records: Experience of the use of the VIPS-model. *Journal of Advanced Nursing, 24*, 853–867.

Empirica. (2007). eHealth for safety. *Impact of ICT on patient safety and risk management in healthcare.* Retrieved from www.ehealth-for-safety.org/. Accessed on March 22, 2014.

Empirica. (2009). *eHealth strategies.* Retrieved from http://www.ehealth-strategies.eu/index.htm

ENS4Care. (2014). *Evidence based guidelines for nurses and social care workers for the deployment of eHealth services.* Retrieved from www.ens4care.eu. Accessed on March 22, 2014.

Ensio, A. (2001). Modelling of nursing interventions. (In Finnish, Hoitotyön toiminnan mallintaminen). Doctoral thesis. Kuopio University (Kuopion yliopiston julkaisuja E. Yhteiskuntatieteet 89. Kuopion yliopiston painatuskeskus), Kuopio, Finland.

Ensio, A., Saranto, K., Ikonen, H., Iivari, A. (2006). The national evaluation of standardized terminology. In Park H-A., Murray P., Delaney C., (Eds.). *Consumer-Centered Computer-Supported Care for Healthy People. Proceedings of NI2006, Seoul. Studies in Health Technology and Informatics.* Amsterdam, The Netherlands: IOS Press. *122*, 749–752.

Ensio, A., Saranto, K., Ikonen, H., Iivari, A. (2006). The national evaluation of standardized terminology. *Studies in Health Technology and Informatics, 122*, 749–752.

EpSOS. (2014). *EpSOS services.* Retrieved from http://www.epsos.eu/epsos-services.html. Accessed on March 22, 2014.

European Commission. (2010). *A digital agenda for Europe.* Retrieved from http://eur-lex.europa.eu/LexUriServ/LexUriServ.do?uri=COM:2010:0245:FIN:EN:PDF

European Commission. (2012). *eHealth Action Plan 2012-2020 - Innovative healthcare for the 21st century.* COM (2012) 736 final. Retrieved from http://eurlex.europa.eu/LexUriServ/LexUriServ.do?uri=COM:2012:0736:FIN:EN:PDF. Accessed on March 22, 2014.

European Commission. (2013). *eHealth – European interoperability framework.* Overall executive summary. Luxembourg: Publications Office of the European Union. Retrieved from http://ec.europa.eu/digital-agenda/en/news/ehealth-interoperability-framework-study

European Commission. (2014a). *eHealth network.* Retrieved from http://ec.europa.eu/health/ehealth/policy/network/index_en.htm. Accessed on March 22, 2014.

European Commission. (2014b). *i2010 subgroup on ehealth.* Retrieved from http://ec.europa.eu/information_society/activities/health/policy/i2010subgroup/index_en.htm. Accessed on March 22, 2014.

European Commission. (2014c). Report from the Commission to the Council. Retrieved from http://ec.europa.eu/health/patient_safety/policy/index_en.htm

European Computer Driving License (ECDL) Foundation. (2014). Retrieved from http://ecdl.com. Accessed on March 22, 2014.

European Union. (2012). Europe in figures. Eurostat yearbook. Retrieved from http://epp.eurostat.ec.europa.eu/cache/ITY_OFFPUB/KS-CD-12-001/EN/KS-CD-12-001-EN.PDF. Accessed on March 22, 2014.

Eysenbach, G. (2001). What is e-health? *Journal of Medical Internet Research, 3*(2), e20.

Fagerström, L., Rainio, A. K., Rauhala, A., Nojonen, K. (2000). Validation of a new method for patient classification, the Oulu Patient Classification. *Journal of Advanced Nursing, 31*(2), 481–490.

Goossen, W. T., Epping, P. J., & Dassen, T. (1997). Criteria for nursing information systems as a component of the electronic patient record: An international Delphi study. *Computers in Nursing, 15*(6), 307–315.

Hämäläinen, P., Doupi, P., & Hyppönen, H. (2008). *eHealth policy and deployment in the European Union. Review and analysis of progress.* Stakes reports 26/2008. Retrieved from http://www.julkari.fi/bitstream/handle/10024/77143/R26-2008-VERKKO.pdf?sequence=1. Accessed on March 22, 2014.

Hämäläinen, P., Reponen, J., Winblad, I., Kärki, J., Laaksonen, M., Hyppönen, H., Kangas, M. (2013). *eHealth and eWelfare of Finland. Checkpoint 2011.* REPORT 5/2013. FinnTelemedicum and National Institute for Health and Welfare, Juvenes Print – Finnish University Print Ltd Tampere, Finland. Retrieved from https://www.julkari.fi/bitstream/handle/10024/104368/URN_ISBN_978-952-245-835-3.pdf?sequence=1

Häyrinen, K., Saranto, K., & Nykänen, P. (2008). Definition, structure, content, use and impacts of electronic health records: A review of the research literature. *International Journal of Medical Informatics, 77*, 291–304.

HOPE. (2013). *Patient safety in practice. How to manage risks to patient safety and quality in European healthcare.* Report on HOPE agora, Hague, June 11–12. Retrieved from http://hope.be/05eventsandpublications/docpublications/94_patient_safety/94_HOPE_Publication-Patient-Safety_December_2013.pdf. Accessed on March 22, 2014.

Hyvis. (2013). *Health and welfare.* (In Finnish). Retrieved from www.hyvis.fi. Accessed on March 22, 2014.

ICF. (2013). *International Classification of Functioning, Disability, and Health.* Retrieved from http://www.who.int/classifications/icf/en/

ICNP – International Council of Nurses. (2013). *Technical Implementation Guide.* International Classification for Nursing Practice (ICNP®). Retrieved from http://www.icn.ch/images/stories/documents/publications/free_publications/ICNP_Technical_Implementation_Guide.pdf. Accessed on March 22, 2014.

ICN – International Council of Nurses. (2013). *International Classification for Nursing Practice (ICNP®)*. Retrieved from http://www.icn.ch/pillarsprograms/international-classification-for-nursing-practice-icnpr/. Accessed on March 22, 2014.

Ikonen, H., Tanttu, K., Hoffren, P., & Mäkilä, M. (2007). Implementing nursing diagnosis, interventions and outcomes in multidisciplinary practice: experiences in Finland. In N. Oud, F. Sheerin, M. Ehnfors, W. Sermeus. (Eds.). Nursing Communication in Multidisciplinary Practice. *Proceedings of the 6th ACENDIO Conference*. Amsterdam, The Netherlands, 183–187.

Imel, M., & Campbell, J. R (2003). *Mapping from a clinical terminology to a classification*. AHIMSA's 75th Anniversary National Convention and Exhibit Proceedings, October 2003. American Health Information Management Association. Retrieved from http://library.ahima.org/xpedio/idcplg?IdcService=GET_HIGHLIGHT_INFO&QueryText=%28mapping+from+a+clinical+terminology+to+a+classification%29%3Cand%3E%28xPublishSite%3Csubstring%3E%60BoK%60%29&SortField=xPubDate&SortOrder=Desc&dDocName=bok1_022744&HighlightType=HtmlHighlight&dWebExtension=hcsp. Accessed on March 22, 2014.

Ingenerf, J., & Pöppl, S. J. (2007). Biomedical vocabularies - The demand for differentiation. In K. Kuhn, J. R. Warren, & T-Y. Leong (Eds.), *MEDINFO 2007 - 12th International Conference on Medical Informatics in Brisbane* (p. 610). Australia, August 20–24. Retrieved from http://vbn.aau.dk/files/12640502/Medinfo2007_part2.pdf. Accessed on March 22, 2014.

International Medical Informatics Association (IMIA). (2014). Retrieved from http://www.imia.org. Accessed on March 22, 2014.

KanTa. (2013a). *National Archive of Health Information, Kanta Services*. Retrieved from http://www.kanta.fi/en/kanta-palvelut. Accessed on March 22, 2014.

KanTa. (2013b). *Timeline of Finnish Healthcare ICT Standardization for Interoperability*. Retrieved from http://www.kanta.fi/documents/12105/3450131/Kanta_ArkkitehtuuriJaAikajana_EN.pdf/d83abeb0-db14-4edf-8877-98b7480e8d59. Accessed on March 22, 2014.

Kaustinen, T. (1995). Development of the nursing intensity classification. (In Finnish, Hoitoisuusluokituksen kehittäminen ja arviointi). Licentiate thesis. University of Oulu, Department of Nursing. University of Oulu, Oulu, Finland.

Kinnunen, U-M., Ensio, A., & Liljamo, P. (2011). Finnish care classification for nursing documentation: Users' voice, in e-health and nursing - How can e-health promote patient safety? ACENDIO 2011. In F. Sheerin, W. Sermeus, K. Saranto, et al. (Eds.), *8th European Conference of ACENDIO* (pp. 250–257). Association for Common European Nursing Diagnoses, Interventions and Outcomes, Dublin, Ohio.

Klazinga, N., Fischer, C., & ten Asbroek, A. (2011). Health services research related to performance indicators and benchmarking in Europe. *Journal of Health Services Research & Policy, 16*, 2.

Lehtovirta, J., & Vuokko, R. (Eds.), (2014). *Terveydenhuollon rakenteisen kirjaamisen opas. Keskeisten kertomusrakenteiden kirjaaminen sähköiseen potilaskertomukseen – Osa I* [Manual for structured data entry in health care. Entering essential patient record structures in the electronic patient record – Part I. Only abstract in English]. National Institute for Health and Welfare (THL). Ohjaus 1/2014. 98 pages. Helsinki 2013. ISBN 978-952-302-108-2 (online). Retrieved from https://www.julkari.fi/bitstream/handle/10024/110913/URN_ISBN_978-952-302-108-2.pdf?sequence=1. Accessed on March 22, 2014.

Liljamo, P., & Kaakinen, P. (2009). Crossmapping the Finnish Classification of Nursing Diagnosis, Nursing Interventions and the Oulu Patient Classification, in Connecting Health and Humans. In K. Saranto, P. Flatley Brennan, H.A. Park, A. Ensio. (Eds.), *Proceedings of NI2009 – The 10th International Congress on Nursing Informatics, Helsinki. Studies in Health Technology and Informatics* (Vol. 146, pp. 774–775).

Liljamo, P., Kaakinen, P., & Ensio, A. (2008). *Opas FinCC -luokituskokonaisuuden käyttöön hoitotyön sähköisen kirjaamisen mallissa*. Kansallisesti yhtenäiset hoitotyön tiedot -hanke 2007–2008. Retrieved from http://www.thl.fi/thl-client/pdfs/53f7c79c-b7db-4a27-914c-aef3899abb78. (In Finnish). Accessed on March 22, 2014.

Liljamo, P., Kinnunen, U-M., & Ensio, A. (2012). *FinCC classification system, user's guide. FiCND 3.0, FiCNI 3.0, FiCNO 1.0*. National Institute for Health and welfare (THL). Classifications, terminologies and statistic guidelines 2/2012, Helsinki. ISSN 1798-0070 (printed); ISSN 1798-0070 (pdf) Retrieved from http://www.julkari.fi/handle/10024/90804 (only abstract in English).

Liljamo, P., & Saranto, K. (2012). Cross-mapping the Finnish Care Classification and the Oulu Patient Classification. In P. A. Abbott, C. Hullin, S. Bandara, L. Nagle, & S. K. Newbold (Eds.), *Proceedings of 11th International Congress on Nursing Informatics* (p. 244), NI2012, American Medical Informatics Association, Nursing Informatics. Retrieved from http://www.ncbi.nlm.nih.gov/pmc/articles/PMC3799112/

MacNeela, P., Scott, P. A., Treacy, M. P., Hyde, A. (2006). Nursing minimum data sets: A conceptual analysis and review. *Nursing Inquiry, 13*, 44–51.

Mantas, J. (1998). *Advances in health telematics education— A NIGHTINGALE perspective*. Amsterdam, the Netherlands: IOS Press.

Mantas, J. (2004). Comparative educational systems. In E. Hovenga & J. Mantas (Eds.), *Global health informatics education* (pp. 8–17). Amsterdam, the Netherlands: IOS Press.

Mantas, J., Ammenwerth, E., Demiris, G., Hasman, A., Haux, R., Hersh, W., ... IMIA Recommendations on Education Task Force. (2010). Recommendations of the

International Medical Informatics Association (IMIA) on education in biomedical and health informatics, first revision. (IMIA Recommendations on Education Task Force). *Methods of Information in Medicine, 49*, 105–120. doi:10.3414/ME5119.

Meyer, I., Hüsing, T., Didero, M., & Korte, W. B. (2009). *eHealth benchmarking*. Final report. Retrieved from http://www.ehealth-benchmarking.eu/results/docu ments/eHealthBenchmarking_Final-Report_2009.pdf. Accessed on March 22, 2014.

Ministry of Social Affairs and Health. (2007). *eHealth roadmap—Finland*. Reports of the Ministry of Social Affairs and Health (Vol. 15). Retrieved from urn.fi/URN:ISBN:978-952-00-2286-0. Accessed on March 22, 2014.

Moen, A., Hackl, O. W., Hofdijk, J., Van Gemert-Pijnen, L., Ammenwerth, E., Nykänen, P., Hoerbst, A. (2012). eHealth in Europe – Status and challenges. *European Journal of Biomedical Informatics, 8*(1), 2–7.

Morris, R., MacNeela, P., Scott, A., Treacy, M.P., Hyde, A., Matthews, A., ...Byrne, A. (2010) The Irish nursing minimum data set for mental health: A valid tool for the collection of standardized nursing data? *Journal of Clinical Nursing, 19*(3–4), 359–367.

NANDA International. (2014). *Defining the knowledge of nursing*. Retrieved from http://www.nanda.org. Accessed on March 22, 2014.

National Council for the Professional Development of Nursing and Midwifery. (2006). *An evaluation of the extent of measurement of nursing and midwifery interventions in Ireland*. Retrieved from http://ncnmpublications.com/pdf/nc102_Evaluation_Report.pdf. Accessed on March 22, 2014.

Onnela, E., & Svenström, R. (1998). *Oulu-hoitoisuusluokituksen kehittäminen Oulun yliopistollisessa sairaalassa 1995–1997*. (In Finnish). Oulu, Finland: Loppuraportti.

Ora-Hyytiäinen, E., Ikonen, H., Ahonen, O., Rajalahti, E., Saranto, K. (2010). Learning by developing, in nursing and informatics for the 21st century. An international look at practice, education and EHR trends. In C. A. Weaver, C. W. Delaney, P. Weber, & R. L. Carr (Eds.), *Nursing and informatics for the 21st century: An international look at practice, education and EHR trends*. (2nd ed., pp. 169–174). Chicago, IL: Healthcare Information and Management Systems Society.

Rajalahti, E., & Saranto, K. (2009). Standardized nursing documentation – Developing together. In K. Saranto, P. Flatley Brennan, H. A. Park, M. Tallberg, A. Ensio (Eds.), *Connecting Health and Humans - Proceedings of NI2009 – The 10th International Congress on Nursing Informatics*, Helsinki.

Rauhala, A., & Fagerström, L. (2004). Determining optimal nursing intensity: The RAFAELA method. *Journal of Advanced Nursing, 45*(4), 351–359.

Saba V. (1992). Home health care classification (HHCC) of nursing diagnoses and interventions. *Caring, 11*, 50–57.

Saba, V. K. (2007). *Clinical Care Classification (CCC) System manual: A guide to nursing documentation*. New York, NY: Springer Publishing Company.

Saba, V. K. (2012). *Clinical Care Classification (CCC) System, version 2.5. User's guide* (2nd ed.). New York, NY: Springer Publishing Company.

Saranto, K., & Kinnunen, U-M. (2009). Evaluating nursing documentation—Research designs and methods: Systematic review. *Journal of Advanced Nursing, 65*(3), 464–476.

Saranto, K., Kinnunen, U-M., Kivekäs, E., Lappalainen, A-M., Liljamo, P., Rajalahti, E., & Hyppönen, H. (2013). Impacts of structuring nursing records: A systematic review. *Scandinavian Journal of Caring Sciences*, 2013. doi: 10.1111/scs.12094. Retrieved from http://onlineli-brary.wiley.com/doi/10.1111/scs.12094/pdf. Accessed on March 22, 2014.

Sermeus, W., Aiken, L. H., Van den Heede, K., Rafferty, A. M., Griffiths, P., Moreno-Casbas, M. T., ... RN4CAST consortium. (2011). Nurse forecasting in Europe (RN4CAST): Rationale, design and methodology. *BMC Nursing, 10*, 6. doi:10.1186/1472-6955-10-6.

Sermeus, W., & Deleise, L. (1997). Development of a presentation tool for nursing data. In R. A. Mortensen (Ed.), *ICNP in Europe: Telenurse*. Amsterdam, the Netherlands: IOS Press.

Sermeus, W., Delesie, L., Van Landuyt, J., Wuyts, Y., Vandenboer, G., & Manna, M. (1994). *The nursing minimum data set in Belgium: A basic tool for tomorrow's health care management*. Leuven, Belgium: Katholieke Universiteit Leuven.

Sermeus, W., van den Heede, K., Michiels, D., Delesie, L., Thonon, O., Van Boven, C., ... Gillet, P. (2005). Revising the Belgian nursing minimum dataset: From concept to implementation. *International Journal of Medical Informatics, 74*(11–12), 946–951.

SSN. (2010). *The Nordic Nurses Federation (NNF)*. Retrieved from http://www.ssn-nnf.no/ikbViewer/page/ssn/english. Accessed on March 22, 2014.

Stroetmann, K. A., Artmann, J., & Stroetmann, V. N. (2011). *European countries on their journey towards national eHealth infrastructures*. Final European progress report. Retrieved from http://www.ehealth-strategies.eu/report/eHealth_Strategies_Final_Report_Web.pdf. Accessed on March 22, 2014.

Tanttu, K., & Rusi, R. (2007). Nursing documentation project in Finland: developing a nationally standardized electronic nursing documentation by 2007, in Nursing Communication in Multidisciplinary Practice. In N. Oud, F. Sheerin, M. Ehnfors, et al. (Eds). *Proceedings of the 6th European Conference of ACENDIO* (pp. 213–217). Amsterdam, the Netherlands: Oud Consultancy.

The International Health Terminology Standards Development Organisation (IHTSDO). (2014). *SNOMED CT. The global language of healthcare*. Retrieved from http://www.ihtsdo.org/snomed-ct/

Thoroddsen, A., Ehrenberg, A., Sermeus, W., & Saranto, K. (2012). *A survey of nursing documentation, terminologies and standards in European countries.* Advancing global health through informatics. In P. A. Abbott, C. Hullin, S. Bandara, L. Nagle, & S. K. Newbold (Eds.), *Proceedings of NI2012.* Retrieved from http://euro pepmc.org/articles/PMC3799179. Accessed on March 14, 2014.

Thoroddsen, A., Saranto, K., & Ehrenberg, A., & Sermeus, W. (2009). Connecting Health and Humans. *Studies in Health Technology and Informatics, 146.*

University of Eastern Finland. (2014). *Department of Health and Social Management.* Retrieved from http://www.uef. fi/en/stj/etusivu. Accessed on March 22, 2014.

van den Heede, K., Michiels, D., Thonon, O., Sermeus, W. (2009). Using nursing interventions classification as a framework to revise the Belgian nursing minimum data set. *International Journal of Nursing Terminologies and Classifications, 20*(3), 122–131.

WHO. (1977). Development of designs in and documentation of nursing process. Report on a Technical Advisory Group. Copenhagen, Denmark: WHO.

WHO. (2013). *Health for All database (HFA-DB),* Updated July 2013. Retrieved from http://data.euro.who.int/hfadb. Accessed on March 22, 2014.

53

Pacific Rim Perspectives

Evelyn J. S. Hovenga / Michelle L. L. Honey / Lucy A. Westbrooke

• OBJECTIVES

1. Describe the development of nursing informatics in some Pacific Rim countries.
2. Identify historical milestones, changes, and trends influencing nurses to embrace informatics.
3. Discuss nursing informatics leadership, international links, education, and research, along with their impact upon the development of nursing informatics as a nursing discipline or specialty.

• KEY WORDS

Information systems
Standards
eHealth
Public policy
Professional organizations

The evolution of nursing informatics (NI) has varied in each of the Pacific Rim countries. The adoption of informatics usually began as a vision by one or more individuals. Such people used any number of opportunities plus their leadership skills to promote and disseminate the use of information technologies to support nurses in all areas of nursing practice. This has and continues to occur in healthcare, educational, and government organizations, as well as within the information technology (IT) industry and via any number of new and existing professional organizations. Events external to the nursing profession frequently became the catalyst stimulating some type of activity by nurses toward the adoption of informatics. International and multi-disciplinary links have assisted these beginnings and its progression. Australia, New Zealand, Korea, and Hong Kong have made considerable progress since the early 1980s followed by Japan, Singapore, Thailand, Taiwan, and China in recent years. Nurses in a number of other countries in the Pacific region have only just begun or have yet to learn about NI.

The Asia Pacific Medical Informatics Association (APAMI) was formed in 1993 as a regional group of the International Medical Informatics Association. APAMI has helped launch national healthcare informatics associations in Malaysia, Indonesia, and the Philippines and has generated awareness about the field in India, Pakistan, Sri Lanka, and Fiji (APAMI, n.d.). Other member nations are Australia, Hong Kong, Japan, Korea, New Zealand, the People's Republic of China, Singapore, Taiwan, and Thailand where APAMI has played a significant role in the promotion of NI (APAMI, n.d.). Significant progress of NI has been made in Taiwan, Hong Kong, and China. Nurses and others with an interest in Health Informatics (HI) and/or NI in these countries who are interested in promoting informatics to their profession need to link up with this network.

Anecdotal evidence suggests that it continues to be a challenge for many nurses in this region to obtain appropriate education in informatics both during their initial nurse education and as a component of post–nurse registration specialist courses with some exceptions. Notwithstanding these conditions, an increase in computer use by practicing nurses in Australia, New Zealand, and other Pacific Rim countries is creating an awareness of the opportunities and gains to healthcare resulting from an increase in the use of computers, information, and telecommunication technologies. Nurses in all health environments are becoming more dependent on electronic information.

This chapter aims to provide an overview of these historical events, primarily from Australia and New Zealand but also from Singapore, Taiwan, China, and Hong Kong relative to national HI, or eHealth, initiatives and trends, and to highlight critical success factors for the benefit of those who have yet to embark on such a journey. The chapter concludes by summarizing significant events and examining their impact on the evolution of nursing informatics in this region.

NATIONAL HEALTH SYSTEM INFRASTRUCTURES

New Zealand's total population is reported as nearly 4.5 million. Approximately three-quarters of these people are found in urban areas. Auckland, the largest city, has over a third of the total population. The population by age indicates that a fifth (20%) are under 15 years of age and 14% are over 65 years of age. The proportion of older people is projected to increase. Ethnicity statistics depicts a diverse population, with the majority of people in New Zealand being European (69%), with Maori, the indigenous people, making up a further 15% of the population (Statistics New Zealand, 2013).

Australia is a federation of eight states and territories. It has a population of over 22 million. Around 9.4% of its gross domestic product (GDP) is spent on health services. Approximately 71% of its households are located in inner and outer urban and provincial areas, mostly near cities on the coast. Australia has one of the lowest population densities outside its major cities. In 2009, there were around 1105 Full-Time Equivalent (38 hours per week) registered nurses and mid-wives per 100,000 population of whom 20% were aged 55 or over (AIHW, 2012, p. 506).

Government's health policies need to address the increased demand for health services imposed by:

- An ageing population
- Increased complexity of need
- A greater incidence of long-term conditions
- Growing consumer demand for choice

- Changing lifestyle factors
- Technological developments
- An increasing focus on partnership between consumers and providers

These pressures are expected to continue to intensify (Ministry of Health and District Health Boards New Zealand Workforce Group, 2007). Every nation needs to target and prioritize where health IT investments are made as judicious use of technology could be the key to the long-term sustainability of a national healthcare service and health outcome improvements.

National Health System Funding Frameworks

In Australia, patient classification system development that describes the case mix serviced by healthcare organizations began collaboratively with Professor Fetter from Yale University during the 1980s. The Australian Refined Diagnosis Related Group (AR-DRG) standard is now in use nationally for costing and funding purposes. This Australian case-mix program relies on data obtained from individual patient records, including the International Statistical Classification of Diseases and Related Health Problems (10th revision), Australian Modification (ICD-10-AM) codes. A number of case-mix systems are in use to suit a variety of patient population types. Service weights to reflect the cost of providing various hospital-based services including nursing are updated from time to time. These are included in various funding formulas adopted around the country. The 2009 review report on Australia's case-mix system states that, "this system reaps benefits to the community of around $4 billion per annum in savings (for bed days) against an estimated annual cost of $10 million" (Commonwealth of Australia, 2009; Commonwealth of Australia, 2010). The government's Web site on case-mix is very informative. This same case-mix system has been adopted by a number of other countries.

Australian taxpayers contribute a 1.5% Medicare levy, and high-income earners who do not have private health insurance pay an additional 1%; this contributed 15% to the Australian Government's total health funding for 2009–2010 (AIHW, 2012, p.474). The taxpayer contributions to Medicare are projected to increase to cover disability services. Spending on cardiovascular diseases was higher than for any other disease, at $7.9 billion (AIHW, 2012, p 477). The Australian government also manages its Pharmaceutical Benefits Scheme (PBS) that is jointly funded by them and non-government sources; it accounts for 14% of recurrent health expenditures (AIHW, 2012, p. 478).

New Zealand also has a publicly funded healthcare system, which means that healthcare is free or heavily subsidized to the consumer (New Zealand Immigration, 2012). The government's Ministry of Health primarily allocates funds to 20 district health boards (DHBs) based on population. The DHBs both purchase and provide healthcare services for their region. DHBs are increasingly working together to ensure the delivery of health services in the most cost-effective and efficient manner to meet national, regional, and local needs.

The New Zealand Accident Compensation Corporation (ACC) provides comprehensive, no-fault personal injury cover for all residents through a range of health benefits and subsidies to assist individuals in the event of an accident (ACC, 2012). In addition the ACC funds injury prevention, early rehabilitation and collects statistics for injuries suffered by the population. The establishment of the ACC has virtually eliminated suing for compensation in the event of an accident. ACC funding is provided through a levy on employers, employees, and vehicle registration. ACC deals with over 1.5 million new claims each year, which is in addition to a significant number of ongoing claims.

Private insurance–funded healthcare is increasing. Given the aging population, improved options of health treatments, increased demands yet limited public budgets, and increased waiting times for elective surgery, this trend is likely to continue. The role of the private sector now accounts for nearly 20% of healthcare (New Zealand Immigration, 2012). The cost of private health insurance is increasing with premiums rising faster than the general cost of living, and consequently there is a widening gap between those who can afford private healthcare to supplement care provided through the public system. This has particularly affected the older population who are most likely to require health services and are less able to pay for private insurance as they move into retirement on reduced incomes.

All prescription-related medicines are regulated by the government through Pharmac. Subsidies are available on a range of medicines, although only a few options within each drug classification may be subsidized by Pharmac. The public can purchase an increasing number of over-the-counter remedies. There is a burgeoning need for drug information for medical practitioners, nurses, and consumers. Pharmac has also recently taken responsibility for medical device management.

Technology and Healthcare Trends

The past decade has seen major changes in technology including the development of cloud services, the maturity of systems integration services, the proliferation of devices and mobile access to applications, and the dramatically enhanced capacity to collect and analyze massive datasets.

Additionally, health service providers have become more capable with respect to ICT development and change management. The healthcare environment is changing at an ever-increasing pace due to this proliferation.

Embracing the advances in technology enables us to deliver healthcare in new and innovative ways. Basic hardware has advanced into multiple components of input and output devices. Development of infrastructures has enabled this technology to be networked. The Internet provides a medium to transmit information nationally and internationally. The physical constraints and boundaries are now so blurred that healthcare delivery can occur and/or be supervised by experts located anywhere at any time.

Some Australian nurses are using personal digital assistants (PDAs) for point-of-care information and clinical documentation for community and acute hospital nursing, hospital-based infection control, and/or wound management. Many new monitoring devices are being connected to information systems for automated data entry. Improvements in portability are now enabling the use of technology in a greater range of settings. Both PDAs and tablets are being used or trialled in the clinical setting by students and healthcare professionals alike.

Changes in healthcare provision in New Zealand have brought a more collaborative approach. Integrating care is now viewed as a priority. This is being supported by technology-enabled information flow (Ministry of Health, 2011). Electronic health event summaries, along with laboratory and radiology data, are now being transmitted between providers and across primary and secondary sectors. In the pharmaceutical area, data are available on prescriptions dispensed.

The Internet and intranets are providing a wealth of information to health providers as well as consumers. This is being supported by increasingly sophisticated national broadband infrastructures. New Zealand has a high proportion of Internet users: 88% of the population (Internet World Stats, 2012). One in two rural homes have broadband access, but 12% of homes still have a dial-up connection, and the most common reason for not switching to broadband is cost (Statistics New Zealand, 2013). The government has put in place two initiatives to improve broadband services—the Ultra-Fast Broadband and the Rural Broadband Initiative, which will bring faster broadband using fiber optic technology to 97.8% of homes, schools, businesses, and hospitals (Ministry of Business Innovation and Employment, 2012).

This increased Internet speed will improve the exchange of information and support the use of new technologies. A survey of New Zealand consumers ($n = 1783$) found 67.9% of participants used a computer to access health information, and the Internet was the third most popular source of health information, after the doctor/health center and nurses (Honey, Roy, Bycroft, Boyd, & Raphael, 2014). This study identified that New Zealand consumers found accessing online health information useful and they could mostly trust the information they found. However, this study also found that consumers were not aware of existing New Zealand health information Web sites and resources and therefore these are under-utilized.

These include the portal Health Navigator (www.healthnavigator.org.nz) which collates, coordinates, and identifies the most useful resources for primary and secondary prevention of long-term conditions; HealthPoint (www.healthpoint.co.nz) which provides local information about what to expect prior to, during and following a referral; Health Topics A-Z (www.agewell.org.nz) which promotes healthy ageing; and Web Health (www.webhealth.co.nz) which aims to connect communities by providing a directory of health and social services. Consumer awareness will be essential for high usage of the planned national telehealth service to provide the public with easy access to comprehensive health advice, support, and information (Ministry of Health, 2013d). New Zealand consumers are increasingly using technology. National strategies have identified the provision of consumer information, patient portals, and shared health records as important developments for the immediate future.

The Web environment and the use of powerful integration engines are now providing contextual views of data that are browser based and single log-on. Placed over multiple health information systems, these connections or portals provide a "single patient-centric view" of data across all applications for use by clinicians. We now have tools that allow ease of messaging and mapping along with products to support the clinical workflow process. Online technologies provide products and services that enhance patient care and improve clinical outcomes through evidence-based health information and decision support systems. Mobile computing, specifically the use of Smart Phones, is increasing in line with global trends.

In March 2013, Horizon research found more adults in New Zealand now use a smart phone than a standard mobile, which was a 13.6% rise over the previous nine months (Horizon Poll, 2013). Mobile computing has also increased with the use of tablets, including iPads. While these are seen in use among consumers and students there is an increase in their use in the healthcare environment as well. For example, in secondary care health professionals may Bring Your Own Device (BYOD) for use in multidisciplinary team meetings. In the community setting the Royal New Zealand Plunket Society is using tablets for point-of-care data entry in the area of well child health (Hardiker & Hynes, 2012).

Another global trend has been the increase in the use of social media, with internationally a 19% rise in the number of social media users in 2012 and a predicted further increase of 16% in 2013 (eMarketer, 2012). Social media can be a platform in healthcare to promote and improve health and as a means of contact with and between consumers. By facilitating interactions online discussion forums can develop communities among those interested in discussing health-related topics (Lu, Zhang, Liu, Li, & Deng, 2013). Two examples illustrate this: A community-based support service for teen parents, Thrive (https://www.facebook.com/pages/Thrive-Teen-Parent-Support-Trust/246635878698248), use Facebook as their main communication tool. A further example involves a service that provides support to families with mental health problems who are using an online forum to extend their service provision (Honey et al., 2013).

New Zealand has one of the highest rates of social media usage with 81% of Internet users using social media to share information (Community Net Aotearoa, 2013). However, the rise of social media use has also caused concern, and the Nursing Council of New Zealand in the nurses Code of Conduct now makes specific mention of the use of social media and electronic communication (Nursing Council of New Zealand, 2012).

Although New Zealand is a small country, it has a surprising number of health IT companies producing software that is not only being used locally but also internationally. Information technology is New Zealand's third largest export behind dairy and tourism, and is the fastest growing, highest per-capita earning industry for the country. On the domestic front, information communication technologies (ICT) contribute nearly $20 billion to New Zealand's economy and employ over 40,000 people (New Zealand Technology Industry Association, 2013). The New Zealand government has identified innovation as one of six priority areas to support and has therefore funneled funding into research and development in ICT (New Zealand Technology Industry Association, 2013).

Standards Development and Adoption

The availability of detailed and clinically relevant data is essential for clinical care decisions and for oversight groups making decisions related to the quality of that care. Today, health information systems are expected to meet a variety of changing demands for data and information to support many purposes, such as:

- Providing immediate feedback to care providers by automated alerts related to relevant best practice guidelines

- Decision support
- Generating data needed for internal and external quality monitoring
- Exchanging critical patient information in a timely manner across the healthcare continuum
- Reducing provider burden associated with current documentation requirements
- Payment policy
- Outcomes research

Health data and information standards, including standardized terminology systems, support the increasing need to safely and securely exchange a wide variety of patient and clinical information between various healthcare providers and IT systems. With point-of-care documentation, technology is now available to build electronic health information systems that will efficiently meet a variety of needs.

National adoption of technical standards is a prerequisite to being able to optimize the use of IT by means of securing semantically interoperable clinical systems and contribute significantly to a sustainable national health system. This can only be accomplished with the universal adoption of appropriate standards. Of particular importance is the design and architecture of any national health information and integration platform based on specific sets of technical standards.

Standards Australia (SA) was persuaded to establish a health informatics committee in 1992 (Standards Australia, n.d.). The SA IT-14 Committee now has several active technical sub-committees and works closely with other similar groups such as HL7 International via HL7 Australia (Health Level Seven, n.d.), the ISO Technical Committee 215, the Comite Europeen de Normalisation (CEN) Technical Committee 251, the Integrating the Healthcare Enterprise (IHE) international organization, the International Health Terminology Standards Development (IHTSDO), and the openEHR Foundation. In Australia, nurses are represented via the Royal College of Nursing although other nurses also contribute from time to time.

The focus in Australia has been in the area of standards development to facilitate data interchange, initially designed to support all types of e-commerce. This later expanded to support the interchange of clinical data. The Systematized Nomenclature of Medicine-Clinical Terms (SNOMED-CT) has been adopted as the national terminology standard. Australia is an active contributor to the development of international standards. This ensures that these standards are able to meet Australian and New Zealand industry needs. Once international standards have been completed and published, the SA IT-14 considers

whether this can be adopted for Australia as is or if we need to develop an implementation guide that meets specific Australian needs. In some instances, Australian standards are being reviewed and modified via the ISO Technical Committee 215 to suit the international market. All Australian standards are freely available in pdf format via the SA's eHealth Web site (www.e-health.standards.org.au). This was made possible by Australian government funding, as IT industry standards compliance is highly valued.

Australia's National eHealth Transition Authority (NEHTA), established in 2005, now works closely with the SA IT-14 Committee to ensure that standards development priorities match its business priorities as detailed in its latest strategic plan (NEHTA, 2013). NEHTA's role is to lead the uptake of eHealth systems of national significance, to coordinate the progression and accelerate the adoption of eHealth by delivering urgently needed integration infrastructure and standards for health information. Its vision is to enhance healthcare by enabling access to the right information, for the right person, at the right time and place. NEHTA publishes several Web sites that collectively provide information to support all stakeholders, including the Clinical Knowledge Manager (http://dcm.nehta.org.au/ckm/); it has adopted five strategic priorities that are guiding their work activities:

1. Deliver, operationalize, and enhance the essential foundations required to enable ehealth.
2. Coordinate the progression of priority ehealth initiatives.
3. Manage the delivery of key components of the Australia Government's PCEHR Program.
4. Accelerate national adoption of ehealth.
5. Lead the further progression of ehealth in Australia.

In 2001, the New Zealand Minister of Health directed that a Ministerial Committee on a Health Information Standards Organisation (HISO) be established to manage health information standards. HISO drew together hitherto disparate health-related groups with a specific interest in producing IT standards for New Zealand. HISO's role included identifying, developing, publishing, and monitoring New Zealand's health information standards. HISO has over the years been governed by different bodies but has been incorporated under the Health IT Board since 2009 (Ministry of Health, 2013a). The purpose of HISO is to support and promote the development, understanding, and use of fit-for-purpose health information standards to improve the New Zealand health system. HISO aims to endorse existing standards if appropriate and only develop standards that are specific to New Zealand or are not currently available internationally.

A key driver for HISO's role is the consistent use of standards. This is aimed at acceptance throughout health and health-related industries of such standards that require the enablement of real-time access to information about the standards (i.e., Which standards are agreed upon? Which are being developed or proposed? What initiatives are taking place? What are the downstream implications?), including where the information may be freely accessed.

eHealth Policy, Governance, and Funding initiatives

In Singapore the Integrated Health Information Systems (IHiS) organization began in 2008 with over 600 staff from their healthcare clusters' IT departments (IHiS, 2014) as an integrated IT enabler. Their aim was to drive greater synergies and high-performing systems by strengthening and consolidating their IT workforce. IHiS provides the full suite of IT services for all public hospitals, national specialty centers, and polyclinics. It has the responsibility to architect and oversee the performance of the health services' clinical, business, and healthcare analytics by standardizing, harmonizing, and optimizing IT resources across the public healthcare sector. Its aim is to maximize synergies from shared systems and ensure cost-effective healthcare delivery. This is collectively managed by their Chief Information Officer, Applications, Architecture, Integration and Development, and Technology Management divisions. This structured collaboration has resulted an aggregation of demand for hardware, software, and projects, interoperable electronic medical records (EMRs) across health clusters, specialized expertise and career paths for IT staff, and a critical mass of IT skills to meet future healthcare demands.

SingHealth hospitals in Singapore have included Heads or Directors of Nursing Informatics within their hospital executive structures who work closely with IHiS staff. A new mobile application to help nurses manage pressure ulcers, prevent patient falls, and enhance medication safety designed by and for nurses was recently launched. The SingHealth Nurses Pal also features an intravenous (IV) drip rate calculator and alarm function (Singapore Health, 2014).

Australia's first national strategic information action plan, Health Online, was initiated in 1999. This was followed by a number of projects initiated by the Australian government: Health*Connect*, Medi*Connect*, the provision of quality health information for consumers known as Health*Insite*, and the national supply chain initiative along with more than 360 projects such as the integration of primary health and hospital care, several shared and coordinated care projects, and the establishment of health call centers. Since 2004, the Australian government has commissioned and received numerous reports with many recommendations. In addition, various state and jurisdiction reports were commissioned such as the NSW Health Garling Report on Acute Services. All such reports made reference to the need for widespread adoption of eHealth. The National Hospitals and Health Reform Commission's (NHHRC) report identified a number of gaps in safety and quality due to sub-optimal information sharing, and proposed health informatics solutions that are expected to result in improvements (Australian Government, 2008).

The term *eHealth* only came into widespread usage a few years ago. By 2005, there was no agreed-upon definition for *eHealth* yet this term is widely used and has various meanings (Oh, Rizo, Enkin, & Jadad 2005). As a consequence, there was a lack of consistency in the population's understanding of and perceptions about the workforce's knowledge and skill requirements and the likely impact of successful eHealth strategy implementations. The World Health Organization (WHO) has adopted the following definition to clarify interpretation for all associated with international trade, foreign policy, diplomacy, and the health industry (WHO, n.d.):

eHealth is the transfer of health resources and healthcare by electronic means. It encompasses three main areas:

- *The delivery of health information, for health professionals and health consumers, through the Internet and telecommunications*
- *Using the power of IT and e-commerce to improve public health services, e.g., through the education and training of health workers*
- *The use of e-commerce and e-business practices in health systems management*

The 2008 National eHealth Strategy reinforced existing collaboration between Commonwealth, State, and Territory Governments on the core foundations of a national eHealth system, and identified priority areas where this can be progressively extended to support health reform in Australia. It also provided sufficient flexibility for individual States and Territories, and the public and private health sectors, to determine how they go about eHealth implementation within a common framework and set of priorities to maximize benefits and efficiencies.

The 2010 federal budget announced the government's intention to fund the adoption of personally held and controlled EHRs (PCEHR). Australia has also initiated a National Broadband Network rollout; the Healthcare Identifiers Bill was passed by the Australian Federal Parliament. Capacity to host multiple healthcare applications including clinical software programs, decision support tools for diagnosis and management, care plans, referral tools, e-prescribing tools, and a range of online training and other administrative and clinical services is improving despite a number of failures around the country. Electronic prescribing and dispensing of medications was introduced in 2011. The eHealth record system launched in June 2012 is now under review. The National eHealth Transition Authority (NeHTA) is jointly funded by the Australian Government and all State and Territory Governments to facilitate the transition to a connected system where every Australian is at the center of healthcare (NEHTA, 2013). Australian Nursing and Midwifery Federation (ANMF, http://anmf.org.au/pages/issue-2-e-news-on-e-health)—telehealth tutorial links to e-news on eHealth.

The new Government (from Sept 2013) is reviewing all past commitments and is making a number of directional changes; its eHealth policy directions are yet to be made public. PCEHR implementation has disappointed many. NIA members are providing feedback around the PCEHR via the Australian College of Nursing. Other HI organizations (HISA, HIMAA, and ACHI) are also providing feedback to the Ministerial PCEHR review. This project has received extensive nursing and other HI expert advice, mostly via NeHTA as appointees to "clinical lead" positions. Expert advice received was often not acted upon.

The new Australian government is expected to develop new health policies based on their view that we need a closer working relationship between GPs and hospitals, better ehealth solutions, and improved coordination of care for people with chronic and complex conditions, including cancer. The pressures faced by most countries that influence eHealth policy and funding initiatives include:

- A growing older population, more people with long-term and complex health conditions.
- Workforce issues including an aging workforce, where nurses comprise the single largest health professional group.
- Health inequalities and the need to address Mâori (the indigenous people of New Zealand) health disparities because of their over-representation in morbidity and mortality data (Connolly et al., 2010). The same is true for Australia's indigenous population.

These pressures exist now and can only be expected to intensify in the next decade. Nations need to target and prioritize where health IT investments are made, as judicious use of technology could be the key to the long-term sustainability of a free healthcare service and improving health outcomes. New Zealand has a desire for a more informed consumer (Davey & Gee, 2002). It also has a history of free health service, consequently there is an

expectation that healthcare will continue to be freely available and that evidence-based best practice will determine the treatments with no consideration of cost. Australia is in similar situation. Nurses are recognized as having enormous potential to advance health and disability outcomes (Nursing and Midwifery Workforce Strategy Group, 2006).

The Health*SMART* program adopted by the Victorian Government is now 10 years old. In late 2012 the Victorian Minister for Health convened a panel to examine the future of health sector ICT and make specific conclusions and recommendations to nominated terms of reference. Panel members appointed to undertake this Ministerial Review of Vic Health Sector ICT (2013) did not include a nurse although opportunities for submissions and discussion forum participation, were made available.

The Auditor General's audit report on the *Clinical ICT Systems in the Victorian Public Health Sector* (October 2013) indicated that poor planning and inadequate understanding of the complex requirements of designing and implementing clinical ICT systems meant that the Department of Health has delivered the Health*SMART* clinical ICT system to only four Victorian health services at a cost of $145.3 million and that some clinical ICT systems have issues that potentially affect patient safety and need to be closely monitored and resolved by the department and relevant health services. This had been projected by outside HI experts and ignored at the time when this decision was made. It was also reported that outside the Health*SMART* program, other clinical ICT systems that have been incrementally developed with strong clinician engagement enjoy wide acceptance and support from end users. Although their functionality is not directly equivalent to the Health*SMART* system, these other systems have involved significantly less capital and ongoing expenditure. Such outcomes again demonstrate the need for HI education and the benefits of engaging with clinical staff.

New Zealand's healthcare is guided by a national health strategy, which has the goal of good health and well-being for all New Zealanders throughout their lives (Ministry of Health, 2000). Furthermore, the New Zealand Health Strategy (2000, p. 29) recognizes the importance of good information management and states: "The ability to exchange high-quality information between partners in healthcare processes will be vital for a health system focused on achieving better health outcomes." The economic downturn which began in 2008 provided the impetus to seriously look at how care was delivered and supported. Following a Ministerial Review in 2009, changes to the health sector occurred with the objective of "better, sooner, more convenient health services" (Ministry of Health, 2011). The National Health IT Board was formed as a health sector leadership group supporting the delivery of high-quality healthcare and providing strategic leadership on health information investments and solutions.

The overall vision for information management in New Zealand was in 2010 in the National Health IT Plan (National Health IT Board, 2010) and subsequently updated for 2013/14 (Ministry of Health, 2013c). The update describes the work that needs to be done to achieve the Government's eHealth vision of all New Zealanders having electronic access to their own core health information and improve the quality, accuracy, and timeliness of health and disability services. Four priorities are identified for 2014 and beyond: electronic medication management, national clinical solutions, regional information platforms, and community-based integrated care initiatives (Ministry of Health, 2013e).

This plan will have been achieved when there are sustainable common platforms managing clinical and administrative information and interoperable systems to securely and seamlessly share information. This can be accomplished with good leadership and governance models that support robust and timely decision-making. It is recognized that in order to achieve the vision there must be a partnership of patients/consumers, health practitioners, health and disability providers, vendors, shared service agencies, the Ministry of Health, and other key partners such as Pharmac and the Health Quality and Safety Commission (Ministry of Health, 2013e).

Although this seems an ambitious plan, significant progress has been made in many areas, including sharing and transfer of records in the primary sector, shared care planning tools, patient portals, sharing of picture archiving and communications systems (PACS), electronic prescription services and commencement of electronic prescribing and administration in hospitals. The core infrastructure of the NHI has been upgraded and now provides enhanced searching, address, and geocoding functions. Telehealth initiatives are also increasing. The need for shared and accessible records from multiple sites was reinforced following the Christchurch earthquakes in 2010 and 2011 when there was major disruption to healthcare delivery. The work that had already occurred in the sharing of information with regional repositories and national systems such as InterRAI proved invaluable (BCS, 2013; InterRAI, n.d.). The challenges of governance, funding, and capability still remain but there is a sector-wide commitment to performance improvement.

Telehealth is a disruptive force and as it becomes a reality it is challenging the traditional way care is delivered and the roles of all participants. The Telehealth Forum has been established under the umbrella of the National IT Health Board to promote the use of telehealth, and

maximize the benefits of the Government's broadband program. The National Health IT Board has funded the establishment of the Forum because it recognizes telehealth is an important component of an integrated model of healthcare (National Health IT Board, 2013). The telehealth pilot and evaluation by the West Coast DHB highlighted the challenges and changes required for successful use of telehealth (Day & Kerr, 2012).

Telehealth is increasingly seen as an enabler to support care delivery. Some DHBs are already providing some telehealth services such as patient consultations, particularly when they have a high proportion of their population rurally based and spread over a wide geographic area (Lucas, Honey, & Day, 2012). The role played in telehealth by each of the DHBs varies. DHBs delivering primary and secondary care to their populations may require the support of tertiary services from some of the other DHBs. For example, multi-site, multi-disciplinary team meetings (MDMs) using videoconferencing are used to support cancer services under the leadership of larger tertiary services. Planning also is underway for a national telehealth service using a multi-channel approach including telephone triage and phone advice, text, e-mail, phone applications, social media, and Web-based services to improve public access to a range of advice, counseling, and referral services (Ministry of Health, 2013d). Remote monitoring of consumers in the home is still limited at this stage but on the increase. There is some remote monitoring of directly observed therapy (DOT) for medication compliance and research on smart homes to support people to remain at home for longer (Suryadevara & Mukhopadhyay, 2013).

Following a Ministerial Review in 2009, changes to the health sector have been instigated with the overall objective of "better, sooner, more convenient health services." The implementation of these changes has been divided into three areas: organization change, implementation of the recommendations of the Ministerial Review Group (MRG) report, and review and amendments to legislation to support the changes.

One of the recommendations of the MRG was the establishment of the National Health Board and the formation of a sub-committee, the National Health IT Board. The MRG made a number of informatics-related recommendations that included strengthening health information technology and clinical leadership, prioritization of new technologies and medical devices, and addressing procurement from a national perspective. The National Health IT Board is seen as a health sector leadership group to support the delivery of high-quality healthcare by providing strategic leadership on health information investments and solutions and to lead a national health IT agenda. The Health IT Board has created a draft National Health IT Plan for consultation, which aims to "drive a culture of innovation, partnership and respect to support health sector leaders to make appropriate health IT investments in the context of the whole sector" (Ministry of Health, 2010) and to work toward the eHealth vision: "To achieve high quality healthcare and improve patient safety, by 2014 New Zealanders will have a core set of personal health information available electronically to them and their treatment providers regardless of the setting as they access health services" (Ministry of Health, 2010).

Although focused on person-centric health systems, there are generic principles that apply to other information systems. The first phase calls for reducing duplication by consolidation of systems in the health sector and leveraging the work already completed by other successful projects. With a more consolidated platform, shared care planning between providers can be enabled. The overall aim is to address New Zealand's most pressing health IT needs and significant issues that continue to form barriers to improving health outcomes and reducing delivery costs. The recent economic downturn is one of the drivers for this new initiative, with the Minister of Health hoping to achieve savings of $700 million over 5 years by having common back-office systems for the country's 20 district health boards. In addition, these strategies form the cornerstone of activity for a strong IT infrastructure to address longer-term issues such as electronic health records.

To date, the development of a national technology infrastructure has proved useful; however, securing appropriate access to relevant clinical and administrative information throughout the health sector remains the greatest challenge. Much progress has been made in primary healthcare. For example, in a comparative study of 11 countries, New Zealand was found to have 92% of community-based practices with advanced electronic health information capacity across functions, including electronic prescribing and ordering of tests; electronic access to test results, prescription alerts, and clinical notes; guidelines, preventive and follow-up care reminders; and computerized lists of patients by diagnosis, medications, due for tests, or preventive care (Schoen et al., 2009).

New Zealand's government health policy has been driving toward a population health management approach. Accordingly, the sector has been slowly moving away from a "bricks and mortar," hospital-centric approach toward integrated healthcare (Ministry of Health, 2001). Although significant gaps remain, the move has proved heavily reliant on collaboration between government, contracting agencies, and delivery units.

Information Governance

The national health information agreements and the establishment of the National Health Data Dictionary in 1993 laid the foundation for consistent health data sets in Australia. This continues to provide the national infrastructure needed to provide high-quality health data. It includes Australia's repository for national metadata standards for health, METeOR, providing online access to a wide range of nationally endorsed data definitions and tools for creating new definitions based on existing already-endorsed components (AIHW, n.d.). Also available via METeOR are the National Data Dictionaries, national minimum data sets, and data set specifications.

An Australian Community Nursing Minimum Data Set was developed during the early 1990s. This has been adopted and extended by the Department of Veteran Affairs (DVA) and is used by them to monitor the provision of community nursing services provided via DVA contracts. The DVA has also developed and adopted a Community Nursing Classification system consisting of four levels based on service type, client type, and clinical care, and technical care. A number of other minimum data sets (MDS) exist such as the palliative care MDS, the nurse practitioner MDS, the NSW State Spinal Cord Injury Service MDS, and health and community care (HACC) MDS. The Royal District Nursing Service (RDNS) in Melbourne makes use of a number of these in their information system via a data-mapping matrix. The RDNS also manages a data warehouse.

Australia's health sector governance is constantly changing. A 2004 review undertaken on behalf of the then newly established National Health Information Group (NHIG) and the Australian Health Information Council (AHIC) identified distributed governance over many jurisdictions as a significant impediment to the provision of better healthcare outcomes, safety, quality, and cost efficiencies (ICT Standards Committee, 2004). A strategic workplan for 2007–08 to 2012–13 (NHIMPC, 2007), and a published model of the national governance structure for Information Management (IM) and Health Information Communication Technology (ICT) changed in 2008, following a change of government. A National Health Information Standards and Statistics Committee (NHISSC) was established in 2008 and continues to provide a national health data governance service despite changes in Governments (NHISSC, n.d.).

Historically, primary care in New Zealand made use of the READ codes, which is continued by the Accident Compensation Corporation (ACC). The ACC describes READ codes as "a hierarchical clinical coding system;

each level provides a more specific diagnosis of an injury" (ACC, 2012; ACC, 2013). Secondary care used the ICD-10 classification system, originating from the World Health Organization as a means of classifying and coding diseases and signs, symptoms, abnormal findings, complaints, social circumstances, and external causes of injury or diseases (World Health Organization, 2010). In addition, Logical Observation Identifiers, Names, and Codes (LOINC) is used for laboratory data and Health Level Seven (HL7) is the favored messaging standard. Both Australia and New Zealand have invested in Systematized Nomenclature of Medicine—Clinical Terms (SNOMED CT®). HISO has endorsed the use of SNOMED-CT as the clinical terminology to be used in New Zealand. However, the uptake of SNOMED-CT has been slow. READ codes are mapped to SNOMED-CT and work is underway to accomplish this mapping also with ICD-10 and LOINC.

The New Zealand Ministry of Health is responsible for national collections and surveys of health and disability information. National collections provide information which contributes to understanding the health needs of New Zealanders. The Ministry of Health hosts 14 national collections including the National Minimum Data Set containing discharge information, the National Non-Admitted Patient Collection, the Program for the Integration of Mental Health Data (PRIMHD), and the National Medical Warning System. Other core systems supporting healthcare also include the National Health Index (NHI), a register of all consumers and the Health Practitioner Index, a register of health providers and facilities, addressing and geo-coding services are also provided (Ministry of Health, 2013b). New Zealand has been fortunate to have an NHI database for registering all consumers of healthcare for more than 25 years. Each person is assigned a unique healthcare identifier, either at birth or on first contact with a healthcare provider, and this NHI number is designed to follow the individual through each healthcare event in his/her life, allowing easier tracking of information through healthcare episodes.

The national data collections have been developed in consultation with health sector representatives and provide valuable health information to support performance monitoring, decision-making, policy formulation, funding, evaluation, and research (Ministry of Health, 2013b). Statutory requirements govern the reporting of certain mandatory items (e.g., maternity events and diseases such as cancer, tuberculosis, and other communicable diseases).

All information collection, storage, access, and retrieval in New Zealand are governed by the Privacy Act (1993), the Health Information Code (1994), and subsequent amendments. The New Zealand Law Commission completed a review of this legislation in 2011 (Privacy Commissioner, 2013) and this act remains one of the most comprehensive pieces of privacy legislation anywhere in the world.

The University of Hong Kong is making good use of a number of standardized assessment instruments for older, frail, or disabled individuals (University of Hong Kong, n.d.). The assessment instruments were made available by interRAI, a collaborative network of researchers in over 30 countries, for their research. The interRAI minimum datasets for nursing home, home care, and mental health are now available in Chinese. Australia and New Zealand's interRAI coordinating center is located and managed by the Center for Geriatric Medicine based at the University of Queensland in Brisbane. A nursing and mid-wifery MDS for human resources for health was developed by two Australian nurses (Jill While and Michele Rumsey) using data collected from 30 countries within the Western Pacific and Southeast Asia WHO Regions during 2006–2008 (WHO, 2008).

Nursing Workforce

A total of 50,060 nurses practicing in New Zealand provide care to its population (Nursing Council of New Zealand, 2013). The nursing workforce in New Zealand is the single largest health professional group and is recognized as having enormous potential to advance health and disability outcomes (Nursing Council of New Zealand, 2011). With most of the nurses and mid-wives practicing in Auckland, this large city has by default become the focus of the drive for greater health informatics awareness. Notable changes have occurred within New Zealand nursing legislation that impact on nursing roles. Firstly, in line with international trends in nursing workforce development, the Nursing Council of New Zealand established the role of nurse practitioner, followed by the legislation enacting nurse prescribing that came into force in 2005. With nurse practitioners and prescribing being in place for less than a decade, there were 110 Nurse Practitioners in 2013. There continues to be a move toward further post-graduate education to attain new and expanded nursing roles (Nursing Council of New Zealand, 2013).

The impact of globalization has seen an increase in the movement of nurses in and out of New Zealand, which increases the challenges for the Nursing Council in terms of ensuring safety to practice at the level expected in New Zealand while not providing unnecessary barriers for overseas nurses. Over a third of those added to the register in 2013 were Registered Nurses who had qualified outside New Zealand (Nursing Council of New Zealand, 2013). As part of ensuring standards of practice the Health Practitioners Competence Assurance Act (2003) requires each health practitioner group to describe its

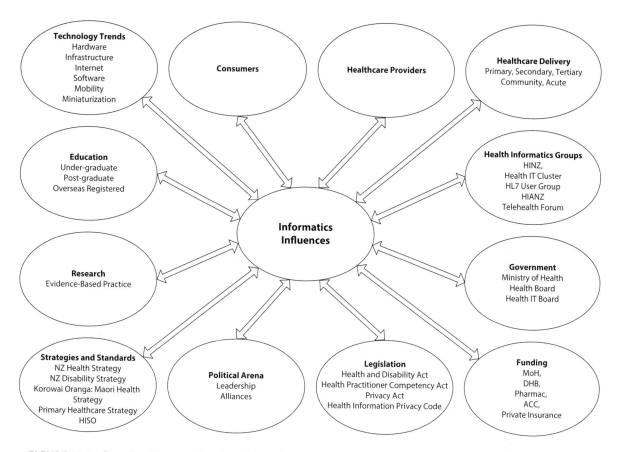

• **FIGURE 53.1.** Overview Diagram Showing Major Influences on Informatics in New Zealand.

profession in terms of scopes of practice. The purpose of scopes of practice is to ensure the safety of the public by defining the health services that health practitioners can perform.

Changes are continuous in the informatics arena. There are many sources and pressures for these. Figure 53.1 describes the major influences on informatics in New Zealand.

REGIONAL DEVELOPMENTS

Health and Nursing informatics developments are highly dependent upon Government and associated industry initiatives and available ICT infrastructures. For example, the International Telecommunication Union (ITU) is a major player in a number of South-East Asian countries with a strong Telemedicine focus with Japan as a leader in the Asia-Pacific region. National Nursing Organizations also

play a major role dependent upon their level of recognition and adoption of Nursing Informatics as a nursing specialty or special interest (National Nursing Organizations, n.d.).

The Asia *e*Health Information Network (AeHIN) was launched in Bangkok in August 2012 as a unique forum to promote better use of information and communication technology (ICT) to achieve better health. The AeHIN is open to all *e*Health, HIS, and civil registration and vital statistics (CRVS) professionals from multiple sectors within South and Southeast Asia—including developed and low- and middle-income countries—to maximize a regional approach for greater country-level health impacts. This came about as a response to several outcomes of the 2011 Asia-Pacific HIS Country Ownership and Leadership Forum (www.hisforum.org), where participants called for increased inter-country collaboration, openness, strategic reuse, and peer-to-peer assistance in better and new ways (AeHIN, 2012a).

AeHIN is well supported by many well-resourced organizations, including WHO, ITU, the Rockefeller Foundation, Australia Aid, US Aid, and more. It is an instrumental node for facilitating the 2013 Global Observatory of eHealth (GoE), a WHO initiative which started in 2005. GoE is about providing countries with strategic information and evidence that will support policies and interventions on eHealth. AeHIN's secretariat is supported by the Medical Informatics Unit, University of the Philippines Manila, whose Director, Dr. Alvin B. Marcelo, is the current AeHIN Chair. AeHIN has a well-developed governance structure, including advisory, management, and scientific committees, and a five-year strategic implementation plan detailing its vision, goals, and strategic action points to address four primary objectives (AeHIN, 2012b):

1. Enhancing leadership and governance
2. Capacity building
3. Peer assistance
4. Promoting standards and interoperability

HI and NI Professional Organizations

Both New Zealand and Australia have many health informatics and related professional organizations and groups advising various government departments and specific projects. There tends to be a considerable overlap of members between these. Health Informatics New Zealand (HINZ)

is working closely with the Australasian College of Health Informatics. Both organizations have many nurses as members and fellows.

There are a number of informatics-related groups in New Zealand, each with a slightly different focus. Table 53.1 identifies and provides a high-level definition of these groups. Health Informatics New Zealand (HINZ) is a national, not-for-profit organization whose focus is to facilitate improvements in business processes and patient care in the health sector through the application of appropriate information technologies (HINZ, 2013). HINZ emerged in September 2000 from two health informatics organizations: Nursing Informatics New Zealand (NINZ) and New Zealand Health Informatics Foundation (NZHiF). HINZ does not compete with existing organizations or activities, but works to assist and network key influential partners to improve the effectiveness of health informatics in New Zealand. Membership is for anyone who has an interest in health and informatics who wants to be part of an organization that can provide relevant up-to-date information about health informatics. HINZ holds an annual conference in collaboration with other health IT organizations.

New Zealand participates in the international health informatics arena through representation in the International Medical Informatics Association (IMIA), International Medical Informatics Association Nursing Informatics group (IMIA-NI), various working groups of IMIA, and the Health Information Management System

TABLE 53.1	New Zealand Health Informatics Groups
Group	**Description**
ACC www.acc.co.nz	The Accident Compensation Corporation (ACC) manages New Zealand's accident compensation scheme, which provides comprehensive no-fault personal accident insurance for all citizens. ACC works to prevent injury, buy health and disability support services to treat, care for, and rehabilitate injured consumers, and collect national accident and injury data.
Health Information Governance Expert Advisory Group (HIGEAG) www.ithealthboard.health.nz/who-we-work/higeag	The Health Information Governance Expert Advisory Group (HIGEAG) was established to develop a health information governance framework for the New Zealand health sector. HIGEAG reports to, and advises, the National Health IT Board (NHITB). Membership of this group in 2013 includes nurses and others active in health informatics.
Health Workforce NZ www.healthworkforce.govt.nz	Health Workforce New Zealand (formed in 2009) provides leadership, coordination, and oversight of planning and development of the workforce across the country's health and disability sector. Their goal is to ensure that staffing is aligned with planning on delivery of services and that the healthcare workforce is fit for purpose.
HIANZ www.hianz.org.nz	Health Information Association of New Zealand (HIANZ) was founded in 1989 and is the networking and support organization for health information personnel, such as those involved in clinical coding, medical records, and health and medical libraries.

(continued)

TABLE 53.1	New Zealand Health Informatics Groups *(continued)*
Group	**Description**
HINZ www.hinz.org.nz	Health Informatics New Zealand (HINZ) is a national, not-for-profit organization whose focus is to facilitate improvements in business processes and patient care in the health sector through the application of appropriate information technologies. HINZ has special interest groups and the HINZ Nursing Informatics group is the most active of HINZ groups.
HISO www.ithealthboard.health. nz/hiso	The Health Information Standards Organisation is the expert advisory group for standards to the National Health IT Board to support and promote the development, understanding, and use of fit-for-purpose health information standards to improve the New Zealand health system.
NZHITC www.healthit.org.nz	The New Zealand Health IT Cluster Inc. (NZHITC), established in 2002, is an independent, representative organization that advocates and represents the health IT industry to decision-makers and leaders in the health sector. The Cluster includes software and solution developers, consultants, health policy-makers, health funders, and infrastructure companies that have agreed to work collaboratively to provide mutual support for local and international business development. The NZHITC mission statement is to "Collaborate to position New Zealand as a world leader in the supply and use of innovative health technology".
NZHUG www.hl7.org.nz	New Zealand Health Level 7 User Group (NZHUG) is the New Zealand arm of the international Health Level 7 (HL7) organization, which has a proven and widely used methodology for standards development that promotes information interoperability in healthcare. The organization comprises technical committees and special interest groups. The technical committees are directly responsible for the content of the standards. Special interest groups serve as a test bed for exploring new areas that may need coverage in HL7's published standards.
New Zealand Telehealth Forum www.ithealthboard.health. nz/who-we-work/new- zealand-telehealth-forum	The New Zealand Telehealth Forum, funded by the National Health IT Board, has been established to promote the use of telehealth, and maximize the benefits of the Government's broadband program.
MoH www.moh.govt.nz	The Ministry of Health plays an important role for the formal intra- and inter-government liaison work it undertakes, its influence on sector policy and strategy, and its funding capability. The Ministry established the National Health Board (NHB) in 2009 to overcome the challenges facing the health system and to improve the quality, safety, and sustainability of healthcare for New Zealanders.
NICLG: National Information Clinical Leadership Group www.ithealthboard.health. nz/who-we-work/national- information-clinical-leader ship-group	This group provides clinical leadership input to the National Health IT Plan and was established in recognition that a key challenge to sharing health information is in advancing the development and use of clinical information systems consistently nationally. Strategic leadership and ownership from clinicians is required in a range of clinical process and information solutions including clinical decision support, safe medications management, safe sharing of information and transfer of care. A number of nurses are members of this group.
NHITB: National Health IT Board www.ithealthboard.health.nz	The National Health Information Technology Board is a sub-committee, the National of Health Board, and has the role of providing leadership on the implementation and use of information systems across the health and disability sector, and to ensure that health sector policy is supported by appropriate health information and IT solutions. In addition this group works to provide leadership across the health sector for IT investments in relation to patient safety and value for money; support for an improved health information model; and set direction for the appropriate and effective use of personal health information.
NIHI http://nihi.auckland.ac.nz/	The National Institute for Health Innovation (NIHI) is based at the University of Auckland and supports research including the use of technologies to support healthcare delivery.
Statistics New Zealand www.stats.govt.nz	Statistics New Zealand (Stats NZ) administers the Statistics Act (1975) producing the official statistics for the nation.

Society Asia-Pacific (HIMSS Asia-Pac) (Westbrooke, Honey, & Carr, 2011).

The history of the formation of medical, health, and nursing informatics groups in Australia reflects the difficulties experienced as a consequence of a federal system of government and vast distances between population centers.

Australia has had a representative to IMIA's Working Group 8 (WG8) (now NI sig) since 1984. Nurses were the second group of health professionals to organize themselves to promote health informatics in Australia. The general practitioners were first, beginning in the late 1970s. The Health Information Managers Association of Australia (HIMAA) has been in existence since 1949, but its integration of informatics is more recent. Nursing informatics is now a special interest group of the Health Informatics Society of Australia (HISA), which came into existence in 1993. It has been a long and torturous path to reach this position, as can be learned from the historical summary that follows.

Australian Historical Milestones

Nursing informatics in Australia began with the Royal Australian Nursing Federation (now ANF) in 1984. A year later, a small group of mid-wives in Victoria, including Joan Edgecumbe, who was the Executive Officer of HISA till 2009, decided to call a general meeting of nurses interested in computer use. About 70 nurses agreed to establish the Nursing Computer Group Victoria (NCGV). This group continued to flourish and hosted the Fourth International Symposium on Nursing Use of Computers and Information Science in Melbourne in 1991. The profits from this conference enabled the formation of the Health Informatics Society of Australia. These and other associated events are summarized in Table 53.2.

In 2003, the HISA NI Sig (NIA) was funded to develop a strategic plan for nursing informatics capacity building, and a plan for the nursing profession's engagement with the Australian government and its informatics agenda. The plan has provided a lot of useful information for various

TABLE 53.2	History of Australian Health Informatics Professional Groups and the Promotion of This Discipline	
Year	**By Whom**	**Purpose**
1949	Health Information Managers Association of Australia (HIMAA)	Established—refer to http://www.himaa.org.au.
1984	Royal Australian Nurses Federation (RANF)	Adoption of position statement on "Computerisation in Health Services – Implications for Nursing" (Royal Australian Nurses Federation, 1984).
1985	RCNA	Seventh National Conference theme, "Information Processing- Challenges and Choices for Nurses," Melbourne. This inspired a small group of mid-wives.
1985	Midwives Association	General meeting of nurses interested in computer use—70 nurses attended. The Nursing Computer Group Victoria (NCGV) was established.
1986	Royal Adelaide Hospital Nurses Education Fund	Sponsored a National Nursing Conference with the theme: "From Lamp to Light Pen – Computers in Nursing" to celebrate their 150 Jubilee. Nurses from Queensland and Western Australia computer groups established the previous year, networked.
1986	Health Commission of Victoria	Government funded the then senior nursing advisor to undertake a world tour to investigate the likely impact on nurses of computer use in the health industry.
1986	Royal Australian College of General Practitioners (RACGP)	National computer committee established following the formation of several State-based medical computing interest groups.
1986	Australian participants at Medinfo'86	Around 20 Australians met in Washington, DC, and decided to form a network with the aim of promoting health informatics among health professionals. This resulted in the formation of a number of computer groups in several States over the years that followed. Meanwhile the Australian Computer Society (ACS) Inc. was the organization that represented Australia at IMIA.
1987	RACGP	Computer Fellow position established in conjunction with Monash University's Department of Community Medicine.
1988	RACGP	Standards for Computerized Medical Records Systems released.

(continued)

TABLE 53.2	History of Australian Health Informatics Professional Groups and the Promotion of This Discipline *(continued)*	
Year	**By Whom**	**Purpose**
1989	Australian Medical Informatics Association (AMIA)	A Western Australia initiative to form AMIA with State-based branches. The inaugural meeting of AMIA (Victorian Branch) was held in Melbourne in 1991. AMIA secured an affiliation with the Australian Computer Society (ACS) and became the ACS medical informatics special interest group.
1990	Australian Health Informatics Association SA	Sixteen health informatics enthusiasts met in South Australia and established AHIA SA. They published six issues of the Health Informatics News and Technology (HINT) annually.
1991	Australian Computer Society (ACS) medical informatics special interest group	The ACS MI SIG organized a one-day health track at the ACS annual conference held in Adelaide that year. This was seen as an opportunity for members of the many disparate groups to meet and discuss the possibility of forming one national organization. Disagreement regarding the name (medical vs. health) and the entry requirements remained unresolved.
1991	Australian Health Informatics Association Qld	A group of health professionals organized regular educational meetings in Brisbane and formed AHIA Qld.
1991	Health Informatics Association New South Wales (HIANSW)	HIANSW was established by 36 people representing a wide range of health and IT professionals, including Nurses. They produces a regular newsletter, Computers in Health Information Processing (CHIP).
1991	Nursing Computer Group Victoria	International Nursing Informatics Symposium held in Melbourne hosted by the NCGV under the auspices of the IMIA Nursing Informatics working group.
1991	NI'91 Post-Conference meeting	Nurses from all States and Territories discussed the formation of a National Nursing Informatics group. Everyone agreed to work together, but the formalization of a new national organization was problematic due to differences between the state-based groups regarding affiliations with other professional nursing organizations. Subsequently, the Nursing Computer Group Victoria changed its name to Nursing Informatics Australia (NIA).
1992	Nursing Informatics Australia (NIA)	Post-conference profits were used to establish a secretariat and launch a new look magazine.
1992	Australian Nursing Informatics Council (ANIC)	One representative from each state-based nursing informatics group was appointed to form ANIC.
1992	Standards Australia	Health Informatics Standards Committee—IT-14 established.
1992	HIANSW Conference	Another attempt at uniting the 23 distinct groups was made at the first HIANSW conference held in Laura, New South Wales, to discuss how to best work together and how health (medical) informatics should be represented at IMIA. This resulted in a resolution to: 1. Form a National Council of Health Informatics Groups. 2. Combine three newsletters/journals, CHIP, HINT, and Nursing Informatics Australia into one national and multi-disciplinary magazine with a national editorial board. The first issue of *Informatics in Healthcare Australia* came out in May 1992 funded by NIA.
1992	AMIA meeting, Melbourne	Discussion paper summarizing deliberations, and a scenario for the development of one new national organization to represent the field of health informatics in Australia was circulated widely.
1992	Australian Nursing Informatics Council (ANIC)	Initiated the idea to organize a national conference in 1993. Several groups supported this idea, and since NIA was the only organization with the necessary funds, this group managed this inaugural conference. This became an annual event known as HIC—Health Informatics Conference.

(continued)

TABLE 53.2	History of Australian Health Informatics Professional Groups and the Promotion of This Discipline *(continued)*	

Year	By Whom	Purpose
1993	Health Informatics Society of Australia (HISA)	A special meeting of representatives from interested groups, facilitated by Dr. Ian Graham, who was the Director, Centre for Health Informatics at the Austin Hospital, was held in Sydney. This meeting produced a draft Constitution for HISA, reflecting an agreed set of principles (refer to www.hisa.org.au).
1993	HISA Victoria	NIA was re-constituted as the HISA Victoria branch.
1993	HISA Inaugural general meeting	The draft constitution was presented to potential HISA members at its inaugural general meeting held in conjunction with the inaugural Health Informatics Conference (HIC '93), and they voted for its adoption. Conference profits were then used to fund the further development of the constitution and incorporation.
1994	HISA Constituted	The NIA (now HISA Vic) secretariat became HISA's secretariat.
1994	HISA Standards SIG	HISA's representative to IT-14 informed the committee of the recommendation for the adoption of HL7 messaging standards, this was accepted.
1995	HISA	HISA became the official group to represent Australia at IMIA.
1996	HISA NI Sig	HISA Nursing Informatics special interest group established. Now known as Nursing Informatics Australia (NIA).
1997	General Practice Computing Group (GPCG)	Established by GPs, funded by the Australian Government Department of Health and Ageing, to provide a strategic and cooperative approach to Australian GP informatics (refer to www.gpcg.org/).
2000	HISA	A new constitution was adopted, making HISA a company limited by guarantee of its members.
2001	Australian College of Health Informatics (ACHI)	Meeting of seven Health Informaticians funded by the Australian Department of Health and Aged Care resulted in the formation of ACHI in 2002 with 18 invited Fellows selected via a peer review and consensus regarding the country's 20 top health informaticians to act as the peak reference body for health informatics in Australia. By 2004 there were 30 Fellows and Members (refer to www.achi.org.au).
2002	HL7 Australia	A Health Level Seven (HL7) user group established. An HL7 International Affiliates meeting held in Melbourne (refer to www.hl7.org.au).
2002	HISA	Hosted an international ISO TC215 meeting in Melbourne.
2003	HISA	A Pathology SIG established.
2004	HISA	An Aged care SIG established.
2007	HISA	Hosted the Medinfo2007 in Brisbane.
2009	Australasian College of Health Informatics (ACHI) http://www.achi.org.au/	ACHI has increased its membership to suitably qualified candidates in New Zealand and Asia. There is an agreement between HINZ and ACHI to work together. ACHI initiated the establishment of the Australian Health Informatics Education Council (AHIEC), continues to provide a secretarial service for this Council, and prepared a strategic workplan for national HI and NI education.
2010	ACHI	ACHI was accepted as a member of the Australian Council of Professions Ltd.
2013	Certification of Health Informatics Australasia (CHIA)	A collaborative project between ACHI, HISA, and HIMAA launched. http://www.healthinformaticscertification.com

bureaucrats, but there has not been a noticeable change in nurses' involvement at senior decision-making levels. Since then NI's contributions have been ad hoc mainly by individual experts or via the Royal College of Nursing. The Coalition of National Nursing Organisations (CoNNO) did develop a Position Statement on Nursing and eHealth under the leadership of its NIA member (CoNNO, 2008). This group meets twice each year to discuss current issues impacting the nursing profession.

It has been a difficult path toward the recognition and professionalization of health (and nursing) informatics as a discipline. We have not yet managed to achieve a unity or consensus regarding how best to operate as one national professional organization to date, although increasingly joint activities are being organized.

HI AND NI RESEARCH

Health-related information has a number of uses. Apart from the direct use of information in the care of clients, there is a growing awareness of the need for timely and accurate data for research. Three specific areas that are gaining more attention within nursing informatics are clinical pathways, evidence-based practice, and nursing service architecture, with the Internet and workplace intranets providing ready access to evidence. As well as drawing on international evidence and guidelines such as The Cochrane Collaboration, International Council of Nurses Evidence-Based Practice Resources, and the National Institute for Health and Clinical Excellence (NICE) guidelines, local and organizational level approaches to the use of evidence-based practice with access to selected resources can be found (Clayton & Bland, 2012; Gilmour, Huntington, Broadbent, Strong, & Hawkins, 2012; Shahtahmasebi, Villa, Nielsen, & Graham-Smith, 2010).

Research in health informatics is varied and tends to follow local trends and developments, often with nurses contributing within multi-disciplinary teams. Mobile health (mhealth), such as the use of mobile phones to provide health promotion, provides an example. Early research in the use of text messages to consumers showed promise and more recent research has included adding video messages (Whittaker et al., 2011), international collaborative research into the longer term effects of smoking cessation delivered via text messages (Free et al., 2011), and the use of a mobile phone youth depression prevention intervention (Whittaker et al., 2012).

Research in health and nursing informatics is supported through highly contested government and other funding, and through Master's and Doctorate programs

in a number of Australian and New Zealand government-funded universities. For example, Auckland University of Technology, Massey University, the University of Auckland, and the University of Otago offer post-graduate education that includes health informatics components as do some Australian Universities.

Funding organizations such as the Australian Research Council and the National Health & Medical Research Council continue to provide funding for HI-related issues. A number of doctoral candidates are funded via their HI research grants. In 2000, the NHMRC's allocation was $311,015 and in 2012 this had increased to $10 million; most of which, $6 million or 36 out of a total of 67 grants, was for bio-informatics projects (NHMRC, 2013). Well-established university-based research centers, such as those located at the University of New South Wales, and the University of Melbourne, tend to be most successful in attracting research funding for various health and nursing informatics projects. Grant allocations are projected to decrease over the next few years.

The main avenues for sharing health informatics research is through internationally indexed conference proceedings and journal publications, plus local professional conferences and workshops such as the Health Informatics New Zealand (HINZ) annual conference and quarterly seminars, workshops, and meetings held by AeHIN, APAMI, and HIMMS-AsiaPac. The Nursing Informatics Australia special interest group of HISA organizes an annual one day preconference to HISA's annual conference, known as HIC, where between 40 and 60 papers are presented each year. Papers presented at this conference are indexed in CINAHL and INFOMIT. They provide a good overview of progress in health informatics in Australia. HISA also organizes topic-specific conferences at other times of the year. In addition, ACHI and HISA sponsor the management of the free *electronic Journal of Health Informatics (eJHI)* (eJHI, n.d.) that is becoming increasingly more popular among scholars and is attracting a good selection of fully refereed papers.

The *Healthcare and Informatics Review Online (HCIRO)* became the official journal of HINZ in 2007 (www.hinz.org.nz/journal). *HCIRO* is dedicated to reviewing and interpreting significant developments in healthcare delivery with a particular focus on health informatics and is the only New Zealand–based journal focusing on health IT issues. The journal has a wide local and international readership, and is gaining credibility in business and academic circles. The focus of the journal is on knowledge gained through the practical experience of managing health issues. Its objectives are to facilitate the exchange of ideas among interested members of the health sector and to develop a widely accessible resource of experience in health delivery. In addition national HI general information about current happenings is shared via a magazine titled PULSE-IT (http://www.pulseitmagazine.com.au/).

HI AND NI EDUCATION

The first Australian experiences of nurses using computers were compiled into an edited text by Graham MacKay and Anita Griffin in 1989 (MacKay & Griffin, 1989). The first Australian textbook on health informatics was published in 1996 (Hovenga, Kidd, & Cesnik 1996), a second edition was published by IOS Press in 2010 followed by a text on Health Data Governance in 2013 (Hovenga, Kidd, Garde, Hullin, 2010; Hovenga & Grain, 2013). Another popular Australian text was edited by the late Moya Conrick, a nurse who has made a significant contribution to nursing informatics in Australia over the years (Conrick, 2006).

Much of nursing informatics education continues to be provided by nursing computer and informatics groups via study days, seminars, and conferences. The Lincoln Institute of Health Sciences (now Latrobe University) provided registered nurses undertaking post-registration degrees with opportunities to include computer studies in their coursework as early as 1979. Central Queensland University introduced nurses to computers in 1989 with a strong commitment to a computer-assisted and -managed learning project (Zelmer, McLees, & Zelmer, 1991). Informatics education for nurses in Australia varies considerably from one university to another (Soar et al., 2003).

A study of 10,000 nurses in Australia (44% response rate) on their use of information technology has clearly identified that nurses recognize benefits of adopting more information technology in the workplace. Hegney et al. (2007) found that nurses surveyed were frustrated by the limitations of access to technology; that software was not always fit for purpose; that there was a lack of opportunities for NI training; and that Nurses felt poorly informed about information technology health initiatives and were poorly consulted about implementation of these initiatives.

Some schools of nursing attempt to integrate informatics into their under-graduate nursing program to some extent. Central Queensland University offered an under-graduate degree program in nursing informatics as a post-registration program, but it was discontinued in 2007. Most University-based nursing programs have one person attempting the impossible, often in environments where fellow nurse academics have little or no knowledge of informatics. In some instances, there is active resistance to its introduction. Anecdotal evidence suggests that this continues to be true in 2013. As from 2014, the Australian

College of Nursing has contracted eHealth Education, a private registered training organization established by senior health informatics educators who had become disillusioned with the university system, to deliver an NI professional development program.

A number of universities in the region are now offering a certificate, post-graduate diploma, or master's degree in health informatics or equivalent. Some of their graduates are now pursuing post-doctoral studies, others are actively engaged in promoting the use of IT in the workplace, and many work in hospital-based nursing informatics positions although they may not be titled as such.

Nursing informatics has been recognized as significant by the Ministries of Health and Education in New Zealand since the early 1990s (Hausman, 1989; Westbrooke & Honey, 2011). Nurses registering for practice in New Zealand complete a three-year under-graduate degree. Much of nursing informatics is integrated into under-graduate curriculum under the guise of other subjects (Honey & Baker, 2004). For example, law and ethics covers the Privacy Act (1993), which emphasizes the importance of the collection, storage, and use of client information, whether stored on paper or computer; evidence-based practice includes the discernment of evidence to ascertain its worthiness to base nursing practice on; and research includes literature searches, and therefore the use of the Internet and access to international nursing literature databases. Thus, under-graduate nurse education reflects the need for computer literacy.

Changes have taken place in under-graduate nursing education, include the credentials with which new nurses qualify, the information and computer literacy of students, and increased use of technology. Nursing Council of New Zealand does not identify any specific computer skills within the competencies that registered nurses are required to attain; yet the competencies involve information management and communication that may be achieved using ICT. The new nursing student, most commonly from secondary school, enters with greater computer skills compared to earlier cohorts. Rather than compulsory computer skills training, optional classes are available for those students who require additional assistance.

There is an increase in technology use within nursing education, with interest in innovative ways to support student learning, such as using wikis (Doherty, Honey, & Stewart, 2012); reusable learning objects (Lim, Doherty, & Honey, 2011); and simulation (Brown et al., 2012; Edgecombe, 2013; Honey, Connor, Veltman, Bodily, & Diener, 2012; Stewart & Davis, 2012). New Zealand, like other western countries, is challenged to provide enough clinical practice and simulation is seen as a means to enhance teaching and learning within a consistent, safe, and realistic environment (Brown et al., 2012). The manner simulation is provided varies, with both low and higher fidelity options, and utilizing technology to a greater or lesser extent, yet there are similarities in terms of scenarios and learning objectives that can be shared among nurse educators (Edgecombe, 2013). Some educators have ventured into virtual worlds to provide simulated experience in both nursing and mid-wifery (Honey et al., 2012; Stewart & Davis, 2012).

The impact of these changes in under-graduate nursing education has had a flow-on effect within post-graduate education. Furthermore, the changes in health service delivery in New Zealand and the establishment of new roles such as the Nurse Practitioner and advanced practice roles have driven the ongoing demand for post-graduate nursing education. These new advanced nursing roles require post-graduate qualifications, yet there have been access barriers for nurses, generally based in urban areas. Nurses are found throughout the country and the nature of nursing necessitates shift work. Nurses in New Zealand are predominantly women, and there are gender issues that make access to post-graduate education problematic. Learning that utilizes the benefits of technology is becoming increasingly common with flexible learning, e-learning, and online courses available for post-graduate nursing education through most Schools of Nursing (Honey, 2007).

Health informatics education in New Zealand has evolved in a different manner than other countries, such as the United States and Great Britain. Separate post-graduate courses in nursing informatics have not been viable perhaps due to the smaller numbers of nurses. Nurses favor health informatics options. New Zealand's five programs which provide post-graduate education in health informatics continue to gain enrollments and are well regarded by students and graduates. These options provide nurses the opportunity to study informatics in a broad context alongside other health professionals.

Competencies and Credentialing

Nursing specialty and other organizations have developed and adopted practice standards, competencies, guidelines for curricula development, and various professional development programs. Australia has more than 50 such specialty national nursing organizations (NNOs), where the Health Informatics Society Australia's nursing informatics special interest group (HISA NI Sig known as NIA) is one of these. Each specialty has developed a set of competencies and provided credentialing services with

Nursing Informatics being an exception despite a number of attempts to do so.

The first study undertaken in Australia to establish NI learning needs was undertaken during the early 1990s (Carter & Axford, 1993). This was followed by a general HI skills Internet/Web-based survey based on IMIA's educational guidelines and the use of Benner's competency levels, from which nurses' responses were separately identified and analyzed (Garde, Harrison, & Hovenga, 2005). The focus of this research was on the perceptions of individual nurses as they relate to their own roles. Self-assessed levels of competent (35%), proficient (33%), and expert (4%) combined was 72%. A later government-funded competency development study was undertaken by Foster and Bryce (2009) under the auspices of the ANMF; however, authorization for publication of the draft report has not been received.

Another survey was undertaken in Western Australia during 2012 to establish nurses existing informatics competency level and knowledge base regarding the five competency domains, computer literacy, information literacy, information management, attitudes and awareness, and governance based on the TIGER NI competencies model and the draft NI Professional competency standards for Australia (Foster & Bryce, 2009). Ellis (2012) noted that:

The importance of nursing informatics competency standards specifically for nurses has been highlighted by numerous studies and reports in order for nurses to maintain the necessary skills to effectively use ICT solutions. Currently no such standards exist in Australia.

A self-assessment methodology based on Benner's five competency levels was used (Ellis, 2012). This local survey of 1465 nurses with a 33% response rate (a representative sample) was undertaken in response to the WA Government's aim to improve the access and integrity of information through new systems and technology. This study found that a quarter of the nurses rated themselves as below competent with enrolled nurses showing the lowest levels of competency. This finding is similar to the results obtained from the 2005 study (Garde et al., 2005). The only statement that the majority of nurses disagreed with was "computer and technology in health will reduce my workload" (52%). This was viewed as being due to "negative past experiences, common misconception or inadequate education leading to inefficient use." A set of draft competency standards for local use resulted from this study.

There continues to be a very significant skills shortage in this area, as was revealed in the numerous Australian government reports commissioned over the last 10 years or so. In an effort to address this, ACHI established an education committee in late 2008, which obtained Government funding in 2009 to establish what is now known as the Australian Health Informatics Education Council (AHIEC). A strategic workplan was developed and published in late 2009 (AHIEC, 2009-2010). This work was continued via a collaborative effort from ACHI, HISA, and HIMAA resulting in the development of an agreed set of HI competencies and the launch of the **Certified Health Informatician Australasia** certification program in July 2013 at HIC (CHIA, 2013).

A 2006 New Zealand study involving an online survey and interviews with the major tertiary education providers offering post-graduate health informatics programs explored the potential for improving the health informatics workforce capability (Kerr et al., 2006). The study found that there was "clearly a role for graduates with a set of competencies that can provide a bridge between the IT specialist working in the health sector and the clinicians assisting with IT developments" (Kerr et al., 2006, p. 5). Despite this study being well received no changes eventuated. However, with the impetus of shared health records by 2014 it became evident that the pressing issue was a lack of informatics aware clinicians (Ministry of Health, 2012). The lack of health informatics awareness is compounded by the increasing number of health professionals not educated in New Zealand.

The HINZ Education Group developed a strategy with three aspects to meet this challenge (Parry et al., 2013). The first was to identify health informatics competencies (Fig. 53.2) and then to indicate which were core competencies needed by everyone and the competencies which depended on the person's role—as clinician, manager, or technical specialist. The second initiative, with funding support from the National Health IT Board, aimed to increase health informatics awareness among existing staff by offering "Introduction to Health Informatics" workshops to clinicians, managers, and technical staff in their place of work. The goal, by taking education to existing staff, was to make the free workshops easily accessible and in a two-hour format that could fit into their work day and in addition, HINZ provides a certificate of attendance. The third aspect is to promote cooperation between New Zealand universities so that those enrolling for further health informatics education will be able to identify the most appropriate educational option whether they have a general interest, are an informatics specialist, or a health professional with an interest in health informatics (Parry et al., 2013). This aspect addresses a recommendation from the 2006 study that national agreement on a post-graduate health informatics curriculum would improve the effectiveness and the marketability of programs (Kerr et al.,

2006). Figure 53.2 represents the required core HI competencies identified by the HINZ Education Group.

IMPACTS ON NI DISCIPLINE DEVELOPMENT

It is clearly evident that professional health, medical, and nursing organizations, along with educational providers and research centers, play a major role in the awareness raising, education, and dissemination of knowledge about the field of health and nursing informatics in the Pacific Rim. This is becoming increasingly complex with the proliferation of government initiatives spanning multiple government departments. This is also a reflection of the multi-disciplinary nature of health informatics. Nurses, as the largest group of health professionals, have a major role to play. This requires sound knowledge about the numerous stakeholders so that nurses can benefit healthcare consumers—our patients, communities, and society as a whole.

Some educational providers, governments, and healthcare providers in this region have recognized this need and taken steps to address issues raised. There is an urgency to develop a critical mass of nurse informaticians. We need to continue to raise widespread awareness of a now well-established fact that nurses can and need to make better use of available technologies and that all applications need to have a strong nursing focus to enable the realization of

Core competencies in Health informatics

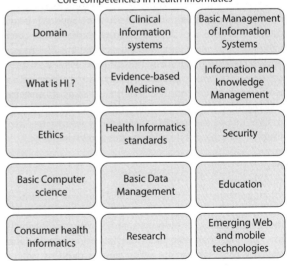

Domain	Clinical Information systems	Basic Management of Information Systems
What is HI ?	Evidence-based Medicine	Information and knowledge Management
Ethics	Health Informatics standards	Security
Basic Computer science	Basic Data Management	Education
Consumer health informatics	Research	Emerging Web and mobile technologies

• **FIGURE 53.2.** Health Informatics Competencies Identified by the HINZ Education Group. (Reproduced, with permission of the HINZ Education Group.)

projected benefits for both patients and the health system as a whole. The overall regional collaboration has been a great development as it enables nurses and others with an interest in developing nursing applications to share experiences.

ACKNOWLEDGMENTS

The authors would like to sincerely thank Polun Chang, PhD, Rung-Chuang Feng, PhD, RN, Ying Wu, PhD, RN, ACNP, ANP, and Ming-Chuan Kuo, MS, RN, for their contribution about events in Taiwan, China, and Hong Kong. More descriptions of Taiwan, China, and Hong Kong are in Chapter 54, Nursing Informatics in Asia, by Park.

REFERENCES

Accident Compensation Corporation (ACC). (2012). *Using Read Codes*. Retrieved from http://www.acc.co.nz/for-providers/lodge-and-manage-claims/prv00037. Accessed on November 20, 2013.

Accident Compensation Corporation (ACC). (2013). *About ACC*. Retrieved from http://www.acc.co.nz/about-acc/index.htm. Accessed on November 20, 2013.

Asia eHealth Information Network (AeHIN). (2012a). *JLN eBook on standards and interoperability released*. Launch workshop. Retrieved from http://www.aehin.org/. Accessed on January 8, 2014.

Asia eHealth Information Network (AeHIN). (2012b). *AeHIN Regional eHealth Strategic Plan: 2012–2017 implementation plan*. Retrieved from http://www.aehin.org/AboutUs/AeHINStrategicPlans.aspx. Accessed on January 8, 2014.

Asia Pacific Association for Medical Informatics (APAMI). (n.d.). Retrieved from http://www.apami.org/. Accessed on January 8, 2014.

Australian Government. (2008). National Health and Hospitals Reform Commission (NHHRC). *A healthier future for all Australians—Interim report*. Retrieved from http://www.health.gov.au/internet/nhhrc/publishing.nsf/Content/interim-report-december-2008. Accessed on January 8, 2014.

Australian Health Informatics Education Council (AHIEC). (2009–2010). *Strategic Workplan 2009-10 and beyond*.

Australian Institute of Health and Welfare (AIHW). (2012). *Australia's health 2012 p.506*. Retrieved from http://www.aihw.gov.au/publication-detail/?id=10737422172. Accessed on January 8, 2014.

Australian Institute of Health and Welfare (AIHW). (n.d.). *METeOR*. Retrieved from http://meteor.aihw.gov.au/content/index.phtml/itemId/181162

BCS. (2013, April). *Interview with Dr Nigel Millar - Health informatics*. Retrieved from http://www.bcs.org/content/ConWebDoc/50633. Accessed on January 8, 2014.

Brown, R. A., Guinea, S., Crookes, P. A., McAllister, M., Levett-Jones, T., Kelly, M., & Smith, A. (2012). Clinical simulation in Australia and New Zealand: Through the lens of an advisory group. *Collegian: The Australian Journal of Nursing Practice, Scholarship and Research, 19*(3), 177–186.

Carter, B. E., & Axford R. L. (1993). Assessment of computer learning needs and priorities of registered nurses practicing in hospitals. *Computers in Nursing, 11*(3), 122–126.

Certified Health Informatics Australasia (CHIA). (2013). *Competencies framework*. Retrieved from http://www.healthinformaticscertification.com/CHIA-Competencies-Framework.pdf. Accessed on January 4, 2013.

Clayton, J., & Bland, M. (2012, September 4–6). *Improving nursing utilisation of evidence to inform clinical practice: A New Zealand case study*. Paper presented at the meeting of NET2012: 23rd International Networking for Healthcare Education Conference, Cambridge, UK.

Coalition of National Nursing Organisations (CoNNO). (2008). *Position Statement – Nursing and eHealth*. Retrieved from http://www.conno.org.au/publications. Accessed on January 4, 2014.

Commonwealth of Australia. (2009). *Casemix review report*. Retrieved from http://www.health.gov.au/casemix

Commonwealth of Australia. (2010). *Building a 21st century primary healthcare system, Australia's first national primary healthcare strategy*. Retrieved from http://www.yourhealth.gov.au/internet/yourhealth/publishing.nsf/content/report-primaryhealth#.Usy3vLSwD5Q. Accessed on January 8, 2014.

Community Net Aotearoa. (2013). 1.8 Million New Zealanders interacting via social networking sites. Retrieved from http://www.community.net.nz/how toguides/socialnetworking/News/nielsenreport.htm. Accessed on November 20, 2013.

Connolly, M., Boyd, M.-A., Kenealy, T., Moffitt, A., Sheridan, N., & Kolbe, J. (2010). *Alleviating the burden of chronic conditions in New Zealand: The ABCC NZ Study workbook 2010*. Auckland, New Zealand: The University of Auckland and Freemason's Unit of Geriatric Medicine. Retrieved from http://dhbrf.hrc.govt.nz/media/docu ments_abcc/ABCC_Study_Workbook_Final.pdf

Conrick, M. (Ed.), (2006). *Health informatics: Transforming healthcare with technology*. Melbourne, Australia: Thomson, Social Science Press.

Davey, J. A., & Gee, S. (2002). *Life at 85 plus: A statistical review*. Wellington, New Zealand: New Zealand Institute for Research on Ageing.

Day, K., & Kerr, P. (2012). Telehealth - Rethinking healthcare roles for smarter care. *Health Care and Informatics Review Online, 2012, 16*(2), 8–16. Retrieved from http://www.hinz.org.nz/journal/2012/11/Telehealth--Rethinking-Healthcare-Roles-for-Smarter-Care/1053. Accessed on December 8, 2013.

Doherty, I., Honey, M., & Stewart, L. (2012, June 21–22). Enhancing the undergraduate experience through a collaborative wiki exercise to teach nursing students discipline specific terminology. In P. Lam (Ed.), *Proceedings of the 7th International Conference on e-Learning (ICEL 2012)* (pp.58–62). Hong Kong, China: Academic Publishing International Limited.

Edgecombe, K. (2013). *Collaboration in clinical simulation: Leading the way*. Wellington, New Zealand: Ako Aotearoa, National Centre for Tertiary Teaching Excellence. Retrieved from http://akoaotearoa.ac.nz/communities/collaboration-clinical-simulation-leading-way. Accessed on December 4, 2013.

Electronic Health Informatics Journal (eJHI). (n.d.). Retrieved from http://www.eJHI.net

Ellis, L. (2012). *Nurses ICT competency survey report*. Retrieved from http://www.smphu.health.wa.gov.au/search.aspx. Accessed on January 8, 2014.

eMarketer. (2012). *Your social media strategy global*. Retrieved from http://www.emarketer.com/Article/Your-Social-Media-Strategy-Global/1009022. Accessed on November 18, 2013.

Foster, J., & Bryce, J. (2009). Australian Nursing Informatics Competency Project 2009. In K. Saranto, P. F. Brennan, H. Park, M. Tallberg, A. Ensio (Eds.), *NI2009 Proceedings* (pp. 556–560). Amsterdam, the Netherlands: IOS Press. Retrieved from http://eprints.qut.edu.au/31927/

Free, C., Knight, R., Robertson, S., Whittaker, R., Edwards, P., Zhou, W., & Roberts, I. (2011). Smoking cessation support delivered via mobile phone text messaging (txt-2stop): A single-blind, randomised trial. *The Lancet, 378*(9785), 49–55. doi:10.1016/S0140-6736(11)60701-0.

Garde, S., Harrison, D., & Hovenga, E. (2005). Skill needs for nurses in their role as health informatics professionals: A survey in the context of global health informatics education. *International Journal of Medical Informatics, 74*(11–12), 899–907.

Gilmour, J. A., Huntington, A., Broadbent, R., Strong, A., & Hawkins, M. (2012). Nurses' use of online health information in medical wards. *Journal of Advanced Nursing, 68*(6), 1349–1358. doi:10.1111/j.1365-2648.2011.05845.x.

Hardiker, N. R., & Hynes, B. (2012, June 23–27). *Guidance on evaluating options for representing clinical data within health information systems*. Paper presented at the 11th International Congress on Nursing Informatics (NI'2012), Montreal, Canada. Retrieved from http://www.ncbi.nlm.nih.gov/pmc/articles/PMC3799132/. Accessed on December 6, 2013.

Hausman, J. P. (1989). *Guidelines for teaching nursing informatics*. Wellington, New Zealand: Ministry of Education.

Health Informatics New Zealand (HINZ). (2013). *About health informatics New Zealand*. Retrieved from http://www.hinz.org.nz/page/about-hinz/about-hinz. Accessed on November 19, 2013.

Health Level Seven (HL7). (n.d.). *Electronic health record functional model and standard*. Retrieved from http://www.hl7.org/ehr

Hegney, D., Buikstra, E., Eley, R., Fallon, T., Gilmore, V., & Soar, J. (2007). *Nurses and information technology - Final report ANMF*. Retrieved from http://anmf.org.au/documents/reports/IT_Project.pdf

Honey, M. (2007). *Teaching and learning with technology as enabler: A case study on flexible learning for postgraduate nurses*. Unpublished doctoral thesis, University of Auckland, Auckland, New Zealand.

Honey, M., & Baker, H. (2004, July 27–29). *Integrated undergraduate curriculum for health informatics*. Paper presented at the HINZ 2004 Third National Health Informatics Conference: Towards a Healthy Nation, Wellington, New Zealand.

Honey, M. L. L., Connor, K., Veltman, M., Bodily, D., & Diener, S. (2012). Teaching with Second Life: Haemorrhage management as an example of a process for developing simulations for Multi-User Virtual Environments (MUVEs). *Clinical Simulation in Nursing, 8*(3), e79–e85. doi:10.1016/j.ecns.2010.07.003.

Honey, M., Dore, E., Yeoman, M., Young, C., McGivern, E., & McIntosh, N. (2013, November 27–29). *An on-line forum to support families with mental health problems*. Paper presented at the 12th National Health Informatics Conference: Engaged patients – Rebalancing the clinical relationship. Rotorua, New Zealand: Health Informatics New Zealand.

Honey, M., Roy, D., Bycroft, J., Boyd, M., & Raphael, D. (2014). *Promoting the meaningful use of health information for New Zealand consumers*. Paper submitted to the 12th International Congress on Nursing Informatics (NI'2014), Taipei, Taiwan.

Honey, M., & Westbrooke, L. (2011). Nursing informatics New Zealand (NINZ). In R. Carr, A. Pistacchi & L. McKay (Eds.), *HINZ: The first ten years 2000-2010* (pp. 6–13). Auckland, New Zealand: Health Informatics New Zealand.

Horizon Poll. (2013). *New Zealanders moving smartly away from standard mobiles*. Retrieved from https://www.horizonpoll.co.nz/page/297/new-zealand. Accessed on November 21, 2013.

Hovenga, E. J. S., & Grain, H. (2013). *Health data governance*. Amsterdam, the Netherlands: IOS Press.

Hovenga, E. J. S., Kidd, M., & Cesnik, B. (1996). *Health informatics: An overview*. South Melbourne, Australia: Churchill Livingstone.

Hovenga, E. J. S., Kidd, M., Garde, S., & Hullin, C. (2010). *Health informatics: An overview*. Amsterdam, the Netherlands: IOS Press.

ICT Standards Committee. (2004). Foundations for the future: Priorities for health information standardisation in Australia, 2004–2008 unpublished working paper.

Integrated Health Information Systems (IHiS) organisation. (2014). Retrieved from https://www.ihis.com.sg/. Accessed on January 5, 2014.

Internet World Stats. (2012). *Internet usage and population in oceania*. Retrieved from http://www.internetworldstats.com/stats6.htm#oceania. Accessed on November 20, 2013.

InterRAI. (n.d.) Retrieved from http://www.interrai.org

Kerr, K., Cullen, R., Duke, J., Holt, A., Kirk, R., Komisarczuk, P., ... Wilson, S. (2006). *Health informatics capability development in New Zealand: A report to the Tertiary Education Commission*. Wellington, New Zealand:

National Steering Committee for Health Informatics Education in New Zealand. Retrieved from http://homepages.mcs.vuw.ac.nz/~peterk/healthinformatics/tec-hi-report-06.pdf. Accessed on November 21, 2013.

Lim, A. G., Doherty, I., Honey, M. L. L. (2011). Creating teaching objects: A case study of delivering recorded narrations in nursing education. *Computers, Informatics, Nursing: CIN, 29*(6 Suppl.), TC114–TC119. doi:10.1097/NCN.0b013e3182285bca.

Lu, Y., Zhang, P., Liu, J., Li, J., & Deng, S. (2013). Health-related hot topic detection in online communities using text clustering. *PLoS ONE, 8*(2), e56221. doi:10.1371/journal.pone.0056221.

Lucas, J., Honey, M., & Day, K. (2012, November 7–9). *Clinicians' perceptions of telemedicine opportunities and barriers: Interim findings of a descriptive study.* Paper presented at the 11th National Health Informatics Conference: Health Informatics into Clinical Practice, Rotorua, New Zealand: Health Informatics. Retrieved from http://www.hinz.org.nz/uploads/file/2012conference/Papers/P5_Lucas.pdf. Accessed on December 6, 2013.

MacKay, G., & Griffin, A. (1989). *Nurses using computers: Australian experiences.* Armidale, New South Wales, Australia: A.C.A.E Publications.

Ministerial Review of Vic Health Sector ICT (2013, August). Retrieved from http://www.health.vic.gov.au/publications/

Ministry of Business Innovation and Employment. (2012). *Ultra-fast broadband initiative.* Retrieved from http://www.med.govt.nz/sectors-industries/technology-communication/fast-broadband/ultra-fast-broadband-initiative. Accessed on November 21, 2013.

Ministry of Health. (2000). *The New Zealand health strategy.* Wellington, New Zealand: Ministry of Health.

Ministry of Health. (2001). *The health and independence report.* Wellington, New Zealand: Ministry of Health.

Ministry of Health. (2010). *IT health board.* Retrieved from http://www.ithealthboard.health.nz/

Ministry of Health. (2011). *Better, sooner, more convenient health care in the community.* Wellington, New Zealand: Ministry of Health. Retrieved from http://www.health.govt.nz/publication/better-sooner-more-convenient-health-care-community. Accessed on December 10, 2013.

Ministry of Health. (2012). *Shared health information – The way of the future.* Wellington, New Zealand: Ministry of Health. Retrieved from http://www.health.govt.nz/system/files/documents/topic_sheets/shared-health-information-seminar-summary.pdf. Accessed on November 20, 2013.

Ministry of Health. (2013a). *Health Information Standard Organisation.* Retrieved from http://www.ithealthboard.health.nz/who-we-work/hiso. Accessed on December 10, 2013.

Ministry of Health. (2013b). *National collections and surveys.* Wellington, New Zealand: Ministry of Health. Retrieved from http://www.health.govt.nz/nz-health-statistics/national-collections-and-surveys. Accessed on November 20, 2013.

Ministry of Health. (2013c). *National Health IT Plan update 2013/14.* Wellington, New Zealand: Ministry of Health. Retrieved from http://www.ithealthboard.health.nz/sites/all/files/national-health-IT-plan-update-2013-14-nov13%20-%202.pdf. Accessed on December 8, 2013.

Ministry of Health. (2013d). *National telehealth services.* Retrieved from http://www.health.govt.nz/our-work/national-telehealth-services. Accessed on December 10, 2013.

Ministry of Health. (2013e). *Presentation on National Health IT Plan update.* Wellington, New Zealand: Ministry of Health. Retrieved from http://www.ithealthboard.health.nz/national-health-it-plan. Accessed on December 8, 2013.

Ministry of Health and District Health Boards New Zealand Workforce Group. (2007). *A career framework for the health workforce in New Zealand.* Wellington, New Zealand: Ministry of Health and District Health Boards New Zealand. Retrieved from http://www.dhbsharedservices.health.nz/Site/Future_Workforce/Default.aspx. Accessed on December 8, 2013.

National eHealth Transition Authority (NEHTA). (2013). *Strategic Plan (2011-2012).* Retrieved from http://www.nehta.gov.au/about-us/our-strategy. Accessed on January 8, 2014.

National Health Information Standards and Statistics Committee (NHISSC). (n.d.). Retrieved from http://www.aihw.gov.au/nhissc/

National Health IT Board. (2010). *National Health IT Plan.* Wellington, New Zealand: National Health IT Board. Retrieved from http://www.ithealthboard.health.nz/sites/all/files/National%20Health%20IT%20Plan%20v11_1.pdf. Accessed on December 8, 2013.

National Health IT Board. (2013). *New Zealand Telehealth Forum.* Retrieved from http://www.ithealthboard.health.nz/who-we-work/new-zealand-telehealth-forum. Accessed on December 8, 2013.

National Health and Medical Research Council (NHMRC). (2013). Retrieved from http://www.nhmrc.gov.au/grants/research-funding-statistics-and-data. Accessed on January 7, 2014.

New Zealand Immigration. (2012). *Excellent healthcare.* Retrieved from http://www.newzealandnow.govt.nz/living-in-nz/family-friendly/excellent-healthcare. Accessed on November 18, 2013.

New Zealand Technology Industry Association. (2013). *Industry overview.* Retrieved from http://www.ict.org.nz/. Accessed on November 21, 2013.

NHIMPC. (2007). *Strategic Workplan 2007–08 to 2012–13.* Retrieved from http://www.ahmac.gov.au/NHIMPC_Strategic_Work_Plan.pdf

Nursing Council of New Zealand. (2011). *The New Zealand nursing workforce.* Wellington, New Zealand: Nursing Council of New Zealand. Retrieved from http://nursingcouncil.org.nz/Publications/Reports. Accessed on December 10, 2013.

Nursing Council of New Zealand. (2012). *Code of conduct for nurses*. Wellington, New Zealand: Nursing Council of New Zealand.

Nursing Council of New Zealand. (2013). *Annual report 2013*. Wellington, New Zealand: Nursing Council of New Zealand.

Nursing and Midwifery Workforce Strategy Group. (2006). *Nursing workforce strategy*. Retrieved from http://www. dhbnz.org.nz/includes/download.aspx?ID=25740

Oh, H., Rizo, C., Enkin, M., & Jadad, A. (2005). What is e-health (3): A systematic review of published definitions. *Journal of Medical Internet Research, 7*(1), e1. Retrieved from http://www.jmir.org/2005/1/e1

Parry, D., Hunter, I., Honey, M., Holt, A., Day, K., Kirk, R., & Cullen, R. The HINZ Education Working Group. (2013). Building an educated health informatics workforce – the New Zealand experience. In H. Grain & L. K. Schaper (Eds.), *Studies in health technology and Informatics 188: Health Informatics: Digital Health Service Delivery - The future is now* (pp. 86–90). Amsterdam, the Netherlands: IOS Press.

Privacy Commissioner. (2013). *Privacy Act and codes*. Retrieved from http://privacy.org.nz/the-privacy-act-and-codes/privacy-law-reform-resources. Accessed on November 20, 2013.

Royal Australian Nurses Federation. (1984). *Computerised patient data and nursing information systems: Some considerations*. Melbourne, Australia: Royal Australian Nurses Federation.

Schoen, C., Osborn, R., Doty, M. M., Squires, D., Peugh, J., & Applebaum, S. (2009, November 5). A survey of primary care physicians in 11 countries, 2009: Perspectives on care, costs, and experiences Commonwealth Fund International Health Policy Survey of Primary Care Physicians. *Health Affairs Web Exclusive*, w1171–w1183.

Shahtahmasebi, S., Villa, L., Nielsen, H., & Graham-Smith, H. (2010). Proposal of a holistic model to support local-level evidence-based practice. *The Scientific World, 10*, 1520–1529. doi:org/10.1100/tsw.2010.144.

Soar, J., Marsault, A., Sara, T., Mount, C., Hardy, J., Swinkels, W., & Yearwoord, J. (2003). *Health informatics education, HISA, & Australian Department of Health and Ageing*. Retrieved from http://www.health.gov.au/internet/hconnect/publishing.nsf/content/7746B10691FA666CCA 257128007B7EAF/$File/hiefrept.pdf

Standards Australia. (n.d.). *eHealth*. Retrieved from http://www.e-health.standards.org.au

Statistics New Zealand. (2013). *Latest releases*. Retrieved from www.stats.govt.nz. Accessed on November 20, 2013.

Stewart, S., & Davis, D. (2012). On the MUVE or in decline: Reflecting on the sustainability of the Virtual Birth Centre developed in Second Life. *Australasian Journal of Educational Technology, 28*(Special issue 3), 480–503.

Suryadevara, N. K., & Mukhopadhyay, S. C. (2013, November 27–28). *A smart healthcare monitoring system for independent living*. Paper presented at the 12th National Health Informatics Conference: Engaged Patients - Rebalancing the clinical relationship, Rotorua, New Zealand: : Health Informatics. Retrieved from http://www.hinz.org.nz/uploads/file/2013conference/ Smart%20Healthcare%20Monitoring%20System%20-%20 Suryadevara.pdf. Accessed on December 10, 2013.

University of Hong Kong. (n.d.). *interRAI coordinating centre*. Retrieved from http://ageing.hku.hk/interrai/ index.html

Westbrooke, L., Honey, M., & Carr, R. (2011). International connections. In R. Carr, A. Pistacchi, & L. McKay (Eds.), *HINZ: The first ten years 2000-2010* (pp. 63–70). Auckland, New Zealand: Health Informatics New Zealand.

Whittaker, R., Dorey, E., Bramley, D., Bullen, C., Denny, S., Elley, C., & Salmon, P. (2011). A theory-based video messaging mobile phone intervention for smoking cessation: Randomized controlled trial. *Journal of Medical Internet Research, 13*(1), e10.

Whittaker, R., Merry, S., Stasiak, K., McDowell, H., Doherty, I., Shepherd, M., & Rodgers, A. (2012). MEMO--a mobile phone depression prevention intervention for adolescents: Development process and post-program findings on acceptability from a randomized controlled trial. *Journal of Medical Internet Research, 14*(1), e13. doi:10.2196/ jmir.1857.

World Health Organisation (WHO). (n.d.). *eHealth Definition*. Retrieved from http://www.who.int/trade/ glossary/story021/en/

World Health Organization (WHO). (2008). *WHO human resources for health minimum data set*. Retrieved from http://www.who.int/hrh/documents/hrh_minimum_ data_set.pdf

World Health Organization (WHO). (2010). *International classification of diseases*. Retrieved from http://www. who.int/classifications/icd/en/. Accessed on December 8, 2013.

Zelmer, L. McLees, M. A., & Zelmer, A. (1991). A progress report on the use of CAL/CML in a three year pre-registration diploma program. In E. Hovenga, K. Hannah, K. McCormick, & J. Ronald (Eds.), *Nursing informatics '91; Proceedings of the fourth international conference on nursing use of computers and information science*. Melbourne, Australia: Springer-Verlag.

54

Nursing Informatics in Asia

Hyeoun-Ae Park

• OBJECTIVES

1. Describe the development of nursing informatics (NI) in selected Asian countries.
2. Identify historic milestones, changes, and trends influencing how nurses embrace informatics, such as government initiatives and international collaborations.
3. Discuss NI practice, education, and research.

• KEY WORDS

Information systems
Standards
Health informatics
Government initiatives

INTRODUCTION

Asia is the world's largest and most populous continent covering 30% of the Earth's land area and hosting 60% of the world's population. Asia is a very vibrant and diverse region in terms of geography, socio-economy, culture, and politics with 49 sovereign countries and 48 official languages. Asian countries face complex language issues when implementing health informatics programs. China, Japan, and Korea have double byte languages, which make the migration to digital records even more challenging.

Asia's size and diversity presents many challenges in the development of health informatics in terms of communication, information sharing, standards implementation, and manpower training. Health informatics development in Asia correlates with socio-economic development and depends on government and industry commitment to health informatics infrastructures.

This chapter provides eHealth initiatives in Asia, academic activities of APAMI, and overview of NI in three countries in Asia including South Korea, Japan, and Taiwan.

eHealth Initiatives in Asia

eHealth collaboration in the APEC region started when APEC leaders recognized the digital divide among member countries and decided to support underprivileged populations within the region in 2000. In 2001, leaders of member countries addressed basic health issues within the region and declared use of ICT to extend healthcare services to a wider community. In 2003, APEC leaders called for health security and established a health surveillance network to monitor disease outbreaks and bio-terrorism. At a ministerial meeting in 2005, ministers underscored the importance of the use of ICT to better face threats to health in the region and welcomed the eHealth Initiatives. In 2006, as part of the eHealth Initiative, an annual APEC eHealth Seminar and Action Project were launched.

Based on the feedback from eHealth Seminars, the APEC eHealth Community was introduced in 2009 to share information, and to exchange human and material resources through a connection between developed and underdeveloped economies in terms of eHealth. The APEC eHealth Community made it possible to promote government participation in the development of policy, legislation, and standards and encourage APEC member country participation by arranging for each member country to take turns hosting seminars under the leadership of the APEC eHealth Community.

The APEC eHealth Community holds an annual meeting called the APEC eHealth Community Forum. Key objectives of the APEC eHealth Community Forum include bridging the gap between APEC member countries through seminars capacity building in information sharing, acknowledging high-value cases related to eHealth, and vitalizing eHealth focused industries within the region. The main activities of the eHealth Community Forum consist of technical presentation, exhibition of eHealth products, and poster presentation. Experts from industries, academia, and research institutes actively participate in these activities.

The APEC eHealth Community Forum supports its member countries with a detailed scheme depending on the current status of eHealth. It will implement the initiative-level plan to share information on the current status of eHealth and promote eHealth awareness, the mid-level plan to develop technology through the attainment of advanced health IT information, and the advanced-level plan to introduce new eHealth technology.

Asia-Pacific Association for Medical Informatics (APAMI)

APAMI was established in 1993 as IMIA regional member of IMIA to promote regional cooperation and development of health informatics. To date, APAMI has 15 society members, including Australia, China, Hong Kong, India, Indonesia, Japan, Korea, Malaysia, New Zealand, the Philippines, Singapore, Sri Lanka, Taiwan, Thailand, and Vietnam.

Activities of APAMI include triennial conferences and working groups. An inaugural triennial conference for APAMI was held in Singapore in 1994. Subsequent APAMI conferences were held in Sydney, Australia, in 1997; Hong Kong, in 2000; Daegu, Korea, in 2003; Taipei, Taiwan, in 2006; Hiroshima, Japan, in 2009; and Beijing, China, in 2012. Working groups within APAMI include the Standardization WG, the Health Informatics for Developing Countries WG, the Decision Support WG, and the Nursing Informatics WG. Each WG hosts a workshop during the APAMI triennial conferences.

Health informatics activities that APAMI actively promotes include telemedicine, bioinformatics, and public health informatics. The Asia-Pacific region is a major player in telemedicine because of the large-sized countries, its low specialist-to-population ratio, affordable cost of technology

and telecommunication, and high penetration rate of ICT for equitable distribution of healthcare services. One such example is oncology center network for telemedicine in Japan, which connects 14 cancer centers throughout Japan. There were more than 130 teleconferences per year with 16,000 participants. High-resolution images are transferred among centers as part of teleconference services. Asia-Pacific countries with active telemedicine projects include China, Korea, Australia, India, Bhutan, Singapore, Indonesia, Hong Kong, and New Zealand.

In addition, many countries in the APAMI region such as China, Hong Kong, Japan, Korea, Singapore, India, Malaysia, Thailand, and the Philippines are actively promoting bioinformatics. China, Hong Kong SAR, Singapore, and Taiwan are especially active in working on public health informatics after the Asian SARS outbreak of 2003. The SARS outbreak provided an opportunity for APAMI to take on this new challenge through public health informatics. APAMI addresses public health informatics research and development such as informatics deployed in contact tracing, epidemiological reporting, and monitoring to tackle acute disease outbreaks such as SARS.

Overview of Nursing Informatics in Asia

Since computers were first introduced into the healthcare sectors of Asian countries in the 1970s, there have been exciting developments in healthcare informatics associated with the rapid growth in information and communication technology. The first applications of information technology in healthcare in Asian countries were in administration, billing, and insurance; now these countries are moving toward implementing paperless electronic health records. The short histories of health informatics varied between the three countries, but all governments have played a very important role in introducing information technology into the healthcare sector by providing funds, developing infrastructure, and introducing policies to promote its use. Professional organizations have also played an important role. In most of these countries computers were first used in nursing during the early 1970s, although the terms health informatics and NI were not introduced until the 1980s or early 1990s following the establishment of professional organizations for health informatics.

The adoption of informatics in these three countries usually began as the vision of a group of individuals involved with the government or a professional organization, who promoted the use of information technology to support nurses in all areas of nursing. This occurred in nursing care practice, education, and research organizations, as well as within the information technology industry and via related government departments and existing professional organizations.

As information technology has become indispensable to the daily activities of healthcare professionals, more and more nursing schools are beginning to realize the importance of providing informatics courses to nurses. Basic computer literacy education is now a part of nursing education in the three countries, and graduate programs majoring in NI are also available now in South Korea and Taiwan.

Reports of research into NI began to appear in the domestic nursing journals of the three countries in the 1990s. In the three countries, information technology first appeared as an educational tool, following by its use in clinical practice in applications such as expert systems and electronic nursing records. This use in clinical practice led to the development of standards becoming a favorite research topic. Current research topics include terminology and classification, decision support systems, mobile computing, and telemedicine.

Events external to the nursing profession frequently catalyzed the adoption of informatics by nurses. International multi-disciplinary informatics links have assisted these beginnings and their progression. The progress in South Korea and Japan has been expedited by the hosting of the International Medical Informatics Association (IMIA) triannual conferences in 1980 and 1997. Moreover, the formation of the Asia-Pacific Association for Medical Informatics in 1993 helped promote national healthcare informatics association in the three countries due to the hosting of triannual conferences in the Pacific Rim. The China, Japan, and Korea Medical Informatics Associations formed in 1999 helped nurses in these three countries to share and exchange experience and knowledge among both experts and users in these countries.

This chapter provides an overview of the historical events in South Korea, Japan, and Taiwan and highlights factors that are critical to success in healthcare informatics for the benefits of those who have yet to embark on such a journey. The chapter concludes by summarizing significant events and examining their impact on the evolution of NI in this region.

SOUTH KOREA

South Korea is located in the Far East of the Asian continent, and its territory consists of the Korean Peninsula extending southward with 4410 islands around it. The area of South Korea is 99,392 km². Mountains account for almost 70% of the territory, and the cultivated area is only 21%. Currently, South Korea is the fourth largest

economy in the Asia-Pacific region and the 13th largest in the world. As of 2009, the population of Korea was about 50 million. The population predominantly lives in urban areas, with more than 41% living in one of the five major cities (Statistics Portal, 2012).

As of 2011, life expectancy in Korea was measured at 81.3, which exceeds the average life expectancy at birth (81.1) across countries measured by the Organisation for Econmic Co-operation and Development (OECD). The number of hospital beds was over 9 per 1000 individuals in 2011, ranking the second highest among OECD countries. With 2.0 physicians per 1000 individuals, Korea ranked 8th lowest. Further, Korea had 4.7 nurses per 1000 individuals which is lower than the average of OECD 8.8 (OECD, 2013).

South Korea introduced universal health insurance in 1989, covering hospital stays, physician visits, and prescription drugs for the whole population. The South Korean healthcare industry is on the growth track. Several new developments are contributing to the changing face of the South Korean healthcare industry. Biotechnology and health informatics are growing segments of the healthcare industry in Korea. In particular, health informatics in South Korea has grown considerably in recent years due to rapid growth of the information technology (IT) sector in Korea and with the help of the professional outreach activities of the Korean Society of Medical Informatics (KOSMI).

History of Nursing Informatics in Korea

The use of computers in South Korean healthcare began in the late 1970s in hospital finance and administration systems to expedite insurance reimbursements. Soon thereafter, the national health insurance system expanded to cover the whole population, and computers became necessary equipment to file reimbursement in healthcare organizations. The terms *health informatics* and *nursing informatics* were first introduced in Korea when the KOSMI was founded in 1987.

A Nursing Informatics Special Interest Group was organized as one of the five special interest groups in the KOSMI in 1993. Since then, the Nursing Informatics Special Interest Group has held its own session at the bi-annual conference of the KOSMI. Nursing has been highly visible in the KOSMI through presenting and publishing papers on the use of computers in nursing at these conferences and in the *Journal of the KOSMI*. Currently, more than 200 of the KOSMI's active members are nurses.

Korean nurses have attended and participated in many international conferences promoted and organized by the International Medical Informatics Association (IMIA) and the International Medical Informatics Association Special Interest Group on Nursing Informatics (IMIA-NI) since the KOSMI was founded in 1987. Korean nurses represented the country at the IMIA-NI for the first time in 1995, since then Korea has sent a representative to the group and participated actively in developing and furthering nursing informatics within the country and outside the country. The IMIA conference MEDINFO98 and the IMIA-NI conference NI2006 held in Seoul provided excellent opportunities for Korean nurses to become acquainted with nursing informatics at the global level.

Further momentum for nursing informatics has been coming from funding for a nursing informatics study group provided by the Korean Science and Engineering Foundations since 1998. Activities of the study group include journal reviews and research activities such as survey studies of nursing informatics education and computer applications in nursing practice in Korean hospitals.

Use of Information Technology in Clinical Practice

According to a report published by the Korean Hospital Association in 2005, 100% of tertiary hospitals, 98.7% of community hospitals, and 95.4% of physician's offices have admission/discharge/transfer systems. Such a high implementation rate is believed to have been initially driven by financial factors associated with medical insurance claims. Eventually, the focus shifted to all areas of patient care as clinicians began to use computers in their practices. This report shows that almost 100% of tertiary hospitals, 84.2% of community hospitals, and 66.9% of physician's offices are using computerized provider order-entry systemsa. In addition, about 90.5% of tertiary hospitals, 78.6% of community hospitals, and 22.6% of physician's offices are equipped with picture archiving and communication systems (PACSs). There has been a great deal of interest among healthcare organizations in acquiring these systems since the Korean government announced high reimbursement rates for diagnostic radiology examinations using PACS in early 2000. Hospitals are now beginning to implement paperless electronic medical record (EMR) systems. As of 2010, 50.2% of tertiary hospitals and 35.0% of general hospitals have either basic or comprehensive EHR systems (Yoon, Chang, Kang, & Park 2012).

The use of computers in clinical nursing practice in Korea began first in medium-sized hospitals. These hospitals initially used computers mainly for administration and billing, as did most hospitals in other countries. These systems allow nurses to view their work list on screens or printouts so that they do not need to copy medication schedules or care activities onto the Kardex, or take

notes on a piece of paper. Nursing information systems were proliferated when large hospitals with more than 1000 beds began opening in the mid-1990s. These new hospitals were equipped with nursing information systems when they first opened. They included unique nursing activities such as nursing assessment, nursing care plans, and patient classifications in addition to nursing activities related to billing, managerial or coordinating activities, and physician-delegated tasks. Hospitals are now beginning to implement paperless electronic nursing record (ENR) systems. A standardized nursing terminology based on the International Classification for Nursing Practice was integrated into the ENR system and introduced at Seoul National University Hospital in Korea in 2003. Since then, nursing data collected with the system have been stored in a clinical data repository. Data stored in the repository are being used for research and clinical practice (Ahn & Park, 2013; Park, Cho, & Ahn, 2012). Currently, detailed clinical model-based electronic nursing records system is being developed in Korea (Park, Min, Jeon, & Chung, 2012).

Nursing Informatics Education

As IT has become indispensable in healthcare, and its impact on the daily activities of healthcare professionals has become significant, nursing schools are beginning to realize the importance of the health informatics education for clinicians. According to a survey on curriculums of Korean nursing schools posted in 2010, about 69% (78/135) of nursing schools with baccalaureate programs offer nursing informatics courses and 40.8% (29/71) of nursing schools with three-year diploma programs offer nursing informatics courses (Lee & Park, 2009). Nursing informatics courses were taught under different course titles, such as nursing informatics, nursing and informatics, nursing informatics and laboratory, medical and nursing informatics, nursing informatics and nursing process, nursing informatics and nursing management, nursing informatics science, and nursing informatics and evidence-based nursing. The course contents in these courses vary a great deal from school to school, and most of the instructors did not receive formal education on nursing informatics, rather they are self-taught instructors on the subject. This indicates that there is a need to identify content to cover in nursing informatics courses for four-year programs and three-year diploma programs, and standardize the programs based on the tasks of healthcare professionals.

Most nursing schools in Korea are adding informatics to the graduate-level curriculum so that students can take informatics courses as an elective. There is only one graduate program specializing in nursing informatics in Korea, which is at Seoul National University College of Nursing. This program started in 2003 and awards master's and doctoral degrees in nursing informatics. This program is playing a very important role in nursing informatics in Korea by producing not only nursing informatics practitioners, but also qualified nursing informatics educators.

Nursing Informatics Research

Since the introduction of the terms *medical informatics* and *nursing informatics* in 1987 in Korea, there have been many research studies on the use of information and technology in the healthcare field. We identified the trends of nursing informatics research since the introduction of medical informatics and nursing informatics in 1989 in Korea by reviewing nursing informatics–related literatures published in Korea (Lee & Park, 2009). We reviewed the abstracts of oral and poster presentations at the KOSMI bi-annual conferences and papers published in the *Journal of Korean Academy of Nursing, Korean Journal of Nursing Query*, and *Journal of Korean Academy of Adult Nursing*. We included all of the abstracts and articles that were either authored by a nurse researcher or had relevance or application to nursing. A total of 192 papers were reviewed to examine the research trend of NI in Korea. We have grouped the NI research into the following seven areas: clinical practice; teaching and learning; decision support; public and consumer health informatics; patient-centered healthcare such as telemedicine and ubiquitous healthcare; standardization activities; and use of IT for nursing research.

The number of NI-related papers published in Korea has increased dramatically over the past 20 years. Early studies on the use of computers for clinical nursing practice in the late 1980s and 1990s focused on attitudes toward or changes in workflow after computerized patient order entry (CPOE) implementation. In the mid-2000s, as terminology-based ENR systems were introduced, the outcomes of ENRs were studied in terms of direct and indirect care time and user satisfaction. Patient safety programs became part of the ENR. Quite a few papers have been published on the use of IT as a tool (e.g., CD-ROM, computer-assisted instruction, and Web-based learning) for learning and education in Korea. In the late 1990s and late 2000s, the popular research was in the area of decision support. With an aging population and increasing numbers of patients with aging-related diseases, there is a need for patient-centered healthcare such as telemedicine. Standardization activities in Korea are widely published and include work such as care plans, nursing practice guidelines and critical pathways, nursing document forms, and the use of nursing terminology for ENR systems.

Information technology has been used for research into nursing and for data analysis, including both qualitative and quantitative research.

The growing interest in IT has been reflected in nursing research in Korea. Over last two decades, the introduction of EMR and ENR systems, health informatics education, and health informatics research have either directly or indirectly influenced the development and expansion of NI research in Korea.

Standardization Activities

There are current efforts to introduce various health informatics standards in healthcare information systems in South Korea. The primary motivation for this is compatibility of data, clinical documentation, and research outcomes across the country. Korean experts are actively involved in standards development activities in different international standards development organizations, such as the International Standards Organization (ISO) and Health Level Seven (HL7).

The Korean Ministry of Health introduced a Health Informatics Standards Committee in 2004 in an attempt to develop a single, integrated healthcare terminology in Korea as part of the National Health Information Infrastructure (Ministry of Health, Labour and Welfare, 2004). This committee is in charge of developing, disseminating, and maintaining healthcare terminologies. There are 14 sub-committees working on healthcare terminologies in 14 different areas, such as medicine, dentistry, public health, and nursing. The Nursing Sub-committee translated the majority of existing nursing terminologies, such as the North American Nursing Diagnosis Association Taxonomy I and II, Nursing Interventions Classifications, Clinical Care Classifications, the Omaha System, and the International Classification for Nursing Practice (ICNP), into Korean. This committee also collected and standardized nursing statements documented in nursing records and mapped them to the ICNP. Outputs from this committee are available for Korean hospitals to access and use in their electronic patient record systems (Park & Cho, 2009).

Government Initiatives

The Korean government initiated information systems planning for the public health sector and the National Health Information Infrastructure in 2005. As part of these initiatives, the Korean government established the Center for Interoperable EHR (CiEHR) in 2005. The role of the CiEHR is to develop core technologies necessary to implement a lifetime electronic health record (EHR), which enables the public to securely access and use their own medical record anytime and anywhere, as necessary, from the cradle to the grave.

Once the lifetime EHR is fully implemented, medical practitioners will be able to provide diagnoses and treatments with enhanced accuracy based upon sufficient patient data. The public benefits by receiving higher-quality medical care. In addition, the lifetime EHR will eventually reduce the costs and risks of medical care and eliminate redundancy in laboratory tests and prescriptions. Ultimately, the EHR promotes public health and chronic disease management, as it establishes the foundation for receiving systematic lifetime healthcare services.

In the first two years, CiEHR has established plans for a national healthcare information system. The center has been engaged in ongoing development of infrastructure for the next-generation EHR system by developing its necessary functions and standards including an integrated medical terminology and data model, administered service management system, and clinical decision support system. Research and development conducted by CiEHR is the outcome of collaboration with the 30 EHR-associated hospitals and 21 participating companies. This effort will be the cornerstone for utilizing health IT in the public healthcare sector and disseminating health IT to the private healthcare sector.

The research outcome of CiEHR creates a synergy effect through collaboration with national health IT projects, and public and private healthcare organizations. The ultimate goal of CiEHR is to enable the nation to conveniently receive healthcare at anytime and anywhere by practicing safe exchange of medical information between healthcare organizations. It aims to produce practical outcomes that can be applied by real users in real situations.

Professional Outreach

Since its inception in 1987, the KOSMI has played a key role in promoting and developing health informatics in Korea by holding bi-annual academic conferences, various seminars, workshops, and open forums, and by publishing journals. KOSMI has also offered educational programs for beginners in health informatics.

Professional organizations such as the Korean Medical Association and the Korean Nurses Association have also played significant roles by including health informatics in their continuing education programs. Another healthcare informatics expert group, the Health Informatics Standardization Committee, serving as the South Korean technical advisory group of the ISO Technical Committee 215, has held open forums and published health information standards.

The IMIA has contributed significantly to furthering the knowledge of South Korean healthcare professionals about worldwide trends in health informatics. South Korean experts in health informatics have attended and participated in many international conferences and meetings promoted or sponsored by the IMIA since 1989.

Technology Trends

The rapid growth in the number of mobile telephone users (currently estimated to be around 92% of the total population) and the advances in wireless local area network technology have led to mobile computing in healthcare becoming a popular issue in South Korea, with many healthcare organizations testing its feasibility in special wards. The main users of mobile computing currently are nurses attending patients at bedsides, but this will soon be extended to other healthcare professionals. Although personal digital assistants (PDAs), tablet PCs, and notebooks are all suitable mobile computing platforms, users favor notebook computers with wireless LAN connections because of their large screen size and easier-to-use interface.

The need for telemedicine continues to grow in Korea with the increasing numbers of elderly patients, patients with chronic diseases, and patients who are discharged early. Many telemedicine systems have been tested over the past 10 years, one of which is a teleconsultation system initiated by the Korean government. Such systems allow, for example, a primary care physician at a health center in a remote area to have a telepathology or a teleradiology consultation with the specialists of a tertiary hospital. Another example of telemedicine is telecare at home, with the Telecare Center of Seoul National University Hospital and the Telemedicine Center of Gil Hospital being among the most active telecare-at-home clinics. Telepractioners at these centers maintain special schedules for their remote clients. They set aside one to two days per week to take care of their clients using virtual reality technology via the Internet. Currently, the teleconsultation fee is reimbursed by health insurance, but the use of telecare-at-home clinics is not covered. In July 2009, the Korean government began permitting telemedicine between healthcare professionals and clients.

Another technical trend in healthcare is called *ubiquitous computing in healthcare*. Ubiquitous healthcare can be defined as the environment where healthcare is available to everyone, everywhere without any dependence on time and location and where the technologies enabling ubiquitous healthcare will be assimilated flawlessly in our daily lives such that the technologies become invisible (Sneha & Varshney, 2006). It is being considered an alternative to traditional face-to-face healthcare services in Korea. Since revision of medical laws to include e-prescriptions and telehealth was passed in 2002, several attempts were made to utilize ubiquitous computing in healthcare in both public and private sectors in Korea. For example, the Korean government initiated various pilot projects to promote ubiquitous computing in healthcare such as the Smart Digital Home, Health Management, and Health Promotion projects that use ubiquitous IT for underprivileged populations; the Ubiquitous Home Healthcare project for the elderly; and the u-City project. The local governments have also initiated various ubiquitous healthcare trials such as health center–based home healthcare, telemedicine in rural underserved regions, telemedicine for the elderly in nursing homes, and tele-emergency services.

The private sector has also made various attempts to utilize ubiquitous computing in healthcare. One example is the B2C ubiquitous healthcare model, which was developed to help manage chronic diseases (e.g., diabetes and hypertension), promote health in the general population (e.g., exercise, diet, and life style management), and support disease prevention in the private sector. Another example is the B2B model, where medical information solutions companies collaborate with healthcare organizations and insurance companies to provide ubiquitous healthcare services.

Recently, major healthcare organizations, leading telecommunication companies, universities and government research institutes, medical device and sensor companies, medical information solutions companies, and the safety and security industries are beginning to collaborate in ubiquitous healthcare in Korea. For example, a consortium of healthcare organizations with life insurance companies, medical information solutions companies, and local governments led by SK Telecom and LG Electronics is developing ubiquitous healthcare models for private clinics and major healthcare organizations. About 8000 patients with diseases such as diabetes, hypertension, cancer, chronic respiratory disease, and metabolic syndrome will participate in this pilot project.

Ubiquitous computing is being used in nursing too. Home care nurses send data measurements of their clients to doctors at health centers. Doctors monitor data measurements sent by the home care nurses and send recommendations to the nurses' PDAs. Nurses, in return, deliver nursing care to home care clients using short message service (SMS) systems or phones. Another example is the use of ubiquitous computing by community health practitioners. Community health practitioners share bioinformation collected from clients with hypertensive and diabetic medications with doctors. Nurses prescribe and dispense medications for the patients based on doctors' orders delivered to them via wireless networks.

Ubiquitous computing is also used in nursing homes; nurses working in nursing homes can consult with doctors at a hospital located remotely via teleconferencing technology. Nurses working in community settings and for vendors are actively involved in different types of ubiquitous healthcare activities as healthcare providers, business model planners, and developers.

JAPAN

The population of Japan is about 127 million, which is about twice that of the United Kingdom and half that of the United States. There are about 10,000 hospitals in Japan, of which about 430 have more than 400 beds. About 852,000 nurses work at these hospitals, including about 220,000 nurse aides (assistant nurses). There are about 278,000 medical doctors, 97,000 dentists, and 253,000 pharmacists (JNAP, 2013; Health and Welfare Statistics Association, 2009). The healthcare delivery system in Japan provides easy access to healthcare. All citizens can choose healthcare institutions and doctors freely, and their financial contribution to health insurance is proportional to their income. The insurance fee is deducted from the monthly salary and pooled by each insurance union. Insured individuals and families pay 20% and 30%, respectively, of all health expenditure, and the publicly funded health insurer pays the rest when a patient receives medical treatment in a hospital. The hospital receives reimbursement for the balance from the National Health Insurance system. The Japanese government will contribute a maximum of 70,000 yen to the medical treatment of a person during a one-month hospital stay. Both the easy access to healthcare and low out-of-pocket cost in Japan help provide the populace with a sense of security.

The total health expenditure of Japan remains lower than that in some other advanced nations, which is partially attributable to healthier dietary habits. The relatively small number of healthcare professionals working in Japan also helps contain healthcare expenditures. The average length of hospital stays has recently been shortened, and thus many newly hospitalized patients are in the acute phase. This increases the probability of medical accidents, which can be offset by utilizing health informatics to improve medical safety.

Health Informatics in Japan

Japan began to pay attention to the use of computers in healthcare during the late 1970s following the increased use of computers in other industries. Japan hosted MEDINFO80, the International Medical Informatics

Association conference in 1980. The Japanese Association of Medical Informatics (JAMI) was founded at that time with the aim of supporting health informatics in Japan. Since then, JAMI has held 24 annual and bi-annual academic conferences, and these conferences have contributed considerably to the progress of health informatics in Japan (Japan Association of Medical Informatics, 1996; Kamiizumi & Ota, 2004). Initially, research was focused on computerized billing systems for medical fees, and the development of the use of personal computers at an individual level. The focus then shifted to research and development of systems at the organizational level, such as hospital and regional information systems, and research into basic information technology for healthcare such as database design, network security, and data-switching technology. The current focuses are ethical issues in health informatics, medical finances, and quality assurance. This illustrates that the scope of health informatics has gradually expanded since it was first introduced into Japan during the 1980s.

Medical information departments in about 50 national university hospitals have made the largest contribution to the development of health informatics in Japan. Each organization has been developing its own hospital information systems for its own applications to clinical practice, education, and research (Japan Association of Medical Informatics, 1980–2003). This work helped Japan to determine the information, information technology, and mechanisms that were needed for healthcare applications, but the independence of these applications has hindered standardization in many healthcare fields. Standardization is one of the many problems in the use of healthcare information technology that needs to be resolved.

History of Nursing Informatics in Japan

The Third International Congress on Medical Informatics, MEDINFO80, organized by the International Medical Informatics Association, was held in Tokyo in 1980. This congress included a special interest group on nursing informatics, which represented the beginning of nursing informatics in Japan (JAMI, 1996; Kamiizumi & Ota, 2004). This did not result in immediate progress in Japanese nursing informatics education, due to schools being vocationally oriented. However, in the late 1990s nursing education in Japan rapidly shifted to a more academic orientation, and there are now more than 100 universities offering baccalaureate programs and 40 universities offering graduate programs. Some baccalaureate programs and graduate schools include nursing informatics courses in their curricula. Nursing informatics was applied more in clinical practice than in academic fields during the 1990s, with more nurses learning about utilizing

computers in nursing practice through the activities of medical information departments in national university hospitals. It was also evident that clinical nurses presented more papers than academic researchers at the annual meetings of the JAMI. The Annual Meeting for Nursing Information Systems that was established as a task force of the JAMI also supports clinical practice, and most of its members are clinical nurses. The Nursing Division of the JAMI was established in 2000 and is managed by a team of clinical nurses and academic researchers. Several textbooks on nursing informatics have been published, but systematized nursing informatics education has not yet been implemented. The Japanese Nurses Association prepared a course on nursing information management as the first step toward a continuing education curriculum for ward managers. The standard textbook was published in March 2004 (Kamiizumi & Ota, 2004). The lecturers are researchers of health informatics and nursing informatics, and clinical nurses working at the hospitals where hospital information systems were introduced.

Nursing Informatics Practice

Becoming a specialist in nursing informatics is useful when hospital information systems and electronic health records are introduced. However, the accreditation program of the Japan Nursing Association does not recognize the training for such specialists. Instead, the training of informatics nurses mainly occurs in hospital settings. In each hospital, nurses working on medical information are active in committees and working groups. Most of them are involved with not only nursing-related work but also medical-information-related work. Their lack of formal technical education often causes difficulties, and hence it is predicted that the importance of nurses with nursing informatics education will increase. The JAMI began an accreditation program for healthcare information technologists in 2003. Hospitals are looking for new healthcare staff with knowledge of both healthcare and information technology who can control information flow. Although a healthcare information technologist is a healthcare professional with such training, it is necessary to distinguish between the roles of the nursing informatics clinical nursing specialist and a healthcare information technologist. Informatics nurses will be expected to expand their activities in healthcare when both professions are introduced to hospitals.

Nursing Informatics Education

As of April 2013, there were 522 professional schools, 27 junior colleges, 218 universities, and 121 graduate schools in Japan, compared with 461 professional schools, 74 junior colleges, and 30 universities in 1994 (JNAP, 2013). This comparison illustrates that nursing education in Japan has shifted from professional schools to universities and postgraduate education in the past six years. However, there are still very few universities with separate nursing informatics programs. The increasing development of hospital information systems in Japan has led to discussions on the utilization of information technology in clinical nursing practice. Continuous education of nursing informatics is being emphasized, along with the promotion of electronic health records. However, it is difficult to conclude that the curricula of nursing schools have reflected the changes in society and clinical fields. Rather, it appears that clinical practice is now more advanced than nursing education.

Universities provided elementary computer literacy education during the first half of the 1990s, but this became unnecessary thereafter due to the introduction of computer education into elementary and junior high schools. Overall, the teaching of computer literacy on document retrieval, utilization of statistical processing, and Web utilization has increased, but barriers to the development of nursing informatics remain in Japan: (1) there are few researchers and educators in nursing informatics, (2) there is little development of educational tools, and (3) the cost of improving the network and computer environments is high. However, the importance of universities providing a satisfactory curriculum is being recognized due to the increasing importance of nursing informatics, with this being more so in graduate schools than in baccalaureate education.

Nursing Informatics Research

The amount of nursing informatics research is increasing in Japan; the two main purposes of which are improving the quality and standardization of nursing practice. Nursing informatics was one of the main subject areas of paper presentations at a recent annual meeting of the Japanese Academy of Nursing (Japan Academy for Nursing Science, 2003), indicating that it is becoming one of the major areas in nursing. There were many reports on research into the use of information technology as an educational tool during the 1990s (Ochiai, Sota, & Ezumi 1997; Kanai-Pak et al., 1997; Muranaka et al., 1997; Yamanouchi, Nakano, & Nojiri, 1997; Majima, 1997; Ezumi, Sota, & Ochiai, 1997), and on the use of information technology in clinical practice, especially on decision support systems for nursing in hospital information systems and electronic health records (JAMI, 2003). There has also been research into the use of information to prevent nursing-related accidents (Kato, Tsuru, & Iizuka, 2013) and into telenursing (Kawaguchi, Azuma, & Ohta, 2004). Research into nursing-practice algorithms using thinking-aloud methods have begun in Japan (Tsuru, et al., 2009, 2010).

Japanese Government Initiatives and Standards Development in Japan

An "e-Japan" strategy encompassing all Japanese ministries and related agencies is progressing now in Japan. The adoption of EHR is one of the main themes in the healthcare sector. The Ministry of Health, Labor, and Welfare announced a grand design for healthcare, and set the following achievement goals for 2006 (Tanaka, 2007): (1) electronic health records will be introduced into 60% of hospitals with more than 400 beds, and into 60% of clinics, and (2) the electronic health expenditure payment system will be introduced into 70% of all hospitals. Standardization of the terminology used in electronic health records is a requirement for achieving this goal, and the Ministry of Health, Labor, and Welfare has begun a project for developing a national standard, which is publicly available on the Internet (The Medical Information System Development Center, 2004). This is especially useful for hospitals introducing hospital information systems for the first time. The following five standards have already been completed: (1) 581 facilities now perform medical diagnoses using the ICD-10; (2) 330 facilities have surgical and medical treatment standards; (3) 5700 clinical tests have been registered in the clinical laboratory test standard; (4) about 38,000 drug names have been registered by 203 enterprises; and (4) about 210,000 medical supplies have been registered by 336 enterprises. Standardized symptoms, physiologic function examinations, imaging tests, dental terminology, and nursing terminology are currently under development, and nursing actions and observation items in nursing terminology will be available to the public by the middle of 2004. The terminology used in nursing practice have been collected, analyzed, and re-designed. About 260 fundamental nursing practices have been identified and named in Japan. They have been categorized into daily-life care, family support, guidance and education, inter-organizational coordination, care in the usage of equipment, and care for the terminally ill and the bereaved family, and others. There are two hospitals utilizing the terminology describing nursing care plan and nursing order and implementation of care. Difference in the nursing care offered to patients became clear. Continuous 24-hour observation of nursing care can be shared, indicating that the use of such a system is very useful for the medical profession.

NURSING INFORMATICS IN TAIWAN, HONG KONG, AND CHINA

Nursing Informatics History

The Taiwan Nursing Informatics Association (TNIA) was established in 2006. Since then NI has become an important nursing professional specialty in Taiwan. TNIA has taken many strategic steps to get supports; its members have learned from international organizations, such as IMIA NI SIG, AMIA NIWG, ANI, TIGER. It has held many international and local conference workshops to inspire many nurses to gain an interest in NI every year.

TNIA's progress resulted in being granted to host the office of National EHR Projects by the Ministry of Health in the early 2010s. Currently, all medical centers and many hospitals in Taiwan have set up NI specialist positions and formed a NIS multi-professional development task force. Nursing information systems have become widely implemented applications within clinical settings. Many creative and award-winning NIS projects such as smart handheld medication administration with strong double-checking safety design were initiated.

With TNIA's responsibility of holding the 12th international congress on nursing informatics (NI2014), the support and blessings received from global NI communities have helped mobilize nursing leaders and various professionals to work together in demonstrating the achievements and visions of NI in clinical nursing, nursing education, research, as well as administration. The local NI2014 committee organization has become the best platform for NI leaders in Taiwan to work together. In terms of results, this active mobilization made Taiwan achieve the first breaking record of submissions. Its submitted papers and posters, covering various topics, outnumbered those from other countries, including the United States. Out of 258 total conference papers and posters, 84 were from Taiwan, compared with 66 from the United States and only 1 from Taiwan for the NI2003 conference. This achievement in Taiwan, within its first 10 years of TNIA's existence, could not be made without the high-quality nurses, hardworking hospital IT personnel, and committed nurse leaders. Taiwan is making its strategic plan to join the global NI community to work with other countries to develop their NI professionals.

The Republic of China inaugurated its Nursing Informatics group at the Asia-Pacific Association for Medical Informatics (APAMI) meeting held in Beijing in 2012. Dr. Ying Wu, the Dean of School of Nursing, Capital Medical University, successfully organized the first China National Nursing Informatics Conference in Beijing in October of 2013. She is also the current President of APAMI. Working with Dr. Polun Chang, she began to organize the NI courses and workshops in Beijing.

The National Institute of Hospital Administration (NIHA) is the main governmental organization in China. NIHA has the largest mobilization and impact in the formation of national as well as local policy of developing hospital information systems, including nursing information systems. It is working with the China Hospital Information Management Association (CHIMA) to hold their national conferences, called the Chinese Hospital Information Networking Conference (CHINC), which attracts more than 3000 attendants nationwide every year. CHIMA organized the largest nursing team to promote nursing informatics, thanks to the long leadership of Dr. Baoluo Li and Dr. Yu-Xiu Gong, who are currently editing the first nursing informatics textbook in China. The other NIHA leader, Dr. Li Yao, has taken another route to affect the development of nursing informatics by educating the national nursing leaders. Outside the hospital context, the China Medical Informatics Association (CMIA), via its Chinese IMIA representative, is playing the other driving force in promoting nursing informatics.

As from 2012, Dr. Polun Chang and Ming-Chuan Kuo had actively participated at various national and local conferences, training workshops in China on behalf of NI2014 and TNIA, to demonstrate the meanings and values of nursing informatics, as well as the global trends such as the case of Technology Informatics Guiding Education Reform (TIGER). TNIA also invited leaders from China to attend the conference in Taiwan to exchange insights and build connections. Nursing informatics communities in China, Taiwan, and Hong Kong have worked well together. We believe that future cooperation will be closer and better. Fully and sincerely supported by the TNIA, a special China Nursing Informatics Forum is set up for NI2014 to link the nursing informatics expertise cross China, Taiwan, Hong Kong, and global NI community. In June 2014, the TNIA hosted NI2014, the successful 12th international congress on nursing informatics in Taipei.

Hong Kong hospitals have a well-established Clinical Management and numerous other associated systems widely used by nurses. Hong Kong nurses established NURSINFO (HK) Ltd. (http://www.nursinfo.hk/) in 1991, and this organization has enjoyed a consistent increase in membership. They have as their motto, "Nursing Informatics for Excellence in Patient Care." They organize regular educational activities, use a communication network, produce a regular newsletter, and are actively involved with the Hong Kong Society of Medical Informatics and the Hong Kong Computer Society. Together, they participate in the organization of trade exhibits and regular conferences.

The Hong Kong Hospital Authority is responsible for over 40 hospitals and over 50 specialist clinics that are part of a large multi-site, multi-protocol intelligent data network to provide seamless data communications throughout Hong Kong. Implementation began in 1993. This included a clinical management system focusing on patient-oriented data sharing. This system provides longitudinal medical profiles for patients and can be accessed by healthcare professional on a need-to-know basis. Telemedicine and videoconferencing are in use, and multimedia enhancement in the clinical setting with voice recording and imaging now helps speed up the work process and strengthens services in the clinical areas.

Hong Kong's Hospital Authority (HKHA) system has been widely accepted as part of the hospital infrastructure. With support from the Hong Kong Authority under the great leadership of Dr. Eric Chan, they are implementing a strategic action to bring their public hospital information systems into one single platform. The building of nursing care and documentation system was clearly highlighted as a key component for this action in their five-year plan for clinical system development and in their nurse manager meetings. Their private sector is also actively implementing e-hospital integrated medical solutions based on standards such as HL7, CDA, and IHE to provide clinical professionals a united portal for data assessing. Mobile clinical solutions for unit dose medication administration were also implemented.

The HKHA's Health Informatics Web site (http://www3.ha.org.hk/hi/) has not been updated since 2007. Individual nurse informaticists do publish as informatics has been fully integrated supporting their daily practice. Neither the College of Nursing in Hong Kong nor the Hong Kong Society of Medical Informatics makes any mention of nursing informatics via their websites.

The Singapore Nurses' Association has recognized Nursing Informatics as a specialty and established a Specialty Chapter accordingly. The Thai nurses also began with a Nursing Informatics special interest group.

Use of Computers in Clinical Practice

According to a recent survey, about 60% of healthcare organizations plan to set up a nursing information system. Every large healthcare organization in Taiwan already uses information systems in nursing environments. With the increasing popularity of mobile nursing stations, nursing information systems, barcode medication administration, and RFID, it is evident that nursing information systems are growing rapidly (Chang, Lin, & Lee, 2008). Currently, many hospitals have already implemented nursing information systems.

Since 1992, computerized care plan systems have been used in clinical settings. Moreover, patient classification systems have been applied in patient assessments, nursing interventions, and staff workload assignments (Hsu, Feng, Lo, & Wang, 1996), and decision support systems have been integrated with medical and nursing diagnoses. Expert systems implemented on PDAs for the emergency room triage system have also been reported (Chang, Tzeng, & Sang, 2003; Lai, Liu, Hsu, & Chen, 2001). In addition, PDAs have recently been used by nurses in their daily practice. Nurses can input and output data including vital signs when caring for patients, as well as access patient laboratory results, medications, and medical records without having to go back to nursing stations (Li, Wang, Hsu, Chen, & Chang, 1998; Lin & Liao, 2003).

In 2005, about 79% of hospitals in Taiwan had 80% of their nursing documentation computerized, including 50% of documentation in the ICU; 82% of the nursing staff were able to input and retrieve patient data from the information system.

Computerized nursing systems have mainly been established to manage patient vital signs, care plans, and medication administration records in acute units, the ICU, and in long-term care units. These systems also contain administrative functions like clinical classification systems, shift arranging (scheduling), personnel management, education and training, quality control, as well as assets and material management.

The Care Information Council was initiated in some hospitals' Departments of Nursing (DON) to develop and integrate the hospital information systems into the relevant nursing processes, including electronic medical record and care planning systems. The learning platform provides nurses with self-designed educational tools, and demonstrates how the nursing information system can apply to clinical and health education.

It is very common to use information technology in nursing practice in Taiwan. It provides wireless and laptop equipment to help nursing staff collect, save, transmit, and manage patient data faster and correctly. Especially after nurses became proficient in the wireless environment, many medical centers and big hospitals widely built mobile nursing stations to provide instant, convenient, and point-of-care nursing.

In 2005, Chang Gung Memorial Hospital Linkou Branch established an RFID operational care system in order to make the operations processes easier. The system includes functions to ensure patient data such as auto-checking, proof of action, and other applications (Chang et al., 2008). Based on the success of the Chang Gung system, other hospitals are expanding RFID technology into units like the emergency room, the delivery room, and the nursery.

Taichung Veterans General Hospital was the first hospital to combine CPOE and RFID into a barcode management administration (BCMA) system. Currently, many hospitals have already implemented BCMA systems.

The Taiwan Nursing Information Council, which is part of the TNIA, has invited 18 hospitals to set up a clinical nursing terminology and share experiences using the platform in an effort to promote nursing information systems and enhance clinical nursing information environments in Taiwan.

Use of Computers in Nursing Education

Many nursing schools in Taiwan provide NI courses and some have set up NI programs. The nursing school of National Yang Ming University, led by Drs. Shu Yu, I-Ju Chen, Polun Chang and supported by Dr. Connie Delaney, the Dean of School of Nursing at the University of Minnesota (USA), launched its formal NI graduate program in 2013. Together with the NI group, led by Dr. Polun Chang, at the Institute of Biomedical Informatics, School of Medicine, this development makes the National Yang-Ming University one of the largest and best NI programs in Asia.

In 2013, the Nanyang Polytechnic (NYP), Singapore, and the Healthcare Information and Management Systems Society (HIMSS) have established a Centre of Excellence to provide their students with hands-on training on innovative systems equipping them with skills and honing their abilities to adopt IT solutions. Nurses will be prepared to use and manage electronic medical record systems, the wireless vital signs monitoring, and the closed loop medication management system used in many Singapore hospitals.

One of nine learning objectives of the Nursing Science program at the First International University in Thailand, Assumption University indicates that its nurse graduates need to: "Have ability and skills in nursing informatics, numerical and statistics analysis." The Rangsit University's (RSU) Four-Year Bachelor of Nursing Science has Nursing Informatics as one of its foundation subjects.

Computer-assisted instruction programs have been developed by the Ministry of Education for nursing vocational education programs since 1986. The content includes diet education for diabetic patients, biostatistics, maternal child health, stress management, and patient nutrition (Chen, 1992). Although a formal master's program focusing on NI was not available until 2001, the elective courses in baccalaureate and master's programs had started in the late 1990s. All baccalaureate programs included at least one or two computer courses. Currently, some nursing students act as assistants for faculty in designing distance-learning classes.

The growth of the Internet has led to the integration of distance education into nursing curricula. Online courses are available for baccalaureate programs in counseling, teaching principles and strategies, and long-term care. In addition, some schools provide multimedia self-testing systems. Students are videotaped when tested for nursing skills such as injections or enemas, and then the content is sent online to the instructor for grading. Schools provide an environment with simulated patients for students to practice before taking the test (Chang, Shu, & Chang, 2002).

At least eight graduate programs in health or biomedical/medical informatics provide informatics training at the master's level for students with a nursing background, including the National Yang-Ming University, the National Taipei College of Nursing, the Chung-Cheng University, Taipei Medical University, Chang-Gung University, and Tzu-Chi University. A total of about 10 master's students with nursing backgrounds will graduate from these informatics programs every year. Among these eight universities, the National Yang-Ming University, the Chung-Cheng University, Taipei Medical University, and Tzu-Chi University have doctoral programs with about 10 students with nursing backgrounds enrolled, although no PhDs have been awarded yet.

In mid-2003, the TNIA conducted a series of seminars and training courses in NI that have been run continuously since then by the National Yang-Ming University, the Taipei College of Nursing, the National Union of Nurses' Associations, and the Chang-Gung Institute of Technology. Therefore, nursing informatics programs have been integrated into more universities and hospital institutions. The clinical application of office tools and information skills were very helpful for solving unique problems within the nursing field.

Use of Computers in Nursing Research

Based on the development of the TNIA, growing interest in NI has been reflected in nursing research. The number of studies related to NI has increased exponentially in the past 10 years. Nursing research, especially that pertaining to NI, can empower evidence-based practice. Knowledge building creates the expertise to conduct comparative studies of nursing care. And those NI research studies, presentations, and publications empower Taiwan to be visible in the international NI community.

Standardized terminologies such as existing nursing diagnosis classification systems and the ICNP have been translated for clinical use, and tested for their reliability and validity (Lu, 1998; Chiang, 1998). Users' perceptions and satisfaction toward computer use in daily practice also have been analyzed. Qualitative approaches such as interviews have been used to explore how well nurses will accept the change from manual charting to computerized documentation (Lee, Yeh, & Ho, 2002). Quantitative approaches such as surveys have been applied to investigate the attitude toward and satisfaction with the use of PDAs for charting and the storage of nursing records (Lai & Chen, 2003), along with factors affecting the use of nursing information (Lee, Lin, & Chang, 2005).

After 2006, more and more nursing personnel have joined in conducting NI research, and these research studies have been published in national and international nursing journals. Some of the NI research has focused on security (Hsu, Lin, & Tseng, 2009). Another research focus has been quality improvement in utilization of information technology in nursing care (Chang, 2007) including surveys of the factors related to nurses' acceptance of the use of mobile nursing stations in hospitals (Chang et al., 2008). The scope of NI studies included system development (Tai et al., 2009), nursing continuing education (Liu, Chang, Hsu, & Lai, 2007), and literature review (Chu, Tsai, Huaa, & Chen, 2010). Currently, studies are focused on radio-frequency identification (RFID) applications in medical and health industry pilot projects (Shao, 2010) and the feasibility of the role of nurse informatics specialists.

Professional Outreach

- The TNIA organized an international symposium and joined the Joint Conference of Medical Informatics in Taiwan (JCMIT) to conduct an annual national NI academic conference, in addition to conducting bi-annual NI congresses, seminars, and workshops.

- The TNIA initiated a Nursing Informatics (NI) Roundtable Alliance to discuss NI issues and share experiences and knowledge among institutions.

- The TNIA has played a very important role in disseminating informatics by including nursing informatics as a required course for any continuing education programs that were accredited and offered by the TWNA in 2005. Since 2000, the TNIA has also offered educational programs for those who have no background in informatics.

- The TNIA played a leadership role in the development of the electronic medical record starting in 2010.

- The TNIA is proposing that an informatics nurse specialty be recognized as one of the clinical nursing specialties.

Future Directions

- Expand the role of the informatics nurse specialist to take a more active part in developing nursing information systems in health institutions.

- Establish the nursing terminology system and communication platform in Taiwan.

- Improve and upgrade the level of nursing informatics education to include nursing informatics and computer courses in nursing programs.

- Strengthen relationships with other international nursing informatics organizations.

- Establish the Chinese Nursing Terminology Center to develop computerized literature databases so that researchers can conduct searches at any time and in any place.

SUMMARY

The healthcare environment in Asian countries is becoming inhospitable due to high healthcare costs, increasing competition among healthcare organizations, decreased funding from the government, and consumers with more sophisticated demands. The introduction of information technology and information systems can help healthcare organization survive under these difficult circumstances.

Healthcare informatics and the use of information technology has proceeded rapidly in Asian countries, with exciting development in the areas of clinical practice, informatics research, and informatics education over the past two decades. All of these developments have improved—either directly or indirectly—the productivity of healthcare professionals, the efficacy of the healthcare industry, and also the education of healthcare professionals.

It is clear that professional organizations play a major role in raising awareness, educating, and disseminating knowledge in health informatics. This is becoming increasingly complex with the proliferation of government initiatives spanning multiple government departments, which is a reflection of the multi-disciplinary nature of health informatics. Nurses, as the largest group of health professionals, have a major role to play. A sound knowledge of the many stakeholders will ensure that nurses can coordinate their efforts to ultimately benefit the healthcare consumer, communities, and society as a whole.

ACKNOWLEDGMENTS

The author would like to thank InSook Cho for contributing the section on Korea; Satoko Tsuru for contributing the section on Japan; and Rung-Chuang Feng, Ming-Chuan

Kuo, Li-Ping Fang, Xiang-Fen Lai, Ming-Xiang Tu, and Polun Chang for contributing the section on Taiwan.

REFERENCES

Nursing Informatics in Korea

Ahn, H., & Park, H.-A. (2013). Adverse-drug-event surveillance using narrative statements in electronic nursing records. *CIN: Computers, Informatics, Nursing, 31*(1), 45–51.

OECD (2013), *Health at a Glance 2013: OECD Indicators, OECD Publishing*. Retrieved from http://dx.doi.org/10.1787/health_glance-2013-en.

Lee, M. K., & Park, H. A. (2009). *Research trends in nursing informatics in Korea*. Poster presented at APAMI 2009, Hiroshima.

Park, H. A., & Cho, I. (2009). Education, practice, and research in nursing terminology: Gaps, challenges, and opportunities. *IMIA Yearbook of Medical Information 2009*, 103–108.

Park, H.-A., Cho, I., & Ahn, H. (2012). Use of narrative nursing records for nursing research. *Nurs Inform.* 2012, Jun 23;2012:316. eCollection 2012.

Park, H.-A., Min, Y. H., Jeon, E., & Chung, E. (2012). Integration of evidence into a Detailed Clinical Model-Based Electronic Nursing Record System. *Healthcare Informatics Research, 18*(2), 136–144.

Sneha, S., & Varshney, U. (2006). Ubiquitous healthcare: A new frontier in e-health. *AMCIS 2006 Proceedings*. Paper 319. Retrieved from http://aisel.aisnet.org/amcis2006/319

The Statistics Portal. (2012). *South Korea: Total population from 2004 to 2014 (in million inhabitants)*. Retrieved from http://www.statista.com/statistics/263747/total-population-in-south-korea/ (English)

Yoon, D., Chang, B. C., Kang, S. W., & Park, R. W. (2012). Adoption of electronic health records in Korean tertiary teaching and general hospitals. *International Journal of Medical Informatics, 81*(3), 196–203.

Nursing Informatics in Japan

Ezumi, H., Sota, Y., & Ochiai, H. (1997). Teaching method and evaluation of information education in Shimane Nursing College. *Studies in Health Technology and Informatics, 46*, 601.

Health and Welfare Statistics Association (Tokyo). (2009). *Journal of Health and Welfare Statistics, 56*(9). (Japanese).

Japan Association of Medical Informatics. (1980–2003). *Japan Journal of Medical Informatics Supplement.* (Japanese).

Japan Association of Medical Informatics. (1996). *Nursing information system workshop. Information system for nursing.* Tokyo, Japan: Japanese Nursing Association Publishing Company. (Japanese).

Japanese Nursing Association Publishing (JNAP). (2013). *Statistical data on nursing service in Japan.* Tokyo, Japan: Japanese Nursing Association Publishing Company. (Japanese).

Kamiizumi, K., & Ota, K. (2004). *Nursing information management.* Tokyo, Japan: Japanese Nursing Association Publishing Company. (Japanese).

Kanai-Pak, M., Hosoi, R., Arai, C., Ishii, Y., Seki, M., Kikuchi, Y., ... Sato, K. (1997). Innovation in nursing education: Development of computer-assisted thinking. *Studies in Health Technology and Informatics, 46*, 371–375.

Kato, S., Tsuru, S., & Iizuka, Y. (2013), A structural model for patient fall risk and method for determining countermeasures, *Journal of Quality, 20*(5), 503–520.

Kawaguchi, T., Azuma, M., & Ohta, K. (2004). Development of a telenursing system for patients with chronic disease. *Journal of Telemedicine and Telecare, 10*(4), 239–244.

Majima, Y. (1997). Application of the Internet for nursing education, in nursing informatics. *Studies in Health Technology and Informatics, 46*, 587.

Ministry of Health, Labour and Welfare. (2004). *Welcome to Ministry of Health, Labour and Welfare.* Retrieved from http://www.mhlw.go.jp/english/index.html

Muranaka, Y., Fujimura, R., Yamashita, K., Furuhashi, Y., Yamamoto, S., & Arita, K. (1997). Development of a CAI program entitled "Introduction to Nursing Process." Requirement for nursing education in Japan. *Studies in Health Technology and Informatics, 46*, 487–491.

Ochiai, N., Sota, Y., & Ezumi, H. (1997). Self-study program on HTML browser–application to clinical nursing general remarks course. *Studies in Health Technology and Informatics, 46*, 360–363.

Tanaka H. (2007), Current status of electronic health record dissemination in Japan. *JMAJ, 50*(5):399–404.

The Medical Information System Development Center. (2004). *MEDIS-DC.* Retrieved from http://www.medis.or.jp. (Japanese).

Tsuru, S., Iizuka, Y., & Munechika, M. (2009). Structuring clinical nursing knowledge using PCAPA - patient condition adoptive path system. *Stud Health Technol Inform, 146*:391–395.

Tsuru, S., Nakanishi, M., Kawamura, S., et al. (2010). Nursing function and nursing knowledge in clinical practice from acute care to home care. *Japan Journal of Medical Informatics Supplement 2010*, 219–224. (Japanese).

Yamanouchi, K., Nakano, M., & Nojiri, M. (1997). A small intranet for teaching how to use Internet. *Studies in Health Technology and Informatics, 46*, 585.

Nursing Informatics in Taiwan

Chang, W. (2007). Information technology application and patient safety. *Journal of Healthcare Quality, 1*(4), 16–19. (Chinese).

Chang, M., Lin, J. S., & Lee, T. T. (2008). Applications of nursing Informwation systems: Sharing the experience of implementation in a hospital. *The Journal of Nursing, 55*(3), 75–80.

Chang, P. J., Shu, T. H., & Chang, C. B. (2002). Current status and future development of multimedia web-based learning in the nursing department of the National Taipei College of Nursing. *Journal of Health Science, 4*(3), 265–272.

Chang, P., Tzeng, Y. M., & Sang, Y. Y. (2003). The development of wireless PDA support systems for comprehensive and intelligent triage in emergency nursing. *Journal of Nursing, 50*(4), 29–40.

Chen, W. L. (1992). Application of computer assisted instruction in nursing education. *Journal of Nursing, 39*(4), 118–123.

Chiang, L. C. (1998). Nursing diagnosis development in Taiwan: Now and future. *Journal of Nursing, 45*(2), 28–39.

Chu, K. C., Tsai, M. Y., Huaa, C. Y., & Chen, K. H. (2010). *Nursing informatics - Current state and future trends.* (Chinese). Retrieved from http://libir.tmu.edu.tw/bitstream/987654321/22253/1/23_S1616561

Hsu, N. L., Feng, R. C., Lo, H. Y., & Wang, P. W. (1996). The establishment of factor type patient classification systems. *Journal of Nursing, 43*(3), 23–35.

Hsu, C. L., Lin, Y. C., & Tseng, K. C. (2009). A real-time interactive healthcare platform preserving security and privacy. *Journal of Taiwan Occupational Therapy Research and Practice, 5*(2), 156–171. (Chinese).

Lai, H., & Chen, L. (2003). Nurse satisfaction with the clinical use of personal digital assistant. *Tzu Chi Medical Journal, 15*(2), 97–103.

Lai, Y. H., Liu, L., Hsu, C. Y., & Chen, J. S. (2001). Medical diagnosis assisted nursing process support system. *New Taipei Nursing Journal, 3*(1), 67–78.

Lee, T., Lin, K. G., & Chang, P. (2005). Factors affecting the use of nursing information systems in Taiwan. *Journal of Advanced Nursing, 50*(2), 170–178.

Lee, T. T., Yeh, C. H., & Ho, L. H. (2002). Application of a computerized nursing care plan system in one hospital: Experiences of ICU nurses in Taiwan. *Journal of Advanced Nursing, 39*(1), 61–67.

Li, T. Z., Wang, R. H., Hsu, S. S., Chen, L. F., & Chang, H. Y. (1998). Information technology and nursing: Using PDAs in clinical nursing care. *Journal of Nursing, 45*(1), 69–76.

Lin, J. S., & Liao, Y. C. (2003). A study of nurses' attitude and satisfaction toward using personal digital assistant in nursing practice. *New Taipei Journal of Nursing, 5*(2), 3–12.

Liu, S. C., Chang, P., Hsu, C. L., & Lai, H. F. (2007). From analyzing the nursing informatics courses in schools to improving the nursing informatics competencies. *The Journal of Taiwan Association for Medical Informatics, 16*(1), 79–92. (Chinese).

Lu, Z. Y. (1998). Current status and future development of ICNP. *Journal of Nursing, 45*(2), 35–39.

Shao, K. N. (2010). *A government project research in Taiwan: RFID applications in the medical and health industry pilot project.* (Chinese, unpublished project).

Tai, H. L., Lin, H. W., Chang, C. C., Lin, S. A., Ko, S. H., & Chang, P. (2009). Nurses developing an end-user-computing process research of information system—taking the hemodialysis nursing information system as an example. *VGH Nursing, 26*(3), 244–253. (Chinese).

55

Nursing Informatics in South America

Heimar de Fatima Marin

- OBJECTIVES

1. Describe nursing informatics development in South America.
2. Provide examples related to the use of information technology and communication in clinical practice and education.
3. Describe educational and distance learning efforts.

- KEY WORDS

South America
Nursing informatics
Training and education
Distance learning

South America is a subcontinent that comprises 13 countries in three territories, with a total area of 17,819,100 km^2 covering 12% of Earth's surface; it contains 6% of the world's population. The most populated country is Brazil (201,033.000) followed by Colombia (47,130.000) and Argentina (41,350.000). The official language for most of the countries is the Spanish; in Brazil, it is the Portuguese. In 1991, Argentina, Brazil, Paraguay, and Uruguay signed the Treaty of Asunción to create the southern common market (MERCOSUR). The primary objective was the integration of the four States parties through the free movement of goods, services, and productive factors, the establishment of a Common external tariff (TEC), the adoption of a common commercial policy, the coordination of macro-economic and policies, and the harmonization of legislation in the relevant areas. In 2012, Venezuela was integrated to MERCOSUR. To achieve its primary objective, a Fund for Structural convergence of MERCOSUR (FOCEM) was created in 2004 to finance programs to promote structural convergence, developing competitiveness, and promote social cohesion, in particular in the economies of smaller economies and regions whose development is lagging behind; support the

functioning of the institutional structure and the strengthening of the integration process. Brazil is the biggest contributor, providing 70% of Fund resources followed by Argentina (27%) (available at http://www.mercosul.gov.br/saiba-mais-sobre-o-mercosul).

The health systems in South American countries vary, although six countries including Brazil consider health as a universal right at the Constitution. Other countries refer to this right in general terms, related to social determinants of health or even as a right to access health services. Also, in South America, unlike European countries, the universalization of social protection in health is not completed in a uniform manner. Although, in some cases, formal coverage reach the entire population, the systems are generally fragmented and segmented (Giovanella, Feo, Faria, & Tobar, 2012).

Nursing education occurs mostly in public or private universities. Most countries implemented graduate programs focused on different and local needs such as Women Health, Prenatal Care, and Intensive Care. Nursing Informatics has been based more on activities of individuals than on a global policy established by governments or national efforts. The levels of development and deployment of technological resources are varied across countries in South America; however, the use of technology has enabled a significant evolution in health and nursing education, practice, research, and administration. Among all regions of the world, South America has consistently seen the highest growth in information technology for the past 25 years. However, there are still significant factors that impact a broad adoption and deployment of health IT resources for consumers and professionals in certain countries and regions within South America, including infrastructure and human resources.

Information and communication technology (ICT) in healthcare is used to improve quality of life, health conditions, and professional performance, transforming not only the daily lives and health conditions of the general population, but also the practice of healthcare professions. Among all healthcare providers across the world, nurses have progressively incorporated information systems and educational resources in their practice (Marin & Lorenzi, 2010).

South American countries show a consistent use of ICT resources related to the evolution of technology in the region. Most developed regions of the country have better access and ability to implement health IT services and applications in nursing care and education. In the last years, governmental bodies and stakeholders have realized that additional investments are necessary to change this situation, and more activities are being implemented to optimize educational and health resources in underdeveloped regions.

Although computers and ICT resources are widely recognized as an important tool to support nurses taking care of patients and to organize nursing service and nursing education, the adoption has varied in the countries or even in the regions of the same country. The use of the Internet and wireless communication is also a definitive trend in this field and most of universities and educational institutes are using to promote distance learning programs. Consequently, hospitals also are exploring ways to introduce new resources in order to facilitate the process of patient care and promote quality and safety.

The objective of this chapter is to present an overview and provide examples of the development of nursing informatics in South America, identifying some initiatives and progress in the field, including discussion of the current use of distance education programs, and initiatives to disseminate nursing informatics resources in the region. The examples are concentrated to some South American countries. It was also decided to include Cuba, which is a Caribbean country (Latin America and The Caribbean) that also presents a consistent evolution in the use of technology in healthcare.

Although, even with growing initiatives in South American countries, it is necessary to emphasize that the inclusion of nursing elements of practice in the patient record is the responsibility of nurses. They need to be involved with the programmers, vendors, and developers to drive the professional requirements. Taking care of patients is the primary focus for nurses. Therefore, it is essential to ensure that all information required to perform nursing care is existent in a clear and comprehensive manner at the health information systems. Consequently, nursing education programs are also essential to prepare the new generation of professionals.

Additionally, at the last three years, congresses, conferences, workshops, education, and training programs were organized throughout South American countries and also to assemble several different countries from South America and abroad. The main objectives are to share experiences and information in nursing informatics and search for solutions that could enhance the delivery of patient care.

BACKGROUND

Nursing has been identified around the world as an emerging profession for over 100 years. In 2010, the 100th anniversary of the death of Florence Nightingale, widely considered the pioneer who established nursing as a profession, was celebrated. Since her work in the Crimean War, the professional has been continuously evolving based on the influences of science and technology. There are several examples of the use and development of computer applications in healthcare impacting the nursing profession, and nurses can be considered the primary users of technology in healthcare (Safran, Slack, & Bleich, 1989).

Historically, nurses are accustomed to facing challenges, adapting new tools into their practice to improve performance, and creating new models to enhance patient care. Technology represents a unique opportunity for nurses to face further challenges, discover ways to innovate, and possibly re-design their methods of care (Marin, 1996).

Today's technology significantly modifies human activities and, consequently, the way we learn and work. The traditional methods of teaching, managing, and practicing the healthcare professions do not support the requirements of modern life anymore. Education is achieved through a continuous and diverse process, and its value is enduring. Teaching and learning are critical to maintaining a high quality of life and designing our future.

In the healthcare area, information is the key element for the decision-making process. The more specific information is available to support clinical decisions, the better care can be delivered to the patient. The quality of care is related to the scope of knowledge and information that health providers can access on which to base their clinical decisions. Thus, technology plays an important role in facilitating access to this information; for the information to be useful and meaningful, it has to be easily available.

Currently, health systems around the world face considerable challenges in providing healthcare services, and more systems in the global health sector are seeking improvement in the overall health situation, enhancing the operative capacity of the national health programs, decreasing mortality and morbidity rates, and improving the quality of life through informatics-based systems (Marin & Lorenzi, 2010).

Recognizing that computers and all information and communication technology (ICT) resources are powerful instruments, each country is gradually becoming aware of the potential for applying IT to enhance the quality of care of clients and patients. While the lack of national policies delays the process, cultivating awareness of the capabilities of ICT is the first step toward adopting these technologies.

There is a clear trend toward computerization of health records. In addition, more people are able to connect to the Internet, which is a telecommunication resource that has no comparison when it comes to fast exchange of data and information. As a result, we can expect to see better-informed healthcare providers and consumers (Pan America Health Association & World Health Organization, 2001).

Considering trends in healthcare informatics, and to facilitate the process in South American countries, the Pan American Health Organization (PAHO) has published guidelines and protocols to orient the development and deployment of information and communication technology in Latin America and the Caribbean (Pan America Health Association & World Health Organization, 1998, 2001, 2003).

It is also important to emphasize that the South American region ranks third in information technology expenditure. The Information Society Index (www.idc.com/groups/isi/main.html), which measures the use of information, computers, and social infrastructure, identified that countries in the region are rapidly evolving.

In April 2013, the Economic Commission for Latin America and the Caribbean (ECLAC) organized a working meeting in Chile to endorse ICT in the region, according to the Pan American Health Organization eHealth Strategy and Plan of Action (2012–17). The objective is to guarantee sustainable development of the Member States' health systems. Adoption of the eHealth Strategy and Plan of Action is envisaged as a means of improving health services access and quality, based on the use of ICTs, the development of digital literacy and ICTs, access to information based on scientific evidence and ongoing training, and the use of various methods. This will facilitate progress toward the goal of societies that are more informed, equitable, competitive, and democratic. In such societies, access to health information is considered a basic right of the people (available at http://www.paho.org/ict4health/). The ECLAC meeting provided a list of some indicators to facilitate the process, such as number of hospitals and primary care centers with Internet access, level computer, and Internet use to manage patient information.

NURSING INFORMATICS INITIATIVES

In South American countries, as in any other country in the world, the initial motivation to develop computer systems in the healthcare area was driven by financial and administrative concerns. The hospital sector can be considered the area better served by information systems. Countries like Brazil, Argentina, Colombia, Chile, and Paraguay have implemented clinical information systems in hospitals or health institutes.

Although clinical information systems are being used in some ways to support clinical care and management, a few hospitals or healthcare institutes have developed applications for nursing documentation where nursing data can be processed. In general, patient data that are also used for nursing administration are integrated in the system or nurses have to collect and analyze nursing data separately.

Hospitals have been working to design their own systems in order to attend to specific needs and policies. More recently, national and international software industries have become more represented in the South American healthcare market. Consequently, they provide a broader range of solutions with systems that address patient care documentation. In Brazil, for instance, the balance of economy opened doors for several international industries that are commercializing products to attend local needs. Most of private hospitals of the country are adopting these products and working to customized all applications according to the national rules and legislation.

Many additional initiatives are spread throughout Latin American countries. It can be observed that the use of computers as an instrument to support nurses' activities in taking care of patients still needs considerable investment of human and material resources. Clinical systems based on the nursing process are not common in these countries, even though very requested by all clinicians at the bedside.

Most of the computer systems implemented intended to control administrative data. The most frequently implemented and used applications still are the nursing orders and some functionality for documenting nursing notes, but with no structure or format. Using free-text documentation, it is more difficult to perform analysis and evaluation of nursing care. In one sense, we have a large amount of nursing data, but not necessarily a large amount of information to design nursing care plans to be delivered at the patient's bedside.

In spite of this, nurses are more involved with the design, implementation, and evaluation of clinical information systems. Vendors and developers recognize that the success of a computer system requires nursing input and collaboration. In addition, as an open and evolving market, international developers are making investments to sell and implement computer systems in South America, because South America represents one of the most promising markets in the world of technology.

Argentina

In Argentina, most of the health computer systems in use were acquired from the health software industry, although some applications were also locally developed. In both cases, there are only a small number of applications that include resources for nursing activities. Furthermore, Argentina was one of the first countries in South America to introduce topics related to health informatics in the formal education of physicians. It is estimated that the formal organization of the nursing informatics movement in South America began in 1991. Since then, interest in nursing informatics has been growing, and it has become an important topic at congresses and conferences. In 2008, the II Argentine Symposium of Nursing Informatics was held within the II Latin American Congress of Medical Informatics with more than 100 participants from different South American countries (Leonzio & Barrios, 2010).

Nursing Informatics Group is affiliated of Argentina Association of Medical Informatics (AAIM) which is a country member of IMIA and also a representative member at IMIANI SIG, recognized as the major Working Group in the field of Nursing Informatics, regardless of their participation in any other working group in the region. In this last period, the focus was to develop the Project FAENET which is the Virtual network of nursing Argentina of the Federation Argentina of Nursing. This virtual network connects nurses across the country. The objective of the project also includes developing and providing information management tools for nurses in the country stimulating experience exchange, education, investigation, and networking.

Recently, Argentinian nurses are deeply involved as a founder with the Working Group of Nursing informatics at IMIA-LAC, a network established to serve as a forum to congregate Spanish spoken nurses to share experiences and initiatives on nursing informatics.

Brazil

Nursing Informatics in Brazil initiated around 1985 focusing on education and practice. Since then, several nursing schools and universities managed to include nursing informatics content in the curriculum, considering that education is achieved through a continuous and diverse process, and its value is enduring. Although educational strategies have changed over time, the essence and fundamental principles remain; education is a process that cultivates the development of values and civilization as a whole.

Furthermore, technology can transform not only nursing practice, but also nursing training and educational models. With the introduction of computers into the healthcare area, nurses became primary users, responsible for data input. Consequently, they had to become computer-literate in order to use computer technology in an efficient manner. To meet educational and training needs, nursing schools and hospitals initiated programs to prepare nurses to use computers. In addition to instruction on how to use computer applications, course instructors also began to consider the use of computers to teach nursing content.

Computer applications in nursing education are also causing a shift from a passive teaching model to an active learning process. Computers enable students to work at the time that best meets their specific needs. Usually, the programs are very interactive and easy to use and offer immediate feedback about students' performance.

A grant from the Fogarty International Center of the National Institutes of Health (U.S.) promoted the establishment of a bilateral consortium of health informatics faculty. A program was designed to enhance training in Brazil by augmenting the teaching resources of local faculty. This training program was based on the experience of the Brazilian faculty and some lessons learned from an existing training program in Boston (U.S.), which involved faculty from Harvard University and its affiliated hospitals (Marin, Massad, Marques, & Machado, 2004; Marin & Ohno-Machado, 2012). During the development and implementation of this training program, different regions of Brazil were reached, delivering courses that were previously given in São Paulo, Rio de Janeiro, and Manaus. By the end of 2003, it was found that around 1724 professionals were involved as either faculty members or students in the program. The program continued to provide the certificate program, and the graduate program stimulated students to participate in national and international conferences. At the end of 2009, the grant was once again renewed to fund the program for five more years. The latest term of the grant is dedicated to support the certificate program based on distance education, where Maputo University (Mozambique, Africa) was involved. Two onsite courses were delivered at Eduardo Mondlane University in Maputo for over 40 healthcare and computer science professionals. The program is coordinated and delivered by faculty of the Health Informatics Department and the Nursing School at Universidade Federal de São Paulo, which also offers the graduate program (master's and doctoral) in economics and health informatics (Marin & Ohno-Machado, 2012).

In 2008, the Ministry of Education and the Universidade Aberta do Brasil created a program of distance learning provided by UNIFESP that offers a specialized degree in healthcare informatics for 500 professionals at 10 different centers throughout Brazil. There has been a trend toward distance learning program development in South America. Computer technology is providing students living in distant regions and having difficulties in accessing the main educational centers the opportunity to improve their personal knowledge base. A contributing factor to the development and success of these programs is the distance between countries and cities due to the geographic characteristics of South America. In 2013, the program included several poles in São Paulo State supported by the Secretary of Health comprising 806 students. Other than Health Informatics Specialization course, several programs are offered in the country such as Nursing Management, Prenatal care, Environment Education, and Indigenous Health (more information available on http://portaluab.unifesp.br).

In 2006, an important information and communication technologies project named the RUTE network was deployed in Brazil. The infrastructure was developed by the University Network of Telemedicine and Telehealthcare of the Science and Technology Ministry (MCT), which is coordinated by the National Network of Teaching and Research and the National Program of Telehealthcare for primary healthcare. The RUTE network integrates teaching hospitals and basic healthcare networks. By 2013, the RUTE network integrates approximately 131 healthcare institutions throughout the country and hundreds of basic healthcare units in their respective states, covering all Brazilian states. In addition, RUTE handles integrating multi-professional healthcare into the community, and this infrastructure has improved access to healthcare and health information for the populations that live in regions that are remote and difficult to reach. (For additional information the RUTE network, see rute.rnp.br/sobre/instituicoes.)

The RUTE network also opened an ongoing channel for the development of research studies and interchange of specialized health knowledge. This has resulted in the growth of scientific collaboration, increased enrollment in healthcare training courses, and improved access to continuing education with the introduction of e-learning on a national level. Currently, 64 Special Interest Groups (SIG) are established and develop a weekly agenda to promote discussion, second-opinion diagnoses and treatments, and conferences. Currently, over 300 healthcare institutes are involved and participating on the activities developed by these SIGs. (For addition information, see www.rnp.br/index.php).

Since its creation, the RUTE network has been used by nurses across states to promote meetings and scientific discussions. The available telecommunication resources can also be used as a tool by nurses to support activities in patient care delivery such as monitoring medications, fluids, and feedings; documenting physiologic examinations; clarifying instructions; and helping patients understand medical procedures and treatments, thereby reducing anxiety and promoting better treatment adherence.

As mentioned and acknowledged, distance learning can be used to train large numbers of nurses in different geographic locations and work settings. To take advantage of the available resources in information technology, nurses should have a minimum of computer-based education established in their educational curriculum. Nurses with little or no previous experience in data standards and computer technology should receive basic training in the use of computer-supported nursing information systems or computer applications in nursing practice.

In February 2009, in an effort to stimulate participation of nurses within the country, the first online social network for nursing informatics and telenursing was created. It will be an ongoing source for nurses and other professionals to share information and innovations, as well as network with specialists for the development of the nursing profession (Sasso, Silveira, Peres, & Marin, 2010). Since 2010, several courses were organized focusing on nursing care (trauma, intensive care, prenatal care, management and administration, terminologies, and nursing process) and nursing informatics.

TIGER Brazil. Although Nursing informatics training and education has been in place since 1990 when Schools of Nursing started to introduce contents and specific courses in the nursing curriculum, the content was basically based on faculty experience and available with no formal structure. Recently, with the initiative of TIGER, the Nursing Informatics Special Interest Group of the Brazilian Health Informatics Society (SBIS-NI) two conferences were organized in the national congress to promote the harmonization of the content to be included on the nursing curriculum as well as the definition of competencies for nursing informatics in the country.

The TIGER Initiative, an acronym for Technology Guiding Education Reform, was founded in 2004 to develop a shared vision, strategies, and specific actions for improving nursing practice, education, and the delivery of patient care through the use of health information technology. It has emerged as a grassroots effort in 2006 the United States to allow informatics tools, principles, theories, and practices to be used by inter-disciplinary providers and consumers; interweave enabling technologies into practice, education, and research to improve outcomes, patient safety and reduce costs; and prepare workforce to use technology and informatics for improvement of patient care (Ball, Skiba, & Marin, 2013).

In 2013, a group of faculty and nurses from private and public hospitals organized an invited meeting during the e-Health 2013 Conference hosted by the Brazilian Health Informatics to initiate the development of a strategy and action plan for Tiger Brazil. The initial phase decided was to elaborate a curriculum content related to the Nursing Informatics Competencies to be integrated into the nursing curriculum and continuous education programs.

Connected to the education programs are the research activities which continue to be incremented. A search was performed in the electronic directory of the National Research Council for Science and Technology (CNPq) of Brazil in 2013 and founded 608 research groups included in this directory; approximately 91 groups developed some type of study and research in ICT and healthcare. More specifically, there are 21 research groups in nursing informatics in the country; the pioneer was the Nursing Informatics Research Group at the Federal University of São Paulo (NIEn-UNIFESP). However, there is a growing research movement in this field, which is evidenced by the several groups that have been established in the last 10 years across the country, such as the Research Group in Technology, Information, Health, and Nursing Informatics at the Federal University of Santa Catarina, and the GEPETE at the Nursing School at São Paulo University, a research group in information technology and nursing work process (Sasso et al., 2010; CNPq, 2014).

Efforts also have been made in the area of Nursing Terminology, and various clinical vocabularies are available; however, building a vocabulary that standardizes the clinical nomenclature for use in clinical practice and that fulfils all requirements is a challenge. In Brazil, the dissemination of the International Classification of Nursing practice (ICNP) started around 1996, when NIEn/UNIFESP became a sponsoring partner in the Telenurse

Consortium, a project led by Randi Mortensen, director of the Danish Institute for Health and Nursing Research. The paper and electronic forms of the Brazilian version of the ICNP (www.epm.br/enf/nien/cipe) have been available since September 1997. Later, the ICNP Beta 2 became available in a Brazilian Portuguese version (Conselho Internacional de Enfermagem, 2003). In 2007, ICNP Version 1 was published in Brazil; Version 2 was published in 2011 (CIPE, 2007; CIPE, 2011).

Other terminologies are also being used in the country, including the Home Health Care Classification (HHCC) System developed by Virginia Saba (Saba, 1992), which is also available on the Internet (www.sabacare.com) in a Brazilian Portuguese version and the Clinical Care Classification (CCC) System, translated and published in Portuguese in 2008 (Saba, 2008). In 2008, during the National Congress in Health Informatics (CBIS2008) organized by the Brazilian Society of Health Informatics, the Nursing Informatics Special Group (SBIS-GIE) hosted a symposium on nursing informatics where Dr. Virginia Saba presented the Clinical Care Classification System. The symposium was attended by over 120 participants and was followed by a celebration to launch the CCC book, along with the third edition of Introduction to Nursing Informatics written by Marion Ball, Kathryn Hannah, and Margaret Edward, which was also translated by members of the SBIS-GIE.

The most frequently used vocabularies may not necessarily be the best ones, but they may reflect the demands of insurance companies and other payers. Although there are quantitative differences in terms of breadth of coverage and internal representational structure, no clinical vocabulary has been elected so far as the ultimate solution for clinical documentation, automated retrieval, and rapid communication. Several obstacles have yet to be surpassed before nursing communities embrace a standardized vocabulary that proves useful in a variety of tasks and settings: regional, national, and international (Marin & Machado, 1996).

The task is a challenge, and continuous studies must be done to reach the balance that will facilitate nursing practice documentation around the world. Historically, nurses have faced several problems obtaining nursing documentation. Currently, with the expansion of health knowledge and information, the quantity of nursing documentation has certainly increased; however, the same cannot necessarily be said about the quality of the information documented. Health data rarely become health information.

ISO 18104—Health Informatics: Categorical structures for representation for nursing diagnoses and nursing actions in terminological systems. In 1999, under the leadership of

Virginia Saba, then president of the International Medical Informatics Nursing Informatics—Special Interest Group (IMIA NI SIG)—along with the International Council of Nurses (ICN), the development of the ISO (International Standard Organization) standards was begun to cover several terminologies of nursing documentation, supporting the mapping and recording of nursing data. This standard was presented to the Technical Committee—ISO/TC 215—health informatics and was approved as ISO 18104:2003—Health Informatics: Integration of a Reference Terminology Model for Nursing (Saba, Hovenga, Coenen, McCormick, & Bakken, 2003).

The aim of this international standard was to establish a reference terminology model for nursing aligned with the goals and objectives of other health-specific terminology models to provide a more unified terminology reference model. It included the development of terminology reference models for diagnosis and nursing actions, relevant terminologies, and definitions for implementation (Saba et al., 2003).

Considered an international standard to be reviewed periodically, in 2009 began the reviewing process. The draft version was renamed as ISO/DIS18104-Health Informatics: Categorial structures for representation of nursing diagnosis and nursing actions in terminological support systems. The document currently available is registered as in Final Draft stage Information Standards (FDIS), expecting to be approved as international standard, in accordance with the protocols established by the ISO Committee (ISO, 2013).

To verify adequacy of the model with nursing documentation in the country, a study was conducted using data from in two teaching hospitals that use different nursing terminologies for nursing diagnoses documentation and nursing actions or interventions. From the institutions' database, it was randomly selected expressions for nursing diagnoses documentation and nursing interventions, without considering other electronic records or accessing the records' identity. The proposed structure and the study findings showed that all records for nursing diagnoses had focus, judgment, or clinical finding. This finding indicates that nurses recognize the importance of giving a name to the phenomena they observe and of representing the care domain in which they are responsible. A few uses of terms for potential risk or chance were also observed; it could be inferred that the study sample considered this observation, because data derived from inpatient units, in other words, an environment that is supposed to be controlled and which has the aim of managing all risks or threats to patient safety. In summary, different terminologies used could be mapped in the categorical proposal, showing that the record does not need an exclusive terminology: the

structure and form used for describing the phenomenon are important and must have a communication potential among all members of health team (Marin, 2009; Marin, Peres, & Dal Sasso, 2013).

Chile

The introduction of information and communication technology into healthcare was established by the Ministry of Health by the Digital Agenda Initiative. This initiative has the objective to contribute to healthcare development through the use of technology in order to increase competitiveness, equality of opportunities, quality of life, efficiency, and transparency to the public sector (Munoz, 2010).

In 2010, it was created by the Computer Health Center at the Faculty of Health Sciences in the University Central of Chile, with nursing leadership. The mission was the generation and dissemination of scientific and inter-disciplinary knowledge in informatics in healthcare discipline, the application in the health system, and the development of networks to pursue sustainability and become a leading entity in Chile and Latin America. Its objective is to attend the need of continuous education for healthcare professionals and engineers, promoting courses and certificate programs (Spanish language only) using distance education resources. In addition, the Center also provides infrastructure to conduct research in health informatics and nursing, promoting collaboration between public and private sectors to develop applications to facilitate management and decision-making process in clinical and administrative area.

The projects include the digital literacy of students and The Project FONDEF (Fondo de Fomento al Desarrollo Científico y Tecnológico del Gobierno de Chile) which develops a mobile solution of electronic clinical record for homecare dedicated to patients in vulnerable conditions of health. This project not only innovates, but also develops a strong sense of humanization of care using the technology. In addition, it also provides funding for the master program in nursing informatics.

It is worthwhile also to highlight the *Red de Enfermería Informática de Chile* (REICH) led by Luisa Sepulveda Moreno. It was originated in 2013 as a working group of the Health Computer Association of Chile to support the International Nursing Group of the Pan American Health Organization. This group mission is to promote cooperation between the Chilean nurses interested in facilitating the development of nursing informatics as a tool for the management of care. The REICH has promoted the development of the discipline through conferences and seminars, both face to face and virtual, in collaboration with countries such as Cuba, Venezuela, Argentina, Peru, and

Uruguay. The Faculty of Sciences of the University Central of Chile has around 500 nursing students who perform clinical practice in hospitals and family healthcare centers. The practice is required to all students in order to learn how to provide safe and quality care.

To support practice activities, in 2011 a Clinical Simulation Center was established to support the training of students promoting the development of technical skills, learning skills and abilities as the communication and teamwork. An important component is also the technology and the use of electronic clinical record, mobile health, and telemedicine, among others. This Center has allowed the integration of clinical simulation into nursing care classes as a practice, prior to perform activities in a real environment. In addition, it allows nursing care services in hospitals and institutes to utilize the center for training their staff assuring continuous education in safety and welfare of the patient. It has been incorporated in teaching of nursing informatics, consistent to the concept of eHealth, where the use of ICTs is key to access, safety, quality, and continuity of care for individuals, families, and communities.

The Center provides clinical simulation, establishing different scenarios of care within hospitals, healthcare centers, and homecare. Also, it integrates concepts from basic sciences through the use of laboratories of Anatomy, chemistry, microbiology, pharmacology, and physiology. The work is promoted in a multi-professional team, enhancing the undergraduate programs, for which there are laboratories of orthotics, medical technology, chiropractic and nursing care in such a way that students can understand the different roles of each professional in the healthcare team.

Considering the initial applications, nursing informatics in Chile has had a vertiginous development in the past five years, emphasizing mobile-health projects which are very important due to the geographic disposition of the country, as informed by Erika Caballero Munoz, Luiza Sepulveda Moreno, and Elizabeth Fornet Langerfeldt (Universidad Central, Santiago de Chile), renowned leaders in the country.

Cuba

Nursing informatics in Cuba has been evolving since the initial application and early incorporation of computing as subject in the curriculum (1976). Since the end of the 1980s, the use of some Computer-Assisted Instruction (CAI) applications has been quite commonplace. At the end of the 1990s, with the assimilation of multimedia tools and with the Cuban link to the Internet (1996), the CAI improved and many alternatives were developed on virtual form to support education, including some sources for continuing education, such as The Virtual University of Health, and its Virtual Clinic.

Nursing Informatics courses are offered at a basic level including basic computer courses, training on specific applications, and preliminary aspects of the efficient integration of informatics in nursing. It is a goal to work toward offering an NI degree at the diploma, credit, master's, and doctoral levels in nursing in Cuba. The Health Informatics Masters course at CECAM has been important, allowing nurses to be educated in this field. The existing HIT systems are focused on clinical systems in the hospitals, and within the community health system. Clinical systems have been developed in hospitals to focus on individual and providing definitions and guidelines on nursing care in accordance with the medical diagnosis. The Emergency Units are equipped with automated systems for nursing assessment and intervention. Intranets are frequently used to strengthen and support nursing management. The availability of statistical tools, data collections, and specialized software have been essential for nurses (IMIA NI, 2012).

Cuba also established the network of Nursing Informatics (REDENFI) that is a group of technicians and nurses, based on a strategy of joint and scientific cooperation for the development of the required infrastructure and to exchange experiences, information, and knowledge to the benefit of the profession (http://www.sld.cu/sitios/redenfermeria/). The group, led by Niurka Vialart Vidal and Xaily Gavilondo Marino, congregates over 160 participants. The objectives are to apply technological tools for improving and strengthening nursing professionals, create practice groups on specific topics allowing interchange of information and knowledge, facilitate the coordination between members, connecting nursing activities to other healthcare specialties.

The group has been very active in the promotion of Nursing Informatics. Several conferences and workshops were organized during 2013. Publications and reports from meetings and conferences are available at http://www.sld.cu/sitios/redenfermeria/.

THE WGNI IMIA-LAC—WORKING GROUP OF NURSING INFORMATICS AT IMIA-LAC

The WGNI IMIA-LAC was established in 2008 during the IMIA LAC conference held in Argentina. It is still in process of organization and development, focusing on activities to organize a dynamic workforce and build strategies to promote nursing informatics in the region. Since its foundation, it was understood that the Group has its organizational scope within IMIA-LAC but it is under IMIA NI SIG coordination. The main goal is to integrate activities and avoid parallel tasks where the strengths and efforts would be duplicated. The WGNI IMIA-LAC is also responsible for the coordination of the International Network of Nursing Informatics of PAHO (Red Internacional de Enfermería Informática de OPS—RIEI).

WGNI IMIA-LAC and RIEI work together to create resources for collaboration between nurses and others professionals who are interested to facilitate nursing informatics development and deployment. It aims to share knowledge, experiences, and ideas for nursing practice through ICT resources. WGNI IMIA-LAC principles are based on solidarity, transparency, trust, and intercultural respect, following the IMIA Code of Ethics (http://www.imia-medinfo.org/new2/node/39).

The coordinating group is under Patricia Abbott (USA), Erika Caballero (Chile), Hugo Leonzio (Argentina); Niurka Vialart (Cuba) and Jose Angel Sanguino (Venezuela) are also key collaborators. Currently, participating countries are Argentina, Cuba, Brazil, Chile, Colombia, Cuba, United States, Mexico, El Salvador, Panama, Mexico, Peru, Venezuela, and Uruguay.

SUMMARY

Nursing informatics as an integrated part of healthcare follows the progress that has been made in the whole sector of health informatics. Because of the significant variation among countries and even within larger countries, the development of nursing informatics is conducted on a case-by-case basis, taking into consideration the specific requirements of each region. Furthermore, the development and deployment of nursing informatics is dependent on national priorities and policies, human capabilities, and continuous efforts and research to optimize resources and discover new models to enhance the quality of care delivered.

The healthcare reforms currently occurring worldwide are closely related to the political and economic development of each country. However, the nature of these worldwide changes in healthcare delivery requires that nurses and allied professionals be prepared for leading and managing in a global healthcare environment, either in the re-design of nursing care delivery or by assuming new roles and positions. In any event, nurses must participate in this process of transformation by providing expertise and knowledge to planning, management, education, and care delivery (Marin & Lorenzi, 2010).

Technological advances give nurses the opportunity to drive their own professional destinies. Adapting technological resources into practice helps nurses see emerging trends in the healthcare field as challenges and unique opportunities for career growth. There are new roles, new areas, and new jobs demanding experts in every country. There are a vast number of opportunities available for those who have decided to incorporate information technology into their daily practice and the process of taking care of patients.

Nurses must stand out in the use and selection of technology, anticipate needs, and have the data and the information available before you might need. The speed of the process is important and therefore is necessary to "hide" the technological complexity, making simple "front end" of the system that will be used by providers at the point of care delivery. Usability is critical to the success of any technology resource deployment. Technology cannot itself be more important than the care and assistance in healthcare—it is a means, a resource to promote and increase the quality of the service (Marin, 2012).

REFERENCES

Ball, M., Skiba, D., Marin, H. F. et al. (2013). TIGER initiative: Activities and future plans. In C. U. Lehman, E. Ammenweth, & C. Nohr (Eds.), *MEDINFO 2013. Proceedings* (p. 1250). IOS Press.

CIPE Versão 1. (2007). *Classificação Internacional para a Prática de Enfermagem* Conselho Internacional de Enfermeiros. Translated by Heimar F. Marin. São Paulo: Algol Editora.

CIPE Versão 2. (2011). *Classificação Internacional para a Prática de Enfermagem* Conselho Internacional de Enfermeiros. Translated by Heimar F. Marin. São Paulo: Algol Editora.

CNPq. (2014). Conselho Nacional de Desenvolvimento Científico e Tecnologico. *Diretorio de Grupos de Pesquisa no Brasil*. Retrieved from http://dgp.cnpq.br/buscaoperacional/. Accessed on January 21, 2014.

Conselho Internacional de Enfermagem. (2003). *Classificação internacional para a prática de enfermagem beta 2*. tradução: Heimar de F. Marin, São Paulo, SP.

Giovanella, L., Feo, O., Faria, M., & Tobar, S. (2012). *Health Systems in South America: Challenges to the universality, integrity and equity* (pp. 27–46). Rio de Janeiro, Brazil: ISAGS.

IMIA NI. (2012). Bid to host NI 2012, the Thirteenth International Congress on Nursing Informatics. Proposed prepared by Patricia Abbott, Chair of NI 2012, Montreal, Canada, p. 32.

International Organization for Standardization— ISO. (2013). *Health informatics: Categorial structures for representation of nursing diagnoses and nursing actions in terminological systems, FDIS 18104*. Geneva: ISO; [cited 2013 May 22]. Retrieved from

http://www.iso.org/iso/home/store/catalogue_ics/
catalogue_detail_ics.htm?csnumber=59431

Leonzio, C. H., & Barrios, C. (2010) A historical account and current status of hursing informatics in Argentina. In C. A. Weaver, C. W. Delaney, P. Weber, & R. L. Carr (Eds.), *Nursing and informatics for the 21st century: An international look at practice, education and EHR trends* (2nd ed., pp. 332–336). Chicago, IL: HIMSS.

Marin, H. F. (1996). Nursing informatics applications. In N. Oliveri, M. Sosa-Iudicissa, & C. Gamboa (Eds.), *Internet, telematics and health* (p. 265). Amsterdam, The Netherlands: IOS Press.

Marin, H. F. (2009). Terminologia de referência em enfermagem: a Norma ISO 18104. *Acta Paul Enferm, 22*(4), 445–448.

Marin, H. F. (2012). Prioridades, Informática e cuidado em saúde. In SPDM & Interfarma (Ed.), *A sáude no Brasil em 2021 – reflexões sobre os desafios da próxima década.São Paulo* (pp. 193–198).

Marin, H. F., & Lorenzi, N. M. (2010). International initiatives in nursing informatics. In C. A. Weaver, C. W. Delaney, P. Weber, & R. L. Carr (Eds.), *Nursing and informatics for the 21st century: An international look at practice, education and EHR trends* (2nd ed.). Chicago, IL: HIMSS.

Marin, H. F., & Machado, L. O. (1996). Introduction to clinical vocabularies: What does the clinician need to know? *Proceedings of the eight national conference on clinical computing in patient care: Capturing the clinical encounter*, Boston, MA.

Marin, H. F., Massad, E., Marques, E. P., & Machado, L. O. (2004). International training in health informatics: A Brazilian experience. *MEDINFO 2004*, San Francisco, CA.

Marin, H. F., & Ohno-Machado, L. (2012). Biomedical informatics experience in Brazil and Mozambique. In Mantas J et al. (Eds.), *Quality of life through quality of information, Proceedings of MIE 2012*. IOS Press, MIE2012 / CD / Short Communications (Oral).

Marin, H. F., Peres, H. H. C., & Dal Sasso, G. T. M. (2013). Categorical structure analysis of ISO 18104 standard in nursing documentation. *Acta Paulista de Enfermagem*. [serial on the Internet]. 2013 [cited 2013 Oct 01]; *26*(3), 299–306. Retrieved from http://www.scielo.br/scielo.php?script=sci_arttext&pid=S0103-21002013000300016&lng=en. http://dx.doi.org/10.1590/S0103-21002013000300016

Munoz, E. M. C. (2010). The electronic health record in Chile. In C. A. Weaver, C. W. Delaney, P. Weber, & R. L. Carr (Eds.), *Nursing and informatics for the 21st century: An international look at practice, education and EHR trends* (2nd ed.). Chicago, IL: HIMSS.

Pan America Health Association, & World Health Organization. (1998). *Information systems and information technology in health: Challenges and solutions for Latin America and the Caribbean*. Health Services Information Systems Program. Washington, DC: Division of Health Systems and Services Development.

Pan America Health Association, & World Health Organization. (2001). *Building standard-based nursing information systems*. Washington, DC: Division of Health Systems and Services Development.

Pan America Health Association, & World Health Organization. (2003). *O Prontuário eletrônico do paciente na assistência, informação e conhecimento médico*. Washington, DC: Division of Health Systems and Services Development.

Saba, V. K. (1992). The classification of home healthcare classification of nursing diagnoses and interventions. *Caring Magazine, 11*, 50–56.

Saba, V. K. (2008). *Sistema de Classificação de Cuidados Clínicos – CCC*. Translated by Heimar F. Marin, São Paulo: Algol Editora.

Saba, V. K., Hovenga, E., Coenen, A., McCormick, K., & Bakken, S. (2003, September). Nursing language – Terminology models for nurses. *ISO Bulletin*, 16–18.

Safran, C., Slack, W. V., & Bleich, H. (1989). Role of computing in patient care in two hospitals. *M.D. Computing, 6*, 141–148.

Sasso, G. T. M., Silveira, D. T., Peres, H. H. C., & Marin, H. M. (2010). Brasil: Case study 14G. In C. A. Weaver, C. W. Delaney, P. Weber, & R. L. Carr (Eds.), *Nursing and informatics for the 21st century: An international look at practice, education and EHR trends* (2nd ed., pp. 343–346). Chicago, IL: HIMSS.

56

Nursing Informatics in South Africa

Irene van Middelkoop / Susan Meyer

• OBJECTIVES

1. Introduce the history of nursing informatics in South Africa.
2. Identify the problems of implementing computerization in a resource-constrained environment.
3. Describe the barriers to establishing a nursing informatics speciality.
4. Describe nursing informatics from a South African perspective.

• KEY WORDS

Nursing informatics
South Africa
Computers
History
Barriers

INTRODUCTION

South Africa, the most southern country at the tip of the African continent, has been through some dramatic changes in recent years. Historically, it has been a country characterized by numerous conflicts. In 1652, Dutch settlers arrived to establish a refreshment post for the ships traveling the route from Europe to the East around the African Continent. The British also arrived and conflict between the two resulted in the Boer War at the turn of the twentieth century. However, animosity was put aside and by 1910, the Union of South Africa was established under joint rule. In 1961, South Africa became a republic. In 1948, the National Party implemented a policy of apartheid, which led to a period of fear and protests and culminated in the first multi-racial election in 1994. This election resulted in the African National Congress coming into power (CIA, 2010). A number of imbalances that had evolved during the apartheid regime now had to be corrected; one of which was the provision of healthcare.

HEALTHCARE IN SOUTH AFRICA

Healthcare in South Africa consists mainly of a very large public sector and a smaller private sector (SouthAfrica. info, 2010a). The public sector caters to those who have insufficient funds for treatment and those who do not have medical insurance (known in South Africa as Medical Aid), which is about 72% of the population (SouthAfrica. info, 2010b). Nearly half of the state's expenditures are spent on health, catering to almost 80% of the population. This has created yet another imbalance: the public sector is under-staffed and over-utilized. During the 2012/2013 budget year, the health budget was R121 billion, but in 2011, 8.3% of the GDP was spent on health, a total of R248.6 billion (approximately $23 billion). Of this 48.5% was spent in the private sector, which accounts for 16% of the population, whereas 49.2% was spent on the public sector (84% of the population) (SouthAfrica. Info, 2014).

THE HISTORY OF NURSING INFORMATICS

In 1978, an International Medical Informatics Association (IMIA) working conference was held in Cape Town on hospital information systems, led by Dr. Marion J. Ball (Safran, 2003). Thereafter, in 1988, the first nursing informatics workshop was held in Rustenburg, which was attended by a number of nurses keen to take on the specialty of nursing informatics. The Western Cape province of South Africa was, at that time, the focus area for health informatics, with an informatics department being established at the Groote Schuur Hospital, which had active participation from its members.

At MEDINFO 95, a paper was presented titled "Recognizing Nursing Informatics," which emphasized the need for nursing informatics to be separated from medical informatics (Babst & Isaacs, 1995). Sadly, the status quo remains, with no further advancement in the South African nursing informatics environment.

However, there has been very little progress as far as nursing informatics is concerned. Nursing informatics is defined as combining healthcare, information science, and computer science (Lanciault, 2014), and if that is anything to go by, South Africa sure has a long way to go, regarding career paths and implementation of the speciality. The emphasis currently is to find enough nursing and medical staff to provide the basic healthcare, and although there are hospital information systems in certain hospitals, the staff implementing the systems could be from any discipline in the hospital, not necessarily having nursing or medical staff having input into the implementation.

The South African Health Informatics Association (SAHIA) is keen to start a chapter for those working in or interested in nursing informatics but it is slow to get off the ground.

NURSING EDUCATION

The National Strategic Plan for Nursing Education, Training, and Practice was launched in February 2013, which deals with the assignment of nurses, and specifies the requirements for the various categories of nurses (South African Government News Agency, 2013).

Currently, nursing education in South Africa offers three main programs: a four-year nursing degree, a four-year nursing diploma, and the two-year enrolled nurse's course. There are also the auxiliary nurses who are very much practical nurses.

These courses are, however, currently undergoing change with an emphasis on degree nurses, which is due

to be implemented in 2015. The new curriculum includes some hours of computer usage providing basic training. This may assist with the use of computer technology involved in nurses' work, which could be a hospital information system or a simple database in a rural clinic. The Government is encouraging computer training by providing training courses, but there is little chance of practice as when the nurses return to their place of work, there are no computers available for them to work on and become proficient (Asah, 2013). The number of personal computers in South Africa lags far behind the rest of the first-world countries. Frequently when new employees start work, they are confronted with a computer and are expected to be able to use it. Nurses are no different. Thus, the inclusion of even a basic computer course as a compulsory subject in all nursing education programs should be compulsory.

Needless to say, nursing informatics is not even mentioned in any list of nursing specialities, and thus there are no specific qualifications, although post-graduate qualifications in medical (or health) informatics and telemedicine are offered at certain universities. These, however, do not focus on nursing. There is no career path in nursing informatics, and those nurses who do work in an informatics department are self-taught and do the best they can under the circumstances. The fact that nursing informatics is not regarded as a speciality and is not even recognized is a demoralizing factor for those who are passionate about the discipline and strive for a high standard.

eHEALTH STRATEGY IN SOUTH AFRICA

In 2012, the Government released the document "National eHealth Strategy, South Africa 2012/2013-2016/2017" (Department of Health, 2012) which details the strategy to reach the vision of "enabling a long and healthy life for all South Africans" (Department of Health, 2012, p. 8) with the aims being to:

- Support the medium-term priorities of the public health sector
- Pave the way for future public sector eHealth requirements
- Lay the requisite foundations for the future integration and coordination of all eHealth initiatives in the country (both public sector and private sector) (Department of Health, 2012, p. 8)

This is the first eHealth strategy that has been published, and it details many aspects which need correcting, improving, and implementing. For example, one of the very basic items which needs consensus from all parties is a common identifier for patients. Currently each province has their own identifying numbering system, and these may even differ in the various hospitals in the province. This is due to the lack of interoperability between various hospital information systems (or other systems such as a stand-alone pharmacy system) in place. Hence the transfer of data is a problem. It will be a long haul to standardize all systems, and to attain consensus among all the parties.

To have a successful rollout of a national health plan, it will be essential that the information technology aspects are well coordinated and implemented, and that there is adequate knowledgeable and competent staff to do so. The emphasis of this seems to be at provincial level, and not so much at the hospital or clinic level.

According to Vital Wave Consulting, which has done an analysis of health information systems in developing countries, South Africa is placed at Stage 3, which is "migration of traditional district health information systems to electronic and storage" (Department of Health, 2012, p. 13). However, the aim is to move to stages 4 and 5, with stage 5 being a fully comprehensive and integrated national health information system.

Standardization and interoperability are the areas which need to be worked on for a centralized system to work. To this end, the following areas are being focused upon:

- Pharmaceutical coding
- Diagnostic Coding Schema
- Procedural Coding Schema
- Diagnostic Related Grouping
- Standards for Clinical Content (Department of Health, 2012, p. 16)

There is some work being done locally by the South African Bureau of Standards (SABS) on two standards which have been adopted locally, namely ISO/TS 18308:2004 (SANS 18308 Health Informatics—Requirement for an EHR Architecture) and ISO/TR 20514:2005 (SANS 20514 Health Informatics—EHR—Definition, scope, and context) (Department of Health, 2013, p. 16). However, this road of standardization needs to be taken further.

HOSPITAL INFORMATION SYSTEMS IN SOUTH AFRICA

Healthcare in South Africa is still in a major state of flux in that there is a massive drive to get the National Health Insurance scheme set up and working. This has been in the pipeline for a number of years now and is gaining impetus.

As recent as 26 February 2014, the Budget Speech presented by the Minister of Finance, Mr. Pravin Gordhan, spoke to the issue of National Health Insurance. Herewith an excerpt:

> *National Health Insurance*
> *This administration has also launched a far-reaching reform to make quality healthcare affordable to all South Africans. The Department of Health's white paper on NHI and a financing paper by the National Treasury have been completed and will be tabled in Cabinet shortly. The unfolding of NHI is premised on two pillars being put in place. Improvements have to be made in public sector health delivery, and the high cost of private health care has to be reduced. This approach is supported by the World Health Organisation.*
>
> *NHI pilot districts have been established in every province, supported by funding for NHI as a conditional grant. In addition to hospital and clinic building and refurbishment programmes, R1.2 billion has been allocated for piloting general practitioners' contracts. An Office of Health Standards Compliance has been established to ensure that public healthcare provision meets the required standards. A new funding framework for the National Health Laboratory Services and associated research activities has been agreed. But the improvements to this country's health system over the past five years are best seen in our rising life expectancy, the reduction in infant, child and maternal mortality and the changed lives of 2.5 million people who now have access to anti-retrovirals. Over the period ahead, enrolment in the HIV treatment programme will expand by about 500 000 a year,* (Gordhan, 2014, p. 13)

There have been many discussions surrounding this topic as it has far reaching consequences. The main aspect is to align the Public and Private Healthcare situations. Public—meaning services delivered by the Government, and Private—is healthcare provided to persons who have Healthcare Insurance (in South Africa, it is referred to as Medical Aids) and is much more expensive than Public Healthcare.

The implementation of the National Health Insurance is currently underway, albeit slowly. The main aim is to improve the access to and improvement of the quality of healthcare for all South Africans (Matsoso & Fryatt, 2013). Pilot sites have been identified and set up in all of the nine provinces with the objective. It has been proven to be an ambitious project with its challenges, one of which is the number of doctors and nurses. To combat this in the long run, the number of medical student places at medical schools have been increased, as well as the increase of the number of Cuban medical specialists recruits, and contracting of private doctors to provide services in the under-serviced communities (Matsoso & Fryatt, 2013).

To ensure improved health outcomes as well as service delivery, technology will be used, although the cost-effectiveness of such technology is still to be investigated (Matsoso & Fryatt, 2013). This will also be a major challenge especially in rural areas where computer expertise is minimal and many of the destined users are computer illiterate. Even the provision of stable electricity is problematic in some of the very rural areas. The National Health Insurance plan will be looking to an effective information system for standardization across private and public sector systems. Although there is at least one information system registered for each province in the public sector, only about a third of the public hospitals have a functional EMR system (Department of Health 2012, p. 14).

Many of the tasks will fall on the shoulders of the nurses especially in the rural areas as extensive use is made of primary healthcare nurses. The ratio of population to nurses varies from province to province, from a ratio of 165:1 to 303:1. These numbers include registered and enrolled nurses as well as auxiliary nurses (SANC, 2013).

However, what still has to be dealt with, is the additional burden of AIDS and tuberculosis. In a country already struggling to provide a quality health service to its people, the prevalence of the HIV pandemic has placed an enormous burden on government resources. There has been the "brain drain," whereby thousands of healthcare workers—mainly nurses—have departed for "greener pastures" in countries such as Australia, Canada, the United Kingdom, and even countries in the Middle East. It is appropriate to ask why they have left; some of the main reasons include crime, fear of degradation of the public health and education systems, general feelings of insecurity, as well as the lure of a better income in first-world countries.

All this has contributed to a dearth of nurses in a country that is crying out for more nurses in their (mainly) nurse-driven clinics as well as in hospitals (Douglas-Sweet, 2008). South Africa needs to determine how to better facilitate the remaining nurses' work by providing tools that can access information in the form of electronic patient data. This may also lure nurses back to South Africa.

STANDARDS

A mechanism whereby the basic standards that are required for Public Health Institutions resulted in the establishment of the Board of the Office of Health Standards Compliance; this in turn will assist to facilitate the implementation of the National Core Standards.

This in itself is an enormous undertaking as the state of Public Health in South Africa has been placed under tremendous strain in the last few years and the Government is constantly playing catchup, especially in dealing with the increased patient loads; the high costs of professional salaries; the increased costs of materials for maintaining an institution in good functional order.

Hence, the introduction of the National Core Standards program. The current Minister of Health in South Africa, Dr. Aaron Motsoaledi, stated that "*the importance of providing quality health services is non-negotiable. Better quality of care is fundamental in improving South Africa's current poor health outcomes and in restoring patient and staff confidence in the public and private health care system. If quality is defined as "getting the best possible results within available resources", then these National Core Standards set out how best to achieve this.*" (Department of Health, 2011, p. 5)

The National Core Standards also fits in with the National Department of Health's 10 Point Plan (2009–2014) which is to try and bring about "*a long and healthy life for all South Africans*" and part of the Service Delivery Agreement between the President and the various Provincial Governments and other stake holders, are the following key aspects:

- Improve life expectancy.
- Improve mother and child health and survival.
- Reduce the impact of HIV/Aids and TB.
- Improve health systems effectiveness (Department of Health, 2011, p. 8).

Within the National Core Standards framework, the levels or requirements for each health facility to attain are fairly universal in that it is looking at the lowest common denominator now so that the levels of improvement will occur, which in turn strengthens the notion that we go from a minimum acceptable level of care that must address vital areas of care delivery, especially those patients who are at high risk or are extremely vulnerable. The next level within this framework then progresses to the essential areas of care delivery, which carries a medium risk with the goal of optimum care, where the levels become developmental and carry a lower risk of susceptibility.

This is expressed in the seven Domains of the National Core Standards:

Domain 1: Patient Rights

Domain 2: Patient Safety—Clinical Governance and Clinical Care

Domain 3: Clinical Support Services

Domain 4: Public Health

Domain 5: Leadership and Corporate Governance

Domain 6: Operational Management

Domain 7: Facilities and Infrastructure (Department of Health, 2011, p. 10)

This is furthermore boosted by the six Priority Areas in an attempt to expedite the immediate improvement of quality service delivery, namely:

1. Values and attitudes of staff
2. Cleanliness
3. Waiting times
4. Patient safety and security
5. Infection prevention and control
6. Availability of basic medicines and supplies (Department of Health, 2011, p. 15.)

In an attempt to implement these baseline requirements, it is important to note that they are independent of the Health System that is in place, and in South Africa, there are still only a handful of institutions that have computerized information systems. Even fewer have fully integrated computer systems. Despite a national drive to implement an eHealth strategy, the need and demand for effective healthcare supersede the computerization of the clinical workplace.

This is obviously a dilemma that is faced as those of us who find ourselves in Nursing Informatics in South Africa try to overcome on a continual basis. The merging of the paper environment to the computer environment in the health sector is, indeed, a major challenge.

The new Nursing Curriculum that was introduced this year for the first time addresses the need for computer education for nursing professionals. There is still a very long road to travel to bring the levels of understanding of what it means to have a computerized hospital information system to fruition. All that we can do currently as Nursing Informaticians is keep the torch flying, keep motivating clinical staff to see that IT in Healthcare is a very powerful tool at their disposal, and also how to use it effectively. There is an enormous burden that we carry in reminding nurses, especially, that it is always about the patient.

As mentioned in the Finance Minister's speech that the improvements over the past five years are reflected already in a life expectancy that is rising, that there is a decrease in the mortality rates for infants and mothers, as well as millions of patients affected and infected with HIV/AIDS now having access to appropriate treatment—this all happen under sometimes exceptionally trying circumstances and with a threadbare nursing staff complement, and is indeed a major achievement. By utilizing computerized hospital information systems, this improvement will be the reward seen in accurate records, up-to-date patient information, and the appropriate coding of patients according to the International Classification of Diseases (ICD-10). The application of Early Warning Scoring Systems for vulnerable patients, and if documented, provides the necessary alerts to occur.

The abuse of current manual systems—for example—seen with the increasing trend to "sell" HIV medication can also be closely monitored by the application of a fully integrated computerized information system that provides for medication dispensing and stock management. Closing the gap electronically keeps everyone honest and more importantly, the patient is protected with all the allergy checks, drug interactions, and dosing. With the implementation of the National Core Standards, the need for monitoring and evaluation is a prime requirement, and what better way is there than to have appropriate computerized systems in place that take an enormous load off a depleted staff complement and an overburden healthcare system that is hugely fragmented. We have a long way to go still to achieve these goals, but at least we are making progress.

CONCLUSION

A concerted effort is required by the informatics community to bring nursing informatics to the attention of educators and to the nursing community at large. More information needs to be disseminated so that the importance of nursing informatics, especially concerning the use of systems for information and patient management, is directed to the right sectors. It is the way of the future, but without skilled and trained nurses who are able to use the tools available to provide optimum patient care, the benefit of having such first-class technology may be lost.

REFERENCES

Asah, F. (2013). Computer usage among nurses in rural health-care facilities in South Africa: Obstacles and challenges. *Journal of Nursing Management, 21*, 499–510.

Babst, T. A., & Isaacs, S. (1995). Recognizing nursing informatics. *Medinfo, 8*(2), 1313–1315.

CIA. (2010). *CIA - The world factbook.* Retrieved from https://www.cia.gov/library/publications/the-world-factbook/geos/sf.html

Department of Health. (2011). *National core standards for health establishments in South Africa.* Tshwane, South Africa: Department of Health, South Africa.

Department of Health. (2012). *National ehealth strategy South Africa 2012/2013-2016/2017.* South Africa: Department of Health.

Department of Health. (2013). *The National Strategic Plan for Nurse Education, Training and Practice 2012/13 - 2016/17*. Retrieved from http://www.sanc.co.za/archive/archive2013/NursingStrategy2013.html

Douglas-Sweet, V. A. (2008). The storm after the calm: South Africa moves to a primary healthcare model. *Advanced Practice Nursing eJournal*. Retrieved from http://www.medscape.com/viewarticle/572044

Gordhan, P. (2014). *Budget speech*. Retrieved from http://www.sanews.gov.za/south-africa/2014-budget-speech

Lanciault, T. (2014). *What is nursing informatics? - NurseTogether*. Retrieved from http://www.nursetogether.com/what-is-nursing-informatics

Matsoso, M. P., & Fryatt, R. (2013). National health insurance: The first 16 months. *South African Medical Journal, 103*(3), 156–158. Retrieved from http://www.samj.org.za/index.php/samj/article/view/6601. Accessed on April 26, 2014. doi:10.7196/samj.6601.

Safran, C. (2003). Presentation of Morris F. Collen Award to Dr. Marion J. Ball. *Journal of the American Medical Informatics Association, 10*(3), 287–288.

SouthAfrica.info. (2010a). *Health care in South Africa*. Retrieved from http://www.southafrica.info/about/health/health.htm#.UzbZlK2OGF8

SouthAfrica.info. (2010b). *NHI: Decent healthcare for all*. Retrieved from http://www.southafrica.info/news/nhi-010709.htm

SouthAfrica.info. (2014). *Health care in South Africa*. Retrieved from http://www.southafrica.info/about/health/health.htm#.VJe7vCAGA

South African Government News Agency. (2013). *Strategic plan to revitalise nursing profession*. Retrieved from http://www.sanews.gov.za/south-africa/strategic-plan-revitalise-nursing-profession

South African Nursing Council (SANC). (2013). *SANC geographical distribution 2013*. Retrieved from http://www.sanc.co.za/stats/stat2013/Distribution%202013xls.htm

Overview of Clinical Care Classification (CCC) System

Virginia K. Saba / Luann Whittenburg

• OBJECTIVES

1. Describe the Clinical Care Classification (CCC) System.
2. Describe the coding structure of the CCC System Terminologies.
3. Describe documenting a Nursing Plan of Care (PoC) using the CCC System and based on the nursing process.
4. Understand how the Nursing Diagnoses, Interventions, and Outcomes are linked together for ease of use.

• KEYWORDS

Nursing terminology
Clinical Care Classification System
Nursing diagnoses
Nursing outcomes
Nursing interventions
Expected and actual outcomes
Nursing action types
Nursing plan of care
Nursing standard

INTRODUCTION

This Appendix provides an overview of the Clinical Care Classification (CCC) System version 2.5. It also includes Table A.4 which serves as a Work Sheet and Guide for the development of an electronic Nursing Plan of Care (PoC) and/or documentation of Professional Nursing Practice.

The CCC Systems consists of two inter-related terminologies: CCC of Nursing Diagnoses and Outcomes and the CCC of Nursing Interventions and Actions, both of which are classified by 21 Care Components to form one integrated system. The CCC System is a nursing terminology

standard with structured, coded, nursing concepts designed to electronically document nursing practice and/or Nursing PoC based on the six phases of the nursing process (ANA, 2010). (See also a PoC Use Case in Chapter 26.)

BACKGROUND

Traditionally, nurses remain responsible for patient care 24 hours a day, 7 days per week, 365 days a year in most acute healthcare facilities, and even though they "spend a great deal of time managing and documenting patient care data/information" (Moss, Andison, & Sobko, 2007, p. 543), they never fully record many of their nursing interventions, actions, and other services, which are written as narrative progress notes. Nurses continue to rely on their caring skills based on intuition or trial-and-error methodologies for evidence-based care protocols. Nurses have not fully adapted to the age of databases and cloud computing. The documentation of nursing practices is not "visible" in the majority of healthcare information technology (HIT) applications or electronic healthcare record (EHR) systems.

Further, nursing departments are not revenue-generating centers, primarily because nursing services are not electronically coded while medical and ancillary healthcare services are reimbursed based on the International Classification of Diseases (ICD-9; ICD-10) (WHO, 1992), Current Procedural Terminology (CPT) (AMA, 2014), or other specialty service such as radiology, laboratory, pharmacology code sets. Nursing salaries remain bundled into the inpatient facility's room rate and not based on coded actions or relative value units (RVUs). As a result, nursing service costs are critical missing pieces of information generating a huge gap in the national healthcare cost of care equation.

As an integral member of the healthcare team, professional nursing, and the body of professional nursing knowledge, must be updated and visible in the electronic health record. Nurses must require that HIT/EHR systems document their care using coded nursing concepts in a nursing terminology framework designed for electronic processing, namely, the Clinical Care Classification (CCC) System. With such a documentation system, nurses can begin to investigate their own nursing practices and generate new nursing knowledge to improve patient care and measure healthcare outcomes. Then, as a profession, we can better demonstrate that evidence-based nursing practice is indispensable to the effective delivery of quality healthcare. And nursing will increase the *evidence* as to why appropriate nursing staffing levels are important and have the data to influence local, state, national, and international policies regarding the *scope of nursing practice*.

The CCC System provides the *essence of care* essential for conducting the vital research and generating the evidence necessary for nursing professional practices. The use of nursing data with a professional information framework to quantify evidence-based practice can demonstrate the contribution of nurses in improving patient care and their outcomes. Thus discrete nursing care data will become *visible* as an essential member of the healthcare team. The CCC System will allow nursing to document, at the point of care, their nursing care diagnoses, interventions/actions, and outcomes. Using such a standardized nursing terminology with standardized coded concepts (data

elements) nurses will be able to describe the *essence of care* without requiring the pre-or post-coordination of concepts needed from a reference (not user friendly) terminology. Using the CCC System, which is an interface (user friendly) terminology, was developed and designed for use by nurses and allied health professionals to electronically document patient care and nursing workflow at the point of care. Further, it has been proven that the CCC of Nursing Interventions Actions can be used to cost out their nursing services based on RVUs as well as describe a full range of nursing practice across all healthcare settings and can be adapted to provide nursing resource costs (Saba & Arnold, 2004). Lastly, the CCC System allows patient care documentation from nurses to be stored in HIT and EHR Systems, in databases for comprehensive data analyses, and aggregated for Big Data repositories (Saba, 2012; Saba & Taylor, 2007; Whittenburg, 2009).

CCC SYSTEM

The CCC System has been and is currently the *only* coded nursing terminology standard with coded concepts based on the nursing process framework to electronically document nursing practice and Nursing PoCs. The CCC System was developed by federally funded research which was empirically developed from live patient care data collected nationwide. The CCC System was specifically designed for computer-based processing. In 2007 and 2008, the CCC System was selected as the first national interoperable nursing terminology standard by the Secretary of the Department of Health and Human Services as meeting the nursing documentation needs of the EHR. The CCC System has also been "recognized" by the American Nurses Association (ANA) as a standardized nursing terminology designed for electronic documentation of nursing practice. The CCC System is available for use by copyright permission without licensing fees. Nurses know that medical diagnoses alone cannot explain nor generate nursing care of patients' data. The CCC System's standardized terminology framework and standardized concepts allow the CCC System to efficiently and effectively code and electronically process professional nursing practices as well as create nursing and inter-disciplinary plans of care.

CCC SYSTEM DESCRIPTION

The CCC System consists of two inter-related nursing terminologies: CCC of Nursing Diagnoses and Outcomes and CCC of Nursing Interventions/Actions. Each is classified using the 21 Care Components representing one single system (Saba & Taylor, 2007; Saba, 2012). The CCC

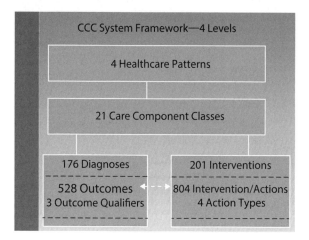

• **FIGURE A.1.** CCC System Framework. (Reproduced, with permission, from SabaCare, Inc.)

System is represented by a *four-level* framework which allows nursing data to be aggregated upward, as well as parsed downward to atomic level concepts (Fig. A.1).

First-Level Healthcare Patterns and Second-Level Care Components

The CCC System framework's *first level* consists of four Healthcare Patterns: (a) Physiological, (b) Psychological, (c) Functional, and (d) Health Behavioral. They are also used to categorize the *second level*, which consists of 21 Care Components. A Care Component represents *"a cluster of data elements that depict four healthcare patterns and represent a holistic approach to patient care"* (Saba, 2012, p. 5). The CCC Care Components also provide the framework for the electronic processing of the nursing POCs. The Care Components are used to classify the two CCC Nursing Terminologies, and link the six phases of the nursing process. Also they are used to link the two terminologies together, as well as link them to other standardized terminologies such as SNOMED CT, ICD-9/10, International Classification of Nursing Practice (ICNP), etc. The Care Components are represented by Name, Code (one letter) with its Definition in the first column in the CCC System Guide shown in Table A.4. The comparison of the ANA's Six Phases of the Nursing Process is mapped to the six steps of the CCC System Nursing Plan of Care (PoC) using the CCC System, as illustrated in Table A.1.

Third Level—Two Terminologies

CCC of Nursing Diagnosis. The *third level* consists of the two CCC System (Version 2.5) terminologies: (a) CCC of

Nursing Diagnoses and Outcomes and (b) CCC of Nursing Interventions/Actions. The CCC of Nursing Diagnoses consists of 176 Nursing Concepts that represent 60 major categories and 116 subcategories concepts. A diagnosis is defined by the ANA as:

> *A clinical judgment about the healthcare's consumer response to actual and potential health conditions or needs. The diagnosis provided the basis for the determination of a plan to achieve expected outcomes....* (ANA, 2010, p. 64)

The Nursing Diagnoses provide the basis for the Nursing PoC and the selection of CCC Nursing Interventions. The Nursing Diagnoses are listed by Care Component by Name, Code (1 Alpha and 2/3 digits), with its Definition in the second column of the CCC System Guide shown in Table A.4.

CCC of Nursing Interventions. The CCC of Nursing Interventions is the other terminology at the framework's *third level*. The CCC of Nursing interventions consist of 201 Core CCC Nursing Interventions/concepts represented by 77 major categories and 124 subcategories that depict nursing interventions, procedures, treatments, activities, and/or services provided to a patient. A Nursing Intervention is defined as:

> *A single nursing action designed to achieve an outcome for a diagnosis (medical/nursing) for which the nurse is accountable* (Saba, 2012, p. 99).

The Core Nursing Interventions are listed by each Care Component by Name, Code (1 Alpha and 2/3 digits), with its Definition in the third column of the CCC

TABLE A.1 Comparison of the ANA's Six Phases of Nursing Process Mapped to the Six Steps of the CCC Nursing Plan of Care (PoC)

ANA Six Phases of Nursing Process	CCC System Six Steps of Nursing PoC
Assessment	Care Components
Diagnosis/Problem	Nursing Diagnoses
Outcome Identification	Expected Outcomes/Goals
Planning	Nursing Interventions
Implementation	Intervention Action Types
Evaluation	Actual Outcomes

System Guide, as shown in Table A.4. Note: there are more Nursing Interventions than Nursing Diagnoses listed for each Care Component. This occurs because caring for a patient generally involves more than one nursing service to treat a patient's medical/nursing diagnosis or problem. In the original research every patient listed three to five medical/nursing diagnoses to eight to 10 nursing interventions/actions (Saba, 1992).

Fourth Level—Two Qualifiers

Nursing Diagnosis Outcomes. The *fourth level* is represented by two sets of qualifiers: (a) Nursing Diagnoses and Outcomes and (b) Nursing Interventions/Actions, both of which are listed at the top of the CCC System Guide, as shown in Table A.4 (columns two and three).

The three Expected Outcomes and/or Actual Outcomes shown in Table A.2 represent the patient's condition on admission and are used to indicate the Goals/Expected Outcomes of the nursing care planned for the patient's diagnosis or problem, whereas the Actual Outcomes represent the results of the patient care by the nurse. Each of the 176 CCC Nursing Diagnoses/Problems *must* be combined with at least one of the three Nursing Outcome Qualifiers totaling 528 unique Expected Outcomes or Actual Outcomes. Each refers to the status of the patient's condition being treated. This combination represents a unique structure to the CCC System; in that, the Outcome Qualifiers listed in the PoCs are documented and coded separately, providing unique specific data for the Comparison of the CCC Nursing Expected Outcomes and/or Actual Outcomes.

Nursing Intervention Action Types. At the top of the third column in the CCC System Guide shown in Table A.4, which consists of the 201 CCC Nursing

Interventions, are four qualifiers represented by the four Action Types:

1. *Assess or Monitor*: Collect, analyze, and monitor data on health status.

2. *Perform/Care or Provide*: Perform a therapeutic action.

3. *Teach or Instruct*: Provide knowledge and education.

4. *Manage or Refer*: Coordinate the patient care process.

The four Action Types focus on the specific action needed to carry out the core Nursing Intervention. Each of the 201 Core CCC of Nursing Interventions *must be* combined with at least one of the four Action Types totaling 804 unique CCC of Nursing Interventions/Actions. This combination is mandatory and represents a unique structure for the CCC System; in that, the Action Types provide a new concept with a new definition and expand the focus of the scope of the Nursing Interventions listed in the PoCs. It uses a one-digit code which is documented and coded separately, providing specific unique data about the CCC Nursing Interventions. The Action Types also provide the measures used to determine status of the care processes, provide the evidence for clinical decision-making, and used, with its RVUs, to cost out care (Saba, 2012).

Note: A CCC Nursing Diagnosis shall be supported with at least one CCC Nursing Intervention; a CCC Nursing Intervention shall be supported with at least one Nursing Diagnosis. Each provides the logic and rationale for implementing nursing care actions and generating outcomes. This care process follows the nursing process for professional practice in a Nursing PoC.

CCC SYSTEM FRAMEWORK STRUCTURE

The CCC System's *four level* framework and coding structure supports the inter-relationships among and feedback between the data elements as shown in the CCC System Information Model in Fig. A.2. The Structure of the CCC System has several unique features:

Level 1: Four Healthcare Patterns

Level 2: 21 Care Components

Level 3: Two Nursing Terminologies

    176 CCC Nursing Diagnoses

    201 CCC Nursing Interventions

Level 4: Two Sets of Qualifiers:

    Three Expected Outcomes and Three Actual Outcomes

    Four Action Qualifiers: Four Action Types

TABLE A.2	Three Qualifiers for Expected Outcomes & Actual Outcomes	
Expected Outcome/Goals Qualifiers	**Actual Outcome/Care Qualifiers**	
1. To/Will Improve: Change or Resolve	1. Improved: Did Change or Resolved	
2. To/Will Stabilize: Stay the same	2. Stabilized: Did Not Change—Same	
3. To/Will Deteriorate: Worsen and/or Die	3. Deteriorated: Did Get Worse—Died	

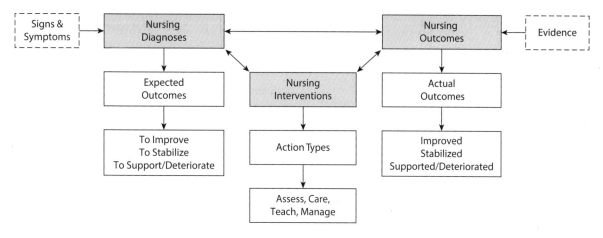

• **FIGURE A.2.** CCC System Information Model. (Reproduced, with permission, from SabaCare, Inc.)

Together they make the design, development, and documentation of nursing practice and PoCs and interdisciplinary plans of care *"Ready to Use."*

CCC CODING STRATEGY

The CCC System uses a five-character alphanumeric structure to code the constructs of the two terminologies, making standardized, coded nursing documentation possible to link and track the patient care process for a health condition (Saba, 2012). The CCC coding structure is based on the code format of the *International Statistical Classification of Diseases and Related Health Problems: Tenth Revision: Volume 1, WHO, 1992 (ICD-10).* "The coding strategy for each terminology consists of the following:

- First Position: One alphabetic character code for Care Component (A to U);

- Second, Third, & Fourth Positions: Either a Two-digit code for a core concept (major category) with a decimal point, and/or followed by a third-digit code for a subcategory.

- Fifth position: One-digit code for: either a) one of three Expected or Actual Outcomes and /or b) one of four Nursing Intervention Action Types" (Saba, 2012, p. 88)

CCC SYSTEM NURSING POC EXAMPLE

An example of the CCC System's Coding Structure for a Nursing PoC is shown in Table A.3. It represents the *essence of care.*

TABLE A.3	Example of the CCC System's Coding Structure for a Nursing PoC
Assessment (S/S):	**Activity Component: (A)**
Nursing Diagnosis:	Physical Mobility Impairment: (A01.5)
Expected Outcome/Goal:	Patient's Condition (will) Improve: (A01.5.**1**)
Planning: 2 Core Interventions	Ambulation Therapy: (A03.1)
	Rehabilitation Exercise: (A05.0)
Nursing Intervention/ Action:	Teach: Ambulation Therapy: (A03.1.**3**)
Nursing Intervention/ Action:	Perform Rehabilitation Exercise: (A05.0.**2**)
Actual Outcome:	Patient's condition (has) Improved: (A01.5.**1**)

Reproduced, with permission of Springer Publishing Company via Copyright Clearance Center.

CCC POC SYSTEM EXAMPLE: DATA ANALYSES

The data generated for the coded Nursing PoC provide the specific nursing care information as well as outcomes in the example as follows:

Evidenced-Based: Number and Frequency of Nursing Diagnoses and Core Nursing Interventions

Care Measures: Comparison of Expected Outcomes to Actual Outcomes

Workload and Resources: Number of Action Types for Clinical Condition, Patient, Nurse, or Nursing Unit

Cost: Number of Action Types by Time with Predetermined Relative Value Units (RVUs) for specific Nursing Interventions

Numerous other reports can be generated and/or aggregated for the different levels of administration.

NURSING PLAN OF CARE (POC) TYPES

An end user can develop at least three different types of PoCs: (1) Standardized PoC is a predetermined plan of care for a specific disease and/or healthcare condition (traditional care plan); (2) Individualized PoC is configured for an individual patient with a specific disease and/or healthcare condition (clinical practice guideline; critical path); and (3) Interactive PoC is dynamically entered based on a specific patient in response to specific branching logic and menu-driven options. Examples of these three types of PoCs can be seen on the Web site www.clinicalcareclassification.com or in *Clinical Care Classification (CCC) System Version 2.5 User's Guide (2012), pp. 92–93.*

SUMMARY

This Appendix serves as a reference and resource on the use of standardized nursing data and the use of the CCC System nursing terminology standard as an integrator to achieve the exchange of nursing outcomes, resources, and workload between and among health systems and enables nurses' contributions to patient outcomes to be evaluated. The CCC System gives nursing the data that are urgently needed to generate new nursing information, knowledge, and wisdom (Englebardt & Nelson, 2002) and the evidence to improve patient care and healthcare outcomes. The use of coded standardized nursing concepts based on the CCC System's Information Framework, provided the *essence of care* essential for conducting research to generate the evidence necessary

for the evaluation and recognition of nursing's contribution to patient care and outcomes. The CCC System is a nursing terminology standard for data interoperability for healthcare planning, coordination, and continuity of care. The CCC System was created for all healthcare settings to "name nursing phenomena and to document and code nursing practice" (Saba, 2007, p. 14). It is envision that it serves as the ICD and CPT terminologies for Nursing Practice (Taylor, 2007).

CCC SYSTEM "READY-TO-USE" GUIDE

Use Table A.4 as a beginning CCC System *"Ready-to-Use"* Guide for developing a Nursing PoC using the CCC System. It has been determined that during any given shift, a nurse will address one to three patient problems, representing the *essence of care.* This means nurses begin to develop a PoC based on the identification of the CCC Nursing Diagnoses derived from the patient's Assessed Signs and Symptoms guided by the Care Component. Each selected Nursing Diagnosis requires a Care Goal or Expected Outcome, and each Nursing Diagnosis also requires the selection of one or more Nursing Interventions from the list of CCC of Nursing Interventions for the same Care Component Classes. The Nursing Interventions Guide the selection of Nursing Intervention/Action Types used for the nursing and inter-professional coordination of patient care. This process is repeated for each identified Nursing Diagnosis, which forms the PoC for a given patient.

Once the PoC is developed, nurses document the care provided by selecting the Intervention Action Types planned/performed for each shift or workday. At this point a patient status can be provided on request or for the "change-of-shift" report. You will have to determine an Actual Outcome for each Nursing Diagnosis at a given point in time, meaning determine a point at which the Nursing Diagnosis was Improved, Stabilized, Deteriorated on, or before Discharge. The codes used for the PoC are now in the background of an electronic system and available to be summarized for outcomes and analysis.

TABLE A.4	Clinical Care Classification System, Version 2.5: CCC of Nursing Diagnoses and Outcomes and the CCC of Nursing Interventions/Actions with Definitions, Classified by 21 Care Components[a,b]	
Care Components (A–U)	**Nursing Diagnoses and Outcomes**	**Nursing Interventions/Actions**
Coding structure consists of five alphanumeric digits First—A to U: **CC** Second/third—major category Fourth—subcategory Fifth—qualifier	**Expected Outcomes and Actual Outcomes** To improve (.1) or improved (.1) To stabilize (.2) or stabilized (.2) Deterioration (.3) or deteriorated (.3) *Example: Expected Outcome: Activity Alteration—To Improve—A01.0.1* *Example: Actual Outcome: Activity Alteration Improved—A01.0.1*	**Nursing Intervention—Action Types** Assess or monitor (.1) Perform or care (.2) Teach or instruct (.3) Manage or refer (.4) *Example: Assess Activity Care—A01.0.1* *Example: Perform Activity Care—A01.0.2* *Example: Teach Activity Care—A01.0.3* *Example: Manage Activity Care—A01.0.4*

A. Activity Component
Cluster of elements that involve the use of energy in carrying out musculoskeletal and bodily actions
	Activity Alteration—A01.0
	Change in or modification of energy used by the body
	    Activity Intolerance—A01.1
	    Incapacity to carry out physiological or psychological daily activities
	    Activity Intolerance Risk—A01.2
	    Increased chance of an incapacity to carry out physiological or psychological daily activities
	    Diversional Activity Deficit—A01.3
	    Lack of interest or engagement in leisure activities
	    Fatigue—A01.4
	    Exhaustion that interferes with physical and mental activities
	    Physical Mobility Impairment—A01.5
	    Diminished ability to perform independent movement
	    Sleep Pattern Disturbance—A01.6
	    Imbalance in the normal sleep/wake cycle
	    Sleep Deprivation—A01.7
	    Lack of a normal sleep/wake cycle
	Musculoskeletal Alteration—A02.0
	Change in or modification of the muscles, bones, or support structures
		Activity Care—A01.0
		Activities performed to carry out physiological or psychological daily activities
		    Energy Conservation—A01.2
		    Actions performed to preserve energy
		Fracture Care—A02.0
		Actions performed to control broken bones
		    Cast Care—A02.1
		    Actions performed to control a rigid dressing
		    Immobilizer Care—A02.2
		    Actions performed to control a splint, cast, or prescribed bed rest
		Mobility Therapy—A03.0
		Actions performed to advise and instruct on mobility deficits
		    Ambulation Therapy—A03.1
		    Actions performed to promote walking
		    Assistive Device Therapy—A03.2
		    Actions performed to support the use of products to aid in caring for oneself
		    Transfer Care—A03.3
		    Actions performed to assist in moving from one place to another
		Sleep Pattern Control—A04.0
		Actions performed to support the sleep/wake cycle
		Musculoskeletal Care—A05.0
		Actions performed to restore physical functioning
		    Range of Motion—A05.1
		    Actions performed to provide active and passive exercises to maintain joint function
		    Rehabilitation Exercise—A05.2
		    Actions performed to promote physical functioning
		Bedbound Care—A61.0
		Actions performed to support an individual confined to bed
		    Positioning Therapy—A61.1
		    Process to support changes in body positioning
		Diversional Care—A77.0
		Actions performed to support interest in leisure activities or play

(continued)

TABLE A.4	Clinical Care Classification System, Version 2.5: CCC of Nursing Diagnoses and Outcomes and the CCC of Nursing Interventions/Actions with Definitions, Classified by 21 Care Components[a,b] *(continued)*

Care Components (A–U)	Nursing Diagnoses and Outcomes	Nursing Interventions/Actions

B. Bowel/Gastric Component
Cluster of elements that involve the gastrointestinal system
	Bowel Elimination Alteration—B03.0
	Change in or modification of the gastrointestinal system
	    Bowel Incontinence—B03.1
	    Involuntary defecation
	    Diarrhea—B03.3
	    Abnormal frequency and fluidity of feces
	    Fecal Impaction—B03.4
	    Feces wedged in intestines
	    Perceived Constipation—B03.5
	    Impression of infrequent or difficult passage of hard, dry feces without cause
	    Constipation—B03.6
	    Difficult passage of hard, dry feces
	Gastrointestinal Alteration—B04.0
	Change in or modification of the stomach or intestines
	Nausea—B04.1
	Distaste for food/fluids and an urge to vomit
	Vomiting—B04.2
	Expulsion of stomach contents through the mouth
		Bowel Care—B06.0
		Actions performed to control and restore the functioning of the bowel
		    Bowel Training—B06.1
		    Actions performed to provide instruction on bowel elimination conditions
		    Disimpaction—B06.2
		    Actions performed to manually remove feces
		    Enema—B06.3
		    Actions performed to give fluid rectally
		    Diarrhea Care—B06.4
		    Actions performed to control the abnormal frequency and fluidity of feces
		Bowel Ostomy Care—B07.0
		Actions performed to maintain the artificial opening that removes bowel waste products
		    Bowel Ostomy Irrigation—B07.1
		    Actions performed to flush or wash out the artificial opening that removes bowel waste products
		Gastric Care—B62.0
		Actions performed to control changes in the stomach and intestines
		    Nausea Care—B62.1
		    Actions performed to control the distaste for food and desire to vomit

C. Cardiac Component
Cluster of elements that involve the heart and blood vessels
	Cardiac Output Alteration—C05.0
	Change in or modification of the pumping action of the heart
	Cardiovascular Alteration—C06.0
	Change in or modification of the heart or blood vessels
	    Blood Pressure Alteration—C06.1
	    Change in or modification of the systolic or diastolic pressure
	    Bleeding Risk—C06.2
	    Increased chance of loss of blood volume
		Cardiac Care—C08.0
		Actions performed to control changes in the heart or blood vessels
		Cardiac Rehabilitation—C08.1
		Actions performed to restore cardiac health
		Pacemaker Care—C09.0
		Actions performed to control the use of an electronic device that provides a normal heartbeat

D. Cognitive/Neuro Component
Cluster of elements involving the cognitive, mental, cerebral, and neurological processes
	Cerebral Alteration—D07.0
	Change in or modification of mental processes
	    Confusion—D07.1
	    State of being disoriented (mixed up)
	Knowledge Deficit—D08.0
	Lack of information, understanding, or comprehension
	    Knowledge Deficit of Diagnostic Test—D08.1
	    Lack of information on test(s) to identify disease or assess health condition
		Behavior Care—D10.0
		Actions performed to support observable responses to internal and external stimuli
		Reality Orientation—D11.0
		Actions performed to promote the ability to locate oneself in an environment

(continued)

TABLE A.4	Clinical Care Classification System, Version 2.5: CCC of Nursing Diagnoses and Outcomes and the CCC of Nursing Interventions/Actions with Definitions, Classified by 21 Care Components[a,b] *(continued)*

Care Components (A–U)	Nursing Diagnoses and Outcomes	Nursing Interventions/Actions
	Knowledge Deficit of Dietary Regimen—D08.2 *Lack of information on the prescribed diet/food intake* **Knowledge Deficit of Disease Process—D08.3** *Lack of information on the morbidity, course, or treatment of the health condition* **Knowledge Deficit of Fluid Volume—D08.4** *Lack of information on fluid volume intake requirements* **Knowledge Deficit of Medication Regimen—D08.5** *Lack of information on prescribed regulated course of medicinal substances* **Knowledge Deficit of Safety Precautions—D08.6** *Lack of information on measures to prevent injury, danger, or loss* **Knowledge Deficit of Therapeutic Regimen—D08.7** *Lack of information on regulated course of treating disease* **Thought Process Alteration—D09.0** *Change in or modification of thought and cognitive processes* **Memory Impairment—D09.1** *Diminished ability or inability to recall past events*	**Wandering Control—D63.0** *Actions performed to control abnormal movability* **Memory Loss Care—D64.0** *Actions performed to control a person's inability to recall ideas and/or events* **Neurological System Care—D78.0** *Actions performed to control problems of the neurological system*
E. Coping Component *Cluster of elements that involve the ability to deal with responsibilities, problems, or difficulties*	**Dying Process—E10.0** *Physical and behavioral responses associated with death* **Community Coping Impairment—E52.0** *Inadequate community response to problems or difficulties* **Family Coping Impairment—E11.0** *Inadequate family response to problems or difficulties* **Disabled Family Coping—E11.2** *Inability of family to function optimally* **Individual Coping Impairment—E12.0** *Inadequate personal response to problems or difficulties* **Adjustment Impairment—E12.1** *Inadequate adjustment to condition or change in health status* **Decisional Conflict—E12.2** *Struggle related to determining a course of action*	**Counseling Service—E12.0** *Actions performed to provide advice or instruction to help another* **Coping Support—E12.1** *Actions performed to sustain a person dealing with responsibilities, problems, or difficulties* **Stress Control—E12.2** *Actions performed to support the physiological response of the body to a stimulus* **Crisis Therapy—E12.3** *Actions performed to sustain a person dealing with a condition, event, or radical change in status* **Emotional Support—E13.0** *Actions performed to maintain a positive affective state* **Spiritual Comfort—E13.1** *Actions performed to console, restore, or promote spiritual health*

(continued)

TABLE A.4	Clinical Care Classification System, Version 2.5: CCC of Nursing Diagnoses and Outcomes and the CCC of Nursing Interventions/Actions with Definitions, Classified by 21 Care Components[a,b] *(continued)*

Care Components (A–U)	Nursing Diagnoses and Outcomes	Nursing Interventions/Actions
	Defensive Coping—E12.3 *Self-protective strategies to guard against threats to self* **Denial—E12.4** *Attempt to reduce anxiety by refusal to accept thoughts, feelings, or facts* **Post-trauma Response—E13.0** *Sustained behavior related to a traumatic event* **Rape Trauma Syndrome—E13.1** *Group of symptoms related to a forced sexual act* **Spiritual State Alteration—E14.0** *Change in or modification of the spirit or soul* **Spiritual Distress—E14.1** *Anguish related to the spirit or soul* **Grieving—E53.0** *Feeling of great sorrow* **Anticipatory Grieving—E53.1** *Feeling great sorrow before the event or loss* **Dysfunctional Grieving—E53.2** *Prolonged feeling of great sorrow*	**Terminal Care—E14.0** *Actions performed in the period surrounding death* **Bereavement Support—E14.1** *Actions performed to provide comfort to the family/friends of the person who died* **Dying/Death Measures—E14.2** *Actions performed to support the dying process* **Funeral Arrangements—E14.3** *Actions performed to direct the preparation for burial*
F. Fluid Volume Component *Cluster of elements that involve liquid consumption*	**Fluid Volume Alteration—F15.0** *Change in or modification of bodily fluid* **Fluid Volume Deficit—F15.1** *Dehydration or fluid loss* **Fluid Volume Deficit Risk—F15.2** *Increased chance of dehydration or fluid loss* **Fluid Volume Excess—F15.3** *Fluid retention, overload, or edema* **Fluid Volume Excess Risk—F15.4** *Increased chance of fluid retention, overload, or edema* **Electrolyte Imbalance—F62.0** *Higher or lower body electrolyte levels*	**Fluid Therapy—F15.0** *Actions performed to provide liquid volume intake* **Hydration Control—F15.1** *Actions performed to control the state of fluid balance* **Intake—F15.3** *Actions performed to measure the amount of fluid volume taken into the body* **Output—F15.4** *Actions performed to measure the amount of fluid volume removed from the body* **Hemodynamic Care—F79.0** *Actions performed to support the movement of solutions through the blood* **Intravenous Care—F79.1** *Actions performed to support the use of infusion equipment* **Venous Catheter Care—F79.2** *Actions performed to support the use of a venous infusion site* **Arterial Catheter Care—F79.3** *Actions performed to support the use of an arterial infusion site*

(continued)

| TABLE A.4 | Clinical Care Classification System, Version 2.5: CCC of Nursing Diagnoses and Outcomes and the CCC of Nursing Interventions/Actions with Definitions, Classified by 21 Care Components[a,b] *(continued)* |

Care Components (A–U)	Nursing Diagnoses and Outcomes	Nursing Interventions/Actions

G. Health Behavior Component
Cluster of elements that involve actions to sustain, maintain, or regain health
	Health Maintenance Alteration—G17.0
	Change in or modification of ability to manage health-related needs.
	   Failure to Thrive—G17.1
	   Inability to grow and develop normally
	Health-Seeking Behavior Alteration—G18.0
	Change in or modification of actions needed to improve health state
	Home Maintenance Alteration—G19.0
	Inability to sustain a safe, healthy environment
	Noncompliance—G20.0
	Failure to follow therapeutic recommendations
	   Noncompliance of Diagnostic Test—G20.1
	   Failure to follow therapeutic recommendations on tests to identify disease or assess health condition
	   Noncompliance of Dietary Regimen—G20.2
	   Failure to follow the prescribed diet/food intake
	   Noncompliance of Fluid Volume—G20.3
	   Failure to follow fluid volume intake requirements
	   Noncompliance of Medication Regimen—G20.4
	   Failure to follow prescribed regulated course of medicinal substances
	   Noncompliance of Safety Precautions—G20.5
	   Failure to follow measures to prevent injury, danger, or loss
	   Noncompliance of Therapeutic Regimen—G20.6
	   Failure to follow regulated course of treating disease or health condition
		Community Special Services—G17.0
		Actions performed to provide advice or information about special community services
		   Adult Day Center—G17.1
		   Actions performed to direct the provision of a day program for adults in a specific location
		   Hospice—G17.2
		   Actions performed to support the provision of offering and/or providing care for terminally ill persons
		   Meals on Wheels—G17.3
		   Actions performed to direct the provision of a community program of delivering meals to the home
		Compliance Care—G18.0
		Actions performed to encourage adherence to care regimen
		   Compliance with Diet—G18.1
		   Actions performed to encourage adherence to diet/food intake
		   Compliance with Fluid Volume—G18.2
		   Actions performed to encourage adherence to therapeutic intake of liquids
		   Compliance with Medical Regimen—G18.3
		   Actions performed to encourage adherence to physician's/provider's treatment plan
		   Compliance with Medication Regimen—G18.4
		   Actions performed to encourage adherence to prescribed course of medicinal substances
		   Compliance with Safety Precaution—G18.5
		   Actions performed to encourage adherence with measures to protect self or others from injury, danger, or loss
		   Compliance with Therapeutic Regimen— G18.6
		   Actions performed to encourage adherence with plan of care
		Nursing Contact—G19.0
		Actions performed to communicate with another nurse
		   Bill of Rights—G19.1
		   Statements related to entitlements during an episode of illness
		   Nursing Care Coordination—G19.2
		   Actions performed to synthesize all plans of care by a nurse
		   Nursing Status Report—G19.3
		   Actions performed to document patient condition by a nurse

(continued)

TABLE A.4	Clinical Care Classification System, Version 2.5: CCC of Nursing Diagnoses and Outcomes and the CCC of Nursing Interventions/Actions with Definitions, Classified by 21 Care Components[a,b] *(continued)*	
Care Components (A–U)	**Nursing Diagnoses and Outcomes**	**Nursing Interventions/Actions**

		Physician Contact—G20.0
		 Actions performed to communicate with a physician/provider
		    Medical Regimen Orders—G20.1
		    Actions performed to support the physician's/ provider's plan of treatment
		    Physician Status Report—G20.2
		    Actions performed to document patient condition by a physician/provider
		 Professional/Ancillary Services—G21.0
		 Actions performed to support the duties performed by health team members
		    Health Aide Service—G21.1
		    Actions performed to support care services by a health aide
		    Social Worker Service—G21.2
		    Actions performed to provide advice or instruction by a social worker
		    Nurse Specialist Service—G21.3
		    Actions performed to provide advice or instruction by an advanced practice nurse or nurse practitioner
		    Occupational Therapist Service—G21.4
		    Actions performed to provide advice or instruction by an occupational therapist
		    Physical Therapist Service—G21.5
		    Actions performed to provide advice or instruction by a physical therapist
		    Speech Therapist Service—G21.6
		    Actions performed to provide advice or instruction by a speech therapist
		    Respiratory Therapist Service—G21.7
		    Actions performed to provide advice or instruction by a respiratory therapist

H. Medication Component
 Cluster of elements that involve medicinal substances
	Medication Risk—H21.0
	 Increased chance of negative response to medicinal substances
	    Polypharmacy—H21.1
	    Use of two or more drugs together
		Chemotherapy Care—H22.0
		 Actions performed to control and monitor antineoplastic agents
		 Injection Administration—H23.0
		 Actions performed to dispense medication by a hypodermic
		 Medication Care—H24.0
		 Actions performed to support use of prescribed drugs or remedies regardless of route
		    Medication Actions—H24.1
		    Actions performed to support and monitor the intended responses to prescribed drugs
		    Medication Prefill Preparation—H24.2
		    Actions performed to ensure the continued supply of prescribed drugs

(continued)

TABLE A.4	Clinical Care Classification System, Version 2.5: CCC of Nursing Diagnoses and Outcomes and the CCC of Nursing Interventions/Actions with Definitions, Classified by 21 Care Components[a,b] *(continued)*

Care Components (A–U)	Nursing Diagnoses and Outcomes	Nursing Interventions/Actions
		Medication Side Effects—H24.3 *Actions performed to control adverse untoward reactions or conditions to prescribed drugs* **Medication Treatment—H24.4** *Actions performed to administer/give drugs or remedies regardless of route* **Radiation Therapy Care—H25.0** *Actions performed to control and monitor radiation therapy*
I. Metabolic Component *Cluster of elements that involve the endocrine and immunologic processes*	**Endocrine Alteration—I22.0** *Change in or modification of internal secretions or hormones* **Immunologic Alteration—I23.0** *Change in or modification of the immune system*	**Allergic Reaction Care—I26.0** *Actions performed to reduce symptoms or precautions to reduce allergies* **Diabetic Care—I27.0** *Actions performed to support the control of diabetic conditions* **Immunologic Care—I65.0** *Actions performed to protect against a particular disease*

J. Nutritional Component
Cluster of elements that involve the intake of food and nutrients
	Nutrition Alteration—J24.0
	Change in or modification of food and nutrients
	  Body Nutrition Deficit—J24.1
	  Less than adequate intake or absorption of food or nutrients
	  Body Nutrition Deficit Risk—J24.2
	  Increased chance of less than adequate intake or absorption of food or nutrients
	  Body Nutrition Excess—J24.3
	  More than adequate intake or absorption of food or nutrients
	  Body Nutrition Excess Risk—J24.4
	  Increased chance of more than adequate intake or absorption of food or nutrients
	  Swallowing Impairment—J24.5
	  Inability to move food from mouth to stomach
	Infant Feeding Pattern Impairment—J54.0
	Imbalance in the normal feeding habits of an infant
	Breastfeeding Impairment—J55.0
	Diminished ability to nourish infant at the breast
		Enteral Tube Care—J28.0
		Actions performed to control the use of an enteral drainage tube
		  Enteral Tube Insertion—J28.1
		  Actions performed to support the placement of an enteral drainage tube
		  Enteral Tube Irrigation—J28.2
		  Actions performed to flush or wash out an enteral tube
		Nutrition Care—J29.0
		Actions performed to support the intake of food and nutrients
		  Feeding Technique—J29.2
		  Actions performed to provide special measures to provide nourishment
		  Regular Diet—J29.3
		  Actions performed to support the ingestion of food and nutrients from established nutrition standards
		  Special Diet—J29.4
		  Actions performed to support the ingestion of food and nutrients prescribed for a specific purpose
		  Enteral Feeding—J29.5
		  Actions performed to provide nourishment through a gastrointestinal route
		  Parenteral Feeding—J29.6
		  Actions performed to provide nourishment through intravenous or subcutaneous routes
		Breastfeeding Support—J66.0
		Actions performed to provide nourishment of an infant at the breast
		Weight Control—J67.0
		Actions performed to control obesity or debilitation

(continued)

TABLE A.4	Clinical Care Classification System, Version 2.5: CCC of Nursing Diagnoses and Outcomes and the CCC of Nursing Interventions/Actions with Definitions, Classified by 21 Care Components[a,b] *(continued)*

Care Components (A–U)	Nursing Diagnoses and Outcomes	Nursing Interventions/Actions
K. Physical Regulation Component *Cluster of elements that involve bodily processes*	**Physical Regulation Alteration—K25.0** *Change in or modification of somatic control* **Autonomic Dysreflexia—K25.1** *Life-threatening inhibited sympathetic response to noxious stimuli in a person with a spinal cord injury at or above T7* **Hyperthermia—K25.2** *Abnormally high body temperature* **Hypothermia—K25.3** *Abnormally low body temperature* **Thermoregulation Impairment—K25.4** *Fluctuation of temperature between hypothermia and hyperthermia* **Infection Risk—K25.5** *Increased chance of contamination with disease-producing germs* **Infection—K25.6** *Contamination with disease-producing germs* **Intracranial Adaptive Capacity Impairment—K25.7** *Intracranial fluid volumes are compromised*	**Infection Control—K30.0** *Actions performed to contain a communicable disease* **Universal Precautions—K30.1** *Practices to prevent the spread of infections and infectious diseases* **Physical Healthcare—K31.0** *Actions performed to support somatic problems* **Health History—K31.1** *Actions performed to obtain information about past illness and health status* **Health Promotion—K31.2** *Actions performed to encourage behaviors to enhance health state* **Physical Examination—K31.3** *Actions performed to observe somatic events* **Clinical Measurements—K31.4** *Actions performed to conduct procedures to evaluate somatic events* **Specimen Care—K32.0** *Actions performed to direct the collection and/or the examination of a bodily specimen* **Blood Specimen Care—K32.1** *Actions performed to collect and/or examine a sample of blood* **Stool Specimen Care—K32.2** *Actions performed to collect and/or examine a sample of feces* **Urine Specimen Care—K32.3** *Actions performed to collect and/or examine a sample of urine* **Sputum Specimen Care—K32.5** *Actions performed to collect and/or examine a sample of sputum* **Vital Signs—K33.0** *Actions performed to measure temperature, pulse, respiration, and blood pressure* **Blood Pressure—K33.1** *Actions performed to measure the diastolic and systolic pressure of the blood* **Temperature—K33.2** *Actions performed to measure the body temperature* **Pulse—K33.3** *Actions performed to measure rhythmic beats of the heart* **Respiration—K33.4** *Actions performed to measure the function of breathing*

(continued)

TABLE A.4	Clinical Care Classification System, Version 2.5: CCC of Nursing Diagnoses and Outcomes and the CCC of Nursing Interventions/Actions with Definitions, Classified by 21 Care Components[a,b] *(continued)*		
Care Components (A–U)	**Nursing Diagnoses and Outcomes**		**Nursing Interventions/Actions**

L. Respiratory Component
Cluster of elements that involve breathing and the pulmonary system

Respiration Alteration—L26.0
Change in or modification of the breathing function

    Airway Clearance Impairment—L26.1
    Inability to clear secretions/obstructions in airway

    Breathing Pattern Impairment—L26.2
    Inadequate inhalation or exhalation

    Gas Exchange Impairment—L26.3
    Imbalance of oxygen and carbon dioxide transfer between lung and vascular system

Ventilatory Weaning Impairment—L56.0
Inability to tolerate decreased levels of ventilator support

Oxygen Therapy Care—L35.0
Actions performed to support the administration of oxygen treatment

Pulmonary Care—L36.0
Actions performed to support pulmonary hygiene

    Breathing Exercises—L36.1
    Actions performed to provide therapy on respiratory or lung exertion

    Chest Physiotherapy—L36.2
    Actions performed to provide exercises for postural drainage of lungs

    Inhalation Therapy—L36.3
    Actions performed to support breathing treatments

    Ventilator Care—L36.4
    Actions performed to control and monitor the use of a ventilator

Tracheostomy Care—L37.0
Actions performed to support a tracheostomy

M. Role Relationship Component
Cluster of elements involving interpersonal work, social, family, and sexual interactions

Role Performance Alteration—M27.0
Change in or modification of carrying out responsibilities

    Parental Role Conflict—M27.1
    Struggle with parental position and responsibilities

    Parenting Alteration—M27.2
    Change in or modification of nurturing figure's ability to promote growth

    Sexual Dysfunction—M27.3
    Deleterious change in sexual response

    Caregiver Role Strain—M27.4
    Excessive tension of one who gives physical or emotional care and support to another person or patient

Communication Impairment—M28.0
Diminished ability to exchange thoughts, opinions, or information

    Verbal Impairment—M28.1
    Diminished ability to exchange thoughts, opinions, or information through speech

Family Process Alteration—M29.0
Change in or modification of usual functioning of a related group

Sexuality Pattern Alteration—M31.0
Change in or modification of a person's sexual response

Socialization Alteration—M32.0
Change in or modification of personal identity

Communication Care—M38.0
Actions performed to exchange verbal/nonverbal and/or translation information

Psychosocial Care—M39.0
Actions performed to support the study of psychological and social factors

    Home Situation Analysis—M39.1
    Actions performed to analyze the living environment

    Interpersonal Dynamics Analysis—M39.2
    Actions performed to support the analysis of the driving forces in a relationship between people

    Family Process Analysis—M39.3
    Actions performed to support the change and/or modification of a related group

    Sexual Behavior Analysis—M39.4
    Actions performed to support the change and/or modification of a person's sexual response

    Social Network Analysis—M39.5
    Actions performed to improve the quantity or quality of personal relationships

(continued)

TABLE A.4	Clinical Care Classification System, Version 2.5: CCC of Nursing Diagnoses and Outcomes and the CCC of Nursing Interventions/Actions with Definitions, Classified by 21 Care Components[a,b] *(continued)*

Care Components (A–U)	Nursing Diagnoses and Outcomes	Nursing Interventions/Actions
	Social Interaction Alteration—M32.1 *Change in or modification of inadequate quantity or quality of personal relations* **Social Isolation—M32.2** *State of aloneness, lack of interaction with others* **Relocation Stress Syndrome—M32.3** *Excessive tension from moving to a new location*	
N. Safety Component *Cluster of elements that involve prevention of injury, danger, loss, or abuse*	**Injury Risk—N33.0** *Increased chance of danger or loss* **Aspiration Risk—N33.1** *Increased chance of material into trachea–bronchial passage.* **Disuse Syndrome—N33.2** *Group of symptoms related to effects of immobility* **Poisoning Risk—N33.3** *Exposure to or ingestion of dangerous products* **Suffocation Risk—N33.4** *Increased chance of inadequate air for breathing* **Trauma Risk—N33.5** *Increased chance of accidental tissue processes* **Fall Risk—N33.6** *Increased chance of conditions that result in falls* **Violence Risk—N34.0** *Increased chance of harming self or others* **Suicide Risk—N34.1** *Increased chance of taking one's life intentionally* **Self-Mutilation Risk—N34.2** *Increased chance of destroying a limb or essential part of the body* **Perioperative Injury Risk—N57.0** *Increased chance of injury during the operative processes* **Perioperative Positioning Injury—N57.1** *Damages from operative process positioning* **Surgical Recovery Delay—N57.2** *Slow or delayed recovery from a surgical procedure* **Substance Abuse—N58.0** *Excessive use of harmful bodily materials* **Tobacco Abuse—N58.1** *Excessive use of tobacco products* **Alcohol Abuse—N58.2** *Excessive use of distilled liquors* **Drug Abuse—N58.3** *Excessive use of habit-forming medications*	**Substance Abuse Control—N40.0** *Actions performed to control substances to avoid, detect, or minimize harm* **Tobacco Abuse Control—N40.1** *Actions performed to avoid, minimize, or control the use of tobacco* **Alcohol Abuse Control—N40.2** *Actions performed to avoid, minimize, or control the use of distilled liquors* **Drug Abuse Control—N40.3** *Actions performed to avoid, minimize, or control the use of any habit-forming medication* **Emergency Care—N41.0** *Actions performed to support a sudden or unexpected occurrence* **Safety Precautions—N42.0** *Actions performed to advance measures to avoid danger or harm* **Environmental Safety—N42.1** *Precautions recommended to prevent or reduce environmental injury* **Equipment Safety—N42.2** *Precautions recommended to prevent or reduce equipment injury* **Individual Safety—N42.3** *Precautions to reduce individual injury* **Violence Control—N68.0** *Actions performed to control behaviors that may cause harm to oneself or others* **Perioperative Injury Care—N80.0** *Actions performed to support perioperative care requirements*

(continued)

TABLE A.4	Clinical Care Classification System, Version 2.5: CCC of Nursing Diagnoses and Outcomes and the CCC of Nursing Interventions/Actions with Definitions, Classified by 21 Care Components[a,b] *(continued)*

Care Components (A–U)	Nursing Diagnoses and Outcomes	Nursing Interventions/Actions

O. Self-Care Component
Cluster of elements that involve the ability to carry out activities to maintain oneself
	Bathing/Hygiene Deficit—O35.0
	Impaired ability to cleanse oneself
	Dressing/Grooming Deficit—O36.0
	Inability to clothe and groom oneself
	Feeding Deficit—O37.0
	Impaired ability to feed oneself
	Self-Care Deficit—O38.0
	Impaired ability to maintain oneself
	  Activities of Daily Living Alteration—O38.1
	  Change in or modification of ability to maintain oneself
	  Instrumental Activities of Daily Living Alteration—O38.2
	  Change in or modification of more complex activities than those needed to maintain oneself
	Toileting Deficit—O39.0
	Impaired ability to urinate or defecate for oneself
		Personal Care—O43.0
		Actions performed to care for oneself
		  Activities of Daily Living—O43.1
		  Actions performed to support personal activities to maintain oneself
		  Instrumental Activities of Daily Living—O43.2
		  Complex activities performed to support basic life skills

P. Self-Concept Component
Cluster of elements that involve an individual's mental image of oneself
	Anxiety—P40.0
	Feeling of distress or apprehension whose source is unknown
	Fear—P41.0
	Feeling of dread or distress whose cause can be identified
	Meaningfulness Alteration—P42.0
	Change in or modification of the ability to see the significance, purpose, or value in something
	  Hopelessness—P42.1
	  Feeling of despair or futility and passive involvement
	  Powerlessness—P42.2
	  Feeling of helplessness or inability to act
	Self-Concept Alteration—P43.0
	Change in or modification of ability to maintain one's image of self
	  Body Image Disturbance—P43.1
	  Imbalance in the perception of the way one's body looks
	  Personal Identity Disturbance—P43.2
	  Imbalance in the ability to distinguish between the self and the nonself
	  Chronic Low Self-Esteem Disturbance—P43.3
	  Persistent negative evaluation of oneself
	  Situational Self-Esteem Disturbance—P43.4
	  Negative evaluation of oneself in response to a loss or change
		Mental Healthcare—P45.0
		Actions taken to promote emotional well-being
		  Mental Health History—P45.1
		  Actions performed to obtain information about past or present emotional well-being
		  Mental Health Promotion—P45.2
		  Actions performed to encourage or further emotional well-being
		  Mental Health Screening—P45.3
		  Actions performed to systematically examine emotional well-being
		  Mental Health Treatment—P45.4
		  Actions performed to support protocols used to treat emotional problems

(continued)

TABLE A.4	Clinical Care Classification System, Version 2.5: CCC of Nursing Diagnoses and Outcomes and the CCC of Nursing Interventions/Actions with Definitions, Classified by 21 Care Components[a,b] *(continued)*

Care Components (A–U)	Nursing Diagnoses and Outcomes	Nursing Interventions/Actions

Q. Sensory Component
Cluster of elements that involve the senses, including pain
	Sensory Perceptual Alteration—Q44.0
	Change in or modification of the response to stimuli
	    Auditory Alteration—Q44.1
	    Change in or modification of diminished ability to hear
	    Gustatory Alteration—Q44.2
	    Change in or modification of diminished ability to taste
	    Kinesthetic Alteration—Q44.3
	    Change in or modification of diminished balance
	    Olfactory Alteration—Q44.4
	    Change in or modification of diminished ability to smell
	    Tactile Alteration—Q44.5
	    Change in or modification of diminished ability to feel
	    Unilateral Neglect—Q44.6
	    Lack of awareness of one side of the body
	    Visual Alteration—Q44.7
	    Change in or modification of diminished ability to see
	Comfort Alteration—Q45.0
	Change in or modification of sensation that is distressing
	Pain—Q63.0
	Physical suffering or distress; to hurt
	    Acute Pain—Q63.1
	    Severe pain of limited duration
	    Chronic Pain—Q63.2
	    Pain that persists over time
		Pain Control—Q47.0
		Actions performed to support responses to injury or damage
		    Acute Pain Control—Q47.1
		    Actions performed to control physical suffering, hurting, or distress
		    Chronic Pain Control—Q47.2
		    Actions performed to control physical suffering, hurting, or distress that continues longer than expected
		Comfort Care—Q48.0
		Actions performed to enhance or improve well-being
		Ear Care—Q49.0
		Actions performed to support ear problems
		    Hearing Aid Care—Q49.1
		    Actions performed to control the use of a hearing aid
		    Wax Removal—Q49.2
		    Actions performed to remove cerumen from ear
		Eye Care—Q50.0
		Actions performed to support eye problems
		    Cataract Care—Q50.1
		    Actions performed to control cataract conditions
		    Vision Care—Q50.2
		    Actions performed to control vision problems

R. Skin Integrity Component
Cluster of elements that involve the mucous membrane, corneal, integumentary, or subcutaneous structures of the body
	Skin Integrity Alteration—R46.0
	Change in or modification of skin conditions
	    Oral Mucous Membrane Impairment—R46.1
	    Diminished ability to maintain the tissues of the oral cavity
	    Skin Integrity Impairment—R46.2
	    Decreased ability to maintain the integument
	    Skin Integrity Impairment Risk—R46.3
	    Increased chance of skin breakdown
	    Skin Incision—R46.4
	    Cutting of the integument/skin
	    Latex Allergy Response—R46.5
	    Pathological reaction to latex products
		Pressure Ulcer Care—R51.0
		Actions performed to prevent, detect, and treat skin integrity breakdown caused by pressure
		    Pressure Ulcer Stage 1 Care—R51.1
		    Actions performed to prevent, detect, and treat stage 1 skin breakdown
		    Pressure Ulcer Stage 2 Care—R51.2
		    Actions performed to prevent, detect, and treat stage 2 skin breakdown
		    Pressure Ulcer Stage 3 Care—R51.3
		    Actions performed to prevent, detect, and treat stage 3 skin breakdown
		    Pressure Ulcer Stage 4 Care—R51.4
		    Actions performed to prevent, detect, and treat stage 4 skin breakdown

(continued)

TABLE A.4	Clinical Care Classification System, Version 2.5: CCC of Nursing Diagnoses and Outcomes and the CCC of Nursing Interventions/Actions with Definitions, Classified by 21 Care Components[a,b] *(continued)*

Care Components (A–U)	Nursing Diagnoses and Outcomes	Nursing Interventions/Actions

	Peripheral Alteration—R47.0
	Change in or modification of neurovascular-
	ization of the extremities
		Mouth Care—R53.0
		Actions performed to support oral cavity
		problems
		   Denture Care—R53.1
		   Actions performed to control the use of
		   artificial teeth
		Skin Care—R54.0
		Actions to control the integument/skin
		   Skin Breakdown Control—R54.1
		   Actions performed to support tissue integrity
		   problems
		Wound Care—R55.0
		Actions performed to support open skin areas
		   Drainage Tube Care—R55.1
		   Actions performed to support wound drain-
		   age from body tubes
		   Dressing Change—R55.2
		   Actions performed to remove and replace a
		   new bandage on a wound
		   Incision Care—R55.3
		   Actions performed to support a surgical wound
		Burn Care—R81.0
		Actions performed to support burned areas
		of the body

S. Tissue Perfusion **Component** *Cluster of elements that* *involve the oxygenation* *of tissues, including the* *circulatory and vascular* *systems*	**Tissue Perfusion Alteration—S48.0** *Change in or modification of the oxygenation of* *tissues*	**Foot Care—S56.0** *Actions performed to support foot problems* **Perineal Care—S57.0** *Actions performed to support perineal problems* **Edema Control—S69.0** *Actions performed to control excess fluid in tissue* **Circulatory Care—S70.0** *Actions performed to support the circulation of* *the blood (blood vessels)* **Vascular System Care—S82.0** *Actions performed to control problems of the* *vascular system*

T. Urinary Elimination
  Component
Cluster of elements that
involve the genitourinary
systems
	Urinary Elimination Alteration—T49.0
	Change in or modification of excretion of the
	waste matter of the kidneys
	   Functional Urinary Incontinence—T49.1
	   Involuntary, unpredictable passage of urine
	   Reflex Urinary Incontinence—T49.2
	   Involuntary passage of urine occurring at
	   predictable intervals
	   Stress Urinary Incontinence—T49.3
	   Loss of urine occurring with increased
	   abdominal pressure
		Bladder Care—T58.0
		Actions performed to control urinary drainage
		problems
		   Bladder Instillation—T58.1
		   Actions performed to pour liquid through a
		   catheter into the bladder
		   Bladder Training—T58.2
		   Actions performed to provide instruction on
		   the care of urinary drainage

(continued)

TABLE A.4	Clinical Care Classification System, Version 2.5: CCC of Nursing Diagnoses and Outcomes and the CCC of Nursing Interventions/Actions with Definitions, Classified by 21 Care Components[a,b] *(continued)*

Care Components (A–U)	Nursing Diagnoses and Outcomes	Nursing Interventions/Actions

	Urge Urinary Incontinence—T49.5
	Involuntary passage of urine following a sense of urgency to void
	Urinary Retention—T49.6
	Incomplete emptying of the bladder
	Renal Alteration—T50.0
	Change in or modification of kidney function
		Dialysis Care—T59.0
		Actions performed to support the removal of waste products from the body
		  Hemodialysis Care—T59.1
		  Actions performed to support the mechanical removal of waste products from the blood
		  Peritoneal Dialysis Care—T59.2
		  Actions performed to support the osmotic removal of waste products from the blood
		Urinary Catheter Care—T60.0
		Actions performed to control the use of a urinary catheter
		  Urinary Catheter Insertion—T60.1
		  Actions performed to place a urinary catheter in bladder
		  Urinary Catheter Irrigation—T60.2
		  Actions performed to flush a urinary catheter
		Urinary Incontinence Care—T72.0
		Actions performed to control the inability to retain and/or involuntarily retain urine
		Renal Care—T73.0
		Actions performed to control problems pertaining to the kidney
		Bladder Ostomy Care—T83.0
		Actions performed to maintain the artificial opening to remove urine
		  Bladder Ostomy Irrigation—T83.1
		  Actions performed to flush and wash out the artificial opening to remove urine

U. Life Cycle Component
Cluster of elements that involve the life span of individuals
	Reproductive Risk—U59.0
	Increased chance of harm in the process of replicating or giving rise to an offspring/child
	  Fertility Risk—U59.1
	  Increased chance of conception to develop an offspring/child
	  Infertility Risk—U59.2
	  Decreased chance of conception to develop an offspring/child
	  Contraception Risk—U59.3
	  Increased chance of harm preventing the conception of an offspring/child
	Perinatal Risk—U60.0
	Increased chance of harm before, during, and immediately after the creation of an offspring/child
	  Pregnancy Risk—U60.1
	  Increased chance of harm during the gestational period of the formation of an offspring/child
		Reproductive Care—U74.0
		Actions performed to support the production of an offspring/child
		  Fertility Care—U74.1
		  Actions performed to increase the chance of conception of an offspring/child
		  Infertility Care—U74.2
		  Actions performed to promote conception by the infertile client of an offspring/child
		  Contraception Care—U74.3
		  Actions performed to prevent conception of an offspring/child
		Perinatal Care—U75.0
		Actions performed to support the period before, during, and immediately after the creation of an offspring/child
		  Pregnancy Care—U75.1
		  Actions performed to support the gestation period of the formation of an offspring/child (being with child)

(continued)

| TABLE A.4 | Clinical Care Classification System, Version 2.5: CCC of Nursing Diagnoses and Outcomes and the CCC of Nursing Interventions/Actions with Definitions, Classified by 21 Care Components[a,b] *(continued)* |

Care Components (A–U)	Nursing Diagnoses and Outcomes	Nursing Interventions/Actions
	Labor Risk—U60.2 *Increased chance of harm during the period supporting the bringing forth of an offspring/child* **Delivery Risk—U60.3** *Increased chance of harm during the period supporting the expulsion of an offspring/child* **Postpartum Risk—U60.4** *Increased chance of harm during the period immediately following the delivery of an offspring/child* **Growth and Development Alteration—U61.0** *Change in or modification of age-specific normal growth standards and/or developmental skills*	**Labor Care—U75.2** *Actions performed to support the bringing forth of an offspring/child* **Delivery Care—U75.3** *Actions performed to support the expulsion of an offspring/child at birth* **Postpartum Care—U75.4** *Actions performed to support the period immediately after the delivery of an offspring/child* **Growth and Development Care—U76.0** *Actions performed to support age-specific normal growth standards and/or developmental skills*

[a]Clinical Care Classification (CCC) System, Version 2.5 [previously known as (a) Clinical Care Classification (CCC) System, Version 2.0, Copyright © 2004, and (b) Home Healthcare Classification (HHCC) System, Version 1.0, Copyright © 1994] pending Copyright © 2012 by Virginia K. Saba, EdD, RN, FAAN, FACMI, LL, may be used ONLY with written Permission by Dr. Virginia K. Saba. (Permission Form available from Web site http://www.sabacare.com)
[b]Revised 1992, 1994, 2004, 2006, and 2011.

REFERENCES

American Medical Association. (2014). *Current procedural terminology*. Chicago, IL: AMA.

American Nurses Association. (2010). *Nursing: Nursing scope and standards of practice*. Silver Spring, MD: ANA.

Englebardt, S. P., & Nelson, R. (2002). *Health care informatics: An interdisciplinary approach*. St. Louis, MO: Mosby Incorporated.

Moss, J., Andison, M., & Sobko, H. (2007, November). *An analysis of narrative nursing documentation in an otherwise structured intensive care clinical documentation system*. Paper presented at the 2007 meeting of the American Medical Informatics Association. Washington, DC: AMIA.

Saba, V. K. (1992). The classification of home health care nursing diagnoses and interventions. *Caring, 10*(3), 50–57.

Saba, V. K. (2007). *Clinical Care Classification (CCC) System Manual, Version 2.0: A guide to nursing documentation*. New York, NY: Springer Publishing.

Saba, V. K. (2012). *Clinical Care Classification (CCC) System, Version 2.5: User's guide*. New York, NY: Springer Publishing.

Saba, V. K., & Arnold, J. M. (2004). Clinical care costing method for the Clinical Care Classification System. *International Journal of Nursing Terminologies and Classifications, 15*(3), 69–77.

Saba, V. K., & Taylor, S. L. (2007). Moving past theory: Use of a standardized coded nursing terminology to enhance nursing visibility. *CIN: Computers, Informatics, Nursing, 25*(6), 324–331.

Taylor, S. (2007). Foreword. In V. K. Saba (Ed.), *Clinical Care Classification (CCC) System: A guide to nursing documentation*. New York, NY: Springer Publishing.

Whittenburg, L. (2009) Nursing terminology documentation of quality outcomes. *Journal of Healthcare Information Management, 23*(3), 51–55.

World Health Organization (WHO). (1992). *International statistical classification of diseases and related health problems: Tenth revision: Volume 1 (ICD-10)*. Geneva, Switzerland: WHO.

INDEX

Page numbers followed by f or t indicate figures or tables, respectively.

ASDs. *See* Application-Specific
   Devices (ASDs)
Asia, nursing informatics in, 801–813
Asia eHealth Information Network
   (AeHIN), 787–788
Asia-Pacific Association for Medical
   Informatics (APAMI),
   777–778, 802
Assembler language, 49, 49f
Association for Common European
   Nursing Diagnosis,
   Interventions, and Outcomes
   (ASCENDIO), 763–764
Association for Nomenclature,
   Taxonomy, and Nursing
   Diagnoses (AENTDE), 764
ASTM. *See* American Society for
   Testing and Materials (ASTM)
ATA. *See* American Telemedicine
   Association (ATA)
ATLAS.ti software, 676
Audiotaping, qualitative research, 675
Audit control, security technology
   safeguards, 150f, 156t–157t,
   158
Australia
   competencies and credentialing
      in nursing informatics in,
      795–796
   eHealth policy and governance in,
      782–785
   health and terminology standards
      in, 780–782
   history of nursing informatics in,
      790, 790t–792t, 793
   information governance in,
      785–786
   national healthcare in, 778–787
   nursing education in, 794–796
   nursing informatics in, 242–243,
      786–797
   nursing research in, 793–794
   professional informatics
      organizations in, 788,
      788t–789t, 790, 790t–792t,
      793
Authentication protocols, security
   technology safeguards, 150f,
   156, 156t–157t, 158
Auto-ID systems, 413, 413t
Automated dispensing cabinets
   (ADCs), 438–443

Automated inventory control, 439
Automated performance measures,
   evidence-based practice, 562
Availability issues, health information
   technology security, 150f, 155
Avatars, in experiential learning,
   645–646
Awareness of information technology
   threats, 150f, 152

B
Bachelor of science in nursing
   (BSN), learning and practice
   structures for, 349–352,
   349f–350f, 351t, 352f
Backup utilities, software, 47
Barcoded-assisted medication
   administration (BCMA),
   435–438, 493–494
   in Asia, 811–813
Barcoding technology, medications,
   431
Basic input/output system (BIOS), 46
Battery life, advanced hardware
   systems and, 38
BCMA. *See* Barcoded-assisted
   medication administration
   (BCMA)
Beacon Community Program, 263
Behavioral science
   information-*seek*ing behavior of
      nurses, 688–689
   nursing informatics and, 238–240
   web-based cognitive behavioral
      interventions, 681
Belgian nursing minimum data set
   (B-NMDS), 760
Benchmarking, 97
Benefits analysis
   project management, 173
   vendor assessment, 312–313
Berkeley International Name Domain
   (BIND), 67
Best-of-breed vendor assessment
   model, 311–312
Best practices. *See also* Evidence-
   based practice
   Magnet model, 451–455
   scheduling and staffing issues and,
      327–328
Bibliographic retrieval systems,
   689–694, 690t, 699

Bi-directional connectivity, medical
   devices, 414
Big bang theory, project
   management, 181
Big data, 96
   evidence-based practice and,
      561–562
   genetics and genomics, 712–713
   physiologic data, 670
Binary large objects (BLOBs), object-
   oriented database model, 91
BIND. *See* Berkeley International
   Name Domain (BIND)
Bioinformatics
   data sharing, 715
   data validation, 715
   ethical and legal issues, 715–718,
      717f
   future trends in, 715
   genetics/genomics profile and,
      712–713
   standards, 714–715
   toolkits for, 713–714
Biomedical text mining (BioNLP),
   51–52
BioNLP. *See* Biomedical text mining
   (BioNLP)
BIOS. *See* Basic input/output system
   (BIOS)
Bits (binary digit), 33
BLOBs. *See* Binary large objects
   (BLOBs)
Blogs, 634–635, 703
Blueprint for Nursing Genomic
   Science, 718–722, 719t–721t
Bluetooth, 38–39
Blu-ray, 27t, 28, 28f
B-NMDS. *See* Belgian nursing
   minimum data set (B-NMDS)
Bologna Process in European nursing
   education, 761–762
Boolean Logic, 78
Boolean operators, database
   organization case study, 78
BPM. *See* Business Performance
   Management (BPM)
Brazil, nursing informatics in,
   820–823
Bring Your Own Device (BYOD),
   41–42
   Australian and New Zealand
      healthcare and, 780

GS. *See* Google Scholar (GS)
GT.M database engine, 67–68

H
H1N1 flu epidemic, 475–478
Hadoop platform, 714
Handheld computers, 31–32. *See also*
    Personal digital assistants
Hard drive, 27, 27f, 27t
  size of, 33
Hardin Meta Directory of Internet
    Health Sources, 698
Hardware
  advanced systems, 37–43
  components, 24–29
    CPU chip, 25, 25f
    input and output devices, 26
    memory, 25–26
    motherboard, 24–25, 24f
    storage media, 27–29, 27f, 27t
  computer architecture and,
    23–24, 24f
  computer power, 33
  computer speed, 33–34
  computer types, 29–32
    handheld computers, 31–32
    mainframes, 29–30
    microcomputers (persona
      computers), 30–31, 31b
    supercomputers, 29
  connectivity, compatibility, and
    incompatibility issues, 32–33
  defined, 23
  historical development of, 4–8
  network hardware, 34
  peripherals, 24, 27, 31
  project management requirements,
    175
  standards and protocols, 39
  wireless communication systems,
    38–39
Healthcare analytics
  data validity, 518, 518t
  database administrator, 523
  quality metrics, 520, 521
  population health, 514t
  value-based purchasing, 519, 521
Healthcare Effectiveness Data and
    Information Set (HEDIS), 540,
    543
Healthcare facilities, mHealth
    inside, 42

Healthcare informatics, defined,
    232. *See also* Nursing
    informatics (NI)
Healthcare Informatics Standards
    Panel (HITSP), 388
Healthcare Information and
    Management Systems Society
    (HIMSS)
  electronic health records, 10–11, 166
  healthcare project management
    and, 166
  healthcare reform and, 257
  nursing informatics and, 11t,
    233–234, 730–731
  Nursing Informatics Community,
    242
  public health policy and, 285–286
  Standards Work Group, 108f
  usability testing and, 199
Healthcare information systems
    (HISs)
  historical development of, 5
  home health care and, 379
  open source software/free software
    applications in, 68–71
Healthcare information technology
    (HIT), 593–594
  historical evolution of, 5–8
  nursing education standards in,
    9–10, 593–605
  nursing terminology standards and,
    115–125
  overview, 3–4
  software, 379
Healthcare Information Technology
    Standards Panel (HITSP),
    387–388
Healthcare policy
  changes in, 251–253
  consumer-centered engagement in,
    502–503
  defined, 283, 283f
  future issues in, 267
  government reforms and, 249–251
  information technology and,
    594–595
  mHealthcare, 43
  nursing informatics and, 265–267,
    281–289
  reform of, 372
Health Professional Education,
    643–644, 645, 647

Healthcare project management
  analysis phase, 170–173
  communications systems for,
    299, 301
  documentation, 170
  environmental assessment, 169–170
  feasibility study, 169
  governance issues, 224
  implementation, evaluation,
    maintenance and support,
    180–181, 182f, 183–184
  legacy systems data conversion,
    176–177, 177f
  management skills, 224
  planning phase, 166–168, 166f, 167f
  professional staff for, 224
  Project Management Plan,
    defined, 165
  resource planning, 170
  scope of development project,
    168–170
  steering committee, 167, 167f
  system design, development and
    customization, 174–176
  team structure, 167–168, 168f
  timeline, 170
  web resources for, 224
Healthcare reform, 296, 298, 302, 304.
    See also Healthcare Policy,
    reform of; HIMSS, healthcare
    reform and
Health data. *See* Data and data
    processing
Health information exchanges (HIEs),
    110, 251
  communication systems, 303–304
  eHealth applications, 338
  future challenges, 260
  interoperability, 256
  state programs, 262–263
Health Information Standards
    Organisation (HISO) (New
    Zealand), 781–782
Health information technology. *See*
    Information technology
Health Information Technology for
    Economic and Clinical Health
    (HITECH) Act, 7, 10, 102,
    250, 252, 253, 255, 257, 260,
    262, 263, 264, 265, 266, 592
  computerized provider order entry
    and, 401–407

T

Tablet PCs, 32
  clinical care using, 681
  healthcare applications, 41–43
  online learning, 620–621
Taiwan, nursing informatics in,
    810–813
Taiwan Nursing Informatics
    Association (TNIA), 810–813
Task analysis and composition,
    human-computer interaction
    usability, 138–141
TCO. *See* Total cost of ownership
    (TCO)
TCP/IP. *See* Transfer Control
    Protocol/Internet
    Protocol (TCP/IP) standards
Teaching. *See* Faculty in nursing
    education; Nursing education
Technical analysis, project
    management, 171
Technical differentiators, vendor
    assessment, 314–315
Technical Experts Panels (TEPs), 286
Technical specifications
  project management, 175
  vendor assessment, 316–317, 317t
Technology Informatics Guiding
    Educational Reform (TIGER)
    initiative, 609
  Asian nursing informatics and,
    810–813
  in Brazil, 821–823
  invitational summit, 611
  nursing education reforms, 597
  nursing informatics and, 241,
    243, 600
  public health policy and, 286
  system usability and clinical
    application design, 205–206
  TIGER Initiative Foundation, 612
Technology lifecycle. *See also* System
    life cycle (SLC)
  decision-making and, 276–280, 276f
Telehealth
  applications, 335–337
  basic principles, 334
  eHealth and informatics, 727–736,
    732–733
  emergency preparedness and
    response and, 339

historical context of, 333
  in New Zealand, 784
  trends in, 41–42
Telemedicine
  basic principles, 334
  decision support tools, 336–337
  historical context of, 333–334
  international organizations for,
    730–731
  Pacific regional developments in,
    787–793
TELENURSING consortium
    (Europe), 759, 763–764
Teletriage, 337
TEPs. *See* Technical Experts Panels
    (TEPs)
Term, defined, 120
Terminology
  advanced terminology systems,
    119–125
  in Australian and New Zealand
    healthcare, 781–782
  Clinical Care Classification System,
    835–836
  coding structure and, 119
  complex adaptive systems, 530,
    530t–531t
  in Europe, 758–761
  evidence-based practice, 572–573,
    573t
  international organizations for,
    730–731
  nursing terminologies, 115–125
    coding structure, 119
    computers and, 116, 119
    current data sets, 116, 118f
    health terminologies, 116,
      117t, 118f
    historical background, 116
    summary and implications, 125
  quality measurement and, 546
  research on, 670–671
  standards, 104–106
Testimony, health IT transformation
    and, 266–267
Testing
  challenges and barriers, 201
  clinical system elements, 192–194,
    193f
  genetic and genomic testing,
    715–718, 717f

human-computer interaction
    usability, 139–140
  models and methodologies,
    190–191, 191t
  ONC tools for, 110
  online learning, 621–623
  project management and, 179–180
  strategy and process, 191–192
  system functional testing, 189–201
  types of, 194, 195t–196t, 196–197,
    198f, 199, 200f, 201
Text formatting languages, 52
Texting, in nursing education and
    practice, 634–635
Text scanning, qualitative
    research, 675
Theory, 229, 235–240
Therapeutics, genomics and, 710–711
Third-generation languages, 49–50
Third-generation (3G) networks,
    wireless communication
    systems, 38–39
TIGER. *See* Technology Informatics
    Guiding Educational Reform
    (TIGER)
TLS. *See* Transport Layer Security
    (TLS)
TNIA. *See* Taiwan Nursing
    Informatics Association
    (TNIA)
ToC. *See* Transitions of Care (ToC)
    initiative
Tolven system, 70
Total cost of ownership (TCO),
    open source software/free
    software, 61
TPIR. *See* Translating practice into
    research (TPIR)
TPO. *See* Treatment, payment, and
    healthcare operations (TPO)
TPS. *See* Transactional processing
    systems (TPS)
Tracking systems, disaster electronic
    medical records, 481–482
Trajectory human-computer
    interaction, 134–135, 135f
Transactional processing systems
    (TPS), 29, 518–519
Transfer Control Protocol/Internet
    Protocol (TCP/IP) standards,
    39, 104